Principles and Practice of
Geriatric Psychiatry

Principles and Practice of
Geriatric Psychiatry

Second Edition

Edited by

John R. M. Copeland

Liverpool University Department of Psychiatry, Liverpool, UK

Mohammed T. Abou-Saleh

St George's Hospital Medical School, London, UK

Dan G. Blazer

Duke University Medical Center, Durham, North Carolina, USA

JOHN WILEY & SONS, LTD

Other Wiley Editorial Offices

John Wiley & Sons, Inc., 605 Third Avenue,
New York, NY 10158-0012, USA

WILEY-VCH Verlag GmbH, Pappelallee 3,
D-69469 Weinheim, Germany

John Wiley & Sons Australia Ltd, 33 Park Road, Milton,
Queensland 4064, Australia

John Wiley & Sons (Asia) Pte Ltd, 2 Clementi Loop #02-01,
Jin Xing Distripark, Singapore 129809

John Wiley & Sons (Canada) Ltd, 22 Worcester Road,
Rexdale, Ontario M9W 1L1, Canada

British Library Cataloguing in Publication Data

A catalogue record for this book is available from the British Library

ISBN 0-471-98197-4

Typeset in 9/10pt Times from the authors' disks by Dobbie Typesetting Limited, Tavistock, Devon.
Printed and bound in Great Britain by Antony Rowe Ltd, Chippenham, Wiltshire.
This book is printed on acid-free paper responsibly manufactured from sustainable forestry,
in which at least two trees are planted for each one used for paper production.

Contents

List of Contributors   xi
Preface   xix
Preface to First Edition   xxi

PART A   HISTORICAL BACKGROUND   1

1   A Conceptual History in the Nineteenth Century   3
    G. E. Berrios
2   Scope and Development in the Twentieth Century   7
    E. W. Busse
3   The Development in Britain   9
    Tom Arie
4a The Development in the USA, 1600–1900   13
    W. A. Achenbaum, C. Cederquist, V. Kahl
    and K. Rosenberg
4b In the Beginning   15
    The Late F. Post

PART B   NORMAL AGEING   17

B1   Theories of Ageing
5   General Theories of Aging   19
     E. W. Busse

BII   Brain Ageing
6   Structural Changes in the Aging Brain   23
     G. Mazeika and P. M. Doraiswamy
7   Anatomy of the Ageing Brain   25
     J. T. Campbell III and C. E. Coffey
8   Quantitative Structural Changes in the
     Ageing Brain   45
     Bente Pakkenberg, Lisbeth Regeur and
     Hans Jørgen G. Gundersen
     Potential Regeneration of the Ageing Brain   47
     S. B. Dunnett
     Hippocampal Changes and Memory Impairment
     in Normal People   49
     J. T. O'Brien
9   Neuroendocrinology of Ageing   51
     R. A. Burns and M. T. Abou-Saleh

10   Neurophysiology of Ageing as Reflected by
     Electroencephalogram (EEG) and Event-related
     Potentials (ERPs)   57
     D. H. R. Blackwood, W. J. Muir and H. Forstl
11   Pharmacokinetic and Pharmacodynamic
     Considerations in Old Age Psychopharmacology   61
     F. Schifano

BIII   Psychology of Ageing
12   Normal Ageing—A Problematical Concept   65
     D. B. Bromley
     Cohort Studies   68
     P. Rabbitt
13   Chronological and Functional Ageing   71
     J. M. Guralnik and D. Melzer
     Health Expectancy: Monitoring Changes in
     Population Health   74
     C. Jagger
14   Life Satisfaction   75
     L. K. George

BIV   Sociology of Ageing
15   The Normal Aged among Community-dwelling
     Elders in the UK   79
     C. Victor
     Do Life Events Seem Less Stressful to the Old?   82
     A. D. M. Davies
     Support Networks   83
     G. C. Wenger
16   World Statistical Trends and Prospects   87
     G. C. Myers
     Demography of the Old: Implications of
     Recent Trends   90
     E. Grundy

PART C   ABNORMAL AGEING   93

17   The Influence of Social Factors on Mental Health   95
     D. Mechanic and D. D. McAlpine
18   The Natural History of Psychiatric Disorders:
     Early-onset Disease in Late Life and
     Late-onset Illness   99
     J. Hays
19   Mortality and Mental Disorders   103
     M. E. Dewey

20 Long-term Outcome Studies of Psychiatric
    Disorders: Methodological Issues and Practical
    Approaches to Follow-up   105
    A. Stueve, J. Toner and A. V. Quismorio

PART D   DIAGNOSIS AND ASSESSMENT   109

DI   Epidemiology, Diagnosis and Nosology
21 **The Importance of Multidimensional Assessment
    in Clinical Practice   111**
    M. R. Eastwood and A. Desai
22 **Classification of Dementia and Other Organic
    Conditions in ICD-10   113**
    A. Jablensky and J. E. Cooper
23 **Psychiatric Diagnosis and Old Age: New
    Perspectives for "DSM-IV-TR" and Beyond   117**
    E. D. Caine

DII   Clinical Assessment
24 **History and Mental Status Examination   123**
    H. N. Richards and G. J. Maletta
25 **The Physician's Role   127**
    L. Young

DIII   Standardized Methods and Rating Scales
26 **Needs and Problems   133**
    B. J. Gurland
27 **Non-computerized Assessment Procedures:
    Fundamental Assessment Issues   137**
    P. Logue
    Short Assessment Scales
    Mini-Mental State Examination   140
    J. Cockrell and M. Folstein
    IQCODE: Informant Interviews   141
    A. F. Jorm
    Staging Dementia   142
    *B. Reisberg, G. Gandrota, A. Zaidi
    and S. H. Ferris*
    Psychogeriatric Assessment Scales   146
    A. F. Jorm
28 **Computer Methods of Assessment of
    Cognitive Function   147**
    T. W. Robbins and B. J. Sahakian
29 **The Assessment of Depressive States   153**
    T. R. Thompson and W. M. McDonald
    **The Geriatric Depression Scale:
    Its Development and Recent Application   157**
    R. O'Hara and J. A. Yesavage
    **Center for Epidemiologic Studies Depression Scale:
    Use among Older Adults   158**
    D. G. Blazer
30 **The Development of the EURO-D Scale   159**
    M. Prince

31 **Interviews Aimed at Differential Psychiatric
    Diagnosis
    GMS–HAS–AGECAT Package   161**
    J. R. M. Copeland
    CAMDEX   162
    D. W. O'Connor
32 **Assessment of Daily Living   165**
    K. H. Asberg
33 **Rating Scales Designed for Nurses and
    Other Workers   169**
    K. C. M. Wilson, B. Green and P. Mottram
34 **Comprehensive Interviews
    OARS Methodology   173**
    G. G. Fillenbaum
    **The Comprehensive Assessment and Referral
    Evaluation (CARE): An Approach to Evaluating
    Potential for Achieving Quality of Life   174**
    B. Gurland and S. Katz

PART E   ORGANIC DISORDERS   177

EI   Delirium
35 **Delirium—An Overview   179**
    A. F. Fairburn
    Delirium in Institutions   182
    B. Kamholz and C. Colenda
    Prognosis of Delirium   183
    A. Treloar

EII   Dementia
36 **Nosology of Dementia   185**
    I. Skoog and J. R. M. Copeland
    **Cross-national Inter-rater Reliability of
    Dementia Diagnosis   189**
    D. W. O'Connor
37 **Early Detection   191**
    S. Henderson
38 **Dementia Epidemiology: Prevalence and Incidence   195**
    A. F. Jorm
39 **Case-control Studies   199**
    S. Henderson
    **Results from EURODEM Collaboration on
    the Incidence of Dementia   200**
    *L. J. Launer, for the EURODEM Incidence
    Research Group*
    MRC/DoH Cognitive Function and Ageing Study   202
    *J. Nickson, C. F. M. McCracken and C. Brayne,
    on behalf of MRC CFAS*
40 **The Epidemiology of Alzheimer's Disease:
    An Update   205**
    L. J. Launer
    The Lundby Study, 1947–1997   208
    *P. Nettelbladt, O. Hagnell, L. Öjesjö,
    L. Otterbeck, C. Mattisson, M. Bogren,
    E. Hofvendahl and P. Toräker*

Nutritional Factors in Dementia 210
D. N. Anderson and M. T. Abou-Saleh

EIII   Alzheimer's Disease
41 **The Genetics of Alzheimer's Disease** 213
B. L. Plassman and J. C. S. Breitner
The Role of Presenilins in Alzheimer's Disease 217
D. M. A. Mann
Apolipoprotein-E (Apo-E) 218
D. G. Blazer
**Down's Syndrome and Alzheimer's Disease:
Update** 219
D. W. K. Kay and B. Moore
**International Criteria for Alzheimer's Disease
and Their Problems—ICD-10, DSM-IV and
NINCS–ADRDA** 221
K. Rockwood
42 **The Neuropathology of Alzheimer's Disease** 223
D. M. A. Mann
**Oxford Project to Investigate Memory and
Ageing (OPTIMA): A Longitudinal
Clinicopathological Study of Dementia
and Normal Ageing** 227
A. D. Smith
**Consortium to Establish a Registry for
Alzheimer's Disease (CERAD)** 228
G. G. Fillenbaum and A. Heyman
43 **Neurotransmitter Changes in Alzheimer's Disease:
Relationships to Symptoms and Neuropathology** 229
P. T. Francis and E. K. Perry
44 **Antemortem Markers** 233
*S. J. Van Rensberg, F. C. V. Potocnik
and D. J. Stein*
45 **Clinical Features of Senile Dementia and
Alzheimer's Disease** 237
B. Pitt
46 **Assessment and Management of Behavioural and
Psychological Symptoms of Dementia (BPSD)** 241
R. McShane and N. Gormley
Eating Disorders in Alzheimer's Disease 245
P. E. Cullen and C. Ballard

EIV   Vascular Dementia
47 **Pathology of Vascular Dementia** 247
J. M. MacKenzie
**International Criteria for Vascular Dementia and
Their Problems: ICD-10, DSM-IV, ADDTC
and NINDS–AIREN** 249
J. V. Bowler and V. Hachinski
48 **Vascular Dementia** 251
P. Humphrey
**Vascular Dementia Subgroups: Multi-infarct
Dementia and Subcortical White Matter Dementia** 255
I. Skoog
The Role of Blood Pressure in Dementia 256
I. Skoog

EV   Other Dementias
49 **Neuropathology: Other Dementias** 259
J. M. MacKenzie
50a **Dementia and Parkinson's Disease** 265
R. B. Godwin-Austen
Clinical Criteria for Dementia with Lewy Bodies 268
I. G. McKeith
50b **Subcortical Dementia** 269
J. R. Burke
50c **Early-onset Dementias** 273
G. Mazeika
51a **Creutzfeldt–Jakob Disease and Other
Degenerative Causes of Dementia** 277
T. F. G. Esmonde
51b **Frontotemporal Dementia (Pick's Disease)** 281
J. R. Hodges
52 **Alcoholic and Other Toxic Dementias** 285
E. M. Joyce
53 **Reversible Dementias** 289
M. Philpot and J. Pereira

EVI   Clinical Diagnosis of the Dementias
54 **Differential Diagnosis of Dementia** 293
C. Busby and A. Burns
55a **Distinguishing Depression from Dementia** 297
W. E. Fox and D. C. Steffens
55b **Benign Senescent Forgetfulness, Age-associated
Memory Impairment and Age-related Cognitive
Decline** 303
K. A. Welsh-Bohmer and D. J. Madden

EVII   Outcome of the Dementias and Subtypes
56 **Minor Cognitive Impairment** 305
K. Ritchie and J. Touchon
Alzheimer's Disease—One or Several? 307
C. Holmes and A. H. Mann
Prognosis of Dementia 308
B. Reisberg, A. Kluger and E. Franssen

EVIII   Treatment and Management of Dementias
57 **Acute Management of Dementia** 313
B. Pitt
58a **Present and Future Treatments of Alzheimer's
Disease** 317
L. J. Whalley and J. M. Starr
58b **Possible Future Treatments and Preventative
Strategies for Alzheimer's Disease** 325
S. Lovestone
59a **Psychological and Psychosocial Interventions** 327
E. Miller
59b **Informal Carers and Their Support** 331
D. Buck
The Role and Influence of the Alzheimer's Society 334
N. Graham

EIX   Conditions Associated with, or Sometimes
Mistaken for, Primary Psychiatric Conditions

60 **The Psychiatric Manifestations of**
CNS Malignancies 335
M. Glantz and E. W. Massey

61 **Peripheral Neuropathy and Peripheral Nerve**
Lesions 341
J. M. Massey and E. W. Massey

EX   Investigations of Organic States and Dementia

62 **Electroencephalography (EEG)** 345
The Late G. W. Fenton

63 **Computed Tomography (CT)** 351
A. Burns and G. Pearlson

64 **Magnetic Resonance Imaging (MRI)** 355
K. R. R. Krishnan

65 **Functional Magnetic Resonance Imaging (MRI)** 357
K. R. R. Krishnan

66 **Positron Emission Tomography (PET)** 359
P. F. Liddle and C. L. Grady

67 **Single-photon Emission Computed**
Tomography (SPECT) 363
M. T. Abou-Saleh

PART F   AFFECTIVE DISORDERS 369

FI   Nosology and Classification

68 **Nosology and Classification of Mood Disorders** 371
D. G. Blazer

FII   Depression, Dysthymia, Bereavement and
Suicidal Behaviour

69 **Genetics of Affective Disorders** 375
J. L. Beyer and D. C. Steffens

70a **Environmental Factors, Life Events and**
Coping Abilities 379
T. C. Antonucci and J. S. Jackson

70b **The Aetiology of Late-life Depression** 381
M. Prince and A. Beekman
Risk Factors and the Incidence of Post-stroke
Depression 386
P. W. Burvill

71 **Epidemiology of Depression: Prevalence**
and Incidence 389
D. G. Blazer
Epidemiological Catchment Area Studies of
Mood Disorders 392
D. G. Blazer
EURODEP—Prevalence of Depression in Europe 393
J. R. M. Copeland
Depression in Older Primary Care Patients:
Diagnosis and Course 393
J. M. Lyness and E. D. Caine

72 **Neurochemistry** 397
L. S. Schneider, updated by M. T. Abou-Saleh

73 **Neuro-imaging**
Neuro-imaging Studies of Depression 403
M. T. Abou-Saleh
Is Imaging Justified in the Investigation
of Older People? 404
D. McWilliam

74 **Clinical Features of Depression and Dysthymia** 407
D. G. Folks and C. V. Ford
Outcome of Depressive Disorders: Findings of
a Longitudinal Study in the UK 413
V. K. Sharma
Longitudinal Studies of Mood Disorders
in the USA 415
D. G. Blazer
Outcome of Depression in Finland 416
S.-L. Kivelä

75a **Physical Illness and Depression** 417
M. E. Evans
Physical Illness and Depression:
A Number of Conundrums 423
M. R. Eastwood

75b **Depression after Stroke** 425
P. Knapp and A. House
Treatment of Depression in Older People
with Physical Disability 427
S. Banerjee and F. Ruths

76 **Acute Management of Late-life Depression** 429
V. Gardner and D. C. Steffens

77 **Electroconvulsive Therapy (ECT)** 433
D. G. Wilkinson

78 **Pharmacological Treatment of Depression** 439
M. T. Abou-Saleh
Treatment-resistant Depression 442
A. J. Flint

79 **Psychotherapy of Depression and Dysthymia** 445
T. R. Lynch and C. M. Vitt

80 **Long-term Management of Affective Disorders** 453
M. T. Abou-Saleh

81 **Laboratory Diagnosis: Dexamethasone**
Suppression Test 461
M. T. Abou-Saleh

82 **Bereavement** 465
R. Kastenbaum

83 **Suicidal Behaviour** 469
H. Cattell

FIII   Mania

84 **Genetics and Aetiology** 473
T. Thompson and W. McDonald

85 **Epidemiology and Risk Factors** 477
S. Lehmann and P. Rabins

86 **Mania: Clinical Features and Management** 479
S. Lehmann and P. Rabins

87 **Prognosis** 481
M. M. Husain

88   The Management of Acute Mania   483
      J. L. Beyer and K. R. R. Krishnan

PART G   SCHIZOPHRENIC DISORDERS AND
MOOD-INCONGRUENT PARANOID STATES   491

89   Late-life Psychotic Disorders:
      Nosology and Classification   493
      L. T. Eyler Zorrilla and D. Jeste
90   Clinical Assessment and Differential Diagnosis   497
      D. N. Anderson
91   Aetiology, Genetics and Risk Factors   503
      D. J. Castle and R. M. Murray
      Brain Imaging in Schizophrenia-like and
      Paranoid Disorders in Late Life   508
      R. Howard
92   Schizophrenic Disorder and Mood-incongruent
      Paranoid States: Epidemiology, Prevalence,
      Incidence and Course   511
      R. Howard
93   The Fate of Schizophrenia with Advancing
      Age: Research Findings and Implications for
      Clinical Care   513
      R. Howard
94   Rehabilitation and Long-term Management   517
      R. Pugh
95   Treatment of Late-onset Psychotic Disorders   521
      E. M. Zayas and G. T. Grossberg
96   Risk Factors for Dyskinesia in the Elderly   527
      T. R. E. Barnes

PART H   NEUROSES   535

97   Nosology and Classification of
      Neurotic Disorders   537
      D. Bienenfeld
98   Epidemiology of Neurotic Disorders   541
      D. G. Blazer
99   Stress, Coping and Social Support   545
      L. R. Landerman and D. Hughes
100   Clinical Features of Anxiety Disorders   551
      E. L. Cassidy, P. J. Swales and J. I. Sheikh
101   Prognosis of Anxiety Disorders   555
      P. J. Swales, E. L. Cassidy and J. I. Sheikh
102   Acute Management of Anxiety and Phobias   559
      J. I. Sheikh, E. L. Cassidy and P. J. Swales
103   Psychopharmacological Treatment of Anxiety   563
      J. L. Beyer and K. R. R. Krishnan
104   Obsessive–Compulsive Disorder   571
      J. Lindesay
105   Hypochondriacal Disorder   575
      A. Allen and E. W. Busse
106   Other Neurotic Disorders   579
      J. J. Schulte and D. Bienenfeld

PART I   PERSONALITY DISORDERS   585

107   Personality Disorders: Aetiology and Genetics   587
      V. Molinari, T. Siebert and M. Swartz
108   Theoretical and Management Issues   593
      R. C. Abrams

PART J   MENTAL AND BEHAVIOURAL
DISORDERS DUE TO PSYCHOACTIVE
SUBSTANCES   599

109   Alcohol Abuse in the Elderly   601
      H. Kyomen and B. Liptzin
110   Epidemiology of Alcohol Problems and
      Drinking Patterns   607
      C. F. Hybels and D. G. Blazer
111   Drug Misuse in the Elderly   613
      P. Bown, A. H. Ghodse and M. T. Abou-Saleh
      Benzodiazepam Use and Abuse in the
      Community: Liverpool Studies   619
      K. Wilson and P. Mottram

PART K   LEARNING AND BEHAVIOURAL
DISORDERS   621

112   Old Age and Learning Disability   623
      O. Raji and S. Hollins
113a Elderly Offenders   627
      J. M. Parrott
113b Sleep and Ageing: Disorders and Management   631
      H. Chiu
      Rating Scale for Aggressive Behaviour
      in the Elderly   633
      L. C. W. Lam
114   Sexual Disorders   635
      J. M. Kellett
115   Phenomenology of Wandering   637
      A. Habib and G. T. Grossberg

PART L   THE PRESENTATION OF MENTAL
ILLNESS IN ELDERLY PERSONS IN
DIFFERENT CULTURES   639

116a Problems of Assessing Psychiatric Symptoms
      and Illness in Different Cultures   641
      M. Abas
116b Depression in the Indian Subcontinent   645
      V. Patel
116c Dementia in the Indian Subcontinent   647
      S. Rajkumar, M. Ganguli and D. Jeste
117   Dementia and Depression in Africa   649
      O. Baiyewu
118   Mental Illness in South America   651
      S. L. Blay

**PART M   THE PRACTICE OF
PSYCHOGERIATRIC MEDICINE   653**

119   Psychiatry of the Elderly—the WPA/WHO
      Consensus Statements   655
      C. Katona

MI   The British Model of the Organization of Services
120   Development of Health and Social Services in
      the UK in the Twentieth Century   657
      J. P. Wattis
121   The Pattern of Psychogeriatric Services   661
      J. P. Wattis
      Organization of Services for the Elderly
      with Mental Disorders   664
      E. Chiu
122   The Multidisciplinary Team   667
      H. Rosenvinge
123   Community Care: The Background   671
      C. Godber
      Health Care of the Elderly:
      The Nottingham Model   673
      Tom Arie
124   The Development of Day Hospitals and
      Day Care   677
      R. Jenkins and D. J. Jolley
125   Day Care   681
      J. M. Eagles and J. Warrington
126   New Technology and the Care of
      Cognitively Impaired Older People   685
      A. Sixsmith

*MII   The North American Model of the
      Organization of Services*
127   The United States System of Care   689
      C. C. Colenda, S. J. Bartels and G. L. Gottlieb
128   Community-based Psychiatric Ambulatory Care:
      The Private Practice Model in the USA   697
      E. M. Stein and G. S. Moak
129a The Psychiatrist's Role in Linking
      Community Services   705
      D. Johnston, K. A. Sherrill and B. V. Reifler
129b The Medical Psychiatry Inpatient Unit   709
      D. G. Folks and F. C. Kinney
130   The Psychiatrist in the Nursing Home   713
      W. E. Reichman
      Patient Autonomy vs. Duty of Care—
      the Old Age Psychiatrist's Dilemma   715
      A. Treloar
131   Psychiatric Services in Long-term Care   717
      I. R. Katz, K. S. Van Haitsma and J. E. Streim
132   Care in Private Psychiatric Hospitals   723
      *K. G. Meador, M. M. Harkleroad
      and W. M. Petrie*
133   Quality of Care and Quality of Life in
      Institutions for the Aged   727
      M. Powell Lawton

MIII   Liaison with Medical and Surgical Teams
134   Liaison with Medical and Surgical Teams   731
      S. A. Mann
135   Education and the Liaison Psychogeriatrician   737
      D. N. Anderson

MIV   Rehabilitation and General Care
136   Rehabilitation   739
      R. Jones
137   Anaesthetics and Mental State   743
      D. G. Seymour
138a Nutritional State   749
      D. N. Anderson and M. T. Abou-Saleh
      Mental Illness in Nursing Homes and
      Hostels in Australia   752
      D. Ames
138b Caregivers and Their Support   755
      K. C. Buckwalter, L. Garand and M. Maas
      The Sydney Dementia Carers'
      Training Program   762
      H. Brodaty
138c Elder Abuse—Epidemiology, Recognition
      and Management   771
      M. J. Vernon
138d The Care of the Dying Patient   775
      R. E. Nelson and K. G. Meador

MV   Prevention of the Mental Disorders of Old Age
139a Prevention in Mental Disorders of Late Life   779
      B. D. Lebowitz and J. L. Pearson
139b A Damning Analysis of the Law and the
      Elderly Incompetent Patient—
      Rights, What Rights?   783
      P. Edwards
139c Older People, Clinicians and Mental
      Health Regulation   789
      E. Murphy

MVI   Education
140   Training Requirements for Old Age
      Psychiatrists in the UK   791
      S. M. Benbow
      Old Age Psychiatrists and Stress   793
      S. M. Benbow
141   Developing and Maintaining Links between
      Service Disciplines: The Program for
      Organizing Interdisciplinary
      Self-education (POISE)   795
      J. A. Toner
142   Appendix: International Psychogeriatric
      Association   799
      B. Reisberg and F. F. Finkel

Index   801

Contributors

M. Abas Department of Psychiatry and Behavioural Science, University of Auckland, Private Bag 92019, Auckland, New Zealand

M. T. Abou-Saleh Department of Addictive Behaviour and Psychological Medicine, St George's Hospital Medical School, Cranmer Terrace, London SW17 0RE, UK

R. C. Abrams Department of Psychiatry, New York Presbyterian Hospital, Box 140, 525 East 68 Street, New York, NY 10021, USA

W. A. Achenbaum Institute of Gerontology, University of Michigan, 300 North Ingalls, Ann Arbor, MI 48109-2007, USA

A. Allen Dorothea Dix Hospital, Raleigh, NC, USA

D. Ames Associate Professor of the Psychiatry of Old Age, Department of Psychiatry, 7th Floor, Charles Connibere Building, Royal Melbourne Hospital, Parkville, Victoria 3050, Australia

D. N. Anderson North Mersey Community NHS Trust, EMI Directorate, Sir Douglas Crawford Unit, Mossley Hill Hospital, Park Avenue, Liverpool L18 8BU, UK

T. C. Antonucci Institute for Social Research, University of Michigan, Ann Arbor, MI 48106-1248, USA

T. Arie Ageing and Disability Research Unit, The Medical School, Queen's Medical Centre, Nottingham NG7 2UH, UK

K. Hulter-Asberg University of Uppsala, Gotgatan 3, S-753 15 Uppsala, Sweden

O. Baiyewu Department of Psychiatry, University of Ibadan, College of Medicine, PMB5116, Ibadan, Oyo State

C. Ballard MRC Neurochemical Pathology Unit, Newcastle General Hospital, Westgate Road, Newcastle upon Tyne NE4 6BE, UK

S. Banerjee Section of Mental Health and Ageing, Health Services Research Department, Institute of Psychiatry, De Crespigny Park, London SE5 8AF, UK

T. R. E. Barnes Professor of Clinical Psychiatry, Imperial College School of Medicine, Academic Centre, St Bernard's Site, Ealing Hospital, Uxbridge Road, Ealing UB1 3EU, UK

S. J. Bartels Department of Psychiatry, Dartmouth Medical School, Hanover, NH, USA

A. Beekman Institute of Psychiatry, De Crespigny Park, London SE5 8AF, UK

S. M. Benbow Wolverhampton Health Care NHS Trust, Penn Hospital, Penn Road, Wolverhampton WV4 5HA, UK

G. E. Berrios Department of Psychiatry, Addenbrooke's Hospital, Box 189, Hills Road, Cambridge CB2 2QQ, UK

J. L. Beyer Department of Psychiatry, Duke University Medical Center, Box 3519, Durham, NC 27710, USA

D. Bienenfeld Department of Psychiatry, Wright State University School of Medicine, PO Box 927, Dayton, OH 45401-0927, USA

D. H. R. Blackwood Royal Edinburgh Hospital, Edinburgh, UK

S. L. Blay Serviço Público Federal, Universidade Federal de São Paulo, Escola Paulista de Medicina, Rua Botucatu 740, CEP 04023-900 São Paulo, Brazil

D. G. Blazer Department of Psychiatry and Behavioral Sciences, Box 3003, Duke University Medical Center, Durham, NC 27710, USA

M. Bogren Department of Clinical Neuroscience, Division of Psychiatry, The Lundby Study, Lund University Hospital, St Lars, SE-221 85 Lund, Sweden

J. V. Bowler Department of Neurology, Royal Free Hospital, Pond Street, London NW3 2QG, UK

P. Bown Department of Addictive Behaviour and Psychological Medicine, St George's Hospital Medical School, Cranmer Terrace, London SW17 0RE, UK

C. Brayne Department of Public Health and Primary Care, University of Cambridge, Forvie Site, Robinson Way, Cambridge CB2 2SR, UK

J. C. S. Breitner Professor and Chair, Johns Hopkins University, School of Hygiene and Public Health, Department of Mental Hygiene, 624 Broadway, Baltimore, MD 21205-1999, USA

H. Brodaty Academic Department of Psychogeriatrics, University of New South Wales, Prince Henry Hospital, Little Bay, NSW 2036, Australia

D. B. Bromley Department of Psychology, University of Liverpool, Eleanor Rathbone Building, Liverpool L69 3BX, UK

D. Buck Department of Primary Care, Whelan Building, Brownlow Hill, University of Liverpool, Liverpool L69 3GB, UK

K. C. Buckwalter University of Iowa, 234 CMAB, Iowa City, Iowa 52242-1121, USA

J. R. Burke Division of Neurology, Department of Medicine, Duke University Medical Center, Box 2900, Durham, NC 27710, USA

A. Burns Academic Department of Psychiatry, University of Manchester, Withington Hospital, West Didsbury, Manchester M20 8LR, UK

P. W. Burvill 35 Gardner Street, Como 6152, Western Australia

C. Busby Academic Department of Psychiatry, University of Manchester, Withington Hospital, West Didsbury, Manchester M20 8LR, UK

E. W. Busse Duke University Medical Center, Durham, NC 27710, USA

E. D. Caine University of Rochester Medical Center, Department of Psychiatry, 300 Crittenden Boulevard, Rochester, NY 14642-8409, USA

J. J. Campbell III Department of Psychiatry, Henry Ford Health System, 1 Ford Place, Detroit, MI 48202, USA

E. L. Cassidy Stanford University School of Medicine, Department of Psychiatry and Behavioral Sciences/ TD-114, Stanford, CA 94305-5723, USA

D. J. Castle Mental Health Research Institute & University of Melbourne, 155 Oak Street, Parkville, Victoria 3052, Australia

H. Cattell Wrexham Maelor Hospital, 1 Croesnewydd Rd, Wrexham LL13 7TD, UK

C. Cederquist Institute of Gerontology, University of Michigan, 300 North Ingalls, Ann Arbor, MI 48109-2007, USA

E. Chiu Academic Unit for Psychiatry of Old Age, St George's Hospital Medical Service, University of Melbourne, 283 Cotham Road, Kew, Victoria 3101, Australia

H. Chiu Department of Psychiatry, The Chinese University of Hong Kong, Prince of Wales Hospital, Shatin NT, Hong Kong

F. Cleveland Kinney University of Alabama School of Medicine, Birmingham, AL, USA

J. R. Cockrell Department of Psychiatry, Medical University of South Carolina, Charleston, SC 29401, USA

C. C. Colenda Department of Psychiatry, College of Human Medicine, Michigan State University, East Lansing, MI 48824-1316, USA

J. E. Cooper Department of Psychiatry and Behavioural Science, Medical Research Foundation Building, Level 3 Rear, 50 Murray Street, Perth, WA6000, Australia

J. R. M. Copeland Department of Psychiatry, Royal Liverpool University Hospital, Liverpool L69 3GA, UK

P. E. Cullen Bushey Fields Hospital, Russells Hall, Dudley, West Midlands DY1 2LZ, UK

A. D. M. Davies Department of Psychology, Eleanor Rathbone Building, Bedford Street South, Liverpool L69 7ZA, UK

A. Desai Department of Psychiatry, St Louis University Medical School, 1221 South Grand Boulevard, St Louis, MO 63104, USA

M. Dewey Trent Institute for Health Services Research, Medical School, Queen's Medical Centre, Nottingham NG7 2UH, UK

P. M. Doraiswamy Department of Psychiatry, Duke University Medical Center, Box 3018, Durham, NC 27710, USA

S. Dunnet School of Biosciences, Cardiff University, Biomedical Sciences Building, Museum Avenue, Cardiff CF10 3US, UK

J. M. Eagles Block A, Clerkseat Building, Royal Cornhill Hospital, Aberdeen AB25 2ZH, UK

M. R. Eastwood 18 Montague Road, Cambridge CB4 1BX, UK

P. C. Edwards Ventura House, Market Street, Hoylake CH47 2AE, UK

T. F. G. Esmonde Department of Neurology, Ward 21, Quin House, Royal Victoria Hospital, Grosvenor Road, Belfast BT12 6BA, UK

M. E. Evans Elderly Mental Health Directorate, Wirral and West Cheshire Community NHS Trust, Clatterbridge Hospital, Bebington, Wirral L63 4JY, UK

L. T. Eyler Zorrilla Department of Psychiatry and Neurosciences, Division of Geriatric Psychiatry, University of California at San Diego, VA San Diego Healthcare System (116A-1), 3350 La Jolla Village Drive, San Diego, CA 92161, USA

A. F. Fairburn Consultant in Old Age Psychiatry, Castleside Unit, Centre for the Health Care of the Elderly, Newcastle General Hospital, Newcastle upon Tyne NE4 6BE, UK

S. H. Ferris Department of Psychiatry, New York University School of Medicine, 550 First Avenue, New York, NY 10016, USA

G. G. Fillenbaum Division of Medical Psychology, Department of Psychiatry and Behavioral Sciences, Box 3003, Duke University Medical Center, Durham, NC 27710, USA

F. F. Finkel Department of Psychiatry, New York University School of Medicine, 550 First Avenue, New York, NY 10016, USA

A. J. Flint Toronto General Hospital, 8 Eaton North Room 238, 200 Elizabeth Street, Toronto, Ontario, Canada M5G 2C4

D. G. Folks Department of Psychiatry, University of Nebraska College of Medicine, Omaha, NE 68198-5575, USA

M. F. Folstein New England Medical Center, Department of Psychiatry, Box 1007, 750 Washington Street, Boston, MA 02111, USA

C. V. Ford Department of Psychiatry and Behavioral Neurobiology, University of Alabama School of Medicine, Birmingham, AL, USA

H. Förstl Department of Psychiatry and Psychotherapy, Technical University of Munich, Ismaninger Strasse 22, D-81675 München, Germany

W. E. Fox Department of Psychiatry, Duke University Medical Center, Box 3903, Durham, NC 27710, USA

P. T. Francis Centre for Neuroscience, GKT School of Biomedical Science, King's College London, Hodgkin Building, Guy's Campus, St Thomas Street, London SE1 1UL, UK

E. Franssen Department of Psychiatry, New York University School of Medicine, 550 First Avenue, New York, NY 10016, USA

G. Gandrota Department of Psychiatry, New York University School of Medicine, 550 First Avenue, New York, NY 10016, USA

M. Ganguli Department of Epidemiology, University of Pittsburgh Graduate School of Public Health, Western Psychiatric Institute and Clinic, 3811 O'Hara Street, Pittsburgh, PA 15213-2593, USA

L. Garand School of Nursing, University of Pittsburgh, PA, USA

V. Gardner Department of Psychiatry, Duke University Medical Center, Box 3903, Durham, NC 27710, USA

L. K. George Department of Psychiatry, Box 3003, Duke University Medical Center, Durham, NC 27710, USA

A. H. Ghodse Department of Addictive Behaviour and Psychological Medicine, St George's Hospital Medical School, Cranmer Terrace, London SW17 0RE, UK

C. Gilleard Springfield University Hospital, 61 Glenburnie Road, London SW17 7DJ, UK

M. Glantz 710 Robinson Road, PO Box 665, Hinsdale, MA 01235, USA

C. Godber Elderly Mental Health Service, Moorgreen Hospital, Botley Road, West End, Southampton SO30 3JB, UK

R. Godwin-Austen Department of Neurology, University Hospital, Queen's Medical Centre, Nottingham NG7 2UH, UK

N. Gormley Section of Old Age Psychiatry, Institute of Psychiatry, De Crespigny Park, Denmark Hill, London SE5 8AF, UK

G. L. Gottlieb Department of Psychiatry, Harvard University School of Medicine, Boston, MA, USA

C. L. Grady Rotman Research Institute, Baycrest Centre for Geriatric Care, University of Toronto, 3560 Bathurst St, Toronto, Ontario, Canada M6A 2E1

N. Graham 27 St Alban's Road, London NW5 1RG, UK

B. Green Academic Unit, University of Liverpool, EMI Directorate, St Catherine's Hospital, Derby Road, Birkenhead L42 0LQ, UK

G. T. Grossberg Department of Psychiatry, St Louis University Medical School, 1221 South Grand Boulevard, Suite 202, St Louis, MO 63104, USA

E. Grundy Centre for Population Studies, London School of Hygiene and Tropical Medicine, 49–51 Bedford Square, London WC1B 3DP, UK

H. J. G. Gundersen Stereological Research Laboratory, Aarhus University, Århus, Denmark

J. M. Guralnik Epidemiology, Demography and Biometry Program, National Institute on Aging, Gateway Building, Room 3C309, 7201 Wisconsin Avenue, Bethesda, MD 20892, USA

B. J. Gurland The Columbia University Stroud Center, 100 Haven Avenue, Tower 3, 30th Floor, New York, NY 10032, USA

A. Habib Department of Psychiatry, St Louis University Medical School, 1221 South Grand Boulevard, Suite 202, St Louis, MO 63104, USA

V. Hachinski Department of Clinical and Neurological Sciences, London Health Sciences Centre, 399 Windermere Road, London, Ontario, Canada N6A 5A5

O. Hagnell Department of Clinical Neuroscience, Division of Psychiatry, The Lundby Study, Lund University Hospital, St Lars, S-221 85 Lund, Sweden

K. Hall Department of Psychiatry, Indiana University School of Medicine, Clinical Building 394A, 541 Clinical Drive, Indianapolis, IN 46202-5111, USA

M. M. Harkleroad Parthenon Pavilion, Memory Disorders Center, Nashville, TN, USA

J. Hays Division of Geriatric Psychiatry, Department of Psychiatry and Behavioral Sciences, Box 3003, Duke University Medical Center, Durham, NC 27710, USA

A. S. Henderson NHMRC Psychiatric Epidemiology Research Centre, Australian National University, Canberra, ACT 0200, Australia

H. C. Hendrie Department of Psychiatry, Indiana University School of Medicine, Clinical Building 394A, 541 Clinical Drive, Indianapolis, IN 46202-5111, USA

A. Heyman Division of Medical Psychology, Department of Psychiatry and Behavioral Sciences, Box 3003, Duke University Medical Center, Durham, NC 27710, USA

J. R. Hodges MRC Brain and Cognitive Sciences Unit, 15 Chaucer Road, Cambridge CB2 2EF, UK

E. Hofvendahl Department of Clinical Neuroscience, Division of Psychiatry, The Lundby Study, Lund University Hospital, St Lars, SE-221 85 Lund, Sweden

S. Hollins Department of Psychiatry of Disability, St George's Hospital Medical School, University of London, Cranmer Terrace, London SW17 0RE, UK

C. Holmes Department of Psychiatry, Section of Epidemiology and General Practice, De Crespigny Park, Denmark Hill, London SE5 8AF, UK

A. House Academic Unit of Psychiatry and Behavioural Sciences, 15 Hyde Terrace, Leeds LS2 9LT, UK

R. Howard Section of Old Age Psychiatry, Institute of Psychiatry, De Crespigny Park, Denmark Hill, London SE5 8AF, UK

D. Hughes Duke University Medical Center, Box 3003, Durham, NC 27710, USA

P. Humphrey The Walton Centre for Neurology and Neurosurgery, Lower Lane, Fazakerley, Liverpool L9 7LJ, UK

M. M. Husain Psychiatry Division, University of Texas, Dallas, TX 75390-8898, USA

C. F. Hybels Department of Psychiatry and Behavioral Sciences, Box 3003, Duke University Medical Center, Durham, NC 27710, USA

A. Jablensky Department of Psychiatry and Behavioural Science, Medical Research Foundation Building, Level 3 Rear, 50 Murray Street, Perth, WA 6000, Australia

J. S. Jackson Institute for Social Research, University of Michigan, Ann Arbor, MI 48106-1248, USA

C. Jagger Department of Epidemiology and Public Health, University of Leicester, 22–28 Princess Road West, Leicester LE1 6TP, UK

R. Jenkins Department of Old Age Psychiatry, Mental Health Directorate, Penn Hospital, Penn Road, Wolverhampton, West Midlands WV4 5HN, UK

D. V. Jeste Department of Psychiatry and Neurosciences, Division of Geriatric Psychiatry, University of California at San Diego, VA San Diego Healthcare System (116A-1), 3350 La Jolla Village Drive, San Diego, CA 92161, USA

D. Johnston Department of Psychiatry and Behavioral Medicine, Wake Forest University School of Medicine, Bowman Gray Campus, Medical Center Boulevard, Winston-Salem, NC 27157-1087, USA

D. J. Jolley Department of Old Age Psychiatry, Mental Health Directorate, Penn Hospital, Penn Road, Wolverhampton, West Midlands WV4 5HN, UK

R. Jones Section of Old Age Psychiatry, Nottingham University, A Floor, South Block, Queen's Medical Centre, Nottingham NG7 2UH, UK

A. F. Jorm NHMRC Psychiatric Epidemiology Research Centre, Australian National University, Canberra, ACT 0200, Australia

E. M. Joyce Division of Neuroscience and Psychological Medicine, Imperial College School of Medicine, Charing Cross Site, St Dunstan's Road, London W6 8RP, UK

V. Kahl Institute of Gerontology, University of Michigan, 300 North Ingalls, Ann Arbor, MI 48109-2007, USA

B. Kamholz Department of Psychiatry, Michigan State University, School of Medicine, East Lansing, MI 48824, USA

R. J. Kastenbaum Hugh Downs School of Human Communication, 208 E. Citation Lane, Tempe, AZ 85284, USA

C. Katona Department of Psychiatry and Behavioural Science, Royal Free and University College London, Wolfson Building, 48 Riding House Street, London W1N 8AA, UK

I. R. Katz Section of Geriatric Psychiatry, University of Pennsylvania, 3600 Market Street, RM 758, Philadelphia, PA 19104, USA

S. Katz The Columbia University Stroud Center, 100 Haven Avenue, Tower 3, 30th Floor, New York, NY 10032, USA

D. W. K. Kay 8 Grosvenor Place, Newcastle upon Tyne NE2 3RE, UK

J. M. Kellett Division of Geriatric Medicine, St George's Hospital Medical School, Level 01, Jenner Wing, Cranmer Terrace, London SW17 0RE, UK

T. B. L. Kirkwood Biological Gerontology Group, The School of Biological Sciences and Department of Geriatric Medicine, 3.239 Stopford Building, University of Manchester, Oxford Road, Manchester M13 9PT, UK

S.-L. Kivelä Department of General Practice, University of Oulu, Department of Public Health Science and General Practice, P.B. 5000, 90401, Oulu, Finland

A. Kluger Department of Psychiatry, New York University School of Medicine, 550 First Avenue, New York, NY 10016, USA

P. Knapp Academic Unit of Psychiatry and Behavioural Sciences, 15 Hyde Terrace, Leeds LS2 9LT, UK

K. R. R. Krishnan Department of Psychiatry, Duke University Medical Center, Box 3950, Durham, NC 27710, USA

H. H. Kyomen McLean Hospital, 115 Mill Street, Belmont, MA 02478, USA

L. C. W. Lam Department of Psychiatry, The Chinese University of Hong Kong, Prince of Wales Hospital, Shatin NT, Hong Kong

H. R. Lamb USC Department of Psychiatry, IRD 715, 2020 Zonal Avenue, Los Angeles, CA 90033, USA

L. R. Landerman Duke University Medical Center, Box 3003, Durham, NC 27710, USA

L. J. Launer Epidemiology, Biometry and Demography Program, National Institute on Aging, National Institutes of Health, Gateway Building, Room 3C-309, 7201 Wisconsin Avenue, Bethesda, MD 20892, USA

B. D. Lebowitz Adult and Geriatric Treatment and Preventive Interventions Research Branch, National Institute of Mental Health, 6001 Executive Boulevard, Rm 7160, MSC 9635, Bethesda, MD 20892-9635, USA

S. Lehmann Department of Psychiatry and Behavioral Sciences, Johns Hopkins Medical Institutions, 600 North Wolfe Street, Asolf Meyer Building, Room 279, Baltimore, MD 21287-7279, USA

P. F. Liddle Department of Psychiatry, University of British Columbia, Vancouver, BC, Canada

J. Lindesay Division of Psychiatry for the Elderly, Department of Psychiatry, University of Leicester, Leicester General Hospital, Gwendolen Road, Leicester LE5 4PW, UK

B. Liptzin Baystate Medical Center, Department of Psychiatry, Springfield, MA 01199, USA

P. Logue Duke University Medical Center, Box 3427, Durham, NC 27710, USA

S. Lovestone Section of Old Age Psychiatry, Institute of Psychiatry, De Crespigny Park, Denmark Hill, London SE5 8AF, UK

T. R. Lynch Department of Psychiatry and Behavioral Sciences, Duke University Medical Center, Box 3362, Durham, NC 27710, USA

J. M. Lyness Department of Psychiatry, University of Rochester Medical Center, 300 Crittenden Boulevard, Rochester, NY 14642, USA

M. Maas College of Nursing, University of Iowa, Iowa City, IA, USA

J. M. MacKenzie Department of Pathology, Grampian University Hospitals NHS Trust, Link Building, Foresterhill, Aberdeen AB25 2ZD, UK

D. J. Madden Box 2980, Duke University Medical Center, Durham, NC 27710, USA

G. J. Maletta VA Medical Center, 1 Veterans Drive, Minneapolis, MN 55417, USA

A. H. Mann Department of Psychiatry, Section of Epidemiology and General Practice, De Crespigny Park, Denmark Hill, London SE5 8AF, UK

D. M. A. Mann Clinical Neuroscience Research Group, 1st Floor, Stopford Building, Department of Medicine, University of Manchester, Oxford Road, Manchester M13 9PT, UK

S. A. Mann Mental Health Administration, Clacton and District Hospital, Clacton-on-Sea, Essex CO15 1LH, UK

E. W. Massey Duke University Medical Center, Box 3909, Durham, NC 27710, USA

J. M. Massey Duke University Medical Center, Box 3909, Durham, NC 27710, USA

C. Mattison Department of Clinical Neuroscience, Division of Psychiatry, The Lundby Study, Lund University Hospital, St Lars, S-221 85 Lund, Sweden

G. Mazeika Department of Psychiatry, Duke University Medical Center, Durham, NC 27710, USA

C. F. M. McCracken Department of Public Health and Primary Care, University of Cambridge, Forvie Site, Robinson Way, Cambridge CB2 2SR, UK

W. M. McDonald Emory University School of Medicine, Fuquay Center for Late Life Depression, 1841 Clifton Road NE, Atlanta, GA 30329-5120, USA

I. G. McKeith Department of Old Age Psychiatry, Institute for Health of the Elderly, Wolfson Research Centre, Newcastle General Hospital, Westgate Road, Newcastle upon Tyne NE4 6BE, UK

R. McShane Fulbrook Centre, Churchill Hospital, Oxford OX3 7JU, UK

D. McWilliam Consultant Psychiatrist, Ribbleton Hospital, Miller Road, Preston PR2 6LS, UK

K. G. Meador Duke University, Department of Psychiatry and Behavioral Sciences, Durham, NC 27708, USA

D. Mechanic Institute for Health, Health Care Policy and Aging Research, 30 College Avenue, New Brunswick, NJ 08901, USA

D. Melzer Department of Community Medicine, Institute of Public Health, University of Cambridge, Cambridge, UK

E. Miller Centre for Applied Psychology, University of Leicester, University Road, Leicester LE1 7RH, UK

G. S. Moak Department of Psychiatry, University of Massachusetts Medical School, 55 Lake Avenue North, Worcester, MA 01655, USA

V. Molinari Houston VAMC Psychology Service 116B, 2002 Holcombe Blvd, Houston, TX 77030, USA

B. Moore Department of Psychiatry, University of Newcastle upon Tyne, UK

J. T. Moroney Consultant Neurologist, Department of Neurology, Beaumont Hospital, Beaumont Road, Dublin 9, Ireland

P. Mottram Academic Unit, University of Liverpool, EMI Directorate, St Catherine's Hospital, Derby Road, Birkenhead L42 0LQ, UK

W. J. Muir Royal Edinburgh Hospital, Edinburgh, UK

E. Murphy North East London Health Authority, 81 Commercial Road, London E1 1RD, UK

R. M. Murray Institute of Psychiatry, De Crespigny Park, Denmark Hill, London SE5 8AF, UK

G. C. Myers Center for Demographic Studies, Duke University Medical Center, Durham, NC 27710, USA

R. E. Nelson Duke Institute of Care at the End of Life, Duke University, Durham, NC, USA

P. Nettelbladt Department of Clinical Neuroscience, Division of Psychiatry, The Lundby Study, Lund University Hospital, St Lars, SE-221 85 Lund, Sweden

J. Nickson Department of Public Health and Primary Care, University of Cambridge, Forvie Site, Robinson Way, Cambridge CB2 2SR, UK

J. T. O'Brien Wolfson Research Centre, Institute for the Health of the Elderly, Newcastle General Hospital, Westgate Road, Newcastle upon Tyne NE4 6BE, UK

D. W. O'Connor Aged Mental Health Research Group, Kingston Centre, Monash University, Warrigal Road, Cheltenham 3192, Melbourne, Victoria, Australia

R. O'Hara Department of Psychiatry and Behavioral Sciences, Stanford University School of Medicine, Stanford, CA 94305, USA

L. Öjesjö Department of Clinical Neuroscience, Magnus Huss Clinic, Karolinska Institute, SE-171 76 Stockholm, Sweden

L. Otterbeck Department of Clinical Neuroscience, Division of Psychiatry, The Lundby Study, Lund University Hospital, St Lars, SE-221 85 Lund, Sweden

B. Pakkenberg Research Laboratory for Stereology and Neuroscience, Bispebjerg University Hospital, Bispebjerg Bakke 23, DK 2400 Copenhagen NV, Denmark

J. M. Parrott Director of Specialist Mental Health, The Bracton Centre, c/o Bexley Hospital, Bexley Lane, Bexley, Kent DA5 2BW, UK

V. Patel Sangath Centre, 841/1 Alto Porvorim, Goa 403521, India

G. Pearlson Johns Hopkins Hospital, Baltimore, MD, USA

J. L. Pearson Adult and Geriatric Treatment and Preventive Interventions Research Branch, National Institute of Mental Health, 6001 Executive Boulevard, Rm 7160, MSC 9635, Bethesda, MD 20892-9635, USA

M. A. Pericak-Vance Center for Human Genetics, Duke University Medical Center, Box 3445, 026 CARL Building, Durham, NC 27710, USA

J. Pereira Department of Mental Health for Older Adults, South London and Maudsley NHS Trust, Maudsley Hospital, Denmark Hill, London SE5 8AZ, UK

E. K. Perry MRC Building, Centre of Development and Chemical Brain Aging, Newcastle General Hospital, Westgate Road, Newcastle upon Tyne, UK

W. M. Petrie Parthenon Pavilion, Memory Disorders Center, Nashville, TN, USA

M. Philpot Department of Mental Health for Older Adults, South London and Maudsley NHS Trust, Maudsley Hospital, Denmark Hill, London SE5 8AZ, UK

B. Pitt Palmers House, Maltings Drive, Epping, Essex CM16 6SG, UK

B. L. Plassman Box 41, 905 W. Main Street, Suite 25D, Duke University Medical Center, Durham, NC 27710, USA

The Late F. Post Formerly Emeritus Physician, The Bethlem Royal Hospital and Maudsley Hospital, Denmark Hill, London SE5 8AZ, UK

F. C. V. Potocnik University of Stellenbosch, Tygerberg 7505, South Africa

M. Powell Lawton Polisher Research Institute, Philadelphia Geriatric Center, 5301 Old York Road, Philadelphia, PA 19141, USA

M. Prince Institute of Psychiatry, De Crespigny Park, Denmark Hill, London SE5 8AF, UK

R. Pugh Consultant Psychiatrist, St Luke's–Woodside Hospital, Woodside Avenue, London N10 3HU, UK

A. V. Quismorio Center for Geriatrics and Gerontology, The Columbia University Stroud Center, 100 Haven Avenue, Tower 3, 30th Floor, New York, NY 10032, USA

P. Rabbitt Age and Cognitive Performance Research Centre, University of Manchester, Oxford Road, Manchester M13 9PL, UK

P. Rabins Department of Psychiatry and Behavioral Sciences, Johns Hopkins Medical Institutions, 600 North Wolfe Street, Asolf Meyer Building, Room 279, Baltimore, MD 21287-7279, USA

O. Raji St George's Hospital Medical School, Cranmer Terrace, London SW17 0RE, UK

S. Rajkumar Newcastle Mental Health Service, 20 Stewart Avenue, Newcastle, NSW 2303, Australia

L. Regeur Research Laboratory for Stereology and Neuroscience, Bispebjerg University Hospital, Bispebjerg Bakke 23, DK 2400 Copenhagen NV, Denmark

W. E. Reichman Department of Psychiatry, Robert Wood Johnson Medical School, University of Medicine and Dentistry of New Jersey, 671 Hoes Lane, Piscataway, NJ 08855-1392, USA

B. V. Reifler Department of Psychiatry and Behavioral Medicine, Wake Forest University School of Medicine, The Bowman Gray Campus, Medical Center Boulevard, Winston-Salem, NC 27157-1087, USA

B. Reisberg Department of Psychiatry, New York University School of Medicine, 550 First Avenue, New York, NY 10016, USA

H. N. Richards VA Medical Center, 1 Veterans Drive, Minneapolis, MN 55417, USA

K. Ritchie INSERM E99-30, Epidemiology of Central Nervous System Pathologies, CRLC Val d'Aurelle, 34298 Montpellier cedex 5, France

T. W. Robbins Department of Experimental Psychology, University of Cambridge, Downing Street, Cambridge CB2 3EB, UK

K. Rockwood Dalhousie University, 1421–5955 Jubilee Road, Halifax, NS, Canada B3H 2E1

K. Rosenberg Institute of Gerontology, University of Michigan, 300 North Ingalls, Ann Arbor, MI 48109-2007, USA

H. Rosenvinge University of Southampton, Thornhill Unit, Moorgreen Hospital, Botley Road, West End, Southampton SO30 3JB, UK

E. A. Ruths South London and Maudsley NHS Trust, Queen's Resource Centre, Queen's Road, Croydon, Surrey, UK

B. J. Sahakian Department of Experimental Psychology, University of Cambridge, Downing Street, Cambridge CB2 3EB, UK

F. Schifano St George's Hospital Medical School, Cranmer Terrace, London SW17 0RE, UK

L. S. Schneider USC Geriatric Studies Center, 1975 Zonal Avenue, KAM 400, University of Southern California, Los Angeles, CA 90033, USA

J. J. Schulte Department of Psychiatry, Wright State University School of Medicine, PO Box 927, Dayton, OH 45401-0927, USA

D. G. Seymour Medicine for the Elderly, University of Aberdeen, Foresterhill Health Centre, Westburn Road, Aberdeen AB9 2AY, UK

V. K. Sharma Victoria Central Hospital, Wirral and West Cheshire Community NHS Trust, Mill Lane, Wallasey CH44 5UF, UK

J. I. Sheikh Stanford University School of Medicine, Department of Psychiatry and Behavioral Sciences/TD-114, Stanford, CA 94305-5723, USA

K. A. Sherrill Department of Psychiatry and Behavioral Medicine, Wake Forest University School of Medicine, The Bowman Gray Campus, Medical Center Boulevard, Winston-Salem, NC 27157-1087, USA

T. Siebert Duke University Medical Center, Box 3903, Durham, NC 27710, USA

A. J. Sixsmith Shelley's Cottage, University of Liverpool, Liverpool L69 3BX, UK

I. Skoog Institute of Clinical Neuroscience, University of Göteborg, Sahlgrenska University Hospital, SE-413 45 Göteborg, Sweden

A. D. Smith University Department of Pharmacology, Mansfield Road, Oxford OX1 3QT, UK

J. M. Starr Department of Geriatric Medicine, University of Edinburgh, Edinburgh, UK

D. C. Steffens Department of Psychiatry, Duke University Medical Center, Box 3903, Durham, NC 27710, USA

D. J. Stein University of Stellenbosch, Tygerberg 7505, South Africa

E. M. Stein 4300 Alton Road, Suite 360, Miami Beach, FL 33140, USA

J. E. Streim Polisher Research Institute, Philadelphia Geriatric Center, 5301 Old York Road, Philadelphia, PA 19141, USA

A. Stueve Center for Geriatrics and Gerontology, The Columbia University Stroud Center, 100 Haven Avenue, Tower 3, 30th Floor, New York, NY 10032, USA

P. J. Swales Veteran Affairs, Palo Alto Health Care System, Palo Alto, CA, USA

M. Swartz Duke University Medical Center, Box 3903, Durham, NC 27710, USA

T. R. Thompson Emory University School of Medicine, Fugua Center for Late Life Depression, 1841 Clifton Road NE, Atlanta, GA 30329-5120, USA

J. A. Toner Center for Geriatrics and Gerontology, The Columbia University Stroud Center, 100 Haven Avenue, Tower 3, 30th Floor, New York, NY 10032, USA

P. Toråker Department of Clinical Neuroscience, Division of Psychiatry, The Lundby Study, Lund University Hospital, St Lars, SE-221 85 Lund, Sweden

J. Touchon INSERM E99-30, Epidemiology of Pathologies of the CNS, CRLC Cal d'Aurelle, 34298 Montpellier cedex 5, France

A. Treloar Community Mental Health Team for Older Persons, Memorial Hospital, Shooters Hill, London SE18 3RZ, UK

K. S. Van Haitsma Mental Illness Research Education and Clinical Center, Philadelphia VA Medical Center, PA, USA

S. J. van Rensburg University of Stellenbosch, PO Box 19113, Tygerberg 7505, South Africa

M. J. Vernon Department of Elderly Medicine, Burton House, Withington Hospital, Nell Lane, West Didsbury, Manchester M20 8LR, UK

C. R. Victor Department of Public Health Sciences, St George's Hospital Medical School, Hunter Wing, Level 6, Cranmer Terrace, London SW17 0RE, UK

C. M. Vitt Department of Psychiatry and Behavioral Sciences, Duke University Medical Center, Box 3362, Durham, NC 27710, USA

J. Warrington Block A, Clerkseat Building, Royal Cornhill Hospital, Aberdeen AB25 2ZH, UK

J. P. Wattis Leeds Community and Mental Health Services, The Mansion, Meanwood Park Hospital, Tongue Lane, Leeds LS6 4QB, UK

K. A. Welsh-Bohmer Department of Psychiatry, Duke University Medical Center, Box 3503, Durham, NC 27710, USA

C. Wenger Centre for Social Policy, Research and Development, School of Sociology and Social Policy, University of Wales, Bangor, Gwynedd LL57 2DG, UK

L. J. Whalley Department of Psychiatry, University of Aberdeen, Aberdeen, UK

P. J. Whitehouse Alzheimer Center, University Hospital of Cleveland, 1220 Fairhill Road, Suite C357, Cleveland, OH 44120-1013, USA

D. G. Wilkinson Moorgreen Hospital, Botley Road, West End, Southampton SO30 3JB, UK

K. C. M. Wilson Academic Unit, University of Liverpool, EMI Directorate, St Catherine's Hospital, Derby Road, Birkenhead L42 0LQ, UK

B. Winblad Karolinska Institute, Department of Clinical Neuroscience, Occupational Therapy and Elderly Care Research (NEUROTEC), Division of Geriatric Medicine, Huddinge Hospital B84, S-141 86 Stockholm, Sweden

J. A. Yesavage Veterans Administration, Palo Alto Health Care System, Palo Alto, CA, USA

L. Young Broadbeck, Leazes Villas, Burnopfield, Newcastle upon Tyne NE16 6HW, UK

A. Zaidi Department of Psychiatry, New York University School of Medicine, 550 First Avenue, New York, NY 10016, USA

E. M. Zayas Department of Psychiatry, St Louis University Medical School, 1221 South Grand Boulevard, Suite 202, St Louis, MO 63104, USA

Preface

The editors were very gratified that the first edition of this textbook was generally well received and that a second edition has been called for. It is now seven years since the original book appeared, and there have been many more advances in the subject. In spite of new sections and some wholesale rewriting, it has been possible once again, to contain the information in one volume. Very sadly some of our original contributors have died. New authors have replaced them while others have been added in an endeavour to keep the text authoritative and up-to-date. The helpful criticisms of the first edition have been carefully considered in the preparation of this one. Having so many distinguished authors with such a breadth of interest, while greatly enhancing the book, has led to a long gestation period, but we believe that it has been worthwhile. Much of the original format has been retained in order to continue to stimulate lively debate and exchange of views. If the book contributes to the growing strength of Geriatric Psychiatry internationally, it will have done its work.

John R. M. Copeland
Mohammed T. Abou-Saleh
Dan G. Blazer

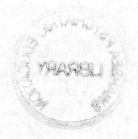

Preface to First Edition

The discipline of the psychiatry of old age has moved rapidly in recent years and the number of practitioners has expanded worldwide. An authoritative text is required which draws on the knowledge of these experts and which reflects both new scientific advances and innovations in service development.

In a comparatively new subject many of the issues are still contentious and on some of these we have tried to provide the opportunity for the expression of different points of view. Readers are asked to judge the issues for themselves from the evidence set out.

Here and there short, special articles have been commissioned which present research findings in more detail and describe new aspects of care. They are intended to enliven the text and their choice has been dependent on timing and opportunity.

We have also tried to give a "feel" for what is happening in developing countries and the scope of the problems experienced by local practitioners.

Even a book of this size can never be complete and no doubt gaps in the coverage of subjects will be identified. We would be glad to have them pointed out. The more comprehensive a book aims to be the longer it takes to come to publication and in a fast-moving area of knowledge this can be a problem. Many of our authors have been kind enough to update their contributions at a late stage, which we hope has overcome this difficulty to some extent.

In the early stages of the development of a subject there is insufficient corpus of knowledge to assemble in book form. This situation has changed dramatically for geriatric psychiatry in recent years. We hope that the knowledge gathered here from our distinguished international panel of authors bears this out.

John R. M. Copeland
Mohammed T. Abou-Saleh
Dan G. Blazer

Part A

Historical Background

A Conceptual History in the Nineteenth Century

G. E. Berrios

Department of Psychiatry, Addenbrooke's Hospital, Cambridge, UK

The history of geriatric psychiatry can be written from two viewpoints. The "externalist" approach focuses on the social and political variables that have controlled attitudes towards abnormal behaviour in old age, and on the professionalization of those charged with the care of the mentally infirm elderly. The "internalist" approach—to be followed in this chapter—concentrates on the origin of the scientific language of psychogeriatrics. An adequate historical account should include information on theories of ageing, both physical and mental, brain sclerosis and the formation of a viable concept of mental illness. On the first rubric much research has been done[1-9]; far less work exists on the other two. On psychogeriatric care before the nineteenth century[10,11] there is very little: this may simply reflect a historical reality.

VIEWS ON AGEING BEFORE THE NINETEENTH CENTURY

Like most other aspects of human life, ageing has also been portrayed in terms of metaphors. Classical views, following the nature—nurture controversy, conceived of ageing as resulting from either internal instructions or from the buffeting of foreign factors[4,8].

The "wear and tear" view happened to be popular during the early nineteenth century, the period on which this chapter will concentrate. It was based, as it had always been, on the ageless observation that all natural objects, whether animate or not, are subject to the ravages of time. Surprisingly enough, the "wear and tear" view has not always generated an understanding attitude. In fact, across times and cultures great ambiguity has existed in regard to the treatment of old folk. Fortunately, a realistic acceptance seems to have predominated although there is plenty of evidence of hostility. The Hebrew tradition, and indeed its Christian offshoot, encouraged much reverence towards the wisdom and value of old age. But even in societies which have made great play of this view, veneration has been reserved for those in positions of power or influence[12]. Little is known about attitudes towards elderly women or old men in humbler stations[11].

So, it can be concluded that, all in all, a view seems to have predominated that ageing was undesirable and that the identification of wear factors was important to devising ways of prolonging life[5,13].

A second ambiguity can be detected in these earlier writings. It concerns the extent to which the ageing process necessarily involves the human mind. Whilst it was a palpable fact that all human frames decayed, not everyone accepted that this had necessarily to affect the soul or mind. Extant descriptions of the psychological changes brought about by old age suggest that people were aware that the mind also underwent a decline. However, theory and religion encouraged the view that the spirit could or did escape wear and tear, and that human beings grew ever more wise and useful, thanks to the accumulation of experience and knowledge. This belief must have been available in all those societies that felt the need to create adequate spaces for all manner of intellectual and/or sociopolitical gerontocracies[2]. Some seem even to have separated chronological age and functional age in order to justify such concessions. From the point of view of the history of psychogeriatrics, it would be useful to know to what extent this belief was undermined by the occasional case of dementia amongst those elderly in positions of power[1] Historical evidence seems to show that these situations were neither more nor less perturbing than mental illness occurring at other periods of life. Indeed, fail-safe devices seem to have been available in these societies to cope with the upheavals created by such occurrences.

Men like Buffon, Darwin and Goethe reshaped ideas on ageing during the eighteenth century. Buffon[14] wrote: "All changes and dies in Nature. As soon as it reaches its point of perfection it begins to decay. At first this is subtle and it takes years for one to realise that major changes have in fact taken place" (p. 106). Buffon put this down to an "ossification" process similar to that affecting trees: "this cause of death is common to animals and vegetables. Oaks die as their core becomes so hard that they can no longer feed. They trap humidity, and this eventually makes them rot away" (p. 111).

Erasmus Darwin's views resulted from the application of yet another metaphor, namely, that ageing results from a breakdown of "communication" between man and his environment[15]. Darwin suggested that such breakdown followed a loss of irritability (a property of nerve fibres) and a decreased response to sensation:

"It seems our bodies by long habit cease to obey the stimulus of the aliment, which support us . . . three causes may conspire to render our nerves less excitable: 1. If a stimulus be greater than natural, it produces too great an exertion of the stimulated organ, and in consequence exhausts the spirit of animation; and the moving organ ceases to act, even though the stimulus is continued. 2. If excitations weaker than natural be applied, so as not to excite the organ into action, they may be gradually increased, without exciting the organ into action, which will thus acquire a habit of disobedience to the stimulus. 3. When irritative motions continue to be produced in consequence of stimulus, but are not succeeded by sensation . . ." (p. 365).

Principles and Practice of Geriatric Psychiatry, 2nd edn. Edited by J. R. M. Copeland, M. T. Abou-Saleh and D. G. Blazer

VIEWS ON AGEING DURING THE NINETEENTH CENTURY

In 1807 Sir John Sinclair[16] published a major compendium on ageing and longevity which included references to most pre-nineteenth century sources. It was, in a way, the last grand glance to the past. Soon afterwards work started by those who, like Léon Rostan (1791–1866), based their claims on empirical findings. Rostan, one of the most original members of the Paris school, published in 1819 his *Recherches sur le Ramollissement du Cerveau*[17], where the view commenced that vascular disorders might be as important as parenchymal ones in brain ageing. Even more important was his uncompromising anti-vitalistic position enshrined in the claim that all diseases were related to pathological changes in specific organs[18,19].

During the 1850s Reveillé-Parise[3] saw his task as writing on "the history of ageing, that is, mapping the imprint of time on the human body, whether on its organs or on its spiritual essence" (p. v). In regard to ageing itself he wrote: "the cause of ageing is a gradual increase in the work of decomposition . . . but how does it happen? What are the laws that control the degradation that affects the organization and mind of man?" (p. 13). Reveillé-Parise dismissed the toxic view defended by the Italian writer Michel Lévy[20] according to which there was a gradual accumulation of calcium phosphates that led to petrification, to an "anticipation of the grave". This view, he stated, had no empirical foundation and was based on a generalization from localized findings. Reveillé-Parise supported the view that ageing results from a negative balance between composition and elimination which equally affected the cardiovascular, respiratory and reproductive organs.

Finally, the views should be mentioned of J. M. Charcot, who in 1868 offered a series of 24 lectures on the diseases affecting the elderly[21]. Charcot dedicated Lecture 1 to the "general characters of senile pathology"; he started by saying that all books on geriatrics up to his time had "a particularly literary or philosophical turn [and had been] more or less ingenious paraphrases of the famous treatise De Senectute" (p. 25). He praised Rostan for his views on asthma and brain softening in the elderly, and predictably also mentioned Cruveilhier, Hourman and Dechambre, Durand-Fardel and Prus. He criticized Canstatt and other German physicians because in their work, "imagination holds an immense place at the expense of impartial and positive observation" (p. 26). Charcot's own contribution was based on the general principle that "changes of texture impressed on the organism by old age sometimes become so marked, that the physiological and pathological states seem to merge into one another by insensible transitions, *and cannot be clearly distinguished*" (p. 27).

THE DEVELOPMENT OF THE NOTION OF BRAIN SCLEROSIS

When in 1833 Lobstein[22] described the basic pathology of arteriosclerosis, he did not imagine that it would, during the second half of the century, become the mechanism of "senility" *par excellence*[14,23,24]. Motor and sensory deficits, vertigo, delusions, hallucinations and volitional, cognitive and affective disorder were all attributed to the effect of arteriosclerosis[25,26]. They related to the brain via a two-stage speculative pathophysiology: parenchymal and/or vascular disorders could affect the brain, and the distribution of the lesions could be diffused or focal. Vascular changes included acute ischaemia (on which clinical observation was adequate)[27,28] and chronic ischaemia, invented as a separate syndrome by extrapolating from the symptoms and signs observed during the acute states[24]. The role of arteriosclerosis as a causal and prognostic factor in relation to the involutional psychoses was challenged early in the twentieth century[29] but this paper remained unnoticed. Hence, some of the old notions, such as that of "arteriosclerotic dementia", remained active well into the 1960s[30].

Alienists during the same period, however, were already able to distinguish between states where a putative chronic and diffuse reduction in blood supply had taken place from focalized damage, i.e. what they called "multifocal arteriosclerotic dementia" and was equivalent to what is currently called multi-infarct dementia[24,31,32].

NINETEENTH CENTURY VIEWS ON MENTAL DECAY IN THE ELDERLY

It is against this background that the history of the language and concepts dedicated to understanding mental disorders in the elderly must be understood. In addition to these neurobiological frameworks, a psychological theory that explained the manner of the decline was required. Such a psychopathology was provided by the heuristic combination of associationism, faculty psychology[33], and statistics[34] that characterized the early and middle part of the nineteenth century.

Yet another perspective, originating in clinical observation, was added during the 1830s. It led to the realization that, in addition to the well known forms of mental disorder, the elderly might exhibit specific forms of deterioration, and that these could be related to recognizable brain changes. There is only space in this chapter to deal with two examples: one typifying a "specific" disorder of old age, namely the history of chronic cognitive failure or dementia; the other illustrating the effect of a general mental disorder (melancholia) on the elderly.

THE FORMATION OF THE CONCEPT OF SENILE DEMENTIA

The history of the word and concept of dementia before the nineteenth century has been touched upon elsewhere[35]. Suffice it to say here that, at the beginning of the last century, "dementia" had a "legal" and a "medical" meaning and referred to most acquired states of intellectual dysfunction that resulted in serious psychosocial incompetence. Neither age of acquisition nor reversibility was part of its definition. These two dimensions were only incorporated during the nineteenth century and completely changed the semantic territory of the dementia concept.

Anecdotal observation of cases of senile dementia abound both in the fictional literature and in historical documents[36], but the concept of "senile dementia", as it is currently understood, only took shape during the latter part of the nineteenth century. Indeed, it could not have been otherwise, as the neurobiological and clinical language that made it possible only became available during this period[37,38]. But even after the nosological status of senile dementia had become clearer, there were many who, like Rauzier[39], felt able to state: "it may appear either as a primary state or follow most of the mental disorders affecting the elderly" (p. 615). Following Rogues de Fursac[40], Adrien Pic—the author of one of the most influential geriatric manuals during this period[41]—defined senile dementia as: "a state of intellectual decline, whether or not accompanied by delusions, that results from brain lesions associated with ageing" (pp. 364–365). It was against this background that the concept of Alzheimer's disease, which became the prototype for all senile dementias, was created during the first decade of the twentieth century[37]. Recent work has shown that its "discovery" was controlled by ideological forces well beyond what could be described as "scientific"[37,42]. These forces also introduced unwarranted clinical strictures, such as the exclusion of non-cognitive symptoms[43,44] and false age boundaries, which took many years to disappear.

THE FORMATION OF THE CONCEPT OF INVOLUTIONAL MELANCHOLIA

The concept of "senile or involutional psychoses", which featured so prominently in Kraepelin's early classification, included: presenile delusional insanity, senile dementia, late catatonia and involutional melancholia[45,46]. The reasons that led Kraepelin to separate this group were mostly theoretical, to wit, that they appeared during a period of life when "sclerotic" changes were beginning to occur; the same factor accounted for their bad prognosis[46].

The general history of melancholia and depression has been analysed elsewhere[47-49]. Suffice it to say here that by the 1860s depression was considered to be an independent syndrome resulting from a primary disorder of affect. This meant that hallucinations, delusions and cognitive impairment were secondary to the pathological feelings. This conviction was particularly strong towards the end of the century, when emotional mechanisms became popular in the explanation of most forms of mental disorder[50]. By the end of the century the metaphor of depression as a form of "reduction" or "loss" had become firmly established. No better example can be found than the fact that up to 1893 (fourth edition) Kraepelin felt obliged to classify all forms of agitated depression as mania![51].

KRAEPELIN AND INVOLUTIONAL MELANCHOLIA

Much of the current confusion on the meaning of involutional melancholia can be explained if attention is given to the circumstances of its historical development (for a full analysis of this process and list of references, see reference 52). The conventional story[53-56] is that up to the seventh edition of his textbook Kraepelin considered involutional melancholia as a separate disease, and that when confronted by the evidence collected by Dreyfus[57], he decided to include it, in the eighth edition, under the general heading of manic depressive insanity. Indeed, this account was first offered by Kraepelin himself (see reference 57, p. 169).

The story is, however, more complex and it is unlikely that the findings of Dreyfus alone caused Kraepelin's change of heart. For example, Thalbitzer[58] claimed that his own work had also been influential (p. 41). In the eighth edition Kraepelin abandoned not only involutional melancholia but the entire group of "senile psychoses". A recent statistical analysis of Dreyfus's old series has also shown that his conclusion that the natural history of involutional melancholia was no different from that of depression affecting younger subjects was wrong[51].

CONCLUSIONS

This short chapter, providing a historical vignette on the origin of the language of old age psychiatry, suggests that it was born during the nineteenth century from three conceptual sources: theories of ageing, neurobiological hypotheses concerning brain sclerosis, and the realization that specific forms of mental disorder might affect the elderly. Two clinical illustrations were provided, one pertaining to the origins of the concept of senile dementia, and the other to the notion of involutional melancholia.

REFERENCES

1. Huber J-P, Gourin P. Le vieillard dément dans l'Antiquité classique. *Psychiatrie Française* 1987; **13**: 12–18.
2. Minois G. *Histoire de la Vieillesse. De l'Antiquité à la Renaissance.* Paris: Fayard, 1987.
3. Reveillé-Parise JH. *Traité de la Vieillesse.* Paris: Baillière, 1853.
4. Grmek MD. *On Ageing and Old Age.* Den Haag: W Junk, 1958.
5. Legrand MA. *La Longévité à Travers les Âges.* Paris: Flammarion, 1911.
6. Freeman JJ. *Aging. Its History and Literature.* New York: Human Sciences Press, 1979.
7. Kotsovsky D. Le problème de la vieillesse dans son développement historique. *Riv Biol* 1931; **13**: 99–111.
8. Grant RL. Concepts of aging: an historical review. *Persp Biol Med* 1963; **6**: 443–78.
9. Bastai P, Dogliotti GC. *Physiopathologie de la Vieillesse.* Paris: Masson, 1938.
10. Robinson DR. The evolution of geriatric psychiatry. *Med Hist* 1972; **16**: 184–93.
11. Kastenbaum R, Ross B. Historical perspectives on care. In Howells J, ed., *Modern Perspectives in the Psychiatry of Old Age.* Edinburgh: Churchill Livingstone, 1975, 421–49.
12. Cicero. *De Senectute, De Amicitia, De Divinatione.* Translated by W A Falconer, London: Loeb, 1923.
13. Gruman GJ. A history of ideas about the prolongation of life. *Trans Am Phil Soc* 1966; **56**: 1–97.
14. Buffon M le Comte, Georges Louis Leclerc. *Histoire Naturelle de l'Homme, de la Vieillesse et de la Mort. Vol 4 Histoire Naturelle de l'Homme.* Paris: De L'imprimerie Royale, 1774.
15. Darwin E. *Zoonomia; or, the Laws of Organic Life.* 2 Vols. London: Johnson, 1794–1796.
16. Sinclair Sir J. *The Code of Health and Longevity.* Edinburgh: Constable, 1807.
17. Rostan LL. *Recherches sur le Ramollissement du Cerveau.* Paris, 1819 and 1823.
18. Rostan LL. Jusqu à quel point l'anatomie pathologique peut-elle éclairer la thérapeutique des maladies. Thèse de concours. Paris, 1833.
19. Chereau A. Rostan. In Dechambre A, Lereboullet L, eds, *Dictionnaire Encyclopédique des Sciences Médicales*, Vol 84. Paris: Masson, 1877, 238–40.
20. Lévy M. *Traité d'hygiène Publique et Privée.* Paris: Baillière 1850.
21. Charcot JM. *Clinical Lectures on Senile and Chronic Diseases.* Translated by William S Tuke. London: The New Sydenham Society, 1981.
22. Lobstein JG. *Traité de Anatomie Pathologique*, Vol 2. Paris: Baillière, 1838.
23. Demange E. *Étude Clinique et Anatomopathologique de la Vieillesse.* Paris: Ducost, 1886.
24. Potain C. Cerveau (Pathologie). In Dechambre A, Lereboullet L, eds, *Dictionnaire Encyclopédique des Sciences Médicales*, Vol 14. Paris: Masson, 1873, 214–345.
25. Marie A. Démence. Paris: Doin, 1906.
26. Albrecht T. Manischdepressives Irresein und Arteriosklerose. *Aligem Zeitschr Psychiat* 1906; **63**: 402–447.
27. Schiller F. Concepts of stroke before and after Virchow. *Med Hist* 1970; **14**: 115–31.
28. Fields WS, Lamak NA. *A History of Stroke.* New York: Oxford University Press, 1989.
29. Walton GL. Arteriosclerosis probably not an important factor in the etiology and prognosis of involution psychoses. *Boston Med Surg J* 1912; **167**: 834–836.
30. Weitbrecht HJ. *Psychiatrie im Crundriss.* Berlin: Springer, 1968.
31. Ball B, Chambard E. Démence. In Dechambre A, Lereboullet L, eds, *Dictionnaire Encyclopédique des Sciences Médicales*, Vol 26. Paris: Masson, 1882, 559–635.
32. Spielmeyer W. *Die Psychosen des Rückbildungs und Creisenalters.* Leipzig: Deuticke, 1912.
33. Berrios GE. Historical background to abnormal psychology. In Miller E, Cooper PJ, eds, *Adult Abnormal Psychology.* Edinburgh: Churchill Livingstone, 1988, 26–51.
34. Birren JE. A brief history of the psychology of ageing. *Gerontologist* 1961; **1**: 69–77.

35. Berrios GE. Dementia during the seventeenth and eighteenth centuries: a conceptual history. *Psychol Med* 1987; **17**: 829–37.

36. Torack RM. The early history of senile dementia. In Reisberg B, ed, *Alzheimer's Disease*. New York: Free Press, 1983, 23–8.

37. Berrios GE. Alzheimer's disease: a conceptual history. *Int J Geriat Psychiat* 1990; **5**: 355–65.

38. Schwalbe J. Dementia senilis. In *Lehrbuch der Greisenkrankheiten*. Stuttgart: Enke, 1909, 479–89.

39. Rauzier G. *Traité des Maladies des Vieillards*. Paris: Baillière, 1909.

40. Rogues de Fursac J. *Manual de Psiquiatría* (translation of 5th French edition by J Peset). Valencia: Editorial Pubul, 1921.

41. Pic A. *Précis des Maladies des Vieillards*. Paris: Doin, 1912.

42. Dillman R. *Alzheimer's Disease. The Concept of Disease and the Construction of Medical Knowledge*. Amsterdam, Thesis Publishers, 1990.

43. Berrios GE. Non-cognitive symptoms and the diagnosis of dementia. Historical and clinical aspects. *Br J Psychiat* 1989; **154** (Suppl 4) 11–16.

44. Berrios GE. Memory and the cognitive paradigm of dementia during the 19th century: a conceptual history. In Murray RM, Turner TH, eds, *Lectures on the History of Psychiatry*. London: Gaskell, 1990, 194–211.

45. Cabaleiro Goas M. Los sindromes psicóticos de la presenilidad. *Acta Luso-Española de Neurología y Psiquiatrla* 1955; **14**: 17–26.

46. Cabaleiro Goas M. Psicosis preseniles no orgánicocerebrales y su prevención. In *Proceedings of I Congreso Nacional de Geronto- Psiquiatría preventiva. Xl Reunión de la Sociedad Española de Psiquiatría*. Madrid: Liade, 1974, 117–42.

47. Berrios GE. Melancholia and depression during the 19th century: a conceptual history. *Br J Psychiat* 1988; **153**: 298–304.

48. Berrios GE. Depressive and manic states during the 19th century. In Georgotas A, Cancro R, eds, *Depression and Mania*. New York: Elsevier, 1988, 13–25.

49. Berrios GE. The history of the affective disorders. In Paykel ES, ed. *Handbook of Affective Disorders*, 2nd edn. Edinburgh: Churchill Livingstone, 1992, 43–56.

50. Berrios GE. The psychopathology of affectivity: conceptual and historical aspects. *Psychol Med* 1985; **15**: 745–58.

51. Kraepelin E. *Psychiatrie*, 4th edn. Leipzig: Meixner, 1893.

52. Berrios GE. Affective symptoms in old age: a conceptual history. *Int J Geriat Psychiat* 1991; **6**: 337–46.

53. Sérieux P. Review of Dreyfus's Melancholie. *L'Encéphale* 1907; **2**: 456–8.

54. Post F. *The Clinical Psychiatry of Late Life*. Oxford: Pergamon, 1965.

55. Kendell RE. *The Classification of Depressive Illness*. Oxford: Oxford University Press, 1968.

56. Jackson SW. *Melancholia and Depression. From Hippocratic Times to Modern Times*. New Haven, CT: Yale University Press, 1985.

57. Dreyfus GL. *Die Melancholie. Ein Zustandsbild des manisch-depressiven Irreseins*. Jena: Gustav Fischer, 1907.

58. Thalbitzer S. *Emotions and Insanity*. London: Kegan Paul, Trench, Trubner, 1926.

2

Scope and Development in the Twentieth Century

Ewald W. Busse

Duke University Medical Center, Durham, NC, USA

Interest in the health and well-being of the elderly has existed since antiquity; over the centuries some remarkable observations were made regarding the health, the mental changes, and the care of the elderly. Some explanations were offered for age changes that were reasonable and some were fanciful, limited by existing scientific knowledge[1]. During the twentieth century, many biological and behavioral theories of aging have been advanced and tested, emphasizing that aging is a multidimensional phenomenon.

To understand the rapid emergence of the psychiatry of old age during the twentieth century, one must appreciate that around the year 1900, the age composition of the population began to change. Life expectancies for both males and females were being extended, particularly for females. This was paralleled by a rapid expansion in science and technology.

Although the term "gerontology" has been around for many years, the term "geriatrics" was not coined until 1914 by Nascher. In that year he published the book *Geriatrics. The Diseases of Old Age and Their Treatment*[2]. A prolific writer, Nascher's last publication in 1944 was *The Aging Mind*[3]. He observed that chronic brain syndrome was likely to be familial and he believed that it was an accelerated primary aging process that was influenced by heredity. Seven years prior to Nascher, Alzheimer published his landmark report, which described what is now known as Alzheimer's disease and is sometimes referred to as "the disease of the century"[4]. In the 1960s, books on aging and psychiatry began to appear. Among the best known of those in the English language were *The Clinical Psychiatry of Late Life*[5] by Felix Post and *Behavior and Adaptation in Late Life*[6]. In the ensuing years, many important publications have appeared that reflect rapid advances in scientific knowledge and clinical practice. In the 1940s, gerontological and geriatric societies were organized in many countries in Europe and in North America. Early in 1950 the International Association of Gerontology was founded in London, UK, with the support of the Nuffield Foundation. The first international congress of gerontology was held in Liège, Belgium, July 9–12, 1950[7]. The International Psychogeriatric Association was founded in 1980 and held its first meeting in Cairo in 1982[8].

GERIATRIC MEDICINE AND GERIATRIC PSYCHIATRY

For the past several decades, psychiatry and geriatrics have been experiencing what is called by many an "identity crisis"[9]. This crisis in identity centers on the sphere of professional activity that is the proper task of psychiatrists and geriatricians and whether their activity produces a source of self-esteem to the physicians.

The geriatric psychiatrist is making a significant contribution to solving this so-called identity crisis. The geriatric psychiatrist must often function as a primary care physician and his/her skills include proficiency in psychiatry, geriatric medicine, neurology and the social sciences. Geriatric psychiatrists are very aware that many of the disorders they treat can be cured or prevented but the resulting suffering can be relieved and the disability reduced. The situation does encourage the clinician to make observations that contribute to a better understanding of the course of chronic illness and to look for hidden clues that can lead to investigations which may, in the future, bring improved convalescence or even eradication of chronic disease and disability.

TECHNOLOGY

Advances in technology have widened the scope of old age psychiatry. For example, biochemical changes in the brain are distorted by the dying process and postmortem events. Routine postmortem examinations have limited usefulness, although rapid autopsies have improved the situation. *In vivo* brain imaging has enhanced our ability to observe biochemical processes and alterations in the aging brain[10].

PSYCHOPHARMACOLOGICAL APPROACH

The psychopharmacological approach is currently the dominant treatment for mental and emotional symptoms in elderly people. Psychotropic medications often reduce or eliminate symptoms, but do not alter the cause of the disorder. Consequently, very critically needed and exciting opportunities for research lie ahead for the geriatric psychiatrist.

Because of the possible multiple etiology of many psychiatric disorders of late life, it is highly likely that the geriatric psychiatrist will have to have a broad knowledge base and therapeutic skills including the use of medications, psychotherapeutic techniques, and procedures to reduce risks inherent in the socioeconomic status and environment.

PSYCHOTHERAPY

It is unfortunate that in 1905 Freud expressed the view that patients "near or above the fifties" were not suitable subjects for psychoanalysis[11]. For many years, this undoubtedly affected therapists' attitudes towards all psychotherapy for the elderly. Fortunately, a number of prominent psychoanalysts challenged

Principles and Practice of Geriatric Psychiatry, 2nd edn. Edited by J. R. M. Copeland, M. T. Abou-Saleh and D. G. Blazer

this Freudian view and reported psychotherapeutic success with older patients[12]. Beginning in the mid-twentieth century, a number of psychotherapeutic techniques were described and clinically evaluated for their effectiveness. Some are particularly applicable to the elderly psychiatric patient and include both behavioral and cognitive forms of psychotherapy. In Europe and North America psychotherapeutic approaches have been successfully used for elderly outpatients with depression and/or hypochondriasis.

THE SUBSPECIALTY OF GERIATRIC PSYCHIATRY

Geriatric consultants have served in the National Health Service in the UK for many years. A geriatric consultant is not a primary care physician and sees patients by referral, usually from general practitioners[13]. The geriatric consultant is likely to be hospital-based. Psychogeriatric long-term care beds are increasing in number and the responsibility is usually assigned to a consultant psychiatrist specializing in the psychiatry of old age. In 1985, the Royal College of Physicians of London conducted their first examination of candidates for a diploma in geriatric medicine. Although the Board of Examiners of the College includes representatives from general practice and from psychogeriatrics, the future of old age psychiatry as an area of specialization in the UK remains uncertain. In 1989 the British Department of Health recognized psychogeriatrics as an official subspecialty.

In Canada, the Royal College of Physicians and Surgeons in 1981 conducted examinations for special competence in geriatric medicine. Although geriatric psychiatry is not recognized as a subspecialty, the College has encouraged the development of programs in geriatric psychiatry. Since 1988 in the USA, the American Board of Internal Medicine, in collaboration with the American Board of Family Practice, has offered by examination a certificate of added qualifications in geriatrics. The examination is administered to candidates from both Boards at the same time in the same testing centers and the criteria for qualification are identical for both Boards[14].

Geriatric psychiatry was the first subspecialty area for which the American Board of Psychiatry and Neurology offered an examination for added qualifications. The first examination was given in April 1991 to 661 candidates and the second year to 578 candidates. Since the first examination 3435 certificates have been issued[15]. The next examination was scheduled for the year 2000 and the first re-certification in 2000 as well. All added qualifications in geriatric psychiatry will be time-limited to 10 years. In most European countries an examination is not required for qualification in a medical specialty. However, Sweden is moving to the examination as a requirement.

Recently there has been a rapid development of professional organizations concerned with geriatric psychiatry. Two of the most active are the American Association of Geriatric Psychiatry and the International Association of Geriatric Psychiatry. The American association has made available geriatric psychiatry self-assessment.

For many years, it was believed that many physicians are reluctant to become involved in geriatrics. Numerous explanations have been offered, including relatively low monetary compensation, the lack of satisfactory treatment outcomes and lack of personal satisfaction and scientific challenge[16]. This view has rapidly changed and considerable interest and satisfaction is evident among medical students as well as physicians in training and practice. A recent study of those who completed geriatric fellowships in geriatric medicine or psychiatry and have now been in practice for at least 3 years found that 93% were satisfied with their career choice, 80% felt that they had maintained professional status and prestige, 71% were satisfied with their incomes and 96% found personal gratification in taking care of elderly patients[17].

REFERENCES

1. Busse FW, Blazer DG. The future of geriatric psychiatry. In Busse FW, Blazer DG, eds, *Geriatric Psychiatry*. Washington, DC: American Psychiatric Press, 1989, 671–95.
2. Nascher IL. *Geriatrics: The Diseases of Old Age and Their Treatment*. Philadelphia, PA: Blakistons, 1914.
3. Nascher IL. *The Aging Mind*. Medical Record No. 157, 1944, 662.
4. Reisberg B. Preface. In Resiberg H, ed., *Alzheimer's Disease*. New York: The Free Press (Macmillan Inc), 1983.
5. Post F. *The Clinical Psychiatry of Late Life*. Oxford: Pergamon, 1965.
6. Busse EW, Pfeiffer I. *Behavior and Adaptation in Late Life*. Boston, MA: Little, Brown, 1969; 2nd edn, 1977.
7. Busse EW. International Association of Gerontology. In Maddox GL, editor-in-chief, *Encyclopedia of Aging*. New York: Springer, 1987, 359–60.
8. Bergener M. International Psychogeriatric Assocation. In Maddox GL, editor-in-chief, *Encyclopedia of Aging*. New York: Springer, 1987, 365.
9. Detre T. The future of psychiatry. *Am J Psychiat* 1987; **144**: 621–5.
10. Procter A, Doshi B, Bowen D, Murphy E. Rapid autopsy brains for biochemical research: experience in establishing a programme. *Int J Geriatr Psychiatry* 1990; **5**(5): 287–94.
11. Freud S. On Psychotherapy. In *Collected Papers*, Vol 1. London: Hogarth. First published 1905; reprinted 1949.
12. Abraham K. The applicability of psycho-analytic treatment to patients at an advanced age. In Abraham K, ed., *Selected Papers of Psychoanalysis*. London: Hogarth, 1949.
13. Brocklehurst JC. The evolution of geriatric medicine. *J Am Geriatr Soc* 1978; **26**: 433–9.
14. Certification in Geriatric Medicine. American Board of Internal Medicine and the American Board of Family Practice. Philadelphia, PA, 1999.
15. Juul D. Subspecialty certification in geriatric psychiatry. Personal communication, 1999.
16. Busse EW. Presidential address: there are decisions to be made. *Am J Psychiat* 1972; **129**: 33–41.
17. Siu AL, Beck JC. Physician satisfaction with career choices in geriatrics. *Gerontologist* 1990; **30**(14): 529–34.

3

The Development in Britain

Tom Arie

University of Nottingham, UK

Psychogeriatrics, the psychiatry of old age, was born as a service activity some 25 years ago; in 1989 it became an official specialty in the National Health Service (NHS). Until the 1960s interest in the mental disorders of old age had been largely confined to research, but today special psychiatric services for old people are widely established, and the care of mentally ill old people is recognized as a major issue by professional workers, governments and the lay public, not only in developed countries but also in the Third World. Britain has led this movement.

ORIGINS

At the end of the 1960s, about half-a-dozen psychiatrists were running psychogeriatric services. Now there are some 450 and most health districts have such a service[1]. This movement has the backing of government and of the relevant professional and voluntary bodies. The origins of this service specialty are five-fold:

1. Pressure of the increase in the numbers of the aged, particularly of the very aged.
2. Growth in psychiatry's capacity to treat conditions previously regarded as hopeless[2].
3. The movement of psychiatry from mental hospitals into people's homes, and into the general hospital.
4. The effectiveness of geriatrics in British medicine.
5. The writings and teaching in the 1960s of a small group of figures such as Sir Martin Roth and David Kay in Newcastle, Felix Post in London, and the pathologist Nicholas Corsellis at Runwell, on epidemiology[3], clinical features and prognosis[4-6] and pathology of the mental disorders of old age[7].

In 1966 a paper from Newcastle[8] emphasized the intertwining of physical, mental and social factors in the psychosyndromes of old age, and called for general hospital facilities for collaborative assessment of these complex disorders. Other writers were concerned with the possibly damaging effects of "misplacement" of old people in units of the "wrong" specialty, and Duncan Macmillan, a great psychiatric innovator, with his colleagues set up an early assessment unit and took a special interest in the assessment and care of old people[9,10].

THE PSYCHOGERIATRIC MOVEMENT

A symposium at the end of the 1960s[11] stands as a statement of what had then been achieved, and of the directions in which people were looking. Half-a-dozen younger psychiatrists were meeting as a "coffee house group", sharing their experiences of setting up local services. They established contacts with government and with national bodies and they wrote, lobbied and spoke at innumerable meetings. Above all, they influenced younger colleagues[12].

In 1973 they formed a Group within the Royal College of Psychiatrists and in 1978, as numbers grew, the Group achieved the status of a Specialist Section. The Section has provided guidance on development of services, norms for staff and facilities and advice on changing issues. Successive chairmen of the Section have reflected the development of the specialty through three "generations" of workers.

By 1985–1986 some 250 psychiatrists were running local psychiatric services specifically for the aged[13], in a variety of different styles but with a common philosophy; there have been many reports describing such services (reviewed in ref. 14). Currently, it is likely that some 450 consultant psychiatrists are primarily engaged in this work.

From the late 1970s, international networks were established, both personally and through bodies such as the World Health Organization, the Geriatric Psychiatry Section of the World Psychiatric Association, and the International Psychogeriatric Association. For a decade a course on psychogeriatrics has been run in Nottingham for the British Council, with participants from over 30 countries; versions of this have been "exported" to Australia, Israel, Poland and Portugal. An apparatus of education is established, and the Royal College of Psychiatrists sets standards for training. There are full professors of psychogeriatrics at some seven UK universities and academic posts are established in most medical schools.

A TYPICAL SERVICE

Principles for providing such services, and accounts of resources needed, have been the subject of publications by individual workers, by the Royal College of Psychiatrists and by the government (reviewed in ref. 14). *The Rising Tide* from the NHS Health Advisory Service[15] has also been influential.

Developments have generally been around a group of core workers and facilities, the latter often determined by what happened to be available in the locality. One, and preferably two, psychiatrists will have special responsibility for the aged, working with nursing (including community nursing), remedial, social services, psychology and housing department staff, and with family doctors and their teams, with geriatric medical services and with voluntary and private facilities. The service generally deals with all forms of mental illness in old age, of which the commonest is depression, and the most exacting is dementia; but old age psychiatry spans virtually the whole of psychiatry—few problems

Principles and Practice of Geriatric Psychiatry, 2nd edn. Edited by J. R. M. Copeland, M. T. Abou-Saleh and D. G. Blazer
©2002 John Wiley & Sons, Ltd

abate with age, and many become more intricate, with the admixture of physical and social problems.

The main thrust of a service is to maintain function, independence and choice. Staff strive to bring services to people in their homes, but hospital admission must be available for those who need it, as must a consultative service for other departments. Most services see patients initially at home and much follow-up takes place there or in the day hospital. Many units run special services, such as "memory clinics" or relatives' support groups, or collaborate in running stroke, continence or "orthogeriatric" services.

Standard facilities comprise an admission unit, which should be in the district hospital, outpatient clinics and day hospitals. A close relationship should exist with geriatrics, and in a few cases (especially where geriatrics and psychogeriatrics are located apart from each other) there are joint "psychogeriatric assessment units", in which psychiatrists and geriatricians collaborate. In Nottingham's Department of Health Care of the Elderly, geriatricians, psychogeriatricians and related staff have worked together in one department.

Longer-stay units, also offering respite admission, nowadays are smaller and more "domestic", and often close to their local communities. Much long-stay care is now private. Long-stay care remains the "Achilles heel" of the care of the elderly; the government's reaction to the report of its Royal Commission on Long-stay Care is still awaited[16], whilst a series of National Required Standards on all aspects of long-stay care are currently about to go out to consultation[17].

Wattis' analysis gives some support to the claim that services for older people provided by specialist psychogeriatricians are stronger than those provided by general psychiatrists who spend only a minority of their clinical time in old age psychiatry[8]. Such specialist services have significantly more consultant and non-medical staff time per thousand elderly served and are more likely to have acute beds on a district general hospital site and long-stay beds within the catchment area served. Their consultants are more likely to be involved in educational activities and to report research interests.

Voluntary Organizations

There has been a great growth of public awareness of the problems of mentally ill older people and of those who look after them. Bodies such as the Alzheimer's Disease Societies (now active in many countries) form a generally vigorous alliance with the professions as pressure groups, sources of information or support, or as fund-raisers.

Research[8]

There is nowadays hardly a relevant university department that is not concerned with the mental disorders of old age; biological research on the dementias has moved fast, as has clinical research and research on services and on carers. National and international collaboration in clinical and epidemiological studies is growing. A major longitudinal study of cognitive change in old people under the auspices of the Medical Research Council has been completed. The advent of journals such as the *International Journal of Geriatric Psychiatry* and *International Psychogeriatrics* reflects the clearer identity of the field and the growth of research activity.

Education and Entry to the Specialty[4]

Demands for teaching come from the health professions and beyond (e.g. police, clergy, architects, designers). Teaching in old

Table 3.1. What does a psychogeriatric service do?

Assessment
Diagnosis
Hospital liaison
"Rehabilitation"
Continuing care
Long-term and intermittent care
Support for carers
Planning
Advocacy, liaison and fund-raising
Other services
  Voluntary
  Private
  Non-health professions
  Government
  "The public"
  The media
Advice (e.g. financial, legal, "ethical")
Education
Research

age psychiatry is now common in the training of most of the health professions, and post-qualification courses are increasingly available. Day symposia abound. To enter the specialty in the UK, doctors need first to complete the 3 year basic training in psychiatry before taking the MRCPsych diploma of the Royal College of Psychiatrists, which will usually include 6 months in a psychogeriatric unit. Following the examination, higher trainees, in psychogeriatrics will spend 2 years in a psychogeriatric service and 2 years in general psychiatry, usually maintaining links with the former through clinical work or research and obtaining special experience (e.g. in geriatric medicine, neurology or management). Such training will qualify the doctor for a post as a psychogeriatrician, i.e. a psychiatrist devoting all or the bulk of his/her time to the psychiatry of old age. Higher trainees in general psychiatry may opt to spend a year in psychogeriatrics, and would then be qualified to take a "special interest" post, such as may exist in small districts. Many "doctors with domestic commitments" have trained part-time in psychogeriatrics.

Training arrangements will need to be adjusted for doctors who, having opted to do a year in psychogeriatrics, decide that they want this to become their main activity and so will wish to complete the full 2 years. In a new specialty there need to be clear standards and carefully monitored training, along with flexibility. Table 3.1 summarizes the range and scope of the work.

INTERNATIONAL DEVELOPMENTS

Psychogeriatric services are now in being in most developed countries, and there is activity in this field in the Third World too[20]. The International Psychogeriatric Association is a thriving body, as is the World Psychiatric Association's Geriatric Psychiatry Section, which has lately published a series of broadly-based Consensus Statements on the content of the specialty, on Organization and on Education[21].

ACKNOWLEDGEMENT

This chapter was originally based, with permission, on: Arie T. Emerging specialties: Psychogeriatrics. *Br J Hosp Med* 1990; **44**: 70–1.

REFERENCES

1. Arie T. Martin Roth and the psychogeriatricians. In Davison K, Kerr A, eds, *Contemporary Themes in Psychiatry: A Festschrift for Sir Martin Roth*. London: Gaskell, 1989.
2. Post F. Then and now. *Br J Psychiat* 1978; **133**: 83–6.
3. Kay DWK, Beamish P, Roth M. Old age mental disorders in Newcastle upon Tyne. *Br J Psychiat* 1964; **110**: 146–68, 668–82.
4. Roth M. The natural history of mental disorder in old age. *J Ment Sci* 1955; **101**: 281–301.
5. Post F. *The Significance of Affective Symptoms in Old Age*. Maudsley Monograph No. 10. London: Oxford University Press, 1962.
6. Post F. *Persistent Persecutory States of the Elderly*. London: Pergamon, 1966.
7. Corsellis JAN. *Mental Illness and the Ageing Brain*. Maudsley Monograph No. 9. London: Oxford University Press, 1951.
8. Kay DWK, Roth M, Hall MRP. Special problems of the aged and the organisation of hospital services. *Br Med J* 1966; **ii**: 967–72.
9. Morton EVB, Barker ME, Macmillan D. The joint assessment and early treatment unit in geriatrics. *Gerontol Clin* 1968; **10**: 65.
10. Macmillan D. Preventive geriatrics. *Lancet* 1960; **ii**: 1439.
11. Kay DWK, Walk A (eds). *Recent Developments in Psychogeriatrics: A Symposium*. Royal Medico-Psychological Association. Ashford, Kent: Headley Brothers, 1971.
12. Jolley DJ. Psychiatrist into psychogeriatrician. *Br J Psychiat News Notes* 1976; November: 11–13.
13. Wattis JP. Geographical variations in the provision of psychiatric services for old people. *Age Ageing* 1988; **17**: 171–80.
14. RCP and RCPsych. *Care of Elderly People with Mental Illness. Specialist Services and Medical Training*. London: Royal College of Physicians of London and Royal College of Psychiatrists, 1999.
15. NHS Health Advisory Service. *The Rising Tide*. Sutton, Surrey: Health Advisory Service, 1982.
16. *Royal Commission on Long-stay Care with Respect to Old London*. London: HMSO, 1999.
17. Centre for Policy on Ageing. *National Required Standards for Residential and Nursing Homes for Older People*. London: Centre for Policy on Ageing, 1999.
18. Wattis JP. A comparison of 'specialized' and 'non-specialized' psychiatric services for old people in the United Kingdom. *Int J Geriatr Psychiat* 1989; **4**: 59–62.
19. Arie T (ed.). *Recent Advances in Psychogeriatrics*, 2nd edn. Edinburgh: Churchill Livingstone, 1992.
20. Arie T, Jolley DJ. Psychogeriatrics. In Freeman H (ed.), *A Century of Psychiatry*. London: Mosby-Wolfe, 1999.
21. World Health Organization and World Psychiatric Association. *Lausanne Technical Consensus Statements on Psychiatry of the Elderly*. Geneva: WHO, 1999.

The Development in the USA, 1600–1900

W. Andrew Achenbaum, Crystal Cederquist, Vicki Kahl, Kathryn Rosenberg

University of Michigan, Ann Arbor, MI, USA

There is a dearth of information about the care of mentally ill older persons in the USA from the seventeenth through the nineteenth centuries. Despite an extensive literature on the history of the various stages of the mental health movement during the period, little is known about the treatment of the aged, members of ethnic and religious minority groups, or of women of any age who became ill between 1600 and 1900. Much reported here refers to a largely white, male, New England data set. Virtually no evidence comes from the south or from west of the Mississippi.

In colonial times the mentally ill, along with other classes of dependents, were treated as a local responsibility, primarily placed with their own or other families. Clergy and physicians alike subscribed to a belief in demoniacal possession that was widespread in seventeenth century America. Few colonial doctors investigated other possible causes of mental disorders; no "scientific" theory for dealing with the mentally ill was yet in vogue.

Legal cases involving persons suffering from mental illness were decided on an individual basis. In 1639, the Massachusetts General Court was empowered to determine settlement for wandering individuals. Six years later, as a result of the need for such rulings, three men were selected to form a committee to consider provisions of a law for "disposing of inmates and settling impotent aged persons and vagrants"[1]. It is probable that a significant minority of the people affected by this law were mentally ill, but the extant records do not yield adequate documentation to verify the incidence or treatment of such cases.

The "violent" insane among public dependents were ordinarily treated as common criminals. The harmless mentally ill were treated almost the same as other paupers. Records have been found as early as 1676 of the levy of a small tax on a village in Massachusetts to help one man build and maintain a small block house for his son, who was "bereft of his natural senses"[2].

In an effort to deal with its indigent and insane citizens, Boston in the late 1600s established the first almshouse in New England. Following English custom (which was to continue in America well into the nineteenth century), indigents and petty offenders were herded indiscriminately into this poorhouse—the sick and well, the able-bodied and impotent, and law-breaking and law-abiding, young and aged, "worthy poor" and vagrants, sane and insane. In 1736, the "Poor-House, Work-House, and House of Corrections of New York City" was built in Manhattan. Elsewhere, poorhouses and houses of corrections also served as repositories for the mentally ill. The founding of the Pennsylvania Hospital in 1752 (with its special section for the insane in the basement) and in 1773 the opening of the Virginia Eastern Asylum (the first American institution exclusively for mental patients) at Williamsburg, Virginia, provided crucial steps in a more humane treatment orientation for the mentally ill. No special treatment for the elderly on account of their age, however, was instituted.

Besides attempts to effect reforms to help the insane during the Revolutionary period (*c.* 1765–1820), a few Americans challenged prevailing beliefs. Dr Benjamin Rush, who joined the staff of physicians at Pennsylvania Hospital in 1783, became known as the Father of American Psychiatry, in part because he advanced the humane and intelligent treatment of the insane. In addition to studying the effects of the moon on mental illness, Rush proposed that ill women and men engage in meaningful work, a forerunner of occupational therapy. He wanted patients to write down all that troubled their minds. Rush believed in kind treatment: asylums were to hire intelligent men and women to attend the patients. All visitors who had a disturbing effect on patients were to be excluded.

Rush's views on mental health in late life are worth mentioning, because they anticipated later views and because so few of his contemporaries took an interest in the subject. Older people, he felt, were naturally protected against certain maladies; madness, he observed, tended to attack mainly between the ages of 20 and 50. In his *Medical Inquiries and Other Observations on Diseases of the Mind*[3], Rush claimed that "the moral faculties, when properly regulated and directed, never partake of the decay of the intellectual faculties in old age, even in persons of uncultivated minds". Potential, not just decline, characterized even those past 80 years of age.

Ironically, the "enlightened" view that older persons did not suffer as greatly as younger people from the scourges of mental impairment justified, for many Americans, the view that it was acceptable to treat elderly persons who did need help as "invisible lunatics". This perception was reinforced by two trends. First, in the wake of the Revolution, a rising tide of humanitarianism dominated reformist thought in the early 1800s. Officials removed restraints in mental hospitals in the expectation that more humane treatment would facilitate recovery. This "moral treatment" concept dominated psychiatric practice for over 20 years until the 1830s, when it was abandoned. Karl Menninger[4] attributes its decline to the influx of immigrants crowding the hospitals and the emergence of a new scientific perspective. Second, physicians such as Dr Weir Mitchell and Dr Pliny Earle assembled a battery of statistics to convince the medical profession that mental illness was incurable[5,6]. If so, lifetime follow-ups would inevitably disclose recurrences of mental illness in a patient. This prognosis struck a death blow at moral treatment, and ushered in a long era of therapeutic nihilism. "Psychiatrists tended more and more," claims Gerald Grob, America's foremost scholar of the history of mental illness, "to disregard the psychogenic aspects of mental illness and to emphasize its somatic etiology"[7].

Principles and Practice of Geriatric Psychiatry, 2nd edn. Edited by J. R. M. Copeland, M. T. Abou-Saleh and D. G. Blazer

In this context, there seemed to be little sense in doing much for the old. The elderly were discouraged from care in the state psychiatric hospitals, because they were thought, by virtue of their age, to be untreatable. If there were low probability that insanity could be cured even if detected early and treated aggressively, the elderly should not be allowed to take up valuable space that could be used to treat the curable. Therefore, custodial care for the elderly insane was the best that could be provided by families, almshouses, or prisons[8,9].

The elderly, nevertheless, represented a significant proportion of the institutionalized population. A comprehensive survey of insanity among the general population of Massachusetts conducted in 1854, for instance, revealed that insane people in asylums aged 60 and above made up 9.8% of the inmates. Nearly one out of every five insane persons in Massachusetts was over 60 years old. Despite such data, Rosenkrantz and Vinovskis[10] maintain that the pervasiveness of insanity among the elderly was not recognized by nineteenth century physicians; the elderly insane remained the least likely age group to be institutionalized.

A lack of systematic record-keeping concerning mental health admissions of the aged prior to 1900 makes it hazardous to generalize about trends. Even so, based on nineteenth century data from Massachusetts, the following propositions seem warranted. On the one hand, admission rates fluctuated from one decade to the next, which suggests that those who ran institutions had considerable power to determine who could enter. On the other hand, men outnumbered women in asylums, probably because families found older women more deserving of support and less disruptive or threatening in behavior. Alcohol abuse, it is worth noting, was more likely to be cited as a diagnosis of insanity for males[8].

Because of the prevailing nihilism, the dependent elderly were generally sent to local almshouses rather than mental institutions prior to 1890[11]. Superintendents may have discouraged the admission of elderly patients, considering them a threat to the therapeutic mission of the hospital. However, records showed that patients over 70 were not troublesome and were kindly tolerated. They did receive less specific medical therapy than younger inmates. Curiously, given the rampant nihilism, what care they received apparently proved efficacious: more than half of those in institutions in their seventh decade were discharged due to recovery or improvement. The rest, however, usually stayed until death.

Because a significant proportion of mental patients aged in place, it is not surprising that the percentage of the elderly in institutions was greater than that in the general population. In 1880, there were 140 public and private mental hospitals caring for nearly 41 000 patients; 9300 were kept in almshouses; the rest were cared for in their own homes. The Census of 1880 showed 91 997 insane persons out of a total American population of 50 000 000; 52% were female, 71% native born, and 93% white. Responsibility for the aged insane was usually divided between local almshouses and mental hospitals. Between 1880 and 1890, insane persons constituted nearly a quarter of the total almshouse population. Between 1851 and 1890 nearly 10% of California's institutionalized insane were 60 years or older; in Arizona in 1900 the figure was only 1.71%; and in Massachusetts in the 1880s it was 12.1%. Most of the aged insane were said to be suffering from some form of senility.

The increasing use of the term "senility" to characterize impairments in mental health in later years signals the emergence of new scientific views of senescence. William James in *Principles of Psychology*[12] and George Beard in *American Nervousness*[13] contended that the majority of the elderly invariably experienced a decline in mental faculties and a decreased ability to learn new materials and/or to adapt to changing circumstance. Charles Brown-Séquard hypothesized that the decline resulted from "diminishing action of the spermatic glands". W. A. N. Dorland[14] believed that people's "creativity" declined after age 60. Metchnikoff's attribution of old age to a chronic disease process is indicative of the pessimistic thought regarding the well-being of the elderly in general[15]. In view of such thought, it is not surprising that the elderly mentally ill were regarded as quite hopeless and undeserving of efforts at rehabilitation. Indeed, there was so little interest in this population that "geriatrics" did not become a medical specialty until the twentieth century under the influence of Dr I. L. Nascher[16].

As basic processes of aging became a focus of scientific inquiry for a growing number of researchers, others tried to understand the etiology of more late-life disorders. Alois Alzheimer established (in a 1907 report) a histologic picture of the disease that would later bear his name. But there was not much interest in old age-associated dementia until increases in adult life expectancy started to change the demographic make-up of industrial societies[17].

REFERENCES

1. Hurd H, ed. *The Institutional Care of the Insane in the United States and Canada*, Vol. 1. Baltimore, MD: Johns Hopkins Press, 1916, 81.
2. Deutsch A. *The Mentally Ill in America*. New York: Columbia University Press, 1949, 66.
3. Rush B. *Medical Inquiries and Other Observations on Diseases of the Mind*. New York, 1812. Hafner Reprints, 1962.
4. Menninger K. *The Vital Balance*. New York: Viking, 1963, 402.
5. Brody JB. The *Journal of Nervous and Mental Disease*, the first 100 years. *J Nerv Ment Dis* 1974; **159**: 1–11.
6. Olverholser W. Founding of the Association. In Hall JK, Zilbourg B, Bunker HA, eds. *One Hundred Years of American Psychiatry*. New York: Columbia University Press, 1944.
7. Grob C. *The State and the Mentally Ill*. Chapel Hill, NC: The University of North Carolina Press, 1966.
8. Achenbaum WA. *Old Age in the New Land*. Baltimore, MD: Johns Hopkins University Press, 1978.
9. Haber C. *Beyond Sixty-Five*. New York: Cambridge University Press, 1983, 89.
10. Rosenkrantz B, Vinovskis MA. Invisible lunatics. In Spicker S, Van Tassel D, Woldwald K, eds. *Aging and the Elderly*. Atlantic Highlands: Humanities Press, 1978, 96–123.
11. Grob G. *Inner World of American Psychiatry*. New Brunswick, NJ: Rutgers University Press, 1985.
12. James W. *Principles of Psychology* (2 vols). New York: Henry Holt, 1885.
13. Beard GM. *American Nervousness*. New York: GP Putnam, 1881.
14. Dorland WAN. *Age of Mental Virility*. New York: Century Co., 1908.
15. Metchnikoff E: *Prolongation of Life*. New York: GP Putnam, 1908.
16. Nascher IL. *Geriatrics*. Philadelphia, PA: P. Blakiston, 1914.
17. Iqbal K, Wisniewski HM, Winblad B (eds). *Alzheimer's Disease and Related Disorders*. New York: Alan R. Liss, 1989, 1–2.

4b

In the Beginning

The Late Felix Post

In 1943, after a year's early training as one of the war-time refugees of the Maudsley Hospital, Professor Aubrey Lewis passed me on to Professor D. K. Henderson and the Royal Edinburgh Hospital for Nervous and Mental Diseases, where I initially worked in the private department. During one of his rounds, Henderson said to me: "Post, do you see all these old people here? Why don't you write 'em up?" This I obediently did, and my article appeared in the *Journal of Mental Science*[1]. The article started by demonstrating that the admission rate of patients over 60 to the Royal Edinburgh Hospital had risen between 1901 and 1941 more steeply than the proportion of this age group in the Scottish population. Interestingly, at this early date, I had found no difficulties in the differential diagnosis of my colleagues' and my own patients. There were 22 senile, arteriosclerotic and presenile dementia patients, 20 manic–depressive patients, 25 patients suffering from involutional or senile melancholia and 51 patients with schizophrenia. Assuming that the functional psychoses were the concern of general psychiatry, the rest of the paper dealt with the dementias and with an attempt to link the type associated with delusions and hallucinations to earlier personality characteristics. I noted that a high proportion of dementia admissions had been precipitated by terminal confusional states, and that of 111 patients admitted over the preceding 4 years with organic psychoses, only 23 were still occupying beds. I made the false prediction that in the future the main burden of the hospital services would be represented by the chronicity and survival of melancholic and paranoid patients. I did not anticipate that electroconvulsive therapy (ECT) and antidepressive drugs, while producing lasting recoveries in only 25% of cases, would make at least temporary discharge from inpatient care possible in most cases.

Aubrey Lewis was more farsighted. He had published, with a psychiatric social worker[3] a paper describing the psychiatric and social features of the patients in the Tooting Bec Hospital for Senile Dementia, London, UK, and in 1946 predicted, in the *Journal of Mental Science*[3] that ageing and senility would become a major problem of psychiatry.

After army service, I consulted Lewis about possible positions and he recommended me for the post of assistant physician at the Maudsley Hospital. I flattered myself that in me Lewis had seen a future brilliant psychiatrist, but was soon to be disillusioned. Even before the Bethlem Royal and Maudsley Hospitals were united in 1948, Lewis had conceived the idea of using some of the Bethlem beds to establish a unit for patients over the age of 60. After a heated discussion with the Bethlem matron, Lewis obtained agreement for the admission of senile patients to a hospital which, like the Maudsley, had previously admitted only patients thought to be recoverable. Uncovering his batteries, he asked me to take on the development of this Geriatric Unit. Once again, I obeyed (to say without enthusiasm would be an understatement) and, right up to my retirement, I continued also to run a unit and outpatient clinic for younger adults.

A report in the *Bethlem Maudsley Gazette*[4] demonstrated that both the Bethlem staff and I had "caught fire". The article started with a tribute to Professor Aubrey Lewis and his almost revolutionary idea of including experience in geriatric psychiatry within postgraduate training. The article went on to describe how patients over 60 had gradually infiltrated the Bethlem wards to emerge as a unit for 26 women and 20 men. The two wards were staffed by the same number of senior and junior nurses as the other adult wards, with two trainee psychiatrists changing every 6 months to other departments. There was one psychiatric social worker (PSW), later usually assisted by a trainee. The occupational therapy department had collaborated with the nursing staff to devise and carry out a daily occupational programme as well as socializing activities. The PSW ran a weekly afternoon of handicrafts, tea and talk near the Maudsley, where throughout my tenure I conducted a weekly follow-up and supportive clinic. The first year during which the unit had been in full swing was 1952, and it was recorded that during that year there had been 3.00 admissions to each geriatric bed compared to 3.74 admissions to each general psychiatric place. Patients who had been dementing, but whose home care was no longer possible had been excluded from admission, though not rigidly, as well as patients with recurring illnesses that had been adequately treated at the Bethlem-Maudsley or other hospitals. Of 133 patients, nine died, only four had to be transferred to their regional mental hospitals, seven were resettled in homes for the elderly, while 113 could be returned to family care. One year after discharge, information was successfully obtained about 121 of 124 cases. Seven patients had died, including one suicide of a woman who had discharged herself. Thirty ex-patients had to be readmitted to our or other hospitals, thirty-five were still outside hospital but by no means symptom-free, but 45 patients would be classified as recovered. These relatively favourable results were due to 89 patients having suffered from affective illnesses: 24 had symptoms associated with brain damage, 10 were mainly paranoid and 10 were regarded as having psychoneurosis. In spite of 4–6 weeks of conservative management 52 patients had to be given ECT. I concluded the article by pointing to research needs and by opining that with 30–40% of patients admitted to British mental hospitals being over the age of 60, training in the special problems of this age group was essential for all entrants to general psychiatry.

The history of the beginning would be incomplete without a brief account of further developments. My little textbook (rightly out of print) and publications on the long-term outcome of

Principles and Practice of Geriatric Psychiatry, 2nd edn. Edited by J. R. M. Copeland, M T. Abou-Saleh and D. G. Blazer
©2002 John Wiley & Sons, Ltd

affective, paraphrenic and schizo-affective illnesses were largely my own work, but many of the junior psychiatrists made contributions and they and clinical psychologists, as well as social workers, instigated their own researches. Many later made a name for themselves, and some became leading psychogeriatricians. Among them were Tom Arie, the late L. K. Hemsi, David Jolley, Robin Jacoby, David Kay, Kenneth Shulman and, last but certainly not least, Raymond Levy. After the Bethlem-Maudsley had accepted a district commitment and the admission of involuntary (sectioned) patients, Raymond Levy and my successor, Klaus Bergmann (not a Bethlem trainee), managed to move the Geriatric Unit to the Maudsley, so much closer to the patients' family homes. Raymond Levy succeeded in establishing an Academic Department of Old Age Psychiatry, which has continued to conduct research into the dementias of late life, that most important subject, previously neglected on account of admission restrictions before the hospital abandoned its ivory tower to accept a district commitment. With similar developments elsewhere, psychogeriatrics became a world movement, and Sir Aubrey Lewis would be pleased.

REFERENCES

1. Post F. Some problems arising from a study of mental patients over the age of sixty years. *J Ment Sci* 1944; **90**: 554–65
2. Lewis AJ, Goldschmidt H. Social causes of admission to a mental hospital for the aged. *Sociol Rev* 1943; **365**: 86–98.
3. Lewis AJ. Ageing and senility: a major problem of psychiatry. *J Ment Sci* 1946; **92**: 150–70.
4. Post F. Geriatric Unit (a report on progress made, with special reference to 1952). *Bethlem Maudsley Hosp Gaz* 1955; **1**: 270–1.

Part B

Normal Ageing

BI   Theories of Ageing

BII   Brain Ageing

BIII Psychology of Ageing

BIV   Sociology of Ageing

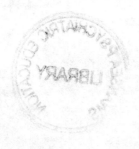

General Theories of Aging

Ewald W. Busse

Duke University Medical Center, Durham, NC, USA

INTRODUCTION

There is no satisfactory composite theory of aging, but numerous theories have been advanced to explain how and why living organisms age and die[1,2]. Given the multidimensionality of human beings, many theories of aging, some familiar and some overlapping, have been developed. Theories of aging are usually grouped by biological, psychological, or sociological sciences. A comprehensive review of theories of aging is beyond the scope of this chapter. However, the selected theories that are to be reviewed are particularly relevant to the psychiatry of old age.

Depending on the discipline, the phenomenon of aging takes on different definitions. Biologic aging is made up of a number of undesirable processes. There are multiple processes of aging that result in a decline in efficiency of the organism and end in its death. Aging, particularly in the psychosocial sciences, often includes a desirable process of maturation, that is, acquiring a desirable quality such as wisdom.

THE BIOLOGICAL THEORIES OF AGING

Biological theories of aging can be broken down into two broad categories: the developmental genetic theories (primary aging) and the stochastic theories (secondary aging processes)[3,4]. Primary aging refers to those declines in function that are genetically controlled, while secondary (stochastic) aging consists of random changes resulting from acquired disease and trauma. If the hostile events related to secondary aging could be prevented, life would be extended but, because of primary aging, decline and death are inevitable.

Deliberate Biological Programming

Hayflick and Moorhead[5] made an important contribution to our understanding of cellular aging. They demonstrated that human mitotic cells would divide a finite number of times and then the cell culture would die. Numerous studies demonstrated that the "normal" cells have a memory for the number of duplications, which is believed to be encoded in the genetic material. In contrast, cancer cells have abnormal chromosomes and have the capacity for dividing endlessly.

The capacity for a programmed cell death that exists in mitotic (dividing) cells is also present in postmitotic (non-dividing) cells. Cells incapable of dividing, such as neurons, do age and die. Certain types of brain cells, such as those located in the hypothalamus, appear to be much more vulnerable than others. In aging, not only are neurons lost, but there are alterations of neuronal synapses and networks[6].

Apoptosis is a "physiological normal process by which multicellular organisms get rid of injured, infected or developmentally unnecessary cells"[7,8]. Apoptosis is similar, if not identical, to a programmed cell death. The term is derived from Greek and means the dropping of petals from flowers or leaves from trees. The term "necrosis" is also commonly used to describe another kind of cell death. Necrosis is a type of cell death that is the result of the failure of nutrients to reach the cell. Death by necrosis is quite different from death by apoptosis. In necrosis the cells blow up, spill their contents and start an immune response. In apoptosis, however, the cells seem to condense, but develop blebs that separate and form "apoptosis bodies". Apoptosis bodies undergo rapid phagocytosis; thus, in apoptosis the cells die with little observable reaction, while when they die of necrosis they produce a widespread inflammatory response.

Genetics of Human Aging

In humans and in many other animal species, females outlive males and this difference can be attributed to genetic factors, as the male has a Y and an X chromosome and the female has two X chromosomes. The small Y chromosome does not appear to contain sufficient genetic material for the normal development or well-being of a human. Its primary function is to provide male characteristics[9]. Chromosomes contain the vast majority of genes, but a few exist within the mitochondria. Mitochondrial genes are important to aerobic respiration and age changes. All mitochondrial genes are inherited from the mother[10].

The Aging Clock

Miller provides a working definition of aging as follows: "Aging is a process that converts fit adults into frail adults with a progressive increased risk of illness, injury and death"[11]. He favors as an explanation for aging the existence of a single aging clock. This aging clock is in turn linked to many of the observed biological clocks that are seen in both humans and animals. Miller holds that a useful way of determining biological age will eventually emerge rather than depending upon chronological age. He supports the view that the genetic control of lifespan should be considered relatively minor. He believes that it influences lifespan at no more than 15–35%. Living in a favorable environment and having favorable living habits influence most of the lifespan.

Inherent in our functioning are the biological rhythms observed at the hormonal levels. Many of the biological rhythms are synchronized by control centers within the brainstem. The hypothalamus plays a particularly important role in the losses of homeostatic mechanisms in the body. The responsible nuclei (clusters of cells within the hypothalamus) change with aging. These cells decline not only in number but also in efficiency. Sleep changes in late life are clearly associated with alteration of control centers within the brainstem. Van Gool and Mirmiran[12] propose that our biological rhythms become desynchronized as we age.

The Free Radical Theory

A free radical is often considered a molecular fragment, as it has an unpaired electron. It is unstable and highly reactive. Free radicals are ubiquitous in living substances and are produced by normal metabolic processes as well as by external causes such as ionizing radiation, ozone and chemical toxins. Free radicals have been linked to DNA damage, the cross-linkage of collagen and the accumulation of age pigments[13,14].

The Accumulation of Waste

With the passage of time, certain pigments such as lipofuscin accumulate in neurons and other cells. While there is no direct evidence that these pigments may be harmful to these cells, there is an association with the wear and tear of aging. Interestingly, the accumulation of lipofuscin is limited to the cells that are capable of dividing[15].

The Immune System and Aging

The autoimmune theory of aging was proposed by Burnett[16], Walford[17] and Comfort[18]. It was suggested that a small number of immunologically competent cells may mutate in such a fashion as to lose their tolerance to their host antigen and subsequently give rise to a clone of "renegade" cells[19], producing antibodies that might result in death or damage in a large number of cells, including neurons. "Anti-brain antibodies" are believed to be related to neuronal injury in senile dementia of the Alzheimer type. Autoimmunity to vascular antigens has also been reported[20].

The immune system is a complex network, but it has been found that restoring certain components can improve immunity. Interleukin-2 (IL-2) declines with age and it appears that the administration of IL-2 may retard the human aging processes[21].

Caloric Restriction and Aging

It is well established that physical inactivity and overeating contribute to obesity, which in turn increases morbidity and mortality[22]. Determining the pathophysiology of overeating is being given considerable attention. It appears that oxidative stress associated with excess caloric intake results in damage that impacts on the process of senescence and various diseases common in late life. In contrast, a calorie-restricted diet in laboratory animals results in an increase in average lifespan. However, it is unclear whether further caloric restrictions in non-obese humans will add to life expectancy.

Other Biological Theories of Aging

The disposable soma theory holds that nature's demand for reproduction takes precedence over a demand for longevity[23]. Nature gives a priority to those traits that are inherent in the organism that favor reproductive success—traits that enhance their fecundity. Hence, somatic cells are disposed of after achieving reproductive success. However, it appears that the selection of traits that are favorable for reproduction may indirectly influence lifespan because the increased reserve capacity to carry an animal to and through a longer reproductive life also adds to the animal's capacity to live longer.

The brain–body weight theory is based on evidence that the heavier the brain when compared to the weight of the body, the more likely the organism is to be inclined to longevity[24]. This relationship of brain and body is called "the index of cephalization". Naturally there are deviations from this correlation and this in turn has made the theory of limited validity.

Biophysicists have proposed a theory of aging that aims to explain why larger living organisms tend to live longer than smaller organisms. One explanation is that "lifespan tends to lengthen and metabolism slows down in proportion to the quarter power of the animal's body weight", or what might be called a "scaling theory" of aging[25]. The theory is sometimes linked to the system of distributing nutrients. The rate of a heartbeat is relevant to the distribution of nutrients. For example, the elephant lives much longer than the chicken and has a much slower heart rate. However, the capillaries of elephants are the same size as those found in the chicken.

PSYCHOLOGICAL THEORIES OF AGING

Psychologists have accumulated a wealth of information regarding mental stability and change in late life. As in biology, this information has not been integrated into a viable comprehensive theory. The main areas that have been studied by psychologists can be placed in three broad categories: cognition, personality and coping mechanisms.

Cognitive Psychology

The term "cognition" subsumes the range of human intellectual functioning[26]. Cognition is to perceive, to remember, to reason, to make decisions, to solve problems and to integrate complex knowledge. Measures of various types of cognition are influenced by chronological age, environment, task characteristics and other influences. With advancing age, individual differences in cognitive functions seem to increase. A comprehensive coverage of the studies on intelligence and memory in old age is beyond the scope of this chapter and will be presented at greater length in Section BIII, while basic concepts in those areas will be introduced in this chapter. In general, adults with high intelligence and education will show minimum decline in their performances with increasing age, while a significant decline is observed in adults with lower intelligence and age. However, older adults in general tend to perform less well in new or novel situations[26].

Loss of memory is a common complaint of old age and has received considerable attention by psychologists. There are several theoretical models of memory functioning. Such theories attempt to define various stages of information processing. Often attempts are made to distinguish short-term from long-term memory. Other theorists talk about primary, secondary and tertiary memory.

Research on intellectual functioning has been under way for many years and has been productive. Intellectual performance seems to be strongly influenced by physical health. However, patterns of stability and change across the life cycle vary according to the ability that is being measured[26]. Perlmutter[27] crystallizes the issue of psychological change and stability by positing a "multiprocess phenomenon conception", as opposed to Baltes' "dual process phenomenon conception" of development followed by decline[28]. Perlmutter sees decline as neither inevitable nor universal and says that some cognitive skills may improve or may be acquired as one ages. However, as one reaches the point of "terminal drop"[29], which is a curvilinear decline related to the distance of death rather than old age itself, there will be a decline in intellectual functioning.

Schaie's 30 stage theory of adult cognitive development attempts to formulate four cognitive stages in sequence. The first stage in childhood and adolescence is "acquisitive", which is followed by the "achievement" stage in young adulthood, then by the "responsible and executive" stage in the middle-aged individual, and finally the "reintegrative" stage in old age. The shift is translated essentially from "What should I know?" to "How should I use what I know?" to "Why should I know?"

Ribot[31] advanced the "cognitive regression hypothesis" which hypothesized that the structures first formed are the last ones to degenerate in old age. This has not been proved to be a constant feature, depending on what components of cognition are being studied. Essentially, no adult age differences have been found in conservation, egocentrism and concept attainment[32]. However, when it comes to constructing classification, young children and the elderly tend to have a holistic perception, while older children and younger adults are more analytic[33–35]. The fact that older adults have an easier time learning dated items and retrieving dated items follows Ribot's law. In regard to free recall, older adults as well as younger children use motoric encoding and real-life objects and do not score as well as young adults, who perform better on standard memory tasks[36].

Personality Theories

Thomae and Lehr[37] have proposed an antistage theory of aging, where personality, development and adjustment are affected by the historical events throughout the life cycle. This theory is in partial conflict with the eight-stage theory of Erikson[38], which is a stage theory of ego development through the life cycle, culminating with the stage of maturity, as the elderly person may find either ego integrity through satisfaction with his past life, or despair and disgust over past failures. Bortwinick[39] has noted increasing cautiousness with advancing age, with the degree of cautiousness being influenced by the type of problem and its timing. Okun et al.[40] point out that cautiousness is not strictly an age effect, but that differences can be attributed to cohort influence.

According to Neugarten and Gutman[41], people maintain their personality characteristics in late life. When personality changes occur, they appear to be related to losses, particularly those involving health and social support systems. Some sex differences are noted; men are more affiliative and more nurturant, women are more individualistic and more aggressive as they become older.

Costa and McCrae[42], in their literature review on personality stability throughout the life cycle, also report that series of longitudinal studies show stability of personality traits in adulthood. The variables studied have included anxiety, introversion, conservatism, irritability or apathy. Costa and McCrae themselves have proposed five broad factors in personality traits: neuroticism, extroversion, openness to experience, agreeableness and conscientiousness. While there is stability of personality throughout the lifespan of an adult, there are generational differences, secondary to cohorts. Personality changes may be very tightly woven with mastery and the ability to cope.

SOCIAL THEORIES OF AGING

Broadly, the sociological theories of aging can be broken down into those that examine the relationship of the older person to society and those that study the role and status of the elder. In their disengagement theory, Cumming and Henry[43] claimed that the withdrawal of the elderly from their previous societal roles with reduction in all types of interaction, essentially a shift of attention from the outer world to the inner world, was desirable and helped the elderly to maintain life satisfaction. With their exchange theory of aging, Homans[44] and Blau[45] also suggested that elderly people withdrew from social interaction. Ongoing social exchanges had become more costly in old age and therefore less rewarding.

In contrast to the disengagement theory, the activity theory[46,47] proposed that activity contributes to health and life satisfaction. Undoubtedly, the selection of activities to be pursued by the elderly is limited by the decline that accompanies aging. However, remaining active is felt to be good for the elderly.

Neugarten and Gutman[41] sought a compromise in the continuity theory, by noting that older adults tend to behave in a pattern established in their earlier life as they cope and make adaptive choices. At times the person may disengage and at other times remain active. Atchley[48] felt that the continuity theory was an illusive concept because aging produces changes that cannot be completely offset, so that there is no going back to a prior state.

Age and sex stratification provide different perspectives about aging by looking at different age and sex groups with different roles and expectations. As each group moves through time, it responds to changes in the environment[49]. Riley[50] describes a cohort effect or "cohort flow", where a group of people born at the same time in history are together and have certain common experiences and characteristics. The status of the aged is high in static societies and tends to decline with rapid social change[51]. This ties in with Cowgill and Holmes'[52] modernization theory, which suggests that the status of the aged in any society is inversely related to the level of industrialization within that society. With industrialization, the powers and prestige of the elderly are reduced. In a primitive society aging can be a liability, but older people who continue to perform useful and valued roles have a higher standing and are well treated[52]. These sociological theories have varying degrees of validity. In sociology, as well as in biology and psychology, there are no overarching theories that incorporate the theories described above.

REFERENCES

1. Busse EW, Blazer DG. The theories and processes of aging. In Busse EW, Blazer DG, eds, *Handbook of Geriatric Psychiatry*. New York: Van Nostrand Reinhold, 1980, 3–27.
2. Moody HR. Toward a critical gerontology: the contribution of the humanities to the theories of aging. In Birren JE, Bengtson VL, eds, *Emergent Theories of Aging*. New York: Springer, 1988, 19–40.
3. Cristofulo VJ. An overview of the theories of biological aging. In Birren JE, Bengtson VL, ed, *Emergent Theories of Aging*. New York: Springer, 1988, 118–27.
4. Busse EW. The myth, history, and science of aging. In Busse EW, Blazer DG, eds, *Geriatric Psychiatry*. Washington, DC: American Psychiatric Press, 1989, 3–34.
5. Hayflick L, Moorhead PS. The serial cultivation of human diploid cells. *Exp Cell Res* 1961; **25**: 585–621.

6. Vogel FS. Neuroanatomy and neuropathology of aging. In Busse EW, Blazer DG, eds, *Geriatric Psychiatry*. Washington, DC: American Psychiatric Press, 1989, 79–96.

7. Than PB, Miller RS. Apoptosis death and transfiguration. *Sci Med* 1999; **6**: 8–34.

8. Weiner A, Maizele N. A deadly double life. *Science* 1999; **284**: 63–4.

9. Busse EW. Clinical characteristics of normal ageing. In Meier-Ruge W, ed, *Teaching and Training in Geriatric Medicine. Vol. 1: The Elderly Patient in General Practice*. Basel, Switzerland: Karger, 1987, 59–163.

10. Palca J. The other human genome. *Science* 1990; **249**: 1104–1105.

11. Miller RJ, Kleemeier A. Are there genes for aging? *J Gerontol Biol Sci* 1999; **54**: B297–307.

12. Van Gool WA, Mirmiran M. Ageing and circadian rhythms. In Schwab DS, Sliers E, Murmiran M, Von Hearen S, eds, *Progress in Brain Research*. Vol. 70. Amsterdam: Elsevier, 1976, 255–77.

13. Fridovich L. The two faces of oxygen: benign and malignant. *Duke Univ Lett* 1979; **3**: 1–4.

14. Harman D. The aging process. *Proc Natl Acad Sci USA* 1981; **78**: 7124–8.

15. Nandy K. Morphological changes in the aging brain. In Nandy K, ed, *Senile Dementia: A Biomedical Approach*. Amsterdam: Elsevier, North Holland, 1978, 19–29.

16. Burnet M. Autoimmune disease, 11: pathology of the immune response. *Br Med J* 1959; **ii**: 720–25.

17. Walford RL. Autoimmunity and aging. *J Gerontol* 1962; **17**: 281–5.

18. Comfort A. Mutation, autoimmunity and aging. *Lancet* 1963; **ii**: 138–40.

19. Rennie J. The body against itself. *Sci Am* 1990; **263**(6): 106–15.

20. Fillit H. Immune mechanisms of microvascular and neuronal injury in dementia. In Hasegawa K, Homma A, eds, *Psychogeriatrics: Biomedical and Social Advances*. Amsterdam: Excerpta Medica, 1990, 76–9.

21. Pahwu R, Chatila T, Grod R, *et al.* Recombinant interleukin-2 therapy in severe combined immunodeficiency disease. *Proc Natl Acad Sci USA* 1989; **86**: 569–73.

22. Weindruch R, Schol RS. Caloric intake and aging. *New Engl J Med* 1997; **337**: 286–9.

23. Kirkwood TBL, Rose MR. Evolution of senescence: late survival sacrifice for reproduction. *Phil Trans R Soc Lond* 1991; **332**: 5–24.

24. Scaker GA. Longevity, aging and death: an evolutionary perspective. *Gerontologist* 1978; **18**: 112–120.

25. Mackensie D. New clues to why size equals destiny. *Science* 1999; **284**: 1607–9.

26. Siegler IC, Poon IW. The psychology of aging. In Busse EW, Blazer DG, eds, *Geriatric Psychiatry*. Washington, DC: American Psychiatric Press, 1989.

27. Perlmutter MI. Cognitive potential throughout life. In Birren JE and Bengston VL, eds, *Emergent Theories of Aging*. New York: Springer, 1988, 249–68.

28. Baltes PB, Dittman-Kohli F, Dixon RA. New perspectives on the development of intelligence in adulthood: toward a dual-process conception and a model of selective optimization with compensation. In Baltes PB, Brim Jr OB, eds, *Life Span Development and Behavior*. Vol 6. New York: Academic Press, 1984, 34–76.

29. Kleemeier R. Intellectual changes in the senium. *Proc Soc Stat Sect Am Stat Assoc*, Washington, DC, 1962, 290–5.

30. Schaie KW. Toward a stage theory of adult cognitive development. *Int J Aging Hum Dev* 1977; **8**: 129–33.

31. Ribot T. *Diseases of Memory*. New York: Appleton, 1882.

32. Backman I. Applications of Ribot's law of life span cognitive development. In Maddox GL, Busse LW, eds, *Aging: The Universal Human Experience*. New York: Springer, 1987, 403–10.

33. Vygotsky LS. *Thought and Language*. Cambridge, MA: MIT Press, 1962.

34. Kinsbourne M. Attentional dysfunctions and the elderly: theoretical models and research perspectives. In Poon LW, Fozard JL, Cermak LS, *et al.*, eds, *New Directions in Memory and Aging*. Hillsdale, NJ: Erlbaum, 1980.

35. Bourne LE. An inference model for conceptua 28. Bo rule learning. In Solso RL, ed, *Theories in Cognitive Psychology*. The Loyola Symposium, Potomac: Erlbaum, 1974.

36. Backman L, Nilsson LG. Aging effects in free recall: an exception to the rule. *Human Learning* 1984; **3**: 53–69.

37. Thomae H, Lehr U. Stages, crises, conflicts and life-span development. In Sorensen AB, Weinert FE, Sherrod LR, eds, *Human Development and the Life Course: Multidisciplinary Perspectives*. Hillsdale, NJ: Erlbaum, 1986, 429–44.

38. Erikson EH. Identity and the life cycle. In *Psychological Issues, I*. New York: International Universities Press, 1959, 120.

39. Botwinick J. Cautiousness with advanced age. *J Gerontol* 1966; **21**: 347–53.

40. Okun MA, Siegler IC, George LK. Cautiousness and verbal learning in adulthood. *J Gerontol* 1978; **33**: 94–7.

41. Neugarten BI, Gutmann DL. Age–sex roles in personality in middle age: a TAT study. In *Personality in Middle and Later Life*. New York: Atherton, 1964, 44–89.

42. Costa PT Jr, McCrue RR. The case for personality stability. In Maddox GL, Busse EW, eds, *Aging: The Universal Human Experience*. New York: Springer, 1987.

43. Cumming EH, Henry WE. *Growing Old: The Process of Disengagement*. New York: Basic Books, 1961.

44. Homans GC. *Social Behavior: Its Elementary Forms*. New York: Harcourt Brace Jovanovich, 1961.

45. Blau PM. *Exchange and Power in Social Life*. New York: Wiley, 1964.

46. Cavan RS, Burgess EW, Havighurst RJ, Goldhamer H. *Personal Adjustment in Old Age*. Chicago: Science Research Associates, 1949.

47. Havighurst R. Successful aging. In William R, Tibbitts C, Donuhue W, eds, *Processes of Aging*. New York: Atherton, 1963.

48. Atchley RC. A continuity theory of normal aging. *Gerontologist* 1989; **29**(2): 183–90.

49. Palmore E. *Social Patterns in Normal Aging: Findings from the Duke Longitudinal Study*. Durham, NC: Duke University Press, 1981.

50. Riley MW. Social gerontology and the age stratification of society. *Gerontologist* 1971; **11**: 79–87.

51. Ogburn WP, Nimkoff MF. *Sociology*. Boston: Houghton Mifflin, 1940.

52. Cowgill DO, Holmes LD. *Aging and Modernization*. New York: Appleton Century Crofts, 1972.

53. Simmons LW. *The Role of the Aged in Primitive Society*. New Haven, CT: Yale University Press, 1945.

Structural Changes in the Aging Brain

Gandis Mazeika and P. Murali Doraiswamy

Duke University Medical Center, Durham, NC, USA

It has long been recognized that aging is associated with progressive changes in brain structure. The extent to which the brain is affected by aging is determined by a complex interplay of environmental and genetic factors. Little information is currently available on the influence of specific factors on brain aging; however, a significant amount of work has been done describing the aggregate of changes in the aging brain[1].

Methods applied to the study of brain aging have included anatomic studies and neuroimaging. Each method has specific strengths and weaknesses, leading at times to confusing and even contradictory results when comparing studies using different techniques. For instance, anatomic studies are subject to fixation artifacts and have rarely controlled for subjects' cranial size. On the other hand, magnetic resonance imaging (MRI) volumetry suffers from distortion effects due to imperfections in the magnetic field and from difficulty in precisely gauging the gray matter–white matter junction[2-4]. Furthermore, no consensus exists regarding the definition of normal brain aging. Attempts at a definition have been confounded by various problems, such as difficulties in screening out individuals with subclinical neurodegenerative disease, and difficulties in conducting adequate longitudinal studies.

Despite these shortcomings, some information is available on the regional distribution of age-associated atrophy. A general principle of brain aging that has emerged is that phylogenetically newer structures, such as neocortex and neostriatum, tend to show more age-associated atrophy than phylogenetically older structures, such as the hippocampus and brainstem.

NEUROIMAGING STUDIES

Studies using various neuroimaging techniques have repeatedly demonstrated progressive age-related volume loss in widespread areas in the brain. The overall loss of tissue volume averages 0.2%/year, starting in mid-adulthood. Changes are manifested primarily by increases in ventricular volume and by cortical atrophy, as measured by increased sulcal markings[9,10].

These changes have significant clinical consequences. Increases in ventricular volume result in decreased cerebral compliance, rendering the aging brain less resilient to changes in intracranial pressure. Cortical atrophy, on the other hand, causes the brain parenchyma to pull away from the skull table, lengthening cortical bridging veins and increasing vulnerability to subdural hemorrhages.

In neuroimaging studies, gray matter volume loss has been found to be typically greater than white matter loss. Most affected is the pre-frontal cortex, with a rate of volume loss of about 0.5%/ year. Areas of moderate volume loss include the temporal, parietal and cerebellar cortex. The occipital cortex is relatively spared, while pons, tectum and hippocampus show minimal changes with normal aging[9].

Various explanations for these differences in rate of atrophy have been offered, including regional differences in calcium homeostasis and expression of inflammatory mediators, such as 5-lipoxygenase. None of these hypotheses has been verified. Another important consideration is that distortions associated with image acquisition, such as movement artifact and inhomogeneities in the magnetic field, may result in insufficient precision to accurately measure volume changes in smaller structures, such as the pons.

The relative absence of hippocampal changes in normal aging stands in contrast to the dramatic decline in hippocampal volumes observed during the course of Alzheimer's disease, frontotemporal dementia and certain other disorders, such as mesial temporal sclerosis. Some researchers have attempted to exploit this difference as a means to assist in the diagnosis of Alzheimer's disease; however, hippocampal volumetry remains an experimental technique at present[2].

Aside from changes in volume, neuroimaging has revealed other interesting structural changes with aging. The most intensely studied of these changes is the increasing prevalence of leuko-araiosis, or periventricular white matter hyperintensities. The significance of leuko-araiosis is uncertain, but is thought to be related to tissue damage as a consequence of microvascular disease. Leuko-araiosis tends to be more prominent in individuals with hypertension or diabetes, although some degree of perivascular white matter changes are found in most individuals above age 65. To date, no strong relationship has been found between leuko-araiosis and cognitive decline[3,4].

Other noteworthy age-related changes include accumulation of iron in the striatum, deep cerebellar nuclei and motor cortex and the deposition of calcium in the pineal gland, choroid plexus and in the walls of the basilar and middle cerebral arteries. The clinical significance of these changes is also uncertain.

POST-MORTEM STUDIES

One important question that cannot be addressed by neuroimaging studies is the extent of actual cell loss occurring with brain atrophy. A sizable number of gross and microanatomical post mortem studies have been conducted to investigate this and other types of anatomical changes that occur in the brain with aging, although so far very few studies have attempted to compare neuroimaging with histologic data in the same individuals[5].

Post-mortem volumetric studies have confirmed the findings from the neuroimaging literature that the frontal lobe shrinks proportionately more than the temporal, parietal and occipital lobes. In contrast to neuroimaging findings, however, is the observation that white matter volume loss appears to be greater than that found in gray matter. One possible explanation for this discrepancy is that aging seems to increase the water content of the gray matter–white matter junction, possibly distorting its apparent location on MRI imaging[5].

Post-mortem ultrastructural studies have shed light on a variety of questions regarding changes at the microscopic and cellular level. Typical findings within normal aging brains include dilated perivascular spaces (Virchow–Robin spaces), mild demyelination, reactive gliosis and appearance of vacuoles and lipofuscin within neuronal and glial cell bodies. While many of these changes are attributed to age-associated "wear and tear", the overall degree of white matter disorganization is mild when compared with that seen in arteriosclerotic brain disease[5–7].

An important finding confirmed in most ultrastructural studies is that most of the age-associated change in brain volume is attributable to decreases in the volumes of individual cells rather than to dropout of neurons and glia. Studies have repeatedly confirmed that the proportion of small cortical neurons increases with age. There is also some evidence for simplification of dendritic arborization with age[5].

However, evidence also exists for at least a small degree of cell loss in various regions of the brain during normal aging, including parts of the substantia nigra, the locus coeruleus and the suprachiasmatic nucleus of the hypothalamus. Some cell loss has also been demonstrated in the cortex, specifically in layers 2 and 4[6].

Other findings reported in ultrastructural studies or aging are that neurofibrillary tangles, but not amyloid plaques, appear in the CA1 cortex of the hippocampus and layer II of the entorhinal cortex. Aging also appears to affect the terminal first-order sympathetic axons, as manifested by swollen axons with neurofilamentous aggregates adjacent to the second-order sympathetic neuronal bodies[2].

SUMMARY

While there is no current consensus on the definition of normal brain aging, certain patterns have been tentatively identified. These include the observation that phylogenetically newer structures seem to atrophy at a faster rate than older structures such as the hippocampus, diencephalon and brainstem, and that most of the atrophy observed with normal aging can be attributed to cell shrinkage and dearborization, rather than to cell loss. The clinical consequences of these changes include decreased resilience to changes in intracranial pressure and increased vulnerability to subdural hemorrhages. Areas of observed significant cell loss include the substantia nigra, locus coeruleus and suprachiasmatic nucleus of the hypothalamus.

Many important unanswered questions remain regarding normal aging, including:

1. What is the relationship between structural changes in brain tissue and age-related changes in other organ systems?
2. To what extent does apoptosis affect the brain in normal aging?
3. What are the environmental and genetic determinants of the rate at which the brain ages?
4. To what extent do gender differences affect cerebral aging?
5. To what extent does cell loss in the substantia nigra, locus coeruleus and suprachiasmatic nucleus impact on the changes in balance, gait, mood and sleep pattern that are observed with aging? Is cell loss within these areas truly "normal" or does it represent pathology with a high degree of penetration, such as might be seen with an environmental toxin or with a ubiquitous viral infection?

REFERENCES

1. Brody H. The nervous system and aging. *Adv Pathobiol* 1980; **7**: 200–9.
2. Troncoso JC, Martin LJ *et al.* Neuropathology in controls and demented subjects from the Baltimore Longitudinal Study of Aging. *Neurobiol Aging* 1996; **17**(3): 365–71.
3. Golomb J, Kluger A *et al.* Non-specific leukoencephalopathy associated with aging. *Neuroimag Clin N Am* 1995; **5**(1): 33–44.
4. Scarpelli M, Salvolini U *et al.* MRI and pathological examination of post-mortem brains: the problem of white matter signal areas. *Neuroradiology* 1994; **36**(5): 393–8.
5. Terry RD, DeTeresa R *et al.* Neocortical cell counts in normal human adult aging. *Ann Neurol* **21**(6): 530–9.
6. Troncoso JC, Sukhov RR *et al. In situ* labeling of dying cortical neurons in normal aging and in Alzheimer's disease: correlations with senile plaques and disease progression. *J Neuropathol Exp Neurol* **55**(11): 1134–42.
7. Unger JW. Glial reaction in aging and Alzheimer's disease. *Microsc Res Techn* 1998; **43**(1).
8. Anglade P, Vyas S *et al.* Apoptosis in dopaminergic neurons of the human substantia nigra during normal aging. *Histol Histopathol* **12**(3): 603–10.
9. Coffey CE, Wilkinson WE *et al.* Quantitative cerebral anatomy of the aging human brain: a cross-sectional study using magnetic resonance imaging. *Neurology* 1992; **42**(3,pt 1): 527–36.
10. Doraiswamy PM, Figiel GS *et al.* Aging of the human corpus callosum: magnetic resonance imaging in normal volunteers. *J Neuropsychiat Clin Neurosci* 1991; **3**(4): 392–7.

7

Anatomy of the Aging Brain

John J. Campbell III[1] and C. Edward Coffey[1,2]

Departments of [1]Psychiatry, and [2]Neurology, Henry Ford Health System, Detroit, MI, USA

INTRODUCTION

Knowledge of the spectrum and extent of changes in brain morphology that occur with 'normal aging' is critical to any understanding of age-related illnesses, such as dementia. Prior to the recent introduction of advanced brain imaging techniques, post mortem studies served as the only source of information regarding the anatomy of the aging human brain. A common finding among them was a reduction of brain size with age, consisting initially (in the seventh decade) of atrophy of the gray matter (widening of sulci and thinning of gyri), followed by a decline in the volume of the white matter (in the eighth and ninth decades of life)[1]. The cortical atrophy appeared to be most prominent in the frontal and parietal parasagittal areas and consisted of a decrease in the volume rather than in the number of individual neurons[2]. Ventricular enlargement was also observed, but the degree of the dilatation was variable among the different studies[1,3].

There are several sources of error inherent to post mortem studies. Most of the studies included subjects with very different causes of death, which themselves can lead to a variety of changes in brain morphology; in particular, the cause of death may be quite different for young vs. elderly cohorts. Another disadvantage of the post mortem measurements is that the brain can be altered in unpredictable ways prior to tissue processing, as well as during the process of fixation[4,5].

Many of these problems have now been obviated by the development of imaging techniques, such as computed X-ray tomography (CT) and magnetic resonance imaging (MRI), which have provided an opportunity to examine the human brain *in vivo*[105]. In this chapter, we critically review those brain imaging studies that have investigated age-related changes in brain anatomy. Any understanding of these data must begin, however, with a discussion of relevant methodological issues.

ISSUES OF METHODOLOGY

Study Design

Studies of the aging brain can be classified as either cross-sectional or longitudinal. Cross-sectional studies select subjects from all age groups and examine them during roughly the same time period. Subject recruitment is relatively easy and large amounts of data can be acquired and analyzed in a short period of time. Two main limitations are inherent to cross-sectional studies; the secular or generation effect and the survivor or cohort effect. The secular effect refers to differences among successive generations with respect to variables that could influence brain anatomy. For example, differences between elderly and non-elderly cohorts with respect to nutrition or socioeconomic status could be associated with differences in brain morphology that have nothing to do with aging *per se*. The survivor effect refers to the biased selection of very healthy individuals, since those with underlying diseases usually die earlier and do not have the chance to be selected for study.

Longitudinal studies follow the same subjects with repeated examinations over time. Data acquisition is very labor-intensive and takes place over long periods of time. Longitudinal studies are limited by a period effect (changes over time in the methodology of the study) and an attrition effect (dropouts), in which the participants available at the end of the study may be quite different from the sample recruited initially.

Sample Selection

Age-related changes in brain morphology will obviously depend critically upon the criteria used to select the population under study. 'Normal' volunteers from the community may differ markedly from patients with 'clinically normal' brain CT or MRI scans with respect to variables that may influence brain anatomy. Medical and psychiatric illness, smoking, alcohol consumption, nutrition, education, environment, sex and height are just some of the variables that must be considered when comparing brain anatomy among individuals. Population heterogeneity is especially great among the elderly, and Rowe and Kahn[6] have suggested a distinction between 'usual aging' (no clinically obvious brain disease) and 'successful aging' (minimal decline in neurobiologic function in comparison with young subjects). The increased variability of measures of brain anatomy seen in 'normal' elderly populations may be due in part to the relative mix of subjects with usual vs. successful aging.

Imaging Technology

Brain imaging techniques differ in their safety, sensitivity and anatomic resolution. One of the oldest methods for *in vivo* brain imaging is pneumoencephalography (PEG). PEG is unsuitable ethically for the study of the normal brain, due to its associated discomfort and high morbidity rate. The procedure itself may also directly affect the size of the cerebrospinal fluid (CSF) spaces[7]. These problems limit the application of this technique to patients with sufficient neurologic symptomatology to warrant such an

Principles and Practice of Geriatric Psychiatry, 2nd edn. Edited by J. R. M. Copeland, M. T. Abou-Saleh and D. G. Blazer

invasive procedure. As a result, the 'normality' of the sample in studies using PEG can be easily criticized.

With advances in computer technology, two new brain imaging methods have been recently introduced, computed X-ray tomography (CT) and magnetic resonance imaging (MRI). The major advantage common to both techniques is the opportunity to study both the CSF spaces and the brain parenchyma in great detail. Computed X-ray tomography is a relatively simple and inexpensive technique, with the advantage of short study acquisition times. The method is limited, however, by low spatial and density resolution, partial volume artifacts (the effect of the coexistence of multiple tissue and fluid components in the same volume unit) and bone-hardening artifacts (false elevation of brain CT numbers adjacent to the skull)[5,8]. These technical problems have limited the ability of CT to quantitate brain changes with aging.

Magnetic resonance imaging takes advantage of the magnetic characteristics of tissue protons to study the brain. The main advantages of this technique are the excellent resolution of gray matter, white matter and CSF and the high sensitivity to disease processes, due to the fact that multiple factors (proton density, proton environment, etc.) contribute to the signal characteristics of each structure. The images are free of bone artifacts and the brain can be examined across all three major planes (i.e. axial, coronal and sagittal). Another advantage of MRI technology is that it does not utilize ionizing radiation. Disadvantages of MRI are the partial volume artifacts, the relatively longer study acquisition times and the fact that claustrophobic subjects cannot tolerate the examination due to the physical characteristics of the equipment[9,10].

Method of Image Analysis

Anatomical studies of the aging brain have used either qualitative or quantitative measures of brain morphology. In *qualitative studies*, raters employ various scales to examine the parameters of interest including, for example, the degree of cortical atrophy and ventricular enlargement. Qualitative ratings are relatively easy to use, are clinically relevant[11], do not depend on advanced instrumentation and sophisticated computations, and may display significant correlations with more quantitative methods[12]. On the other hand, the accuracy of these ratings depends on the skill of the raters and, as such, it is difficult to compare the results of studies from different authors using different scales. In addition, the sensitivity and resolution of the scales are limited by the number of rating categories (usually three to five)[13].

The *quantitative measurements* can be categorized as volumetric, planimetric (area measurement of regions of interest) or linear (distance measurement between points of interest) (Table 7.1). Volumetric methods are very accurate (according to validation studies on phantoms) and are very sensitive to changes

in brain size[8,14,15]. The accuracy of the volume measurements is increased by obtaining relatively thin imaging slices (< 5 mm), by reducing the interscan gap (contiguous slices are preferred) and by scanning the entire extent of the structure of interest.

Planimetric studies have the advantage of being less laborintensive than volumetric measures and, although they correlate reasonably well with volumetric measurements, at least for structures with regular shape[12,15], their overall accuracy and sensitivity is not as good. Thus, for a simple three-dimensional structure, a doubling of the volume will result in only a 1.5-fold increase in the area of a cross-section. For more complicated shapes with irregular configurations, the correlation of planimetric to volumetric measurements is much worse.

Linear measurements are the least accurate and least sensitive, primarily because they have a non-linear relationship to volume measurements. As a result, small but potentially important changes in volume may be underestimated by linear measurements, even when used in combination[15]. Finally, it is important to note that the size of various brain structures or regions might be expected to vary with the size of the subject's brain; e.g. subjects with larger brains might be expected to have larger ventricles. Any morphometric study of brain structures across individuals should therefore take into consideration intergroup differences in brain size[15–17].

LITERATURE REVIEW

This section summarizes the effects of aging on CSF space size, size of brain parenchyma, ventricular size, and incidence of subcortical hyperintensities as reported in the literature.

Table 7.2 reviews the reported changes in the size of brain parenchyma with aging. The proportion of sulcal CSF volume to cranial volume (an indirect measure of cortical gray matter atrophy) increases from approximately 3% at the second decade of life to approximately 10% in the ninth decade. This age-related increase in sulcal CSF volume appears to accelerate after the sixth decade. Studies that have directly measured brain parenchyma have reported a 15–25% decrease in cortical gray matter volume, while the white matter, in most studies, appears to remain stable. However, studies of the corpus callosum consistently demonstrate age-related reductions in total callosal volume, particularly in the anterior regions. Finally, age-associated reductions in the areas of the pituitary and cerebellar vermis, as well as in the volume of the caudate nucleus, have been reported, though attempts at replicating those results have yielded some negative findings.

Some studies have attempted to estimate reductions in brain size indirectly by measuring changes in the volume of CSF spaces (Table 7.3). Results consistently indicate that the size of CSF spaces increases with age. More specifically, ventricular:brain ratio (VBR) may increase in a non-linear manner from 2% to

Table 7.1.   Linear measurements—definitions

Bifrontal ratio Distance between the tips of the frontal horns divided by the distance between the inner tables of the skull. Measured at the slice best showing the caudate[19]

Bicaudate ratio Minimal distance between the caudate indentation of frontal horn divided by the distance between the inner tables of the skull. Measured at the slice best showing the caudate[19]

Lateral ventricular ratio Distance between the lateral walls of the bodies of the lateral ventricles divided by the distance between the inner tables of the skull. Measured at the slice showing the maximum area of bodies of lateral ventricles[16]

Cortical sulci ratio Sum of widths of the four widest sulci divided by the transpineal inner table diameter. Measured in two supraventricular slices cutting through the centrum semiovale[19]

Interhemispheric fissure ratio Maximal width of interhemispheric fissure divided by the transpineal coronal inner table diameter[19]

Sylvian fissure ratio Average of maximal Sylvian fissure width divided by the transpineal inner table diameter[19]

Third (III) ventricle ratio The product of the sagittal and coronal diameters of the IIIrd ventricle, divided by the product of the transpineal and midsagittal inner table diameters; measured at the level of maximum IIIrd ventricle area[19]

Table 7.2. Aging and changes in size of brain parenchyma

Study	Subjects	Imaging and measurement technique	Findings
Haug 1977[18]	170 Scans 0–75 years old. Subjects with 'normal neurological findings' complaining of headaches	CT, linear (maximum width of interhemispheric fissure)	Cortical atrophy increased with age; width of interhemispheric fissure increased approximately 5-fold (0.5–2.8 mm) from age 16–30 to age 61–75, in a continuous fashion
Jacoby et al., 1980[19]	50 Healthy elderly volunteers, 62–88 years old, 10 M, 40 F. No history of significant psychiatric or neurologic illness. Handedness not specified	CT. Ratings (four-point scale) of cortical atrophy from films by single blinded rater; five regions rated (frontal, parietal, temporal, insular and occipital) and scores summed	Age correlated with total cortical atrophy score. Interactions with sex or laterality not reported. Adjusting for age, no relation between any CT measure and performance on the Hodkinson test of memory and orientation
Cala et al., 1981[20]	115 Volunteers, 15–40 years old, 62 M, 53 F. No history of migraine, head trauma, or excessive alcohol intake (no additional details provided). All but eight subjects right-handed	CT ($n = $ two scanners). Ratings (five-point scale) of cortical atrophy (no additional details provided). Axial slices (13 mm thick)	Age apparently associated with increased frequency of mild (grade 2) atrophy of frontal lobes and cerebellar vermis, but no statistical analysis reported. Interactions with sex or laterality not reported
Zatz et al., 1982[12]	123 Normal volunteers, 20–90 years old. Unequal sex distributions among different age groups, with more women in the old group. Excluded: history of neurological problems or major medical diseases	CT. Planimetry (sulcal fluid area in two supraventricular slices divided by cranial size). Volumetric (total fluid volume in temporo-Sylvian area divided by total cranial volume). Axial slices ($n = 9$) 10 mm thick, with 10 mm interscan gap; lowest slice at the level just above the petrous pyramids and orbital roofs	Increased cortical atrophy with age. Area of sulcal fluid in supraventricular levels was stable until the seventh decade then increased four-fold from age 60 to 80+ Volume of fluid in temporo-Sylvian area was stable until age 60; then increased by 30% from age 60 to age 80+
Gado et al., 1983[14]	12 normal volunteers 64–81 years old. Excluded: subjects with dementia	CT. Sulcal volumetric ratio (ratio of sulcal to cranial volume). Axial slices ($n = 7$), including three sections above the roof of the lateral ventricle and four below it	Increased cortical atrophy with age; cortical sulcal volume ratio increased by 13.3% in 1 year follow-up
Gomori et al., 1984[21]	148 Neurologically intact patients (subjects with minor neurological symptoms and patients with lung, breast, prostate or colon cancer but no CNS involvement. All subjects had normal neurological examinations), 28–84 years old	CT. Linear (cortical sulci ratio, frontal interhemispheric fissure ratio, Sylvian fissure ratio)	Cortical atrophy increased with age; age correlated with Sylvian fissure, interhemispheric fissure and cortical sulci ratios ($r = 0.53$, 0.4 and 0.2, respectively). Sylvian fissure ratio increased 1.6-fold between ages 28–49 and 80–84 continuously; interhemispheric fissure ratio increased five-fold across the same age groups continuously
Laffey et al., 1984[11]	212 Normal volunteers living independently, 65 years old and older. Sex distribution same in all groups (52% M, 48% F). Excluded: alcoholism and history or findings of neurological illness	CT. Qualitative rating (five-point scale) of cortical atrophy by two experienced radiologists. Axial slice at the mid-ventricular level	Trend (not significant) for increased cortical atrophy with age; mean rating of 0.83 at age 65–69 to 1.4 at age 80–89. Males showed higher scores for cortical atrophy in all age groups
Schwartz et al., 1985[5]	30 Healthy male volunteers 21–81 years old. No history of major medical, neurologic or psychiatric illness. Handedness not specified	CT. Volume measurements derived from computer-assisted segmentation technique (ASI-II program). Axial slices ($n = 7$) starting from the plane of the inferior orbitomeatal line (10 mm thick, 7 mm interscan gap)	Adjusting for intracranial volume (IV), age negatively correlated with volume of gray matter and with volume of gray plus white matter, but not with white matter volume. Subjects more than 60 years old ($n = 11$) had smaller volumes of thalamus, lenticular nuclei and total gray matter than younger subjects ($n = 19$). Effects similar for both hemispheres
Pfefferbaum et al., 1986[13]	57 Normal volunteers 20–84 years old, 27 M, 30 F	CT. Sulcal volumetric ratio (ratio of total sulcal volume to total cranial volume). Axial slices ($n = 12$) with 8 mm interscan gap, starting from the level of the superior roof of the orbit and proceeding upwards	Increased cortical atrophy with age; volume ratio increased seven-fold from the third to the eighth decade. The increase was faster after age 60
Stafford et al., 1988[22]	79 Normal male volunteers, 31–87 years old. Excluded: alcoholism, psychiatric illness, learning disability, severe head trauma, epilepsy, hypertension, chronic lung disease, renal disease, coronary artery disease, cancer	CT. Planimetry: ratio of cortical sulcal area to cranial area. Axial slice at supraventricular levels	Cortical atrophy increased with age; cortical sulci area ratio increased 1.8-fold between ages 30–39 and 70+ (0.012–0.022), faster after the sixth decade
Golomb et al., 1993[23]	154 Healthy volunteers with MMSE > 27, 55–88 years old (70 ± 8 years), 73 M, 81 F. No evidence of active medical, neurologic, or psychiatric illness. Handedness not specified	CT ($n = 51$); MR imaging ($n = 81$); both CT and MR imaging ($n = 22$). Blinded ratings (4-point scale) of hippocampal atrophy as defined by dilatation of transverse choroidal fissure on films, by raters ($n = ?$) with established reliabilities	Subjects with hippocampal atrophy (rating of 2 or greater in either hemisphere; $n = 50$) significantly older than those without atrophy. More males (41%) than females (25%) with hippocampal atrophy

continues overleaf

Table 7.2 *continued*

Study	Subjects	Imaging and measurement technique	Findings
Meyer *et al.*, 1994[24]	81 Healthy volunteers, 27–90 years old, 44 M, 37 F. No major neurologic or psychiatric illness	CT (*n* = 2 scanners). Blinded measure of tissue density (densitometry) and regional brain volume (trace methodology) from axial slices (8 mm thick)	Age associated with decreased tissue density in cortical gray matter (frontal, temporal, parietal, and occipital) and in white matter (frontal only), but not in subcortical gray matter (caudate, putamen, or thalamus). Age associated with decreased ratios of cortical gray matter volume to IV and subcortical gray matter volume to IV, but not with white matter volume to IV. Interactions with sex or laterality not reported
Elwan *et al.*, 1996b[25]	88 Healthy 'lower middle class' volunteers, 40–76 years old (54.8 ± 9.6 years), 57 M, 31 F. No major medical, neurologic, or psychiatric illness. All right-handed	CT. Multiple linear measurements (no additional details provided)	No correlation between age and maximal bifrontal distance, bifrontal index, maximal bicaudate distance, maximal septum–caudate distance, or cella media index. Interactions with sex or laterality not reported
Yoshii *et al.*, 1986[26]	33 Normal volunteers, 24–82 years old	Magnetic resonance (MR) imaging. Planimetry	No significant correlation between corpus callosum area and age. Trend for decline in the area of anterior half of corpus callosum with age (*r* = 0.31, *p* = 0.8)
Simon *et al.*, 1987[27]	48 Subjects, including normal volunteers and patients with normal MR imaging studies, 11 months to 64 years old, 25 M, 23 F. Excluded: periventricular high signal areas, anomalous development of the corpus callosum, pre-scan diagnosis of multiple sclerosis	MR imaging (0.15 tesla). Planimetry; midsagittal slice, 5 mm thick	Corpus callosum area did not change after the 18th year of age
Uematsu *et al.*, 1988[28]	17 normal male volunteers, mean age 31.5 years old, SD 5.5 years. Physically healthy	MR imaging (0.5 tesla). Planimetry; midsagittal slice 10 mm thick	No significant correlation between corpus callosum area and age
Condon *et al.*, 1988[29]	40 Volunteers, 20–60 years old, 20 M, 20 F. No additional details provided	MR imaging (0.15 tesla). Volume measurement (two raters) derived from computer-assisted pixel segmentation of contiguous sagittal slices (variable slice thickness and number)	For males but not females, age negatively correlated with ratio of total brain volume to IV. Interactions with laterality not reported
Yoshii *et al.*, 1988[30]	58 Volunteers, 21–81 years old, 29 M, 29 F. Neurologic and psychiatric histories not reported. Handedness not specified	MR imaging (1.0 tesla). Mathematically derived estimate of brain volume from inversion recovery films, based on planimetric area measurement made on single slice (10 mm thick) at level of foramen of Monro. Blinded global ratings of cortical atrophy from films (axial slices, [*n* = ?], 10 mm thick, 3 mm interscan gap). Number of raters and rater reliabilities not specified	No correlation between age and brain volume. Age significantly correlated with ratings of cortical atrophy for both males and females
Hayakawa *et al.*, 1989[31]	143 Patients and seven normal volunteers, 0–60 years old. All with normal MR imaging scans	MR imaging (0.35 tesla). Planimetry; midsagittal slice 10 mm thick	Decrease in size of brain structures with age. Pituitary area decreased progressively after 20 years of age. Trend for decrease in cerebellar vermis area after the fifth decade; pontine and corpus callosum area remained stable during the adult life
Hauser *et al.*, 1989[32]	25 normal volunteers, mean age 37 years old, SD 8.6 years, 14 M, 11 F. Excluded: history of medical or psychiatric illness	MR imaging (0.5 tesla). Planimetry; midsagittal section	Corpus callosum area did not correlate with age
Jernigan *et al.*, 1990[33]	58 Healthy volunteers, 8–79 years old, 35 M, 23 F. No history of neurologic, psychiatric, or medical illness (diabetes mellitus, heart disease). Handedness not specified	MR imaging (1.5 tesla). Volume estimates (one of two raters) derived from computer-assisted pixel classification of multiple spin-echo axial images (5 mm thick, 2.5 mm interscan gap)	Age negatively correlated with ratios of cerebral volume to IV and of gray matter volume to IV. Among gray matter structures, age negatively correlated with ratios of cortical gray matter volume to IV, caudate volume to IV, and diecephalon volume to IV; but not with thalamus volume to IV or anterior cingulate volume to IV. No correlation between age and ratio of white matter volume to IV. Interactions with sex or laterality not reported

continued

Table 7.2 *continued*

Study	Subjects	Imaging and measurement technique	Findings
Krishnan *et al.*, 1990[34]	39 Healthy volunteers, 24–79 years old, 17 M, 22 F. No evidence of major medical, neurologic, or psychiatric illness. Handedness not specified	MR imaging (1.5 tesla). Stereological measurement (one of two raters) of axial slices (variable number, 5 mm thick, 2.5 mm interscan gap) from intermediate and T_2-weighted films	Age negatively correlated with total caudate volume (males = females). Caudate volume was less in subjects older than 50 years ($n = 22$). No adjustments for cranial size
Doraiswamy *et al.*, 1991[35]	36 Healthy volunteers (overlap with subjects Krishnan *et al.*, 1990), 26–79 years old, 16 M, 20 F. No evidence of major medical, neurologic, or psychiatric illness. Handedness not specified	MR imaging (1.5 tesla). Area measurement of T_1-weighted midsagittal image using computer-assisted trace methodology. Rater reliabilities not reported	Age negatively correlated with corpus callosum area in males but not in females
Escalona *et al.*, 1991[36]	37 Healthy volunteers (overlap with subjects Krishnan *et al.*, 1990), 24–79 years old, 16 M, 21 F. No evidence of major medical, neurologic, or psychiatric illness. Handedness not specified	MR imaging (1.5 tesla). Stereological measurement (one of two raters) of axial slices (variable number, 5 mm thick, 2.5 mm interscan gap) from intermediate and T_2-weighted films. Good rater reliabilities	No association between age and volume of cerebellar hemispheres
Gur *et al.*, 1991[37]	69 Healthy volunteers, 18–80 years old, 34 M, 35 F. No neurologic or psychiatric illness; 66 right-handed; three left-handed	MR imaging (1.5 tesla). Volume measurements (any two of four raters) derived from segmentation technique based on two-feature pixel classification of multiple spin-echo axial images (5 mm thick, contiguous)	Older ($\geqslant 55$ years) subjects ($n = 26$) had smaller whole brain volumes than younger subjects (males = females)
McDonald *et al.*, 1991[38]	36 Healthy volunteers (subjects also included in Krishnan *et al.*, 1990), 24–79 years old, 13 M, 23 F. No evidence of major medical, neurologic or psychiatric illness	MR imaging (1.5 tesla). Same as Krishnan *et al.*, 1990 (above)	Age negatively correlated with total putamen volume (males = females; left = right), but no adjustments for cranial size
Shah *et al.*, 1991[39]	36 Healthy volunteers (overlap with subjects in Krishnan *et al.*, 1990), 26–79 years old, 16 M, 20 F. No evidence of major medical, neurologic, or psychiatric illness	MR imaging (1.5 tesla). Computer-assisted measurements from T_1-weighted midsagittal films by single rater with established intra-rater reliabilities	Increasing age associated with decreasing midbrain area (males > females?). No age effects on areas of pons, medulla, anterior cerebellar vermis or 4th ventricle
Tanna *et al.*, 1991[40]	16 Healthy volunteers, 52–86 years old, 5 M, 11 F. No evidence of major medical, neurologic, or psychiatric illness. Handedness not specified	MR imaging (1.5 tesla). Volume measurements (one of two raters with established reliabilities) derived from segmentation techniques based on two-feature pixel classification of multiple spin-echo axial images (5 mm thick, 2.5 mm interscan gap)	Age negatively correlated with ratio of total brain volume to total CSF plus total brain volume. Interactions with sex or laterality not reported
Coffey *et al.*, 1992[41]	76 Healthy volunteers, 36–91 years old, 25 M, 51 F. No lifetime history of neurologic or psychiatric illness. All right-handed	MR imaging (1.5 tesla). Volume measurements (one of three blinded raters with established reliabilities) using computer-assisted trace methodology of T_1-weighted coronal images ($n = 30$–35, 5 mm thick, contiguous). Blinded clinical ratings (five-point scale) of 'cortical atrophy' (average score of two raters)	Age associated with decreased total volumes of the cerebral hemispheres (0.23%/year), the frontal lobes (0.55%/year), the temporal lobes (0.28%/year), and the amygdala–hippocampal complex (0.30% per year); all effects similar for males and females, and for both hemispheres. Increasing age associated with increasing odds (8.9%/year) of 'cortical atrophy', from 0.08 at age 40 to 2.82 at age 80
Doraiswamy *et al.*, 1992[42]	75 Healthy volunteers (overlap with subjects in Krishnan *et al.*, 1990), 21–82 years old (52.5 ± 18 years), 34 M, 41 F. No neurologic or psychiatric illness	MR imaging (1.5 tesla). Blinded stereological measurements of volume and linear measurements of size of midbrain on T_2-weighted axial films (no additional details provided)	Age negatively correlated with midbrain volume and anteroposterior diameter, but not with red nucleus size. Effects similar for both males and females
Jack *et al.*, 1992[43]	22 Healthy elderly volunteers, 76.3 ± 11.3 years old, 10 M, 12 F. No major medical or neurologic illness; no depression. Handedness not specified	MR imaging (1.5 tesla). Volume estimates (single rater) derived from computer-assisted pixel classification of T_1-weighted coronal images (4 mm thick, contiguous). Intra-rater reliabilities not reported	Age associated with decreased ratio of hippocampal volume to IV and of anterior temporal lobe volume to IV. Interactions with sex or laterality not reported
Lim *et al.*, 1992[44]	14 Healthy male volunteers, eight young (21–25 years old) and six elderly (68–76 years old). No evidence of significant medical or psychiatric illness. Handedness not specified	MR imaging (1.5 tesla). Blinded volume measurements derived from semi-automated pixel segmentation of intermediate and T_2-weighted axial images ($n = 8$, 5 mm thick, 2.5 mm interscan gap)	Compared to younger males, older males had lower ratio of gray matter volume to IV (49.7% vs. 38.7%). No group difference in ratio of white matter volume to IV (47.2% vs. 41.2%). Interactions with laterality not reported

continues overleaf

Table 7.2 *continued*

Study	Subjects	Imaging and measurement technique	Findings
Murphy *et al.*, 1992[45]	27 Healthy male volunteers, 19–92 years old. No major medical, neurologic or psychiatric illness. Handedness not specified	MR imaging (0.5 tesla). Blinded volume measurements using computer-assisted trace methodology of proton density axial images ($n = 36$, 7 mm thick, contiguous). Manual tracing of subcortical from enhanced images. Rater reliabilities were established, but number of raters not reported	Older males (>60, $n = 17$) had smaller ratios of total, left, and right hemisphere volume to IV than younger males. Older males had smaller ratios of total caudate volume to IV and of total lenticular nuclei volume to IV than younger males; no difference in ratio of total thalamus volume to IV. Reductions in caudate and lenticular volumes also found when the volumes were normalized to total brain volume, suggesting a differential effect of aging on these structures. Older males exhibited a R > L asymmetry in lenticular nuclei; the reverse was true in younger males.
Doraiswamy *et al.*, 1993[46]	Same as Doraiswamy *et al.*, 1992	MR imaging (1.5 tesla). Blinded linear measurements of interuncal distance on T_1-weighted axial image (no additional details provided)	Age associated with larger interuncal distance (NB: this measure was not correlated with amygdala volume in a follow-up study [Early *et al.*, 1993]). Interactions with sex or laterality not reported
Raz *et al.*, 1993a,b,c[47,48,49]	29 Healthy volunteers, 18–78 years old (43.8 ± 21.5 years), 17 M, 12 F. No history of medical, neurologic, or psychiatric illness. All right-handed	MR imaging (0.3 tesla). Volume measurements using computer-assisted trace methodology of digitized images from the films, by two blinded raters with high reliabilities. T_1-weighted axial slices ($n = 9$, 4.2 mm thick, 6.0 mm interscan gap). T_2-weighted coronal slices ($n = 17$–21, 6.6 mm thick, 8.6 mm interscan gap)	After controlling for head size, age associated with decreased volumes of caudate and visual cortex (females > males). No association between age and volumes of dorsolateral prefrontal cortex, anterior cingulate gyrus, prefrontal white matter, hippocampal formation, postcentral gyrus, inferior parietal lobule or parietal white matter
Christiansen *et al.*, 1994[50]	142 healthy volunteers, 21–80 years old, 78 M, 64 F. No major medical or neurologic illness	MR imaging (1.5 tesla). Area and volume measurements using computer-assisted trace methodology of T_2-weighted axial slices ($n = 15$, 4 mm thick, 4 mm interscan gap). Number of raters, their 'blindness' and their reliabilities not specified	Age associated with decreased volume of cerebral hemispheres. Interactions with sex or laterality not reported
Cowell *et al.*, 1994[51]	130 healthy volunteers (overlap with subjects in Gur *et al.*, 1991), 18–80 years old, 70 M, 60 F. No major medical, neurologic or psychiatric illness. All right-handed	MR imaging (1.5 tesla). Volume measurements using a combination of computer-assisted trace methodology and pixel segmentation of 3D images reconstructed from T_2-weighted axial images (5 mm thick, contiguous). Good rater reliabilities, but 'blindness' not specified	Ratio of frontal lobe to IV was smaller in males over 40 years old than in younger males; no such group difference in females. In contrast, the R > L asymmetry of frontal lobe to IV was larger in older females than younger females; no such group difference in males. Ratio of temporal lobe to IV was also smaller in males over 40 years old than in younger males; no such group difference in females; no interactions with laterality. Ratio of the remaining brain volume to IV was smaller in older than younger subjects for both sexes; no interactions with laterality
DeCarli *et al.*, 1994[52]	30 Healthy male volunteers, 19–92 years old. No major medical, neurologic, or psychiatric illness. 29 Right-handed	MR imaging (0.5 tesla). Volume measurements using computer-assisted trace methodology of T_1-weighted coronal images (6 mm thick, contiguous) through temporal lobe, by single (blind?) rater	Age associated with decreased ratio of frontal lobe volume to IV but not with temporal lobe volume to IV. No interactions with laterality
Pfefferbaum *et al.*, 1994[53]	73 Healthy male volunteers (included in Pfefferbaum *et al.*, 1993), 21–70 years old (44.1 ± 13.8 years). No major medical, neurologic, or psychiatric illness. Left handers included (n not specified)	MR imaging (1.5 tesla). Blinded volume measurements derived from semi-automated pixel segmentation of intermediate and T_2-weighted axial images ($n = 17$–20, 5 mm thick, 2.5 mm interscan gap)	Adjusting for head size, age associated with decreased cortical gray matter volume (0.7 ml/year), but not with cortical white matter volume. Interactions with laterality not reported
Soininen *et al.*, 1994[54]	32 Healthy volunteers from the community, all with MMSE scores >25, 16 with age-associated memory impairment (AAMI) (67.7 ± 7 years; 4 M, 12 F), 16 controls (70.2 ± 4.7 years; 6 M, 10 F) without AAMI. All but one right-handed	MR imaging (1.5 tesla). Blinded volume measurements using computer-assisted trace methodology of T_1-weighted coronal images (1 mm thick, contiguous) through temporal lobe, by single rater with established reliabilities	No group differences in hippocampal volumes, although controls (but not AAMI subjects) exhibited significant R > L asymmetry. No group differences in amygdala volume or asymmetry

continued

Table 7.2 *continued*

Study	Subjects	Imaging and measurement technique	Findings
Blatter *et al.*, 1995[55]	194 Healthy volunteers, 16–65 years old, 89 M, 105 F. No history (by questionnaire) of any neurologic or psychiatric illness. 95% Right-handed	MR imaging (1.5 tesla). Volume measurements derived from semi-automated pixel segmentation and trace methodologies of intermediate and T_2-weighted axial images (5 mm thick, 2 mm gap). High rater reliabilities (blinded status?)	Adjusting for head size, age associated with decreased total brain volume and gray matter volume, but not white matter volume. Correlations tended to be higher for males than females, but these apparent differences were not analyzed. However, only females showed significant age-related reductions in gray matter. Interactions with laterality not reported
Convit *et al.*, 1995[56]	37 Healthy adult volunteers, 27 older (14 M, 13 F; 69.2 ± 8.3 years old), 10 younger (5 M, 5 F; 26.1 ± 4.1 years old). No evidence of stroke or major medical or psychiatric illness	MR imaging (1.5 tesla). Blinded volume measurements by single rater (reliabilities?) using computer-assisted trace methods of T_1-weighted coronal images (4 mm thick, 10% gap)	Controlling for sex and head size, age associated with volume loss in lateral temporal lobe (especially fusiform gyrus) and medial temporal lobe (especially hippocampus and parahippocampus)
Hokama *et al.*, 1995[57]	15 Healthy male community volunteers. 20–55 years old. No lifetime history of major medical, neurologic or psychiatric illness. All right-handed	MR imaging (1.5 tesla). Volume measurements of basal ganglia using semi-automated computer assisted trace methodology from T_1-weighted coronal and axial sections (1.5 mm thick, contiguous) by raters with established reliabilities	Age associated with decreased volumes of caudate and putamen, but not of globus pallidus. No correlation between basal ganglia volumes and IQ as estimated by WAIS-R information subscale
Parashos *et al.*, 1995[58]	80 Healthy volunteers (overlap with subjects in Coffey *et al.*, 1992), 30–91 years old, 28 M, 52 F. No lifetime history of neurologic or psychiatric illness. All right-handed	MR imaging (1.5 tesla). Blinded area measurements using computer-assisted trace methodology of T_1-weighted midsagittal image (5 mm thick), made by single rater with established rater reliabilities	Adjusting for IV, increasing age associated with smaller total and regional callosal areas, especially of anterior regions (males = females)
Fox *et al.*, 1996[59]	11 Adult volunteers with no evidence of memory impairment on testing, 5 M, 6 F; 51.3 ± 5.9 years old. No additional details provided	MR imaging (1.5 tesla). Volume measurements using computer-assisted pixel segmentation of T_1-weighted coronal images (1.5 mm thick, contiguous). Scanning repeated at 12.8 ± 4.3 months and volume differences determined from subtraction images	Over the follow-up period, brain volume decreased by 0.05% (~ 0.03 ml)
Janowsky *et al.*, 1996[60]	60 Healthy elderly volunteers, 66–94 years old (mean 78.2), 15 M, 45 F. No major medical, neurologic, or psychiatric illness. Handedness not specified	MR imaging (1.5 tesla). Area measurement of corpus callosum derived from computer-assisted trace methodology. Number of raters and their 'blindness' not specified	Age associated with decreased total callosal area, anterior callosal area and middle callosal area. Interactions with sex not reported
Murphy *et al.*, 1996[61]	69 Healthy volunteers. 35 M (44 ± 23 years old); 34 F (50 ± 21 years old). No major medical or psychiatric illness. All right-handed	MR imaging (0.5 and 1.5 tesla). Blinded volume measurements using computer-assisted segmentation and trace methodology of contiguous coronal images (5–6 mm thick). Number of raters not specified	Relative to 'young' subjects (age 20–35 years), 'old' subjects (60–85 years) had smaller brain matter volume ratios of cerebellum to IV (males = females), cerebrum to IV (males > females), frontal lobe to IV (males > females), temporal lobe to IV (males > females), parietal lobe to IV (females > males), parieto-occipital lobe to IV (males = females), parahippocampal gyrus to IV (males = females), amygdala to IV (males = females), hippocampus to IV (females > males), thalamus to IV (males = females), lenticular nucleus to IV (males = females), and caudate to IV (males = females). For the frontal lobe, the right side decreased more than the left with age in males, but in females the left side decreased more than the right. For all other regions, there were no interactions with laterality
Deshmukh *et al.*, 1997[62]	10 Healthy male volunteers, 50.1 ± 13.8 years old. No evidence of major medical, neurologic or psychiatric illness. Nine right-handed; one left-handed	MR imaging (1.5 tesla). Volume measures using semi-automated computer-assisted trace methodology from 3D T_1-weighted sagittal sections, realigned in the axial plane, by raters with established reliabilities	Age associated with decreased volume of cerebellar lobules VI–VII

continues overleaf

Table 7.2 *continued*

Study	Subjects	Imaging and measurement technique	Findings
Jack *et al.*, 1997[63]	126 Healthy elderly volunteers 51–89 years old (79.15 ± 6.73 years), 44 M, 82 F. No active neurologic or psychiatric illness. Handedness not specified	MR imaging (1.5 tesla). Blinded volume measurements using computer-assisted trace methodology of T_1-weighted 3D volumetric images (1.6 mm thick, contiguous, $n = 124$) by single rater with established reliabilities	Age associated with decreased volume ratio of hippocampus to IV (45.63 ml/ year), amygdala to IV (20.75 ml/year), and parahippocampal gyrus to IV (46.65 ml/year); effects similar for males and females. Effects were similar for the two hemispheres, except for the parahippocampal gyrus (L > R)
Kaye *et al.*, 1997[64]	30 Healthy elderly volunteers from the community, with MMSE ≥ 24. All ≥ 84 years old; 14 M, 16 F. No evidence of major medical, neurologic or psychiatric illness	MR imaging (1.5 tesla). Blinded volume measurements using computer-assisted trace methodology of T_1-weighted coronal images (4 mm thick, contiguous) by raters with established reliabilities. Scanning repeated annually over a mean of 42 months	No group differences in rate of volume loss in hippocampus (about 2%/year) or parahippocampus (about 2.5%/year)
O'Brien *et al.*, 1997[65]	40 Healthy community volunteers, 55–96 years old, 20 M, 20 F. No evidence of major medical or neurologic illness, or of depression or drug abuse	MR imaging (0.3 tesla). Ratings of amygdala–hippocampal atrophy from T_1-weighted coronal images (5.1 mm thick, 0.5 mm gap) by two raters with established reliabilities, blind to cognitive scores	Age associated with presence of amygdala–hippocampal atrophy
Raz *et al.*, 1997[66]	148 Healthy volunteers, 18–77 years old, 66 M (47.39 ± 18.07 years old); 82 F (45.72 ± 6.48 years old). No major medical, neurologic or psychiatric illness. All right-handed	MR imaging (1.5 tesla). Blinded volume measurements (digital planimetry) from scans of T_1-weighted reformatted coronal images (1.3 mm thick, contiguous). Good rater reliabilities among eight raters	Adjusted for height, age significantly related to smaller volumes of whole brain (males = females), prefrontal gray matter (males = females), inferior temporal cortex (males > females), fusiform gyrus (males = females), hippocampal formation (males = females), primary somatosensory cortex (males = females), superior parietal cortex (males = females), prefrontal white matter (males = females), and superior parietal white matter (males = females). No age effects were found for anterior cingulate cortex, parahippocampal cortex, primary motor cortex, inferior parietal cortex, visual cortex, and precentral, postcentral or inferior parietal white matter. No interactions with laterality
Salat *et al.*, 1997[67]	76 Healthy elderly volunteers, 65–95 years old (mean 77.7 years), 31 M, 45 F. No major medical or neurologic illness, and no depression. All right-handed, except one left-handed F	MR imaging (1.5 tesla). Area measurements (one of three raters with established reliabilities) of corpus callosum, pons, and cerebellum using trace methodology of T_1-weighted midsagittal image	Age associated with decreased total, anterior, and middle callosum areas in females but not males. No relation of age to pons or cerebellum areas
Coffey *et al.*, 1998[68]	330 Elderly volunteers living independently in the community, 66–96 years old (74.98 ± 5.09), 129 M, 201 F. No history of neurologic or psychiatric illness. All right-handed	MR imaging (1.5 tesla, $n = 248$; 0.35 tesla, $n = 82$). Blinded volume measurements (one of two raters with established reliabilities) using computer-assisted trace methodology of T_1-weighted axial images (5 mm thick, no interscan gap)	Adjusting for IV, age associated with decreased cerebral hemisphere volume (−2.79 ml/year) (males = females), frontal region area (−0.13 ml/year) (males = females), temporal–parietal region area (−0.13 ml/year) (males = females), and parietal–occipital region (males > females, −0.31 vs. −0.09 ml/ year, respectively). All effects similar in both hemispheres
Davatzikos and Resnik 1998[69]	114 Healthy volunteers 56–85 years old, 68 M (70.9 ± 7.6 years), 46 F (69.4 ± 8.0 years old). All right-handed. No additional details provided	MR imaging (1.5 tesla). Quantitative morphometry of the corpus callosum using computer-assisted trace methodology of T_1-weighted midsagittal image (1.5 mm thick). Morphometry was quantitated using a template and deformation function. No additional details provided	Age associated with decreased total and regional callosal size (males = females), with exception of anterior and posterior extremes

continued

Table 7.2 *continued*

Study	Subjects	Imaging and measurement technique	Findings
Gunning-Dixon *et al.*, 1998[70]	Same as Raz *et al.*, 1997	MR imaging (1.5 tesla). Blinded volume measurements (digital planimetry) from scans of T_1-weighted reformatted coronal images (1.3 mm thick, contiguous). Good rater reliabilities among eight raters	Age associated with decreased caudate volume (L > R in males, R > L in females), decreased putamen volume (R > L, males = females), and decreased globus pallidus volume (males only)
Gur *et al.*, 1998[71]	17 Healthy volunteers (overlap with subjects in Gur *et al.*, 1991 and Cowell *et al.*, 1994) 31.9 ± 8.9 years old, 13 M, 4 F	MR imaging (1.5 tesla). Volume measurements using a combination of computer-assisted trace methodology and pixel segmentation of 3D images reconstructed from T_2-weighted axial images (5 mm thick, contiguous). Good rater reliabilities, but 'blindness' not specified. Scanning repeated an average of 32 months later.	No significant change over follow-up period in whole brain, CSF or frontal lobe volumes. Significant volume loss was observed for L (7.5%) and R (7.2%) temporal lobes
Guttmann *et al.*, 1998[72]	72 Healthy volunteers, 18–81 years old, 22 M, 50 F. No history of psychiatric illness, epilepsy, or severe head trauma. Handedness not specified	MR imaging (1.5 tesla). Blinded volume measurements using computer-assisted segmentation and trace methodology of contiguous axial images (3 mm thick). Good interrater reliabilities	Age associated with decreased ratio of total white matter volume to IV and decreased total gray matter volume to IV. Interactions with sex or laterality not reported
Jack *et al.*, 1998[73]	24 Elderly volunteers, 70–89 years old (81.04 ± 3.78 years), 8 M, 16 F. No active neurologic or psychiatric illness. Handedness not specified	MR imaging (1.5 tesla). Blinded volume measurements using computer-assisted trace methodology of T_1-weighted 3D volumetric images (1.6 mm thick, contiguous, $n = 124$) by single rater with established reliabilities	Over a 12 month interval, mean hippocampal volume decreased by 1.55% and mean temporal horn volume increased by 6.15% (males = females, L = R)
Laakso *et al.*, 1998[74]	42 cognitively normal healthy elderly community volunteers, 64–79 (72 ± 4) years old, 19 M, 23 F	MR imaging (1.5 tesla). Volume measures using computer-assisted trace methods from T_1-weighted coronal images (~ 2 mm thick, contiguous) by a single blinded rater with established reliabilities	No relation between age and hippocampal atrophy
Mueller *et al.*, 1998[75]	46 Healthy elderly volunteers 65–74 years old (6 M, 5 F), 75–84 years old (8 M, 7 F) and 85–93 years old (9 M, 11 F). All functionally independent, MMSE ≥ 24, and free of major medical and neurologic illness, as well as depression. Handedness not specified	MR imaging (1.5 tesla). Volume measurements (non-blind?) using computer-assisted pixel segmentation of contiguous coronal images (4 mm thick). Excellent interrater reliabilities. Scanning repeated annually or biannually over 3–9 year follow-up	Adjusting for IV, age associated with decreased volumes of total brain, hemispheres, frontal lobes, temporal lobes, basilar–subcortical region, hippocampus, and hippocampal gyrus. Interactions with sex not reported. Over the follow-up period, significant volume decreases were seen in hippocampus (~ 0.02 ml/year), parahippocampal gyrus (in youngest group only, ~ 0.05 ml/year), parietal–occipital region (in middle and oldest age groups, ~ 3 ml/year), and basilar region (in middle group only, ~ 0.5 ml/year). No volume decreases were seen in hemispheres, frontal lobes or temporal lobes
Oguro *et al.*, 1998[76]	152 Healthy adults, 81 M, 71 F, age range 40s–70s. No evidence of neurological disease	MR imaging (0.2 tesla). Linear and area measurements using computer-assisted trace methodology from T_1-weighted midsagittal image (7 mm thick) and T_2-weighted axial images (no details), by raters ($n = ?$) with established reliabilities	Age associated with decreased linear measures of midbrain tegmentum (males only), midbrain pretectum (males and females), and base of pons (males only), but not with pontine tegmentum or fourth ventricle. Age associated with decreased area of cerebellar vermis (males only), but not of pons. Age associated with decreased ratio of cerebrum to IA (males and females) at level of third ventricle and at level of body of lateral ventricles. Interactions with laterality not reported
Pfefferbaum *et al.*, 1998[77]	28 Healthy male volunteers (overlap with Pfefferbaum *et al.*, 1994), 21–68 years old (51 ± 13.8 years). No major medical, neurologic, or psychiatric illness. Left-handers included (n not specified)	MR imaging (1.5 tesla). Blinded volume measurements derived from semi-automated pixel segmentation of intermediate and T_2-weighted axial images ($n = 17$–20, 5 mm thick, 2.5 mm interscan gap). Scanning repeated at 5 year follow-up	Over the follow-up interval, significant decrease in total gray matter volume and in regional gray matter volume (pre-frontal gray ~ 2 ml, or 7%; posterior parieto-occipital gray ~ 1 ml, or 3.5%) (no change in frontal, anterior superior temporal, posterior superior temporal, or anterior parietal regions gray matter volume). Interactions with laterality not reported
Raz *et al.*, 1998[78]	146 Healthy volunteers (overlap with Raz *et al.*, 1997), 18–77 years old, 64 M (48 ± 18 years); 82 F (46 ± 17 years). No evidence of major medical, neurologic or psychiatric illness. All right-handed	MR imaging (1.5 tesla). Blinded volume measurements (digital planimetry) from scans of T_1-weighted reformatted coronal and sagittal images (0.8 mm thick, 1.5 mm thick). Good rater reliabilities	Age associated with volume loss in cerebellar hemispheres (~ 2%/decade), vermis, vermian lobules VI and VII (~ 4%/decade), and posterior vermis (lobules VIII–X; ~ 2%/decade), but not in anterior vermis (lobules I–V) or pons

Table 7.3.   Aging and changes in size of CSF spaces

Study	Subjects	Imaging and measurement technique	Findings
Barron et al., 1976[7]	135 Volunteers, 9 months–90 years old, equal gender distribution in all age groups (8 M, 7 F per decade). No history of neurological disease; psychiatric history not reported. Handedness not specified	Computed tomography (CT). Planimetric determination of ventricular–brain ratio (VBR) by single rater (average of three measurements) from Polaroid photograph	Age associated with increased VBR and with increased variability in VBR. Interactions with sex or laterality not reported
Earnest et al., 1979[79]	59 Volunteer retirees, 60–99 years old, 11 M, 48 F. Living independently and free of neurological disease. Handedness not specified	CT. Linear and planimetric measures of ventricular size at three different levels, from photographs. Linear measurements of four largest sulci. No additional data provided	Subjects 80 years or older ($n = 29$) had larger ratio of ventricular size to intracranial size than did younger subjects ($n = 30$). The sum of the widths of the four sulci was greater in older subjects than in younger subjects. Interactions with sex or laterality not reported
Jacoby et al., 1980[19]	50 Healthy elderly volunteers, 62–88 years old, 10 M, 40 F. No history of significant psychiatric or neurologic illness. Handedness not specified	CT. Ratings (small, normal, enlarged) of ventricular size from films by single blinded rater (rater reliability not reported). Planimetric determination of ventricular–skull ratio and Evans's ratio from films by single rater (average of three measurements) with established reliabilities	8 (16%) Subjects were rated as having 'enlarged' lateral ventricles. No significant correlation between age and ventricular–skull ratio or Evans's ratio. Interactions with sex or laterality not reported. Adjusting for age, no relation between any CT measure and performance on the Hodkinson test of memory and orientation
Meese et al., 1980[80]	160 Healthy 'volunteers', 1–71 years old, 10 M and 10 F in each decade. No additional data provided	CT. Linear measurements of ventricular size and sulcal width from four axial slices (no additional data provided)	Apparent age-related changes in some measures of ventricular size and sulcal width, but these changes not analyzed statistically. Interactions with sex or laterality not reported
Cala et al., 1981[20]	115 Volunteers, 15–40 years old, 62 M, 53 F. No history of migraine, head trauma, or excessive alcohol intake (no additional details provided). All but eight subjects right-handed	CT. ($n =$ two scanners). Planimetric measurements of ventricular–skull ratio at level of frontal horns (no additional details provided). Axial slices (13 mm thick)	No relationship between age and ventricular–skull ratio. Interactions with sex or laterality not reported
Soininen et al., 1982[81]	85 Volunteers, 53 from community and 32 from nursing home, 75 ± 7 years old, 23 M, 62 F. No neurological disease (no additional details provided)	CT. Linear measurements (from films?) of ventricular and sulcal size. Axial slices ($n = 8$–12, 8 mm thick). No additional details provided	Age correlated with ratios of ventricular width to skull width (frontal horn index and cella media index). Age correlated with mean width of four largest sulci. Correlations were found between a composite neuro-psychological test score and the size of the lateral and IIIrd ventricles, the left Sylvian fissure, and the right temporal horn, but the effects of age were not controlled. Interactions with sex or laterality not reported
Zatz et al., 1982a[12]	123 Volunteers, 10–90 years old, 49 M, 74 F. No history of neurological or major medical disease. Handedness not specified	CT. Volume measurement derived from computer-assisted pixel segmentation technique (ASI-II program). Axial slices ($n = 9$, 10 mm thick, 10 mm interscan gap)	Age significantly associated with increased ventricular volume (males = females), even after controlling for intracranial volume (IV). Increased variability of ventricular size with age. Age associated with increased sulcal CSF volume, even after controlling for IV
Gado et al., 1983[14]	12 Elderly volunteers, 64–81 years old, 9 M, 3 F. No additional clinical data provided	CT. Volume measurements derived from computer-assisted pixel segmentation technique (seventh axial slices, 8 mm thick). Linear measurements from axial images. Number of raters and rater reliabilities not specified	During 1 year follow-up, ratio of ventricular volume to IV increased significantly by an average of 3.7%. No significant changes in linear measures of ventricular size (VBR, IIIrd ventricular ratio, frontal horn ratio). During 1 year follow-up, ratio of sulcal volume to IV increased significantly by an average of 13%. Interactions with sex or laterality not reported
Laffey et al., 1984[11]	212 Elderly volunteers, 65–89 years old, 110 M; 102 F. No evidence of alcoholism, dementia, or neurologic illness	CT. Qualitative rating (six-point scale) of ventricular enlargement and sulcal widening from films, by two experienced radiologists with established reliabilities	Age associated with increased ventricular size. No association between age and ratings of sulcal widening. Interactions with sex or laterality not reported

continued

Table 7.3 *continued*

Study	Subjects	Imaging and measurement technique	Findings
Gomori *et al.*, 1984[21]	148 Neurologically intact volunteers, 28–84 years old. Subjects with minor neurological symptoms, patients with lung, breast, prostate, colon cancer but no CNS involvement. Neurologic exam normal	CT. Linear (sum of bicaudate and Sylvian fissure ratios)	CSF space increased with age; age correlated with the sum of the two ratios (bicaudate and Sylvian fissure, $r = 0.64$). The sum of the ratios increased two-fold between ages 28–49 and 80–89, faster after the fifth decade
Takeda *et al.*, 1984[82]	980 Patients scheduled for CT, 10–88 years old, 483 M, 497 F. Included patients with hypertension, diabetes mellitus, ischemic heart disease, lung disease and renal disease. Excluded subjects with abnormal CT	CT. Volumetric. Axial slices ($n = 7$) starting at the supraorbitomeatal line (10 mm thick, contiguous sections)	CSF space increased with age; CSF space volume displayed five-fold increase from age 40 (21.0 cm^3) to 90 (124.3 cm^3). Brain atrophy index (BAI) showed similar increase. Both CSF space volume and BAI were stable before age 40. Brain atrophy was accelerated in males during the fourth decade and the rate decreased afterwards, while atrophy in females proceeded with a stable rate throughout the lifespan. Increased variability with age
Schwartz *et al.*, 1985[5]	30 Healthy male volunteers, 21–81 years old. No history of major medical, neurologic, or psychiatric illness. Handedness not specified	CT. Volume measurements derived from computer-assisted pixel segmentation technique (ASI-II program). Axial slices ($n = 7$) starting from the plane of the inferior orbito-meatal line (10 mm thick, 7 mm interscan gap)	Age correlated with areas and volumes of lateral and IIIrd ventricles, even after adjusting for height and intracranial area. Age correlated with VBR. Increased variability of ventricular size with age. No laterality effects. Age correlated with CSF volume (ventricular plus basal cisterns), even after controlling for IV. Increased variability of CSF volume with age
Pfefferbaum *et al.*, 1986[13]	57 Healthy volunteers, 20–84 years old, 27 M, 30 F. No additional data provided	CT. Volume measurements derived from computer-assisted pixel segmentation technique (modification of Gado *et al.*, 1983). Contiguous axial slices ($n = 5$), starting at the level of the superior roof of the orbits	Age associated with increased ratio of ventricular volume to IV. Increased variability in ventricular volume with age. Interactions with sex or laterality not reported. Age associated with increased ratio of sulcal CSF volume to IV (from single axial slice [8 mm thick] approximately 48 mm from the level of the superior roof of the orbits). Age associated with increased variability of sulcal CSF volume to IV
Nagata, *et al.*, 1987[83]	500 Patients with head CT, 10–90 years old. Excluded: subjects with abnormal CT	CT. Volumetric. Axial slices ($n = 6$), beginning at the level of the basal cistern (10 mm thick)	CSF space increased with age; four-fold increase in BAI between ages 50 (2.3%) and 80 (10%). BAI was stable before the sixth decade. Increased variability with age
Stafford *et al.*, 1988[22]	79 Healthy male volunteers, 31–87 years old. No severe medical or psychiatric illness. Handedness not specified	CT. Volume measurements derived from computer-assisted pixel segmentation technique (ASI-II program). Axial slices ($n = 3$) at mid-, high- and supraventricular levels	Age associated with increased ratio of ventricular–brain volume. Age associated with increased ratio of supraventricular CSF–brain volume. Interactions with laterality not reported. Inverse correlation observed between a discriminant function of ventricular volume measures and a discriminant function of neuropsychological tests of naming and abstraction
Pearlson *et al.*, 1989[84]	31 Healthy elderly volunteers, 68.3 ± 1.2 years old, 15 M, 16 F. No major medical, neurologic, or psychiatric illness. Handedness not specified	CT. Planimetric determination of VBR from films by one of two raters, each with established reliabilities	Age correlated with VBR. Interactions with sex or laterality not reported
Kaye *et al.*, 1992[85]	107 Healthy volunteers, 64 M (21–90 years old); 43 F (23–88 years old). No major medical, neurologic, or psychiatric illness. Handedness not specified	CT. Volume measurements derived from computer-assisted pixel segmentation technique (ASI-II program). Axial slices (10 mm thick, 7 mm interscan gap)	Age associated with increased ventricular volume in both males and females (about 20% per decade); precipitous increases observed beginning in the fifth decade in males and in the sixth decade in females. Interactions with laterality not reported

continues overleaf

Table 7.3. *continued*

Study	Subjects	Imaging and measurement technique	Findings
Sullivan *et al.*, 1993[86]	114 Healthy volunteers, 21–82 years old (51.2±17.7 years), 84 M, 30 F. No history of major medical, neurologic, or psychiatric illness. 90% Right-handed	CT. Volume measurements derived from computer-assisted pixel segmentation technique (modification of Gado *et al.*, 1983). Axial slices ($n = 10$, 10 mm thick). 10 neuropsychological tests (MMSE, Trail Making Test A and B, WAIS-R subtests—Information, Digit Span, Vocabulary, Digit Symbol, Picture Completion, Block Design, and Object Assembly)	Age correlated with total and third ventricular volume, even after adjustments for head size (males=females). No correlation between age related changes in total or third ventricular volume and performance on 10 neuropsychological tests. Age correlated with increased CSF volume in Sylvian fissure and in vertex, frontal and parieto-occipital sulci (males=females).
Shear *et al.*, 1995[87]	35 Healthy volunteers (included in Sullivan *et al.*, 1993), 67.4±7.4 years old, 23 M, 12 F. No history of major medical, neurologic, or psychiatric illness	CT. Longitudinal within-subject follow-up, using blinded volume measurements per technique of Sullivan *et al.*, 1993. High rater reliabilities	Over mean (±SD) follow-up of 2.6 (±0.96) years, increases were observed in CSF volumes of frontal sulci (0.31 ml/year), Sylvian fissure (0.58 ml/year), parieto-occipital sulci (0.05 ml/year), and ventricular system (0.61 ml/year). Interactions with sex not reported
Elwan *et al.*, 1996[88]	88 Healthy 'lower middle class' volunteers, 40–76 years old (54.8±9.6 years), 57 M, 31 F. No major medical, neurologic, or psychiatric illness. All right-handed	CT. Multiple distance measurements (no additional details provided)	Age correlated with maximum width of IIIrd ventricle. Interactions with sex or laterality not reported
Grant *et al.*, 1987[89]	64 Healthy volunteers, 18–64 years old, 25 M, 39 F. No history of neurological disease; psychiatric history not reported. Handedness not specified	Magnetic resonance (MR) imaging (0.15 tesla). Mathematically derived estimate of ventricular volume and CSF volume from signal intensity measurements made on single sagittal slice (number of raters not specified)	Age associated with increased ventricular volume in males, but not females; however, this apparent gender difference was not tested statistically. Interactions with laterality not reported. Age associated with increased total (ventricular plus cisternal) cranial CSF volume (males=females). No control for size of brain or head
Condon *et al.*, 1988[29]	40 Volunteers, 20–60 years old, 20 M, 20 F. No additional details provided	MR imaging (0.15 tesla). Volume measurement (two raters) derived from computer-assisted pixel segmentation of contiguous sagittal slices (variable slice thickness and number)	For males but not females, age correlated with ratio of total ventricular volume to IV, total CSF volume to IV, and total sulcal CSF volume to IV
Yoshii *et al.*, 1988[30]	58 Healthy volunteers, 21–81 years old, 29 M, 29 F. Neurologic and psychiatric histories not reported. Handedness not specified	MR imaging (1.0 tesla). Blinded global ratings (four-point scale) of lateral ventricular enlargement from inversion recovery films (axial slices, n unspecified, 10 mm thick, 3 mm interscan gap). Numbers of raters and rater reliabilities not specified	Age correlated with ratings of lateral ventricular enlargement (males=females). Interactions with laterality not reported
Jernigan *et al.*, 1990[33]	58 Healthy volunteers, 8–79 years old, 35 M, 23 F. No neurologic, psychiatric, or medical (e.g. diabetes mellitus and heart disease) illness. Handedness not specified	MR imaging (1.5 tesla). Volume estimates (one of two raters) derived from computer-assisted pixel classification of multiple spin-echo axial images (5 mm thick, 2.5 mm interscan gap)	Age associated with increased ratio of ventricular CSF volume to IV. Age associated with increased ratio of sulcal CSF volume to IV. Interactions with sex or laterality not reported
Wahlund *et al.*, 1990[90]	24 Healthy elderly volunteers, 75–85 years old (mean = 79 years), 8 M, 16 F. No evidence of neurologic or psychiatric illness. Handedness not specified	MR imaging (0.02 tesla). Visual ratings (5-point scale) of CSF spaces on T_2-weighted axial films (slice = 10 mm thick, no gap) by 2 raters (blind?) with established reliabilities. Area measurements based upon computer-assisted pixel classification technique, from single axial section at level of basal ganglia	No correlation between age and visual ratings or area measurements of sulcal CSF or lateral ventricle CSF size
Gur *et al.*, 1991[37]	69 Healthy volunteers, 18–80 years old, 34 M, 35 F. No neurologic or psychiatric illness. 66 Right-handed; three left-handed	MR imaging (1.5 tesla). Volume measurements (any two of four raters) derived from segmentation technique based on two-feature pixel classification of multiple spin-echo axial images (5 mm thick, contiguous)	Older (≥ 55 years) subjects ($n = 26$) had larger total CSF volume (males > females), larger ratio of ventricular CSF volume to IV (males=females), and larger ratio of sulcal CSF volume to IV (males > females). Effects of age on ratio of ventricular CSF volume to IV were asymmetric (L > R) in males but not in females

continued

Table 7.3 *continued*

Study	Subjects	Imaging and measurement technique	Findings
Tanna et al., 1991[40]	16 Healthy volunteers, 52–86 years old, 5 M, 11 F. No evidence of major medical, neurologic or psychiatric illness. Handedness not specified	MR imaging (1.5 tesla). Volume measurements (one of two raters with established reliabilities) derived from segmentation techniques based on two-feature pixel classification of multiple spin-echo axial images (5 mm thick, 2.5 mm interscan gap)	Age significantly correlated with ratio of ventricular CSF volume to total CSF plus total brain volume. Trend (non-significant) for age to be associated with increasing ratio of sulcal CSF volume to total CSF plus total brain volume. Interactions with sex or laterality not reported
Coffey et al., 1992[41]	76 Healthy volunteers, 36–91 years old, 25 M, 51 F. No lifetime evidence of neurologic or psychiatric illness. All right-handed	MR imaging (1.5 tesla). Volume measurements (one of three blinded raters with established reliabilities) using computer-assisted trace methodology of T_1-weighted coronal images ($n = 30$–35, 5 mm thick, contiguous). Blinded clinical ratings (five-point scale) of lateral ventricular enlargement from films (average score of two experienced raters)	Adjusting for IV, age associated with increased volumes of the third (2.8%/year) and lateral (3.2%/year) ventricles (males = females). Age associated with increased odds (7.7%/year) of at least mild lateral ventricular enlargement, from 0.10 at age 40 to 2.22 at age 80 (males = females). No interactions with laterality
Lim et al., 1992[44]	14 Healthy male volunteers, 8 young (21–25 years old), 6 elderly (68–76 years old). No evidence of significant medical or psychiatric illness. Handedness not specified	MR imaging (1.5 tesla). Blinded volume measurements derived from semi-automated pixel segmentation of intermediate and T_2-weighted axial imaging ($n = 8$, 5 mm thick, 2.5 mm interscan gap)	Compared with younger males, older males had higher percentage of CSF volume to IV (8% vs. 20.1%)
Matsubayashi et al., 1992[91]	73 Healthy volunteers, 59–83 years old, 24 M, 49 F. No history of major medical, neurologic, or psychiatric illness	MR imaging (0.5 tesla). Planimetric determination of ventricular–parenchymal ratio (VPR). No additional details provided	Age correlated with VPR. Interactions with sex or laterality not reported
Murphy et al., 1992[45]	27 Healthy males, 19–92 years old. No major medical, neurologic, or psychiatric illness. Handedness not specified	MR imaging (0.5 tesla). Blinded volume measurements derived from semi-automated pixel segmentation of proton density axial images ($n = 36$, 7 mm thick, contiguous). Rater reliabilities established, but number of raters not specified	Compared with younger males (under 60 years old; $n = 10$), older males ($n = 17$) had larger ratios of lateral ventricular volume to IV, larger ratio of third ventricular volume to IV, and larger ratios of peripheral CSF volume (total CSF volume minus ventricular volumes) to IV. No interactions with laterality
Raz et al., 1993a[47]	29 Healthy volunteers, 18–78 years old, 17 M, 12 F. No major medical, neurologic, or psychiatric illness. Self-reported right-handers	MR imaging (0.30 tesla). Blinded volume measurements from films using digital planimetry of T_1-weighted and proton density sagittal and coronal images. Good rater ($n = 2$) reliabilities	Controlling for head size, age associated with increased lateral ventricular volume (males = females). Interactions with laterality not reported
Christiansen et al., 1994[50]	142 Healthy volunteers, 21–80 years old, 78 M, 64 F. No major medical or neurologic illness	MR imaging (1.5 tesla). Volume measurements using manual tracing of T_2-weighted axial images (4 mm thick, 4 mm interscan gap). No additional details provided	Age associated with increased lateral ventricle volume in males (134%) and females (66%), but these apparent gender differences were not statistically compared. Interactions with laterality not reported
DeCarli et al., 1994[52]	30 Healthy male volunteers, 18–92 years old. No major medical, neurologic, or psychiatric illness. 29 Right-handed	MR imaging (0.5 tesla). Volume measurements of T_1-weighted coronal images (6 mm thick, contiguous) by single rater using computer-assisted pixel segmentation techniques. Good rater reliabilities	Age associated with increased volume of sulcal CSF to IV (1.3%/decade), central CSF to IV (0.3%/decade), and third ventricle CSF to IV (0.04%/decade). For all measures, no interactions with laterality
Pfefferbaum et al., 1994[53]	73 Healthy male volunteers (included in Pfefferbaum et al., 1993), 21–70 years old (44.1 ± 13.8 years). No major medical, neurologic, or psychiatric illness. Left-handers included (n not specified)	MR imaging (1.5 tesla). Blinded volume measurements of T_2-weighted axial slices (5 mm thick, 2.5 mm interscan gap) by four raters using computer-assisted pixel segmentation techniques. Good rater reliabilities	Age associated with increased cortical CSF volume to IV (0.6 ml/year) and ventricular volume to IV (0.3 ml/year). Interactions with laterality not reported
Blatter et al., 1995[55]	194 Healthy volunteers, 16–65 years old, 89 M, 105 F. No history (by questionnaire) of any neurologic or psychiatric illness. 95% Right-handed	MR imaging (1.5 tesla). Volume measurements derived from semi-automated pixel segmentation and trace methodologies, of intermediate and T_2-weighted axial images (5 mm thick, 2 mm gap). High rater reliabilities (blinded status?)	Adjusting for IV, age associated with increased subarachnoid CSF volume, and lateral and IIIrd ventricular volumes, but not IVth ventricular volume; correlations tended to be higher for males than females, but these apparent differences were not analyzed. Interactions with laterality not reported

continues overleaf

Table 7.3 *continued*

Study	Subjects	Imaging and measurement technique	Findings
Murphy *et al.*, 1996[61]	69 Healthy volunteers, 35 males (mean ± SD age = 44 ± 23 years); 34 females (mean ± SD age = 50 ± 21 years). No major medical or psychiatric illness. All right-handed	MR imaging (0.5 and 1.5 tesla). Blinded volume measurements using computer-assisted segmentation and trace methodology of contiguous coronal images (5–6 mm thick). Number of raters not specified	Relative to younger subjects (age 20–35 years), older subjects (60–85 years) had larger ratios of lateral ventricular volume to IV (males = females), third ventricular volume to IV (females > males), and peripheral CSF volume to IV (males = females). No interactions with laterality
Salonen *et al.*, 1997[92]	61 Healthy volunteers, 30–86 years old, 30 M, 31 F. No neurological symptoms or disease; psychiatric history not specified. Handedness not specified	MR imaging (1.0 tesla). Qualitative ratings (five-point scale) of sulcal and lateral ventricular enlargement. Linear measurement of maximum width of third ventricle. T_1-weighted axial slices (5 mm thick, 1 mm interscan gap). Number of raters and rater reliabilities not specified	Age associated with increased ratings of sulcal widening and lateral ventricular enlargement, and with width of IIIrd ventricle. Interactions with sex or laterality not reported
Yue *et al.*, 1997[93]	1488 Healthy elderly volunteers from the Cardiovascular Health Study, 65–80 + years old, numbers of males and females not specified. Handedness not specified. No major medical or neurologic illness (psychiatric illness not assessed)	MR imaging (0.35 or 1.5 tesla). Blinded ratings of sulcal prominence (10-point scale) and ventricular size (10-point scale) from T_1-weighted axial images. Good to excellent rater reliabilities, but number of raters not specified	Age associated with increased sulcal prominence and ventricular enlargement (males = females)
Coffey *et al.*, 1998[68]	330 Elderly volunteers living independently in the community, 66–96 years old (74.98 ± 5.09), 129 M, 201 F. No history of neurologic or psychiatric illness. All right-handed	MR imaging (1.5 tesla, *n* = 248; 0.35 tesla, *n* = 82). Blinded volume measurements (one of two raters with established reliabilities) using computer-assisted trace methodology of T_1-weighted axial images (5 mm thick, no interscan gap)	Adjusting for IV, age associated with increased peripheral (sulcal) CSF volume, lateral fissure CSF volume, lateral ventricular volume (0.95 ml/year), and IIIrd ventricular volume (0.05 ml/year). Males showed greater age-related changes than females for peripheral CSF (2.11 ml/year vs. 0.06 ml/year, respectively) and lateral fissure volumes (0.23 ml/year vs. 0.10 ml/year, respectively). No interactions with laterality
Guttmann *et al.*, 1998[72]	72 Healthy volunteers, 18–81 years old, 22 M, 50 F. No history of psychiatric illness, epilepsy, or severe head trauma. Handedness not specified	MR imaging (1.5 tesla). Blinded volume measurements using computer-assisted segmentation and trace methodology of contiguous axial images (3 mm thick). Good interrater reliabilities	Age associated with increased ratio of total CSF volume to IV. Interactions with sex or laterality not reported
Mueller *et al.*, 1998[75]	46 Healthy elderly volunteers. 65–74 years old (6 M, 5 F), 75–84 years old (8 M, 7 F), and 85–95 years old (9 M, 11 F). All functionally independent, MMSE ≥ 24, and free of major medical and neurologic illness, as well as depression. Handedness not specified	MR imaging (1.5 tesla). Volume measurements (non-blind?) using computer-assisted pixel segmentation of contiguous coronal images (4 mm thick). Excellent interrater reliabilities. Scanning repeated annually or biannually over 3–9 year follow-up	Adjusting for IV, age associated with increased temporal horn volume, but not with total CSF, sulcal CSF, or lateral ventricle volumes. Interactions with sex not reported. Over the follow-up period, significant increases were seen only in total CSF volume (∼1.5 ml/year, females > males) and in lateral ventricular volume (∼1.4 ml/year) (males = females)
Pfefferbaum *et al.*, 1998[77]	28 Healthy male volunteers (overlap with Pfefferbaum *et al.*, 1994) 21–68 years old (51 ± 13.8 years). No major medical, neurologic, or psychiatric illness. Left-handers included (*n* not specified)	MR imaging (1.5 tesla). Blinded volume measurements derived from semi-automated pixel segmentation of intermediate and T_2-weighted axial images (*n* = 17–20, 5 mm thick, 2.5 mm interscan gap). Scanning repeated at 5 year follow-up	Over the follow-up interval, significant increase in volume of lateral (∼5 ml, or 20%) and third ventricles, but not of cortical sulcal CSF volume

17% over the first nine decades of life. Studies using linear measurements show a two-fold enlargement while volumetric studies report a four- to five-fold volume increase. The changes in the size of CSF spaces are accelerated after midlife (60 years). The variance in measures of CSF spaces also increases with age.

The majority of the studies report a progressive enlargement of the lateral and third ventricles with age, which ranges from less than one to three times their initial sizes. No relationship has been found thus far between aging and fourth ventriclar size. As expected, studies using linear measurements show the smallest changes, while studies using planimetric and volumetric measurements agree in finding relatively greater enlargement. The increase in ventricular size is relatively minimal until the sixth decade, after which it becomes more pronounced. Finally, the variability of the measurements of ventricular size increases with age.

Table 7.4. Aging and incidence of subcortical hyperintensities (SH)

Study	Subjects	Imaging and measurement technique	Findings
George et al., 1986[94]	47 Normal volunteers; two age groups: <45 years (n = 35) and 46–78 years (n = 12)	MR imaging (0.3 tesla). Qualitative rating (5-point scale) of subcortical hyperintensities (white and gray matter). Axial slices (n = 7) 8 mm thick with 1.2 cm interscan gap	Subcortical hyperintensities increased with age; no subject under 45 had foci of increased signal; 8/12 subjects over 46 showed single or multiple foci of increased signal
Fazekas, 1989[95]	87 Normal volunteers, 31–83 years old, 40 M, 27 F. Excluded patients with cardiovascular or cerebrovascular disease, hypertension, hyperglycemia, and neurologic or psychiatric illness	MRI (1.5 tesla). Qualitative rating (four-point scale) of subcortical hyperintensities. Axial slices (n = 7) intermediate and T_2-weighted, 5–8 mm thick	The incidence and severity of subcortical hyperintensities increased with age and in the presence of risk factors for vascular disease
Hendrie et al., 1989[96]	27 normal volunteers, 63–86 years old, 10 M, 17 F	MRI (1.5 tesla). Consensus rating (four-point scale) by two blinded raters; axial slices (T_2-weighted) 10 mm thick	Of the population 56.7% had SH; mean age increased with severity of SH
Jernigan et al., 1991[33]	58 Normal volunteers, 8–79 years of age, 35 M, 23 F. Excluded: diabetes mellitus, heart disease, substance abuse, developmental intellectual abnormality, psychiatric illness	MRI (1.5 tesla). Volumetric (ratio of volume of white and grey matter subcortical hyperintensities divided by cranial volume, as derived from computer-assisted pixel classification system). Axial slices of entire brain with thickness 5 mm and interscan gap 2.5 mm	SH volume ratio increased curvilinearly with age (especially after 55 years of age) from slightly over 0% at age 55 to 25% of the supratentorial volume at age 80. Increased variability with age
Matsubayashi et al., 1992[91]	73 Healthy volunteers, 59–83 years of age, 24 M, 49 F. No major medical, neurological or psychiatric illness	MRI (0.5 tesla). Rating (four-point scale) of periventricular SH on T_2-weighted axial slices (no additional details reported)	Subjects with highest SH rating (n = 19) significantly older than other groups
Boone et al., 1992[97]	100 Healthy volunteers, 45–83 years of age, 36 M, 64 F. No major medical, neurological or psychiatric illness	MRI (1.5 tesla). Computer-assisted area measurements of SH from T_2-weighted axial sections by single rater (additional rater information not reported)	Age greater in those subjects with the largest lesion areas
Almkvist et al., 1992[98]	23 Healthy volunteers, 75 years of age and older, 9 M, 14 F. No major medical, neurological, or psychiatric illness	MRI (0.02 tesla). Area measurements of SH from T_2-weighted axial sections by single blinded rater (reliabilities not reported)	No correlation between age and SH area
Coffey et al., 1992[41]	76 Healthy volunteers, 36–91 years old, 25 M, 51 F. No history of neurological or psychiatric illness. All right-handed	MRI (1.5 tesla). Consensus ratings of SH from intermediate and T_2-weighted axial films (four-point scale) by two blinded raters with established reliabilities	Increasing age associated with increased odds of SH in the deep white matter (6.3%/year) and pons (8.1%/year)

Table 7.4 summarizes the effects of aging on the incidence on MRI of foci of T2-signal hyperintensity in the subcortical white matter and gray matter nuclei ('subcortical hyperintensities'). While the studies are difficult to compare because of differences in the definition/rating of subcortical hyperintensity, it is clear that the changes increase with age as well as in the presence of risk factors for vascular disease (e.g. smoking, hypertension, diabetes mellitus, coronary/peripheral vascular disease). In our study of 75 healthy adults[41], subcortical hyperintensity was present in the deep white matter in 64.0% of subjects, in the periventricular white matter in 12.0%, in the basal ganglia in 12% and in the pons in 21.3%. The odds of having subcortical hyperintensity increased from 5% to 9% per year, depending on the anatomic region involved.

QUANTITATIVE MRI AT THE HENRY FORD AGING PROGRAM

One specific aim of our Neuropsychiatry Program at Duke University Medical Center has been to examine brain structure and function in normal aging and in patients with various psychiatric illnesses, particularly affective disorders[41,99–102]. All participants are strongly right-handed and each receives an extensive medical and neuropsychiatric history interview and examination. The normal subjects have no history or clinical evidence of any psychiatric disorder or any illness referable to the brain. The majority of these 'normal' subjects are also free of medical illness, so that our cohort is felt to reflect primarily 'successful' rather than 'usual' aging[38].

The MRI scans of the brain are performed on high-field strength (1.5 tesla) systems. Spin-echo pulse sequences are used to produce T1-weighted (TR = 500 ms, TE = 20 ms), intermediate (TR = 2500 ms, TE = 40 ms) and T2-weighted (TR = 2500 ms, TE = 80 ms) brain images. Slices are interleaved, relatively thin (1–5 mm) and cover the entire extent of the brain in all imaging planes. Structures of interest are outlined using computer-assisted edge detection and trace methodology (Figure 7.1). The area (cm^2) within the outline is calculated automatically and volume (ml) can be determined by multiplying the area by the slice thickness and summing over the multiple slices in which the structure appears[29,38].

The intermediate and T2-weighted MRI images are obtained because they are more sensitive to some forms of pathologic tissue than the T1-weighted scans and because they permit an assessment of subcortical hyperintensities. Both the intermediate and T2-weighted scans are acquired in the axial plane of orientation. The hard copies of these scans are coded and randomized, intermixed with scans from other patient populations, and then formally rated for subcortical hyperintensities[26] by

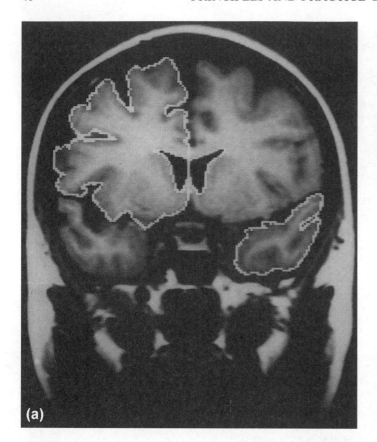

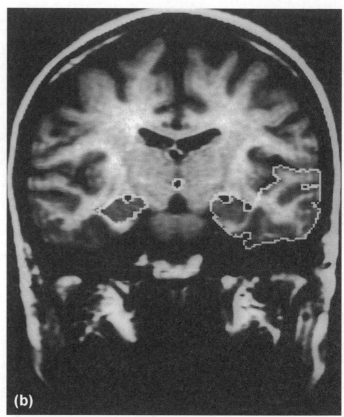

Figure 7.1 Typical coronal MRI images (TR = 500 ms, TE = 25 ms) illustrating anatomic landmarks and computer-assisted measurement of regional brain areas (A) Coronal section at level of optic chiasm, illustrating measurement of the right frontal lobe, the lateral ventricles and the left temporal lobe. (B) Coronal section at the level of the interpeduncular cistern, illustrating measurement of the left temporal lobe, the third ventricle and the right amygdala–hippocampal complex

an experienced research team that is blind to the subject's age and group status (i.e. normal control vs. patient).

These studies are ongoing, and several important findings have emerged[41,99–104]. First, our quantitative imaging and measurement techniques provide highly accurate and reliable assessments of brain size. For example, intraclass correlation coefficients for interrater reliability range from 0.88 to 0.99, depending upon the particular brain region under study. The intraclass correlation coefficients for intrarater reliability range from 0.93 to 0.99. Second, regional brain volume clearly changes with age, with a predilection for the frontal lobes. We have observed a rate of decline of about 0.23%/year for cerebral hemisphere volume. Yet the rate of decrease we have observed for the frontal lobes is twice as great (0.55%/year). Our data also indicate that age related changes in regional cerebral volume is greater for ventricular regions than for parenchymal regions (3%/year vs. 0.23–0.55%/year). Thus, ventricular enlargement may prove to be a more sensitive index of brain aging than cortical atrophy. Third, formal assessments of cortical atrophy and ventricular enlargement suggest that the statistically significant age-related changes in brain volume may not be clinically significant. That is to say, anything more than mild cortical atrophy or mild ventricular enlargement appears to be distinctly uncommon in a medically healthy sample of elderly community volunteers. Fourth, the incidence of subcortical hyperintensity increases with age, but again it is uncommon for such changes to be severe[39,96]. Fifth, the relationship between aging and changes in brain size is not a

simple one, in that it may be affected by a number of covariates (e.g. sex, height, years of education) that can modify the main effects of aging[38]. For instance, we recently found that age-related changes in brain size were significantly greater in men than women for peripheral (sulcal) CSF volume, the lateral (Sylvian) fissure CSF volume, and the parieto-occipital region area[103]. In addition we have observed significant effects of years of formal education on peripheral CSF volume, a marker of cortical atrophy[104]. In a sample of healthy elderly volunteers living independently in the community and Mini Mental State Examination (MMSE) scores of at least 24, each year of education was associated with an increase in peripheral CSF volume of 1.77 ml. These findings are consistent with the 'reserve hypothesis', which posits that education (or factors for which it is a surrogate) provides a protective buffer against the injurious effects of age-related brain changes.

SUMMARY

Advanced brain imaging techniques produce highly accurate anatomic information and provide exciting opportunities to examine *in vivo* the effects of aging on the human brain. Our review of the existing literature indicates that normal aging is associated with cortical and subcortical atrophy, enlargement of the lateral and third ventricles, and an increase in subcortical hyperintensities. The extent of these anatomic changes can now be quantitated with computer-assisted techniques and predictions can be made regarding the amount of change in tissue structure with advancing age. An important goal of future research will be to relate these anatomic changes to functional, neuropsychological and brain metabolic changes that accompany normal aging and age-related diseases of the brain.

ACKNOWLEDGEMENTS

This work was supported in part by grants from the Allegheny Singer Research Institute, the Mental Illness Research Association (Detroit, MI) and the National Institutes of Health, USA.

REFERENCES

1. Powers R. Neurobiology of aging. In *Textbook of Geriatric Neuropsychiatry*. Washington, DC: American Psychiatric Press, 2000.
2. Haug H. Are neurons of the human cerebral cortex really lost during aging? A morphometric examination. In Traber J, Gispen WH, eds. *Senile Dementia of the Alzheimer Type*. Berlin, Heidelburg: Springer-Verlag, 1985; 150–63.
3. Drayer BP. Imaging of the aging brain. Part 1. Normal findings. *Radiology* 1988; **166**: 785–96.
4. Caviness VS Jr, Filipek PA, Kennedy DN. Magnetic resonance technology in human brain science: blueprint for a program based upon morphometry. *Brain Dev* 1989, **11**: 1–13.
5. Schwartz M, Creasey H, Grady CL et al. Computed tomographic analysis of brain morphometrics in 30 healthy men, aged 21 to 81 years. *Ann Neurol* 1985; **17**: 146–57.
6. Rowe JW, Kahn RL. Human aging: usual and successful. *Science* 1987; **237**: 143–9.
7. Barron SA, Jacobs L, Kinkel WR. Changes in size of normal lateral ventricles during aging determined by computerized tomography. *Neurology* 1976; **26**: 1011–13.
8. De Carli C, Kaye JA, Horwitz B, Rapoport S. Critical analysis of the use of computer-assisted transverse axial tomography to study human brain in aging and dementia of the Alzheimer type. *Neurology* 1990; **40**: 872–83.
9. Brant-Zawadzki M. MR imaging of the brain. *Radiology* 1988; **166**: 1–10.
10. Andreasen NC. Nuclear magnetic resonance imaging. In Andreason NC, ed. *Brain Imaging: Applications in Psychiatry*. Washington, DC: American Psychiatric Press, 1989; 67–121.
11. Laffey PA, Peyster RG, Nathan R et al. Computed tomography and aging: results in a normal elderly population. *Neuroradiology* 1984; **26**: 273–8.
12. Zatz LM, Jernigan TL, Ahumada AJ. Changes on computed cranial tomography with aging: intra-cranial fluid volume. *Am J Neuroradiol* 1982; **3**: 1–11.
13. Pfefferbaum A, Zatz LM, Jernigan TL. Computer-interactive method for quantifying cerebrospinal fluid and tissue in brain CT scan: effects of aging. *J Comp Assist Tomogr* 1986; **10**(4): 571–8.
14. Gado M, Hughes CP, Danziger W, Chi D. Aging, dementia, and brain atrophy: a longitudinal computed tomographic study. *Am J Neuroradiol* 1983; **4**: 699–702.
15. Penn RD, Belanger MG, Yasnoff WA. Ventricular volume in man computed from CAT scans. *Ann Neurol* 1987; **3**: 216–23.
16. Zatz LM, Jernigan TL. The ventricular–brain ratio on computed tomography scans: validity and proper use. *Psychiat Res* 1983; **8**: 207–14.
17. Woods BT, Matthysse S. A simple method for conversion of area ratio measurements of cerebral structures to volume estimates. *Biol Psychiat* 1989; **26**: 748–52.
18. Haug G. Age and sex dependence of the size of normal ventricles on computed tomography. *Neuroradiology* 1977; **14**: 201–4.
19. Jacoby RJ, Levy R, Dawson JM. Computed tomography in the elderly: 1. The normal population. *Br J Psychiatry* 1980; **136**: 249–55.
20. Cala LA, Thickbroom GW, Black JL et al. Brain density and cerebrospinal fluid space size: CT of normal volunteers. *Am J Neuroradiol* 1981; **2**: 41–7.
21. Gomori JM, Steiner I, Melamed E, Cooper G. The assessment of changes in brain volume using combined linear measurements: a CT scan study. *Neuroradiology* 1984; **26**: 21–4.
22. Stafford JL, Albert MS, Naeser MA et al. Age-related differences in computed tomographic scan measurements. *Arch Neurol* 1988; **45**: 409–15.
23. Golomb J, de Leon MI, Kluger A et al. Hippocampal atrophy in normal aging: an association with recent memory impairment. *Arch Neurol* 1993; **50**: 967–73.
24. Meyer JS, Takashima S, Terayama Y et al. CT changes associated with normal aging of thc human brain. *J Neurol Sci* 1994; **123**: 200–208.
25. Elwan OH, Baradah OH, Madkour O et al. Parkinson's disease, cognition and aging: clinical, neuropsychological, electrophysiological and cranial computerized tomographic assessment. *J Neurol Sci* 1996; **143**: 64–71.
26. Yoshii F, Barber W, Apicella A et al. Measurements of the corpus callosum (CC) on magnetic resonance (MR) scans: effects of age, sex, handedness, and disease. *Neurology* 1986; **36**(suppl 1): 133.
27. Simon JH, Schiffer RB, Rudick RA, Herndon RM. Quantitative determination of MS-induced corpus callosum atrophy *in vivo* using MR imaging. *Am J Neuroradiol* 1987; **8**: 599–604.
28. Uematsu M, Kaiya H. The morphology of the corpus callosum in schizophrenia: An MRI study. *Schizophren Res* 1988; **1**: 391–8.
29. Condon B, Grant R, Hadley D, Lawrence A. Brain and intracranial cavity volumes: *in vivo* determination by MRI. *Acta Neurol Scand* 1988; **78**: 387–93.
30. Yoshii F, Barker WW, Chang JY et al. Sensitivity of cerebral glucose metabolism to age, gender, brain volume, brain atrophy and cerebrovascular risk factors. *J Cerebr Blood Flow Metab* 1988; **8**: 654–66.
31. Hayakawa K, Konishi Y, Matsuda T et al. Development and aging of brain midline structures: assessment with MR imaging. *Radiology* 1989; **172**: 171–7.
32. Hauser P, Dauphinais ID, Berrettini W et al. Corpus callosum dimensions measured by magnetic resonance imaging in bipolar affective disorder and schizophrenia. *Biol Psychiat* 1989; **26**: 659–68.
33. Jernigan TL, Press GA, Hesselink JR. Methods for measuring brain morphologic features; validation and normal aging. *Arch Neurol* 1990; **47**: 27–32.
34. Krishnan KR, Husain MM, McDonald WM et al. *In vivo* stereological assessment of caudate volume in man: effect of normal aging. *Life Sciences* 1990; **47**: 1325–9.
35. Doraiswamy PM, Figiel GS, Husain MM et al. Aging of the human corpus callosum: magnetic resonance imaging in normal volunteers. *J Neuropsychiat Clin Neurosci* 1991; **3**: 392–7.
36. Escalona PR, McDonald WM, Doraiswamy PM et al. *In vivo* stereological assessment of human cerebellar volume: effects of gender and age. *Am J Neuroradiol* 1991; **12**: 927–9.
37. Gur RC, Mozley PD, Resnick AM et al. Gender differences in age effect on brain atrophy measured by magnetic resonance imaging. *Proc Natl Acad Sci USA* 1991; **88**: 2845–9.
38. McDonald WM, Husain M, Doraiswamy PM et al. A magnetic resonance image study of age-related changes in human putamen nuclei. *NeuroReport* 1991; **2**: 41–4.
39. Shah SA, Doraiswamy PM, Husain MM et al. Assessment of posterior fossa structures with midsagittal MRI: the effects of age. *Neurobiol Aging* 1991; **12**: 371–4.
40. Tanna NK, Kohn MI, Harwich DN et al. Analysis of brain and cerebrospinal fluid volumes with MR imaging: impact on PET data correction for atrophy. *Radiology* 1991; **178**: 123–30.
41. Coffey CE, Wilkinson WE, Weiner RD, et al. Quantitative cerebral anatomy in depression: a controlled magnetic resonance imaging study. *Arch Gen Psychiat* 1992; **50**: 7–16.
42. Doraiswamy PM, Na C, Husain MM et al. Morphometric changes of the human midbrain with normal aging: MR and stereologic findings. *Am J Neuroradiol* 1992; **13**: 383–6.
43. Jack CR, Petersen RC, O'Brien PC et al. MR-based hippocampal volumetry in the diagnosis of Alzheimer's disease. *Neurology* 1992; **42**: 183–8.
44. Lim KO, Zipursky RB, Watts MC et al. Decreased gray matter in normal aging: an *in vivo* magnetic resonance study. *J Gerontol* 1992; **47**: B26–B30.
45. Murphy DGM, DeCarli C, Schapiro MB et al. Age-related differences in volumes of subcortical nuclei, brain matter, and cerebrospinal fluid in healthy men as measured with magnetic resonance imaging. *Arch Neurol* 1992; **49**: 839–45.

46. Doraiswamy PM, McDonald WM, Patterson L et al. Interuncal distance as a measure of hippocampal atrophy: normative data on axial MR imaging. Am J Neuroradiol 1993; 14: 141–3.

47. Raz N, Torres IJ, Spencer WD et al. Pathoclysis in aging human cerebral cortex: evidence from in vivo MRI morphometry. . Psychobiology 1993; 21: 151–60.

48. Raz N, Torres IJ, Spencer WD et al. Neuroanatomical correlates of age-sensitive and age-invariant cognitive abilities: an in vivo MRI investigation. Intelligence 1993; 17: 407–22.

49. Raz N, Torres IJ, Acker JD. Age, gender, and hemispheric differences in human striatum: a quantitative review and new data from in vivo MRI morphometry. Neurobiol Learning Memory 1993; 63: 133–42.

50. Christiansen P, Larsson HBW, Thomsen C et al. Age-dependent white matter lesions and brain volume changes in healthy volunteers. Acta Radiol 1994; 35: 117–22.

51. Cowell PE, Turetsky BI, Gur RC et al. Sex differences in aging of the human frontal and temporal lobes. J Neurosci 1994; 14: 4748–55.

52. DeCarli C, Murphy DGM, Gillette JA et al. Lack of age-related differences in temporal lobe volume of very healthy adults. Am J Neuroradiol 1994; 15: 689–96.

53. Pfefferbaum A, Mathalon DH, Sullivan EV et al. A quantitative magnetic resonance imaging study of changes in brain morphology from infancy to late adulthood. Arch Neurol 1994; 51: 874–87.

54. Soininen HS, Partanen K, Pitkanen A et al. Volumetric MRI analysis of the amygdala and the hippocampus in subjects with age-associated memory impairment. Neurology 1994; 44: 1660–8.

55. Blatter DD, Bigler ED, Gale SD et al. Quantitative volumetric analysis of brain MR: normative database spanning five decades of life. Am J Neuroradiol 1995; 16: 241–51.

56. Convit A, de Leon MJ, Hoptman MJ et al. Age-related changes in brain. I. Magnetic resonance imaging measures of temporal lobe volumes in normal subjects. Psychiat Qu 1995; 66: 343–55.

57. Hokama H, Shenton ME, Nestor PG et al. Caudate, putamen, and globus pallidus volume in schizophrenia: a quantitative MRI study. Psychiat Res Neuroimag 1995; 61: 209–29.

58. Parashos IA, Wilkinson WE, Coffey CE. Magnetic resonance imaging of the corpus callosum: predictors of size in normal adults. J Neuropsychiat Clin Neurosci 1995; 7: 35–41.

59. Fox NC, Freeborough PA, Rossor MN. Visualisation and quantification of rates of atrophy in Alzheimer's disease. Lancet 1996; 348: 94–7.

60. Janowsky JS, Kaye JA, Carper RA. Atrophy of the corpus callosum in Alzheimer's disease versus healthy aging. J Am Geriat Soc 1996; 44: 798–803.

61. Murphy DGM, DeCarli C, McIntosh AR, et al. Sex differences in human brain morphometry and metabolism: an in vivo quantitative magnetic resonance imaging and positron emission tomography study on the effect of aging. Arch Gen Psychiat 1996; 53: 585–94.

62. Deshmukh AR, Desmond JE, Sullivan EV et al. Quantification of cerebellar structures with MRI. Psychiat Res 1997; 75: 159–71.

63. Jack CR, Petersen RC, Xu YC et al. Medial temporal atrophy on MRI in normal aging and very mild Alzheimer's disease. Neurology 1997; 49: 786–94.

64. Kaye JA, Swihart T, Howieson D et al. Volume loss of the hippocampus and temporal lobes in healthy elderly persons destined to develop dementia. Neurology 1997; 48: 1297–304.

65. O'Brien JT, Desmond P, Ames D et al. Magnetic resonance imaging correlates of memory impairment in the healthy elderly: association with medial temporal lobe atrophy but not white matter lesions. Int J Ger Psychiat 1997; 12: 369–74.

66. Raz N, Gunning FM, Head D et al. Selective aging of the human cerebral cortex observed in vivo: differential vulnerability of the prefrontal gray matter. Cerebr Cortex 1997; 7: 268–82.

67. Salat D, Ward A, Kaye JA et al. Sex differences in the corpus callosum with aging. Neurobiol Aging 1997; 18: 191–7.

68. Coffey CE, Lucke JF, Saxton JA et al. Sex differences in brain aging: a quantitative magnetic resonance imaging study. Arch Neurol 1998; 55: 169–79.

69. Davatzikos C, Resnick SM. Sex differences in anatomic measures of interhemispheric connectivity: correlations with cognition in women but not men. Cerebr Cortex 1998; 8: 635–40.

70. Gunning-Dixon FM, Head D, McQuain J et al. Differential aging of the human striatum: a prospective MR imaging study. Am J Neuroradiol 1998; 19: 1501–7.

71. Gur RE, Cowell P, Turetsky BI et al. A follow-up magnetic resonance imaging study of schizophrenia. Arch Gen Psychiat 1998; 55: 145–52.

72. Guttmann CRG, Jolesz FA, Kikinis R et al. White matter changes with normal aging. Neurology 1998; 50: 972–8.

73. Jack CR, Petersen RC, Xu Y et al. Rate of medial temporal lobe atrophy in typical aging and Alzheimer's disease. Neurology 1998; 51: 993–9.

74. Laakso MP, Soininen H, Partanen K et al. MRI of the hippocampus in Alzheimer's disease: sensitivity, specificity, and analysis of the incorrectly classified subjects. Neurobiol Aging 1998; 19: 23–31.

75. Mueller EA, Moore, MM, Kerr DCR et al. Brain volume preserved in healthy elderly through the eleventh decade. Neurology 1998; 51: 1555–62.

76. Oguro H, Okada K, Yamaguchi S et al. Sex differences in morphology of the brain stem and cerebellum with normal aging. Neuroradiology 1998; 40: 788–92.

77. Pfefferbaum A, Sullivan EV, Rosenbloom MJ et al. A controlled study of cortical gray matter and ventricular changes in alcoholic men over a 5-year interval. Arch Gen Psychiat 1998; 55: 905–12.

78. Raz N, Dupuis JH, Briggs SD et al. Differential effects of age and sex on the cerebellar hemispheres and the vermis: a prospective MR study. Am J Neuroradiol 1998; 19: 65–71.

79. Earnest MP, Heaton RK, Wilkinson WE et al. Cortical atrophy, ventricular enlargement and intellectual impairment in the aged. Neurology 1979; 29: 1138–43.

80. Meese W, Kluge W, Grumme T et al. CT evaluation of the CSF spaces of healthy persons. Neuroradiology 1980; 19: 131–6.

81. Soininen H, Puranen M, Riekkinen PJ. Computed tomography findings in senile dementia and normal aging. J Neurol Neurosurg Psychiat 1982; 45: 50–4.

82. Takeda S, Matsuzawa T. Brain atrophy during aging: a quantitative study using computed tomography. J Am Geriatr Soc 1984; 32: 520–4.

83. Nagata K, Basugi N, Fukushima T et al. A quantitative study of physiological cerebral atrophy with aging: a statistical analysis of the normal range. Neuroradiology 1987; 29: 327–32.

84. Pearlson GD, Rabins PV, Kim WS et al. Structural brain CT changes and cognitive defects in elderly depressives with and without reversible dementia (pseudodementia). Psychol Med 1989; 19: 573–84.

85. Kaye JA, DeCarli C, Luxenberg JS et al. The significance of age-related enlargement of the cerebral ventricles in healthy men and women measured by quantitative computed X-ray tomography. J Am Geriat Soc 1992; 40: 225–31.

86. Sullivan EV, Shear PK, Mathalon D et al. Greater abnormalities of brain cerebrospinal fluid volumes in younger than in older patients with Alzheimer's disease. Arch Neurol 1993; 50: 359–73.

87. Shear PK, Sullivan EV, Mathalon DH et al. Longitudinal volumetric computed tomographic analysis of regional brain changes in normal aging and Alzheimer's disease. Arch Neurol 1995; 52: 392–402.

88. Elwan O, Hassan AAH, Naseer MA et al. Brain aging in normal Egyptians: neuropsychological, electrophysiological and cranial tomographic assessment. J Neurol Sci 1996; 136: 73–80.

89. Grant R, Condon B, Lawrence A et al. Human cranial CSF volumes measured by MRI: sex and age influences. Magnet Reson Imag 1987; 5: 465–8.

90. Wahlund LO, Agartz I, Almqvist O et al. The brain in healthy aged individuals: MR imaging. Radiology 1990; 174: 675–9.

91. Matsubayashi K, Shimada K, Kawamoto A et al. Incidental brain lesions on magnetic resonance imaging and neurobehavioral functions in the apparently healthy elderly. Stroke 1992; 23: 175–80.

92. Salonen O, Autti T, Raininko R et al. MRI of the brain in neurologically healthy middle-aged and elderly individuals. Neuroradiology 1997; 39: 537–45.

93. Yue NC, Arnold AM, Longstreth WT et al. Sulcal, ventricular, and white matter changes at MR imaging in the aging brain: data from the cardiovascular health study. Radiology 1997; 202: 33–9.

94. George AE, de Leon MJ, Kalnin A et al. Leukoencephalopathy in normal and pathologic aging. 2. MRI of brain lucencies. Am J Neuroradiol 1986; 7: 567–70.

95. Fazekas F. Magnetic resonance signal abnormalities in asymptomatic individuals: their incidence and functional correlates. Eur Neurol 1989; 29: 164–8.

96. Hendrie HC, Farlow MR, Guerrino-Austrom M *et al.* Foci of increased T2 signal intensity on brain MR scans of healthy elderly subjects. *Am J Neuroradiol* 1989; **10**: 703–7.

97. Boone KB, Miller BL, Lesser IM *et al.* Neuropsychological correlates of white matter lesions in healthy subjects. *Arch Neurol* 1992; **49**: 549–54.

98. Almkvist O, Wahlund LO, Andersson-Lundman G, *et al.* White matter hyperintensity and neuropsychological functions in dementia and healthy aging. *Arch Neurol* 1992; **49**: 626–32.

99. Coffey CE, Figiel GS, Djang WT *et al.* Subcortical hyperintensity on magnetic resonance imaging: a comparison of normal and depressed elderly subjects. *Am J Psychiat* 1990; **147**: 187–9.

100. Coffey CE, Weiner RD, Djang WT *et al.* Brain anatomic effects of ECT: a prospective magnetic resonance imaging study. *Arch Gen Psychiat* 1991; **48**: 1013–21.

101. Coffey CE, Wilkinson WE, Parashos IA *et al.* Quantitative cerebral anatomy of the aging human brain: a cross-sectional study using magnetic resonance imaging. *Neurology* 1992; **42**: 527–36.

102. Coffey CE. Brain morphology in primary mood disorders: implications for ECT. *Psychiat Ann* 1996; **26**: 713–16.

103. Coffey CE, Lucke JF, Saxton JA *et al.* Sex differences in brain aging: a quantitative magnetic resonance imaging study. *Arch Neurol* 1988; **55**: 169–79.

104. Coffey CE, Saxton JA, Ratcliff G *et al.* Relation of education to brain size in normal aging: implications for the reserve hypothesis. *Neurology* 1999; **53**: 189–96.

105. Coffey CE. Anatomic imaging of the aging human brain. In *Textbook of Geriatric Neuropsychiatry*. Washington, DC: American Psychiatric Press, 2000.

8

Quantitative Structural Changes in the Ageing Brain

Bente Pakkenberg, Lisbeth Regeur, Hans Jørgen G. Gundersen*

Neurological Research Laboratory, Kommunehospitalet, Copenhagen, and
*Stereological Research Laboratory, Århus University, Århus, Denmark

Estimates of the total number of human neocortical cells in both hemispheres range from 10 to 100 billions (10^9), but only two major studies describe how to estimate total neuron number. Reduction in the number of cells per unit volume of human cerebral cortex with age has been found in seven distinct neocortical brain regions from newborn to 95 year-old individuals[2]. Haug[3] estimated neuron density in 10–20 rows arranged perpendicular to the pial surface of the cortex in two to four areas per brain, multiplied by the assumed neocortical volume, and found an average of 15×10^9 neurons in the human neocortex. Haug found no decrease in total neuronal number with age and no difference in total numbers between males and females.

The three steps in estimating the total neuronal number in any defined brain region include: (a) delineation and estimation of the region's volume; (b) uniform sampling of the complex and irregularly shaped neocortex; and (c) estimation of the neuronal numerical density.

Based on unbiased principles, the Cavalieri method for the estimation of volume using systematic sampling and point-counting can be applied to any organ that can be cut into slices—physically or by means of optical or other scanning devices—and is independent of size or shape of the organ[4,5]. In a recent study by Regeur[6], neocortical volume, cortical thickness and volume of archicortex, the ventricular system, the central grey matter and white matter were estimated using stereological methods on brains from 28 old females (mean age 81.8 years) with increasing degrees of senile dementia, and brains from 13 (mean age 82.7 years) non-demented control females. Brains from the demented patients [14 Alzheimer's disease (AD) cases and 14 non-AD cases] had a smaller cortex volume and neocortical thickness was significantly reduced in the demented patients, with the highest degree of reduction in the most demented patients, as were the volumes of archicortex. No statistically significant differences were found in the volumes of cortex, white matter, central grey structures, ventricular volume or archicortex between the AD demented cases compared with the non-AD demented cases. The ventricular volume increased with increasing degree of dementia, but the difference between the demented group and the control group did not reach statistical significance. Surface area did not change in the demented patients, and no significant reductions were found in the volumes of white matter or central grey matter structures in the demented patients compared with controls.

In 1984 the dissector method was described, in which three-dimensional particles (e.g. neurons) are sampled with a constant probability without regard to size, shape and orientation of the particles, provided that two requirements are fulfilled: (a) the complete set of particle profiles hit by the dissector's planar transects should be identifiable; (2) the dissector positions are uniformly random in the complete reference region[7]. The method relies on the fact that one can, without any other assumptions at all, count a cell nucleus or any defined particle within a defined reference volume if it is present in a relatively thin section but not in the previous member of a pair of adjacent sections. Particles of arbitrary size and shape can only be sampled with equal probability using a three-dimensional probe, such as the dissector. Systematically sampling a subset of dissectors from the wide range possible in a serially sectioned brain region or central nucleus, taking each with a constant but arbitrary probability, is sufficient for the estimation of the total particle number or, as in this instance, nerve cells (for practical details and analyses of sampling design, *see* refs 5, 8–11). Williams and Rakic[12,13] have applied the same technique using the three-dimensional counting frame[14,15] to obtain estimates of neuronal numerical densities.

A method for uniform sampling in human neocortex combined with a modification of the dissector principle, the optical dissector, has been introduced[16]. With the optical dissector the procedure is performed in thick rather than thin sections, which makes it many times more efficient. Using this method, 94 normal brains were studied, 32 females and 62 males in age-groups 20–90 years[17]. An unbiased estimate of the total number of neurons in the neocortex was obtained simply by multiplying the Cavalieri estimate of the neocortical reference volume by the numerical density obtained with the optical dissector. The number of neocortical neurons in females was 19.3 billion, and in males 22.8 billion, a difference of 16%. The difference in the total number of neocortical nerve cells over the observed range of 70 years was 9.5%, providing an average "loss" of neurons of about 85 000/day. This possible age effect was the same for both sexes. The total number of neocortical neurons in the material varied more than a factor of 2 with a range of 118% (14.7–32.0 billion neurons) (see Figure 8.1). The natural variability in neuron number of 19% ($CV = SD/mean = 0.19$) in normal Danes thus represents a variance of more than eight times the variance of body height [CV (height) = 0.065]: $(0.19/0.065)^2 \approx 8$.

On average, there were 186 million more neurons in the left hemisphere than in the right and this difference was the same in the two sexes. Sex differences were found in the total volume, total surface and thickness of the neocortex, white matter volume, central grey structure and brain weight. With advanced age,

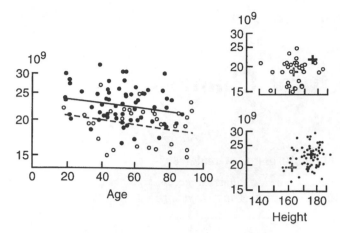

Figure 8.1 The number of neocortical neurons in normal Danes as a function of sex (●, males, ○, females) and age (left). The two orthogonal regression lines are indicated. To the right is illustrated the (absence of a) relation between the total number of neurons and the body height (cm) for each sex separately. The bivariate means for both sexes are shown in each diagram. All axes except the age axis are logarithmic

permanent structural brain changes. More information will help us to be able to separate the changes in normal ageing from those of neurodegenerative disorders and thereby understand the age conditioned functional deficits.

reductions occurred in neocortical volume, surface area, white matter, archicortex volume and brain weight, concomitant with a large increase in the ventricular system, while no change was found in grey matter volume and neocortical thickness. After sex and age were accounted for, neocortical neuron number was a dominating factor in determining the size of other brain structures. Neuronal density was not a function of sex or age.

A major problem in the interpretation of these data is evidently that one must take secular changes into account. Body height in Danish males has increased by approximately 9–10 cm from 1920 to 1980. Precisely *how* to correct for such changes is not known.

In conclusion, age may account for changes in both neocortical neuron number and neocortical volume without any effect on neuronal density. The reduction in cortical volume is seen without concomitant reduction in neocortical thickness, but only with consequence for surface area, a condition rather different from, for example, AD and AIDS, where the equally large atrophy only affects the neocortical thickness[17]. The largest changes in brain volumes are found in the brain white matters, with a reduction of ≈30%. In a recent paper by Tang et al.[18], the total length of the myelinated fibres in five elderly women of 86 000 km was statistically significantly decreased by 27%, compared with 118 000 km in five younger females. As expected, the ventricular volumes increased by 50%, which could at least in part be a white matter volume reduction.

More research is needed to give us knowledge of possible changes during development, ageing and disease. Serious development defects and diseases, such as mental retardation, AD, schizophrenia and AIDS, have all been shown to involve

REFERENCES

1. Blinkov SM, Glezer II. *The Human Brain in Figures and Tables: A Quantitative Handbook*. New York: Plenum, 1968, 201–13.
2. Brody H. Organization of the cerebral cortex. *J Comp Neurol* 1955; **102**: 511–56.
3. Haug H. Brain sizes, surfaces, and neuronal sizes of the cortex cerebri: a stereological investigation of man and his variability and a comparison with some mammals (primates, whales, marsupials, insectivores, and one elephant). *Am J Anat* 1987; **180**: 126–42.
4. Pakkenberg B, Boesen J, Albeck M, Gjerris F. Unbiased and efficient estimation of total ventricular volume of the brain obtained from CT-scans by a stereological method. *Neuroradiology* 1989; **31**: 413–17.
5. Gundersen HJG, Jensen EB. The efficiency of systematic sampling in stereology and its prediction. *J Microsc* 1987; **147**: 229–63.
6. Regeur L. Increasing loss of brain tissue with increasing dementia—a stereological study of postmortem brains from old females (in press).
7. Sterio DC. The unbiased estimation of number and sizes of arbitrary particles using the dissector. *J Microsc* 1984; **134**: 127–36.
8. Gundersen HJG, Bendtsen TF, Korbo L et al. Some new, simple and efficient stereological methods and their use in pathological research and diagnosis. *Acta Path Microbiol Immunol Scand* 1988; **96**: 379–94.
9. Gundersen HJG, Bagger P, Bendtsen TF et al. The new stereological tools: dissector, fractionator, nucleator, and point-sampled intercepts and their use in pathological research and diagnosis. *Acta Path Microbiol Immunol Scand* 1988; **96**: 857–81.
10. Pakkenberg B, Gundersen HJG. Total number of neurons and glial cells in human brain nuclei estimated by the dissector and the fractionator. *J Microsc* 1988; **150**: 1–20.
11. West MJ, Gundersen HJG. Unbiased stereological estimation of the number of neurons in the human hippocampus. *J Comp Neurol* 1990; **296**: 1–22.
12. Williams RW, Rakic P. Three-dimensional counting: an accurate and direct method to estimate numbers of cells in sectioned material. *J Comp Neurol* 1988; **278**: 344–52.
13. Williams RW, Rakic P. Erratum and Addendum. Three-dimensional counting: an accurate and direct method to estimate numbers of cells in sectioned material. *J Comp Neurol* 1989; **281**: 335.
14. Gundersen HJG. *Stereologi—Eller Hvordan Tal for Rumlig Form og Indhold Opnås ved Iagttagelse af Strukturer på Snitplaner*. Copenhagen: Lægeforeningens Forlag, 1981, 1–25 (in Danish).
15. Howard V, Reid S, Baddeley A, Boyde A. Unbiased estimation of particle density in the tandem scanning reflected light microscope. *J Microsc* 1985; **138**: 203–12.
16. Gundersen HJG. Stereology of arbitrary particles. A review of unbiased number and size estimators and the presentation of some new ones, in memory of William R. Thompson. *J Microsc* 1986; **143**: 3–45.
17. Pakkenberg B, Gundersen HJG. Neocortical neuron number in humans: effect of sex and age. *J Comp Neurol* 1997; **384**: 312–20.
18. Tang Y, Nyengaard JR, Pakkenberg B, Gundersen HJG. Age-induced white matter changes in the human brain: a stereological investigation. *Neurobiol Aging* 1997; **18**: 609–15.

Potential Regeneration of the Ageing Brain

Stephen B. Dunnett

School of Biosciences, Cardiff University, Wales, UK

The brain does not spontaneously regenerate. As long ago as 1928, Cajal recorded that "once development was ended, the founts of growth and regeneration of axons and dendrites dried up irrevocably. In adult centres . . . everything may die, nothing may be regenerated"[1]. Although it remains the case that the damaged mammalian central nervous system (CNS) does not generally generate new nerve cells in response to disease or injury, the intervening 70 years have identified a considerable plasticity of axons to remodel nerve connections and a limited degree of neurogenesis, which opens new opportunities for promoting regeneration and repair in the damaged, diseased or ageing nervous system (see Figure 1).

COLLATERAL SPROUTING

The first clear evidence that Cajal's dictum was overly pessimistic in relation to the mammalian CNS came from the demonstration that if a septal cell loses some of its normal axonal inputs, then other afferent axons can sprout into the vacated spaces to form

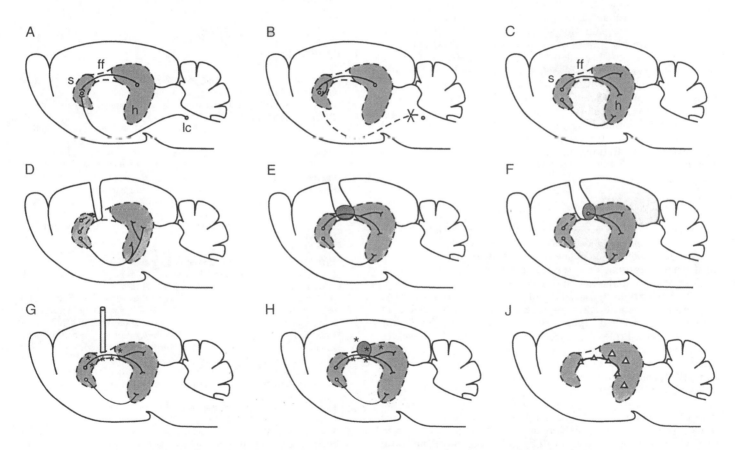

Figure 1. Schematic illustration of examples of regeneration and repair in the septo–hippocampal system of rats. (A) Normal synaptic inputs onto septal cells arising in the hippocampus and brainstem locus coeruleus. (B) Collateral sprouting of afferents from hippocampus following removal of afferents from the brainstem by a lesion of the medial forebrain bundle. (C) Normal septal projections into the hippocampus via dorsal and ventral pathways. (D) Compensatory collateral sprouting of ventral afferents following lesion of afferents to the dorsal hippocampus by transection of the fimbria-fornix bundle. (E) Implantation of hippocampal or glial grafts provides a substrate for regenerative growth of host septal axons back to the hippocampus. (F) Implantation of septal grafts provides a cholinergic reinnervation of the deafferented hippocampus. (G) Chronic injection of NGF molecules (triangles) diffusing via the lateral ventricles provides trophic support of cholinergic septo–hippocampal neurones in aged animals. (H) Implantation of cells engineered to secrete NGF provides similar neuroprotection in aged animals. (J) Neuronal stem cells in subventricular zone have the capacity to divide and differentiate in the adult brain. Whether they can also migrate to repopulate areas of cell loss in the aged brain remains speculative. ff, fimbria-fornix; h, hippocampus; Ic, locus coeruleus; s, septum; small circles, neurones; small triangles, neuronal stem cells; asterisks, growth factor molecules

new synaptic connections with the target cell (Figure 1A,B)[2]. If the new inputs are from a different source, they are by and large not functional. However, collateral sprouting of spared fibres of the same systems can sustain functional recovery in a number of model circuits of the brain (Figure 1C,D)[3,4].

REGENERATIVE SPROUTING

A major problem for extensive axonal reorganization in the adult brain is that although axons can undergo a degree of local sprouting, they do not typically retain the developmental capacity for long-distance growth through the CNS to distant targets[5]. Long-distance growth of axons can nevertheless be promoted by providing an alternative substrate for growth, such as Schwann cells from the PNS, which can be used to bridge a gap caused by a lesion cutting a pathway or be implanted as a track along which new axons can grow (Figure 1E)[6].

NEURAL TRANSPLANTATION

When essential populations of neurons are lost, they may be replaced by transplantation. The techniques are now well established for transplantation of embryonic cells derived from the CNS into the aged brain of experimental animals (Figure 1F) and such grafts have been demonstrated to survive, repopulate areas of denervation, replace deficient innervations and restore lost functions in a wide variety of model systems[7]. There is now compelling clinical evidence that such grafts can provide a substantial alleviation of symptoms in Parkinson's disease[8], and clinical trials are now underway in Huntington's disease, spinal cord injury and stroke[9-11]. It remains a matter of speculation whether neuronal transplantation can alleviate the more diffuse and widespread degeneration associated with ageing and the dementias.

TROPHIC SUPPORT

Neuronal connections are dependent upon trophic support from their targets, and neurodegenerative diseases of ageing may in part be attributable to a decline in growth factor support[12]. Thus, an alternative approach to prevention of progressive neurodegeneration, and to induction and guidance of regenerative axon growth, is to apply or replace identified trophic factors explicitly. For example, central cholinergic neurones, which decline in ageing, are dependent upon nerve growth factor (NGF) for trophic support. Prolonged injections of NGF into the ventricles of ageing rats can inhibit the progressive atrophy of septal cholinergic neurones and block the functional decline in the animals' learning abilities (Figure 1G)[13]. A similar strategy involving chronic central infusions of NGF has been attempted in a pilot experiment in Alzheimer's disease with only modest success[14]. A major issue to be resolved is how to deliver large trophic factor molecules—which do not cross the blood–brain barrier—to defined targets in the brain; the most powerful experimental techniques to date involve implantation of cells that are engineered to secrete the particular trophic factor molecule (Figure 1H)[15].

ADULT NEUROGENESIS

It was believed until very recently that all neurones of the mature nervous system are born in early development, so that once lost they are not replaced. It is now clear that there exists in the adult human brain a small population of resting "neuronal stem cells" with the capacity to both undergo further cell division and differentiate into both neurones and glia (Figure 1J)[16]. This opens the hope that such cells may be recruited for repair, either by isolation, expansion and differentiation into defined neuronal cell types *in vitro* and reimplantation, or by finding the means to induce their spontaneous division, migration to areas of cell loss and local differentiation into appropriate neuronal phenotype to replace lost target cells *in vivo*. However, it must be recognized that substantial technical and theoretical problems remain in translating such procedures into applications for repair in human ageing.

Although the repair of neurodegenerative damage associated with ageing remains experimental, rapid advances are being made in the techniques for inhibiting degeneration, promoting regenerative growth and replacing lost populations of cells. The pessimism that has for long surrounded the poor prognosis of brain damage in ageing and disease is being transformed to an optimism that these novel experimental approaches may find direct clinical application in the neurodegenerative diseases of ageing. Nevertheless, formidable technical problems still need to be overcome to transform theoretical prospects into practical therapies.

REFERENCES

1. Cajal SR. *Degeneration and Regeneration of the Nervous System.* Oxford: Oxford University Press, 1928.
2. Raisman G. Neuronal plasticity in the septal nuclei of the adult rat. *Brain Res* 1969; **14**: 25–48.
3. Bohn MC, Cupit L, Marciano F, Gash DM. Adrenal grafts enhance recovery of striatal dopaminergic fibers. *Science* 1987; **237**: 913–16.
4. Gage FH, Björklund A, Stenevi U, Dunnett SB. Functional correlates of compensatory collateral sprouting by aminergic and cholinergic afferents in the hippocampal formation. *Brain Res* 1983; **268**: 39–47.
5. Fawcett JW. Factors responsible for the failure of structural repair in the central nervous system. In Hunter AJ, Clark M, eds *Neurodegeneration.* New York: Academic Press, 1992, 81–96.
6. Brecknell JE, Fawcett JW. Axonal regeneration. *Biol Rev* 1996; **71**: 227–55.
7. Barker RA, Dunnett SB. *Neural Repair, Transplantation and Rehabilitation.* Hove, UK: Psychology Press, 1999.
8. Lindvall O. Neural transplantation: a hope for patients with Parkinson's disease? *NeuroReport* 1997; **8**: iii–x.
9. Bachoud-Lévy AC, Bourdet C, Brugières P *et al.* Safety and tolerability assessment of intrastriatal neural allografts in Huntington's disease patients. *Exp Neurol* 2000; **161**: 194–202.
10. Falci S, Holtz A, Åkesson E *et al.* Obliteration of a posttraumatic spinal cord cyst with solid human embryonic spinal cord grafts: first clinical attempt. *J Neurotrauma* 1998; **14**: 875–84.
11. Kondziolka D, Wechsler L, Goldstein S *et al.* Transplantation of cultured human neuronal cells for patients with stroke. *Neurology* 2000; **55**: 656–9.
12. Hefti F. Is Alzheimer's disease caused by a lack of nerve growth factor? *Ann Neurol* 1983; **13**: 109–10.
13. Fischer W, Wictorin K, Björklund A *et al.* Amelioration of cholinergic neuron atrophy and spatial memory impairment in aged rats by nerve growth factor. *Nature* 1987; **329**: 65–8.
14. Seiger Å, Nordberg A, Von Holst H *et al.* Intracranial infusion of purified nerve growth factor to an Alzheimer patient: the first attempt of a possible future treatment strategy. *Behav Brain Res* 1993; **57**: 255–61.
15. Martinez-Serrano A, Fischer W, Söderström S *et al.* Long-term functional recovery from age-induced spatial memory impairments by nerve growth factor gene transfer to the rat basal forebrain. *Proc Natl Acad Sci USA* 1996; **93**: 6355–60.
16. Eriksson PS, Perfilieva E, Björk-Eriksson T *et al.* Neurogenesis in the adult human hippocampus. *Nature Med* 1998; **4**: 1313–17.

Hippocampal Changes and Memory Impairment in Normal People

John T. O'Brien

Wolfson Research Centre, Newcastle upon Tyne General Hospital, UK

INTRODUCTION

The nature of age-related cognitive deficits and their relationship to what is "normal", such as Alzheimer's disease (AD), remains a controversial area. It has long been recognized that decline in many aspects of cognitive performance occurs in the majority of individuals as they age. Most interest has focused on memory and various labels have been used, including "benign senescent forgetfulness (BSF)", "age-associated memory impairment (AAMI)", "aging-associated cognitive decline (AACD)"[1] and, most recently, "mild cognitive impairment (MCI)"[2]. MCI describes the condition whereby a subjective memory complaint is accompanied by objective evidence of deficits, usually 1.5 standard deviations below age-corrected norms for a standardized test. Such individuals are known to "convert" to clear AD at a rate of about 15% per year[3], in contrast to previous categories, such as BSF, when progression over time does not occur[4]. However, potential entities such as BSF, AAMI, AACD and MCI are still the subject of criticism, since it is unknown whether they represent a true disorder or a spectrum of the normal population mixed with those with early, and as yet undiagnosed, AD[5,6].

ROLE OF THE HIPPOCAMPUS

The hippocampus has long been known to be central to the human ability to learn new information, particularly for so-called episodic memory, i.e. memory for discrete events, and declarative memory, which is memory requiring conscious retrieval[7]. This contrasts with the role of the hippocampus in animals, which is known to be primarily involved in the formation of spatial memories. Recent evidence suggests that in humans the hippocampus does seem important in the acquisition of new spatial memories, as well as episodic memory, but is not the actual site of such spatial maps once they have been formed[8]. Differential functional organization of the hippocampus in time and space has been demonstrated[7], giving support to the view that the main role of the hippocampus in memory formation is in forming new memories by capturing the event itself, coding it in time and space and binding it together for subsequent processing. Other brain areas (particularly the parahippocampal cortex and the frontal cortex) are also important in forming new memories, especially for encoding[9]. In contrast, other aspects of human memory (e.g. semantic memory) appears not to be dependent on the hippocampus[10] although areas such as the anterior temporal pole and frontal lobe may be important[11].

RELATIONSHIP BETWEEN MEMORY IMPAIRMENT AND HIPPOCAMPAL CHANGES

While this has been reasonably well established for AD, the same is not yet true for using the memory impairment associated with ageing and conditions such as AACD, AAMI and MCI. An age-related decline in temporal lobe and hippocampal volume is found in most, although not all, studies[12–14]. Reductions in medial temporal lobe and hippocampal volumes and reduced perfusion and functional imaging in normal individuals with memory impairment have been described by some groups[15,16] but not others[17], while the excellent spatial memory of taxi drivers has been related to enlargement of the posterior hippocampus in one study[18]. Further research is clearly needed. Similarly, some find a strong correlation between the degree of memory impairment in normal elderly people and volumetric change on magnetic resonance imaging, while others do not[14,16,17]. More consistent is the finding that amongst those who already have memory impairment, reduced temporal and hippocampal volumes do predict those who will decline to develop dementia, as opposed to those who will not[19–22]. However, whether this is simply a reflection of the "contamination" of normal memory-impaired individuals and those with early AD remains unresolved.

Neuropathological data are limited, although MCI individuals may have Alzheimer-type pathology intermediate between those with AD and normals[23]. Another candidate for the cause of any hippocampal damage during ageing would be excessive cortisol excretion associated with ageing, which is known to be toxic to the hippocampus in animals and possibly in humans[24–26]. These remain important avenues for future research. However, other possibilities exist for the neurobiological basis of memory and other cognitive impairments in healthy individuals. Generalized brain atrophy is known to occur with ageing[27,28], whilst an increase in white matter burden, presumably reflecting vascular pathology, occurs and has been linked with cognitive impairment in some studies[29].

CONCLUSION

Despite the hippocampus being central to new learning in humans and the evidence that memory impairment and hippocampal changes occur with ageing, further evidence linking the two is still needed. Undoubtedly, new views on hippocampal function and topographical organization, the better definition of the role of other structures, such as the parahippocampal gyrus and frontal lobe, in different memory functions, combined with further longitudinal clinical, electrophysiological, imaging and pathological studies, will provide a clearer answer to this important question in the near future.

REFERENCES

1. Ritchie K, Touchon J. Mild cognitive impairment: conceptual basis and current nosological status. *Lancet* 2000; **355**: 225–8.
2. Petersen RC, Smith GE, Waring SC *et al*. Mild cognitive impairment: clinical characterization and outcome [published erratum appears in *Arch Neurol* 1999 Jun; **56**(6): 760]. *Arch Neurol* 1999; **56**: 303–8.
3. Petersen RC, Smith GE, Waring SC *et al*. Aging, memory, and mild cognitive impairment. *Int Psychogeriat* 1997; **9**: 65–9.
4. O'Brien J, Beats B, Hill K *et al*. Do subjective memory complaints precede dementia? A 3 year follow-up of patients presenting with benign memory problems. *Int J Geriat Psychiat* 1992; **7**: 481–6.
5. Milwain E. Mild cognitive impairment: further caution [letter]. *Lancet* 2000; **355**: 1018.

6. O'Brien JT, Levy R. Age-associated memory impairment [Editorial] [see comments]. *Br Med J* 1992; **304**: 5–6.

7. Eichenbaum H. Neurobiology. The topography of memory [news, comment]. *Nature* 1999; **402**: 597–9.

8. Teng E, Squire LR. Memory for places learned long ago is intact after hippocampal damage. *Nature* 1999; **400**: 675–7.

9. Rugg MD. Memories are made of this [comment]. *Science* 1998; **281**: 1151–2.

10. Vargha-Khadem F, Gadian DG, Watkins KE *et al.* Differential effects of early hippocampal pathology on episodic and semantic memory [see comments] [published erratum appears in *Science* 1997 Aug 22; 277 (5329): 1117]. *Science* 1997; **277**: 376–80.

11. Mummery CJ, Patterson K, Price CJ *et al.* A voxel-based morphometry study of semantic dementia: relationship between temporal lobe atrophy and semantic memory. *Ann Neurol* 2000; **47**: 36–45.

12. Barber R, Gholkar A, Ballard C *et al.* MRI Volumetric study of dementia with Lewy bodies, Alzheimer's disease and vascular dementia. *Neurology* 2000; **54**: 1304–9.

13. Jack CR Jr, Petersen RC, Xu YC *et al.* Medial temporal atrophy on MRI in normal aging and very mild Alzheimer's disease [see comments]. *Neurology* 1997; **49**: 786–94.

14. Petersen RC, Jack CR Jr, Xu YC *et al.* Memory and MRI-based hippocampal volumes in aging and AD. *Neurology* 2000; **54**: 581–7.

15. Golomb J, de Leon MJ, Kluger A *et al.* Hippocampal atrophy in normal aging. An association with recent memory impairment. *Arch Neurol* 1993; **50**: 967–73.

16. Golomb J, Kluger A, de Leon MJ *et al.* Hippocampal formation size in normal human aging: a correlate of delayed secondary memory performance. *Learning Memory* 1994; **1**: 45–54.

17. Ylikoski R, Salonen O, Mantyla R *et al.* Hippocampal and temporal lobe atrophy and age-related decline in memory. *Acta Neurol Scand* 2000; **101**: 273–8.

18. Maguire EA, Gadian DG, Johnsrude IS *et al.* Navigation-related structural change in the hippocampi of taxi drivers [see comments]. *Proc Natl Acad Sci USA* 2000; **97**: 4398–403.

19. Convit A, de Asis J, de Leon MJ *et al.* Atrophy of the medial occipitotemporal, inferior, and middle temporal gyri in non-demented elderly predict decline to Alzheimer's disease. *Neurobiol Aging* 2000; **21**: 19–26.

20. Jack CR Jr, Petersen RC, Xu YC *et al.* Prediction of AD with MRI-based hippocampal volume in mild cognitive impairment. *Neurology* 1999; **52**: 1397–403.

21. Kaye JA, Swihart T, Howieson D *et al.* Volume loss of the hippocampus and temporal lobe in healthy elderly persons destined to develop dementia. *Neurology* 1997; **48**: 1297–1304.

22. Visser PJ, Scheltens P, Verhey FR *et al.* Medial temporal lobe atrophy and memory dysfunction as predictors for dementia in subjects with mild cognitive impairment. *J Neurol* 1999; **246**: 477–85.

23. Mufson EJ, Chen EY, Cochran E *et al.* Entorhinal cortex beta-amyloid load in individuals with mild cognitive impairment. *Exp Neurol* 1999; **158**: 469–90.

24. O'Brien JT. The "glucocorticoid cascade" hypothesis in man. *Br J Psychiat* 1997; **170**: 199–201.

25. Sapolsky RM, Krey LC, McEwen BS. The neuroendocrinology of stress and aging: the glucocorticoid cascade hypothesis. *Endocr Rev* 1986; **7**: 284–301.

26. Sheline YI, Sanghavi M, Mintun MA, Gado MH. Depression duration but not age predicts hippocampal volume loss in medically healthy women with recurrent major depression. *J Neurosci* 1999; **19**: 5034–43.

27. Fox NC, Freeborough PA, Rossor MN. Visualisation and quantification of rates of atrophy in Alzheimer's disease [see comments]. *Lancet* 1996; **348**: 94–7.

28. Jack CR Jr, Petersen RC, Xu Y *et al.* Rate of medial temporal lobe atrophy in typical aging and Alzheimer's disease. *Neurology* 1998; **51**: 993–9.

29. DeCarli C, Murphy DG, Tranh M *et al.* The effect of white matter hyperintensity volume on brain structure, cognitive performance, and cerebral metabolism of glucose in 51 healthy adults. *Neurology* 1995; **45**: 2077–84.

9

Neuroendocrinology of Ageing

R. A. Burns and Mohammed T. Abou-Saleh

Department of Addictive Behaviour and Psychological Medicine, St George's Hospital Medical School, London, UK

INTRODUCTION

Neuroendocrinology is the study of interactions between the nervous and endocrine systems. Such interactions occur via complex mechanisms involving the cerebral cortex, limbic system, brain stem, hypothalamus, pituitary and periphery with regulatory feedback by many hormones to the pituitary, hypothalamus and probably higher centres such as the hippocampus. Observations of neuroendocrine dysfunction and disorders of behaviour have helped to improve our understanding of mental illness and will be discussed later in this chapter.

Despite a surge of research over the last 25 years, many gaps remain in our understanding of neuroendocrinology, especially that of central secretion and neural control of hormone release. The complex interrelationships between monoamines, neuropeptides and hormones have not been elucidated[1]. Hormones such as insulin and cortisol, once thought to exist only peripherally, are now believed to have central functions as neurotransmitters or neuromodulators[2]. Neuropeptides such as opioids and vasoactive intestinal peptide (VIP) are found centrally and peripherally and some, such as thyrotropin releasing hormone (TRH), can be secreted from the same nerve terminals as classical neurotransmitters, thus also acting as neuromodulators[3]. Some neurotransmitters, once thought to act solely via the hypothalamus, may directly affect the pituitary, bypassing the hypothalamus[4]. The hypothalamus remains the fulcrum of neuroendocrine activity. In response to primarily central stimuli, the hypothalamus acts either: (a) via release of neuropeptide releasing or inhibiting factors into the portal circulation to the anterior pituitary; or (b) via the direct release of neuropeptides to the posterior pituitary. Thus adrenocorticotrophic hormone (ACTH), thyroid stimulating hormone (TSH), growth hormone (GH), follicle stimulating hormone (FSH), luteinizing hormone (LH) and prolactin are released from the anterior pituitary and vasopressin (antidiuretic hormone (ADH)) and oxytocin from the posterior pituitary. There is an intricate multilevel system of feedback mechanisms between adjacent and even distant steps in the process of hormonal secretion. Description of peripheral endocrine effects are beyond the scope of this chapter.

Like other systems, the neuroendocrine system undergoes a degree of decline during senescence, although by varying degrees and different mechanisms. Ageing may affect the neural control of hormones; the endocrine cells themselves, their hormones, hormone receptors and post-receptor events in target cells[5]. Most commonly there is a reduction in receptor cell numbers but hormone-receptor coupling mechanisms have also been implicated[6,7]. As some symptoms of hormonal disorder mimic the symptoms of advancing age it is not surprising that the hypothalamus and endocrine system have been linked as causative agents to the ageing process. Such organ system-based theories of ageing assume the presence of an "organal pacemaker" for ageing which initiates the chain of events seen in senescence[8]. The failure of organ systems, with the loss of homeostasis, is important to many of these theories. Some ideas have focused on more peripheral endocrine glands, e.g. the hypothyroid hypotheses, but there has been a more recent shift to central structures, such as the hypothalamus[9]. Dilman and others have proposed that an elevated hypothalamic threshold to negative feedback is an important element in the "deviation of homeostasis" after the completion of growth, and that a relative hypersecretion of, among others, growth hormone renders the internal environment inconsistent with survival by altering glucose and fatty acid metabolism and resulting in vascular disease, diabetes mellitus and other forms of morbidity[10]. Work by Frolkis *et al*[11] in Kiev has shown that the hypothalamo–pituitary axis plays a role in the regulation of RNA synthesis and in the induction of some enzymes of carbohydrate and protein metabolism. They found that these functions deteriorated with age and their work suggests that homeostatic and repair mechanisms may be influenced, which gives some support for an aetiological role for the neuroendocrine system in ageing. Possibly a more integrated theory involves a more circular mechanism. Genetic programming combines with the internal and external environment to result in impairment of all cells with ageing, including cells of the endocrine system. Impairment of the endocrine system alters homeostatic function and thus accelerates impairment of the remainder of the organism[4]. Given the complexity of the interrelationships within the internal environment, it is unlikely that the debate generated by these theories will be resolved in the near future.

Much of the initial research on ageing and endocrine function was with animal studies which, although helpful, may not be entirely applicable to humans, as there are important differences[12,13]. However, techniques such as immunoassay have enabled us to measure hormone levels directly in humans, but even with this technique a high level of quality control is essential, as is the reliability of measurement. In human studies, too, we must remember that most samples are cross-sectional and we are therefore measuring age *differences* rather than age *changes*; longitudinal studies are therefore desirable. Nevertheless, in spite of these difficulties, greater sophistication and reliability in our measurement techniques, as well as the ability to synthesize hypothalamic releasing factors, have enhanced our understanding of neuroendocrinology and the effect of ageing.

Principles and Practice of Geriatric Psychiatry, 2nd edn. Edited by J. R. M. Copeland, M. T. Abou-Saleh and D. G. Blazer
©2002 John Wiley & Sons, Ltd

AGEING AND NEURAL CONTROL OF ENDOCRINE FUNCTION

As previously mentioned, the neural control of hypophyseal secretion is complex and involves both classical neurotransmitters and neuropeptides, with good evidence that different neurotransmitter systems interact to modulate neurosecretion. Noradrenaline, dopamine, 5-hydroxytryptamine (5-HT), acetylcholine, γ-aminobutyric acid (GABA) and opioid peptides may all directly affect hypophyseal secretion mechanisms, whilst cholecystokinin, vasopressin and other neuropeptides have facilitatory or inhibitory roles[14].

With ageing the secretion of neurotransmitters and receptor binding and *sensitivity* are altered[15]. Animal studies have suggested that the facilitatory effects of Ca^{2+} in neurotransmission may be reduced[16]. The overall brain content of noradrenaline is reduced, with many hypothalamic noradrenergic nuclei showing reduced noradrenaline concentrations with age, and adrenergic receptor sensitivity also appears to decline[17]. Dopamine receptor numbers are reduced, especially in the nigrostriatum. Acetylcholine metabolism also shows reduction[18] and, although reports of reductions of brain 5-HT concentrations have not been fully substantiated, there does appear to be a reduced amplitude of circadian serotonin rhythm and a gradual decrease of 5-HT_2 receptors with age in the cerebral cortex[19]. It is likely that changes occur in other neurotransmitter systems with ageing, further altering the balance of neuronal control of endocrine function. In addition, neuronal sensitivity to feedback loop mechanisms may be altered, as reductions in the concentration of rat hippocampal cortisol receptors have been reported[20]. Exactly how the effects of ageing upon neural mechanisms alter the functioning of subservient endocrine axes is not clear, but age-related changes in each neuroendocrine axis will be described below, with reference made to neural control mechanisms where appropriate.

AGEING AND HYPOTHALAMIC–PITUITARY PERIPHERAL ENDOCRINE AXIS

Morphologically age-related changes of the hypothalamus and pituitary are relatively minor. Calcification of the sella turcica may occur and animal studies have suggested an increase in intracellular lipofuscin, with a reduction in the volume of neuronal end swelling as well as in the number of hypothalamic neurosecretory granules[21]. Fibrosis with loss of basophil cells—hypophysis naviculare—may occur in the anterior pituitary. Functionally, changes may be more pronounced and for the sake of clarity we will deal with each hormonal axis separately, as age-related change is differential.

HYPOTHALAMO–SOMATOTROPH–SOMATOMEDIN AXIS

The secretion of growth hormone (GH) declines in ageing humans[22] with dampening of pulsatile GH release and loss of sleep- and exercise-induced swings. In addition, provocation tests suggest reduced GH reserve. The age-related changes, less pronounced in females, are due at least in part to reduced pituitary sensitivity to hypothalamic growth hormone releasing hormone (GHRH) and reduction of somatotroph numbers. However, reduction in sensitivity of α2 receptors is also implicated, as evidenced by a blunted response to clonidine, an α2 agonist[23]. Peripheral α2 receptor numbers have been found to be diminished. Altered catechol aminergic activity has been implicated in rats as administration of L-dopa reversed both mean and pulsatile GH levels[24]. Somatomedin levels also fall, and it has been postulated that reductions in GH and somatomedin may play a role in osteoporosis and other degenerative diseases in the elderly[25,26].

HYPOTHALAMO–HYPOPHYSO–THYROID (HPT) AXIS

The HPT axis also undergoes changes coincident with ageing with a balanced decline in thyroid hormone production and degradation[27]. In the elderly male, the overall secretion of thyroid stimulating hormone (TSH) is reduced and the response to thyrotropin releasing hormone (TRH) is blunted. This reduction is not marked and in females TSH levels may even increase with age[25]. Pulsatility of TSH is maintained and, although results are inconsistent more recent findings have suggested that diurnal variation is also preserved[29]. Healthy ambulatory ageing subjects show only a slight decrement in serum thyroxin (T4) levels. Thyroid binding globulin levels are unchanged but serum triiodothyronine (T3) concentration may be reduced by 10–20%, partly due to the age-related reduction in conversion of T4 to T3[30].

HYPOTHALAMIC–PITUITARY–GONODAL (HPG) AXIS

The HPG axis also undergoes gradual decline with age[31]. In men, primary testicular failure, possibly a result of reduced testicular perfusion, leads to a gradual reduction in testosterone levels, which becomes more marked after 60 years. Maximally stimulated testosterone, free testosterone and tissue testosterone are also reduced. Despite widespread variation, it is likely that such change is purely related rather than due to sedentariness or minor illness[32]. Reduced testosterone levels and elevated oestradiol (as a result of testosterone degradation in the skin and liver) may account for feminizing features, such as gynaecomastia, which may be seen in old men. Reduction of the feedback testosterone results in elevated levels of luteinizing hormone (LH) and follicle stimulating hormone (FSH) with age. However, sensitivity to negative feedback is increased at the hypothalamic level. The amplitude and frequency of pulsatile gonadotropin releasing hormone (GnRH) and luteinizing hormone releasing hormone (LHRH) are reduced, possibly as a result of neurotransmitter and neuromodulator changes, and pituitary sensitivity to releasing factors also appears to diminish. In ageing females, primary ovarian dysfunction occurs with shortening of the cycle length, depleted oestrogen and elevated FSH[33]. Oestrogen levels fall to around 20% of the premenopausal level and then remain relatively stable, with the primary source of oestrogens being from androgen conversion in adipose tissue as ovarian androgens continue to be secreted[34]. After the menopause, serum FSH and LH levels greatly increase to peak between 51 and 60 years and gradually decline thereafter. Animal studies have suggested increased pituitary sensitivity to LHRH but in humans it is not known whether the increased bioactivity of LH and FSH is as a result of greater pituitary sensitivity or high LHRH levels[35].

In both males and females, the production of adrenal androgens is reduced with senescence. Although prolactin levels are elevated in ageing rats and mice, it is unclear whether this is the case with humans, although recent evidence suggests a slight increase in elderly men and a slight fall in ageing women until the age of 80[36].

HYPOTHALAMIC–PITUITARY–ADRENAL (HPA) AXIS

The HPA axis is the best known and most studied of the neuroendocrine axes because of its intimate involvement in the response to stress[37] (see below). Overall, findings suggest a mild reduction, if any, in basal functioning but with an altered regulatory capacity, an important factor in the stress response. Plasma total cortisol, plasma cortisol binding, plasma and urinary free cortisol and plasma ACTH are unchanged. Diurnal variation of cortisol secretion persists but may occur later in the day. Both ACTH and cortisol show decreased responsivity to provocative stimulation in older individuals and a degree of loss of the inhibitory feedback response[38]. Several studies have shown attenuation of the cortisol response to ACTH, possibly as a result of altered functioning of ACTH-stimulated cAMP gluco-corticoid receptors, whose numbers also diminish with age[39].

POSTERIOR PITUITARY

Morphologically, animal studies have revealed subcellular changes in the posterior pituitary. In humans, earlier evidence suggesting non-alteration of posterior pituitary hormones[40] must be tempered by the more recent evidence of a tendency to increased secretion of vasopressin in the elderly with elevated basal levels. Diminished secretion by ageing hypophyseal tissue is offset by elevation of vasopressin levels as a result of a reduction in renal tubule sensitivity to vasopressin[41]. Animal studies suggest that ageing may result in the loss of a particular group of hippocampal cells normally inhibitory to vasopressin secretion. Oxytocin levels also decrease with age.

AGEING AND STRESS

"Stress" may be defined in many ways but implies demands upon an organism threatening to overwhelm it and resulting in a physiological response. Human physiological responses to stress, either physical or psychological, are characteristic and involve initial adrenal medullary sympathetic activity which is later superseded by activity of the HPA axis during the "adaptation" phase. The HPA axis and its response to stress is outlined in Figure 9.1. Thus, in situations of stress, there is centrally stimulated hypersecretion of ACTH and cortisol, along with facilitatory vasopressin. The HPA axis also plays a major role in the homeostasis of stress and it has been postulated that it achieves this by blunting the organism's persisting and potentially harmful physiological reaction to stress. The repeated aetiological linkage of stress to psychiatric illness has led over the last 25 years to much investigation of the HPA axis in stress and psychiatric illness, resulting in a mushrooming of the concept of psychoneuroendocrinology or behavioural endocrinology and the search for neuroendocrine markers for psychiatric illness. The concept of the neuroendocrine interface as "the window into the brain", although not fulfilling initial expectations, has led to neuroendocrinological techniques becoming powerful research tools and valuable diagnostic aids in psychiatry[42].

With ageing it appears that the physiological stress mechanism becomes compromised and there is also evidence that stressful stimuli can accelerate ageing[43]. At the neurochemical level, rat experiments have suggested changes in monoamine metabolism and poor habituation to stress occurring with increasing age[44]. Such a loss of habituation may be a result of an age-induced reduction of benzodiazepine binding sites[45] (thus increasing vulnerability to anxiety-induced mechanisms) or may be a consequence of a reduction of inhibitory hippocampal cortisol receptor numbers[46]. Despite inconsistent findings there appears to be a diminished maximal response of the HPA axis to stressful stimuli, denoting a reduction in reserve capacity in ageing humans.

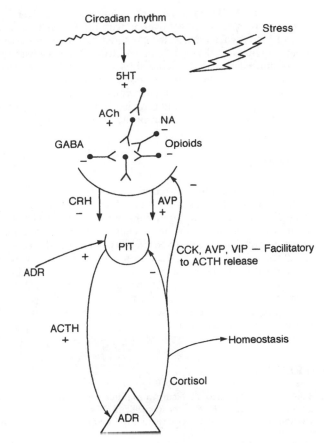

Figure 9.1 The HPA axis and its response to stress. 5-HT, 5-hydroxytrytamine; ACh, acetylcholine; NA, noradrenaline; GABA, γ-aminobytyric acid; CRH, corticotrophin releasing hormone; CCK, cholecystokinin; AVP, arginine asopressin; VIP, vasoactive intestinal peptide; ACTH, adrenocorticotropin; ADR, adrenal gland

AGE AND PSYCHONEUROENDOCRINE MARKERS

As a result of research carried out over the last 25 years, it is now firmly established that mental illness is associated with a high incidence of endocrine abnormality in both young and old. The most commonly investigated endocrine axis in psychological disturbance is the HPA axis, which in depression characteristically shows hyperactivity with elevated circulating ACTH-cortisol and non-suppression by dexamethasone, a powerful synthetic steroid that, in normal individuals, inhibits the secretion of ACTH and hence cortisol. In younger individuals, dexamethasone non-suppression is not truly specific for depression and is common in other affective psychosis and acute schizophrenia, with a lower incidence in anxiety, panic disorder and anorexia nervosa[47]. Dexamethasone suppression is also influenced by age (among other variables), with the healthy elderly showing a tendency towards non-suppression. However, non-suppression is more pronounced in the elderly depressed and those with Alzheimer's disease. In the elderly, as in the young, the dexamethasone suppression test (DST) is still a useful aid when used with careful clinical assessment[48]. It is helpful in differentiating depressive illness from minor psychiatric conditions and chronic schizo-phrenia, and reports have also suggested uses in identifying depressive pseudodementia and demented patients with depression[49]. In depression, the DST is a good predictor of long-term outcome, with greater risk of relapse in non-suppressors[50]. The

TSH response to TRH is also frequently blunted in depression but once again there is considerable overlap with other psychoses and there is an increased tendency to a blunted response in healthy senescent individuals[51]. Reports that blunted TRH responses are more pronounced in elderly depressives have not been entirely confirmed[52]. Growth hormone response to clonidine, an α2 agonist, is blunted in depression, Alzheimer's disease and ageing. Recent data suggest that this blunting is again more pronounced in elderly mentally ill subjects than in the normal elderly[53].

CONCLUSION

Overall, although it is only in recent years that neuroendocrine function in the elderly has been studied in depth, it has been established that significant alterations in function occur with ageing in humans. Some of those changes may approximate endocrine abnormalities observed in younger individuals with mental illness, most notably depression. As yet our knowledge remains limited in the realm of behavioural neuroendocrinology, but such similarities in function of the aged and depressed have led to speculation of some common mechanism underlying age and mental illness. Hopefully research into such speculation will provide further enlightenment.

REFERENCES

1. Tuomisto J, Mannisto P. Neurotransmitter regulation of anterior pituitary hormones. *Pharmacol Rev* 1985; **37**: 249.
2. Hokfelt T, Johannson O, Goldstein M. Chemical anatomy of the brain. *Science* 1984; **225**: 1326.
3. Muller EE. Chairman's concluding remarks. In Valenti G, ed., *Psychoneuroendocrinology of Ageing: Basic and Clinical Aspects*. Fidia Research Series, Vol 16. Padova: Liviana Press, 1988.
4. Valenti G (ed.). *Psychoneuroendocrinology of Ageing: Basic and Clinical Aspects*. Padova: Liviana Press, 1988; 2–5.
5. Sartine JL. Endocrine physiology. In Rotstein M, ed., *Review of Biological Research in Ageing*. 1983; **1**: 181–93, New York: Alan R. Liss.
6. Pritchett JF, Sartin JL, Marple DN *et al*. Interaction of ageing with *in vitro* adrenocortical responsiveness to ACTH and cyclic AMP. *Horm Res* 1979; **10**: 96–103.
7. Albrecht ED. Effect of ageing and adrenocortico-trophin on adrenal 5-3-hydroxysteroid dehydrogenase activity in male rats. *Exp Ageing Res* 1981; **7**: 11–15.
8. Gusseck DJ. Endocrine mechanisms and ageing. *Adv Gerontol Res* 1972; **4**: 105–66.
9. Everitt AV. The neuroendocrine system and ageing. *Gerontology*, 1980; **26**: 108–19.
10. Dilman VM. Hypothalamic mechanisms of ageing and of specific age pathology. A model for the mechanism of human specific age pathology and natural death. *Exp Gerontol* 1979; **14**: 278–300.
11. Frolkis VV, Beyukov VV, Muradian KK. Hypothalamic–pituitary–adrenocortical regulation of RNA synthesis in ageing. *Exp Gerontol* 1979; **14**: 77–85.
12. Green M. *Endocrinology and Ageing*. Philadelphia: WB Saunders, 1981.
13. Meites J. The neuroendocrinology of hypothalamic ageing. In Muller EE, MacLeod RM, eds. *Neuro-endocrine Perspectives*, Vol 5. Amsterdam: Elsevier, 1986; 179–89.
14. Janowsky DS, Risch SC, Overstreet DH. Psychopharmacologic–neurotransmitter–neuroendocrine interactions in the study of the affective disorders. In Halbreich U, ed., *Hormones and Depression*. New York: Raven, 1987.
15. Veith RC, Raskind MA. The neurobiology of ageing: does it predispose to depression? *Neurobiol Ageing* 1988; **9**: 101–17.
16. Meyer EM, Crews FT, Otero DH, Larsen K. Ageing decreases the sensitivity of rat cortical synaptosomes to calcium ionophore-induced acetylcholine release. *J Neurochem* 1986; **47**: 1244–6.
17. Simkins JW, Millard WJ. Influence of age on neurotransmitter function. *Endocrinol Metab Clin* 1987; **16**: 893–917.
18. Bartus RT, Dean RL III, Bear B, Lippa AS. The cholinergic hypothesis of geriatric memory dysfunction. *Science* 1982; **217**: 408–17.
19. Wong DF, Wagner HN, Dannals RF *et al*. Effects of age on dopamine and serotonin receptors measured by positron tomography in the living human brain. *Science* 1984; **226**: 1393–6.
20. Sapolsky RM, Krey LC, McEwen BS. The neuroendocrinology of stress and ageing: the glucocorticoid cascade hypothesis. *Endocrinol Rev* 1986; **7**: 284–301.
21. Davies E, Goddard C, Davidson Y, Faragher EB. Age-related changes in the neuronal subcellar compartments in the hypothalamus. In Courstais *et al.*, eds, *Modern Trends in Ageing Research*, Vol 147. London: Libbey, 1986; 525–31.
22. Zadik Z, Chalew SA, McCarter RJ *et al*. The influence of age on the 24-hour integrated concentration of growth hormone in normal individuals. *J Clin Endocrinol Metab* 1985; **60**: 513–16.
23. Bursztyn M, Bresnahan M, Gavras I, Gravas H. Effect of ageing on vasopressin, catecholamines and α2-adrenergic receptors. *J Am Geriatr Soc* 1990; **38**(6): 628–32.
24. Sonntag WW, Forman LJ, Miki N *et al*. L-Dopa restores amplitude of growth hormone pulses in old male rats to that observed in young male rats. *Neuroendocrinology* 1982; **34**: 163–8.
25. Hoffman AR, Griffin C, Kalinyak J *et al*. The hypothalamic–somatroph–somatomedin axis and ageing. In Valenti G, ed., *Psychoneuroendocrinology of Ageing: Basic and Clinical Aspects*, Fidia Research Series, Vol 16. Padova: Liviana, 1988.
26. Rudman D, Feller AG, Nagraj HS *et al*. Effects of human growth hormone in men over 60 years old. *N Engl J Med* 1990; **323**(1): 1–6.
27. Emerson CH, Weiner R. Psychoneuroendocrine control of pituitary TSH secretion and ageing. In Valenti G, ed., *Psychoneuroendocrinology of Ageing: Basic and Clinical Aspects*, Fidia Research Series, Vol 16. Padova: Liviana, 1988.
28. Van Coevorden A, Laurent E, Decoster C *et al*. Decreased basal and stimulated thyrotropin secretion in healthy elderly men. *J Clin Endocrinol Metab* 1989; **69**(1): 177–85.
29. Spaulding SW. Age and the thyroid. *Endocrinol Metab Clin* 1987; **16**: 1013–25.
30. Noth RH, Mazzaferri EL. Age and the endocrine system. *Clin Geriat Med* 1985; **1**: 223–50.
31. Vermeulen A. Ageing of the hypothalmo–pituitary axis in man. *Mod Trends Ageing Res* 1986; **147**: 87–91.
32. Deslypere JP, Vermeulen A. Leydig cell function in normal men: effect of age, life-style, residence, diet A and activity. *J Clin Endocrinol Metab* 1984; **59**: 955–61.
33. Judd HL, Korenman SG. Effects of ageing on reproductive function in women. In Korenman SG, ed., *Endocrine Aspects of Ageing*. New York: Elsevier Biomedical, 1982.
34. Ackerman GE, Smith ME, Mendelson CR *et al*. Aromatization of androstenedione by human adipose tissue stromal cells in monolayer culture. *J Clin Endocrinol Metab* 1981; **53**: 412–17.
35. Cetel NS, Rivier J, Vale W *et al*. The dynamics of gonadotropin inhibition in women induced by an antagonistic analog of gonadotropin-releasing hormone. *J Clin Endocrinol Metab* 1983; **57**: 62–5.
36. Sawin CT, Carlson HE, Geller A *et al*. Serum prolactin and ageing: basal values and changes with oestrogen use and hypothyroidism. *J Gerontol* 1989; **44**(4): M131–5.
37. Sachar EJ. Hormonal changes in stress and mental illness. In Kreiger DT, Hughes JC, eds, *Neuroendocrinology*. Sunderland, MA: Sinauer, 1980; 177–83.
38. Reus VI. Behavioural implications of hypothalamic–pituitary–adrenal dysfunction. In Halbreich U, ed., *Hormones and Depression*. New York: Raven, 1987; 385–401.
39. Sapolsky RM, Armanini M, Packan D, Tombaugh G. Stress and glucocorticoid in a being. *Clin Endocrinol Metab* 1987; **16**: 965–79.
40. Everitt AV. Ageing and its hypothalamic–pituitary control. In Everitt AV, Burgess JA, eds, *Hypothalamus, Pituitary and Ageing*. Springfield, IL: Thomas, 1976; 676–99.
41. Legros JJ. Physiological ageing brain and psychoneuroendocrine control of ADH secretion. In Valenti G, ed. *Psychoneuroendocrinology of Ageing: Basic and Clinical Aspects*, Fidia Research Series, Vol 16. Padova: Liviana, 1988.

42. Halbriech U (ed.). Hormones and depression. *Conceptual Transitions in Hormones and Depression.* New York: Raven, 1987; 1–20.

43. Selye H, Tuchweber B. Stress in relation to and disease. In Everitt AV, Burgess JA, eds., *Hypothalamus, Pituitary and Ageing.* Springfield, IL: Thomas, 1986; 533–59.

44. Sapolsky RM, Krey LC, McEwen BS. The adrenocortical stress response in the aged male rat: impairment of recovery from stress. *Exp Gerontol* 1983; **18**: 55–64.

45. Algeri S, Aita I, Perego C *et al.* Some adaptive mechanisms in the monoaminergic systems of the senescent brain. *Mod Trends Ageing Res* 1986; **147**: 515–24.

46. Sapolsky RM, Krey LC, McEwen BS. The neuro-endocrinology of stress and ageing: the glucocorticoid cascade hypothesis. *Endocr Rev* 1986; **7**: 284–301.

47. Arana GW, Baldessarini RJ. Development and clinical application of the dexamethasone suppression test in psychiatry. In Halbreich U, ed., *Hormones and Depression.* New York: Raven, 1987; 113–33.

48. Abou-Saleh MT. Dexamethasone test in psychiatry: is there a place for an integrated hypothesis? *Psychiat Dev* 1985; **3**: 275–306.

49. Katona CLE, Aldridge CR. The dexamethasone suppression test and depressive signs in dementia. *J Affect Disord* 1985; **8**: 83–9.

50. Abou-Saleh MT. How useful is a dexamethasone suppression test. *Curr Opin Psychiat* 1988; **1**: 60–5.

51. Abou-Saleh MT, Coppen A. Thyrotropin response to TRH stimulation in depression: effect of endogenicity. *Psychiat Res* 1988; **23**: 115–16.

52. McCracken JT, Rubin RT. Neuroendocrine aspects of depression in elderly patients. In Valenti G, ed., *Psychoneuroendocrinology of Ageing: Basic and Clinical Aspects*, Fidia Research Series, Vol 16. Padova: Liviana, 1988; 127–49.

53. Gilles C, Ryckaert P, DeMol J *et al.* Clonidine-induced growth hormone secretion in elderly patients with senile dementia of the Alzheimer type and major depressive disorders. *Psychiat Res* 1989; **27**(3): 277–86.

10

Neurophysiology of Ageing as Reflected by Electroencephalogram (EEG) and Event-related Potentials (ERPs)

D. H. R. Blackwood, W. J. Muir and H. Förstl*

*Royal Edinburgh Hospital, Edinburgh, UK, and *Technical University, Munich, Germany*

INTRODUCTION

The electroencephalogram (EEG), which represents the electrical activity of the brain as recorded from electrodes placed at various positions on the scalp, is essential for the diagnosis of the epilepsies and the study of sleep disorders. It can also be a useful non-invasive aid for the detection and localization of structural brain abnormalities and the diagnosis of diffuse encephalopathies in patients with fluctuating levels of consciousness. Many of these conditions are common in the elderly population and it is therefore important to have a full understanding of the effects of normal ageing on the EEG, so that the significance of abnormal findings in elderly subjects can be more clearly interpreted.

ROUTINE EEG

Using standard procedures[1], electrodes, prepared with conductive jelly, are placed on the scalp and positioned in rows over frontal, temporal, parietal and occipital regions, according to the International 10-20 System[2]. Most recording equipment permits an easy selection of different montages of electrode pairs and the filtered and amplified potential differences between pairs of electrodes are then recorded on paper trace (qEEG) and stored for quantitative analysis. Recordings are usually obtained from several scalp regions and under different physiological conditions. The resting EEG is recorded with the subject's eyes open and for a period with the eyes closed to test the responsiveness of background activity. Routine inspection of the EEG waveform takes account of changes in frequency, amplitude and response to activation procedures such as hyperventilation, which may be employed to accentuate certain EEG abnormalities. The presence or absence of paroxysmal activity will be noted. For the detection of brain abnormalities, changes in frequency are generally more reliable than changes in amplitude. By convention, four frequency bands are described: EEG waveforms in the range 8–13 Hz denote the alpha range, which is commonly observed in occipital brain regions of young persons during wakefulness when the eyes are closed (alpha is attenuated by visual attention). There is wide normal variation in the alpha rhythm, and slowing occurs with normal ageing, delirious states and metabolic disorders. If frequencies greater than 13 Hz are present, the EEG is said to show beta rhythm. Such fast activity may be found in normal people but is also increased by some drugs, including benzodia-

zepines and barbiturates. At the lower end of the spectrum, activity in the range 4–7 Hz is termed theta. Theta activity can be marked in young children, becoming less by the time of puberty. Frequencies below 4 Hz are grouped as delta activity. Theta and delta activity occur during sleep and are commonly found in neurological disorders whose slow wave abnormality may only be diffusely recorded, as, for example, in encephalopathies. Such slow wave bands also prevail when localized at electrodes overlaying space-occupying lesions.

THE ORIGIN OF THE EEG

The scalp-recorded rhythmic activity of the EEG is believed to be generated in the cerebral cortex, especially in large pyramidal neurones orientated vertically toward the surface of the scalp. However, rhythmic activity arising in subcortical regions, in particular in the thalamus, can be imposed on and modify the activity of these cortical cells via thalamo-cortical projections[3,4], so that the scalp-recorded EEG reflects changes in both cortical and sub-cortical structures. Much of the EEG variation usually detected can be attributed to hereditary factors. The early twin studies by Lennox et al.[5], showing that brain electrical cerebral activity is strongly influenced by genetic factors, have been amply confirmed[6,7].

EEG CHANGES WITH AGEING

The most widely reported changes in the EEGs of elderly subjects are the slowing of alpha activity and the onset of focal theta and delta waves over the temporal regions[8–12]. The changes are complex, as they affect the alpha, the slow wave and the fast frequency bands regarding both power and topographic distribution[13–15]. Other reported changes corresponding to age include a much diminished slow wave response to hyperventilation and an increase in the occurrence of spike paroxysms in elderly subjects with no clinical evidence of a seizure disorder.

It is not clear, however, which if any of these changes are the result of a neuronal ageing process *per se*, rather than being manifestations of mild subclinical degenerative brain disease, including, for example, cerebrovascular disease, which is more common in the elderly. Quantitative EEG changes of power or complexity can be employed for highly successful statistical discrimination between demented patients and elderly controls[16,17]. Subtle cognitive impairment has been related to the presence of EEG abnormalities in some groups of otherwise healthy elderly subjects, supporting the view that many of the changes found in the EEGs of elderly subjects are due to specific subclinical pathologies[18]. No changes are observed in highly select groups of 'successfully aged' individuals[14,19].

NORMAL AGEING

In an early study on an elderly population, Silverman et al.[20] recorded EEGs of 90 healthy subjects aged over 60 and reported a diffuse slowing of the background rhythm in 26% and focal abnormalities in 43% of the subjects. These findings have been confirmed more recently[10,21,22]. The slowing of the alpha rhythm with age was clearly demonstrated by Hughes and Cayaffa[23], who recorded the EEGs of 420 subjects aged 5–80 years. All subjects had been hospitalized and had undergone extensive neurological assessment in order to exclude the presence of brain pathology. In this group, the alpha peak frequency, which, up to the age of 60, had been between 10–11 Hz, fell to 9–10 Hz in subjects aged over 60. Some authors, however, claim a decreased slow and an increased fast activity with ageing[24]. The annual changes in non-demented elderly are minimal compared to the alterations of alpha and theta power in demented individuals[25]. There is no correlation between alpha and theta power and the degree of brain atrophy in the non-demented elderly[26].

Hubbard et al.[27] examined the EEGs of 10 centenarians aged 100–105, seven of whom were healthy, with no clinical evidence of degenerative brain disease. In this group, posterior dominant rhythms were in the lower part of the alpha range, and slow wave foci over temporal regions were common. These changes were similar to those found in subjects aged 80, and the study provided no evidence for a progressive decrease in alpha frequency or for an increase in focal temporal slow waves in subjects aged 80–100 years.

Changes in the EEG of elderly subjects, which have been attributed to early cerebrovascular insufficiency, include a diminished response of slow-wave activity to hyperventilation and the development of focal abnormalities, particularly over the anterior temporal regions. In a young person, hyperventilation for a period of 3 or 4 minutes usually produces a gradual increase in diffuse slow activity in the theta and delta range, which settles back to standard level within approximately 1 minute after cessation of over-breathing. This response is age-dependent and is most striking in children, who display delta activity at very high voltages. In contrast, old people show diminished or absent response to over-breathing, which may, in part, be due to diminished alteration in P_{CO_2} when hyperventilating[42].

Bursts of rhythmic theta activity over the temporal regions frequently appear in late adulthood, and these are associated with cognitive and memory deterioration[18,28]. In a recent study, Visser et al.[29] measured the EEG and performed computed tomography (CT) brain scans in a group of clinically healthy subjects aged 65–83 years. In this group of elderly subjects, those with focal EEG delta wave activity, recorded over the left anterior temporal region, performed poorly on neuropsychological tests of word fluency (thought to address temporal lobe function) and also had significant ventricular dilatation measured on the CT scan. It was concluded that such left-sided temporal slow-wave abnormalities found in the EEGs of some elderly subjects may be a valuable early indicator of temporal lobe pathology.

The probability that the EEGs of average adults do not change much throughout life and may, indeed, be relatively normal in otherwise healthy centenarians is thus raised[27]. The slowing of EEG frequency with age could be explained by changes in cerebral blood flow. Regional cerebral blood flow shows a strong inverse correlation with the appearance of EEG slow waves and is directly correlated with posterior alpha activity[30,31]. A direct causal relationship between a reduced cerebral blood flow, an increase in slow waves and a reduced alpha frequency in the EEG of elderly subjects could, therefore, be postulated[32].

EVENT-RELATED POTENTIALS (ERPs) AND AGEING

Electrical cerebral responses to discrete stimuli, such as visual, acoustic or contact stimuli, cannot, by and large, be detected in the scalp-recorded EEG. Electrical response to such events is small in comparison to their cerebral background activity, and averaging techniques are required for their visualization. Such techniques have proved of enormous value to neurologists and psychiatrists studying brainstem and higher cerebral function, by permitting the detection of tiny voltages generated in response to specific stimuli. To extract the time-locked activity generated by a given stimulus, a repeated series of stimuli is presented, and epochs of EEG, captured after each presentation, are summed and standardized/averaged. The random background EEG will tend to decrease in amplitude on summation, whereas the desired event-related potential will remain the same in size.

EXOGENEOUS EVENT-RELATED POTENTIALS

ERPs offer a means to assess peripheral nerve and brainstem function by using different sensory modalities. Early evoked potentials, generated within about 80 milliseconds (ms) after a stimulus, are described as exogenous because they seem to depend on the nature of the stimulus itself rather than any subjective response the subject may make to the stimulus. Auditory brainstem potentials, generated within the first 10 ms after a clicking sound, are evoked in a routine procedure to provide information about the functioning of auditory nerve and brainstem structures in the auditory pathway. Somatosensory event-related potentials (ERPs), evoked by electrical stimulation of, for example, the median nerve at the wrist, include the median nerve action potential, recorded at the brachial plexus, and activity generated in neurones of the spinal dorsal horn and dorsal column. Later peaks probably reflect activity in the medial lemniscus and primary somatosensory cortex. Early visual evoked responses to light flashes reflect activity in the visual path between the retina and the visual striate cortex.

From the second to the ninth decade of life, there is a linear increase in the latency of exogenous potentials[33]. The latency of the median nerve compound action potential, recorded at the brachial plexus (the 'N10 waveform'), increases from an average of 10 ms in the second decade to approximately 12 ms in octogenarians. With few exceptions, a similar rise in latency with increasing age is found in all exogenous potentials of all three sensory modalities addressed and renders age corrections clinically important. The central conduction time of auditory evoked potentials (AEPs) increases by 1–4 ms/year, the latencies of visual evoked potentials (VEPs) by 2–4 ms/decade after age 40 years[34]. Many age-related anatomical, physiological and biochemical changes may contribute to the slowing of nerve conduction implied by these latency delays.

ENDOGENOUS EVENT-RELATED POTENTIALS

ERPs generated more than 80 ms after a stimulus may reflect the psychic condition of an individual. Such responses are termed "endogenous" because their latency and amplitude are hardly influenced by the physical characteristics of the stimulus such as its intensity or frequency, but reflect how attentive the subject is. They also give an indication of the degree of complexity inherent in a cerebral cognitive or memory operation performed on exposure to a stimulus. The P300 response is one endogenous ERP that has been extensively studied, as it is thought to reflect the mental processes of selective attention, learning and memory. To generate a P300 response to an auditory stimulus, the subject is required to attend to a series of low-pitched (non-target) tones, randomly interspersed with high-pitched (target) tones. The recognition of these target tones generates a positive potential, which can be recorded widely over the scalp at approximately 300 ms after the auditory stimulus. The P300 response to the target stimuli is much more explicit, and it is generated only when the subject concentrates on the task; its amplitude is thought to reflect the level of attention and its latency the processing time involved in the recognition of a target tone.

EFFECT OF AGE ON LONG LATENCY EVENT-RELATED POTENTIALS

The latencies of all endogenous event-related potential components appear to increase with age from the second decade onward, a fact that led to extensive research activity in relation to the auditory P300 component[35-41]. Some authors have reported a linear increase of P300 latency with age up to senescence with an increase of 1–2 ms/year. However, comparative studies, comprising large numbers of controls, have found an exponential ageing effect with a much higher rate of increase (of up to 4 ms/year) in P300 latency in subjects older than 60 years as compared to younger adults[37,39,41]. P300 latency is also increased in the presence of a variety of brain pathologies, including the dementias of Alzheimer's disease and cerebrovascular disease. In elderly subjects, it is difficult to separate the effect of ageing *per se* from the effects of subclinical degenerative or vascular changes on endogenous event-related potentials, and this is equally true for routine EEG. In a clinical environment, where P300 measurements may be useful, for example in dementia and schizophrenia, it is essential to carefully match individuals for age, particularly if elderly individuals are concerned.

REFERENCES

1. Binnie CD. Recording techniques: montages, electrodes, amplifiers and filters. In Halliday AM, Butler SR, Paul R, eds, *A Textbook of Clinical Neurophysiology*. Chichester: Wiley, 1987; 3–22.
2. Jasper HH. Report of the Committee on Methods of Clinical Examination in Electroencephalography. *Electroencephalogr Clin Neurophysiol* 1958; **10**: 370.
3. Jasper HH. Diffuse projection system: the integrative action of the thalamic reticular system. *Electroencephalogr Clin Neurophysiol* 1949; **1**: 405–11.
4. Andersen P, Andersson SA. Thalamic origin of cortical rhythmic activity. In Creutzfeldt O, ed, *Handbook of Electroencephalography and Clinical Neurophysiology*. Amsterdam: Elsevier, 1974, 90.
5. Lennox WG, Gibbs EL, Gibbs FA. The brain-wave pattern, a hereditary trait. Evidence from 74 'normal' pairs of twins. *J Heredity* 1945; **36**: 233–43.
6. Vogel F. The genetic basis of the normal human electroencephalogram. *Hum Genet* 1970; **10**: 91–114.
7. Stassen HH, Lykken DT, Propping P, Bomben G. Genetic determination of the human EEG. *Hum Genet* 1988; **80**: 165–76.
8. Obrist WD. The electroencephalogram of normal aged adults. *Electroencephalogr Clin Neurophysiol* 1954; **6**: 245–52.
9. Friedlander W. Electroencephalographic alpha rate in adults as a function of age. *Geriatrics* 1958; **13**: 29–31.
10. Otomo E, Tsubaki T. Electroencephalography in subjects sixty years and over. *Electroencephalogr Clin Neurophysiol* 1966; **20**: 77–82.
11. Wang HS, Busse E. EEG of healthy old persons—a longitudinal study. Dominant background activity and occipital rhythm. *J Gerontol* 1969; **24**: 419–26.
12. Mankovsky N, Beconog R. Aging of the human nervous system in the electroencephalographic aspect. *Geriatrics* 1971; **26**: 100–8.
13. Klass DW, Brenner RP. Electroencephalography of the elderly. *J Clin Neurophysiol* 1995; **12**: 116–31.
14. Ihl R, Besthorn C, Förstl H. EEG. In Förstl H, ed, *Textbook of Old Age Psychiatry*. Stuttgart: Enke, 1997; 117–22.
15. Dustman RE, Shearer DE, Emmerson RY. Life-span changes in EEG spectral amplitude, amplitude variability and mean frequency. *Clin Neurophysiol* 1999; **110**: 1399–409.
16. Besthorn C, Zerfass R, Geiger-Kabisch *et al*. Discrimination of Alzheimer's disease and normal aging by EEG data. *Electroencephalogr Clin Neurophysiol* 1997; **103**: 241–8.
17. Claus JJ, Strijers RLM, Jonkman EJ *et al*. The diagnostic value of electroencephalography in mild senile Alzheimer's disease. *Clin Neurophysiol* 1999; **110**: 825–32.
18. Drachman DA, Hughes JR. Memory and the hippocampal complexes. Aging and temporal EEG abnormalities. *Neurology* 1971; **21**: 1–14.
19. Shigeta M, Julin P, Almkvist O *et al*. EEG in successful aging, a 5-year follow-up study from the eighth to the ninth decade of life. *Electroencephalogr Clin Neurophysiol* 1995; **95**: 77–83.
20. Silverman AJ, Busse BW, Barnes RH. Studies in the processes of ageing: electroencephalographic findings in 400 elderly subjects. *Electroencephalogr Clin Neurophysiol* 1955; **7**: 67–74.
21. Roubicek J. The EEG in the middle aged and the elderly. *J Am Med Soc* 1977; **25**: 145–52.
22. Torres F, Faoro A, Loewenson R, Johnson E. The electroencephalogram of elderly subjects revisited. *Electroencephalogr Clin Neurophysiol* 1983; **56**: 391–8.
23. Hughes JR, Cayaffa JJ. The EEG in patients at different ages without organic cerebral disease. *Electroencephalogr Clin Neurophysiol* 1977; **42**: 776–84.
24. Duffy FH, McAnulty GB, Albert MS. The pattern of age-related differences in electrophysiological activity of healthy males and females. *Neurobiol Aging* 1993; **14**: 73–84.
25. Förstl H, Sattel H, Besthorn C *et al*. Longitudinal cognitive, electroencephalographic and morphological brain changes in ageing and Alzheimer's disease. *Br J Psychiat* 1996; **168**: 280–86.
26. Förstl H, Besthorn C, Sattel H *et al*. Volumetric estimates of brain atrophy and quantitative EEG in normal aging and Alzheimer's disease. *Nervenarzt* 1996; **67**: 53–61.
27. Hubbard O, Sunde D, Goldensohn ES. The EEG in centenarians. *Electroencephalogr Clin Neurophysiol* 1976; **40**: 407–17.
28. Duffy FH, Albert MS, McAnulty G, Garvey AJ. Age-related differences in brain electrical activity of healthy subjects. *Ann Neurol* 1984; **166**: 430–8.
29. Visser SL, Hooijer C, Jonker C *et al*. Anterior temporal focal abnormalities in EEG in normal aged subjects; correlations with psychopathological and CT brain scan findings. *Electroencephalogr Clin Neurophysiol* 1987; **66**: 1–7.
30. Ingvar D, Baldy-Moulinier M, Sulag I, Horman S. Regional cerebral blood flow related to EEG. *Acta Neurol Scand* 1965; **41** (suppl 14): 179–82.
31. Sulg I, Ingvar D. Regional cerebral blood flow and EEG frequency content. *Electroencephalogr Clin Neurophysiol* 1967; **23**: 395–401.
32. Sokoloff L. Cerebral circulatory and metabolic changes associated with ageing. *Res Publ Assoc Nerv Mental Disord* 1966; **41**: 237–54.
33. Allison T. Normal limits in the evoked potential: age and sex differences. In Halliday AM, Butler SR, Paul R, eds, *A Textbook of Clinical Neurophysiology*. Chichester: Wiley, 1987; 155–71.
34. Gilmore R. Evoked potentials in the elderly. *J Clin Neurophysiol* 1995; **12**: 132–8.
35. Goodin DS, Squires VC, Henderson HB, Starr A. Age related variations in evoked potentials to auditory stimuli in normal human subjects. *Electroencephalogr Clin Neurophysiol* 1978; **44**: 447–58.

36. Pfefferbaum A, Ford JM, Wenegrat BG *et al*. Clinical application of the P3 component of event-related potentials. I. Normal Aging. *Electroencephalogr Clin Neurophysiol* 1984; **59**: 85–103.

37. Brown WS, Marsh JT, Larue A. Exponential electro-physiological aging: P3 latency. *Electroencephalogr Clin Neurophysiol* 1983; **55**: 277–85.

38. Picton TW, Stuss DT, Champagne SC, Nelson RF. The effects of age on the human event-related potential. *Psychophysiology* 1984; **21**: 312–25.

39. Gordon E, Kraiuhin C, Harris A *et al*. The differential diagnosis of dementia using P300 latency. *Biol Psychiatry* 1986; **21**: 1123–32.

40. Polich J, Howard L, Starr A. Effects of age on the P300 component of the event-related potential from auditory stimuli: peak definition, variation and measurement. *J Gerontol* 1985; **40**: 721–6.

41. Blackwood DHR, St Clair DM, Muir WJ *et al*. The development of Alzheimer's disease in Down's syndrome, assessed by auditory event-related potentials. *J Mental Deficiency Res* 1998; **32**: 439–53.

42. Binnie CD, Coles PA, Margerison JH. The influence of end-tidal carbon dioxide tension on EEG changes during routine hyperventilation in different age groups. *Electroencephalogr Clin Neurophysiol* 1969; **27**: 304.

11

Pharmacokinetic and Pharmacodynamic Considerations in Old Age Psychopharmacology

Fabrizio Schifano

St George's Hospital Medical School, Department of Addictive Behaviour and Psychological Medicine, London, UK

The elderly have the highest incidence of medical and psychiatric disorders. These conditions frequently occur simultaneously and are often chronic, lasting the lifetime of the individual. Consequently, the elderly require more medication than younger patients and even consumption of "over-the-counter" drugs is considerable among the aged[1]. Because of this multiple drugs administration, they frequently experience adverse side effects. Psychotropic drugs have often been involved in such interactions, and cause twice the incidence of side effects in elderly patients as they do in younger patients[1]. Drug interaction can produce a change in the pharmacological effect of a drug by altering activity at the site of action (a pharmacodynamic interaction), or by changing the plasma concentrations of a drug (a pharmacokinetic interaction), or both.

On the other hand, there has been a tendency of drug studies to focus on younger age groups and to exclude patients with co-morbidity or polypharmacy[2]. As a result, the generalization of current drug trials is a problem in old age psychiatry. Moreover, older adults respond less predictably than younger adults to most medication and this unpredictability is particularly evident among the frail elderly, who often suffer from central neurodegenerative disorders[3].

For these reasons, physicians treating patients with multiple medications may be overly concerned about the potential risks of treatment and deny the patient the chance of recovery[4]. Physicians should, however, remember that response is generally good for elderly people who have specific psychiatric disorders, as is the case with major depressive episodes, and that the risks of leaving the client untreated could be greater than the potential risks of treatment.

Although treatment of the elderly may be complex, with some knowledge of both the pharmacodynamics and pharmacokinetics basics it is something that is both manageable and rewarding. In this chapter, the changes in the effect of psychotropic drugs with aging in general terms will be highlighted.

PHARMACOKINETICS

With aging, changes can occur in one or more of the different pharmacokinetic parameters; absorption, distribution, metabolism and excretion.

Absorption may be slower in the elderly or delayed in onset and this is due to several factors: reduction in gastric pH, diminution of the size of the intestinal absorption area, reduced mesenteric blood flow (in general, the flow to all organs is diminished because of a decreased cardiac output). As a final consequence, the oral bioavailability of drugs may decrease in the elderly[5].

Distribution is grossly influenced by the composition of the body; the volume of distribution may be increased in elderly patients due to a greater percentage of adipose tissue[6]. Most of the psychotropic drugs (and especially sedatives, such as benzodiazepines) are stored in fat tissues and this constitutes a contributory factor for the significant elimination half-life increase that is usually observed in the elderly. In fact, the elimination half-life is determined by clearance (which is the rate of drug removal per unit of plasma concentration) and by volume of distribution itself. The higher the volume of distribution and/or the smaller the clearance, the longer will be the elimination half-life. Moreover, both the lean body mass and the bodily water[7] are decreased, so that ethanol (which is usually distributed across the bodily fluids) will show a higher concentration in the elderly than in younger groups[8]. Plasma protein binding is decreased in the elderly[1] because albumin concentration falls significantly. As a result, an increase in the free (non-bound) drug fraction in the plasma (the one that is able to pass the blood–brain barrier, but also the one that can determine the possible side effects) is observed. On the other hand, distribution of drugs into the brain may be decreased simply because cerebral blood flow (especially in arteriosclerotic patients) is usually diminished.

Metabolism. For psychotropics (lithium being the only notable exception), the most important metabolic processes are carried out in the liver (and elimination of metabolites will be made with faeces). As happens with most organs, the hepatic blood flow is diminished with age. The *metabolic transformation* processes are carried out by the microsomal enzymes in two different ways: hydroxylation and demethylation (processes that are significantly reduced with age) and conjugation with glucuronic acid (a process that is relatively unaffected in the elderly). This explains, for instance, the observation that benzodiazepines such as oxazepam and lorazepam (their major metabolic pathways involve glucuronidation) do not show clinically significant changes in pharmacokinetics with age[9]. On the other hand, chlordiazepoxide, diazepam and all the other pronordiazepam-like compounds (i.e. those that have N-desmethyldiazepam as the major metabolite) will show an increase of elimination half-life with age. In fact, these drugs are not metabolized by glucuronidation in the liver and, as a result, administration of these compounds in the elderly may cause a prolongation of action after a single dose and delayed accumulation on multiple dosing in the elderly[10].

Metabolic interactions usually take place in the liver and are of special interest, as multiple drugs prescription is common in advanced age. The genetically polymorphic cytochrome P450 2D6 (CYP2D6) is responsible for the metabolism of several psychotropics. CYP2D6 activity does not change with age[11]. CYP2D6 activity may be impaired by inhibitors such as paroxetine and fluoxetine[12], which can result in non-linear plasma drug concentration kinetics, as well as drug interaction when other drugs metabolized by CYP2D6 (such as desipramine, nortriptyline, neuroleptics, carbamazepine) are co-administered. Differently from paroxetine, fluoxetine and norfluoxetine (fluoxetine major metabolite), with sertraline the same pharmacokinetic parameters are found in both the young and the aged. Moreover, sertraline has much weaker inhibitory effects on CYP2D6[12].

Average dose adjustments for the aged can be derived from a simple equation and mean pharmacokinetic parameters from older and younger adults. However, individual dose adjustments (large variations in the decline of organ functions is possible) can be obtained from the drug clearance in a particular patient, where clearance/fractional bioavailability may be calculated from the area under the curve (AUC) of the drug in question[5].

Excretion.   Advanced age reduces renal function[6], with important implications for lithium prophylaxis. The most important pharmacokinetic change in old age is a decrease in the *excretory capacity* of the kidney, so that the elderly should be considered as renally insufficient patients[5]. Since lithium is excreted in the urine, guidelines for lithium prescription recommend using a single bedtime dosing regimen[13]. Due to these considerations, an implementation of specialized clinics to manage and monitor elderly patients maintained on lithium has been proposed and discussed.

PHARMACODYNAMICS

Provided that pharmacokinetic guidelines for these adjustments are taken into consideration, the same plasma concentration is achieved in the elderly as in the young adults. However, we are frequently confronted with pharmacodynamic changes in old age that alter sensitivity to drugs, irrespective of changes of drug disposition[5].

The central nervous system (CNS) is especially vulnerable. For example, aging can alter the sensitivity of the GABA carrier to some anesthetics (e.g. propofol and etomidate[14]). Moreover, in a well-known study[15] the effects of a single 10 mg dose of nitrazepam were compared with a placebo in healthy young and old people. Elderly people made significantly more mistakes in the psychomotor tests than the young, despite similar plasma concentration and elimination half-lives in both groups. The difference is probably explained by an increased sensitivity of the aging brain to the action of nitrazepam. It has been proposed[16] that, with advancing age, and prematurely in Alzheimer's dementia (AD), the declining mitochondrial ATP synthesis increases GABA synthesis (a factor possibly responsible for forebrain dystrophic axonal varicosities, losses of transmitter vesicles and swollen mitochondria, markers currently regarded as earliest signs of aging and AD). Moreover, the particular vulnerability of the elderly to sedatives could be explained by aging-related changes in the expression of the gamma (2S) and gamma (2L) subunits in various brain regions, which suggest the existence of aging-related changes in the sub-unit composition in the GABA-A receptors, which in turn might lead to changes in receptor pharmacology[17]. Lastly, it seems that the activity of GABA-A transaminase (an enzyme that degrades GABA to succinic semialdehyde) is inhibited, which results in elevation of GABA content in the brain in some age-related neuropsychiatric disorders such as AD[18].

The elderly are particularly sensitive to drug-induced parkinsonism[19], which can reflect decreases with age in *dopamine* (DA) turnover and the suggested[20,21] age-dependent deficit of the dopaminergic system, presumably related to a reduced number/activity of nigrostriatal and mesolimbic neurons. In humans, an age-related decline of binding of a ligand for dopamine transporters, specifically to the striatum, has been found, at the rate of 6.6% per decade[22].

The response to agents with strong anticholinergic properties (tricyclic antidepressants; classical antipsychotics) increases in old age and may be accompanied by impairment of intellectual capabilities, agitation and, ultimately, delirium[23]. However, non-demented elderly patients with psychiatric problems seem to tolerate psychotropic drugs (with respect to the impact on their cognitive competency) much better than patients with AD[24]. Age-related reduced responsivity of the cholinergic system in the hippocampus has been well documented[25], but also disturbances in GABAergic/cholinergic interaction may play a key role in age-related cognitive dysfunction[26]. During aging, higher affinity nicotine binding in the frontal cortex and the hippocampal formation decreases and these reductions may predispose the neo- and archicortex to the loss of nicotine *acetylcholine* receptor proteins observed in age-associated neurodegenerative conditions[27].

Studies in humans and primates suggest that the aged brain is prone to the degeneration of the locus coeruleus (LC)[28]; the ascending dorsal noradrenergic bundle of the LC is involved in cognitive processes such as memory, learning and selective attention. Moreover, a profound *noradrenaline* depletion in the pre-frontal cortex (an area involved in certain cognitive functions, such as prevention of distractability by irrelevant stimuli) has been described in the elderly[29]. Together with the partial loss of CNS noradrenergic neurons, a compensatory activation of remaining CNS noradrenergic neurons has been described[30], which can explain the enhanced responsiveness (both in normal older subjects and with patients with AD) to noradrenergic agents such as yohimbine[31].

The central serotonergic system is also adversely affected by aging, so that it has been proposed that possible reduction in humans of 5-HT$_{2A}$ receptors and *serotonin* reuptake sites may contribute to ethanol consumption, depression and cognitive dysfunctions frequently seen in the elderly. These changes may alter the effectiveness of serotonergic drugs[32,33].

During the normal process of aging a number of changes in the glutamatergic system (involved in processes such as motor behavior, cognition and emotion), and especially a decrease in the density of *glutamate* NMDA receptors, have been described[34]. Glutamate interacts with other neurotransmitters to conform the substrates of specific circuits of the brain that are relevant to aging. Impairment of intracellular energy metabolism associated with hyperactivation of glutamate receptors may contribute to the neuronal death seen in neurodegenerative disorders[35]; the extent of glutamate neurotoxicity in the hippocampus is highly age-dependent, with mature animals' hippocampi more vulnerable to glutamate-induced cell death[36].

On the whole, aging is associated with changes in the regional brain chemistry and the brain multi-chemical networking profile (MCNP). In fact, there is an increase in overall chemical correlation in MCNP within and across all brain regions with increased age. This increased correlation may reflect an adaptive or compensatory response (possibly related to the elongation of the dendrites with aging) to the reduced levels of regional brain chemicals[37]. Lastly, a diminished efficiency of the homeostatic mechanisms has been described in the aging brain, in part because of the reduced activity of various neurotransmitter systems. Counter-regulatory processes are therefore reduced and reactions to drugs may be increased[23].

PRACTICAL ISSUES

Bearing in mind the above-described pharmacokinetic and pharmacodynamic changes of psychotropic drugs in the elderly, a few principles could be recommended as prescribing guidelines[38]: one should become familiar with a number of preparations and preferably administer them; use as few drugs as possible (including drugs for non-psychiatric conditions); 'keep it as simple as possible': give written instructions; avoid depot-forms, the treatment should be started in low dosages (1/5 to 1/4 of average adult dosage) and slowly increased (no sooner than every 5–7 days[39]); the maintenance dosage is about 1/3–1/2[40] of average adult dosage ('start low and go slow'), but some elderly patients might need and can tolerate full doses[8]. The times required to reach steady-state therapeutic levels are longer.

Moreover, it ought to be emphasized that some psychotropics are more suitable for the elderly than others. For the treatment of affective disorders, *tricyclic antidepressants* are efficacious and inexpensive, but *SSRIs* and newer antidepressants are better tolerated and safer in overdose[41]. With respect to the putative diminished 5-HT responsivity in this population, the ability to identify SSRI non-responders via 5-HT challenge in combination with neuroimaging measures may have important clinical utility[33]. Among the SSRIs, preference is possibly given to sertraline[12]. The selective *MAO-A inhibitors* have not been extensively studied in the elderly, but they have definitely overcome the use of the classical MAO inhibitors. *Lithium* is still the mainstay for the treatment of bipolar disorders, but careful dosage and monitoring of plasma concentration are necessarily required. On the other hand, bipolar elderly patient responders to *valproate* ought to achieve higher serum concentrations of valproate itself[42].

The age-related changes in the pharmacokinetics and pharmacodynamics of the *benzodiazepines* (still the most frequently prescribed drugs for anxiety in the elderly) recommend preferential use of those agents that are metabolized via conjugation (oxazepam); *risperidone* (which is better tolerated in the elderly) may be used as an alternative. However, together with the sedation increase, with a sedative/hypnotic prescription a cognitive function decrease is observed in the elderly, with consequent risks of falls and injury (especially if the diazepam-equivalent dosage is higher and if the patient is prescribed with more different drugs)[43]. According to some suggestions[44], because of the high level of co-morbidity between generalized anxiety disorder and major depression in late life and the observation that anxiety is usually secondary to depression, antidepressants constitute the primary pharmacological treatment for many older people. For the treatment of insomnia, both zopiclone and temazepam are to be considered as effective hypnotics, but the first shows a superiority on sleep architecture[45]. New promising agents, such as *cholecystokinin-B receptor antagonists*, seem to be specific, in aged animals, for an improvement of sleep quality[46]. For the treatment of psychotic syndromes, due to the elderly extreme sensitivity to parkinsonian side effects and to the anticholinergic properties of the *classical antipsychotics*, attention is given to the *newer antipsychotics*, but there is still a paucity of data. Clozapine may be a useful drug but adverse effects can occur[47].

Notwithstanding the aforementioned I am in agreement with Jovic[38], who stated that "psychotropic drugs cannot compensate for the lack of human contacts, devotion and intensive relationships, but complement them".

REFERENCES

1. Roberts J, Tumer N. Pharmacodynamic basis for altered drug action in the elderly. *Clin Geriat Med* 1998; **4**: 127–49.
2. Banerjee S, Dickinson E. Evidence-based health care in old age psychiatry. *Int J Psychiat* 1997; **27**: 283–92.
3. Zubenko GS, Sunderland T. Geriatric psychopharmacology: why does age matter? *Harvard Rev Psychiat* 2000; **7**: 311–33.
4. Tourigny-Rivard MF. Treating depression in old age: is it worth the effort? *Psychiat J Univ Ottawa* 1989; **14**: 367–9.
5. Turnheim K. Drug dosage in the elderly. Is it rational? *Drugs Aging* 1998; **13**: 357–79.
6. Rudorfer MV. Pharmacokinetics of psychotropic drugs in special population. *J Clin Psychiat* 1993; **54** (suppl): 50–54.
7. Chang L, Ernst T, Poland RE, Jenden DJ. *In vivo* proton magnetic resonance spectroscopy of the normal aging human brain. *Life Sci* 1996; **58**: 2049–56.
8. Lader M. Neuropharmacology and pharmacokinetics of psychotropic drugs in old age. In Copeland JRM, Abou-Saleh M, Blazer G, eds, *Principles and Practices of Geriatric Psychiatry*, 1st edn. Chichester: Wiley, 1994; 79–81.
9. Greenblatt DJ. Clinical pharmacokinetics of oxazepam and lorazepam. *Clin Pharmacokinet* 1981; **6**: 89–105.
10. Vozeh S. Pharmacokinetics of benzodiazepines in old age. *Schweiz Med Wochenschr* 1981; **111**: 1789–93.
11. Shulman RW, Ozdemir V. Psychotropic medications and cytochrome P450 2D6: pharmacokinetic considerations in the elderly. *Can J Psychiatr* 1997; **42** (suppl 1): 45–9S.
12. Preskorn SH. Recent pharmacological advances in antidepressant therapy for the elderly. *Am J Med* 1993; **94**: 2S–12S.
13. Shulman KI, Mackenzie S, Hardy B. The clinical use of lithium carbonate in old age: a review. *Prog Neuropsychopharmacol Biol Psychiatr* 1987; **11**: 159–64.
14. Keita H, Lasocki S, Henzel-Rouelle D *et al.* Aging decreases the sensitivity of GABA carrier to propofol and etomidate. *Br J Anaesth* 1998; **81**: 249–50.
15. Castleden CM, George CF, Marcer D, Hallett C. Increased sensitivity to nitrazepam in old age. *Br Med J* 1977; **1**: 10–12.
16. Marczinski TJ. GABA-ergic deafferentation hypothesis of brain aging and Alzheimer's disease revisited. *Brain Res Bull* 1998; **45**: 341–79.
17. Khan ZU, Gutierrez A, Miralles CP, De Blas AL. The gamma subunits of the native GABAA/benzodiazepine receptors. *Neurochem Res* 1996; **21**: 147–59.
18. Sherif FM, Ahmed SS. Basic aspects of GABA-transaminase in neuropsychiatric disorders. *Clin Biochem* 1995; **28**: 145–54.
19. Marti Masso JF, Poza JJ. Drug-induced or aggravated parkinsonism: clinical signs and the changing pattern of implicated drugs. *Neurologia* 1996; **11**: 10–15.
20. Miguez JM, Aldegunde M, Paz-Valinas L *et al.* Selective changes in the contents of noradrenaline, dopamine and serotonin in rat brain during aging. *J Neural Transm* 1999; **106**: 1089–98.
21. Woods J, Druse MJ. Effects of chronic ethanol consumption and aging on dopamine, serotonin and metabolites. *J Neurochem* 1996; **66**: 2168–78.
22. Pirker W, Asenbaum S, Hauk M *et al.* Imaging serotonin and dopamine transporters with 123I-beta-CIT SPECT: binding kinetics and effects of normal aging. *J Nucl Med* 2000; **41**: 36–44.
23. Turnheim K. Adverse effects of psychotropic drugs in the elderly. *Wien Klin Wochenschr* 2000; **112**: 394–401.
24. Thienhaus OJ, Allen A, Bennett JA *et al.* Anticholinergic serum levels and cognitive performance. *Eur Arch Psychiatr Clin Neurosci* 1990; **240**: 28–33.
25. Umegaki H, Tanaya N, Shinkai T, Iguchi A. The metabolism of plasma glucose and cathecolamines in Alzheimer's disease. *Exp Gerontol* 2000; **35**: 1373–82.
26. Araki T, Kato H, Fujiwara T, Itoyama Y. Regional age-related alterations in cholinergic and GABAergic receptors in the rat brain. *Mech Aging Dev* 1996; **88**: 49–60.
27. Hellstrohm-Lindahl E, Court JA. Nicotinic acetylcholinic receptors during prenatal development and brain pathology in human aging. *Behav Brain Res* 2000; **113**: 159–68.
28. Tejani-Butt SM, Ordway GA. Effect of age on [3H]nisoxetine binding to uptake sites for norepinephrine in the locus coeruleus of humans. *Brain Res* 1992; **583**: 312–15.
29. Coull JT. Pharmacological manipulations of the α_2 noradrenergic system. Effects on cognition. *Drugs Aging* 1994; **5**: 116–26.
30. Raskind MA, Peskind ER, Holmes C, Goldstein DS. Patterns of cerebrospinal fluid cathecols support increased central noradrenergic

responsiveness in aging and Alzheimer's disease. *Biol Psychiat* 1999; **46**: 756–65.

31. Peskind ER, Wingerson D, Murray S *et al*. Effects of Alzheimer's disease and normal aging on cerebrospinal fluid norepinephrine responses to yohimbine and clonidine. *Arch Gen Psychiat* 1995; **52**: 774–82.

32. Druse MJ, Tajuddin MF, Ricken JD. Effects of chronic ethanol consumption and aging on 5-HT$_{2A}$ receptors and 5-HT reuptake sites. *Alcohol Clin Exp Res* 1997; **21**: 1157–64.

33. Nobler MS, Mann JJ, Sackheim HA. Serotonin, cerebral blood flow, and cerebral metabolic rate in geriatric major depression and normal aging. *Brain Res Brain Res Rev* 1999; **30**: 250–63.

34. Segovia G, Porras A, Del Arco A, Mora F. Glutamatergic neurotransmission in aging: a critical perspective. *Mech Ageing Dev* 2001; **122**: 1–29.

35. Ikonomidou C, Turski L. Neurodegenerative disorders: clues from glutamate and energy metabolism. *Crit Rev Neurobiol* 1996; **10**: 239–63.

36. Liu Z, Stafstrom CE, Sarkisian M *et al*. Age-dependent effects of glutamate toxicity in the hippocampus. *Brain Res Dev Brain Res* 1996; **97**: 178–84.

37. Grachev ID, Swarnkar A, Szeverenyi NM *et al*. Aging alters the multichemical networking profile of the human brain: an *in vivo* (1)H-MRS study of young vs. middle-aged subjects. *J Neurochem* 2001; **77**: 292–303.

38. Jovic N. Ambulatory psychopharmacotherapy of older subjects. *Schweiz Rundsch Med Prax* 1990; **79**: 608–12.

39. Tierney J. Practical issues in geriatric psychopharmacology. *J Ind Med Assoc* 1999; **97**: 145–7.

40. Bauer J. Special characteristics of psychopharmacotherapy of older patients. *Fortschr Med* 1996; **114**: 297–302.

41. Heger U, Moller HJ. Pharmacotherapy of depression in old age. *Nervenarzt* 2000; **71**: 1–8.

42. Niedermeier NA, Nasrallah HA. Clinical correlates of response to valproate in geriatric inpatients. *Ann Clin Psychiat* 1998; **10**: 165–8.

43. Gales BJ, Menard SM. Relationship between the administration of selected medications and falls in hospitalized elderly patients. *Ann Pharmacother* 1995; **29**: 354–8.

44. Flint AJ. Management of anxiety in late life. *J Geriat Psychiat Neurol* 1998; **11**: 194–200.

45. Hemmeter U, Moller M, Bischof R *et al*. Effects of zopiclone and temazepam on sleep EEG parameters, psychomotor and memory functions in healthy elderly volunteers. *Psychopharmacology (Berl)* 2000; **147**: 384–96.

46. Crespi F. Cholecystokinin-B receptor antagonists improve 'aged' sleep: a new class of sleep modulators? *Methods Find Exp Clin Pharmacol* 1999; **21**: 31–8.

47. Pitner JK, Mintzer JE, Pennypacker LC, Jackson CW. Efficacy and adverse effects of clozapine in four elderly psychotic patients. *J Clin Psychiat* 1995; **56**: 180–85.

12

Normal Ageing—A Problematical Concept

D. B. Bromley

Department of Psychology, University of Liverpool, UK

INTRODUCTION

The word "normal" is used to refer to what is statistically normal, that is within the average range. The range can vary somewhat, say from the middle 50% of a normal distribution to perhaps the middle 80%, depending upon one's purpose. The word is also used to refer to prototypical members of a category, members with characteristics that best exemplify the category as a whole. The word is used to refer to what is socially prescribed and expected, such as the usual forms of appearance and behaviour for a given occasion in a community. Another usage refers to a standard pattern or sequence of events that have a high probability of occurrence, such as impairment of vision and hearing in later life.

NORMAL AND PATHOLOGICAL AGEING

With regard to human ageing, the word "normal" is used in all the above senses, depending upon the context. In professional gerontology, however, the phrase "normal ageing" usually implies the existence of a contrasting condition or process, viz. "pathological ageing". Difficulties arise because normal ageing and pathological ageing are conceptually interdependent. The main historical landmark in attempts to distinguish between them was the publication of Korenchevsky's *Physiological and Pathological Ageing*[1]. Korenchevsky drew attention to the fact that some physiological functions in some elderly human subjects were equal to or superior to those of chronologically younger subjects. Psychological research into sensorimotor and cognitive performance often reveals that some elderly subjects perform as well as or better than the average younger subject.

On the basis of evidence that some individuals show relatively little physiological impairment with age, at least until late life, Korenchevsky inferred the existence of primary (non-pathological) ageing. On the basis of evidence that other individuals show substantially greater than average impairment earlier in adult life, he inferred the existence of secondary (pathological) ageing.

These two inferences, however, are simply two versions of the same argument, namely, that ageing is characterized by wide differences between individuals. If we plot the distributions of scores on physiological or psychological functions for several age groups in a cross-sectional study, we often find considerable overlap between even widely spaced age groups. If the distributions of performance scores for the same respondents at different ages in a longitudinal study are compared, we usually find that individuals tend to retain their position (rank order) relative to other respondents. A minority, however, show decline relative to

their position at earlier ages. These are the people who appear to exhibit pathological ageing. Thus, individual differences in normal ageing tend to be maintained, even though there is a decline with age, on average, over the period studied. These differences are brought about by various causes, including genetic characteristics, life-history events, life styles and environmental conditions.

Even among the community-dwelling elderly, there are wide variations in physical and mental health and wide variations in such things as living conditions, social support, stress and coping strategies and health. In a multicultural society, the range of differences between individuals at later ages is likely to be very wide. The process of normal ageing is a social as well as a biological process. That is to say, society *prescribes* or *normalizes* various stages in the life cycle, so that there are typical ages for the completion of full-time education, marriage (or sexual partnership), parenthood, occupational status and retirement. Such arrangements may change from one generation to the next. This, together with secular changes in health, longevity, life styles and so on, make the concept of "normal ageing" a moving target. Flynn has reported substantial secular (cohort) effects on measures of intelligence[2]. Consider how the contraceptive pill and hormone replacement therapy have changed the life styles of women. Consider also how drugs, AIDS, migration and economic factors may affect ageing in sections of the population. These are technical issues for demography and epidemiology.

It is possible to demonstrate general age trends and effects. For example, the sex difference in longevity is well established; there is a differential decline in fluid and crystallized psychological abilities; anatomical and physiological functions have their characteristic normal patterns of change with age. There are some similarities between the normal (common) effects of ageing and the effects of pathologies such as Alzheimer's disease, as shown by neurological and psychological tests. These trends and effects are compatible with the view that ageing is the result of a multiplicity of causes. They are not proof that there are two sorts of ageing: pathological and normal (non-pathological)[3]. On the other hand, there is the question of whether senile dementia of the Alzheimer type or multi-infarct dementia are the end-results of a normal intrinsic ageing process that would affect anyone who lived long enough, or whether they are abnormal conditions induced by genetic faults, life-history factors or specific extrinsic causes, such as infection or exposure to noxious substances. Genetic mutations increase with advancing age, and may affect performance before the obvious signs and symptoms of disease.

The argument in favour of the notion that there are two sorts of ageing—normal and pathological—is supported by evidence that people suffering from identifiable pathologies, such as cancer, heart disease or diabetes, have reduced life expectations and are functionally less competent in some respects (see van Boxtel *et al.*[5]). Moreover, some of these disorders are age-related; some, such as Simmonds' disease, mimic the normal (usual) effects of ageing. Individuals who survive to a late age do not have a history of such disorders. The difficulty with this argument is that it is circular: pathological conditions are conditions that increase the likelihood of functional impairment and death; conditions that increase the likelihood of functional impairment and death are pathological. If an adverse effect commonly associated with age is not attributable to pathology, then, by definition as it were, it is "normal". If the underlying cause is identified, it is then labelled "pathological". Diseases can be regarded as concepts rather than entities (unless a cause can be found), in which case the distinction between normal and pathological ageing is a matter of definition, not an empirical issue. The empirical issue is how to identify and deal with the many age-related causes of impairment, regardless of whether they affect many people or just a few.

In order to demonstrate the existence of pathological ageing (as distinct from pathologies that increase functional impairment and the probability of death), we would need to show stepwise discontinuities in age trends, or departures from the "normal" distribution of differences in performance. Stepwise discontinuities and bimodal distributions are not common in the sorts of samples recruited for cross-sectional or longitudinal research in ageing.

Defining pathology in terms of a marked deviation from normal function means that the cumulative adverse effects of ageing eventually become pathological relative to standards for younger people but not older people—hence the view that there are many normal old people but few healthy ones! Stoller reported a tendency for older people to interpret their symptoms in terms of pain, discomfort and interference with their activities, rather than in terms of a possible medical condition[5].

Improvements in living conditions, diet, exercise and medical treatment have the effect of extending the average span of life, and so have the effect of redefining what we mean by normal and pathological ageing[6]. The distinction between the "young old", and the "old old" is now well established. Normal ageing can be taken to mean that set of intrinsic age-related effects that characterizes the adult life of people who occupy the middle ground of a distribution of age at death, or that characterizes and explains the average elderly person's functional competence. Pathological ageing can be taken to refer to the intrinsic age-related effects that characterize people who die relatively young, or who perform well below comparable people of the same age, as a consequence of these effects. The problem here is to demonstrate a causal connection between age-related ailments and the so-called "intrinsic" effects of ageing.

Normal or intrinsic ageing can be regarded as a species-specific process of degeneration, subject to a degree of variability depending upon initial genetic endowment and subsequent environmental conditions. Pathological ageing is any substantial deviation from the normal (standard or common) pattern of age-related changes.

THE CAUSES OF AGEING

When we examine the distribution of age at death for human populations, we find a relatively "normal" distribution on which is superimposed a "tail" representing infant mortality, accidents and premature deaths in early adult life. A normal distribution is typically the result of a multiplicity of independent contributory causes. The distributions of scores for physiological and psychological functions, obtained from reasonably large samples of the sort usually recruited in studies of ageing, tend to be relatively normal. So the assumption is that these effects, too, are the result of a multiplicity of independent causes. The aim of such studies is to identify the factors that account for most of the observed variation[7,8]. In some research studies, gender, education, health and intelligence account for a substantial part of the variation in psychological performance, leaving chronological age accounting for little.

The existence of trends and effects associated with chronological age does not imply a causal agent—"ageing". As we have seen, ageing is simply a convenient label for a variety of age-related primary and secondary causes of impairment. Some of these causes no doubt interact and produce many sorts of indirect and long-term effects. For example, injuries, stresses, learning experiences and many other eventualities can occur at different ages. They may have different consequences because other age-related changes have or have not taken place, and because of differences in people's biological, psychological and social characteristics. In any event, given the complexity of the processes involved in human ageing and the long periods of time over which the processes occur, a considerable amount of "turbulence" in the effects of ageing is to be expected. Even small differences in initial personal characteristics and circumstances could lead to wide differences, in physical and mental health and performance, between individuals at later ages.

On this view, older people who are physiologically and psychologically very competent are simply those who have a superior biological constitution, have suffered fewer or less serious adverse effects from the many age-related causes of impairment, and have been able to take advantage of circumstances that promote health and well-being. People who survive to very late life with high levels of physiological and psychological competence are sometimes referred to as a "biological elite". Such people occupy, say, the top 10% of a distribution of physiological or psychological performance. They are studied retrospectively in the hope of identifying some of the factors that contribute to longevity and functional competence in late life.

Older people at the other end of the distribution are those who have not had the same benefits, and are regarded as suffering from one or other of the disorders of late life. On this view, the elderly who occupy either the upper or the lower tail of a relatively smooth normal distribution are different only in degree, not in kind, from those that occupy the middle ground. Of course, future research may identify specific positive and negative factors that will help us to account further for the observed variations in longevity, health and performance.

BASIC RESEARCH AND INTERVENTION

Health, education and gender are important variables in basic research in ageing. Controlling for them often substantially reduces the effects of chronological age (the usual index of "ageing"). It is possible to contrast the age trends in physiological or psychological performance for subjects suffering from known pathologies with the age trends for subjects free from such pathologies. Rabbitt[9] reports that when adults with diabetes are compared with subjects who do not have diabetes but are comparable in other respects, including intelligence, the diabetics perform less well on measures of information processing. Rabbitt also reports that moderate deafness can have a similar, indirect, deleterious effect on information processing. This supports the use of specific health measures as co-variates in research on ageing.

One of the difficulties in both cross-sectional and longitudinal studies of ageing is that samples of older respondents are biased in at least two ways. First, volunteer respondents tend to be physically, psychologically and socially advantaged, relative to non-volunteers of the same age. Sampling bias is a major obstacle to research in ageing. It restricts our ability to generalize our findings to the wider population. Second, older respondents, even older volunteers, are more likely than younger respondents to have various physical and psychological impairments that adversely affect their performance: for example, lack of exercise may impair cardiac function; poorer vision or hearing may slow reaction times and increase errors; social isolation may increase anxiety or depression; disuse, as well as irreversible deterioration, may impair performance, as in driving or playing games; training and practice can help compensate for these losses. These and other sampling biases mean that cross-sectional or longitudinal comparisons are likely to be distorted. If we do not have data on relevant background variables, then we cannot take them into account when we try to interpret age-related effects on performance.

A distinction can be drawn between research samples that are actually representative of their age group, and samples of other sorts. People who survive to later ages differ in a number of ways—biologically, psychologically and socially—from non-survivors. Thus, a representative sample drawn from an older population is not directly comparable with a representative sample drawn from a younger population. Matching members of an older sample with members of a younger sample means using samples biased with respect to the parent population. In a longitudinal study, dropouts have the effect of changing the population represented by the remaining sample.

Research samples consist of two main sorts: (a) volunteers recruited by advertising, "snowballing" or other forms of gentle persuasion; and (b) subjects recruited in ways that make it difficult for them not to take part. In the latter sort of recruiting, the benefits of participation are held to be of direct personal benefit, or in the public interest, as with samples based on medical registers. Risch et al.[10] report on the difficulties encountered in recruiting "normal" volunteers for psychiatric research. Systematic psychiatric screening, over the telephone, failed to exclude 25% of unsatisfactory volunteers, as judged by subsequent tests. However, in a smaller subsequent study, a warning that reimbursement would be withheld if their toxicology test proved positive was effective. In reply, Halbreich confirms the need for close examination of research volunteers, but raises questions about how to achieve this, and about the ethical issues involved[11]. He also considers that screening normal volunteers should include a family history.

Most psychological studies of ageing appear to assume, rather than test, that their volunteers are "normal", although there may be routine mention of the fact that the respondents are free of obvious physical or mental impairment. The usual assumption is that volunteer samples are biased towards better-than-average health, ability, education and social status. Todd et al.[12] describe ways of improving volunteer rates. Bromley (op. cit.) describes a number of methodological difficulties encountered in research into normal ageing, including the difficulties associated with sampling and psychological measurement.

The effects of age, cohort and time of measurement are difficult to disentangle. The method of age-matched controls is often used to compare normal with pathological ageing. The problem here, as in selecting a sample of normal respondents, is how to determine which variables need to be controlled. There are numerous biological, psychological, social and environmental factors known or thought to be involved in ageing, and doubtless many unknown factors. The onus is on the investigator to justify the inclusion or exclusion of particular controls, and on the critic to identify other possibilities. Research needs to move beyond superficial and crude controls for gender, socio-economic status and self-reported health. How this move is to be achieved is itself a research issue (see e.g. Fox et al.[13]). Social groups that have experienced specific long-term life styles, for example in relation to diet, exercise, exposure to toxic substances, can be compared with "normal" social groups in relation to ageing.

Interventions designed to improve the functional capacities of the elderly have had some success but leave some questions unanswered. A sense of control and efficacy appears to be an important and modifiable personality characteristic in later life[14], but intervention raises ethical and management issues. Physical exercise is effective in improving physiological functions even late in life, but prospective studies are needed to exclude the effects of sample bias and lack of control subjects[15]. Rubin et al.[16] describe a prospective study of the onset of dementia in apparently normal elderly volunteers.

Training and practice on sensorimotor and cognitive tasks improve the performance of elderly subjects, but improve the performance of younger adults too. The effects may not generalize much beyond the training task or persist long after training is discontinued. The main point, however, is that performance on the first occasion of an unfamiliar task (in a typical laboratory study) is not necessarily indicative of practised performance on a familiar task of the sort encountered in daily life[17,18]. Recently, more interest has been shown in the role of crystallized abilities (acquired mental skills) in adult life[19]. Practice and experience help to explain the maintenance of high levels of performance in many normal old people.

The concept of normal ageing refers not only to humans but also to other animal species, such as flatworms, rats and monkeys. Plants, too, have their characteristic life cycles. Different strains within a species have their characteristic, normal, patterns of ageing. Selective breeding and treatments, such as dietary restriction and brain chemistry, are used to explore the causes of longevity and age-related pathologies.

It is impossible within the scope of a short article to do justice to the numerous and diverse publications on "normal ageing" that a computer-assisted literature search can identify. The concept of "normal ageing" can be used to refer to various phenomena. The key question is, "Normal in respect of what?"

CONCLUSION

Normal ageing can be defined as a cumulative process of adverse changes in physiological, psychological and social functions that, in a general way, characterize average members of successive older cohorts of adults. This process is at present irreversible and to some extent predictable, but it produces a wide range of differences between individuals in age of onset and rate of change. To a limited extent, people can retard and ameliorate these adverse changes.

Normal ageing is a "socially constructed" concept, referring to an accepted range of variation in the health, appearance and performance of adults at different ages. It is also a "scientifically constructed" concept, referring to research findings in gerontology and other disciplines. Gerontologists find the concept of pathological or abnormal ageing useful in identifying exceptions to and deviations from the normal pattern, but the distinction between normal and pathological ageing remains problematical.

REFERENCES

1. Korenchevsky V. In Bourne GH, ed. *Physiological and Pathological Ageing*. New York: Karger, 1961.
2. Flynn JR. Massive IQ gains in fourteen nations: what IQ tests really measure. *Psychological Bulletin* 1987; **101**: 171–91.
3. Bromley DB. *Behavioural Gerontology: Central Issues in the Psychology of Ageing*. Chichester: John Wiley, 1990.
4. van Boxtel MP, Buntix F, Houx PJ *et al.* The relation between morbidity and cognitive performance in a normal ageing population. *J Gerontol A: Biol Sci Med Sci* 1998; **53**(2): M147–54.

5. Stoller EP. Interpretations of symptoms by older people. A health diary study of illness behavior. *J Aging Health* 1993; **5**(1): 58–81.

6. Verbrugge LM. Longer life but worsening health? Trends in health and mortality of middle-aged and older persons. *Milbank Mem Fund Qu/Health Society* 1984; **62**: 475–519.

7. Shock NW, Greulich RE, Andres R *et al. Normal Human Aging: The Baltimore Longitudinal Study of Aging.* Washington, DC: US Government Printing Office, 1984.

8. Busse EW, Maddox GL. *The Duke Longitudinal Studies of Normal Aging, 1955–1980. An Overview of History, Design and Findings.* New York: Springer, 1985.

9. Rabbitt P. Applied cognitive gerontology: some problems, methodologies and data. *Appl Cogn Psychol*, 1990; **4**: 225–46.

10. Risch SC, Lewine RJ, Jewart RD *et al.* Ensuring the normalcy of "normal" volunteers. *Am J Psychiat* 1990; **147**: 682–3.

11. Halbreich U. Dr Halbreich replies. *Am J Psychiat* 1990; **147**: 683.

12. Todd M, Davis KE, Cafferty TP. Who volunteers for adult developmental research? Research findings and practical steps to reach low volunteering groups. *Int J Aging Hum Dev*, 1984; **18**: 177–84.

13. Fox NC, Freeborough PA, Rossor MN. Visualisation and quantification of rates of atrophy in Alzheimer's disease. *Lancet* 1996; **348**: 94–7.

14. Rodin J, Timko C, Harris S. The construct of social control: biological and psychosocial correlates. In Lawton MP, Maddox GL, eds. *Annual Review of Gerontology and Geriatrics*, Vol. 5. New York: Springer, 1985.

15. Thornton EW. *Exercise and Ageing. An Unproven Relationship.* Liverpool: Institute of Human Ageing, 1984.

16. Rubin EH, Storandt M, Miller JP *et al.* A prospective study of cognitive function and onset of dementia in cognitively healthy elders. *Arch Neurol* 1998; **55**(3): 395–401.

17. Plemons JK, Willis SL, Baltes PB. Modifiability of fluid intelligence in aging: a short-term longitudinal approach. *J Gerontol* 1978; **33**: 224–31.

18. Rabbitt PMA. A fresh look at changes in reaction times in old age. In Stein DG, ed. *The Psychobiology of Aging.* New York: Elsevier/North Holland, 1980.

19. Sternberg RJ, Wagner RK (eds). *Practical Intelligence, Nature and Origins of Competence in the Everyday World.* Cambridge: Cambridge University Press, 1986.

Cohort Studies

Patrick Rabbitt

Age and Cognitive Performance Research Centre, University of Manchester, UK

The word "cohort" originally designated a Roman military unit but has now become a technical term in population studies as a collective noun for any peer group, band or sub-set of individuals under investigation. In current usage, a cohort is any group of individuals who are linked in some way. This link may be experience of common life events, such as particular pathologies, or life transitions, such as menopause, or experience of a particular historical event or socio-economic condition. In gerontology the most common defining factor is age group, and this should be assumed unless some other usage is specified. In gerontology, "cohort" has become a more acceptable term to specify chronological age than the often misused "generation", which has an equally precise and different meaning in studies of kinship terminology.

Note that "age group" may be very loosely defined. For example cohort members may have all been born, or died, in the same week, month, year, decade or even century. The defining boundaries of cohorts cause methodological difficulties because the effects of age are confounded with those of birth cohort and period. That is, groups of people born at the same time (birth cohorts) are by definition all of the same age, and have all lived through the same historical period. Groups of the same age (age cohorts) are not necessarily born at the same time, and so may have experienced different historical periods and events such as wars, with attendant differences in social circumstances. Groups of different ages (different age cohorts) also have not shared particular historical events or periods and, to the extent that their experience of a historical event has overlapped, they have been affected by it at different ages.

Cohort analysis is the methodology of designing and analysing studies to make inferences about the behaviour or condition of a particular sub-group without the necessity for studying them again after one or more successive time periods. It is now the most common methodology used to study changes in behaviour or attitudes, biological and cognitive effects of human ageing and social, political and cultural change. Cohort analyses in developmental and ageing studies are distinguished from longitudinal analyses, in which the same birth cohorts are re-examined at intervals over a period of time. A compromise is cross-sequential analyses, in which different age groups and birth cohorts are repeatedly re-examined and compared with themselves and with others at different measurement points.

Unfortunately, although cohort analyses always allow us to identify and study each of these effects, they do not provide any direct way of examining all of them, independently, in a single study. One reason for this is sampling variability. That is, any cohort samples we can obtain and compare are unlikely to be precisely comparable. A related difficulty, which usually guarantees that samples in gerontological comparisons will not be comparable, is sample attrition. As cohorts age, they lose members and so alter in terms of their credibility as representative samples of the populations from which they were initially selected. The most important limitation on cohort analyses is that there is no way to avoid confounding at least two of the three variables in which we are usually interested: age, cohort and period. This imposes very inconvenient restrictions on statistical analysis; for example, in a multivariate regression analysis, all three variables cannot simultaneously be entered as variables in a regression equation. Although many attempts have been made, and much has been written on the subject, there are still no statistical methods that can clearly separate the effects of birth cohort and period from the effects of ageing. Perhaps the most lucid and helpful discussions have been by Costa and McCrae[1] and Palmore[2]. The current consensus is that decisions must rest on scientific judgement as to which two of the three possible effects are likely to be important, so that the third can be omitted. The obligation to carry out exploratory data analyses to ensure that the effect that is to be neglected is in fact, statistically unimportant, should not need emphasis.

The inevitable confound between age, cohort and period effects is awkward because it means that we cannot use this most economical of all research strategies to solve all of the many problems connected with ageing. However, bearing their overriding limitation in mind, it must be stressed that cohort analyses are not merely an economical, but methodologically flawed, substitute for laborious longitudinal studies. They rather provide a means by which we can answer classes of questions that cannot be approached in any other way. The fact that the cohorts need not contain the same individuals is a statistical advantage as well as logistical convenience. For example, it can be very useful to sample quite different populations of the same birth cohort at different times in their lives so as to make an intracohort trend study. There are also unique advantages in comparing *n* quite different age samples of a population recruited at successive periods of time. This allows us to draw up what has become known as a "standard cohort table", in which the different age cohorts are ordered in rows, and the successive years in which these different age groups were sampled are ordered in columns. This allows us, at least, a rapid and convenient way to carry out exploratory analyses of our data. We can pick out intracohort trends, which become apparent by scanning down the diagonals; that is, we can see how members of a particular age group (whether represented by the same individuals followed over time, or by quite different samples) are affected by both the passage of time (and so, among other factors, by their own biological ageing) and also by changes in the social, economic or epidemiological contexts in which they were studied. Within each of these sampling periods we can compare age cohort differences by scanning down the columns. Finally, by scanning along the rows, we can examine period effects which occur as one age cohort replaces another.

No single technique of comparison, whether cohort analysis, longitudinal analysis or even cross-sequential analysis, can provide a universal methodological panacea. Rather, each can solve problems that the others cannot approach, and none save us the effort of carefully thinking through the questions that we wish to ask of our data, and intelligently considering the implications of the comparisons we must make to answer them. To study the effect of ageing we must simultaneously acquire both cross-sectional and multiple longitudinal data and interpret them as sensibly as we can.

REFERENCES

1. Costa PT, McCrae RR. An approach to the attribution of aging, period and cohort effects. *Psychol Bull* 1982; **92**: 238–50.
2. Palmore E. When can age, period and cohort be separated? *Soc Forces* 1978; **57**: 282–95.

13

Chronological and Functional Ageing

Jack M. Guralnik and David Melzer*

National Institute on Aging, National Institutes of Health, Bethesda, MD, USA,
*Department of Community Medicine, Institute of Public Health, University of Cambridge, UK

Chronological age is the major descriptor by which aging is defined. In an effort to characterize the dynamics and variability of the aging process, recent approaches have used measures of functional aging to reflect the observation that individuals may function at a level above or below that expected for their chronological age. The relationship between chronological and functional age has implications for major questions of aging research and public policy. Do humans have a fixed lifespan? How can we maximize functioning for any given age? How is functional aging associated with vulnerability to disease? Should retirement be mandatory at a certain chronological age or should functional age play a role in this decision?

CHRONOLOGICAL VS. FUNCTIONAL AGING

Chronological age is defined as time since birth; its effect is analyzed in virtually all health studies and indeed in nearly all areas of human research. Although chronological aging is strongly associated with mortality and nearly all diseases, it should not be viewed as an etiologic factor. It is rather a proxy for numerous factors that change or accumulate over time, such as cumulative exposure to toxins and trauma, changes in hormone levels, immunological defenses and genetic repair mechanisms. A great deal of work has gone into identifying factors that explain the relationship between chronological age and susceptibility to disease and dysfunction, but much of this relationship remains unexplained. Identifying chronological age as a risk factor may be of little value, not because age is not strongly related to disease incidence but because an intervention to change one's age is not available. For developing prevention strategies, however, understanding an age association may be important, such as the finding that bone loss accelerates for 10–15 years after menopause, slows for a number of years, and again accelerates after age 75.

A number of different concepts, including functional age, biological age and biomarkers of aging, have been developed based on the observation that physiological measures and functional performance show a range of values in a population of a given chronological age. Functional age is a concept that rests on the premise that a measure other than chronological age could better reflect one's position in the aging process. Although biological and functional age have been defined differently, they are frequently used interchangeably. In contrast to chronological aging, which occurs at a universal fixed rate, functional aging has been termed "non-chronological" because its rate may accelerate or decelerate and, in fact, functional age may be greater or less than one's chronological age.

The concept of biomarkers of aging is particularly appealing because it implies that there are biological measures that reflect the rate of aging and that successful interventions on the aging process would have an effect on these markers. It is unclear at this time whether there is an underlying biological state of aging that can be summed up as a single number that indicates how far along in the aging process the individual has progressed. It has been argued that aging is a complex, uncoordinated phenomenon that can not be summed up in such a way[1]. Others believe that, although a well-validated set of biomarkers does not currently exist, there may be techniques developed that can work well as general indicators of biological age[2]. The requirements of a biomarker are not that it simply be different in persons or animals of different ages but that, in a group of subjects of the same age, it has a distribution of values that relates to other age-sensitive traits, such as longevity[2].

Much of the work done on functional aging has focused on physiological changes that are part of normal human aging. Another aspect of functional aging, which may be termed "functional health status", assesses functioning at the level of the whole older person, describing how that person functions in daily life. Functional health status has been found to be related to chronological age, disease and a variety of other modifying factors. Measures of functional health status have also proved valuable for clinical and health services research[3]. The USA's national goal to increase the span of disability-free life exemplifies the high level of interest in the measurement of functional health in recent years[4].

FUNCTION VS. DISEASE IN CHARACTERIZING OLDER PERSONS AND OLDER POPULATIONS

Understanding the functional aspects of aging has been an important part of geriatric medicine for several decades. In the medical model of disease, the clinician gathers symptoms and signs, makes a diagnosis, and bases the therapeutic approach on this diagnosis. Complementing this disease-orientated approach, functional assessment provides an understanding of the impact and consequences of the older person's disease or diseases, giving information on level of independence and prognosis, as well as health care, rehabilitation and social needs. As aging research has increased in recent years, the functional approach has played an important role in its agenda.

Although normal physiological changes with aging may have an impact on the older person, the far greater functional impact comes from the effects of disease. A framework that represents the

Principles and Practice of Geriatric Psychiatry, 2nd edn. Edited by J. R. M. Copeland, M. T. Abou-Saleh and D. G. Blazer

relationship between disease and disability is therefore valuable in developing the concept of functional aging. The World Health Organization has proposed a theoretical pathway progressing from disease to impairment to disability to handicap[5]. An alternative pathway, proposed by Nagi[6] and utilized by the US Institute of Medicine[7], progresses from diseases and conditions to impairment to functional limitation to disability. An effort to operationalize this latter pathway defines "impairment" as dysfunction and structural abnormalities in specific body systems, "functional limitation" as restriction in basic physical and mental actions such as ambulating, grasping and stepping up, and "disability" as difficulty in doing activities in daily life such as personal care, household management, job and hobbies[8]. Although these pathways have remained essentially theoretical, increasing efforts are now under way to use empirical data to document important steps along the pathway[9].

Disease severity and the co-occurrence of multiple diseases (co-morbidity) play an important role in the process of disablement. In a study using data representative of the older US population, it was found that the prevalence of disability increased with increasing number of chronic conditions, after adjusting for age and sex[10]. The synergistic effect of specific pairs of diseases on disability has also been demonstrated. It is also clear that intervening behavioral, environmental and social factors play an important part in modifying the pathway along its entire course and need to be understood more fully[11,12].

DOMAINS OF FUNCTIONING AND MEASURES OF POPULATION DISABILITY

Functional aging is a multidimensional concept for which several domains must be considered to adequately characterize the total older person. Domains central to aging include physical, cognitive, psychological, sensory and social functioning. In the older population it is of value to separate the cognitive and psychological domains, although at times it may be difficult to ascertain whether cognitive impairment is related to a dementing disease or depression. The importance of sensory impairments in limiting overall functioning is receiving increasing attention in ongoing gerontological research. Social functioning, critically important in the lives of older persons, reflects the impact of the other domains on interactions with family, friends and the community.

Physical functioning, to be the focus of the remainder of this chapter, has traditionally been assessed through self-report of the ability to perform specific tasks, including self-care activities such as bathing and dressing (activities of daily living) and activities necessary to maintain independence in the community, such as shopping and food preparation (instrumental activities of daily living)[13–15]. In cases where individuals have severe physical or cognitive impairment, proxies have been successfully employed to assess functional status, although proxies who have limited contact with the subject tend to provide less valid information[16]. Recently, performance measures of functioning, in which the individual is asked to actually perform standardized tasks, have been employed[17].

A number of national surveys have estimated the prevalence of functional disability in the US population[18]. The prevalence of disability in activities of daily living (ADLs) in the non-institutionalized population rises steeply with increasing age and is slightly higher for women compared with men at the older ages (Figure 13.1)[19]. These rates do not reflect that portion of the population residing in nursing homes, where it is estimated that over 90% of residents require help with ADLs[20]. It is important to keep in mind that, although chronological age is strongly related to disability prevalence, many other factors, such as socio-economic status, have large impacts on disability that are independent of age[12].

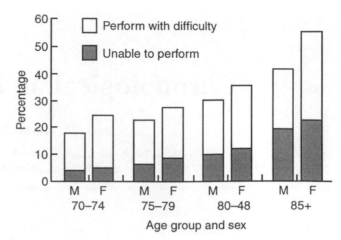

Figure 13.1. Percentage of persons have difficulty or being unable to perform one or more activities of daily living by age and sex, USA, 1995. Activities of daily living include: bathing or showering, dressing, using the toilet, getting in and out of bed or chairs, and eating, walking and getting outside. Source of data: Second Supplement on Aging to the 1995 National Health Interview Survey

COMPRESSION OF MORBIDITY AND THE MEASUREMENT OF ACTIVE LIFE EXPECTANCY

An important issue related to functional aging is the relationship between length of life and the amount of time spent in the disabled state. Life expectancy has increased very substantially in this century. A consequence of this, which is just beginning to be appreciated, however, is that escaping death during the early years from infectious diseases and other causes may mean that many more people survive to ages where they suffer from chronic diseases, which can lead to long-term disability and loss of independence. A major goal of gerontology is to increase longevity without increasing the number of years spent in the disabled or dependent state. Although the recent increase in longevity is well documented, it is not now clear whether these added years of life have been accompanied by years of health and vigor or disease and disability. This question is of particular concern in the coming century, when it is projected that there will be continued increases in life expectancy and unprecedented numbers of old and very old persons. The theory of compression of morbidity predicts a future decrease in the number of years with severe disease and disability[21].

An important tool for evaluating compression of morbidity is what has been termed "active life expectancy" or "disability-free life expectancy"[22]. Active life expectancy is defined as the average number of years an individual at a given age will survive and remain in the active, or non-disabled, state. Most analyses of active life expectancy have employed the ADLs to define disability, with active life expectancy calculated using life table techniques which consider transitions from the active, non-disabled state to both death and disability. The original analysis of active life expectancy considered the transitions to both death and disability as irreversible[22].

However, recent longitudinal studies of aging populations have revealed that a substantial proportion of disabled persons make the transition back to the non-disabled state. Methods to calculate active life expectancy based on these kinds of changes, using multistate life tables, have been developed[23].

The relationship over time between life expectancy and active life expectancy can be used to assess the occurrence of a compression of morbidity. Three possible scenarios for population morbidity in women are illustrated schematically in Figure

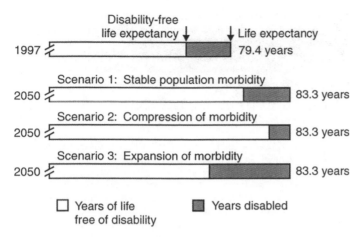

Figure 13.2. Scenarios for change in average burden of population disability level, 1997–2050. Compression of morbidity and alternatives

13.2. The total length of the bars in this figure represent life expectancy observed for 1997 and projected by the Census Bureau for 2050. The length of the unshaded segments of the bars represents active or disability-free life expectancy, and the shaded areas of the bars represent the average number of years in the disabled state. In scenario 1, the onset of disability has been postponed the same number of years as life expectancy has increased, and the number of years spent in the disabled state is unchanged from 1997. In scenario 2, there has been a compression of morbidity. Finally, in scenario 3, although disability-free life expectancy in 2050 has increased compared with 1997, it has not kept pace with increases in life expectancy and there is an expansion of population morbidity.

A vigorous debate over the prospects for a compression of morbidity began with a landmark paper by Fries, in which he made the claim that the compression of morbidity was inevitable in the coming years[21]. He argued that in all species the maximum lifespan is fixed, that human beings are quickly approaching this limit, and that with a stable life expectancy any postponement of disease and disability would result in a compression of morbidity. Although this logic is correct, others have pointed out that life expectancy is probably not going to reach its maximum level for at least the next half century and we must consider that any of the alternative scenarios depicted in Figure 13.2 are possible in the face of increasing life expectancy.

Repeat estimation of active and disabled life expectancy over time using identical techniques in the same target population would allow for a direct assessment of compression of morbidity, but these data are not available. However, disability prevalence, which is not equivalent to disabled life expectancy but reflects a cross-sectional picture of the proportion of the population that is disabled, can be estimated, and a great deal of attention has been focused on longitudinal trends in disability. In the 1970s there was some evidence of a rising prevalence of disability, but in the 1980s rates appear to have declined[24–26].

For example, Manton et al.[24,27] have reported an average annual adjusted decline of 1.1% in the prevalence of a composite measure of severe disability in the population aged 65 and over, from the US National Long Term Care Survey for the period 1982–1994. Freedman and Martin[26] reported similar declines in a more specific measure of difficulty in walking or use of mobility aids from the Survey of Income and Program Participation: for example, the prevalence of disability defined by this criterion declined during the 10 year study period from 30.6% to 27.2% at age 65–79 and at age 80 and over from 44.0% to 40.9%. Although there is a scarcity of longitudinal data from other countries, similar findings have been reported[28] with only a few exceptions where rates have probably been stable.

Possible causes of these declines in disability prevalence include environmental changes making daily tasks easier[8], more intensive use of assistive devices[29] and other social changes, including attitudes to being active in old age. In addition, the proportion of older people who have little education (a potent risk factor for disability) has declined[26,30]. There is also evidence of declining prevalence of some medical conditions in old age, especially cardiovascular disease. Health risk avoidance and improved diagnostic and therapeutic techniques will also have contributed.

The future burden of morbidity and disability in the older population is of great concern to those involved in planning, financing and delivering health care and social services. If current rates of disabling diseases such as Alzheimer's disease and hip fracture remain unchanged, the numbers of older people with these diseases will increase substantially in the next century[31]. Gaining an understanding of factors that have an impact on functional aging is critical if we are to reduce the burden of disability and achieve a compression of morbidity. Ultimately, effective interventions must be developed to prevent the onset and mitigate the consequences of diseases that lead to much of the disability in late life.

REFERENCES

1. Costa PT, McCrae RR. Design and analysis of aging studies. In Masoro EJ, ed. *Handbook of Physiology*, Section 11: *Aging* New York: Oxford University Press, 1995.
2. Miller RA. When will the biology of aging become useful? Future landmarks in biomedical gerontology. *J Am Geriatr Soc* 1997; **45**: 1258–67.
3. Fried LP, Guralnik JM. Disability in older adults: evidence regarding significance, etiology, and risk. *J Am Geriatr Soc* 1997; **45**: 92–100.
4. Public Health Service. *Healthy People 2000: National Health Promotion and Disease Prevention Objectives*. DHHS Publication no. (PHS)79-55701. Washington, DC: US Department of Health and Human Services, Public Health Service, 1990.
5. World Health Organization. *International Classification of Impairments, Disabilities, and Handicaps*. Geneva: World Health Organization, 1980.
6. Nagi SZ. An epidemiology of disability among adults in the United States. *Milbank Mem Fund Q* 1976; **54**: 439–68.
7. Institute of Medicine. Committee on a National Agenda for Prevention of Disabilities. *Disability in America: Toward a National Agenda for Prevention*. Pope M, Taylor AR, eds. Washington, DC: Institute of Medicine, National Academy Press, 1991.
8. Verbrugge LM, Jette AM. The disablement process. *Soc Sci Med* 1994; **38**: 1–14.
9. Jette AM, Assmann SF, Rooks D *et al.* Interrelationships among disablement concepts. *J Gerontol Med Sci* 1998; **53**: M395–404.
10. Guralnik JM, LaCroix AZ, Everett DF, Kovar MG. Aging in the eighties: the prevalence of co-morbidity and its association with disability. Advance Data from *Vital and Health Statistics*, No. 170. Hyattsville, MD: National Center for Health Statistics, 1989.
11. Guralnik JM. Understanding the relationship between disease and disability. *J Am Geriatr Soc* 1994; **42**: 1128–9.
12. Stuck AE, Walthert JM, Nikolaus T *et al.* Risk factors for functional status decline in community-living elderly people: a systematic literature review. *Soc Sci Med* 1999; **48**: 445–69.
13. Branch LG, Meyers AR. Assessing physical function in the elderly. *Clin Geriatr Med* 1987; **3**: 29–51.
14. Applegate WB, Blass JP, Williams TF. Instruments for the functional assessment of older patients. *N Engl J Med* 1990; **322**: 1207–14.
15. Guralnik JM, LaCroix AZ. Assessing physical function in older populations. In Wallace RB, Woolson RF, eds, *The Epidemiologic*

Study of the Elderly. New York: Oxford University Press, 1991: 159–81.

16. Magaziner J, Simonsick EM, Kashner TM *et al.* Patient–proxy response comparability on measures of patient health and functional status. *J Clin Epidemiol* 1988; **41**: 1065–74.

17. Guralnik JM, Branch LG, Cummings SR, Curb JD. Physical performance measures in aging research. *J Gerontol Med Sci* 1989; **44**: M141–6.

18. Weiner JM, Hanley RJ, Clark R, Van Nostrand JF. Measuring the activities of daily living: comparisons across national surveys. *J Gerontol Soc Sci* 1990; **45**: S229–37.

19. Kramarow E, Lentzner H, Rooks R *et al. Health and Aging Chartbook. Health, United States, 1999*. Hyattsville, MD: National Center for Health Statistics, 1999.

20. National Center for Health Statistics, Hing E, Sekscenski E, Strahan G. The National Nursing Home Survey; 1985 summary for the United States. *Vital and Health Statistics*, Series 13, No. 97. DHHS Publication No. (PHS) 89-1758. Washington, DC: US Government Printing Office, 1989.

21. Fries JF. Aging, natural death and the compression of morbidity. *N Engl J Med* 1980; **303**: 130–5.

22. Katz S, Branch LG, Branson MH *et al.* Active life expectancy. *N Engl J Med* 1983; **309**: 1218–24.

23. Land KC, Guralnik JM, Blazer DG. Estimating increment-decrement life tables with multiple covariates from panel data: The case of active life expectancy. *Demography* 1994; **31**: 297–319.

24. Manton KG, Stallard E, Corder LS. The dynamics of dimensions of age-related disability 1982–1994 in the US elderly population. *J Gerontol Biol Sci* 1998; **53**: B59–70.

25. Crimmins EM, Saito Y, Reynolds SL. Further evidence on recent trends in the prevalence and incidence of disability among older Americans from two sources: the LSOA and the NHIS. *J Gerontol Soc Sci* 1997; **52**: S59–71.

26. Freedman VA, Martin LG. Understanding trends in functional limitations among older Americans. *Am J Public Health* 1998; **88**: 1457–62.

27. Manton KG, Corder L, Stallard E. Chronic disability trends in elderly United States populations: 1982–1994. *Proc Natl Acad Sci USA* 1997; **94**: 2593–8.

28. Waidmann T, Manton KG. *International Evidence on Disability Trends among the Elderly*. Washington DC: Office of Disability, Aging and Long Term Care Policy, DHHS, 1998.

29. Manton KG, Corder L, Stallard E. Changes in the use of personal assistance and special equipment from 1982 to 1989: results from the 1982 and 1989 NLTCS. *Gerontologist* 1993; **33**: 168–76.

30. Singer BH, Manton KG. The effects of health changes on projections of health service needs for the elderly population of the United States. *Proc Natl Acad Sci USA* 1998; **95**: 15618–22.

31. Schneider EL, Guralnik JM. The ageing of America: impact on health care costs. *J Am Med Assoc* 1990; **263**: 2335–40.

Health Expectancy: Monitoring Changes in Population Health

Carol Jagger

University of Leicester, UK

The increasing life expectancies experienced by many countries over the last decade have made the debate about the quality and quantity of years lived at older ages particularly relevant for conditions such as dementia, where the prevalence rises steeply with age. Health expectancies were developed to address the question of whether or not longer life is accompanied with a decrease in the quality of life, and they extend the concept of life expectancy to morbidity and disability by providing a means of dividing life expectancy into life spent in various states of good and bad health. Being independent of the size of populations and of their age structure, health expectancies thus allow direct comparison of the different groups that constitute populations: sexes, socioprofessional categories, regions.

As health expectancy combines a life expectancy with a health measure, there are as many possible health expectancies as health measures; for example, disability-free life expectancy, active life expectancy (based on independence in Activities of Daily Living), healthy life expectancy (based on good perceived health) or dementia-free life expectancy. Bone *et al.*[1] reports values for these and other health expectancies for the UK from two longitudinal studies of older people (the Melton Mowbray Ageing Project and the Nottingham Longitudinal Study of Activity and Aging) and from national cross-sectional studies. Dementia-free life expectancy at age 65 years has now been calculated for five countries: France, UK, Belgium, Eire and The Netherlands[2]. Despite difference in life expectancies between countries (ranging for men from 13.5 years in Eire to 15.4 years in France and for women from 16.9 years in Eire to 19.7 years in France), women can expect to live between one and two years and men between 0.5 and 0.7 years of their remaining life with dementia.

Today, estimates of health expectancy (generally disability-free life expectancy) are available for 49 countries[3], although comparisons across time and between countries are still problematic due to the lack of harmonisation of measures and study designs. REVES (Réseau Espérance de Vie en Santé: the International Research Network on Health Expectancy) is an international organization of researchers, clinicians and health planners addressing these issues as well as developing and recommending methods of calculation and furthering the use of health expectancy as a tool for health planning.

REFERENCES

1. Bone MR, Bebbington AC, Jagger C *et al. Health Expectancy and Its Uses*. London: HMSO, 1995.

2. Jagger C, Ritchie K, Bronnun-Hansen H *et al.* Mental health expectancy: the European perspective. A synopsis of results presented at the Conference of the European Network for the Calculation of Health Expectancies (Euro–REVES). *Acta Psychiatrica Scandinavica*, 1998; **98**: 85–91.

3. Robine JM, Romieu I, Cambois E. Health expectancy indicators. *Bull WHO* 1999; **77**(2): 181–5.

14

Life Satisfaction

Linda K. George
Duke University, Durham, NC, USA

Maddox and Wiley[1] suggest that the "relationship between aging and successful adaptation (variously 'morale' or 'life satisfaction' or 'well-being') is perhaps the most persistently investigated issue in the social scientific study of aging". This statement, made a quarter century ago, remains true today. Life satisfaction is variously viewed as a prime indicator of overall life quality, a testimony to the importance of social structure and location for person well-being and one component of "positive mental health"[2]. Life satisfaction research also has helped to balance the vastly overstated crisis orientation that characterized aging research in the past[3]. This chapter examines several facets of life satisfaction in later life: definitional issues, the epidemiology of life satisfaction in later life, major determinants of life satisfaction, mechanisms that may account for age differences in life satisfaction, and some final comments about future directions for life satisfaction research.

WHAT IS LIFE SATISFACTION?

Life satisfaction is most frequently defined as a global assessment of life quality, derived from comparison of one's aspirations to the actual conditions of life[4,5]. Because "life as a whole" or "life in general" is assessed, a long-range time perspective and non-specific life conditions are implied. Life satisfaction is one of a number of concepts that can be subsumed under the more general rubric of subjective well-being. Other indicators of subjective well-being are happiness and mood. Two primary factors underlie the distinctions among these concepts: the ratio of cognitive to affective judgment involved and time frame. Although all subjective well-being measures involve evaluation along a good–bad continuum, life satisfaction is primarily a cognitive assessment of the discrepancy between aspirations and achievements. In contrast, happiness and mood are primarily emotional judgments. In addition, happiness and mood are quite transitory, whereas life satisfaction tends to be stable (although it is sensitive to major events and changes in life conditions). Because it is a more cognitive, stable phenomenon, life satisfaction has been a more attractive candidate for the study of quality of life during old age. Researchers have understandably been more interested in relatively stable judgments of life quality than in indicators that fluctuate widely over brief periods of time.

How life satisfaction is defined has direct implications for methods that can be used to alleviate dissatisfaction. Dissatisfaction represents a significant discrepancy between one's desired life conditions and one's actual life conditions. Consequently, the two major ways to reduce dissatisfaction are either to engage in goal-directed behavior that brings achievements closer to aspirations or to reduce aspirations so that they more closely match the actual conditions of life. As we will see, older adults are especially adept at using the latter strategy to sustain high levels of life satisfaction.

THE EPIDEMIOLOGY OF LIFE SATISFACTION

How satisfied are older adults with their lives? This question has been investigated for 40 years, with consistent results. Studies of samples of both older adults and of adults of all ages consistently document that the vast majority (i.e. typically 85%) are satisfied with their lives[4–7]. Between the 1960s and the 1980s, the life satisfaction of older Americans increased slightly relative to that of the non-elderly[8]. In studies conducted during the 1960s and earlier, older adults were somewhat less satisfied with their lives, on average, than their younger peers. By the mid-1970s, however, this pattern had reversed and has remained stable for more than two decades.

DETERMINANTS OF LIFE SATISFACTION

What are the major determinants of life satisfaction during old age? Research suggests that they fall into two primary categories: (a) objective life circumstances and (b) personality traits and other psychological characteristics.

Objective Life Circumstances

For all adults, regardless of age, the major determinants of life satisfaction include attachments to social structure (especially education, occupation and marital status), personal resources (including health and income), involvement in and support from primary groups (family and friends) and participation in meaningful social and leisure activities[4,5,9–11]. Recent evidence indicates that religious participation also is a robust predictor of life satisfaction[12,13].

Although the same basic set of objective life circumstances underlie life satisfaction for all adults, the meaning and salience of those determinants may vary across ages or stages of the life course. What is highly important for a sense of well-being at one life stage may be less relevant at another. For example, George, Okun, and Landerman[9] found that: (a) marital status is less important for a sense of well-being among young adults than among middle-aged and older adults; (b) income is most important for middle-aged adults and least important for young adults, and intermediate for older adults; (c) health is much more important for older adults than for middle-aged and younger adults; and (d) social relationships are more important for younger and older adults than for the middle-age[9]. The degree to which the determinants of life satisfaction differ across age groups merits further investigation.

Despite evidence that life satisfaction is strongly related to objective life conditions, levels of life satisfaction typically remain stable, even in the face of substantial change in its documented predictors. It is true that significant social losses, especially widowhood and the onset of disability, are associated with decreases in life satisfaction. More surprising, however, is the fact that levels of life satisfaction remain stable in the face of other major changes in life circumstances. For example, although retirement typically results in a 50% reduction in income, there is no evidence that retirement and its accompanying reduced income lessens life satisfaction[14]. Indeed, life satisfaction can be sustained in the midst of potentially devastating chronic stress, as documented in a study of more than 500 family caregivers of demented older adults. Among this sample of caregivers, the average level of psychiatric symptoms was eight times greater than that for random community samples, more than one-third of the caregivers reported using psychotropic drugs, and nearly one-quarter used alcohol on a regular basis to cope. Nonetheless, fully 80% of these caregivers reported that they were satisfied or very satisfied with their lives—a figure only 5% lower than that typically reported in random samples of American adults[15].

These findings testify to the distinctive character of life satisfaction—by definition, life satisfaction refers to subjective perceptions that go beyond the effects of objective life conditions. We need to know more about the cognitive and emotional processes that lead some older people who appear well off in terms of their objective life circumstances to nonetheless find life dissatisfying and burdensome. Similarly, we need to know why it is that many older adults who are less well off than their younger peers—and, indeed, than they were at younger ages—nonetheless find life meaningful and satisfying[16].

Psychological Characteristics

One reason that life satisfaction may be overwhelmingly stable and only partially reflect objective life conditions may be that it reflects, in part, psychological characteristics. Several relatively stable personality traits are significant predictors of life satisfaction: neuroticism, extroversion vs. introversion, and openness to new experience or cognitive flexibility[17–19]. Other social psychological characteristics are related to subjective well-being as well. For example, interpersonal trust is associated with higher life satisfaction[20]. Personal coping strategies also have implications for life satisfaction. Selective optimization with compensation is a coping strategy in which older adults who face limitations due to health problems or diminishing social networks choose to increase their commitments to specific life domains in order to compensate for the inability to invest in other life domains. This strategy for coping with age-related decrements is associated with higher levels of life satisfaction than other coping strategies during late life[21].

EXPLANATORY MECHANISMS

Before examining potential explanatory mechanisms that underlie subjective perceptions of life quality, another age difference in reports of life satisfaction must be noted. There is considerable evidence that older adults are satisfied with life conditions that are objectively worse than those needed to produce perceptions of equivalent life quality among middle-aged and younger adults[8,9]. For example, some economists have observed that older persons often express satisfaction with levels of income that are substantially below those required for minimally adequate food, shelter and medical care[22,23]. Three types of explanatory mechanisms have been suggested as possible explanations for this pattern.

One possible explanation is aspiration theory which, as previously described, has been the basis of most conceptualizations of life satisfaction. From this perspective, some scholars argue that older adults are masters of the art of lowering aspirations to meet realities. A related hypothesis suggests that, because measures of life satisfaction focus on the long term, older persons often view current deprivations as paling in comparison to the dominant patterns of their lives[24,25]. Although aspiration theory can describe plausible ways in which older adults can make peace with less than optimal life conditions, it cannot explain why older adults are willing to lower their aspirations substantially more than younger and middle-aged adults.

Second, other authors have suggested that younger adults use aspiration–achievement comparisons in making judgments about life satisfaction, whereas older persons assess the quality of their lives in terms of perceived equity. Research by Carp and Carp[26] suggests that young and middle-aged adults are satisfied when their achievements closely match their aspirations. In contrast, older adults are satisfied with life when they perceive their life conditions as fair and just (i.e. as matching what they "deserve").

Third, and similar to equity theory, is the theory of relative deprivation, which posits that people will feel deprived only when they see themselves as worse off than others to whom they can appropriately compare themselves[27]. There is strong evidence that most older people see themselves as better off than the "average older person". According to relative deprivation theory, this kind of social comparison will result in high satisfaction. Equity theory and relative deprivation theory share the same problem noted above for aspiration theory. Although each can provide a plausible explanation for why older adults are often satisfied with less than their younger peers, neither explains why many older adults use these strategies to sustain high life satisfaction in the absence of optimal life conditions and most young and middle-aged adults do not.

FINAL THOUGHTS

Much has been learned from a half century of research on life satisfaction. We know and can rejoice in the fact that most older adults find life to be highly satisfying—as do most middle-aged and younger adults. We know that there are robust relationships between objective life conditions and perceptions of life quality. To the extent that this is true, high levels of life satisfaction among older adults confirm that older persons in modern societies share with their younger peers the material and social resources that make life enjoyable and satisfying. We also know, however, that older persons often express satisfaction with levels of resources that are below those necessary for quality of life. In this sense, we cannot deny the possibility that older people are not as well off in important ways as their subjective perceptions would suggest. This possibility—this nagging doubt as to the meaning of older persons' reports of life satisfaction—raises two additional questions that merit increased scrutiny.

First, from a policy perspective, it is prudent to examine the objective life conditions of older adults' lives as well as their ratings of life quality. We do not want, for example, to set standards for the economic resources needed to sustain quality of life on the basis of the thresholds that older people report if they, in fact, report levels that are below those needed to sustain adequate food, shelter and medical care. Similarly, we do not want to ignore the legitimate health and mental health needs of family caregivers of impaired older adults based only on the fact that most caregivers report that their lives are satisfying. A related implication for policy analysis is the utility of life satisfaction measures for assessing the effects of intervention. Given the stability of life satisfaction measures in the face of all but the most major changes in life circumstances, it is probably unwise to evaluate the utility of an intervention on the basis of changes in life satisfaction. Such measures may be so insensitive that meaningful changes in life circumstances would be missed if life satisfaction were the only outcome examined. Moreover, most interventions need not improve life satisfaction to be demonstrably beneficial. For example, interventions that prevent illness or help to alleviate the functional consequences of illness need not improve life satisfaction to be beneficial. It is enough that they make a demonstrable difference in the incidence or functional consequences of disease.

Second, although it may be problematic for policy purposes that perceptions of life quality often stray rather far from objective life conditions, there is something admirable in the fact that most older people find life satisfying despite deprivations in the material and social resources so highly valued in modern societies. We need to investigate the foundations of this phenomenon. Increased understanding of this perplexing facet of life satisfaction is most likely to occur if subjective experience more broadly becomes the focus of investigation. In particular, increased attention should be devoted to studying the life of the self in old age and the sources of meaning that older adults attach to various life domains.

The 15% of the older population who are not able to sustain a sense of well-being also should not be ignored. Although we know that these older adults fare less well than their age peers on measures of income, health, social bonds and leisure participation, we know little else about them. We do not know, for example, whether their dissatisfaction in old age is a life-long pattern or is a response to age-related losses. Given the stability of life satisfaction measures, we also know little about how to facilitate higher levels of satisfaction among these individuals. Modern societies do quite well at providing the social and economic conditions that allow most older adults to find life satisfying. But we still do not know much about how to change life satisfaction. Such knowledge is of high priority, both for the practical purposes of promoting life quality and for gaining a better understanding of its dynamics.

Finally, we must remember that there is important information yet to be learned about life satisfaction. Life satisfaction is not the key barometer of successful aging (as, unfortunately, some of its advocates have implied). But it is important. It is important because it reminds the scientific community that we should be interested in enhancement as well as rehabilitation, in promoting the good life as well as intervening to alleviate bad times. Life satisfaction matters because it demonstrates that social, economic and psychological factors are as important in understanding life's triumphs as its tragedies. Life satisfaction is important because it reminds us to strive for health as well as the absence of disease and to invest in mental health as well as the amelioration of mental illness.

ACKNOWLEDGEMENT

Preparation of this chapter was supported by a grant from the John Templeton Foundation.

REFERENCES

1. Maddox GL, Wiley J. Scope, concepts, and methods in the study of aging. In Binstock RH, Shanas E, eds, *Handbook of Aging and the Social Sciences*, 1st edn. New York: Van Nostrand Reinhold, 1976, 3–34.

2. George LK. Life satisfaction in later life—the positive side of mental health. *Generations* 1986; **10**: 5–8.

3. George LK. Social structure, social processes, and social-psychological states. In Binstock RH, George LK, eds, *Handbook of Aging and the Social Sciences*, 3rd edn. New York: Academic Press, 1990, 186–204.

4. Campbell A, Converse PE, Rodgers WL. *The Quality of American Life*. New York: Russell Sage Foundation, 1976.

5. Andrews FM, Withey SB. *Social Indicators of Well-being*. New York: Plenum, 1976.

6. Rodgers W. Trends in reported happiness within demographically defined subgroups, 1957–1978. *Social Forces* 1982; **60**: 826–42.

7. Mookherjee HN. A comparative assessment of life satisfaction in the United States, 1978–1988. *J Soc Psychol* 1992; **132**: 407–9.

8. Herzog AR, Rodgers WL. Age and satisfaction: data from several large surveys. *Res Aging* 1981; **3**: 142–65.

9. George LK, Okun MA, Landerman R. Age as a moderator of the determinants of life satisfaction. *Res Aging* 1985; **7**: 209–33.

10. George LK, Landerman R. Health and subjective well-being: a replicated secondary analysis. *Int J Aging Hum Dev* 1984; **19**: 133–56.

11. Liang J, Dvorkin J, Kahana E, Mazian F. Social integration and morale: a re-examination. *J Gerontol* 1989; **35**: 746–57.

12. Levin JS, Taylor RJ. Panel analyses of religious involvement and well-being in African Americans: contemporaneous vs. longitudinal effects. *J Sci Study Relig* 1998; **37**: 695–709.

13. Neill CM, Kahn AS. The role of personal spirituality and religious social activity on the life satisfaction of older widowed women. *Sex Roles* 1999; **40**: 310–29.

14. Palmore EB, Fillenbaum GG, George LK. Consequences of retirement. *J Gerontol* 1984; **39**: 109–16.

15. George LK, Gwyther LP. Caregiver well-being: a multidimensional examination of family caregivers of demented adults. *Gerontologist* 1986; **34**: 2553–90.

16. George LK, Clipp EC. Subjective components of aging well. *Generations* 1991; **15**: 57–60.

17. Costa PT, McCrae RR. Influence of extroversion and neuroticism on subjective well-being: happy and unhappy people. *J Pers Soc Psychol* 1980; **38**: 668–78.

18. George LK. The impact of personality and social status factors upon levels of activity and psychological well-being. *J Gerontol* 1978; **33**: 840–7.

19. Okun MA, George LK. Physician- and self-ratings of health, neuroticism, and subjective well-being among men and women. *Personality Individ Diff* 1984; **5**: 523–40.

20. Barefoot JC, Maynard KE, Beckham JC et al. Trust, health and longevity. *J Behav Med* 1998; **21**: 517–26.

21. Freund AM, Baltes PB. Selection, optimization, and compensation as strategies of life management: correlations with subjective indicators of successful aging. *Psychol Aging* 1998; **13**: 531–43.

22. Colasanto D, Kapteyn A, Van der Gaag J. Two subjective definitions of poverty: results from the Wisconsin Basic Needs Survey. *J Hum Resources* 1984; **19**: 127–38.

23. Vaughan DR. *Using Subjective Assessments of Income to Estimate Family Equivalence Scales*. Washington, DC: Social Security Administration, 1980.

24. Oishi S, Diener EF, Lucas RE, Suh EM. Cross-cultural variations in predictors of lie satisfaction: perspectives from needs and values. *Pers Soc Psych Bull* 1999; **25**: 980–90.

25. Holahan CK, Holahan CJ, Wonacott NL. Self-appraisal, life satisfaction, and retrospective life choices over one and three decades. *Psychol Aging* 1999; **14**: 238–44.

26. Carp FM, Carp A. Test of a model of domain satisfactions and well-being: equity considerations. *Res Aging* 1982; **4**: 503–22.

27. Hagerty MR. Social comparisons of income in one's community: evidence from national surveys of income and happiness. *J Pers Soc Psychol* 2000; **78**: 764–71.

15

The Normal Aged among Community-dwelling Elders in the UK

Christina Victor

Department of Public Health Sciences, St George's Hospital Medical School, London, UK

INTRODUCTION

In 1851 there were approximately 1 million people in Britain aged 65 and over, representing 5% of the total population, compared with 9 million or approximately 16% in 1991 and a projected 11 955 000 in 2021[1]. The reasons for this demographic transformation, which is not unique to the UK, have been discussed elsewhere in this book. One very visible manifestation of this change in the structure of our population is the increase in the number of centenarians. At the turn of the century, there were only a handful of British centenarian subjects, 200 at most[2]. As we enter the next millennium there are approximately 6000 Britons aged 100 or more[2]. One feature of population ageing in the next millennium will be the "ageing" of the ethnic minority populations of Britain, which will pose a new set of challenges[3]. Instead of this demographic trend being welcomed as a triumph for public health, population ageing is portrayed as an impending social disaster. Increasingly over the course of this century, old age has been depicted as a "social problem", especially with regard to the health and financial consequences of an ageing population[4,5]. Consequently, research in social gerontology has been dominated by the policy-makers' agenda, which perceived old age as a social problem. The bulk of research has, therefore, concentrated upon defining and enumerating the social problem and pathological aspects of ageing, rather than on enhancing our understanding of "normal" ageing[6]. This is particularly true in the area of health and medicine where, until recently, dementia was seen as a part of "normal" ageing and where there are major debates as to how we are to afford to pay for the health care of older people. It is only recently that researchers have extended the horizons of their research to include research into the non-pathological aspects of later life.

One reason why the prospect of an ageing population is perceived so negatively is because of the prevailing images of the characteristics of the old age and older people generally. These images, beliefs and stereotypes are then transferred to the whole population. Stereotypes about the nature and characteristics of old age and older people abound and reflect a societal ideology which is predominantly youth-centred. To paraphrase the most common beliefs about older age, older people are seen as socially isolated, abandoned by their families, ridden with ill-health and disease (indeed, old age is synonymous with ill-health and disease), consuming excessive amounts of societies' health and social care resources and not contributing in any way to society (i.e. being parasitic upon the young, vigorous working population). Older people are further viewed as being inflexible, lacking vigour, being incapable of learning and shunning innovation and new technology. By inference, an ageing population is seen as being stagnant, uncompetitive and unable to compete or innovate as well as "young" populations. In the rest of this chapter we consider how valid some of these stereotypical images are.

THE LIVING ARRANGEMENTS OF OLDER PEOPLE

One very prevalent image of later life is that of living in institutional care. It is popularly believed that most older people live "in care" (either in a residential or nursing home). Although only approximately 5% of those aged 65+ live in some form of institutional care, this percentage is widely perceived as being much greater[7]. Even for the "oldest old", those aged 90 or more, approximately half are still living in their own homes in the community[8]. For those older people living in the community, another common image is the association of later life with residence in "special" types of housing, such as sheltered housing. Again this is a type of accommodation characteristic of only a minority of older people, with approximately 10% of those aged 75 and over living in such types of housing[1]. Hence, we can conclude that the majority of older people, some 70–99% (depending upon age) live in the community and in "ordinary" housing in the same way as the rest of the population. Home ownership is the main form of tenure, with 68% of those aged 65 and over owning their own homes in 1996/97[1]. A further 27% lived in accommodation rented from the public sector[1]. However across the tenure groups, older people are more likely than other age groups to live in older housing, which typically is in poorer repair, lacking in standard amenities and adequate heating. This is especially true for the minority of older people, approximately 10%, who live in private rented accommodation.

Within Britain, the post-war period has witnessed profound and far-reaching changes in patterns of family formation and household structure. In Britain in 1999, approximately 38% of those aged 65+ lived alone compared with about 10% in 1945[9]. Over the same period, the percentage of older people living with their spouse only has increased to about 50% from 30%. There

Principles and Practice of Geriatric Psychiatry, 2nd edn. Edited by J. R. M. Copeland, M. T. Abou-Saleh and D. G. Blazer
©2002 John Wiley & Sons, Ltd

are, of course, important variations between men and women in terms of living arrangements. At all ages, because of the differential age at marriage between men and women and higher male mortality rates, there are more women living alone than men. For example, 26% of men aged 85 and over live alone, compared with 49% of women of the same age[1]. Simultaneously, the percentage of older people living in larger households of two (or more) generations has decreased to about 10% of those aged 65 and over. Superficially the increase in "solo living" and decrease in the multi-generational household is often interpreted as evidence of the "rejection" of older people by their children and other relatives. However, these changes in household composition are, in fact, the result of much wider social changes, including the trend for younger people to establish independent households on or before marriage, geographical mobility, smaller families and increased rates of marriage combined with the improved financial resources available to older people, which allow them to express a widespread desire for independent living in later life.

SOCIAL NETWORKS AND SOCIAL CONTACT

Older people are often portrayed as a socially isolated group who are neglected by both their families and the wider social world. A key factor in considering the social networks of older people is the availability of kin and especially the marital relationship. The cohort of older women who never married, the post-World War I "spinster generation", has almost died out. Indeed, the percentage of single (never married) women has deceased from 16% of those over 80 in 1972 to 10% in 1999[1]. For the current population of older people, approximately 7% have never married[1]. The percentage of older people who are married varies markedly between men and women. Up to the age of 85 and over, the majority of men are married compared with 16% of women. For women the majority of those aged over 70 are widowed. Hence, for women the loss of a spouse can vastly restrict their social networks. However, the vast majority (97%) report the existence of close relatives and the presence of a close confiding relationship[10,11]. Generally the pattern of contact between older people and their relatives and friends contradicts the image of neglect, as at least 75% of older people report weekly contact with relatives/friends[1]. Amongst older women especially, friendship levels are both extensive and important[12,13]. Furthermore, research has consistently demonstrated that only a minority of older people report that they feel lonely, although this percentage does increase with age and disability[14] but is not synonymous with living alone[14]. Older people are also engaged members of society, as measured by their participation in social, cultural and voluntary activities[1].

HEALTH STATUS

Perhaps the most potent stereotype of all concerning later life relates to the perceived universal prevalence of illness, disability and infirmity. It is widely assumed that chronic ill-health, incontinence and mental impairment is the norm amongst the older age groups. How accurate is this image?

There are a variety of different ways of describing the health status of any given population. One widely used index of health status is mortality data. In Britain, mortality rates show a J-shaped distribution, being high in the first year of life and then decreasing in childhood. Rates then increase with age, so that 75% of deaths in England and Wales of the approximately 500,000 deaths annually were accounted for by those aged 65+[15]. In both Britain and the USA there have been significant reductions in later life mortality rates over the past four decades, which have contributed to increased life expectancy in later life. In 1980, men and women

aged 85 could expect to live, on average, for another 4.3 and 5.8 years, respectively. By 1994 this had increased to 5.3 years and 6.8 years because of decreases in later life mortality rates[1].

Whilst mortality data are useful, they tell us nothing about the health status of those who have not died. However, morbidity data are difficult to collect on a routine basis. One important British source of such data is the General Household Survey, which provides data about the prevalence of acute and chronic health problems amongst the general population of older people resident in the community. For acute self-limiting conditions prevalence rates increase only slightly with age, from 10% for those aged 16–44 to 20% at age 85+[15]. Chronic health problems, as measured by long-standing limiting illness, show a much stronger age gradient, increasing from 12% of those aged 16–44 to 53% at age 80+–91[15]. Although there are variations in disability prevalence estimates between studies, it is clear that chronic health problems are not universal in later life. Again, the last decade has, in Britain, been characterized by an increase in the number of years an older person can expect to live "free from disability"[1]. Hence, the increase in life expectancy has not been accompanied by an increase in the amount of disability experienced by the "average" older person.

Within the elderly population there are important differences in health status, which largely mirror those of the population of working age[15]. For chronic ill-health, women show higher prevalence rates than men of the same age. For example, at 80 and over approximately 48% of men and 55% of women report that they have a long-standing limiting illness[1]. Furthermore, there are significant differences in health status between the social classes. At all ages older people from professional and managerial occupations show rates of chronic ill-health which are significantly lower than their counterparts from the manual occupation groups[16]. Expectation of life at age 65 for men also varies from 16.8 years for those from social class 1 (professional occupations) to 12.6 years for those from unskilled occupations[1]. These differences represent the continuation into later life of the well-documented social class differences in health status observed amongst the pre-retirement age groups.

There are significant methodological problems involved in quantifying the prevalence of dementia and other mental health problems in community samples. The varying methodologies and samples used often account for the varying prevalence rates produced by different studies. For both depression and anxiety there appears to be little significant increase with age. Depressive illness of clinical significance is observed in about 10% of those aged 65+, whilst the prevalence of anxiety is about 11% in those aged 65+[15]. For both conditions prevalence rates are higher in women than men. Dementia prevalence and incidence increase exponentially with age, regardless of the instrument used or sample studied[17]. A meta-analysis of 27 studies suggested that dementia prevalence increased from 1.4% at age 65–69 to 38.6% for those aged 90+[17]. However, even amongst the oldest age groups dementia is not universal.

For both chronic physical and mental impairment there are few data about how prevalence rates may be changing over time. Hence, in making comments about the health status of future cohorts of older people, we are extrapolating current prevalence rates. This may (or may not) be justifiable, as the health status of future cohorts of older people may be improved as a result of better living standards and access to medical care. There are two major stances concerning future patterns of mortality. Fries[19] argues that morbidity will be compressed into the last few years of life, whilst the competing argument suggests that future populations will show increased rates of disability as more and more "frail" people survive into advanced old age[20]. Whilst we cannot be certain if prevalence rates for chronic physical and mental health problems will change, and in what direction, in the future, it is important to remember the limitations inherent in applying current health prevalence rates to succeeding generations.

POVERTY AND SOCIAL INEQUALITY

In contrast to the traditional views of later life as a time of poverty and deprivation[19], there has recently emerged the image of the "Well-Off Older Person (WOOPIE)". This image has portrayed older people as a newly affluent group who are benefiting at the expense of younger people. However, recent studies have illustrated that, for the majority of older people, poverty remains the norm, especially in advanced old age[19]. In Britain, one in three of those living in poverty are older people and rates of poverty increase with age, are higher amongst women than men and amongst those from the manual occupation groups[19]. The explanation of such high rates of poverty amongst older people is the low level of state pensions, the principal source of older people's income, and the lack of access by many older people to additional sources of income, such as occupational and private pensions[20-22].

PATTERNS OF FORMAL AND INFORMAL CARE

Older people are the main users of the formal health and social care services provided in Britain[9]. However, despite this the majority of older people do not regularly use formal care services. For example, 19% of those aged 65+ use hospital inpatient services annually, 6% are visited by a district nurse and 4% by a home help[9]. Even for the potentially most vulnerable (those aged 85+ living alone), the district nurse/health visitor is in contact with less than 15%[9]. For most daily tasks that older people (and indeed other age groups) need help with, the principal source of support comes from the informal sector, usually either a spouse or children[23]. Hence the family is, as it always has been, the major provider of care to the frail older person[23]. However, we still know little about the ties within families that promote the development of the caring relationship[24]. There is comprehensive research evidence which clearly shows that older people are themselves significant providers of care to each other[23] and younger age groups[23].

CONCLUSION

The research evidence now available illustrates that the common stereotypes of later life are both inaccurate and out of date. The majority of older people live in the community, in their own homes, and are integrated within a network of family and social relationships. The health status of older people is considerably better than the popular stereotypes, with chronic physical and mental impairment far from universal, even in the very oldest age groups.

Furthermore, although older people do use the health and social care services, the family remains their principal source of care. Indeed, older people are major contributors to the provision of care.

Moreover, within this less pessimistic review of later life, it is important not to treat older people as a single homogeneous social group. The experience of later life is greatly influenced by important dimensions of social stratification, such as gender, class and, increasingly in the future, ethnicity. It seems likely that such socially differentiating dimensions, especially ethnicity, will become increasingly important in determining the experience of future cohorts of older people.

REFERENCES

1. Matheson J, Summerfield C (eds). *Social Focus on Older People*. London: HMSO, 1999.
2. Thomas R. The demography of centenarians in England and Wales. *Population Trends* 1999; **96**: 5–12.
3. Coleman P, Bond J. Ageing in the twentieth century. In Bond J, Coleman P, eds. *Ageing in Society*. London: Sage, 1990, 1–12.
4. MacIntyre S. Old age as a social problem. In Dingwell R, Heath C, Reid M, Stacey C, eds. *Health Care and Health Knowledge*. London: Croom Helm, 1977, 42–63.
5. Victor CR. Care of the frail elderly: a survey of medical and nursing staff attitudes. *Int J Geriatr Psychiat* 1991; **6**: 743–7.
6. Phillipson C. *Reconstructing Old Age*. London: Sage.
7. Victor CR. *Old Age in Modern Society*, 2nd edn. London: Chapman & Hall, 1994.
8. Bury M, Holme A. *Life after Ninety*. London: Routledge, 1991.
9. Victor CR. *Community Care and Older People*. Cheltenham: Stanley Thornes, 1997.
10. Dale A, Evandrou M, Arber S. The household structure of the elderly population in Britain. *Ageing Soc* 1987; **7**: 37–56.
11. Wenger CG. *The Supportive Network*. London: Allen and Unwin, 1984.
12. Jerrome D, Bond J, Coleman P, eds. *Intimate Relationships in Ageing in Society*. London: Sage, 1991, 181–207.
13. Jerrome D. The significance of friendship for women in later life. *Ageing Soc* 1981; **1**: 175–97.
14. Jones DA, Victor CR, Vetter NJ. The problem of loneliness in the elderly in the community: characteristics of those who are lonely and the factors related to loneliness. *J R Coll Gen Pract* 1985; **35**: 136–9.
15. Victor CR. *Health and Health Care in Later Life*. Buckingham: Open University Press, 1991.
16. Victor CR. Inequality in health in later life. *Ageing Soc* 1991; **11**: 23–39.
17. Kay DWK. The epidemiology of dementia: a review of recent work. *Rev Clin Gerontol* 1991; **1**: 55–67.
18. Joam AF, Korten AE, Henderson AS. The prevalence of dementia; a quantitative integration. *Acta Psychiat Scand* 1985; **71**: 366–79.
19. Fries JF. Ageing, natural death and the compression of morbidity. *N Engl J Med* 1980; **303**(3): 130–5.
20. Vergrugge LM. Longer life but worsening health. *Millbank Mem Fund Qu* 1984; **62**(3): 475–519.
21. Falkingham J, Victor CR. The myth of the Woopie. *Ageing Soc* 1991; **11**: 471–93.
22. Vergrugge LM. Longer life but worsening health. *Millbank Mem Qu* 1984; **62**(3): 475–519.
23. Midwinter E. *Pensioned Off*. Buckingham: Open University Press, 1997.
24. Vincent JA. *Inequality and Old Age*. London: UCL Press, 1995.

Do Life Events Seem Less Stressful to the Old?

A. D. M. Davies

Department of Psychology, University of Liverpool, UK

INTRODUCTION

Problems in defining, measuring and interpreting the impact of a life event have been much discussed[1,2]. Where events occurring to older people are concerned, problems are compounded in that typically, mental health researchers assessing event severity are younger than the people assessed. A "social clock" view of development, however, assumes that the impact of an event depends on whether it is seen as normative or non-normative *for the stage of life*. The paradox is that older people are generally not the group that make the judgements of the severity of events occurring to older adults. A study was therefore carried out to see whether an elderly panel of raters accorded in judgement with a younger panel of four professional raters trained in the Bedford College LEDS scale, and whose ratings had been shown to be consistent and reliable[3].

METHODS

A group of 25 retired university and health service personnel was recruited to rate the severity of the events and difficulties that occurred to a sample of elderly rural people over a 12 month period. The present results refer to the ratings made by a randomly assigned subgroup of 10 (age range 65–82) who were thoroughly trained in the LEDS procedures. Their ratings were compared with those of a (non-elderly) psychologists' rating panel. After training, the panel met for six sessions over a 3 month period to rate 80 life events drawn from a pool of 289 events, which had occurred to an independent sample of 237 rural elderly people living in the community. The events were drawn in a counter-balanced way according to the consensus severity (threat) assigned to the professional panel (I = severely threatening, IV = little or no threat) within each of 20 blocks. Training for the older panel used definitions and guidelines from the Bedford College Manual, together with taped interviews, group discussion and rating practice with feedback about the professional panel's ratings. After all blocks had been rated, five blocks were re-rated to examine reliability (20 events). There was a minimum of 1 week and a maximum of 3 weeks between ratings. All but one participant showed significant agreement between the two ratings (as measured by Kendall's coefficient of concordance). The inconsistent participant's data were excluded from further analysis.

RESULTS

The distribution of severity ratings for the older trained panel over the four levels of event severity were as follows: I, 3; II, 27; III, 34; IV, 16. A one-way analysis of variance (ANOVA) comparing the mean ratings of the old trained panel with those of the professional panel showed that there were significant differences ($F = 5.6$, $P = 0.004$). *Post hoc* comparisons indicated that the old group rated events as less severe than the young group. Cross-tabulations showed that, although there was some agreement of the older and professional panels (weighted kappa = 0.31), the agreement with the professional panel was mainly about which events posed little threat. There was poor agreement for the crucial events of type I (severe threat). Of the 20 "severe threat" events presented, the distribution of ratings for the older panel were: I, 3; II, 6; III, 10; IV, 1. Most of these events concerned deaths of family members which, in general, the older panel (even though they had been trained in the LEDS procedures) did not see as particularly threatening.

CONCLUSION

The results provide support for the view that events such as deaths and severe illness events may be judged less threatening to older people, perhaps because they are seen as "on-time"[4]. Not all death events were rated equally, however. "Death of a spouse" and especially "death of a child" were regarded as more threatening than the death of a sibling or friend. However, in general the older panel rated stressful life events more conservatively.

ACKNOWLEDGEMENT

I would like to thank J. O. E. James and S. J. Wilkinson for their help in the collection of the data reported here.

REFERENCES

1. Davies ADM. Life events, health, adaptation and social support in the clinical psychology of late life. In RT Woods (ed.). *Handbook of the Clinical Psychology of Ageing*. Chichester: Wiley, 1997.
2. Orrell MW, Davies ADM. Life events in the elderly. *Int Rev Psychiat* 1994; **6**: 59–72.
3. Wilkinson SJ, Downes JJ, James O, Davies MG, Davies ADM. Rating reliability for life events and difficulties in the elderly. *Psychol Med* 1986; **16**: 101–5.
4. Neugarten BL. Dynamics of transition of middle age to old age: adaptation and the life cycle. *J Geriat Psychiat* 1970; **4**: 1–87.

Support Networks

G. Clare Wenger

Centre for Social Policy Research and Development, University of Wales, Bangor, UK

It is difficult to find any text in social gerontology which does not refer to social networks, care networks or support networks. In the 1980s, a shift in social gerontology research took place to focus on networks of support rather than whether or not elderly people have contact with each of a range of categories of relationship (spouse, daughter, brother, etc.)[1–6].

Support networks here are defined as those within the larger social network of the individual who regularly provide support in a range of contexts of day-to-day life, and include: members of the same household; relatives seen most frequently; confidant(s); and those people providing, or perceived by elderly respondents to be available to provide, emotional support, instrumental help, personal care or advice. Support networks may range in size from two to 22 but modally cluster around five to seven[4,7,8].

Women have been shown to have more expansive networks than men in a wide range of countries[9]. Research has shown that older people with strong social networks are happier and more likely to perceive themselves to be healthy[10]. Others have suggested that, for people with serious mental illness, social support promotes normality in life styles[11]. A review of the findings on social networks of older people[9] makes the following observations, which have significance for geriatric psychiatry. Dense networks (where a high proportion of members know one another) tend to provide better access to emotional support but may shield or prevent people from seeking professional advice. For example, Veiel[12] found that for some patients, psychological and emotional support in crises received from close relatives was associated with a subsequent increase in depressive symptoms. Loose-knit networks provide better access to resources, including professional care. Residential admissions are less common where there is a close supportive network but this can also be associated with the avoidance of needed professional interventions.

The radius of support networks tends to follow a bimodal distribution, with substantial numbers of older people having either all members within 5 miles or at least one member more than 25 miles away. Support networks typically have a core of family but also include friends, neighbours and home helps. Normative expectations of support for different relationships exist that are well defined but these are likely to be culturally specific. Such expectations are hierarchical. In the UK spouses top the hierarchy, followed by immediate family: daughters/sons and sisters/brothers. Following siblings come friends, and then neighbours. Extended family of grandchildren, nieces/nephews and cousins come below friends and neighbours[13,14]. Expectations are affected by the intervening variables of distance, gender and health. Long-term residents in a community tend to rely on local kin, while retirement migrants are unlikely to have kin nearby and have more diffuse networks[15,16].

The review of the literature referred to above suggests that older people may use different network members in different ways in emergency and non-emergency situations. There is evidence to show that vulnerable or stigmatized groups may be disadvantaged in network terms. Mentally ill people have smaller networks than others and the same is true for dementia sufferers. The more intimate (e.g. bodily care), personal (e.g. washing clothes) or private (e.g. financial concerns) the need of the elderly person (as defined by the culture), the more likely it is that this will be met by a family member. However, non-kin appear to be more important than family for morale, self-esteem and emotional support[17,18]. A high proportion of members of the support networks of elderly people are themselves elderly and/or female. Those who are or have been married tend to concentrate most need for support on one member of their network (usually a spouse or adult child), while those who have not married tend to spread their needs throughout their networks, relying on a wide range of others for one or two types of support.

Based on longitudinal data from the UK[5], it has been shown that, contrary to expectations for largely elderly networks, the size of networks typically remains stable over time, suggesting some form of homeostasis. One exception to this is the support networks of married men, which tend to shrink with widowhood. The average change is equivalent to ± 1–2 over 4 years. However, with increasing physical or mental frailty, networks tend to shift to reflect more reliance on proximate kin, if available, or increasing use of formal services and/or growing social isolation[19].

Loss from networks is predominantly due to death or disability and gains come from the pre-existing social network, with members moving into the supportive core. Tensions in networks may arise from mismatch of expectations between the elderly person and the network member, i.e. where demands exceed normal expectations of the relationship or where different actors define the relationship differently. Mental illness, particularly the resultant cognitive dissonance experienced by network members, can result in network contraction as non-kin withdraw and kin tend to insulate the sufferer from non-kin contacts[19].

Several different typologies of the networks of older people have been developed in Australia[8], the USA[20], the UK[6] and Israel[21]. What is striking is the similarity between them. Each typology: (a) reflects a continuum from close-knit to loose-knit; (b) finds that density is related to the importance of kinship; (c) includes the identification of a household-focused adaptation, based on a privatized life style and a small network; (d) identifies an association with social class (middle-class networks are less dense); and (e) acknowledges the influence of neighbourhood type.

Support networks demonstrate a range of types, which vary in terms of: availability of local kin; levels of interaction with different categories of membership; and the degree of community involvement, as measured by voluntary association. This article focuses on the Wenger support network typology, developed in the UK and subsequently validated in other countries. The Wenger typology identifies five types of network[6], which have distinct parallels with the other network typologies. The five types of networks identified are summarized below. The first three types are based on the presence of local kin; the other two types reflect the absence of local kin:

1. *The local family-dependent support network* has a primary focus on close local family ties, with few peripheral friends and neighbours; it is often based on a shared household with, or close to, an adult child, usually a daughter. Community involvement is generally low. These networks tend to be small and the elderly people are more likely to be widowed, older or in less than good health.

2. *The locally integrated support network* includes close relationships with local family, friends and neighbours. Many friends are also neighbours. It is usually based on long-term residence and active community involvement in church and voluntary organizations in the present or recent past. Networks tend to be larger on average than others.

3. *The local self-contained support network* typically has arm's-length relationships or infrequent contact with at least one relative living in the same or adjacent community, usually a sibling, niece or nephew. Childlessness is common. Reliance is focused on neighbours but respondents with this type of network adopt a household-focused life style and community involvement, if any, tends to be low key. Networks tend to be smaller than average.

4. *The wider community-focused support network* is typified by active relationships with distant relatives, usually children, and high salience of friends and neighbours. The distinction between friends and neighbours is maintained. Respondents with this type of network are generally involved in community or voluntary organizations. This type of network is frequently associated with retirement migration and is commonly a middle-class or skilled working-class adaptation. Networks are larger than average. Absence of local kin is typical.

5. *The private restricted support network* is typically associated with absence of local kin, other than in some cases a spouse, although a high proportion are married. Contact with neighbours is minimal; there are few nearby friends and a low level of community contacts or involvements. The type subsumes two sub-types: independent married couples and dependent elderly persons who have withdrawn or become isolated from local involvement. Networks are smaller than average.

As a result of different network configurations and differing normative expectations for members, some networks are more robust in terms of the provision of the informal support they can provide. Different types of networks react in different ways to the common problems of old age[22,23]. Different network types have different strengths and weaknesses and nature of the risk is related to the type of network[24]. Network types have also been demonstrated to relate to levels of use of domiciliary services and to types of presenting problems[25,26]. Knowledge of network type can, therefore, be a useful tool in planning therapeutic interventions and a measurement instrument for use by practitioners has been developed[22,24]. This makes it possible to identify support network type on the basis of eight questions.

Recent research has paid increasing attention to the significance of network type for professional practice. It has been suggested that to achieve "real improvements in the quality of life", the relationship environment of people with severe, long-term mental health problems needs to be explicitly addressed by practitioners[27]. Other authors[28] make the same point in the context of bereavement. Network type has been shown to be strongly associated with depression but not anxiety[29].

High needs for intervention have been identified in the context of a firm diagnosis of dementia associated with networks that reflect low levels of social support[30]. Admission to long-term care of older people with dementia occurs sooner in all network types other than the family-dependent network. In network types without local kin, the network tends to become private, restricted in the face of dementia[31].

The distribution of network types has been shown to be related to neighbourhood or community. Typically, where population stability is high, those types of networks based on local kin and providing high levels of informal support are found. Where population movement is high, for example in areas where retirement migration is common, the proportion of more vulnerable network types is greater[13,15]. Because of the relationship with coping strategies, knowledge of the distribution of network types can be an important indicator for planning the mix of service provision, in the same way that the identification of the network of an individual can indicate the appropriate type of intervention and potential future outcomes.

REFERENCES

1. Corin E. Elderly people's social strategies for survival: a dynamic use of social networks analysis. *Can Ment Health* 1982; **30**(3): 7–12.
2. Sinclair I, Crosbie D, O'Connor P et al. Networks Project: A Study of Informal Care, Services and Social Work for Elderly Clients Living Alone. London: National Institute for Social Work, 1984.
3. Kendig HL (ed.). *Aging and Families: A Social Networks Perspective*. Sydney, Australia: Allen and Unwin, 1986.
4. Wenger GC. *The Supportive Network: Coping with Old Age*. London: Allen and Unwin, 1984.
5. Wenger GC. A longitudinal study of changes and adaptations in the support networks of Welsh elderly over 75. *J Cross-cultural Gerontol* 1986; **1**(3): 277–304.
6. Wenger GC. Support networks in old age: constructing a typology. In Jefferys M, ed. *Growing Old in the Twentieth Century*. London: Routledge, 1989, 166–85.
7. Stephens RC, Blau Z, Oscar G, Millar M. Ageing, social support systems and social policy. *J Gerontol Soc Work* 1978; **1**(4): 33–45.
8. Mugford S, Kendig H. Social relations: networks and ties. In Kendig H, ed. *Ageing and Families: a Social Networks Perspective*. Sydney, Australia: Allen and Unwin, 1986, 38–59.
9. Wenger GC. Social network research in gerontology: how did we get here and where do we go next? In Minicheillo V, Chappell N, Walker A, Kendig H, eds. *The Sociology of Ageing: International Perspectives*. Melbourne, Australia: International Sociological Association, 1996.
10. Thompson JV. The elderly and their informal social networks. *Can J Aging* 1989; **8**(4): 319–32.
11. Walsh J, Connelly PR. Supportive behaviours in natural support networks of people with serious mental illness. *Health Soc Work* 1996; **21**(4): 296–303.
12. Veiel HOF. Detrimental effects of kin support networks on the course of depression. *J Abnorm Psychol* 1993; **102**(3): 419–29.
13. Wenger GC. A network typology: from theory to practice. *J Aging Stud* 1991; **5**(2): 147–62.
14. Wenger GC, Shahtahmasebi S. Variations in support networks: some social policy implications. In Mogey J, ed., *Aiding and Aging: The Coming Crisis in Support for the Elderly by Kin and State*. New York: Greenwood, 1990, 255–77.
15. Harper, S. The kinship network of the rural aged: a comparison of the indigenous elderly and the retired immigrant. *Ageing Soc* 1987; **7**: 303–27.
16. Wenger GC. The Bangor Longitudinal Study of Ageing. *Generations Rev* 1992; **2**(2): 6–8.
17. Wenger, GC. The special role of friends and neighbours. *J Aging Stud* 1990; **4**(2): 149–67.
18. Wenger GC. Davies R, Shahtahmasebi S. Morale in old age: refining the model. *Int J Geriat Psychiat* 1995; **10**: 993–43.
19. Wenger GC, Scott A. Change and stability in support network type: findings from a UK longitudinal study. *Age Vault: An INIA Collaborating Network Anthology*. Malta: UN International Institute on Ageing, 1992; 105–19.
20. Powers BA. Social networks, social support and elderly institutionalised people. *Adv Nurs Sci* 1988; **10**: 40–58.
21. Litwin H. The social networks of elderly immigrants: an analytic typology, *Journal of Aging Studies* 1995; **9**(2): 155–74.
22. Wenger GC. *The Support Networks of Older People: A Guide for Practitioners*. Brighton: Pavilion Publishing, 1994.
23. Litwin H. Support network type and patterns of help giving and receiving among older people. *J Soc Serv Res* 1999; **24**(3/4): 83–101.
24. Wenger GC. Social networks and the prediction of elderly people at risk. *Aging Ment Health* 1997; **1**(4): 311–30.
25. Wenger GC, Shahtahmasebi S. Variations in support networks: some policy implications. In Mogey J, ed., *Aiding and Ageing: The Coming Crisis*. Westport, CT: Greenwood, 1990, 255–77.

26. Litwin H. Support network type and health service utilization, *Res Ageing* 1997; **19**(3): 274–99.

27. Hatfield B, Huxley P, Mohamed H. The support networks of people with severe, long-term mental health problems, *Practice* 1993; **6**(1): 25–40.

28. Lowenstein A, Rosen A. The relation of locus of control and social support to life-cycle related needs of widows. *Int J Aging Human Dev* 1995; **40**(2): 103–23.

29. Bond J, Gregson B, Smith M *et al*. Outcomes following acute hospital care for stroke or hip fracture: how useful is an assessment of anxiety or depression for older people? *Int J Geriatr Psychiat* 1998; **13**(9): 601–10.

30. Wilcox J, Jones B, Alldrick D. Identifying the support needs of people with dementia and older people with mental illness on a Joint Community Team: a preliminary report. *J Ment Health* 1995; **41**(3): 157–63.

31. Wenger GC. Support networks and dementia. *Int J Geriatr Psychiat* 1994; **9**: 181–94.

32. Wenger GC. The Impact on the family of chronic mental illness in old age. Presented to *WHO Workshop on Mental Health and the Family*, Brussels: Belgium, 17th March, 1989.

16

World Statistical Trends and Prospects

George C. Myers

Center for Demographic Studies, Duke University, Durham, USA

The aging process relates to both individuals and the collective aggregates that they comprise, such as families and nations. The prolongation of human life has resulted in ever-increasing numbers of persons not only reaching the threshold ages defining old age, but living beyond. In most of the world's developed countries, at least four-fifths of the persons born today can expect to reach their 65th birthday and, of these survivors to old age, over 40% will reach 85. At the beginning of this century, only half as many (two-fifths) could expect to reach age 65, with only 14% of the survivors likely to live to age 85. The future will no doubt bring even further extension of life for greater numbers of individuals. A corollary of this development will be increases in the numbers of older persons in our populations, given the large size of future cohorts of persons reaching the older ages.

This remarkable achievement in extending life, largely a phenomenon of the twentieth century, has important consequences for the well-being of individuals and the societies in which they live. Most notably, we must be concerned with the implications of these trends on the life conditions of older persons and their impact on the social, economic, political and health institutions of societies. As many contributions to this volume emphasize, loss of intellectual functioning and the emergence of mental illness are not inevitable concomitants of aging. But the older population does have the highest frequency of cognitive impairments and disruptive behaviors of any age group and are least likely to be seen by mental health specialists[1]. Moreover, these conditions also command high levels of care and support from family and community networks. An increased awareness of the demographic context, both present and future, is necessary for furthering our understanding and treatment of these phenomena.

In this chapter, we provide a statistical treatment of the diverse dimensions of this aging process, particularly population aging, and how it is likely to evolve in the years ahead. Although population aging is truly a world-wide experience, for this volume we focus on conditions within the so-called more developed region (MDR), which include North America, Japan, Europe, Australia and New Zealand. It is in this more developed region that population aging has progressed the most in terms of the proportions of older persons in the population. Moreover, the countries in this region also have experienced major changes in the composition of the aged population itself. The data reported in this chapter are derived from the most recent population projections (medium variant series) of the United Nations, as assessed in 1998[2].

GROWTH OF THE OLDER POPULATION

The older population—persons 65 years and over—is estimated at 171 million for the more developed region in 2000. They represented 14.4% of the total population, about one in every seven persons. The number of older persons has increased by 45 million or 35% since 1980, compared with an increase of only 6% for the under-65 population. By the year 2050, the region's older population is projected to reach nearly 300 million, a numerical increase over the 50-year period of 128 million. As noted in Table 16.1 and Figure 16.1, the growth accelerates after the year 2010, as persons born in the post-World War II period reach the older ages, then subsides somewhat after 2040.

The growth rates for the older population over the total period greatly exceed those of the under-65 population of countries in the region. In fact, the younger population actually declines in number after the year 2010, as newly-aged cohorts advance into

Table 16.1 Population distribution by age group, more developed region, 1980–2050

	0–14	15–64	65–79	80+
1980	243	714	126	22
1990	236	768	144	31
2000	216	801	171	36
2010	196	820	192	50
2020	193	791	232	58
2030	187	749	274	72
2040	182	712	294	92
2050	177	679	299	102

Source: United Nations, *World Population Prospects: The 1998 Revision*, Vol II.

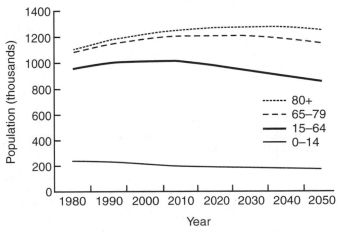

Figure 16.1 Population distribution by age group, more developed region 1980–2050. Source: United Nations, *World Population Prospects: The 1998 Revision*, Vol II

Principles and Practice of Geriatric Psychiatry, 2nd edn. Edited by J. R. M. Copeland, M. T. Abou-Saleh and D. G. Blazer
©2002 John Wiley & Sons, Ltd

the older population and are not fully compensated for by youths. Thus, the proportion of older persons in the total population is expected to steadily increase, reaching nearly 23% in 2030. This aggregate figure masks considerable variation among countries, with Japan (27.3%), and Italy (29.1%) expected to reveal the highest levels and Ireland (17.9%) and New Zealand (18.8%) at the lower end. Nonetheless, the proportion of older persons for all countries in the region is historically unprecedented. An added dimension of these changes in the age composition of the populations is the expectation that by 2015 the proportion of older persons will exceed the proportion of young persons aged 0–14 years, given realization of the assumptions regarding fertility introduced into the projections.

AGE AND SEX COMPOSITIONS OF THE AGED POPULATION

Not only has the region experienced overall population aging, but the older population has itself aged. The growth of the oldest old (persons aged 80 and over) has important implications in terms of the health status of this group of people and their need for health care and social supports. If the assumption is correct that the prevalence of mental health problems increases with age, then these trends toward aging of the older population take on added importance. Moreover, the incidence of the most severe mental disorders (e.g. senile dementia of the Alzheimer's type) is greatly manifested at advanced ages[3]. The percentage of oldest old in the total older population showed a marked rise in the 1980s, when it increased from 17% to 22%. It will steadily rise until the year 2010 (26%) and then will decline slightly to 24% in 2025. The decline reflects the large number of persons who will reach the older ages between 2010 and 2030. Nonetheless, the overall numbers of oldest old will nearly double to 72 million in the region over the 2000 figure.

A noteworthy feature of the older population in the region is the preponderance of women over men. In 2000, there were 153 older women for every 100 men and, among the oldest old, 226 women for every 100 men. These levels for both groups are likely to be somewhat attenuated in the future, as the aged population gains large new cohorts, but the imbalance will still remain.

COMPONENTS OF POPULATION AGING

While the overall age and sex structure of a population is affected by fertility, mortality and migration, the main factors producing changes in the older population result from the relative size of cohorts reaching the older ages and the survival of these older persons to further advanced ages. Although the major source of future growth results from the large baby boom birth cohorts that will enter the older population, as was noted previously, the improved chances of persons reaching old age and surviving to advanced ages have also been a potent force in producing the present and future growth[4].

The average life expectancy of a baby born between 1995 and 2000 and experiencing the age-specific mortality conditions of that period was 71.1 years for a boy and 78.7 for a girl[5]. To gain some perspective on these figures, the following levels were estimated for the period 1970–1975 and projected for future periods:

	Male	Female
1970–1975	67.6	74.7
2020–2025	75.5	81.8
2045–2050	78.2	84.2

There was an increase of 3.5 years for males and 4.0 for females in the 25-year period preceding 1995–2000 and gains of 4.4 and

3.1, respectively, projected for a similar time period to 2020–2025. The reversal in the projected survival by gender can be noted and this is carried over into the next period, when only minor life expectancy gains are forecasted. Aside from this questionable gender reversal, some also view the assumptions underlying the UN projections as rather conservative. In fact, a life expectancy at birth for females of over 84 years has already been attained in Japan and is likely to be exceeded in many other countries by the second decade of the twenty-first century.

The extension of life has meant that the remaining years of life after persons reach age 65 have increased markedly. For the USA, a surviving male could expect to live 15.7 years on average at age 65 in 1996 compared with 11.5 in 1900, a 36% increase[6]. The average female could expect to live an additional 19 years in 1996, a gain of 6.8 years or 55%. Moreover, 76% of men and 86% of women born in 1996 can expect to reach age 65, doubling the percentages in 1900. Thus, not only have more persons reached old age, but an increasing amount of one's life is being spent as an older person.

These improvements in survival have resulted from widespread reductions in communicable diseases and even declines in the lethal progressions of some of the predominant chronic, degenerative diseases. A noteworthy feature of overall mortality trends in the region has been the reductions in death rates at older ages. An emerging issue of considerable policy importance is the extent to which these improvements in longevity have been accompanied by increases in active life expectancy free of major chronic diseases, functional disabilities and institutionalization. While data are lacking to definitively establish past developments, there is evidence that active life expectancy has tended to increase, perhaps even keeping pace with improvements in overall life expectancy[7]. However, with increased population aging, the net result of these developments is the likelihood of increased numbers of persons at old ages with chronic co-morbidities and disabilities and, therefore, in need of long-term care and rehabilitative services.

SUPPORT STRUCTURES

The demographic parameters that relate most directly to these emerging issues concern the households and family conditions of older persons who are likely to need supportive assistance (care-receivers) and those who are potential care-providers. A number of complex demographic and social factors are involved in this matrix.

There has been a steady trend over time toward increased proportions of older persons being married and reduced proportions being single and widowed in the countries of this region[8]. Moreover, this development is true not only for the total aged population, but also for all age groups up to the most advanced. However, it should be noted that a much larger proportion of men than women are likely to be married, with the converse true of widowhood. These trends are a product of both the previous marital experience of persons in cohorts reaching the older ages and improvements in the joint survival of spouses. Nonetheless, there are strong signs that this pattern will change in the next century, as large cohorts of persons who are divorced or have never married enter into the older ages.

Another distinctive trend has been the increasing likelihood of older persons, both married couples and individuals, to live independently from other family members or non-relatives. This pattern of living arrangements reflects the smaller size of families resulting from prior declining fertility, as well as value preferences among older persons for independent living. However, these observations say little about the degree of contact among family

Table 16.2 Generational support ratios, more developed region, 1980–2050

	45–49/65–70	65–69/80+
1980	0.62	2
1990	0.58	1.56
2000	0.64	1.41
2010	0.64	1.1
2020	0.48	1.23
2030	0.41	1.08
2040	0.37	0.8
2050	0.35	0.71

Source: United Nations, *World Population Prospects: The 1998 Revision*, Vol II.

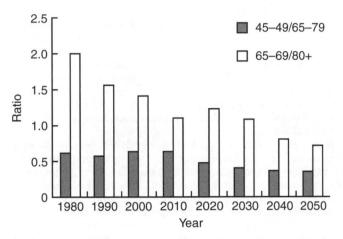

Figure 16.2 Generational support ratios, more developed region, 1980–2050. Source: United Nations, *World Population Prospects: The 1998 Revision*, Vol II

members or the strength of social networks, which appears to have remained strong.

Over the last few decades, increasing numbers of older persons have resided in institutions, although the proportions of such persons have not risen markedly in most developed countries[9]. While only 5–10% of older persons are in institutions at any given time, approximately 40% of persons will be institutionalized at some point in their lifetimes. Future prospects in light of the growing number of older persons living alone have given rise to considerable concern about the social, medical and economic issues of providing non-institutional vs. institutional care. Moreover, there is considerable policy debate over the optimal balance between family and state-provided care, whether in the home or in a more formal setting.

This brief review of trends suggests that there are major developments emerging from the growth of the older population and increased longevity that signal important changes in the potential care burden for vulnerable persons in the aged population. In turn, it raises questions about potential caregivers, most notably members of younger generations. A broad indication of the demographic indicators can be gained from examining ratios of the number of persons who are aged 45–49 to those aged 65–79. The former can be thought of as a group consisting of

children of older persons. A second ratio relates two generations of older persons—those aged 65–69 to those aged 80 and over.

Table 16.2 and figure 16.2 show these two sets of ratios over the period 1980–2050. The importance of these ratios is not in their absolute levels, but in the relative levels over time. The younger generational ratios reveal little meaningful change up to year 2010, but thereafter decline steadily as the baby boom generation enters the older ages. The older generation ratios show more fluctuation. They have declined sharply from 1980 to the present and will continue downward to 2010. They show a rise in 2020, but then slowly decline to below parity through the projection period. In general, the shorter-term trends are somewhat reassuring in terms of the availability of potential caregivers but the longer-term trends reveal the increasing pressures on support systems. It should be noted, however, that such ratios do not inform us about the capacity of younger generations to provide assistance, which can be affected by kin relationships and involvement in employment that precludes extensive assistance.

SUMMARY

Population aging is a pervasive and seemingly irreversible process for countries in the world's more developed region. Not only will older persons increase dramatically in number and as a percentage of total populations, but dynamic forces will modify the socio-demographic and health status composition of aged populations as well. Like the Struldbrugs or Immortals of Swift's *Gulliver's Travels* the advantages of life prolongation have complex consequences, not only for the individuals involved but also for the societies in which they are found.

REFERENCES

1. World Health Organization. *Health of the Elderly: Report of a WHO Expert Committee*. Technical Report Series No. 779. Geneva: World Health Organization, 1989.
2. United Nations. *World Population Prospects: The 1998 Revision*, Vol II. New York: United Nations Secretariat, Department of Economic and Social Affairs, Population Division, 1999.
3. Evans DA. The epidemiology of dementia and Alzheimer's disease: an evolving field. *J Am Geriatr Soc* 1996; **44**: 1482–3.
4. Myers GC. Comparative mortality trends among older persons in developed countries. In Caselli G, Lopez A, eds, *Health and Mortality Among Elderly Populations*. Oxford: Oxford University Press, 1996, 87–111.
5. United Nations. *World Population Prospects: The 1998 Revision*, Vol I. New York: United Nations Secretariat, Department of Economic and Social Affairs, Population Division, 1999.
6. Anderson RN. United States abridged life tables, 1966. *National Vital Statistics Reports*, Vol 47, No. 13. Hyattsville, MD: National Center for Health Statistics, 1998.
7. National Institute on Aging. The declining disability of older Americans. *Research Highlights in the Demography and Economics of Aging*, No. 5, March 1999.
8. Myers GC. Cross-national patterns and trends in marital status among the elderly. In Loriaux M, Remy D, Vilguin E, eds, *Population Agees et Revolution Crise*, Chaire Quetelet 86, Louvain-la-Neuve, Belgium: Institut de Demographie, Universite de Louvain, 1990, 469–81.
9. Kinsella K, Velkoff VA. *An Aging World 1999*. US Bureau of the Census, International Population Reports, Washington, DC: US Government Printing Office, 2000.

Demography of the Old: Implications of Recent Trends

Emily Grundy

London School of Hygiene and Tropical Medicine, London, UK

In most developed countries, at least 10% and in some cases more than 15% of the total population is aged 65 and over[1]. Recent projections suggest that by 2025 the proportion aged 75 and over will lie in this range; by then people aged 65 and over will contribute a quarter of the total in a number of countries including Japan, Italy and Greece, and over one-fifth in most of the rest of Europe. The proportion of "oldest old"—those aged 85 years or more—is increasing particularly rapidly[2]. As the risk of dementia is so strongly age-related, these changes will mean a large increase in the numbers affected unless strategies for prevention and postponement can be identified and implemented. However, there are also other implications of current demographic trends. Here I focus on changes in mortality and survivorship and also consider briefly changes in marriage.

The initial impetus for this ageing of the human world came from the transition to lower fertility that was set in motion in many Western populations in the last quarter of the nineteenth century and is now close to being a global phenomenon. More recently, the pace of population ageing, and the ageing of elderly populations, has been accelerated by marked declines in late age mortality; these are now the predominant motor driving the further ageing of populations with already old age structures[3].

The extent of this change is illustrated for five developed countries in Table 1. In England and Wales, France and the USA,

Table 1 Further expectation of life at age 65, 1900–1995

	1900–1901	1950–1951	1970–1971	1995
Men				
England and Wales	10.1	10.8	11.9	14.8
France	10.0	12.2	13.0	16.1
Japan	10.1	10.9	12.5	16.5
Sweden	12.1	13.5	14.3	16.0
USA	11.4	12.8	13.1	15.3
Women				
England and Wales	11.1	13.4	15.8	18.4
France	10.9	14.6	16.8	20.6
Japan	11.4	13.0	15.4	20.9
Sweden	13.0	14.3	16.9	19.7
USA	12.0	15.1	17.1	19.2

Data from: Government Actuary's Department, Berkeley.
Mortality Database (http://demog.berkeley.edu/wilmoth/mortality); and the Japanese Ministry of Health and Welfare.

Table 2 Survival to age 80 by birth cohort, England and Wales

Year of birth	Survival to age 80 (%)	
	Men	Women
1861	10	16
1881	14	25
1901	17	34
1921*	29	47

*Partly based on projections.
Source: Author's analysis of data from the Government Actuary's Department.

male expectation of life at age 65 increased as much or more between 1970 and 1995 than in the preceding 70 years (or indeed, in the case of England and Wales, in the preceding century[4]). Among women too, the extent of improvement since 1970 is notable. Viewed from a cohort perspective, increases in longevity appear even more remarkable. Table 2 shows the proportion of each birth cohort surviving to the age of 80. Survival to later older age has increased dramatically reflecting not only large improvements in infant and child mortality (still very high in the nineteenth century) but also the more recent improvements in late adult death rates. Today, women of 80 represent not a select group of elite survivors, but *half* their original birth cohort. These improvements are not confined to the "young" elderly; death rates among the oldest old, including centenarians, have also dropped substantially[5,6].

These changes have sparked fierce debate about possible changes in the relationship between mortality and morbidity, the plasticity of the ageing process, possible limits to longevity and, of course, implications for health services. Less frequently considered are the implications for the family and support networks of older people and how these may interact with other changes in, for example, marriage and partnership.

The gender differences in mortality apparent in the tables underlie one of the most notable features of the older population, the preponderance of women. In the UK in 1998 the ratio of women to men at age 60–64 was close to parity (1.04) but rose to 1.85 at age 80–84 and 3.5 in the 90–94 year-old group. One consequence of this gender imbalance, compounded by the common pattern of women marrying men older than themselves, is that 65% of women aged 75 and over are widows, while 62% of men of this age are still married. If the narrowing of sex differentials in mortality continues, as is projected, the proportion of widows in this group will fall to 52% by 2021; however, by then 10% will be divorced (compared with 3% now) and a much larger proportion will have experienced divorce at some point in their lives (21% of those born in 1950 had already experienced divorce by the age of 40[7]). Those who have experienced marital disruption have poorer health in early old age[8], although this may be because of factors associated with both risk of divorce and poor health.

Changes in the age structure of populations also mean change in the age structure of families. Lower mortality increases the availability and duration of "vertical" kin networks. A recent (1999) national survey showed that 74% of people aged 80 and over in Britain were members of three-generation families and over one-third had living children, grandchildren and great-grandchildren[9]. Contacts between older people and their children and grandchildren are frequent; however, there have been very large decreases in the extent of intergenerational co-residence. In 1991 21% of women aged 85 and over lived in two- or three-generational households, compared with 42% 20 years earlier[10]. During the same period (1971–1991) the proportion of older people moving to institutions increased, while the proportion moving to live with relatives fell, suggesting some substitution of the former for family care[11].

Demographic changes of the type and magnitude, which here I have had space to allude to only briefly, require some thinking about roles, relationships and activities throughout the life course.

Most people now spend much longer as the parent of an adult child than they do raising minor children; increasing proportions will have step- and half-kin of various kinds and will live to know their great-grandchildren. However, expectations about these types of relationships may be confused. The increasing diversity of partnering and parenting patterns may also have implications both for mental health in later life and the support of those with mental health problems.

REFERENCES

1. Council of Europe. *Recent Demographic Developments in Europe.* Strasbourg: Council of Europe Publishing, 1998.
2. United Nations. *World Population Prospects, The 1998 Revision.* New York: UN.
3. Preston SH, Himes CL, Eggers M. Demographic conditions responsible for population aging. *Demography* 1989; **26**: 691–704.
4. Grundy E. The health of older adults, 1841–1991. In Charlton J, Murphy M, eds, *The Health of Adult Britain 1841–1991*, Vol II. London: HMSO, 1997; 183–204.
5. Thatcher R. The demography of centenarians in England and Wales. *Population Trends* 1999; **96**: 5–12.
6. Kannisto V. *Development of oldest-old mortality, 1950–1990: evidence from 28 developed countries.* Odense: Odense University Press, 1994.
7. Haskey J. First marriage, divorce, and remarriage: birth cohort analyses. *Population Trends* 1993; **72**: 24–33.
8. Grundy E, Holt G. Adult life experiences and health in early old age in Great Britain. *Social Science and Medicine* 2000; **51**: 1061–74.
9. Grundy E, Murphy M, Shelton N. Looking beyond the household: intergenerational perspectives on living kin and contacts with kin in Great Britain. *Population Trends* 1999; **97**: 33–41.
10. Grundy E. Population review: the population aged 60 and over. *Population Trends* 1996; **84**: 14–20.
11. Grundy E, Glaser K. Trends in, and transitions to, institutional residence among older people in England and Wales, 1971 to 1991. *J Epidemiol Commun Health* 1997; **51**: 531–40.

Part C

Abnormal Ageing

17

The Influence of Social Factors on Mental Health

David Mechanic* and Donna D. McAlpine

Institute for Health, Health Care Policy and Aging Research, Rutgers University, New Brunswick, NJ, USA

Social factors have an enormous influence on the life course, affecting development and socialization, the relative influence of families and peer groups, opportunities for work, recreation and social participation, and patterns of social integration and independence as one reaches the later years. With the rapidity of social change, persons living a normal lifespan are required to modify their expectations and behavior on many occasions if they are to adapt successfully to shifting social conditions. Transformations in technology, sexuality, fertility, family and work life, household structure and many other facets of life, also make it inevitable that different age cohorts will have diverse life experiences.

Almost every aspect of mental health and well-being are influenced by social factors and social institutions[1]. The effectiveness of social institutions, and the extent to which they build supportive relationships, coping capacities and personal commitment, contribute importantly to mental health outcomes. The dynamics of populations, and the distribution of persons at varying ages, also affect the productive capacities of nations, the prevalence of disability and dependence, and the capacity of a society to protect its citizens against the risks of disadvantage. Social attitudes and patterns of community organization can either encourage or inhibit full participation and meaningful roles for children, the elderly, the disabled or other groups, affecting functioning, quality of life and psychological well-being.

The discussion that follows focuses more on severe mental illness than on levels of psychological distress or emotional well-being. The distinction is not clear-cut because even depressive symptoms short of a clinically diagnosable disorder can have devastating effects on functioning and quality of life and are a major source of disability, surpassing in impact many serious chronic diseases[2].

Severe mental disorder, such as depression, bipolar conditions, and schizophrenia results from complex, but poorly understood, interactions between biological vulnerabilities and psychological and social influences. Adverse social and developmental factors may increase susceptibility to serious mental illness, or may contribute to triggering illness among vulnerable persons. Among persons with mental illness, social factors may significantly ameliorate symptoms, influence treatment patterns and enhance or impair quality of life. Most of the major social factors—age, gender, social class, race and ethnicity, familial arrangements and the like—are associated with mental illness, either by contributing to its onset or course or because of social selection factors. Moreover, there are complex interactions among social factors

such that, for example, the impact of socioeconomic status or gender on mental health outcomes may vary by age or by birth cohort.

The epidemiology of illnesses that first occur later in life may be quite different from chronic conditions that persist through much of the life course. Understanding the occurrence of mental illness later in life, however, is complicated by the relationships between physical illness, drug use (commonly prescription drugs) and the occurrence of symptoms consistent with mental illness. Prescription and non-prescription drug use is high in elderly populations because of the prevalence of illness. The inappropriate use of pharmaceuticals among elderly persons is also common and includes physicians over-prescribing to older patients, self-medication and drug interactions[3]. Moreover, drug sensitivity changes with age-related changes in individuals' capacity to absorb and metabolize drugs; therefore, dosages effective in younger patients may be ineffective or excessively high for older patients. There continues to be considerable concern that institutional settings over-use medication in order to sedate and control patients. Drug reactions, including confusion, hallucinations, paranoia and mania, are common and may be inappropriately diagnosed as mental illness.

Schizophrenia typically first occurs in late adolescence or in early adulthood and may have a complex and fluctuating course. Follow-up studies of early-onset schizophrenia indicate that, with aging, the positive symptoms of schizophrenia abate or remain in remission for longer periods of time, and that for a significant minority of persons complete remission is possible, although the processes that lead to such outcomes are not well understood[4]. Selective mortality or the natural course of the disorder may be responsible for the relatively positive outcomes observed among older persons with schizophrenia. It is also possible that lowered personal expectations, the development of coping strategies, improved adaptation and learning how to avoid upsetting stresses also contribute to positive outcomes for persons with schizophrenia. On the one hand, persons with chronic schizophrenia bring into their later years life histories that are likely to be characterized by significant periods of disorder and disruption. On the other hand, they bring an array of skills and coping strategies, developed through dealing with illness over many years, and these may mitigate the potentially negative impact of the illness during later life.

Late-onset schizophrenia is relatively rare and little is known about its course[5,6]. The lack of evidence of late onset of schizophrenia and other psychoses among the elderly may in part result from diagnostic practices that give priority to co-occurring dementia and confusion that are highly prevalent in

*To whom correspondence should be addressed

Principles and Practice of Geriatric Psychiatry, 2nd edn. Edited by J. R. M. Copeland, M. T. Abou-Saleh and D. G. Blazer
©2002 John Wiley & Sons, Ltd

later years. It has only recently been recognized in the USA, and there have been very few community-based studies examining outcomes. There is some suggestion, however, that those persons with onset later in life are able to function better in the community because occupational and social roles have not been interrupted by the disorder earlier in life[5].

There has been more research attention focused on depression during later life and although there have been widespread reports of a high prevalence among this population, epidemiological studies have not confirmed this impression[7]. But it is unclear whether the relatively low rates of depression at older ages are artifacts of epidemiological definitions and methods. Sub-threshold negative affect appears very high in this population, leading many internists and geriatricians who care for the elderly population to believe that epidemiological estimates are biased and do not reflect the real situation. Depression is clearly different in elderly persons than in early and middle adulthood because of complex physical co-morbidities, decrements in function and relationship losses that occur in later life. Older persons are also less likely to acknowledge psychological manifestations of depression, see mental health treatment as more stigmatizing and resist referral to mental health specialists. Assessing depression within the constellation of physical concomitants that might be attributed to a variety of other conditions poses diagnostic challenges for the general physician. There are presently a number of ongoing experimental efforts to improve the recognition and treatment of depression among the elderly in primary care[8].

Most studies examining depression among elderly persons have not dated the onset of the disorder. There is some suggestion, however, that biological or genetic vulnerability may play a lesser role in the etiology of first onset of major depression or bipolar disorders late in life than earlier[9,10]. Late-onset depression and bipolar disorder appear to be triggered more commonly by medical and neurological co-morbidities, while onset earlier in adulthood is more strongly correlated with the occurrence of environmental stressors[10]. Much remains to be learned about the etiology of late-onset disorders but the role of social factors will vary with age.

Recent research reports a gender difference in late-onset schizophrenia, with older women having greater risk[5], although the reason for this difference remains unclear. There is also a gender difference in depression but, unlike schizophrenia, it develops in early adolescence and persists across the life course. The relationship is a complex one and is a matter of continuing controversy. Since abuse of alcohol and drugs and violence are more common among men, and depressed affect more common among women, some explain the two-fold prevalence difference in terms of varying gender-related reaction patterns[11]. Others have argued that the higher rates of reported and diagnosed depressive illness in women result from a greater prevalence of more common and less serious symptoms of depression reported by women, such as sadness and crying, and their greater willingness to report affective symptoms[12]. The issues remain unresolved, with different views depending in part on varying conceptions of the nature of depressive disorders.

Whatever the eventual resolution of these issues, the data do suggest that women in later life are at greater risk for symptoms of schizophrenia and depression than are their male counterparts. At the same time, older women are more likely than older men to be without a partner and they also experience greater economic disadvantage, both of which may exacerbate the negative consequences of mental disorder.

There is a long-established relationship between socioeconomic status and severe mental illness and decades of debate about the relative influence of causative vs. selection factors for explaining the higher prevalence of schizophrenia among those of lower socioeconomic status[13,14]. The weight of the evidence supports the view that the impairment associated with schizophrenia prevents upward mobility comparable to one's age cohort and loss of social position because of difficulties completing one's education and maintaining employment.

Early onset of major depression or bipolar disorder may also impair upward mobility, but socioeconomic status also appears to affect the onset of major depression. A variety of studies suggest that the etiological significance of socioeconomic status in depression relates to the prevalence of major life stresses and persistent difficulties and the lower availability of coping resources and social supports[15].

Disadvantages associated with socioeconomic status put persons with mental illness at risk for a number of negative outcomes that are not directly associated with the illness. Inadequate housing or homelessness remain significant problems for persons with mental illnesses and compromise efforts to provide meaningful services, yet we know very little about these issues in older populations[16]. Economic disadvantage is also a substantial barrier to access to health services and prescription medications in countries without universal health coverage[17]. These problems may be accentuated in later life for those with limited resources.

Socioeconomic status also helps to explain differences in mental health outcomes for different race and ethnic groups in the USA. While there do not appear to be major race/ethnic differences in the prevalence of severe mental illnesses independent of socio-economic status, these factors significantly influence the course of illness. In the USA, rates of services utilization are lower for Mexican Americans, Asian Americans, and African Americans than Whites, when need for services is taken into account[18]. Economic barriers to access to health services contribute to this gap between need and service utilization among certain race and ethnic groups. Cultural differences in attitudes toward mental health services, perceived stigma and discrimination may also play a role[19].

The importance of family for the onset and course of mental illness has been commonly examined. The onset of severe mental disorder early in life increases the likelihood of remaining unmarried, especially for men, and increases the risk of divorce and separation among those who do marry[20]. Thus, many persons with severe mental illness will enter their later years without the benefits of a partner to provide emotional and instrumental support.

Styles of interaction within the family are also important. Most of the research has been focused on schizophrenia and suggests that a highly involved critical orientation to the patient contributes to relapse[21]. Instruction of families based on these principles has been found to be useful in some controlled trials, and offers a conceptual basis for psychoeducational approaches[21,22].

Increasing research in mental health focuses on stress and the coping process and the role of social support in either buffering the effects of stress or independently contributing to emotional well-being. While such factors as stressful events, coping resources, intimate and instrumental relations and self-efficacy have all been found to be associated with variations in psychological distress, their significance for major mental illness is less clear. Moreover, the role of these factors is condition-specific. In schizophrenia, stress acts as a trigger, affecting the occurrence and timing of episodes[23]. In affective disorder, in contrast, stressful events and meanings assigned to these events appear to play a more causative role in conjunction with other factors[12]. There is recent evidence that childhood adversity, such as separation from parents or sexual and physical abuse, may trigger onset of depressive disorders well into adulthood[24].

While, in general, it is believed that social support is important, the forms of social support useful to varying kinds of patients at different stages of their conditions remain unclear[25]. There is much research suggesting especially that intrusive forms of social interaction involving criticism may be detrimental to schizophrenic patients, and the relative protectiveness of intimacy, friendship and instrumental assistance in depression remain unclear. Social support remains a vague concept, having varying operational definitions. Contrasting views of social support explain some of the conflicting research results.

There is increasing research attention being given to the role of religion and religious participation in health outcomes for the elderly and a variety of studies suggest that different aspects of religious involvement play an important role[26]. The pathways through which such effects are manifested remain unclear, although there is increasing suggestion that the social supports and instrumental assistance that might result from religious involvement contribute to better health. Research in this area confronts difficult selection biases, in that persons in better health may be more able and inclined toward religious participation and that persons drawn to varying religious practices may be different in their personalities, attitudes and behaviors than those with lesser or no participation. Nevertheless, the research in this area is gaining rigor and is suggestive of potential pathways.

The focus on coping skills as an important determinant of adaptation in more theoretically orientated studies has found expression in the development of psycho-educational programs to assist chronic mental patients in their rehabilitation. Although the research is modest, it supports the value of problem-orientated educational approaches that assist patients to manage everyday life situations better[27]. Psychosocial research on the importance of self-efficacy has been translated into programs to increase patient empowerment. It has been suggested that such empowerment is an important feature of the success of some commonly studied rehabilitation programs[28]. Increased empowerment may be an important factor, ameliorating the negative impact of highly regimented settings, such as nursing homes and other custodial institutions, but its therapeutic role in the normal range of life settings is yet to be established[29].

Social factors shape the processes through which individuals and families define illness, evaluate its meaning and significance and make decisions about needed care and appropriate practitioners. Epidemiological evidence shows that much serious mental illness is untreated, and those receiving treatment obtain services from a wide variety of practitioners. Processes of help-seeking are influenced by broad social beliefs about the nature of illness and what should be treated, characteristics of the individual and the social contexts in which mental illness occurs, and the organization of services and their physical, social and economic accessibility[1]. Members of varying age cohorts have been socialized differently in relation to the recognition of symptoms, appropriate sources of help and the social stigma of seeking care for particular types of problems. Selection from the community to varying types of service providers is a two-stage process, which depends on general factors affecting the inclination to seek assistance, and other factors more specific to the choice among alternative practitioners. A large proportion of all patients receiving care for a mental illness receive such care exclusively from general medical practitioners, and decisions affecting referral to the specialty mental health sector result not only from personal definitions and inclinations of patients and their families, but also from the organized pathways within a health care system, the ability of generalists to recognize mental illness in their patients and their attitudes to specialty mental health services. Patients with mental illness are referred more readily to specialized services when illness and illness behavior imply social risk and disruption[30]. Diagnosis, itself, is a poor predictor of the referral process.

Patterns of help seeking differ by age. The elderly are less likely to seek psychiatric care than younger adults, and probably are more reluctant to report affective symptoms to interviewers or physicians. In contrast, the elderly complain commonly in general medical settings of diffuse physical symptoms and vegetative symptoms characteristic of depression, and have relatively high rates of receiving prescribed psychoactive drugs. While somatization, as measured more formally, does not seem to vary by age, the elderly are more likely to present distress in a somatic idiom. Interpretation is complicated by the fact that the elderly have higher rates of ill-health and chronic disease than younger individuals, and it is difficult to sort out physical concomitants of chronic disease from somatization of psychosocial distress and depression. Psychoactive drug use also reflects physician behavior, which may be shaped by stereotypes of the elderly and other factors.

The social response to mental illness is influenced by such factors as general attitudes, values and ideologies, concepts of the nature of disorders and their causes, available treatment technologies, the structure of health and welfare services, and the system of social entitlements that a society makes available. The deinstitutionalization of the mentally ill has followed a different course in varying countries, but each of the above factors plays some role in every instance. In the USA, large-scale deinstitutionalization only became possible in the middle 1960s with the expansion of welfare programs that provided subsistence and payment for alternative residential care for mentally ill patients in the community. Some of the evident difficulties in community mental health services reflect cutbacks or fluctuations in welfare and housing entitlements[1].

The magnitude of serious mental illness depends on the distribution of the population, and the numbers of persons in age groups at risk for varying diseases and disabilities. The burden of mental illness depends not only on its magnitude but also on the types of social institutions and programs that help insulate patients, families and communities from its most disruptive stresses. The elderly population, and persons at very old ages, are growing in the USA and many Western countries. The dementias are increasingly important, and patients with such disabilities constitute a growing proportion of the severe mentally ill population. Depending on the constellation of institutional services and home-care programs, patients with dementia are treated in a variety of settings, some placing very large burdens on families and friends. The distribution of such burdens, and the definition of responsibilities, is a political process and a key social policy issue throughout the world.

For the last several decades, the nursing home has been the setting for care of persons who are greatly restricted in the activities of daily living, and a large proportion of persons in these settings have dementia and depression as a secondary condition[31]. Typically, admission to nursing homes occur when individuals are incapable of caring for themselves, when their physical and psychiatric problems create unmanageable burdens for their caretakers, or when community caretakers are no longer available. Admission is often triggered by such events as significant loss of function following trauma, such as hip fractures, confusion and wandering, and incontinence. Relatively few elderly with a primary diagnosis of mental illness, without dementia, are in nursing homes, although nursing home admission often exacerbates confusion, apathy and depression. Most elderly persons resist nursing home admission as long as they can, and increasingly alternative community settings and home-care services are provided to prevent or delay such admission[32].

Nursing homes, like the traditional long-term mental hospital, contribute to an institutional syndrome resulting from vulnerabilites of patients as they respond to decreased social participation, sensory deprivation, loss of efficacy and control over daily life decisions, institutional routinization and the like. There is persuasive evidence that efforts to keep patients involved and participating in valued activities help maintain both mental and physical function. Many nursing homes fail to give these social aspects adequate attention, and patients spend much of their time in isolation and uninvolved. Nursing care may be the best treatment context for some patients who are seriously incapacitated and require a broad range of services difficult to provide in the home or in other community settings, but most impaired elderly benefit from settings that are more successful in sustaining independence and social engagement.

The capacity to cope effectively with mental illness depends on the organization of kinship groups and households, and the existing social institutions in a society. The growing prevalence of divorce, single-person households, small families, high female participation in the workforce, geographic mobility and other trends make it difficult to put increasing reliance on informal social networks for caretaking. Developing alternative structures that are financially viable and humane constitutes a growing challenge everywhere.

REFERENCES

1. Mechanic D. *Mental Health and Social Policy: The Emergence of Managed Care*, 4th edn. Boston: Allyn and Bacon, 1999.
2. Wells KB, Sturm R, Sherbourne CD, Meredith LS. *Caring for Depression*. Cambridge, MA: Harvard University Press, 1996.
3. Lipton HL, Lee PR. *Drugs and the Elderly: Clinical, Social, and Policy Perspectives*. Stanford: Stanford University Press, 1988.
4. Cohen, CI. Outcome of schizophrenia into later life: an overview. *Gerontologist* 1990; **30**: 790–7.
5. Castle DJ, Murray RM. The epidemiology of late-onset schizophrenia. *Schizophr Bull* 1993; **19**: 691–700.
6. Riecher-Roessler A, Loeffler W, Munk-Jorgensen P. What do we really know about late-onset schizophrenia? *Eur Arch Psychiat Clin Neurosci* 1997; **247**: 195–208.
7. Blazer D. Depression in the elderly: myths and misconceptions. *Psychiat Clin N Am* 1998; **20**: 111–19.
8. Unutzer J, Katon W, Sullivan M, Miranda J. Treating depressed older adults in primary care: narrowing the gap between efficacy and effectiveness. *Milbank Q* 1999; **77**: 225–56.
9. Alexopoulos, GS, Young RC, Meyers BS, *et al*. Late-onset depression. *Psychiat Clin N Am* 1988; **11**: 101–15.
10. Yassa, R, Nair NP, Iskandar H. Late-onset bipolar disorder. *Psychiat Clin N Am* 1988; **11**: 117–31.
11. Dohrenwend BP, Dohrenwend BS. Sex differences and psychiatric disorders. *Am J Sociol* 1976; **81**: 1447–54.
12. Newmann JP. Sex differences in symptoms of depression: clinical disorder or normal distress? *J Health Soc Behav* 1984; **25**: 136–59.
13. Mechanic D. *Medical Sociology*, 2nd edn. New York: Free Press, 1976, 214–21.
14. Dohrenwend BP, Levav I, Shrout PE *et al*. Socioeconomic status and psychiatric disorders: the causation-selection issue. *Science* 1992; **255**: 946–52.
15. Brown G, Harris T (eds). *Life Events and Illness*. New York: Guilford, 1989.
16. Cohen CI. Aging and homelessness. *Gerontologist* 1999; **39**: 5–14.
17. Berk ML, Schur CL, Cantor JC. Ability to obtain health care: recent estimates from the Robert Wood Johnson Foundation National Access to Care Survey. *Health Aff* 1995; **14**: 139–46.
18. Pescosolido BA, Boyer CA. How do people come to use mental health services? Current knowledge and changing perspectives. In Horwitz AV, Scheid TL, eds, *A Handbook for the Study of Mental Health: Social Contexts, Theories, and Systems*. New York: Cambridge University Press, 1999, 392–411.
19. Swartz MS, Wagner HR, Swanson JW *et al*. Administrative update: utilization of services. I. Comparing use of public and private mental health services: the enduring barriers of race and age. *Commun Ment Health J* 1998; **34**: 133–44.
20. Kessler RC, Walters EE, Forthofer MS. The social consequences of psychiatric disorders, III: probability of marital stability. *Am J Psychiat* 1998; **155**: 1092–6.
21. Leff J, Vaughn C. *Expressed Emotion in Families*. New York: Guilford, 1985.
22. Falloon IRH, Boyd JL, McGill CW. *Family Care of Schizophrenia*. New York: Guilford, 1984.
23. Brown GW, Birley JL. Crises and life changes and the onset of schizophrenia. *J Health Soc Behav* 1968; **9**: 203–14.
24. Kessler RC, Davis CG, Kendler KS. Childhood adversity and adult psychiatric disorder in the US National Comorbidity Survey. *Psychol Med* 1997; **27**: 1101–19.
25. Thoits PA. Conceptual, methodological, and theoretical problems in studying social support as a buffer against life stress. *J Health Soc Behav* 1982; **23**: 145–59.
26. Idler EL, Kasl SV. Religion among disabled and non-disabled persons II: attendance at religious services as a predictor of the course of disability. *J Gerontol* 1997; **52B**: S306–16.
27. Stein LI, Test MA. *The Training in Community Living Model: A Decade of Experience*. San Francisco, CA: Jossey-Bass, 1985.
28. Rosenfield S. Services organization and quality of life among the seriously mentally ill. In Mechanic D, ed., *Improving Mental Health Services*. San Francisco, CA: Jossey-Bass, 1987, 47–59.
29. Rodin J. Aging and health: effects of the sense of control. *Science* 1986; **233**: 1271–6.
30. Mechanic D, Angel R, Davies L. Risk and selection processes between the general and the specialty mental health sectors. *J Health Soc Behav* 1991; **32**: 49–64.
31. Mechanic D, McAlpine DD. Use of nursing home in the care of persons with severe mental illness: 1985 to 1995. *Psychiatric Services* 2000; **51**: 354–8.
32. Bishop CE. Where are the missing elders? The decline in nursing home use, 1985 and 1995. *Health Aff* 1999; **18**: 146–55.

18

The Natural History of Psychiatric Disorders: Early-onset Disease in Late Life and Late-onset Illness

Judith Hays

Duke University Medical Center, Durham, NC, USA

Is psychiatric pathology fundamentally different depending on when in the life course it emerges? Is the heterogeneity that characterizes late life psychiatric disorders—their risk factors, presentation and course—partly resolved by distinguishing between ages of first onset? This chapter summarizes why studying the onset of psychiatric illness is so difficult and, in spite of that difficulty, what distinguishes the epidemiology of early-onset disease in late life from late-onset illness.

With respect to age of onset, the best-characterized DSM-IV disorder (and our primary focus in this chapter) is major depressive disorder (MDD). Some attention will also be directed to bipolar (BP) disorder and schizophrenia. Much less research has distinguished between early and late onset of dysthymia, "late paraphrenia", or delusional disorder; we touch only briefly on these subtypes. We do not discuss depressive and/or psychotic prodromes of dementia or psychiatric symptoms of other organic etiology, such as cancer or multiple sclerosis, with the exception of disorders related to cerebrovascular infarcts and depression secondary to cardiovascular disease.

Studies of the prevalence and correlates of early-onset vs. late-onset disorders are treacherous for methodological reasons that plague all psychiatric studies and all studies with retrospective designs: determining *who* has *what* disorder and *when* it was first detected. Sometimes there is no consensus on the criteria for a "case", because psychiatric disorders are based on clinical signs and symptoms and represent heterogeneous underlying pathophysiological and psychosocial causes. Subjects may be considered a case according to one set of criteria but not according to another. Elderly persons in particular report significant psychiatric symptoms without meeting diagnostic criteria. Not infrequently, emergent symptoms may alter a diagnosis of long standing. Thus, clinical populations, from which many study samples are drawn, may be non-representative of all affected elders, due to varying patterns of help-seeking, clinical referral and symptom trajectories. All elderly populations in communities and institutions, are subject to survival of the fittest, and early-onset subjects may be systematically absent due to death.

Determining the precise age of onset is also problematical. Recall of specific dates may be compromised by memory lapse or telescoping of events, cognitive impairment or a "reminder effect" associated with multiple episodes. Classification of early-onset vs. late-onset depends on the cut-point chosen, which is often unspecified in diagnostic schema; across various studies, cut-points have ranged between 20 and 60 years of age, although most

use 45 or 50 years. For all of these reasons—diagnostic variability, selection bias, subject attrition and classification issues—estimates of the prevalence and risk of early-onset and late-onset disorders vary dramatically, as described below. Nevertheless, this chapter describes the state of agreement regarding differences in early and late affective and psychotic disorders.

AFFECTIVE DISORDERS

Major Depressive Disorder

The prevalence of affective disorders (MDD/BP) is lower among community-dwelling elders than among younger populations[1,2]. Prevalence estimates of late-life MDD from large studies ($n \geqslant 1000$) range between 1% (USA) to 3.7% (Finland), and prevalence of minor depression ranges from 8.3–23.2%[3–5]. In nursing homes, 5.9–16.5% of patients demonstrate clinically significant depression[6–7]. Among medical outpatients and inpatients, respectively, 5–7% and 10–20% may meet criteria for MDD[8–10]. Of affected elders in the community, van Ojen and colleagues[11] estimated that 70% may have had a first onset after the age of 65, i.e. late-onset depression (LOD) (Amsterdam, Holland). In the ECA (USA) study, the mean age of onset of MDD for subjects older than 65 years was 48.9 years, suggesting a large proportion of patients with late-onset[1].

The most provocative etiological findings regarding age of onset concern structural and functional brain abnormalities among LOD patients. Depressed elderly patients tend to have more abnormalities, particularly in the frontal regions, than do controls, although not universally[12–14]. LOD patients tend to present with more brain lesions than do patients with early onset of depression (EOD)[12], and subcortical and basal ganglia changes have been associated with greater severity in LOD[15]. These results from MRI studies are suggestive when paired with results showing increased vascular medical co-morbidity (e.g. hypertension, stroke and heart disease) among LOD patients[13,16]. Thus, risk of some subtypes of LOD may be attributable to vascular impairment and, by implication, preventable, using heart-healthy strategies such as diet, exercise and stress management. Where these results are heterogeneous, the inclusion or exclusion of subjects with cardiovascular histories may be a major factor[16,17].

At the other end of the modifiability spectrum, genotype may account for differences in the causal webs of EOD and LOD.

Principles and Practice of Geriatric Psychiatry, 2nd edn. Edited by J. R. M. Copeland, M. T. Abou-Saleh and D. G. Blazer
©2002 John Wiley & Sons, Ltd

Krishnan and colleagues[18] found patients with the *ApoE3/4* allele to have later age of onset than those with *2/3* and *3/3*; conversely, Holmes *et al.*[19] showed that *ApoE2* protected against early onset, thus delaying the onset of depression into later life; other studies were inconclusive[20]. Although these findings conflict, the potential to locate common genetic risk factors for depression and dementia in late life continues to receive empirical attention. Pedigree studies have been much more univocal: elders with EOD consistently report more affected close relatives than do elders with LOD[16,21]. Some have suggested recently that age of onset may be a proxy for multiple risk factors, including structural brain changes, vascular medical co-morbidity, neuropsychological impairment, and family history of mood disorders[22].

Evidence of other non-medical risk factors for EOD and LOD is preliminary. Single studies show males and African-Americans at greater risk of LOD than females and Whites, respectively[23,24].

The clinical presentations of early-onset and late-onset disease among elderly patients are not strikingly different, with the possible exceptions of more apathy, anxiety, and psychotic features in LOD[21–25]. Most neurological tests also show no differences, with the possible exception of more impaired executive memory and visual naming ability in LOD[26,27].

On balance, prognosis may be slightly worse for EOD elders, although there are serious methodological difficulties with the evidence and significant heterogeneity of course in late life. Cole[28] summarized conflicting early findings of differential disease trajectories, and studies over the subsequent decade have continued to conflict, some showing EOD elders to have a more relapsing course, more frequent episodes and more treatment refractoriness, and others showing LOD elders to have less favorable treatment response, more cycling in and out of symptoms, and more psychiatric co-morbidity[29–31]. Still other studies demonstrate no difference. However, when treatment and outcome criteria have been standardized, neither LOD nor EOD elders appeared at increased advantage relative to absolute rates of 1 year outcomes (remission, relapse, recovery or recurrence), although weeks to remission were greater in one sample of LOD elders[22].

In a recent comprehensive review of the mortality of depression[32], only one of 57 studies compared mortality by age of onset. Rabins *et al.*[33] found no differences in mortality by age of onset in a small study. More recently, Philibert *et al.*[34] reported lower survival rates for subjects with LOD, especially women with onset later than their 6th decade.

Bipolar Disorder

Manic symptoms and bipolar disorder (BP) I and II are rarer in the population than depressive symptoms or MDD and are most rare late in the life course[35]. Fewer than 1% of US elders in the ECA study reported a 1 week period or more of elevated, expansive or irritable mood; lifetime prevalences of these disorders among persons 65 years and older were 0.1% for BPI and PBII in the same study[1]. Evidence from the UK suggests that the incidence of mania may be bimodal, with a detectable peak after 60 years[36,37]. Among elderly hospitalized psychiatric populations, 3.4–6.4% of all admissions and 12.5% of admissions for affective disorders present with mania; 12–16% of general hospital patients qualify for a bipolar diagnosis[35].

Historically, the two potential causes of mania were thought to be stressful life events and organic disease. Kraepelin[38] first noted the precipitating role of stressful life events in manic depression, and subsequent studies have implicated such events in the incidence of bipolar disease, particularly early-onset mania (EOM)[39]. Late-onset mania (LOM), on the other hand, has long been associated with both vascular and cerebral anomalies and their correlates, including obesity, head injury, EEG changes and

dementia, with confirmatory evidence in more recent studies comparing older vs. younger bipolar patients[40] and LOM vs. EOM patients[39,41]. Yassa *et al.*[35] suggests that where significant life events distinguish LOM patients from aged controls, an organic substrate may have predisposed affected elders to a vulnerability to such events, and they then "react with a 'catastrophic' response (mania)" (p. 126).

A positive family history of bipolar illness has been more characteristically linked with EOM than with LOM patients[39,42–44]. However, methodological problems render this generalization suspect. Retrospective designs, low age-of-onset cut-off points and failure to distinguish between onset of depression vs. onset of mania are a few of the problems limiting the evidence[43]. Evidence of a gender differential in risk of early-onset or late-onset bipolar disorder has also been inconclusive[39]. Interracial comparisons of age of mania onset are not available.

Findings of differential clinical presentations of LOM and EOM in late life have not proved robust. The stereotype that LOM presented more often with "slow and fragmented flights of ideas, more rarely with elated affect, but more often with paranoid and aggressive features (p. 120)" was not confirmed in a summary of studies comparing the phenomenology of LOM and EOM in late life[35].

Prognostic differences by age of first onset of mania are difficult to substantiate[45–47]. In particular, differential survival may underlie the evidence of poor outcomes associated with LOM. To the degree that healthy social interactions are relevant to managing the course of bipolar disorder, recent preliminary findings are noteworthy: age of mania onset was higher among subjects with more positive assessments of social support and receipt of informal instrumental support[39,45].

PSYCHOTIC DISORDERS

Like affective disorders, late life psychoses (LLP) are heterogeneous, and the reach for consensus on diagnostic terminology has been torturous. In this summary we primarily discuss early-onset vs. late-onset schizophrenia (EOS/LOS), with brief mention of delusional disorder and entirely omitting discussion of alternative nomenclature (e.g. late paraphrenia) or subtypes less well characterized with respect to age of onset (e.g. schizoaffective and other psychotic disorders).

The lifetime history of schizophrenia is probably $\leqslant 1\%$ in the elderly community population[48], with annual incidence of three new cases (and 45 relapses) per 100 000 elders[49]. Approximately 25% of elderly schizophrenics experienced a first episode after age 50[50]. Onset of delusional disorder, on the other hand, occurs later, with average onset in the 40s among men and the 60s among women[51]. Late-life incidence of delusional disorder is 15.6/100 000; prevalence in the elderly population is 0.04%[49].

Two powerful risk factors for LOS appear to be cerebral atrophy and brain injury, although a significant number of patients with late-onset LLP present with no apparent cerebral pathology[52,53]. Compared to affective disorders, there is less evidence that EOS and LOS elders present differently with respect to MRI findings[53] or cardiovascular medical co-morbidity. A positive family history of psychosis appears incrementally more likely among, respectively, non-psychotic elderly controls, elders with LOS, and elders with EOS[50]. Findings concerning ApoE differences in onset or phenotype are limited and inconclusive[54]. Female gender and sensory impairment may predispose to LLP[48,55].

There is considerable heterogeneity in the outcome of schizophrenic episodes. A significant number of schizophrenic patients improve and recover fully; others relapse intermittently; others remain chronically symptomatic[56,57]. Long-term studies include mostly EOS patients, who make up the majority of geriatric schizophrenics. LOS, on the other hand, portends generally poor outcomes, although social adaptation may be better in this group, compared to EOS[50,58,59].

CONCLUSION

Overall, there is growing evidence that older patients with late-onset psychiatric disease are different from those who come to late life with a history of early-onset psychiatric illness. Their varying co-morbidity and symptom profiles suggest different (although potentially interacting) etiological factors, with genetic and/or social environmental factors predominating in early-onset disease and behavioral factors in later onset. More work is needed to describe any differential course, but social adaptation appears better for elders whose disease experience has been shorter.

REFERENCES

1. Weissman MM, Bruce ML, Leaf PJ *et al.* Affective disorders. In Robins LN, Regier DA (eds), *Psychiatric Disorders in America: The Epidemiologic Catchment Area Study.* New York: Free Press.

2. Ernst C, Angst J. Depression in old age: is there a real decrease in prevalence? A review. *Eur Arch Psychiat Clin Neurosci* 1995; **245**: 272–87.

3. Blazer DG, Koenig HG. Mood disorders. In Busse EW, Blazer DG, (eds), *The American Psychiatric Press Textbook of Geriatric Psychiatry.* Washington, DC: American Psychiatric Press, 1996, 235–63.

4. Katona CLE. *Depression in Old Age.* Chichester: Wiley, 1994.

5. Ohayon MM, Priest RG, Guilleminault C, Caulet M. The prevalence of depressive disorders in the United Kingdom. *Biol Psychiat,* 1999; **45**: 300–7.

6. Phillips JC, Henderson AS. The prevalence of depression among Australian nursing home residents: results using draft ICD-10 and DSM-III-R criteria. *Psychol Med* 1991; **21**: 739–48.

7. Parmelee PA, Katz IR, Lawton MP. Incidence of depression in long-term care settings. *J Gerontol* 1992; **47**: M189–96.

8. Koenig HG, George LK, Peterson BL, Pieper CF. Depression in medically ill hospitalized older adults: prevalence, characteristics, and course of symptoms according to six diagnostic schemes. *Am J Psychiat* 1997; **154**: 1376–83.

9. Iliffe S, Tai SS, Haines A *et al.* Assessment of elderly people in general practice. 4. Depression, functional ability and contact with services. *Br J Gen Pract* 1993; **43**: 371–4.

10. Evans S, Katona C. Epidemiology of depressive symptoms in elderly primary care attenders. *Dementia* 1993; **4**: 327–33.

11. Van Ojen R, Hooijer C, Jonker C *et al.* Late-life depressive disorder in the community, early onset and the decrease of vulnerability with increasing age. *J Affect Dis* 1995; **33**: 159–66.

12. Ball C, Philpot M. Affective disorders. In Ames D, Chiu E (eds), *Neuroimaging and the Psychiatry of Late Life,* Cambridge: Cambridge University Press, 1997, 172–89.

13. Lavretsky H, Lesser IM, Wohl M, Miller BL. Relationship of age, age at onset, and sex to depression in older adults. *Am J Geriat Psychiat* 1998; **6**: 248–56.

14. Kuman A, Jin Z, Bilker W, Udupa J, Gottlieb G. Late onset minor and major depression: Early evidence for common neuroanatomical substrates detected by using MRI. *Proc Natl Acad Sci USA* 1998; **95**: 7654–8.

15. Soares JC, Mann JJ. The anatomy of mood disorders: review of structural neuroimaging studies. *Biol Psychiat* 1997; **41**: 86–106.

16. Krishnan KRR, Hays JC, Blazer DG. MRI-defined vascular depression. *Am J Psychiat* 1997; **154**: 497–501.

17. Alexopoulos GS, Meyers BS, Young RC *et al.* 'Vascular depression' hypothesis. *Arch Gen Psychiat* 1997; **54**: 915–22.

18. Krishnan KRR, Tupler LA, Ritchie JC *et al.* Apolipoprotein E–ϵ4 frequency in geriatric depression. *Biol Psychiat* 1996; **40**: 69–71.

19. Holmes C, Russ C, Kirov G *et al.* Apolipoprotein E: depressive illness, depressive symptoms, and Alzheimer's Disease. *Biol Psychiat* 1998; **43**: 159–64.

20. Papassotiropoulos A, Bgli M, Jessen F *et al.* Early-onset and late-onset depression are independent of the genetic polymorphism of apolipoprotein E. *Dementia Geriat Cogn Dis* 1999; **10**: 258–61.

21. Baldwin RC, Tomenson B. Depression in later life: a comparison of symptoms and risk factors in early and late onset cases. *Br J Psychiat* 1995; **167**: 649–52.

22. Reynolds CF, Dew MA, Frank E *et al.* Effects of age at onset of first lifetime episode of recurrent major depression on treatment response and illness course in elderly patients. *Am J Psychiat* 1998; **155**: 795–9.

23. Lyness JM, Conwell Y, King DA *et al.* Age of onset and medical illness in older depressed inpatients. *Int Psychogeriat* 1995; **7**: 63–73.

24. Holroyd S, Duryee JJ. Differences in geriatric psychiatry outpatients with early vs. late-onset depression. *Int J Geriat Psychiat* 1997; **12**: 1100–6.

25. Krishnan KRR, Hays JC, Tupler LA *et al.* Clinical and phenomenological comparisons of late-onset and early-onset depression. *Am J Psychiat* 1995; **152**: 785–8.

26. Beats B. The biological origin of depression in later life. *Int J Geriat Psychiat* 1996; **11**: 349–54.

27. Salloway S, Malloy P, Kohn R *et al.* MRI and neuropsychological differences in early- and late-life-onset geriatric depression. *Neurology* 1996; **46**: 1567–4.

28. Cole MG. The prognosis of depression in the elderly. *Can Med Assoc J* 1990; **143**: 336–9.

29. Cole MG. Major depression in old age: outcome studies. In Shulman KI, Tohen M, Kutcher SP (eds), *Mood Disorders Across the Life Span.* New York: Wiley–Liss, 1996, 361–76.

30. Dew MA, Reynolds CF III, Houck PR *et al.* Temporal profiles of the course of depression during treatment: predictors of pathways toward recovery in the elderly. *Arch Gen Psychiat* 1997; **54**: 1016–24.

31. Simpson SW, Jackson A, Baldwin RC, Burns A. Subcortical hyperintensities in late-life depression: acute response to treatment and neuropsychological impairment. *Int Psychogeriat* 1997; **9**: 257–75.

32. Wulsin LR, Vaillant GE, Wells VE. A systematic review of the mortality of depression. *Psychosomat Med* 1999; **61**: 6–17.

33. Rabins PV, Harvis K, Koven S. High fatality rates of late-life depression associated with cardiovascular disease. *J Affect Dis* 1985; **9**: 165–7.

34. Philibert RA, Richards L, Lynch CF, Winokur G. The effect of gender and age at onset of depression on mortality. *J Clin Psychiat* 1997; **58**: 355–60.

35. Yassa R, Nair NPV, Iskandar H. Late-onset bipolar disorder. *Psychiat Clin N Am* 1988; **11**(1): 117–31.

36. Spicer CC, Hare EH, Slater E. Neurotic and psychotic forms of depressive illness: evidence from age-incidence in a national sample. *Br J Psychiat* 1973; **123**: 535–41.

37. Eagles JM, Whalley LJ. Ageing and affective disorders: the age at first onset of affective disorders in Scotland, 1969–1978. *Br J Psychiat* 1985; **147**: 180–7.

38. Kraepelin E. *Manic Depressive Insanity and Paranoia* (trans). Edinburgh: Livingstone, 1921.

39. Hays JC, Krishnan KRR, George LK, Blazer DG. Age of first onset of bipolar disorder: demographic, family history, and psychosocial correlates. *Depression Anxiety* 1998; **7**: 76–82.

40. Steffens DC, Krishnan KRR. Structural neuroimaging and mood disorders: recent findings, implications for classification, and future directions. *Biol Psychiat* 1998; **43**: 705–12.

41. Wylie ME, Mulsant BH, Pollock BG *et al.* Age at onset in geriatric bipolar disorder: effects on clinical presentation and treatment outcomes in an inpatient sample. *Am J Geriat Psychiat* 1999; **7**(1): 77–83.

42. Post F. The management and nature of depressive illnesses in late life: a follow-through study. *Br J Psychiat* 1972; **121**: 393–404.

43. Chen ST, Altshuler LL, Spar JE. Bipolar disorder in late life: a review. *J Geriat Psychiat Neurol* 1998; **11**: 29–35.

44. Leboyer M, Bellivier F, McKeon P *et al.* Age at onset and gender resemblance in bipolar siblings. *Psychiat Res* 1998; **81**: 125–31.

45. Meeks S. Bipolar disorder in the latter half of life: Symptom presentation, global functioning, and age of onset. *J Affect Dis* 1999; **52**: 161–7.

46. Shulman KI. Disinhibition syndromes, secondary mania and bipolar disorder in old age. *J Affect Dis* 1997; **46**: 175–82.

47. Shulman KI, Tohen M. Outcome studies of mania in old age. In Shulman KI, Tohen M, Kutcher SP (eds), *Mood Disorders Across the Life Span*. New York: Wiley–Liss, 1996, 407–10.

48. Henderson AS, Kay DWK. The epidemiology of functional psychoses of late onset. *Eur Arch Psychiat Clin Neurosci* 1997; **247**: 176–89.

49. Copeland JRM, Dewey ME, Scott A *et al*. Schizophrenia and delusional disorder in older age: community prevalence, incidence, comorbidity and outcome. *Schizophren Bull* 1998; **24**: 153–61.

50. Harris MJ, Jeste DV. Late-onset schizophrenia: an overview. *Schizophren Bull* 1988; **14**: 39–55.

51. Jeste DV, Harris MJ, Paulsen JS. Psychoses. In Sadavoy J, Lazarus LW, Jarvik LF, Grossberg GT (eds), *Comprehensive Review of Geriatric Psychiatry II*, 2nd edn. Washington DC: American Psychiatric Press, 1996, 593–614.

52. Symonds LL, Olichney JM, Jernigan TL *et al*. Lack of clinically significant gross structural abnormalities in MRIs of older patients with schizophrenia and related psychoses. *J Neuropsychiat Clin Neurosci* 1997; **9**: 251–8.

53. Howard R, O'Brien J. Paranoid and schizophrenic disorders of late life. In Ames D, Chiu E (eds), *Neuroimaging and the Psychiatry of Late Life*. New York: Cambridge University Press, 1997, 190–203.

54. Arnold SE, Joo E, Martinoli M-G *et al*. Apolipoprotein E genotype in schizophrenia: frequency, age of onset, and neuropathologic features. *NeuroReport* 1997; **8**: 1523–6.

55. Prager S, Jeste DV. Sensory impairment in late-life schizophrenia. *Schizophren Bull* 1993; **19**: 755–72.

56. McGlashan TH. Selective review of recent North American long-term follow-up studies of schizophrenia. In Mirin SM, Gossett JT, Grob MC (eds), *Psychiatric Treatment: Advances in Outcome Research*. Washington, DC: American Psychiatric Press, 1991, 61–105.

57. Harding CM. The interaction of biopsychosocial factors, time, and course of schizophrenia. In Shriqui CL, Nasrallah HA (eds.), *Contemporary Issues in the Treatment of Schizophrenia*. Washington, DC: American Psychiatric Press, 1995, 653–81.

58. Pearlson GD, Rabins P. The late-onset psychoses: possible risk factors. *Psychiat Clin N Am* 1988; **11**(1): 15–32.

59. Jeste DV, Harris MJ, Krull A *et al*. Clinical and neuropsychological characteristics of patients with late-onset schizophrenia. *Am J Psychiat* 1995; **152**: 722–30.

19

Mortality and Mental Disorders

Michael E. Dewey

Trent Institute for Health Services Research, University Hospital, Nottingham, UK

INTRODUCTION

The topic of mortality and mental illness has a long history. Even if we discount the pioneering nineteenth century study of Farr[1] we can still go back as far as the study of Ødegård[2] among the contemporary studies. Both of these were, of course, patient-based and covered all ages.

Why should anyone want to study mortality and its relationship to psychiatric illness in later life? There are many questions we might want to ask:

- Are older people with psychiatric illnesses more likely to die than those without?
- Are older people with psychiatric illnesses more likely to die than younger sufferers after allowing for the general rise in the force of mortality with age?
- If they are more likely to die, in either case, why is this?
- Whether they are more likely to die or not, do they die from different causes?
- What theoretical issues does their risk of mortality raise?
- What implication for service provision does their risk of mortality, elevated or not, have?

There have been some attempts at studying these issues and a small number of relevant reviews. In this chapter there is no attempt to provide a bibliography of all the empirical studies. Instead a number of key references are chosen to illustrate themes.

DEATH CERTIFICATE STUDIES OF MORTALITY

A number of studies have used death certificate data to study mortality and the dementias. The primary goal of these studies has been to estimate prevalence without the expense of performing a community study. Only one study, that of Flaten[3] in Norway, gave estimates of prevalence close to those from community studies, and it has been generally accepted that such studies tell us about the death certification habits of doctors but rather little about the prevalence of dementias or the relationship between the dementias and mortality. There have been no such studies for illnesses other than the dementias.

PATIENT-BASED STUDIES

A full review of these was undertaken by van Dijk and colleagues[4] which should be referred to for details of this work. For reasons outlined in the next section, these studies will not be further discussed here.

COMMUNITY-BASED STUDIES

The primary source of information about the link between mortality and mental illness in this age group is the increasing number of community studies. Careful follow-up of well-defined series of carefully diagnosed cases has its place, but the selection that goes on between primary and secondary care gives rise to the risk that the information cannot be generalized. Since most cases of dementia and depression are managed in primary care, it is there that we must seek information on the mortality of cases of mental disorder. One of the most comprehensive reviews of the past few years was that of Schröppel[5]. She concluded that relatively little was known for either disorder.

The years since Schröppel's review have seen an explosion in studies relevant to dementia and depression. Two recent systematic overviews have synthesized those community mortality studies for dementia[6] and depression[7]. Disappointingly few of the primary studies provide effect sizes that can be combined, but there are enough to warrant the exercise for both disorders. For dementia, meta-analysis of six studies gave an odds ratio for mortality of 2.63 (95% confidence interval 2.17–3.21). There was weak evidence of a higher risk for vascular compared to Alzheimer's, for increasing risk with increasing severity of dementia, and for decreasing relative risk with age. There seemed no evidence of a sex difference. For depression, meta-analysis of 15 cohorts gave an odds ratio of 1.73 (95% confidence interval 1.53–1.95). There was weak evidence that men had a higher relative risk and that studies with longer follow-up have a lower risk.

There have been few studies of other diagnoses in older age, and there has been no systematic review of them. An account is given by Langley in her review[8].

CAUSE OF DEATH

Only one study[9] appears to have addressed the problem of the cause of death in community studies of dementia. Prior to this there had been a number of studies of patient cohorts. Although these doubtless have value, they do not help to solve the problem of the causes of differential mortality. For that we require a direct comparison between the proportion who die of cause X in the demented group with the proportion who die of cause X in the non-demented group. It seems so obvious that this is needed that it is surprising that only Jagger and her colleagues[9] have addressed the issue. They found that, relative to the general population, Alzheimer's disease sufferers had a lower risk due to age, for being manual social class, and for having a history of cancer, and a higher risk for being male. This concords with the meta-analysis quoted above for age, but not for sex.

A detailed editorial[10] discusses issues in research into depression and mortality. In particular there is difficulty in separating association from causation.

METHODOLOGICAL ISSUES

A number of measurement issues have failed to receive appropriate attention. The studies of community samples use different methods of measuring differences in risk. Although for low risks the numerical difference between risk ratios and odds ratios is small, comparison would be simpler if studies reported in a common way.

Patient studies have not really addressed the issue of bias introduced by differential identification of the patient group and the controls. For instance, if date of diagnosis is used as the starting point for survival analysis, there will be a survivor bias and it will be difficult to identify controls in a similar way.

Studies comparing patient groups with the general population have also failed to account for the fact that demented people are part of the population, and if their death rate is very different from that of the population as a whole, and if they form a substantial part of the population, as they will beyond age 85, then the death rate quoted for the general population is an overestimate of that expected for non-demented people.

Few studies have put their results into any clear framework. For instance, the possibilities raised by epidemiologists[11] studying chronic physical illness, and implicit in the textbook relationship between prevalence, incidence and duration of illness, have hardly been explored[12].

DISCUSSION

Mortality has been one of the most studied endpoints in epidemiology, but the reader of the community studies will be struck by the fact that, for few of them, mortality was a primary end point. This has undoubtedly created the patchwork of methods of reporting which bedevils synthesis.

There has been a considerable literature relating mental disorders in younger adults to mortality[13], which has confirmed an increased risk for affective disorders (typical SMR 1.4) and schizophrenias (typical SMR 2.3). The studies quoted here suggest a similar, possibly slightly greater, risk for depression.

There is clearly an elevated risk for both dementia and depression, but there is little that can be confidently asserted beyond that. We do not know whether the risk is modified by other possible explanatory variables like age, sex, physical illness of functional status, neither do we know what causes of death account for the excess cases.

As yet, we do not know what would happen to mortality if we treated depression in older age more vigorously, or what would happen if universally effective treatments for dementia became available and we could treat people with dementia.

REFERENCES

1. Farr W. Report upon the mortality of lunatics. *J Statist Soc Lond* 1841; **4**: 17–33.
2. Ødegård Ø. Excess mortality of the insane. *Acta Psychiat Neurol Scand* 1952; **27**: 353–67.
3. Flaten TP. Mortality from dementia in Norway, 1969–83. *J Epidemiol Commun Health* 1989; **43**: 285–9.
4. van Dijk PTM, Dippel DWJ, Habbema JDF. Survival of patients with dementia. *J Am Geriat Soc* 1991; **39**: 603–10.
5. Schröppel H. Zur mortalität bei dementiellen und depressiven Erkrankungen im Alter. *Zeitschr Gerontopsychol Psychiat* 1994; **7**: 179–93.
6. Dewey ME, Saz P. Dementia, cognitive impairment and mortality in persons aged 65 and over living in the community: a systematic review of the literature. *Int J Geriat Psychiat* 2001; **16**: 751–71.
7. Saz P, Dewey ME. Depression, depressive symptoms and mortality in persons aged 65 and over living in the community: a systematic review of the literature. *Int J Geriat Psychiat* 2001; **16**: 622–63.
8. Langley AM. The mortality of mental illness in older age. *Rev Clin Gerontol* 1995; **5**: 103–12.
9. Jagger C, Clarke M, Stone A. Predictors of survival with Alzheimer's disease: a community-based study. *Psychol Med* 1995; **25**: 171–7.
10. O'Brien JT, Ames D. Why do the depressed elderly die? *Int J Geriat Psychiat* 1994; **9**: 689–93.
11. Haberman S. Mathematical treatment of the incidence and prevalence of disease. *Soc Sci Med* 1978; **12**: 147–52.
12. Dewey ME. Estimating the incidence of dementia in the community from prevalence and mortality results. *Int J Epidemiol* 1992; **21**(3): 533–6.
13. Tsuang MT, Simpson JC. Mortality studies in psychiatry: should they stop or proceed? *Arch Gen Psychiat* 1985; **42**: 98–103.

20

Long-term Outcome Studies of Psychiatric Disorders: Methodological Issues and Practical Approaches to Follow-up

Ann Stueve, John Toner and Anne V. Quismorio

Columbia University Stroud Center, New York, USA

What are the long-term outcomes of various types of psychiatric disorders? How do individuals, interacting with their environments, shape the course and consequences of mental illness? What environmental, personal and illness characteristics are associated with recovery and improvement? Are such characteristics disorder- or life stage-specific? A growing number of long-term follow-up studies have begun to address such questions. Their results both confirm and challenge accepted wisdom. Long-term outcomes of schizophrenia, for example, do seem to be worse on average than those of affective disorders[1]; at the same time, however, outcomes of schizophrenia are remarkably varied, undermining conceptions of its course as progressively deteriorating and chronic[2]. Substantive results from long-term follow-up studies are included in other chapters of this volume (*see* specific disorders). This chapter focuses instead on several basic methodological issues—case identification, co-morbidity, choice of comparison groups, sample representativeness and measurement issues—as they pertain to long-term follow-up studies (*see* refs[3–6] for elaboration). Our purpose is to alert readers to issues that potentially influence the interpretation and comparison of results. Issues associated with the statistical analysis of longitudinal data are beyond the scope of this chapter and are not included (*see* refs[6–8]).

There are two basic types of follow-up investigations: (a) prospective studies, in which the investigator defines a sample on the basis of current attributes (e.g. psychiatric or exposure status) and follows the sample forward in time; and (b) retrospective cohort designs, in which the researchers define the sample on the basis of some past characteristic (e.g. hospital admission during a specified time period, participation in an earlier study) and then reconstruct their subsequent life course up to some later point in time, using records, retrospective interviews, etc.[3] Retrospective cohort (or "catch up") designs require less time to complete than prospective studies covering a similar duration, but are more limited by the availability and quality of extant data and problems of recall. Both types of investigations have been used to elucidate the long-term course[9] and outcomes of psychiatric disorders[1]. The issues discussed below apply to varying degrees to both types of investigation.

CASE IDENTIFICATION

Case identification refers to the criteria and procedures used to determine what constitutes a case of the disorder under study and addresses the question, "long-term outcomes of what?"[10]. Without explicit specification of what constitutes a case, similarities and difference in observed outcomes across studies are difficult to interpret. For example, observed differences may reflect discrepancies in diagnostic practice; observed similarities may be illusory. Case identification is particularly problematic in long-term follow-up studies, where baseline data and diagnoses often predate the introduction of modern diagnostic systems and standardized assessment tools. One way in which investigators have dealt with this problem is to rescore baseline data (e.g. from hospital charts, case notes or interviews) using one or more current diagnostic systems (e.g DSM–III–R, ICD–10) and to select and compare cases based on these newer diagnoses[4]. This practice allows for comparison of outcomes using different nosologies and, insofar as criteria for inclusion and exclusion are reported, facilitates comparison of results across studies. Such benefits of rescoring, however, remain dependent on the quality and comparability of baseline data. Signs and symptoms that were never attended to or recorded obviously cannot be recovered, and their absence potentially introduces error into the rescoring process.

CO-MORBIDITY

A second issue concerns co-morbidity (i.e. the co-occurrence of two or more psychiatric disorders in an individual) and addresses the question, "to what extent are observed outcomes due to psychiatric conditions other than the one under study?"[5,22–25]. What appear to be differences in outcomes of schizophrenia, for example, may be due in part to differences in the prevalence and combination of secondary conditions. Here, too, the assessment of co-morbidity and its ramifications is particularly difficult in long-term follow-up studies, because outcomes may be influenced not only by secondary disorders recorded at baseline but also by the onset and recurrence of other disorders between baseline and follow-up. While some assessment tools [e.g. Schedule for Affective Disorders and Schizophrenia—Lifetime(SADS-L)] generate the data needed to make lifetime diagnoses, sample attrition and reliance on informants may impede reliable assessment of interim conditions for substantial numbers of subjects.

Principles and Practice of Geriatric Psychiatry, 2nd edn. Edited by J. R. M. Copeland, M. T. Abou-Saleh and D. G. Blazer
©2002 John Wiley & Sons, Ltd

CHOICE OF COMPARISON GROUPS

The counterpart of case identification is the designation of comparison groups and addresses the question, "long-term outcomes of disorder X compared with what?" Comparison groups provide benchmarks for interpreting measures of outcome. What comparison groups are appropriate depends, of course, on the research question under investigation and includes, among others, samples of "normal" individuals, of individuals with other psychiatric or medical conditions, or population norms, if available. Comparisons may also be made on the basis of some risk factor (e.g. age of onset) or treatment of interest. What is important to remember when selecting comparison groups and interpreting results is that members of the case, or target, group may differ from those of the comparison group in ways other than the disorder or risk factor of interest, and these "other ways" may account for subsequent differences in outcome and course. Thus, it is important to assess whether comparison groups are comparable to case groups on extraneous dimensions that could influence outcomes.

SAMPLE REPRESENTATIVENESS AND ATTRITION

The representativeness of the sample at baseline and follow-up addresses the question, "to what extent and to whom are results generalizable?" Most current long-term follow-up studies are based on patient samples selected from hospitals, other treatment settings, clinician caseloads or case registries. Selection into treatment, however, is not a random process[11]. Treatment rates have been shown to vary by type of disorder[12], social and demographic characteristics of individuals[12,26], historical period[13], service delivery system and country. In addition, within a catchment area, patients are sorted and filtered into different types of treatment settings (e.g. public vs. private). Thus, the life trajectories of treated subjects may differ not only from those of untreated cases but also from those of patients treated in dissimilar settings.

More significant is the problem of sample attrition, whether due to death, inability to participate, refusal or failure to trace. This is because subjects lost to follow-up tend to differ in systematic ways from those who are located and interviewed[3,14]. Researchers often attempt to assess the type and degree of bias by comparing respondents and non-respondents on baseline characteristics; however, as Kelsey et al.[3] note, "the only way to ensure that bias stemming from loss to follow-up does not distort the study results is to minimize losses through intensive efforts to locate each cohort member" (p. 109). In addition, by reducing sample size, attrition reduces the statistical power of analyses to reliably detect outcome differences. With effort, several long-term follow-up studies have successfully minimized sample attrition[15]; the training and organizational strategies used have been summarized[15,16].

MEASUREMENT OF OUTCOMES

The measurement of outcomes is clearly central to long-term follow-up studies and raises the question, "on what dimensions and how should outcomes be assessed?" Many different measures of outcome have been used in follow-up studies, including measures of symptomatology, hospitalization, role functioning, impairment of social relationships and recovery[1,17,18]. Reliance on single global indices of recovery have proved largely unsatisfactory. Such indices are not only difficult to compare across studies but also imply an overly uniform picture of subjects' functioning. Subjects who fare poorly in one life domain (e.g. employment)

often fare better in others (e.g. symptom profile)[18], and such discrepancies are masked by single global indicators of recovery. Even seemingly objective, domain-specific measures (e.g. unemployment or rehospitalization rates) can be difficult to compare across studies if they are influenced by setting specific economic conditions or social policies[4,19].

Sample attrition further complicates the measurement of outcomes. How should outcomes be assessed for subjects who are deceased or unlocated at follow-up? Investigators often rely on informants and/or records to provide information. However, in addition to raising ethical considerations, informants not only differ from subjects in their access to (and probably recall of) relevant information but also assess subjects' status from different perspectives. Records, too, may not contain the data of interest and, like informant reports, differ in perspective from subjects' self-reports[3,26]. In light of such considerations, it is important to follow the advice of Bromet et al.[4] and ". . . be cautious in comparing results across studies without carefully ascertaining both the definition of outcome and the criteria used in implementing that definition" (p. 154) (see refs[5,17] for elaboration).

MEASURES OF INTERVENING VARIABLES

The longer the time interval between baseline and follow-up, the more likely that intervening events and circumstances play a role in determining outcome status. Measurement of such events and circumstances addresses the question, "what are the interim processes and mechanisms that account for observed outcomes?" Here prospective designs have an advantage over retrospective cohort studies because measurement of potentially mediating and confounding variables can be explicitly built into both baseline and follow-up data collection, and time intervals between follow-ups can be chosen with intervening mechanisms in mind. Retrospective cohort designs are more dependent on the availability of records and/or the recollections of subjects and informants, which are vulnerable to recall and reporting biases[3,20,21,23]. Problems associated with reporting and recall are not avoided by prospective studies, however, especially when intervals between follow-ups are long.

PRACTICAL APPROACHES TO FOLLOW-UP

Smith and Watts[27] provide a thorough summary of methods for locating absent and deceased subjects. Their review of available procedures emphasizes the use of electronic databases as effective means for identifying the location and vital status of lost subjects. Various tools for locating participants lost to follow-up are currently available.

Sources for Locating Patients Assumed Alive

The US Postal Service is a convenient source of information when investigators are faced with outdated addresses. Upon request, an updated address can be obtained as long as the request is made within the year that the individual moved.

Incorrect telephone numbers can be updated by contacting the telephone operator for information on new telephone listings. Unlisted telephone numbers may be obtained, depending on the policy of the telephone company. White-page listings for the entire USA are available for purchase on compact disk (CD-ROM). Compact disks are updated yearly and are relatively affordable. Telephone numbers can also be updated by use of the crisscross (or reverse) directory, which lists telephone numbers by address.

The Internet serves as an effective and cost efficient method of locating absent subjects. Various websites contain an extensive amount of information regarding residential listings. Internet sources differ by the type of information required to perform a search. When utilizing online databases, Smith and Watts[27] suggest that: "It is important that the investigator try each source before moving on to the next site. Failure to locate a number on one site does not mean that a search of another site will be fruitless" (p. 434). Some examples of current websites include:

www.infoseek.com
www.semaphorecorp.com
www.databaseamerica.com
www.four11.com
www.yahoo.com/reference/whitepages
www.angelfire.com
www.yahoo.com/search/people
www.switchboard.com
www.whowhere.com
www.lookupusa.com

The Department of Motor Vehicles can provide useful information on an individual, including one's address, date of birth and social security number, and can select physical characteristics; however, investigators must be cognizant of state-specific limitations and restrictions on public access to information. Similarly, voter registration files are restricted in certain states, yet careful review of files, when available, can produce useful information.

TRW, TRANSUNION and EQUIFAX, the nation's major credit bureaux, can provide vital information on patients, such as current and previous addresses, social security number, birth date, employer and spouse's name. Each of these credit-reporting services offers affordable products for assessing patient status. TRW offers TRW Social Search and TRW Address Update. Transunion offers TRACE, TRACE*plus*, ReTRACE and the ATLAS. Equifax offers DTEC and ID REPORT. Each product can successfully provide essential data but differs by the specific information generated and what is required for initiation of a search. Utilization of these credit bureaux is legal, offering comprehensive, affordable, time- and cost-efficient means for locating patients.

Information brokers may also be of use in attempting to locate missing subjects. Information brokers have access to varied sources of information, yet are typically costly options. As a result, it is recommended that researchers assess the necessity to locate their subjects prior to selecting such alternatives[27,29]. Similar sources of information may be available outside the USA.

Sources for Locating Patients Assumed Deceased

Various services are available for locating individuals who are believed to be dead. The National Death Index (NDI) identifies the states in which death occurred, the corresponding death certificate number and the date of death. The NDI file provides information for all 50 states, the District of Columbia, Puerto Rico and the Virgin Islands. The NDI database is updated annually and begins with deaths occurring in 1979.

NDI users can apply for NDI*plus*, an optional service that, in addition to the aforementioned information, provides details on the underlying and multiple causes of death for deceased patients. Procedures for requesting information through NDI vary by state. Prospective NDI and NDI*plus* users must submit an application form to the National Center for Health Statistics. Information regarding NDI and NDI*plus* can be obtained by contacting:

National Center for Health Statistics, Centers for Disease Control and Prevention, 6525 Belcrest Road, Room 820, Hyatsville, MD 20782-2003, USA.
Tel: (301) 436-8951, ext 109 or 101; fax: (301) 436-7066: e-mail: ROB3@CDC.GOV

The Equifax Nationwide Death Search provides information on deaths since 1955 from data compiled from the Social Security Administration. Search results will produce birthdate, date of death and state and zip code at death. Equifax is updated continuously and is therefore recommended for obtaining data regarding recent deaths. Furthermore, because records are available beginning in 1955, Equifax is potentially more useful for some retrospective cohort designs than the NDI[28].

Other sources for identifying deceased subjects include the Death Master File from the Social Security Index[27,29]. This information can be accessed at www.ancestry.com.

Contact information for additional services includes:

Social Security Administration's Death Master File, US Department of Commerce, Technology Administration, 5285 Port Royal Road, Springfield, VA 22161, USA.
Tel: (703) 487-4630

Equifax Credit Information Services, PO Box 105835, Atlanta, GA 30348-5835, USA.
Tel: (800) 944-6000

Trans Union Corporation, PO Box 8309 File 99506, Philadelphia, PA 19101-8309, USA.
Tel: (610) 690-3126

CONCLUSIONS

Long-term follow-up studies provide a useful vehicle for investigating stability and change in the course and consequences of psychiatric disorders; they raise a number of methodological and practical considerations as well. In this chapter we have tried to highlight basic methodological issues and practical approaches that bear on the interpretation and comparison of research findings and to reference practice approach and texts that address the issues in greater detail.

REFERENCES

1. Tsuang MT, Wooson RF, Fleming JA. Long-term outcome of major psychoses, 1: schizophrenia and affective disorders compared with psychiatrically symptom-free surgical conditions. *Arch Gen Psychiat* 1979; **36**: 1295–301.
2. Carpenter WT, Kirkpatrick B. The heterogeneity of the long-term course of schizophrenia. *Schizophren Bull* 1988; **14**: 645–52.
3. Kelsey JL, Whittemore AS, Evans AS, Thompson WD. *Methods in Observational Epidemiology*. New York: Oxford University Press, 1996.
4. Bromet E, Davies M, Schulz SC. Basic principles of epidemiologic, research in schizophrenia. In Tsuang MT, Simpson JC (eds), *Handbook of Schizophrenia Vol. 3: Nosology, Epidemiology and Genetics*. New York: Elsevier Science 1988, 151–68.
5. McGlashan TH, Carpenter Jr WT, Bartko JJ. Issues of design and methodology in long-term follow-up studies. *Schizophren Bull* 1988; **14**: 569–74.
6. Lawton MP, Herzog AR (eds). *Special Research Methods for Gerontology*. Amityville, NY: Baywood, 1989.
7. Bartko JJ, Carpenter Jr WT, McGlashan TH. Statistical issues in long-term follow-up studies. *Schizophren Bull* 1988; **14**: 575–87.
8. von Eye A (ed.). *Statistical Methods in Longitudinal Research*. San Diego, CA: Academic Press, 1990.
9. Angst J. The course of major depression, atypical bipolar disorder, and bipolar disorder. In Hippus H, Klerman GL, Matussek N, Schmauss M (eds), *New Results in Depression Research*. Berlin: Springer-Verlag, 1986, 26–34.

10. Wing JK. Comments on the long-term outcome of schizophrenia. *Schizophren Bull* 1988; **14**: 669–73.

11. Goldberg DP, Huxley P. *Mental Illness in the Community: The Pathway to Psychiatric Care*. London: Tavistock, 1980.

12. Link B, Dohrenwend BP. Formulation of hypotheses about the ratio of untreated to treated cases in the true prevalence studies of functional psychiatric disorders in adults in the United States. In Dohrenwend BP, Dohrenwend BS, Gould MS *et al. Mental Illness in the United States: Epidemiological Estimates*. New York: Praeger, 1980; 133–49.

13. Kiesler CA, Sibulkin AE. *Mental Hospitalization: Myths and Facts about a National Crisis*. Newbury Park, CA: Sage, 1987.

14. Sharma SK, Tobin JD, Brant LJ. Attrition in the Baltimore Longitudinal Study of Aging during the first twenty years. In Lawton MP, Herzog AR (eds), *Special Research Methods for Gerontology*. Amityville, NY: Baywood 1989, 233–47.

15. Toner J, Stueve A. Methodological issues in long-term follow-up studies of chronic mental illness. In Light E, Lebowitz B (eds), *Chronically Mentally Ill Elderly: Directions for Research*. New York: Springer, 1991; 285–320.

16. Farrington DP, Gallagher B, Morley L *et al.* Minimizing attrition in longitudinal research: methods of tracing and securing cooperation in a 24-year follow-up study. In Magnusson D, Bergman LR (eds), *Data Quality in Longitudinal Research*. Cambridge: Cambridge University Press, 1990, 122–47.

17. Harding CM. Speculations on the measurement of recovery from severe psychiatric disorder and the human condition. *Psychiat J Univ Ottawa* 1986; **11**: 199–204.

18. Strauss JS, Carpenter WT. The prognosis of schizophrenia: rationale for a multidimensional concept. *Schizophren Bull* 1978; **4**: 56–67.

19. Warner R. *Recovery from Schizophrenia: Psychiatry and Political Economy*. London: Routledge & Kegan Paul, 1985.

20. Janson CG. Retrospective data, undesirable behavior, and the longitudinal perspective. In Magnusson D, Bergman LR (eds), *Data Quality in Longitudinal Research*. Cambridge: Cambridge University Press, 1990; 100–21.

21. Raphael K. Recall bias: a proposal for assessment and control. *Int J Epidemiol* 1987; **16**: 167–70.

22. Lyness JM, Bruce M, Koenig HG, *et al.* Depression and medical illness in late life: report of a symposium. *J Am Geriat Soc* 1996; **44**: 198–203.

23. Kessler RC, Nelson B, McGonagle KA *et al.* Comorbidity of DSM–III–R major depressive disorder in the general population: results from the US National Comorbidity Survey. *Br J Psychiat* 1997; **168** (suppl. 30): 17–30.

24. Dixon L. Dual diagnosis of substance abuse in schizophrenia: prevalence and impact on outcomes. *Schizophren Res* 1999; **35**: S93–100.

25. Wittchen HU. Critical issues in the evaluation of comorbidity of psychiatric disorders. *Br J Psychiat* 1996; **168** (suppl. 30): 9–16.

26. Wolfe F. Critical issues in longitudinal and observational studies: purpose, short vs. long term, selection of study instruments, methods, outcomes and biases. *J Rheumatol* 1999; **26**: 469–72.

27. Smith S, Watts HG. Methods for locating missing patients for the purpose of long-term clinical studies. *J Bone Joint Surg* 1998; **80A**: 431–8.

28. Rich-Edwards JW, Stampfer MJ. Test of the National Death Index and Equifax Nationwide Death Search. *Am J Epidemiol* 1994; **140**: 1016–19.

29. Schall L, Marsh GM, Henderson VL. A two-stage protocol for verifying vital status in large historical cohort studies. *JOEM* 1997; **39**: 1097–102.

Part D

Diagnosis and Assessment

DI   Epidemiology, Diagnosis and Nosology

DII   Clinical Assessment

DIII Standardized Methods and Rating Scales

21

The Importance of Multidimensional Assessment in Clinical Practice

M. Robin Eastwood* and Abhilash Desai

(*Formerly at) St Louis University Medical School, St Louis, MD, USA

In many ways, geriatric psychiatry is a paradigm for contemporary medicine. A multidisciplinary team is required to address the complex range of assessment and treatment issues. After all, older people usually have more than one medical illness, are on several medications and may have considerable limitations (vision, hearing, mobility, cognition, finances).

According to Eastwood and Corbin[1], "the problems presented in the assessment and treatment of geriatric psychiatry patients may be best solved by a team composed of members with diverse professional training, meeting frequently to plan investigations, discuss findings and formulate coherent and comprehensive treatment plans. Such a group must function with little overlap of tasks and few interdisciplinary jealousies, be problem-orientated and exercise communication skills in order to be effective and efficient. Although the physician typically chairs team meetings and takes medical and legal responsibility, each member of the team must make a definite contribution, either in direct patient care, or with technical and back-up services", and "Whatever the level of sophistication, a geriatric psychiatry unit should be able to provide an holistic and eclectic approach to assessment of the patient".

For each patient there may be several assessments, each with a definite purpose. Pre-admission assessment in the home is valuable for evaluating functional level and the appropriate level of care. Admission assessment may be necessary to make a diagnosis and treatment plan. Follow-up assessment helps monitored treatment effects and overall outcome. The following health care professionals are required in the therapeutic team:

1. *Psychiatry.* Geriatric psychiatry is best practiced in a short-stay, 10–15 bed unit. Ideally, the unit should be free-standing for the elderly alone. Some would ague, because of the medical risks and need for specialist consultations, that the unit should be in the general hospital. The psychiatrist brings together the psychosocial and biological aspects of medicine and is preferably a geriatric psychiatrist. The amount of training received in a general psychiatry residency is inadequate to qualify as a geriatric psychiatrist. Conversely, a full fellowship is not necessary and a separate 6 month rotation is probably sufficient.
2. *Primary care physician.* It is useful to have a primary care physician on the team. This person can help identify medical problems, and suggest tests and medication to deal with these. They can help in the initial phases of assessment. The pace of research makes it difficult for a psychiatrist to keep up satisfactorily with new medications in other specialties and even for common illnesses like hypertension and diabetes.
3. *Consultation team.* It is useful for the geriatric psychiatry group to offer consultation services to other parts of the hospital. Looking for cases of delirium, dementia and depression to treat or to transfer to the geriatric psychiatry ward is a useful way of doing consultations and sharing good relations with other specialties.
4. *Nursing.* Optimally, the same nurse should be responsible for initial contact, inpatient care and follow-up. With this familiarity, the nurse can be responsive to presenting problems of safety and security, prostheses, fluctuations in daily activity, signs of therapeutic response and drug or other sensitivities.
5. *Social work.* The social worker can assess the strengths and weaknesses of the patient's current social network, and evaluate the potential for benefit from individual, family and group psychotherapy. The social worker should be able to provide individual support to the patient and family members.
6. *Occupational therapy.* The occupational therapist can evaluate the patient's response to social, physical and intellectual stimulation and self-care and instrumental activities of daily living. Occupational and leisure needs can be linked to community agencies upon discharge. This therapist should be able to help patients and their families with activities (music, storytelling, group activities, such as playing various games) that can be used to help cope with problem behaviors and emotional distress.
7. *Psychology.* The psychologist can critically determine global and specific intellectual deficits and help manage certain behaviors.
8. *Pharmacy.* The pharmacist is vital in monitoring drug levels, interactions and reactions in order to avoid the problem of delirium.

It is also advisable to have the consulting services of such specialties as internal medicine, cardiology, neurology, ophthalmology, otolaryngology, urology, physiotherapy and dietary science.

The team faces a variety of diagnostic syndromes. These include dementia, affective disorder, delusional disorder, neurosis and personality disorder, alcohol or drug abuse, and delirium. Each of these requires a standardized diagnostic, treatment and management protocol, all subject to measures of efficiency and efficacy.

REFERENCE

1. Eastwood MR, Corbin SL. Multidimensional assessment in geriatric psychiatry. In Bergener M, ed., *Psychogeriatrics: An International Handbook*. New York: Springer, 1987; 136–7.

22

Classification of Dementia and Other Organic Conditions in ICD-10

A. Jablensky and J. E. Cooper

Department of Psychiatry and Behavioural Science, University of Western Australia, Perth, Australia

The classification of mental disorders in the Tenth Revision of the International Classification of Diseases (ICD-10) is different from its predecessor, ICD-9, in several ways. In addition to a revised content that reflects the most important recent advances in research and clinical practice, it is presented in different versions for different types of professional users. The differences are, however, in degrees of detail and the versions are compatible with each other, since they are all derived from the same basic document (*Clinical Descriptions and Diagnostic Guidelines*, WHO, 1992)[1].

THE USES OF ICD-10

ICD-10 has necessarily retained its historical purpose of facilitating the recording of national and international statistics of morbidity and mortality, but now has the added values of also being designed as a uniquely international aide to clinical work, teaching and research. It achieves these objectives by means of an updated list of diagnostic rubrics, a set of glossary-type definitions of disorders and additional explicit diagnostic criteria. The latter have been developed in two versions: (a) clinical diagnostic guidelines for routine use, allowing sufficient flexibility and discretion in the application of "clinical judgement" in the hospital ward or the outpatient service; and (b) diagnostic criteria for research (ICD-10-DCR), providing stringent decision-making rules to increase the specificity of diagnostic classification and thus ensure a high level of sample homogeneity for the purposes of clinical, biological and other research[2].

As a result of a great deal of collaboration between the advisers to the World Health Organization and the several Task Forces that assembled DSM-IV on behalf of the American Psychiatric Association during the last few years of the preparation of both the classifications, there are very few important differences between them. Since the same body of internationally published research experience and literature was available to both sets of experts during the processes of development, those differences that remain are mainly differences of opinion rather than of fact. Some differences reflect the need for ICD-10 to accommodate a much broader base of international experience and opinions than a national classification. In the development of ICD-10, experts from many different cultures and languages were involved from the earliest stages.

As in ICD-9, Chapter V deals with "Mental and Behavioural Disorders" and is intended for the recording of the clinical syndromes as presented and experienced by the patient. If a specific underlying cause of the disorder is known (or highly probable), additional codes should also be used from other chapters of ICD-10, such as: Chapter I, Infectious and Parasitic Diseases; Chapter II, Neoplasms; or Chapter VI, Diseases of the Nervous System.

DEMENTIA IN ICD-10

In ICD-10, the dementias are embedded in the section on organic and symptomatic mental disorders (codes F00–F09), which contains the following major rubrics:

- Dementia in Alzheimer's disease.
- Vascular dementia.
- Dementia in diseases classified elsewhere.
- Unspecified dementia.
- Organic amnesic syndrome, other than induced by alcohol and drugs.
- Delirium, other than induced by alcohol and drugs.
- Other mental disorders due to brain damage and dysfunction and to physical disease.
- Personality and behavioural disorders due to brain disease, damage and dysfunction
- Unspecified organic or symptomatic mental disorder.

In contrast to ICD-9, the distinction between psychotic and non-psychotic illnesses is of no taxonomic consequence in ICD-10, where disorders of different psychopathological expression are grouped together on the basis of established or presumed common aetiology. In the particular instance of section F0, in which the dementing disorders are included, the underlying classificatory characteristic of "organic" is defined in the sense that "the syndrome so classified can be attributed to an independently diagnosable cerebral or systemic disease or disorder". The subsidiary term "symptomatic" is not used in the titles of individual disorders but it is included in the overall title of the block F00–F09. This is because it is widely used in many countries to indicate those organic mental disorders in which cerebral involvement is secondary to a systemic extra-cerebral disease or disorder. In other words, "symptomatic" in this context is a subdivision of the wider term "organic".

Another feature of ICD-10, as compared to earlier classifications, is the omission of any reference to age as a defining criterion of the disorders accompanied by a cognitive deficit. The terms "senile" and "presenile" are practically absent in the classification, and there is no provision for identifying any mental disorder as necessarily a result of ageing. The classification does, however,

Principles and Practice of Geriatric Psychiatry, 2nd edn. Edited by J. R. M. Copeland, M. T. Abou-Saleh and D. G. Blazer

allow the recording of an unusually early or late onset of the disorder. In other words, the mental disorders occurring in the elderly are no longer considered to belong in a separate category of morbidity. This is very much in line with research conducted in the past two decades, which has demonstrated that the relatively high prevalence of mental morbidity in the elderly in Western cultures is related to a wide range of psychosocial factors (e.g. social isolation, cultural uprooting and institutionalization), as well as to physical co-morbidity, but that the aging process itself does not produce nosologically specific forms of disorders.

If section F0 of ICD-10 is used as a diagnostic decision tree, there is a choice of five entry points at the level of clinical syndrome: (i) dementia; (ii) amnesic syndrome; (iii) delirium; (iv) organic quasi-functional disorder (affective, delusional, halluci-natory or other); and (v) personality or behavioural disorder. Once a disorder is identified at this general syndrome level, the next step is defined by the diagnostic guidelines, which lead into more specific diagnostic categories. The diagnostic decision rules for dementia illustrate the point.

The syndrome of dementia is defined in ICD-10 by "evidence of a decline in both memory and thinking, which is of a degree sufficient to impair functioning in daily living", in a setting of clear consciousness. For a confident diagnosis to be established, such disturbances should have been present for at least 6 months. Deterioration of emotional control, social behaviour and motiva-tion represent significant additional features but the overriding criterion is the presence of memory, learning and reasoning decline. The ICD-10-DCR (research criteria) add anchor points for a grading of the deficits into mild, moderate and severe, separately for memory and intellectual capacity. The overall grading of the severity of dementia is made on the basis of the function which is more severely impaired.

Once the presence of the syndrome of dementia is established, the diagnostic process branches off into the different clinical varieties of dementia typical of Alzheimer's disease, vascular dementia and dementia in diseases classified elsewhere (including Pick's disease, Creutzfeldt–Jakob disease, Huntington's disease, Parkinson's disease, HIV disease and a range of systemic and infectious diseases, such as hepatolenticular degeneration, lupus erythematosus, trypanosomiasis and general paresis). Dementia in Alzheimer's disease is subdivided into Type 1 (onset after the age of 65) and Type 2 (onset before the age of 65). Although the ICD-10-DCR criteria emphasize the ultimate criterion of the neuro-pathological examination and the supporting role of brain imaging, they nevertheless allow for a confident clinical diagnosis to be made if clear evidence of a memory and intellectual performance deterioration has been present for 6 months or more. The ICD-10 criteria for vascular dementia are broader than the corresponding DSM-IV criteria: they include not only multi-infarct (predominantly cortical) vascular dementia but also the subcortical dementias (Binswanger's encephalopathy being an example), as well as the mixed cortical and subcortical forms.

As regards the diagnosis of delirium, ICD-10 has abandoned the distinction between acute and subacute deliria; the condition is defined as "a unitary syndrome of variable duration and degree of severity ranging from mild to very grave", with an upper limit of 6 months' duration and a subdivision into delirium superimposed on dementia and delirium not superimposed on dementia.

The rubric "other mental disorders due to brain damage and dysfunction and to physical disease" includes disorders with "functional" characteristics (e.g. hallucinosis, catatonia, schizo-phrenia-like disorder, and mood disorders) that arise in the context of demonstrable organic illness, such as cerebral disease, systemic disorders and brain dysfunction associated with toxic disorders (other than due to alcohol or drugs). An important, not yet fully validated, addition to this rubric is the "mild cognitive disorder" attributable to physical co-morbidity (including HIV disease), which is defined as transient but nevertheless involving memory and learning difficulties.

Finally, personality and behavioural disorders due to brain disease, damage and dysfunction include familiar conditions such as organic personality disorder (the frontal lobe syndrome, but also other lesions to circumscribed areas of the brain), postencephalitic syndrome, postconcussional syndrome and some new entities, e.g. right hemispheric organic affective disorder (altered ability to express and comprehend emotion without true depression).

In conclusion, two features of ICD-10 should be emphasized. First, as already noted, it does not identify the mental disorders in the elderly as a separate or special category of psychiatric morbidity. In addition to the F0 section listing the organic and symptomatic mental disorders, psychiatric disturbances arising in the elderly population can be classified, according to their presentation and course, in any of the other major sections of ICD-10 (except for F8 and F9, which deal with developmental disorders and behavioural and emotional disorders occurring in childhood and adolescence).

Second, although ICD-10 is not explicitly a multi-axial classification, there are two ways in which multi-axial coding can be achieved if required. The simplest way is to use extra codes from the other chapters of ICD-10 in addition to those in Chapter V; any physical disorders present can be recorded by codes from Chapters I–XIX, and codes from the final two chapters can be used to cover other noteworthy aspects of the clinical picture. These are: Chapter XX, External Causes of Morbidity and Mortality (the X and Y codes, covering drugs causing adverse effects in therapeutic use, and injuries and poisoning); and Chapter XXI, Factors Influencing Health Status and Contact with Health Services (the Z codes, which include a variety of social, family and life-style factors). Another and more comprehensive option is to use the special Multi-axial System now available, which was developed by means of an international collaborative study organized by WHO Geneva[3]. This provides three descriptive axes: Axis I, Clinical Diagnosis; Axis II, Disablements; and Axis III, Contextual Factors. These Axes are a convenient re-arrange-ment of the chapters of ICD-10 listed above, with the addition of a brief set of ratings covering physical disabilities.

PROSPECTS FOR THE FUTURE

It is likely to be many years before the next edition of the international classification is ready for use, but meanwhile there are plenty of issues worthy of debate. Whatever form the classification takes, it seems likely that the principle of recording the clinical picture by means of Chapter V and the underlying physical cause by means of other chapters will remain. Research is now providing many clues about the exact place and the histological nature of the lesions in the central nervous system that give rise to the clinical syndromes, but the clinical syndromes themselves will not change, and will always need to be recorded.

The new non-invasive techniques for brain imaging, such as MRI, SPECT and PET scans, are demonstrating a variety of structural abnormalities in the brains of some (but by no means all) patients with the familiar clinical syndromes that are also present in substantial proportions of normal subjects. These changes are "organic" in a general sense of being something physical, but not in the way the term is used in the ICD (that is, to indicate a concurrent and diagnosable physical disorder). It will probably soon be time to abandon "organic" as a term to be used in a classification, and to develop new terms and concepts that will make these more subtle differentiations clear.

It should be possible to omit the "nested" categories of organically caused syndromes of depression, anxiety and schizophrenia in future versions of Chapter V. Their presence breaks the rule (otherwise followed) that a clinical syndrome should have only one place in the classification. They were included because of a clinical demand for the convenience of being able to specify both a syndrome and its cause by means of only one code. Their omission would cause no loss, while improving the properties of the ICD as a classification. Even desk-top recording systems now have large capacities and increasingly sophisticated software that make them capable of handling many entries for each clinical encounter or spell of patient care.

REFERENCES

1. WHO. *The ICD-10 Classification of Mental and Behavioural Disorders. Clinical Descriptions and Diagnostic Guidelines*. Geneva: World Health Organization, 1992.
2. WHO. *The ICD-10 Classification of Mental and Behavioural Disorders. Diagnostic Criteria for Research*. Geneva: World Health Organization, 1993.
3. WHO. *Multi-axial Presentation of ICD-10 for Use in Adult Psychiatry*. Cambridge: Cambridge University Press, 1997.

23

Psychiatric Diagnosis and Old Age: New Perspectives for "DSM-IV-TR" and Beyond

Eric D. Caine

University of Rochester Medical Center, Rochester, NY, USA

Aging and old age confront the psychiatric clinician and nosologist with special diagnostic problems. Our present syndromology has arisen largely from studying disorders of young and middle-aged adults. It is being challenged now by the general aging of the population in Western as well as many Eastern societies.

Aging reflects evolving biological, psychological, and social processes. Fundamental alterations of central nervous system functioning color the psychopathological and pathophysiological significance of specific symptoms, while the psychosocial meaning of discrete life events changes as one moves across the age spectrum. Old age brings an increase in confounding systemic medical conditions. Thus, we are confronted with an array of yet-to-be-answered questions. What is the relationship between the mentally disordered who have grown old, and the old who develop mental disorders? Does later age of onset connote a fundamentally different disease process, even when the presenting psychopathology is generally similar? How do we separate idiopathic (called "primary" in DSM-IV) psychiatric syndromes from psychopathological conditions caused by defined disease processes? What must the diagnostician and treating clinician do to distinguish those psychopathological symptoms that are amenable to treatment from confounding medical symptoms that reflect systemic illness?

The development of the fourth edition of the American Psychiatric Association's Diagnostic and Statistical Manual (DSM-IV) provided an opportunity to begin considering such issues more formally. These types of questions were almost neglected in previous editions of the DSM, in part due to a lack of meaningful research data, and no doubt reflecting a lack of interest among many American psychiatrists in treating geriatric patients. However, the past 15–20 years have seen a surge in interest in the USA in psychogeriatrics, as evidenced by enhanced clinical training and sharpened clinical identity. The development by the American Board of Psychiatry and Neurology of an "added qualification" in geriatric psychiatry during the past decade crystallized this recognition.

There were relatively few changes in DSM-III or DSM-III-R that pertained to elders. Dementia and delirium were defined more precisely. The term "involutional" was dropped from the classification, due to a paucity of data supporting the qualitative distinctness of involutional melancholia. A criterion had been added in DSM-III to establish a maximum age of onset for schizophrenia at 45 years, but this was deleted in DSM-III-R as more evidence was made available to American writers that schizophrenia-like disorders emerge among older patients and are not solely caused by primary cerebral diseases.

Literature reviews and discussions that were part of the preparation of DSM-IV revealed that there was a continuing lack of rigorous clinical descriptive research in many areas of geriatric psychiatry. There was a dearth of data regarding the natural history of both late-onset disorders and early-onset disorders that persist or recur throughout the life course into old age. It was also apparent that there were insufficient epidemiologic findings to fully define the prevalence or incidence of many later life disorders. In the USA, this may have reflected, in part, an overly rigorous application of DSM-III criteria during the epidemiological catchment area (ECA) studies. Although these were valuable for describing the psychopathology of some elderly patients, the stereotypic use of diagnostic descriptors developed for younger patients had the unintended effect of excluding possible subjects from each of the rubrics. This process was compounded further by employing lay interviewers asking highly structured questions. Many of the critiques regarding traditional approaches to cross-cultural psychiatry (e.g. the problem of "category fallacy"[1]) are equally germane to studies that utilize criteria developed for one age cohort when characterizing the psychopathology evidenced by another. As a result, many recommendations for DSM-IV regarding later life psychiatric disorders were qualitative or impressionistic, more useful for specifying directions for new research but insufficient for substantially revising many of the diagnoses to be included in that new edition.

DSM-IV AND BEYOND

The major innovation of DSM-III was the development of a multiaxial system that provided clinicians with a wider array of descriptive categories for more completely defining their patients' problems. However, there was little evidence in either DSM-III or DSM-III-R that indicated a thorough understanding of the complex multidimensional diagnostic problems posed by aging patients. In contrast, DSM-IV began the process of addressing this deficiency by including for many diagnoses a discussion labeled, "Specific Culture, Age, and Gender Features" or "Specific Age and Gender Features". This approach allows some limited consideration of aging-related issues, but again, the sparse commentary in many of these sections also underscores how little is known about many related questions.

The following discussion reviews each of the DSM-IV axes, considering aging-specific topics. They point to areas of controversy that will need further study before inclusion in a future

Principles and Practice of Geriatric Psychiatry, 2nd edn. Edited by J. R. M. Copeland, M. T. Abou-Saleh and D. G. Blazer
©2002 John Wiley & Sons, Ltd

DSM-V. As well, they will highlight planned alterations for the forthcoming text revision of DSM-IV ("DSM-IV-TR") with regard to the diagnosis and classification of neurodegenerative processes, such as Alzheimer's disease.

Axis I

DSM-III and DSM-III-R continued the tradition of distinguishing between "organic" and "functional" disorders. This conceptual typology had posited a difficult-to-maintain dichotomy, one that was poorly justified in light of modern research[2]. As well, "organic" diagnoses too often had been applied without any clear rationale. Instead, DSM-IV emphasizes a conceptual move away from concerns about the presence of structural pathology, or its absence, to a consideration of etiologic link.

It is more meaningful, both clinically and heuristically, to label a disorder as "primary" (i.e. idiopathic) when its cause is unknown, rather than using a term such as "functional" that implies a specific type of physiological or psychological mechanism. "Organic" arose in the nineteenth century after the detection of organ (i.e. brain) pathology. Research findings of the past 30 years have clouded any hope of using such a criterion for separating alleged psychological from alleged biological disturbances. DSM-IV expects clinicians to clarify whether a disorder is primary (i.e. idiopathic) or "secondary" or "symptomatic". (The text itself avoids using the latter designations, given controversy in the USA regarding their exact definitions.) A lengthy description is provided in DSM-IV to help clinicians reason whether there is sufficient evidence to attribute the etiology of a psychiatric syndrome to a definable disease process. Thus, one might diagnose "mood disorder due to Parkinson's disease" or "psychotic disorder due to Huntington's disease" where there is a decision that the psychopathology is a direct reflection of the fundamental pathophysiological process that causes Parkinson's disease or Huntington's disease.

While DSM-IV includes a chapter describing symptomatic psychiatric conditions, they are distributed throughout the text, grouped with the primary psychiatric disorders with which they share phenomenological features, forcing clinicians to consider differential diagnostic questions directly. Although the impact of this change extends beyond older patients, it has frequent application to elders, given their heightened rates of general medical conditions. Whether geriatric psychiatrists and other clinicians have, in fact, undertaken a more rigorous approach to considering etiological relationships because of the changes in DSM-IV remains to be defined.

Cognitive Disorders

Delirium, dementia and amnestic disorders were clustered together in DSM-IV as "cognitive disorders". DSM-III-R developed, perhaps inadvertently, very restrictive criteria for delirium that excluded a variety of patients whose clinicians were certain about the diagnosis, but unable to use the diagnostic label. Beyond traditional definitions employing attentional dysfunction and fluctuating consciousness, DSM-III-R required the presence of "disorganized thinking", as evidenced by formal thought disturbance. However, mildly delirious patients may not have rambling, irrelevant or incoherent speech. DSM-IV returned to a broader view.

While the successive editions of the DSM have been the primary classification for American psychiatry, ICD-9-CM (*International Classification of Diseases, 9th edn, Clinical Modification*) has been adopted by international treaty as the medical diagnostic coding system used by the US Government for all data collection and reporting regarding morbidity and mortality. In order to receive reimbursement from Medicare, for example, every clinician must report diagnoses in terms of ICD-9-CM codes. These range from 00–0999, and are organized in sections based upon the type of disease process (e.g. infectious and parasitic diseases, 001–139; neoplasms, 140–239), anatomic location (e.g. diseases of the digestive system, 520–579; diseases of the nervous system and sense organs, 320–389) or functional area (e.g. mental disorders, 290–319).

The entire system of diagnostic coding now is being revamped during the development of ICD-10-CM. This is intended to deal with the problem of "double coding" (e.g. diagnosing meningitis as both an infection and a disease of the nervous system) and other shortcomings, most notably an insufficient number of potentially available codes for future classification needs. Beginning with the completion of ICD-10 by the World Health Organization during the early 1990s, the most important change has been the adoption of an alpha-numeric coding system, in which letters are used to indicate the section of the ICD classification from which the code is drawn. Thus, infectious disease codes start with the letter A, neoplasms start with the letter B, etc. Codes formerly contained in the Mental Disorders section (290–309) will start with the letter F, while codes formerly contained in the Diseases of the Nervous System (320–389) will be included under the letter G. The "clinical modification" of ICD-10 currently being developed by the US National Center for Health Statistics, using this alpha-numeric system, will be adopted officially within the next several years. The most significant change for geriatric psychiatry will be the provision in ICD-10-CM of only one code for Alzheimer's disease, G30, instead of the double coding that was part of DSM-IV and ICD-9-CM. Although sufficiently similar to ICD-10 to allow cross-national comparison of health data, ICD-10-CM will have several significant differences in terminology and level of specificity.

Subtypes of dementia of the Alzheimer type (DAT) and vascular dementia (i.e. with delirium, with depressed mood, and with delusions) were first introduced into the DSM-III at a time when these categories were referred to as "primary degenerative dementia" and "multi-infarct dementia". These subtypes were later carried forward into DSM-III-R and DSM-IV. The expressed rationale for adding these subtypes had been parsimony of diagnosis, based on the assumption that these three conditions were fundamental manifestations of dementia. It did not make sense to require a clinician to use an additional diagnosis to describe what were considered to be aspects of the primary clinical condition. But neither DSM-III nor DSM-III-R provided explicit instructions about when to use specific subtypes, and a number of questions arose regarding their use. For example, did "with depressed mood" include full-blown major depressive episodes occurring during the course of Alzheimer's disease, or just milder forms of depression? Should "with delirium" include all forms of superimposed delirium, or just delirium thought to be directly due to Alzheimer's disease or vascular pathology? How should one diagnose delirium secondary to suspected drug toxicity in a demented patient? What should be one's approach to describing other commonly encountered symptoms or signs, e.g. delusions, hallucinations, agitation, or anxiety? When delirium, delusions and depressed mood occur simultaneously, which diagnostic code does one choose?

DSM-IV continued to use this subtyping with three changes. A new subtype, "with behavioral disturbances", was added in order to allow the user to indicate "clinically significant behavioral changes (e.g. wandering)", although this was not codable in any numeric fashion. The "with delusions" subtype required that the delusions be the "predominant feature". Lastly, DSM-IV clarified that depressive presentations meeting criteria for a major depressive episode should be included under the "with depressed mood" subtype, in addition to milder forms.

Even with these changes, the basic reasoning behind the DSM-III, DSM-III-R and DSM-IV subtypes was flawed. Beyond including only a small portion of the array of behavioral, psychological or emotional signs, symptoms or syndromes that can be caused by Alzheimer's disease, the structured hierarchy of the classification implied that these manifestations were a *secondary* or *subordinate feature* of the cognitive symptoms and signs of dementia. Ample data now demonstrate that, when present, they are most often manifestations of fundamental brain pathophysiology, as much as memory or other cognitive dysfunctions. In sum, for a classification that was intended to guide therapeutics as well as communicate information regarding signs, symptoms and prognosis, the system did not work.

A change in coding adopted by ICD-9-CM rendered these subtypes obsolete. In anticipation of planned changes for ICD-10-CM, the October 1997 ICD-9-CM coding recommendations indicated that the preferred diagnostic code for Dementia of the Alzheimer's Type should be 294.1 (for "Dementia in Diseases Classified Elsewhere") instead of 290.xx. Thus, the three subtypes that had been coded with a fifth digit could no longer be captured. These changes are being used to revise the approach in DSM-IV as well.

When a patient has emotional, mood or psychological symptoms or signs that are in need of therapeutic interventions arising from Alzheimer's disease, the clinician will be asked to code these conditions on Axis I as one of the "mental disorders due to a general medical condition". As with other etiologically- or pathologically-defined medical conditions, Alzheimer's disease will be recorded on Axis III. Like other secondary or symptomatic psychiatric conditions, these problems must substantially interfere with a patient's functional integrity to warrant a formal diagnosis.

Beyond dementia itself, the secondary conditions to be coded on Axis I (with an associated Axis III diagnosis of Alzheimer's disease) include psychotic disorder, mood disorder, anxiety disorder, personality change (types include labile, disinhibited, aggressive, apathetic, paranoid, other, combined, and unspecified) and sleep disorder. As there are no data indicating that AD *causes* delirium, despite the frequent occurrence of delirium among patients with dementia of the Alzheimer's type, the clinician will be pressed to define the specific etiology of the delirious condition when possible. Sexual disorders due to AD also should not be diagnosed, again reflecting an absence of clinical or research findings tying Alzheimer's disease to sexual dysfunction. Those patients who are uncontrolled in their sexual behaviors can be captured under the "with behavioral disturbance" subtype. Thus, for a man with AD having dementia and delusions associated with combative behavior, one would use the diagnoses 294.1 and 293.81, the latter for Psychotic Disorder due to Alzheimer's Disease, with Delusions. For a woman with delirium superimposed on DAT, the diagnosis will reflect the presumed etiology of the delirium (e.g. delirium due to anticholinergic use is diagnosed 292.81, Anticholinergic-induced Delirium).

Starting in October 2000, a new fifth digit will allow one to indicate whether the dementia is "with behavioral disturbances" (294.11) or "without behavioral disturbances" (294.10). The inclusion of a codable behavioral descriptor and the conventions regarding the diagnosis of DAT and other symptoms due to Alzheimer's disease will be included in DSM-IV-TR, with an anticipated publication in May 2000. (The DSM-IV text revision project is an empirically-based updating of the text only, without any changes being made to the criteria sets.)

The term "*behavioral and psychological symptoms of dementia*" (BPSD) has not been adopted during the DSM-IV revision process. There are two explanations. The first relates to the label itself. It implies that the signs and symptoms in question are a direct outgrowth of dementia, which is not a fundamental disease process but itself a secondary clinical syndrome, rather than suggesting that the behavioral and psychological symptoms are due to AD-caused brain degeneration. The second reservation reflects a concern that behavioral, psychological and emotional symptoms and signs are not a unitary phenomenon. It is most parsimonious at this time to use the extant, discretely defined "mental disorders due to . . ." and avoid creating yet another unitary diagnostic label that has no established reliability or validity[4].

A major topic for discussion during the development of DSM-IV was a recommendation that "age-associated memory impairment" (AAMI) be included as a diagnostic entity, in keeping with criteria proposed to standardize the definition of aging-associated changes in intellect[5]. Aging-related changes in intellectual ability are robust and demonstrable psychometrically when comparing healthy older subjects with younger control groups, encompass a variety of tasks beyond those related to memory, and are at times troubling for particular individuals. However, doubts were expressed regarding the use of a disease diagnosis for a normative phenomenon. There were no objectively defined standards for establishing a cut-off or threshold to separate it from the earliest manifestations of specific diseases (e.g. the early manifestations of Alzheimer's disease). Indeed, review of available data suggested that mild intellectual declines *relative to age-matched peers* often presaged the development of progressive disease. In contrast, there was clear evidence that AAMI was *not* associated with significant functional or social impairment. Ultimately it was concluded that there were insufficient data to establish a formal psychiatric diagnosis of AAMI[6]. DSM-IV finally included "age-related cognitive decline" as a Z code designation, one of those conditions "not attributable to mental disorders that are a focus of attention or treatment".

Other Axis I Issues

Other Axis I disorders provided focal points for heated debate, but concrete recommendations for classificatory changes were difficult to establish in the absence of well-developed research findings. The problem of mood disorders was illustrative. DSM-III-R criteria amply described many of the features of severe mood disorders seen in elderly patients coming to outpatient clinics or hospital inpatient services. However, they were far less satisfactory for describing the features of affectively impaired patients encountered in the offices of primary care physicians, evaluated in nursing home settings or ascertained through community surveys.

Many suffer "subsyndromal" presentations, either dysthymic states that generally conform phenomenologically to dysthymic disorder but are not sustained for the requisite 2 years, or manifestations that include mood, ideational or somatic features of an affective disorder but without the array of symptoms needed to qualify for a strictly defined diagnosis. A diagnostic system that excludes the majority of potential patients fails to fully serve its descriptive function[7]. But suggestions for change remain incomplete and are not yet supported by a sufficiently large body of careful clinical research. (So-called "minor depression" was added for research purposes to the Appendix of DSM-IV, but it remains uncertain how to apply this construct to the conditions encountered among elders.)

The deletion from DSM-III-R of age 45 years as a cut-off for the onset of schizophrenia removed a major impediment for diagnosing elderly psychotic disorders. However, many clinicians have found unreliable the attempt to distinguish between schizophrenia and delusional (paranoid) disorder, based upon the presence of "bizarre delusions". There is no standard by which one can decide when a delusion becomes "bizarre". Other grounds for distinguishing delusional disorder from schizophrenia are now being considered. Additionally, current criteria for schizophrenia require a significant functional decline during the course of the disturbance, but investigators have noted that many patients with late-onset psychosis maintain stability in their personal and social functioning.

It is rare to encounter elderly patients with pure generalized anxiety disorders. Mixed anxiety–depression is common, but it does not fit easily among mood disorders or among anxiety disorders. Although some continue to advocate consideration of a label such as "mixed dysphoric state", there has been no consensus. Growth in the use of serotonin reuptake inhibitors, and compounds such as extended release venlafaxine, has dampened the debate in practical terms, but their apparent effectiveness for mixed anxiety–depressive states sheds little light that clarifies the nosological confusion.

Regarding obsessive–compulsive disorder, post-traumatic stress disorder and phobias, there are few data available about their occurrence among elders to make any salient recommendations regarding diagnostic classification or modification based on aging-related changes in prevalence, presentation, course, co-morbidity or treatment responsiveness. In a similar vein, there are only a small number of replicated findings regarding the form or frequency of adjustment disorders among older patient groups. However, it has been amply clear that the currently employed 6-month time limit for adjustment disorders is inadequate when one faces a persisting stressful situation, such as a chronic physical disability or the need to care for a spouse with Alzheimer's disease.

While there were some minor text changes in DSM-IV regarding substance use disorders, there has continued to be relatively little attention to specific issues related to older persons. Recent studies[8] have underscored the variety of misconceptions that clinicians hold regarding the frequency and impact of alcohol-related clinical conditions. Many substance abuse problems among elders arise from misuse of prescribed medications; older patients often avoid the adverse social consequences of drug seeking and the medical complications of illicit intravenous administration. Although the abuse/misuse may be physically hazardous, especially as it relates to changes in metabolism or potentials for drug interactions, it is distinct from the jeopardy experienced by younger abusers. Thus, the diagnostic classification must attempt to take into consideration age- and culture-related variations, with an eye to dealing with unsupervised use as well as frank abuse.

Axis II

Consideration of personality factors and related clinical disorders has been hampered by minimal data. Although one may conjecture about the changing presentation of Axis II psychopathology across the age span, there have been remarkably few relevant, systematic studies[9]. Clinicians often recognize residual dysfunctional personality features in older, previously diagnosed patients who later fail to conform to stereotypic descriptions. There are no categories available for denoting such conditions. Similarly, there is no diagnosis of "emergent" personality disorder for describing those patients who, having suffered marginally impairing personality traits throughout their lives, evolve a frank disorder in old age. For example, such a classification would capture those who, having been supported or buffered by others, become dysfunctional following the death of a spouse or parent. This view stresses the setting-dependent nature of disordered personality. Overall, pre-DSM-IV discussions swerved away from issues related to personality and aging, leaving them to be

resolved in future editions. It is clear, however, that the domain of personality dysfunction—even if not captured by current diagnostic categories—is a major component of the geriatric landscape[9], especially when considering problems such as depression in primary care settings[10,11] or suicide in elders[12].

Axis III

As noted previously, DSM-IV includes guidelines for assisting a clinician in discriminating between a primary Axis I disorder and a symptomatic disorder due to a condition diagnosed on Axis III. When there is an etiologic tie, the general medical disorder should be noted as part of the Axis I diagnosis (e.g. "mood disorder due to Alzheimer's disease"), in addition to its notation on Axis III. Despite the presence of guidelines, no rule can be used as an infallible aid to determine whether a condition is truly a manifestation of a fundamental medical disorder or is an unrelated idiopathic ("primary") presentation that occurs by coincidence in the presence of a medical condition that is not tied etiologically to the Axis I psychiatric disorder. Clinical judgment must prevail. Similarly, there are no means available for indicating the current clinical significance of co-morbid conditions, whether they contribute to the patient's overall disability, are confounds of possible treatments, or are merely incidental, coexisting disturbances that have no therapeutic impact or functional implications when considering the primary psychiatric syndromes.

Axis IV

As constituted in DSM-III-R, Axis IV was often unsuitable for use with elders. Its exemplars failed to account for many of the common problems or stresses of later life. Additionally, there was no method provided in the manual for defining the contribution of positive psychosocial factors that mitigated or diminished the contribution of stressors to the development of psychopathology. DSM-IV took another approach, defining what might be called "problem areas". This approach avoided the shortcomings of the previous scale, and included a variety of domains relevant to elders, but it too provided no room for an assessment of compensatory factors, in addition to its problem-definition focus. A psychosocially orientated scale (or set of scales) is necessary, one that reflects a broad conception that includes social supports, occupational and environmental resources, perceived quality of life, as well as stressors, both acute and chronic.

Axis V

Functional ratings may have substantial predictive validity when used with elders, but also have proved unreliable when not used carefully. Current use of Axis V requires an estimation of functional capabilities based upon psychopathology alone. Many commentators question whether one can reliably separate functional deficits due to psychiatric symptoms from those arising from co-morbid physical disorders, especially in elderly patients with multiple diseases. Presently available global functional health measures are psychometrically robust and are excellent predictors of subsequent morbidity and mortality in older patient samples. Two separate rating scales, one devoted to overall global functional capability/disability and a second devoted to severity of psychopathology, would likely show greater utility and reliability than the current Axis V measure. While this approach was discussed for DSM-IV, it was not adopted as it was viewed as untested. Future consideration of how best to rate a patient's functional abilities will be an important issue for DSM-V.

In a similar vein, development of a cognitive rating scale within the overall diagnostic classification would have substantial clinical and heuristic value. Here, too, one confronts substantial controversy. Does the clinician attempt to rate absolute capability or to assess change (i.e. decline)? While a measure reflecting intellectual integrity or decline would assist when considering a wide variety of disorders (including dementia, mood disturbances and psychoses), how should one account for variations in literacy, education, cultural background or country of origin? At present, no single scale has proved suitable for all circumstances. Before inclusion in any formal diagnostic system, such a measure would require substantial testing to ensure both its validity and its reliability.

CONCLUSION

Geriatric psychiatry is only now achieving in the USA the attention and status that it has held for many years in other countries. Historically, clinicians and researchers who have worked in this area have had little impact on the nosologies recorded in the diagnostic manuals of the American Psychiatric Association. This situation is changing dramatically. However, specific suggestions for revision bear only as much weight as the strength of the research base upon which they are built. The rapid growth in North America of research dealing with psychopathology of the elderly is a heartening development, one portending future changes in DSM-V that we may not have yet anticipated.

REFERENCES

1. Kleinman AM. Depression, somatization and the "new cross-cultural psychiatry". *Soc Sci Med* 1977; **11**: 3–10.
2. Reynolds EH. Structure and function in neurology and psychiatry. *Br J Psychiat* 1990; **157**: 481–90.
3. Caine ED, Porsteinsson A, Lyness JM, First M. Reconsidering the DSM-IV diagnoses of Alzheimer's disease: behavioral and psychological symptoms in patients with dementia. *Int Psychogeriat* (in press).
4. Caine ED. Diagnostic classification of neuropsychiatric signs and symptoms in patients with dementia. *Int Psychogeriat* 1996; **8** (suppl 3): 273–9.
5. Crook T, Bartus RT, Ferris SH *et al*. Age-associated memory impairment. *Dev Neuropsychol* 1986; **2**: 261–76.
6. Caine ED. Should aging-associated cognitive decline be included in DSM-IV? *J Neuropsychiat Clin Neurosci* 1993; **5**: 1–5.
7. Lyness JM, Caine ED, King DA *et al*. Psychiatric disorders in older primary care patients. *J Gen Intern Med* 1999; **14**: 249–54.
8. Atkinson RM. Aging and alcohol use disorders. *Psychogeriatrics* 1990; **2**: 55–72.
9. Agronin ME, Maletta G. Personality disorders in late life: understanding and overcoming the gap in research. *Am J Geriatr Psychiat* 2000; **8**: 4–18.
10. Lyness JM, Duberstein PR, King DA *et al*. Medical illness burden, trait neuroticism, and depression in older primary care patients. *Am J Psychiat* 1998; **155**: 969–71.
11. Duberstein PR, Sörensen S, Lyness JM, King DA *et al*. Personality is associated with perceived health and functional status in older primary care patients. *Psychol Aging* (in press).
12. Duberstein PR, Conwell Y. Personality disorders and completed suicide: a methodological and conceptual review. *Clin Psychol Sci Prac* 1997; **4**: 359–76.

24

History and Mental Status Examination

Hallie N. Richards[1] and Gabe J. Maletta[2]

[1]*University of Minnesota Medical School and* [2]*VA Medical Center, Minneapolis, MN, USA*

A successful psychiatric evaluation in the elderly, including a comprehensive mental status examination, involves integrating components of both medical and psychiatric clinical models. The classic medical model pursues symptoms and signs in a problem-orientated fashion, seeking to match them with a single unifying diagnosis and then designing an appropriate treatment strategy leading to a cure. This approach is less useful when dealing with geriatric patients. With these patients, aspects of the psychiatric clinical model are emphasized, i.e. ongoing treatment rather than cure, and chronic rather than acute care given by an inter-disciplinary team. This strategy leads toward maximizing and maintaining individual function and behavior. Geriatric care is involved less with disease and more with disability. This is the case whether the patient has a psychiatric or general medical problem; and treatment goals must address the situation of chronic care needs, in contrast simply to the "fixing" of an isolated problem. Complicated presentations of disease in this age group create problems most successfully approached from an interdisciplinary perspective. Many syndromes manifest themselves with symptoms common to psychiatry, internal medicine and neurology, illustrating the overlap of these disciplines in geriatric care. The unique and challenging aspects of interviewing the elderly requires developing an individualized, functional clinical examination. With this goal in mind, the medical history will be examined and utilized to illustrate how the different medical specialties interact to integrate the art with the science of medicine. A successful blending will result in obtaining the most clinically useful examination possible.

PURPOSE

Obtaining a valid and reliable medical history continues to yield a correct diagnosis in over 80% of clinical situations[1]. This remains true in elderly patients, but accomplishing the task in this age group is often difficult and time-consuming. Perfecting the skills required to interview successfully an old, sick individual is invaluable in understanding an unusual disease process or avoiding costly mistakes in evaluation and treatment[2]. The working, hands-on abilities necessary to effect a successful history fall within two separate realms: fact-finding (science) and empathy (art)[3]. In the first realm, traditional medical training is replete with teaching and experiences. On the other hand, tutelage yielding artful practitioners is much less universal; indeed, it is becoming a rare and treasured experience in a medical residency.

With a view in mind toward expanding the "art" realm, a new look at interviewing elderly people is indicated. The interaction between patient and interviewer becomes much more than the process of collecting facts and related information to make a diagnosis. Gaining medical and social facts pertaining to the individual's problems is a primary but not exclusive goal. Older adults often come to the physician with a complex agenda that may not be obvious by dwelling only on the chief complaint. Conducting the interview by this conventional fact-finding method may not be productive and actually may put one at risk for generating too narrow a differential diagnosis.

In addition to laying the foundation for a satisfying therapeutic relationship, the initial gathering of information should guide the first steps in evaluation. Logical, stepwise investigation of symptoms and signs remains the practical approach to any medical work-up. If this investigation yields nothing, the urge to perform more elaborate tests should be resisted and one should return to the history. Greater dependence on reviewing the history again with the patient is more likely to yield an appropriate plan. The "law of parsimony" is not as useful a guiding principle in the care of geriatric patients as it is in general medicine[4]. A single, unifying diagnosis may not explain satisfactorily a symptom complex responsible for a precipitous functional decline in an elderly individual, and continuing investigation frequently uncovers multiple causes.

An understood but often unstated purpose of the medical interview with old people is getting to know the patient. This requires interviewer empathy (not sympathy or emotional involvement), which may be of the highest importance in the patient's view. Using the initial interview to explore personality and life experiences helps build rapport that is essential to subsequent interactions. Whether a patient's problem is psychiatric or medical, the initial interaction and relationship that grows from it are vital to achieving the goal of proper diagnosis and treatment.

ELEMENTS

Although the components of the medical history in geriatrics do not differ from those in the practice of any other specialty, the order in which they are pursued and their relative importance may be unique. The classic approach of taking a symptom-directed chief complaint, history of present illness, past medical history, review of systems, social history and family history will produce a desired database from which to work. However, mechanically and swiftly following an unbending order or sequence of impersonal questions may provoke successively less and less cooperation if the patient perceives that you are not really "listening". A more effective approach may require the physician to give up some control over the process of the interview, allowing the patient to conduct it on his/her own terms. Valuable information that would otherwise be missed may be hidden in a conversational tangent the patient insists on following.

Review of previous medical records is necessary but they may not be available while you are seeing the patient. Especially in the elderly, a variety of information sources must be accessed in addition to the patient, including reliable family members and others in the social network. Indeed, if these other sources are lacking this should be noted and may itself have significance in the geriatric setting. Even in cognitively intact persons, corroboration is a good idea, as the "facts" may be related differently depending upon one's perspective. Non-medical problems, such as financial stress or social isolation, invariably impact on the elderly patient in unpredictable ways and cannot be ignored while investigating a medical complaint. After thorough investigation of each part of the history, the stories, details and facts are compiled, reviewed and evaluated, resulting in an in-depth, composite picture of the person in relation to the clinical issue at hand.

EXECUTION

For the older patient the first encounter with a physician is very important. Any subsequent interaction will be strongly influenced by the patient's initial impression, e.g. empathetic or distracted, rushed or friendly, interested or detached, confident or tentative. All things will flow from the stage set in the first few minutes of the interview. Therefore, serious thought should go into the initial 5 or 10 minutes of conversation. The physician must approach the situation with confidence, courtesy and the belief that some treatment plan can be developed, no matter how hopeless the situation may initially seem. Indeed, an optimistic stance is often useful when dealing with an elderly patient. The only thing on the physician's mind during the interview should be the patient and the problem at hand.

A skilled interviewer simultaneously questions, interacts (exchange of information), observes and, most importantly, listens. Proficient listening is an active exercise, requiring great concentration. Well placed periods of silence can be fruitful regarding observation or obtaining additional volunteered information, if the atmosphere is supportive and relaxed. It is not necessary to keep a dialogue going non-stop throughout the interview. Silence should be considered as a positive strategy. Sometimes, silent observation is extremely useful, especially with patients who seem to be actively hallucinating or exhibiting abnormal motor movements.

The examiner must function at many levels of interaction simultaneously, which can be physically draining. Making adjustments and modifications for the sensory and sometimes cognitive impairment extant in some patients adds to the interviewer's stress. These modifications include: sitting close; speaking slowly and loudly with frequent repetition; provision of ample time to allow for responses, which often have a prolonged latency; and even, when possible and necessary, use of sound amplifying devices[5].

More active engagement and even providing verbal direction may be a useful and effective tactic during the interview. The personal style of the interviewer is an individual but important trait, and the patient must be convinced that it is genuine. This occurs if the interviewer is truly interested and able to suspend any distracting thought or action. Physical expressions of concern, including touching (e.g. hand holding) are often appropriate with particular geriatric patients and helpful in reinforcing positive rapport.

The best initial tactic is to focus on the chief complaint, but not be limited by it. Know the planned questions and format of the entire interview well, allowing for rearrangement of sections during a particular interview to suit individual situations. This will allow a fluid order without interruption so that an interesting tangent may be followed easily. Open-ended questions may not be productive with the elderly, and if no progress is being made, asking focused, specific questions or using different, sometimes simpler, wording may succeed.

In spite of thoughtfully executed and patiently stated questions, contradictory answers may still be the end result. At that point resist a frustrated summary and probe further, pushing for elaboration. The contradiction will either be resolved directly with new information, or may itself provide new insight when it cannot be explained. Patience is required of both the examiner and patient, and it may be necessary to execute the complete interview in several parts, deferring some material to subsequent sessions.

Astute observation of the patient throughout the entire interaction may yield more information than a multitude of questions. The interviewer, acting as a receiver, uses all senses—eyes, ears and especially immediate feelings—to accept and interpret transmitted information. Much is learned by gazing in the face of an elderly person, e.g. presence or absence of eye contact, facial musculature, position of the head and general affect. Subtle body language, such as hand motion or lack of it, can suggest affective disorder, neurologic or medication problems, or perhaps substantiate complaints of arthritis.

Commenting on objects or memorabilia observed in the surrounding environment serves the dual purpose of providing the opportunity for light conversation and again for building rapport. Reminiscence of earlier times, when the patient was in greater control, can also be a valuable method of gathering data, in addition to putting the patient at ease and strengthening the therapeutic relationship. For the unusually quiet elderly person, try specific "ice-breakers", such as:

"Tell me the story that is your life . . ."

"What was it like to be alive when (some significant event) . . .?"

"When you were my age, how long did you think you would live?"

This particular tactic may even provide the interviewer with insight into cohort differences among different-aged elderly and their impact on disease presentation in individual elderly patients.

Certain problem situations present unique challenges when interviewing the elderly. Unavoidable physical limitations, such as fatigue, hearing or visual impairment and chronic pain, may limit the time of the interview itself or influence the amount of information gained. Cognitive problems, such as memory loss or inability to pay attention, and psychiatric illnesses (temporary or permanent), such as dementia, delirium, generalized anxiety, major affective disorder or even psychosis, may cause difficulties and such diagnoses may only become apparent well into the interview, making all information obtained up to that point suspect. Also, patient biases of many types, such as racial, language and cultural, need to be acknowledged to avoid misinformation and miscommunication. Old patients may view young physicians with distrust, just as age bias may occur in the opposite direction.

Closing the interview successfully is as important in overall impact as is the initial impression[6]. Take care to ensure that all issues on the patient's agenda have been addressed. In any event, a useful strategy is always to end the interview by asking the patient if there are any questions he/she would like to ask the interviewer. Key questions may often be asked by the patient just as the physician closes the encounter, uncovering hidden fears or revealing the real reason (not the stated one) for the visit. Adequate time for patient questions, empathetic listening and thoughtful responses often yield insights missed or left unexplained earlier. A brief statement to the patient at the end of the interview about "where to go from here" can instill confidence that something will be done soon. Later, after time for thoughtful consideration, a detailed explanation of the assessment and treatment plan can be discussed with all interested parties.

The primary goals of psychiatric and general medical treatment merge in the elderly patient[5]. They include the amelioration of symptoms, restoration or maintenance of optimum function, and enhancement of the subjective quality of life. Since curing the elderly of disease is usually not possible, focusing on these goals in a caring manner will enhance the physician–patient relationship and increase the chance of success in treatment.

Once the facts are gathered, one then needs to spend considerable time systematically reviewing and organizing the data into meaningful information, i.e. the formulation. This allows for the development of an integrated diagnosis and treatment plan. The plan is a framework and remains a guide, but can be altered depending on subsequent events and the patient's response to therapy. A well thought out plan also helps avoid costly and often fruitless searching and testing that may lead to over-diagnosis and risky therapeutic choices. Both professional and personal rewards result when extra time and effort are invested in thoroughly examining an elderly person in this manner.

MENTAL STATUS EXAMINATION

The formal mental status examination (MSE) is obtained once a thorough history is obtained. It is a measure of both general psychiatric status and specific cognitive function or dysfunction. Equal time, patience and concentration are required for this portion of the interview, and, especially in the mentally ill elderly, often is a more difficult task for the interviewer. This is because the MSE touches on areas and experiences that may be uncomfortable, embarrassing or even frightening for the patient. Often, parts of the MSE will have already been satisfied by previous observation and interaction while taking the history, e.g.

level of consciousness, appearance and behavior, affect, and parts of the sensorium examination (attention, word-finding).

Table 24.1 displays the components of a formal MSE in the psychiatric interview. The patient's level of consciousness should be described at the outset. Columns 1–4 of Table 24.1 are examples of common descriptors illustrating possible presentations of mental illness. The last four columns suggest areas to consider when investigating sensorium, judgement, insight and risk of causing harm.

At the conclusion of the MSE all acquired information can be recorded in a comprehensive psychiatric database, as outlined below. This serves many purposes, but most importantly it encourages systematic review, comparison with subsequent examinations, and decreases the possibility of overlooking details important to a correct diagnosis. Formulation of an individualized assessment and treatment plan, including functional status, completes the process and, once recorded, allows review and revision at any time. It should be reinforced that psychiatric evaluation of the geriatric patient, including history and MSE, although similar in some ways to examination of younger patients, differs in some key ways. The most important, unique difference for the examiner to understand and appreciate is the need to integrate into the MSE the assessment of concomitant chronic and acute medical conditions and also to augment the historical data obtained from the patient by interviewing other reliable individuals with pertinent information.

Database History

Identification
Informant(s)—determining reliability of the historian is important. It is often useful to supplement the interview by meeting and questioning family and/or friends
Chief complaint
History
Present illness
Past psychiatric

Table 24.1 Components of the mental status examination (MSE)

Appearance and behavior	Affect	Mechanics of thought (speech)	Content of thought	Sensorium (cognitive exam)[6]	Judgment	Insight	Suicidal/homicidal
Grooming	Absent (blank)	(1) Quality:	Preoccupation	Orientation	Decision-making capacity[7]	Ability to understand important components of a situation	Ideation
Dress (gender-appropriate?)	Withdrawn	Rate	Obsession	Memory	Health		Previous attempts
Mannerisms	Sad	Volume	Guilt	Registration	Financial		Family history
Posture	Euphoric	Prosody	Somatic concerns	Recall			Risk factors
Motor activity	Labile	Clarity	Paranoia	Long-term memory			Plan
Interviewer's reaction to patient	Intense	Pressure	Erotica	Attention			
Patient's reaction to interviewer	Constricted	(2) Quantity:	Delusions	Concentration			
	Flat	Spontaneous	Well-organized	Calculation			
	Appropriate to content of talk?	Mono- or polysyllabic	Bizarre	Abstraction			
			Hallucinations (sensory modality)	Comprehension			
				Consequences			
				Planning			
				Foresight			
				Reasoning			
				Problem-solving abilities			
				Language			
				Writing			
				Visual–spatial			

Disciplines other than psychiatry routinely test only orientation to satisfy this section of the MSE. It is important to perform a standard, valid and reliable cognitive examination to achieve an acceptably comprehensive MSE. The Mini-Mental State Examination (MMSE) is a good example of an acceptable test[8]. Also, besides testing cognition, other instruments may be useful in particular patients, especially to evaluate mood and functional capabilities[9]. The interviewer should become familiar and experienced with one or two scales in each area, e.g. Geriatric Depression Scale[10] or Beck's Depression Inventory[11]; Activities of Daily Living[12] Instrumental Activities of Daily Living[13]; Global Deterioration Scale[14]; Cognitive Performance Test[16] Global Assessment of Functioning[17].

Family
Family psychiatric
Personal
Social (including work)
Medical
Current medications
Drug and alcohol
Psychiatric examination (MSE)
Level of consciousness
Appearance and behavior
Affect
Mechanics (stream) of thought
Content of thought
Sensorium
Insight
Judgment
Suicidal/homicidal ideation

A physical examination (including a brief neurologic examination), laboratory evaluation and neuropsychological testing complete the geriatric psychiatric database and are described elsewhere. It is particularly important to evaluate visual and auditory acuity in this age group.

REFERENCES

1. Hampton JR, Harrison MJG, Mitchell JRA *et al.* Relative contributions of history-taking, physical examination, and laboratory investigation to diagnosis and management of medical outpatients. *Br Med J* 1975; **ii**: 486–9.
2. Mader S, Ford A. The Geriatric Interview. In *The Medical Interview*. New York: Springer, 1995; 221–34.
3. Coulehan JL, Block MR. In Lowenthal DT (ed.) *The Medical Interview: A Primer for Students of the Art*. Philadelphia, PA: FA Davis, 1987; chapter 1.
4. Rowe JW, Besdine RW. *Geriatric Medicine*, 2nd edn. Boston: Little, Brown, 1988.
5. Spar JE. Principles of diagnosis and treatment in geriatric psychiatry. In Lazarus L (ed.), *Essentials of Geriatric Psychiatry*. New York: Springer, 1988.
6. Sapira JD. *The Art and Science of Bedside Diagnosis*. Baltimore, MD: Urban & Schwarzenberg, 1990.
7. Applebaum P, Grisso J. Assessing patient's capacities to consent to treatment. *N Engl J Med* 1988; **25**(319): 1635–8.
8. Folstein M, Folstein S, McHugh P. Mini-mental state: a practical method of grading the cognitive state of patients for the clinician. *J Psychiatr Res* 1975; **12**: 189–98.
9. Crook T, Ferris S, Bartus R (eds), *Assessment in Geriatric Psychopharmacology*. New Canaan, CT: Mark Powley, 1983.
10. Yesavage J, Brink T, Rose T *et al.* Development and validation of a geriatric depression screening scale: a preliminary report. *J Psychiat Res* 1983; **17**: 37–49.
11. Beck A. *Depression: Causes and Treatment*. Philadelphia, PA: University of Pennsylvania Press, 1972.
12. Katz S *et al.* Studies of illness in the aged: the index of ADL, a standardized measure of biological and psychosocial function. *J Am Med Assoc* 1963; **185**: 914–19.
13. Lawton M, Brody E. Assessment of older people: self-maintaining and instrumental activities of daily living. *Gerontologist* 1969; **9**: 179–86.
14. Reisberg B, Ferris S, DeLeon M *et al.* The global deterioration scale for assessment of primary degenerative dementia. *Am J Psychiat* 1982; **139**: 1136–9.
15. Cassel C, Riesenberg D, Sorenson L, Walsh J (eds). *Geriatric Medicine*, 2nd edn, New York: Springer, 1990; chapters 33–37.
16. Burns T, Mortimer J, Merchak P. Cognitive Performance Test: a new approach to functional assessment in Alzheimer's disease. *J Geriat Psychol Neurol* 1994; **7**: 46–54.
17. American Psychiatric Association. *Diagnostic and Statistical Manual of Mental Disorders*, 4th edn. Washington, DC: American Psychiatric Association, 1994.

25

The Physician's Role

Lesley Young

The idea that mental disorders may be the result of bodily disease acting on the brain has been current for at least a millennium, since the time of Avicenna[1]. Numerous attempts to relate specific psychological reactions to particular physical disorders have been unsuccessful, however, and it now seems clear that some general mechanism affecting the chemical environment of the brain is responsible[2]. Many descriptive classifications of "organic psychosis" have had to be abandoned and not even the notion of "clouding of consciousness" has always been regarded as a cardinal feature of delirium[3], although the most recent definition of delirium includes "disturbance of consciousness with reduced ability to focus, shift or sustain attention" as a diagnostic criterion[4].

The clinician dealing with a mentally disturbed patient must consider any process capable of interfering with cerebral metabolism or neurotransmission[5,8] as a possible causal factor. Moreover, for reasons still not well understood, the probability of a mental disorder arising from a "physical" cause is greatly increased in old age, so that the psychiatrist will rarely see a mentally ill old person without significant physical disease[6] (and the geriatrician must likewise develop expertise in psychiatry).

The aim of the physician when confronted with a mentally ill patient should be to answer two questions:

- Could there be a physical cause for the mental disturbance?
- Is there any physical condition that is making things worse?

DELIRIUM

"Acute confusional states" are common in old people[7], indeed it is claimed that mental confusion is a far more common herald of physical illness than pain, fever or tachycardias[8]. Delirium may also go unrecognized by attending clinicians[9], or be misdiagnosed as dementia or depression[10], with potentially disastrous consequences[11]. Not only may this mean a denial of personal rights or even permanent incarceration in an institution, but also the underlying cause may go undetected and therefore untreated. Although detailed mental state examination and formal cognitive testing may give some clues, delirium and dementia can only reliably be distinguished by obtaining a full collateral history and by observation of the subsequent course of the illness. However, the serial use of cognitive screening tests, such as the Abbreviated Mental Test score[12] or Mini-Mental State Examination[13], has been shown to be useful in helping to distinguish delirium from dementia. Disorders of attention and alertness are prominent features of delirium, and tests of reaction time and the "face/hand"[14] tests have been claimed to distinguish those whose mental disorder is of recent and rapid onset. Hallucinations and other perceptual disorders are also common and may be found in the absence of any other apparent mental illness, so such phenomena may be under-reported for obvious reasons. Visual hallucinations are said to be particularly common following bereavement[15] and isolated perceptual disorders such as the Charles Bonnet syndrome[16] may be associated with pathology of the sensory system involved, although such phenomena are also seen in cerebrovascular disease[17]. None of these features is unique to delirium, however, and the only reliable way to distinguish delirium from dementia, and sometimes from functional mental illness, is to obtain a detailed history from a third party: the most useful diagnostic tool is the telephone.

If in doubt it should be assumed that the mental disturbance is acute and therefore potentially reversible, so a physical cause should always be sought, a process that may require some detective work. Appropriately enough, the first step is to suspect that the victim has been poisoned. A full drug history, including both prescribed and over-the-counter medication, is necessary. Although drugs acting primarily on the central nervous system, and particularly those affecting the cholinergic neurotransmitter systems, are the most likely to cause problems, any medication should come under suspicion. Numerous drugs have been shown to have cholinergic effects, including many drugs that would not initially appear to exert such an action[18]. Polypharmacy is common in older people[27] and relatively minor cholinergic effects of each individual drug may exert a cumulative effect, thus, the delirium may not be due to one individual drug but rather the combined effect of several. Drugs affecting cardiac output or cerebral blood flow may precipitate memory changes, and diuretics also produce a range of adverse metabolic effects of their own. Long-term use of laxatives may have similar effects. "Minor tranquillizers", such as the benzodiazepines, once thought of as safe alternatives to the barbiturates, are now recognized to cause acute psychiatric disturbance[19] as well as chronic mental impairment, unsteadiness and falls[20]. Opiates, often prescribed together with mild analgesics in combinations such as co-proxamol, may cause acute or long-term problems.

Long-term use of addictive drugs is surprisingly common in the elderly population[21] and is often the result of careless prescription of sleeping tablets or painkillers. Alcoholism is probably an under-recognized problem[27,23] and in this context it should be remembered that delirium may just as easily result from sudden withdrawal of long-term drugs as from their use[24].

Examination of the patient often begins with inspection of the home, looking particularly for evidence of drug or alcohol abuse, poor diet, incontinence and general signs of short- or long-term neglect. The family and neighbours should be interviewed

Principles and Practice of Geriatric Psychiatry, 2nd edn. Edited by J. R. M. Copeland, M. T. Abou-Saleh and D. G. Blazer

wherever possible, mainly to establish the patient's normal mental and physical state and the timing of any change, making use of "landmarks" (such as Christmas) to focus the memory. The patient's current mental state should then be assessed in the light of this information.

Diagnosis and Assessment

When assessing an elderly person with a potential delirium, it is useful to bear in mind the common causes for precipitating delirium, which include infections, biochemical and metabolic derangements, organ failure and drugs. There is frequently more than one potential cause and thus assessment should be continued, even after one "cause" has been identified.

The approach and manner of the clinician towards the patient are of great importance. The aim is to provide a stable and, if possible, familiar sensory environment, so assessment should take place in a well-lit room with a minimum of distracting and misinterpretable stimuli. Physical examination starts with assessment of general hygiene, nutritional state, hydration and superficial signs of injury.

Body temperature must be measured with care: significant infections usually cause fever at any age[25], although it is often missed in elderly patients, where oral or axillary temperature may take longer to equilibrate with core temperature[26]. Suspected hypothermia must be checked by measuring rectal temperature. The relationship between peripheral and core temperature depends mainly on the state of the circulation: cool peripheries are just as likely to indicate arterial shut-down, due to low cardiac output or hypovolaemia, as hypothermia. Other important signs of dehydration or blood loss are a low jugular venous pressure (venous pulsation not visible at the root of the neck with the patient lying at 20° or less to the horizontal) or postural hypotension (a fall of over 20 mmHg systolic and/or 10 mmHg diastolic on sitting or standing up). The latter may, of course, be due to the effect of drugs or autonomic failure, in which case the fall in blood pressure may not be accompanied by reflex tachycardia. High blood pressure has little diagnostic value and should normally be left alone in the acute situation.

Abnormalities of heart rate or rhythm can also seriously affect cardiac output and cerebral perfusion. Heart rate should be assessed by both feeling the pulse and listening over the precordium, where murmurs can also be detected. An electrocardiogram is an essential extension of clinical examination and, as well as documenting heart rhythm, may also show clinically undetectable signs of myocardial infarction. Signs of cardiac failure should be sought, including the presence of a gallop rhythm, fine inspiratory crepitations in the chest and peripheral oedema. The peripheral pulses should be felt. Bruits in the neck are useful, although non-specific, markers of arterial disease.

Abnormalities of respiratory rate or pattern must be noted, as well as the presence of central or peripheral cyanosis. In a delirious patient with cyanosis, warm peripheries and bounding pulses, the characteristic flapping tremor of CO_2 retention should be sought. Focal signs in the chest are useful but non-specific, and a chest X-ray is nearly always required. Any sputum must be examined at the bedside as well as sent for microscopy and culture. Arterial blood gasses are sometimes useful, but both persistent and transient hypoxaemia can be detected non-invasively with a pulse oximeter, although in the presence of signs of hypercapnia measurement of arterial blood gases is preferable.

Examination of the alimentary system begins with nutritional assessment and inspection of the mouth, looking for evidence of sepsis or neoplasm. The abdomen must be carefully examined, as virtually any surgical emergency can present as a change in mental state without apparent abdominal symptoms. Abdominal signs may be far from obvious and many a strangulated hernia in an elderly patient has been missed by the unwary.

Urinary retention and faecal impaction are often detectable per abdomen but a rectal examination should also be done wherever possible. Whether constipation can cause delirium by itself is still a subject of vigorous debate, but most geriatricians and general surgeons are familiar with the elderly patient whose mental and physical state improves dramatically with rehydration and enemas. Examination of the perineum includes inspection of clothing for evidence of incontinence or precautions against it. Incontinence is a frequent finding in patients with delirium[21]; whether as a consequence of the underlying cause or as a direct result of the mental disturbance is not clear.

In the locomotor system, trauma and acute inflammation are important causes of delirium and swelling, warmth, tenderness and pain on movement of any joint should give rise to suspicion. The feet should be carefully examined for signs of ischaemia or sores, and the gait observed.

The most important part of neurological examination is the assessment of conscious level and higher mental function. In a delirious patient this is as much the province of the physician as the psychiatrist and it is important that both terminology and assessment should be standardized. The hard-pressed house physician confronted with an acutely disturbed patient in the middle of the night is unlikely to turn to the Diagnostic and Statistical Manual of Mental Disorders of the American Psychiatric Association for immediate guidance, but she might find a simple standardized assessment of attention, orientation and memory, such as the 10-question Abbreviated Mental Test Score[28] or the Mini-Mental State Examination[13] useful. Such tests are often criticized because they are prone to misuse, a low score being taken as evidence of dementia, but their main value lies in repeated use, when dramatic changes often seen in acute medical patients clearly point[29] to delirium rather than dementia as the cause of poor performance. The routine use of such tests reminds the busy junior doctor to consider the possibility of delirium, and may prompt a search for the underlying cause in those who have a low score. Moreover, routine use of cognitive screening tests can avoid the clinician being fooled by an apparently cognitively intact older person who, in fact, has a significant cognitive deficit but a good "social front", can act as a baseline should the mental status change. It is important to be aware, however, that these tests are merely screening tests, and the scores are influenced by numerous factors other than the current mental disturbance. Including sensory impairments, educational level, social class and language. When applying standardized criteria to patients admitted to a geriatric assessment unit, 18% satisfied DSM-III-R criteria for delirium on admission[29] and the mean duration of the delirium by the same criteria was 7 days. Some deficits persisted longer, however, notably memory impairment, with a mean duration of 28 days. The use of standardized scales will not replace clinical judgement but will undoubtedly lead to greater clarity of thought and discussion, and is essential for progress in research.

Many clinicians place great emphasis on careful neurological examination, looking for focal signs which, if found are usually attributed to cerebrovascular disease. This assumption may often be correct, although the evidence is scant, but it is a mistake to blame everything on acute stroke, since the metabolic disturbance causing delirium may simply be highlighting areas of brain ischaemia. Thus, focal signs may be related to previous stroke damage, where neurological function has largely recovered although perfusion has remained impaired. If this is not appreciated, then the real culprit, which might be a treatable infection, may be missed.

The reliability of subtle focal signs, such as asymmetry in tendon reflexes, should also be regarded with scepticism, given the extent of inter-observer variation in the assessment of the patient with obvious hemiplegic stroke[30,31]. The most reliable signs are those that can be easily reproduced and particularly those that are reflected in the patient's behaviour, such as dysphasia or unilateral neglect. This raises the more general point that the diagnostic assessment does not end with the formal physical examination but must include careful observation of the patient over the next few days. A host of signs that might otherwise have been missed, from episodes of fever, syncope, or fits to a craving for alcohol or opiates, may be revealed. Assessment of vision and hearing are particularly important, as the presence of sensory deficits may increase the risk of developing delirium, and a recent study showed that attention to and correction of sensory deficits may reduce the severity and duration of delirium[32]. Impairments of vision or hearing may also only become clear after a period of observation.

The choice of laboratory tests tends to be determined more by institutional tradition and by habits and attitudes of the clinician than by scientific evidence. The value of any tests depends largely on the prior probability of finding treatable disease. Thus, the urine should always be tested but a computed tomography (CT) scan comes low on the list of priorities. Whilst CT head scans may frequently show minor abnormalities, such as cerebral atrophy, a cause for delirium is rarely found unless there are other features in the history and examination to point to an intracerebral cause, such as new onset of focal neurological signs[33]. Similarly, whilst electroencephalography (EEG) is frequently abnormal in delirium, showing diffuse slow-wave activity[34–36], it is rarely useful as a diagnostic tool unless there is clinical suspicion of epilepsy. Indeed, the very non-specific nature of the EEG changes seen in delirium raises interesting (although under-researched) questions about the pathogenesis of the disorder. Other invasive tests, such as lumbar puncture (LP), have been used in research and numerous abnormalities of neurotransmitters have been identified in delirium, but as a diagnostic test in clinical circumstances, LP is again only useful in those with features of meningism[37,38].

The range of diagnostic possibilities is almost always wide and there may be few clinical clues. This has led to the erroneous and derogatory use of the expression "geriatric screening" to describe the laboratory investigation of elderly patients presenting with non-specific symptoms or functional problems. Screening tests always have a low yield, since the vast majority of subjects have nothing wrong with them, whereas tests done in order to track down the cause of delirium have a high probability of showing an abnormality, and serum calcium, urea and electrolytes, full blood count and glucose should virtually always be done.

DEMENTIA

Delirium and dementia commonly occur together; indeed, the pre-existence of dementia is a major risk factor for the development of delirium[39] and up to 70% of patients presenting with an episode of delirium will have some degree of chronic brain failure as well[40]. There is a clear relationship between the degree of vulnerability of a patient and the size of the insult required to precipitate delirium[39]. The principles of assessing a patient with "decompensated dementia" are similar to those outlined above, with some slight changes in emphasis. A psychological upset or disruption of the normal protective social environment may be enough to precipitate a crisis in a mentally frail person. Whether or not such an episode of decompensation actually constitutes delirium is debatable[41] but it can only be a short step away, as physical complication such as exhaustion, dehydration or hypothermia may quickly supervene. Whether or not the initial

event was some kind of social or psychological trauma, it should not prevent a careful search for physical disease, for in such frail individuals, relatively minor remediable disorders can have dramatic functional consequences.

The distinction between decompensated dementia and delirium is also of practical importance because of the special problems involved in admitting the former group to hospital. A balance must be struck between the patient's need for a stable, familiar and reassuring environment and the availability of facilities for investigation and treatment. The former may be the overriding consideration in the case of decompensated dementia, while in the previously well person with delirium the latter is the main concern. In some (but not all) cases, day hospital facilities may provide a useful compromise.

Physical illness in a person with dementia may also present a decline in physical rather than mental function, with development of non-specific symptoms or signs such as unsteadiness, falls, immobility or incontinence. Again, the sudden appearance of such problems should not be assumed to be due to the progression of dementia or put down to "another stroke" but must be investigated, since timely intervention may prevent irreversible deterioration or even unnecessary institutionalization.

Recent research has highlighted the associations between physical illness and dementia, particularly vascular pathology and risk factors for such conditions. Dementia is thus significantly associated with the presence of atrial fibrillation[42], ischaemic heart disease[43,44], cerebrovascular disease[43,44], hypertension[44,45] and diabetes[46,47]. Moreover, there is suggestive evidence that poor control in some of these conditions may result in accelerated cognitive decline[45]. Therefore, whilst evidence from large-scale prospective studies is not yet available, it would seem sensible for the physician to actively treat such coexisting physical illness in the presence of dementia. Whilst high blood pressure appears to be a risk factor for the development of dementia, the prevalence of low blood pressure and orthostatic hypotension (OH) is also more common in dementia and may have an aetiological role[48,49], and the physician should be alert to the presence of OH and consider appropriate intervention.

Involving physicians in the assessment of patients with dementia is important to help rule out a treatable cause. Clearly no-one can afford to miss "reversible dementia" but unfortunately we have no idea of its true prevalence. Estimates of the frequency of reversibility in series of hospital patients has been reported to be as high as 40%[50], but older studies are hopelessly biased by concentrating on younger "pre-senile" patients from secondary or tertiary referral centres. In the few community-based studies that have been reported, the frequency of "reversible" cases was less than 10%[51]. More recent studies have estimated the prevalence of potentially reversible dementia in the region of 7.2%[52] to 23%[53], although only at best 3% were actually reversed[52,53]. An analogy may be drawn with the frequency of space-occupying lesions in patients presenting with "acute stroke", which was estimated at 15% in a study based at a neurological centre[54], compared to 1.5% in a series of patients admitted to an acute geriatric unit[55] and a similar figure in a community stroke survey[56]. There is an urgent need for equivalent community-based studies of dementia in which all cases are thoroughly investigated. Until then, practice must be based on questionable and possibly ageist assumptions about the likelihood of finding treatable disease in particular groups of patients. Thus, few clinicians would disagree that younger patients should be fully investigated, as well as those of any age whose symptoms are of recent onset or rapidly progressing.

As emphasized above, a careful drug history is of overriding importance, since it is bad enough to miss a treatable disorder but unforgivable to be responsible for causing it or making it worse. As in the case of delirium, all drugs should come under suspicion, including some superficially unlikely offenders such as digoxin, non-steroidal anti-inflammatories and cimetidine. The anticholinergic effects of phenothiazines, tricyclic antidepressants and anti-Parkinsonism drugs commonly cause problems. Longer-acting sulphonylureas may produce a state of chronic befuddlement in elderly patients, contrasting with the acute hypoglycaemic episodes and prominent adrenergic symptoms usually seen in younger diabetics. Stomach remedies, laxatives and diuretics may bring about mental changes through electrolyte disturbances and other mechanisms.

Physical examination is rarely helpful if the patient is "well" but localized neurological signs should obviously raise suspicions of a space-occupying lesion. The association of incontinence and ataxia or gait apraxia with mental disturbance may suggest normal pressure hydrocephalus, but there is considerable overlap with cerebrovascular disease[51]. Similarly, signs of Parkinsonism may be observed in patients with multi-infarct disease or diffuse Lewy body disease, who are unlikely to benefit much from L-dopa. On the other hand, patients with the characteristic extended posture and vertical gaze failure of progressive supranuclear palsy may respond to high doses of dopamine agonists[58]. If the mental deterioration was preceded by a fall or there is evidence of head trauma, no matter how minor, suspicion of subdural haematoma should be aroused.

Some investigations, such as serum B_{12} folate, calcium, thyroid function and screening for syphilis, are cheap to perform and lead to simple, if not always effective, medical treatment if an abnormality is found. It should be remembered that neuropsychiatric disorders caused by cobalamin deficiency[59] or folate deficiency[60,61] can occur in the absence of haematological changes. On the other hand, the scientific evidence on which to base an effective and economically realistic policy for the use of expensive brain imaging techniques in people with dementia is still lacking.

Since the "treatable syndrome" of normal pressure hydrocephalus was first described by Adams et al.[62] in 1965, there has been little agreement about the precise definition of the condition or the indications for treatment. Ventricular enlargement, with or without periventricular leukoaraiosis and various degrees of cortical atrophy, is a common CT finding in mentally normal old people, as well as those with dementia and other neuropsychiatric abnormalities. Clearly, it is not practical to monitor CSF pressure or to perform a lumbar infusion test in all cases, especially as such investigations do not always predict the response to internal shunting[63]. Common sense would suggest that the response to repeated removal of CSF by lumbar puncture might be the best predictor of long-term benefit from surgery, but there again no systematic prospective study, let alone a randomized controlled trial, seems to have been done.

Similar, although less profound, uncertainty surrounds the treatment of subdural haematoma in the elderly. Here at least the CT scan should show a definite abnormality, but the relative merits of surgical and medical treatment (or none at all) are not precisely known. At the time of writing it is not possible to make logical recommendations for the clinical assessment and investigation of elderly people with dementia, since the issues are still surrounded by a fog of confusion and prejudice. The costs of investigation for all may be high, but they must be weighed against the enormous costs of institutional care and the psychological, social and indirect costs of the burden on carers, a substantial part of which might be avoidable. Large-scale, pragmatic outcome trials are urgently needed.

Depression and Functional Illness

In operational terms, if not according to strict definition, the commonest of the reversible dementias is so-called "depressive pseudo-dementia". Here the psychiatrist has more to offer, but the physician is often involved because of the frequency of somatic symptoms and physical disabilities manifested by elderly depressed people. Indeed, when neither physicians nor psychiatrists are involved, people with potentially treatable illness can become heavy consumers of social services[64] or even residential care[65]. In this situation the psychiatric history and mental state examination are of paramount importance, although yet again the possibility of adverse drug effects must be borne in mind. β-Blockers, methyldopa and benzodiazepine are often implicated[66]. Alcohol may be a cause or contributory factor and a simple screening questionnaire, such as the CAGE, should be included in any medical or psychiatric assessment[67]. Physical examination is likely to be less rewarding. Although depression is a common complication of many physical illnesses, the proportion of cases where it is the sole presenting feature is quite small. Nevertheless, the chances of finding physical disease in elderly depressed patients are far higher than in their younger counterparts and its presence has a substantial adverse effect on prognosis: indeed, severe intractable depression in old age is nearly always associated with chronic physical ill-health[68]. Secondary complications of depression, such as dehydration, nutritional deficiencies and constipation, must be identified and treated. It is unlikely that metabolic disturbances such as diabetes or hypothyroidism will be diagnosed clinically, so the appropriate blood tests should be done in all cases. A high ESR or C-reactive protein level should warn of the possibility of tuberculosis, other infection or cancer. An intensive search for occult neoplasia is rarely justified, although a chest X-ray should be done in any patient whose symptoms do not respond rapidly to treatment. Once again, the role of CT scanning will remain unclear until prospective studies of representative groups of old people presenting with clearly defined psychosyndromes have been reported. Finally, it should be remembered that the goal of clinical assessment in elderly patients is rarely to make a single unifying diagnosis. Multiple pathology is the rule rather than the exception and unusual combinations of symptoms or signs are more likely to be due to the combined effects of several common diseases rather than one rare one. The reduced homeostatic reserves of old age also means that a single initial insult (or treatment) often begins a chain of metabolic disturbances that multiply, leading to a cascade of complications. Thus, whatever the primary event, the clinician is often faced with a range of problems as well as pathophysiological diagnoses. Mental disturbance may therefore be seen as just one aspect of a complex multi-system disorder, but few would dispute that it is one of the most interesting and challenging of all.

REFERENCES

1. Lipowski ZJ. In *Delirium: Acute Confusional States.* New York: Oxford University Press, 1990; Ch 1.
2. Engel GL, Romano. Delirium, a syndrome of cerebral insufficiency. *J Chron Dis* 1999; **9**: 60–77.
3. American Psychiatric Association. *Diagnostic and Statistical Manual of Mental Disorders*, 3rd edn. revised. Washington, DC: American Psychiatric Association, 1987.
4. American Psychiatric Association. *Diagnostic and Statistical Manual of Mental Disorders.* 4th edn. Washington, DC: American Psychiatric Association, 1994.
5. Itil T, Fink M. Anticholinergic drug-induced delirium: experimental modification, quantitative EEG and behavioural correlations. *J Nerv Mental Disord* 1966; **143**: 492–507.
6. Arie T. Health care of the very elderly. In *Health Care of the Elderly. Essays in Old Age Medicine, Psychiatry and Services.* London: Croom Helm, 1981.
7. Levkoff S, Cleary P. Epidemiology of delirium: an overview of research issues and findings. *Int Psychogeriat* 1991; **3**(2): 49–67.

8. Hodkinson HM. In *Common Symptoms of Disease in the Elderly*. Oxford: Blackwell Scientific, 1976; **24**.

9. Johnson JC, Kerse NM, Gottlieb G *et al*. Prospective vs. retrospective methods of identifying patients with delirium. *J Am Geriat Soc* 1992; **40**: 16–19.

10. Farrel KR, Ganzini L. Misdiagnosing delirium as depression in medically ill elderly patients. *Arch Intern Med* 1995; **155**: 2459–64.

11. Millard PH. Last scene of all. *Br Med J* 1981; **283**: 1559–60.

12. Jitapunkul S, Pillay I, Ebrahim S. The abbreviated mental test: its use and validity. *Age Ageing* 1991; **20**: 332–6.

13 Anthony JC, LeResche L, Niaz V *et al*. Limits of the MMSE as a screening test for dementia and delirium among hospital patients. *Psychol Med* 1982; **12**: 397–408.

14. Fink M, Green M, Bender MB. The face–hand test as a diagnostic sign of organic mental syndrome. *Neurology* 1952; **2**: 46–58.

15. Olson PR, Suddeth JA, Peterson PJ. Hallucinations of widowhood. *J Am Geriat Soc* 1985; **33**: 543–7.

16. Berrios GE, Brook P. The Charles Bonnet syndrome and the problem of visual perceptual disorders in the elderly. *Age Ageing* 1982; **11**: 17–23.

17. Gold K, Rabins PV. Isolated visual hallucinations and the Charles Bonnet syndrome: a review of the literature and six cases. *Comprehens Psychiat* 1989; **30**: 90–98.

18. Tune L, Carr S, Hoag E, Cooper T. Anticholinergic effects of drugs commonly prescribed in the elderly: potential means for assessing risk of delirium. *Am J Psychiat* 1992; **149**: 1393–4.

19. Oswald J. Triazolam syndrome 10 years on. *Lancet* 1989; **334**: 451–2.

20. Leipzig RM, Cumming RG, Tinetti MF. Drugs and falls in older people: a systematic review and meta-analysis. I. Psychotropic drugs. *J Am Geriat Soc* **47**: 30–39.

21. Morgan K, Dalloso H, Ebrahim S *et al*. Prevalence, frequency and duration of hypnotic drug use among the elderly living at home. *Br Med J* 1988; **296**: 601–2.

22. Bridgewater R, Leigh S, James OFW, Potter JF. Alcohol consumption and dependence in elderly patients in an urban community. *Br Med J* 1987; **285**: 884–5.

23. Saunders PA, Copeland JRM, Dewey ME *et al*. Alcohol use and abuse in the elderly: findings from the Liverpool longitudinal study of continuing health in the community. *Int J Geriat Psychiat* 1989; **4**: 103–8.

24. Beresford TP, Blow FC, Brower KJ *et al*. Alcoholism and ageing in the general hospital. *Psychosomatics* 1998; **29**: 61–72.

25. Darowski A, Najim Z, Weinberg JR, Guz A. The febrile response to mild infection in elderly hospital inpatients. *Age Ageing* 1991; **20**: 193–8.

26. Darowski A, Weinberg JR, Guz A. Normal rectal, auditory canal, sublingual and axillary temperatures in elderly afebrile patients in a warm environment. *Age Ageing* 1991; **20**: 113–19.

27. Hogan DB. Revisiting the O complex: urinary incontinence, delirium and polypharmacy in elderly patients. *Can Med Assoc J* 1997; **15**: 1071–7.

28. Hodkinson HM. Evaluation of a mental test score for assessment of mental impairment in the elderly. *Age Ageing* 1972; **1**: 233–8.

29. Rockwood K. The occurrence and duration of symptoms in elderly patients with delirium. *J Gerontol* 1993; **48**: M162–6.

30. Garraway WM, Akhtar AJ, Gore SM *et al*. Observer variation in the clinical assessment of stroke. *Age Ageing* 1976; **5**: 233–40.

31. Shinar D, Gross CR, Mohr JP *et al*. Inter-observer variability in the assessment of neurological history and examination in the Stoke Data Bank. *Arch Neurol* 1985; **42**: 557–85.

32. Inouye SK, Bogardus ST, Charpentier PA *et al*. A multicomponent intervention to prevent delirium in hospitalised older patients. *N Engl J Med* 1999; **340**: 669–76.

33. Koponen H, Hurri L, Stenback U, Reikkinen PJ. Acute confusional states in the elderly: a radiological evaluation. *Acta Psychiat Scand* 1987; **76**: 126–31.

34. Brenner RP. Utility of EEG in delirium: past views and current practice. *Int Psychogeriat* 1991; **3**(2): 211–29.

35. Jacobsen SA, Lauchter AF, Walter DO. Conventional and quantitative EEG in the diagnosis of delirium among the elderly. *J Neuro Neurosurg Psychiat* 1993; **56**: 153–8.

36. Koponen H. Electroencephalographic indices for diagnosis of delirium. *Int Psychogeriat* 1991; **3**(2): 249–51.

37. Koponen HJ, Leinonen E, Lepola U, Relkkinen PJ. A long-term follow-up study of cerebrospinal fluid somatostatin in delirium. *Acta Psychiat Scand* 1994; **89**: 329–4.

38. Warshaw G, Tanzer E. The effectiveness of lumbar puncture in the evaluation of delirium and fever in the hospitalized elderly. *Arch Fam Med* 1993; **2**: 293–7.

39. Inouye SK. Predisposing and precipitating factors for delirium in hospitalised older patients. *Dementia Geriat Cogn Disord* 1999; **10**: 393–400.

40. Kolbeinsson H, Jonsson A. Delirium and dementia in acute medical admissions of elderly patients in Iceland. *Acta Psychiat Scand* 1993; **87**: 123–7.

41. Lipowski ZJ. In *Delirium: Acute Confusional States*. New York: Oxford University Press, 1990; Ch 6.

42. Ott A, Breteler MM, de Bruyne MC *et al*. Atrial fibrillation and dementia in a population-based study. The Rotterdam Study. *Stroke* 1997; **28**: 316–21.

43. Brayne C, Gill C, Huppert FA *et al*. Vascular risks and incident dementia: results from a cohort study of the very old. *Dementia Geriat Cogn Disord* 1998; **9**: 175–80.

44. Mayer JS, Rauch GM, Crawford K *et al*. Risk factors accelerating cerebral degenerative changes, cognitive decline and dementia. *Int J Geriat Psychiat* **14**: 1050–61.

45. Elias MF. Effects of chronic hypertension on cognitive functioning. *Geriatrics* **53**(suppl 1): 649–52.

46. Tariot PN, Ogden MA, Cox C, Williams TF. Diabetes and dementia in long-term care. *J Am Geriat Soc* 1999; **47**: 423–9.

47. Stewart R, Liolitsa D. Type 2 diabetes mellitus, cognitive impairment and dementia. *Diabet Med* 1999; **16**: 93–112.

48. Passant U, Warkentin S, Gustafson L. Orthostatic hypotension and low blood pressure in organic dementia: a study of prevalence and related clinical characteristics. *Int J Geriat Psychiat* 1997; **12**: 395–403.

49. Guo Z, Vitanen M, Fratiglioni L, Winblad B. Blood pressure and dementia in the elderly: epidemiologic perspectives. *Biomed Pharmacother* 1997; **51**: 68–73.

50. Rabins PV. The reversible dementias. In Arie T ed., *Recent Advances in Psychogeriatrics*. Edinburgh: Churchill Livingstone, 1985; Ch. 7.

51. Clarfield AM. The reversible dementias, do they reverse? *Ann Intern Med* 1988; **109**: 476–86.

52. Farina E, Pomati S, Mariani C. Observations on dementias with potentially reversible symptoms. *Aging* 1999; **11**: 323–8.

53. Freter S, Bergman H, Gold S *et al*. Prevalence of potentially reversible dementias and actual reversibility in a memory clinic cohort. *Can Med Assoc* 1998; **159**: 657–62.

54. Weisberg LA, Nice CN. Intracranial tumors simulating the presentation of cerebrovascular syndromes. Early detection with cerebral CT. *Am J Med* 1977; **63**: 517–24.

55. O'Brien P, Ryder DQ, Twomey C. The role of computerised tomography brain scan in the diagnosis of acute stroke in the elderly. *Age Ageing* 1987; **16**: 319–22.

56. Sandercock P, Molyneux A, Warlow C. Value of computed tomography in patients with stroke: Oxfordshire Community Stroke Project. *Br Med J* 1985; **290**: 193–7.

57. Newton H, Pickard JD, Weller RO. Normal pressure hydrocephalus and cerebrovascular disease: findings of postmortems. *J Neurol Neurosurg Psychiat* 1989; **52**: 804.

58. Jackson JA, Jankovic J, Ford J. Progressive supranuclear palsy: clinical features and response to treatment in 16 patients. *Ann Neurol* 1983; **13**: 273–8.

59. Kindenbaum J, Healton EB, Savage DG *et al*. Neuropsychiatric disorders caused by cobalamin deficiency in the absence of anaemia or macrocytosis. *N Engl J Med* 1988; **318**: 720–8.

60. Snowden DA, Tully CL, Smith CD *et al*. Serum folate and the severity of atrophy of the neocortex in Alzheimer's disease, findings from the Nun study. *Am J Clin Nutrit* 2000; **71**: 993–8.

61. Ebly EM, Schafer JP, Campbell NR, Hogan DB. Folate status, vascular disease and cognition in elderly Canadians. *Age Ageing* 1998; **27**: 485–91.

62. Adams RD, Fisher CM, Hakim S *et al*. Symptomatic occult hydrocephalus with normal cerebrospinal fluid pressure. A treatable syndrome. *N Engl J Med* 1965; **273**: 117–26.

63. Briggs RS, Castleden CM, Elvarez AS. Normal pressure hydrocephalus in the elderly: a treatable cause of dementia? *Age Ageing* 1981; **10**: 254–8.

64. Foster EM, Kay DWK, Bergmann K. Characteristics of old people receiving and needing domiciliary services, the relevance of psychiatric diagnosis. *Age Ageing* 1976; **5**: 245–55.

65. Brocklehurst JC, Carty MH, Leeing JT, Robinson JM. Medical screening of older people accepted for residential care. *Lancet* 1978; **ii**: 141–2.

66. Blazer D. Depression in the elderly. *N Engl J Med* 1989; **320**: 164–6.

67. Beresford TP, Blow FC, Hill E *et al*. Comparison of CAGE questionnaire and computer-assisted laboratory profiles in screening for covert alcoholism. *Lancet* 1990; **336**: 482–5.

68. Baldwin RC, Jolley DJ. The prognosis of depression in old age. *Br J Psychiat* 1986; **149**: 574–83.

26

Needs and Problems

Barry J. Gurland

Columbia University Stroud Centre, New York, NY, USA

Reliable and valid assessment techniques are needed for precision in studying, and communicating about, mental health problems. "Assessment" in this context conventionally refers to questionnaires and performance tests and behavioural observations can also be a part of a mental assessment[1-7].

The content of assessment is usually derived from a clinical experience[8]. However, clinicians may differ from each other, or from one interview to another, in the manner of their interview and their interpretation of the patient's responses. Therefore, reliability in assessment is obtained, in part, by prescribing the order and form of questions and tests (structuring the stimulus) and defining the informative response to be rated (structuring the response)[9]. This structuring of the interview technique enhances reliability, while retaining the focus of a clinically administered interview.

Structuring of mental assessment comes into its own when the condition has to be described in fairly subtle or phenomenological or behavioural terms, or when outcomes are influenced only to a limited degree by treatment or other factors, or where alternative treatments are not obviously different in their benefit and costs. Dramatic outcomes involving, for example, the difference between life and death, or the full recovery of an unusually incurable condition, hardly require precise measurements.

In an effort to reach precision in assessment through structuring of interview, construct validity may suffer. Conditions that are the focus of clinical concern but that cannot be precisely measured by state-of-the-art techniques may be excluded from research attention. Researchers may also choose to select types of patients not posing a problem for measurement. Alternatively, the concept of the condition may be constricted so that it fits within a measurable entity[10]. As the scope of psychiatric treatment expands, assessment techniques may have to follow suit.

A large proportion of elderly patients in institutional settings, and of patients with conditions such as dementia, or long-stay ageing schizophrenics in institutions, are unable to communicate at even a simple level. Testing or performance on cognitive tasks may not be possible, and questioning about inner feelings and thought processes is often completely out of reach. Attempts have been made to address these assessment problems by resort to informants[11,12], observations of reactions to non-verbal stimuli[13] and inferences from responses to fairly straightforward stimuli, such as greeting behaviour. These approaches have not yet been proved to be entirely satisfactory.

The high correlation between mental and physical problems of the elderly makes it inevitable that mental assessment will often be confounded by physical symptoms. Somatic symptoms due to physical illness may register on scales intended to pick up the somatic manifestations of depression. Functional impairment due to physical infirmity[14,15] may spuriously fit criteria for determining the severity of dementia.

Various solutions to the confounding of the mental and physical symptoms have been proposed. Some investigators have chosen to develop instruments that concentrate on the mood state in depression[16,17] or the cognitive state in dementia[18], avoiding the need to attribute somatic or functional symptoms to a mental or physical cause. Other investigators have focused attention on the characteristics of somatic and functional symptoms that are suggestive of a mental rather than physical condition. Nevertheless, the measurement of the physical aspects of mental illness in the elderly still lacks specificity.

Potential users of mental assessment techniques are always concerned about the length of the time taken to administer the interview. Shorter interviews[19-22] are viewed as more acceptable to subjects and less likely to be prematurely terminated, leading to a higher response rate for repeat interviews, cheaper to administer and less prone to error. There is no firm evidence that any of these assertions are true. Brevity has been carried perhaps to an extreme in assessments that serve as screening tools in busy clinical sites. Moreover, little attention has been given to devising interviews that are engrossing, reassuring and even helpful to the subject, so that longer interviews would be welcome.

Lengthening the time available for completing an interview allows more information to be collected on mental health and its associations. For most purposes in research and in clinical applications, there appears never to be enough time for all that might be relevant to study mental illness or clinical management. Brief scales of single dimensions (e.g. depressed mood or cognitive impairment) generally consume up to 10 min of interview time. Inclusion of material bearing upon differential diagnosis[23-25] may extend to 30–40 min for current status and another 30 min or more for history of the illness. A comprehensive assessment[9,25], which covers the possible determinants and consequences of mental illness, may itself require 1 h or more, without exhaustive inquiry into any domain.

Compromises are usually necessary to keep the interview within feasible time limits while maintaining an adequate range of information. In this direction, contingencies may be introduced into the instructions for administration of the interview. Specified areas are probed only if a header question reveals the likelihood of useful information emerging from that area[26]. There is a remarkable absence of empirical data showing that the rationale for these contingencies is well based. Furthermore, the complexity of contingencies may trap the interviewer to errors. Nevertheless, these contingent decision trees do represent the best chance of replicating the efficiencies and productivity of the way an experienced clinician conducts an interview. The advent of

Principles and Practice of Geriatric Psychiatry, 2nd edn. Edited by J. R. M. Copeland, M. T. Abou-Saleh and D. G. Blazer
©2002 John Wiley & Sons, Ltd

computer-assisted technology for governing the conduct of interviews should facilitate the management of elaborate contingencies for driving the interview.

A certain line of questioning or testing may hinge upon a large body of information already gathered, rather than a single item or short set of items. A classic example is the use of an interview as a screen to select subjects for further investigation. Typically the latter investigation is at a separate time and venue, but it could follow straight on the heels of the screening interview at the same session. In either event it is essential to have immediate analysis of the information determining the contingency. Simple additive scoring systems are mainly invoked in these circumstances. Computer methods now allow much more elaborate analyses to determine the flow of sequential interviews or even sequences within a single session interview.

The capacity for rapid retrieval of assessment information on demand greatly enhances the value of mental assessment for supporting clinical decisions. Yet the potential in this respect cannot be fully realized until clinical goals of assessment assume priority over research goals in shaping the form and content of the assessment. Notwithstanding that mental assessment emerged from clinical experience, the current state or nature of mental assessment owes much more to research than clinical interests. A return to the origins of its development is called for, in order to bring assessment into line with clinical as well as research needs[27,28].

Clinical activities, for reasons of practice organization and fiscal considerations, generally take place under pressure of time. The collection and even analysis of information for the review clinician can be delegated to personnel under less time pressure than the physician/psychiatrist. In that arrangement, it becomes essential that the transfer of crucial information to the physician be managed expeditiously. This entails highly discriminating summarization, display and communication of mental assessment information. It also assumes that the physician learns to assimilate the type and form of information and to incorporate it in the planning and monitoring of clinical management. This learning process, like other clinical skills, must be continuously honed through experience assisted by consultation. There are few guidelines as yet as to the assignment, conduct and necessary training for the professional role of marshalling the mental assessment information and communicating it to clinicians.

Much of mental assessment is aimed at documenting the subjective experience or inner states of a patient[29]. The best reporter for this material should be the patient, but the latter may be uncommunicative or give misleading information. An informant may not do much better. Under these circumstances, it would be desirable to turn to objective testing and observation of behaviour[30-32] and laboratory results if these can be obtained. As matters stand, laboratory findings in themselves are at best ambiguous[33] as mental assessment information in the elderly, although there is hope that eventually laboratory tests will play a larger part in mental assessment. In any event, whether intended or not, many subjects in epidemiological studies will not undergo laboratory testing. In the meantime, other ways of achieving objectivity are more likely to be productive. Testing organic mental status is objective in the sense that the task performance of the person is observable and errors can be quantified. Programming is the presentation of the tests through computer software and adds to the objectivity[13,34]. Testing of an objective nature has also evolved for functional performance for tasks involving everyday activities, or simulations of the skill demands entailed in such activities[14,15]. Inefficiencies in carrying out these tasks provide information on the diagnosis of certain mental conditions (e.g. dementia) and the outcomes of a wide range of mental illnesses.

Structuring of testing procedures (backed up by suitable training) allows the results of assessment to be compared with data collected on the same instruments in different studies. It also permits data to be interpreted in the light of accumulated experience on the normal distribution and longitudinal course of levels or patterns of test results in the general population and in specific clinically defined groups. Thus, the value of assessment information is enhanced in diagnoses, prediction of outcomes, selection of treatment and evaluating the significance of changes in levels or patterns of test scores. This full psychometric development warrants the use of the term "standardized" to describe a method (although the term is used to mean structured). However, there are several cautions that must be addressed in attempting to draw upon the potential value of standardization.

Unless an assessment technique is administered in identical fashion in two or more studies, the results of those studies cannot be directly compared and information cannot be transferred from one study to another. Not only must the structure and procedures of the assessment protocol be kept constant, but also the methods of training. Furthermore, adjustments must be made for differences in the characteristics (e.g. age, education and culture) of two populations that might alter the meaning and confound the comparison of results from the same assessment technique[35]. These adjustments may be difficult to make unless standardization has been accomplished on appropriate populations and formulae for interpreting scores have been worked out[36,37]. Attempts are being made to construct culture-free assessments which, in effect, would obviate the need to adjust scores with reference to demographic characteristics.

Most assessment techniques devoted to the classification of mental disorders still rely heavily upon information gathered at one point in time[38], cross-sectional status with or without retrospective historical information. Longitudinal or prospective information is principally regarded as measuring change, course and outcomes. Yet the longitudinal picture of mental health problems offers crucial clues to diagnosis and needs to be incorporated into assessment techniques for classification. In order to meet the demands of longitudinal measurements, assessment techniques must deal with practice effects, ceiling and floor limits to the range of measurement, and the minimization of attrition by maintaining the interest of the subject.

Certain domains of mental ill-health appear well-represented, even over-represented, in current assessment techniques. For instance, there are probably more measures of cognitive impairment[19,25,39-47] and of depressed mood[16,17,48-56] than are strictly needed. Conversely, there are neglected domains. Innovations would be welcome in the measurement of positive mental health, either as a global concept or as applied to specific mental health areas, such as affect[57] and cognition. There is a need to understand the contribution of the measurements of positive states to diagnosis and prognosis.

More generally, the scope of assessment techniques should be expanded and explored so as to fill in gaps in the domains relevant to describing mental health and its associations. Moreover, assessments need to encompass the various perspectives of subject, family member[11,12,58,59], health professional and other parties with a legitimate interest in the subject's mental health. When a complete inventory of domains and perspectives has been captured by assessment techniques, it may become possible to describe a reasonable approximation to the plight of the whole person.

A note on quality of life assessment. The concept and measurement of quality of life has come to fill a prominent place in geriatric health care. Since about 1970 the relevant professional literature on measurement and its applications has steadily increased in volume. Instruments have proliferated and some have assumed ascendancy in terms of widespread use. There is no better indication of the need for measurement of this concept than the many applications to which it has been turned. These include descriptions of the course of illness, comparisons of the outcomes of competing treatments, monitoring of the performance of healthcare systems, accounting for benefits derived from resources allocated to various interventions, assisting decisions on treatment choice, and informing policy formation on development of the health care system and its components.

Yet there are problems of concept and measurement that have emerged for which no satisfactory solutions have yet been found. For example, there are unresolved conflicting advantages and limitations offered by generic or specific measures, by emphases on subjective or objective approaches, by brief or comprehensive assessments, or by combining or segregating status and preferences.

Many of the existing quality of life instruments have adopted scales and indices that had a prior existence as measures of health status. This has created a core of domains that are found in a majority of instruments: this core includes functioning in the activities of daily living, mobility, cognitive status, depression or morale, physical discomfort and self-perceived health. However, there are many other domains that appear in some instruments and not in all, so that the potential cumulative list is lengthy. There is little empirical work to identify which domains are most critical to a good quality of life.

Choosing between the numerous established instruments is a daunting task for the relatively inexperienced researcher or for the clinician wishing to enhance practice standards. An instrument which is widely used may appeal to researchers, reviewers and grant committees on the grounds of its substantial psychometric development, provision of norms, comparison with findings from previous pertinent studies, as well as the credence that comes from the consensus implicit in a large constituency of users.

Nevertheless, there are junctures in the growth of a field within the health sciences at which technological expediency can outstrip the slower work of fundamental understanding. At such points in the history of the maturation of a field the good can pre-empt the excellent. Whether this is the case for the current state of quality of life concept and measurement is a matter of judgment.

REFERENCES

1. Gallo JJ, Reichel W, Andersen L. *Handbook of Geriatric Assessment*. Gaithersburg, MD: Aspen, 1988.
2. Gurland BJ. Mental Health Assessment: assessing mental health in the elderly (Special Supplement Series: Multidisciplinary health assessment of the elderly). *Danish Med Bull* 1989; **7**: 33–7.
3. Kane RA, Kane RL. *Assessing the Elderly: A Practical Guide to Measurement*. Lexington, MA: Lexington Books, 1981.
4. McDowell I, Newell C. *Measuring Health: A Guide to Rating Scales and Questionnaires*. Oxford: Oxford University Press, 1987.
5. Poon L, Crook T, Davis KL *et al*. *Clinical Memory Assessment of Older Adults*. Washington, DC: American Psychological Association, 1986; 1–419.
6. Special Feature. Assessment in diagnosis and treatment of geropsychiatric patients. *Psychopharmacol Bull* 1988; **24**(4): 501–28.
7. Special Supplement Series. Multidisciplinary health assessment of the elderly. *Danish Med Bull* 1989; **7**: 1–86.
8. Wells CE. The differential diagnosis of psychiatric disorders in the elderly. In Cole J, Barrett JE, eds. *Psychopathology in the Aged*. New York: Raven, 1980.
9. Gurland BJ, Wilder DE. The CARE interview revisited: development of an efficient, systematic, clinical assessment. *J Gerontol* 1984; **39**: 129–37.
10. *Diagnostic and Statistical Manual of Mental Disorders*, 3rd edn, revised. Washington, DC: American Psychiatric Association, 1987.
11. Katz MM, Lyerly SB. Methods for measuring adjustment and social behavior in the community: I. Rationale, description discriminative validity and scale development. *Psychol Rep* 1983; **13**: 505–35.
12. Schwartz GE. Development and validation of the Geriatric Evaluation by Relative Rating Instrument (GERRI). *Psychol Rep* 1983; **53**: 479–88.
13. Crook, TH, Larrabee GJ. Interrelationships among everyday memory tests: stability of factor structure with age. *Neuropsychology* 1988; **2**: 1–12.
14. Katz S, Ford AB, Moskowitz RW *et al*. Studies of illness in the aged. The index of ADL: a standardized measure of biological and psychosocial function. *J Am Med Assoc* 1963; **185**: 914–19.
15. Lawton MP, Brody EM. Assessment of older people: self-maintaining and instrumental activities of daily living. *Gerontologist* 1969; **9**: 179–86.
16. Yesavage J, Brink T, Rose T *et al*. Development and validation of a geriatric screening scale: a preliminary report. *J Psychiat Res* 1983; **17**: 37–49.
17. Yesavage J, Brink TL, Terrence LR, Adey M. The Geriatric Depression Rating Scale: comparison with other self-report and psychiatric rating scales. In Crook T, Ferris S, Bartus R, eds, *Assessment in Geriatric Psychopharmacology*. Mark Powley Associates, 1983; 153–68.
18. Pfeiffer E. A Short Portable Mental Status Questionnaire for the assessment of organic brain deficit in elderly patients. *J Am Geriat Soc* 1975; **22**: 433–44.
19. Gurland B, Golden R, Teresis J *et al*. The SHORT-CARE: an efficient instrument for the assessment of depression, dementia and disability. *J Gerontol* 1984; **39**: 166–9.
20. Overall JE, Gorham DR. Introduction—the Brief Psychiatric Rating Scale (BPRS): recent developments in ascertaining and scaling. *Psychopharmacol Bull* 1988; **24**: 97–9.
21. Overall JE, Gorham DR. The Brief Psychiatric Rating Scale (BPRS). *Psychol Rep* 1962; **10**: 799–812.
22. Shader RI, Harmatz JS, Salzman C. A new scale for assessment in geriatric populations: Sandoz Clinical Assessment Geriatric Scale (SCAG). *J Am Geriat Soc* 1974; **22**: 107–13.
23. Endicott J, Spitzer RL. A diagnostic interview for affective disorders and schizophrenia (SADS). *Arch Gen Psychiat* 1978; **35**: 837–44.
24. Roth M, Tym E, Mountjoy CQ *et al*. CAMDEX: a standardised instrument for the diagnosis of mental disorders in the elderly with special reference to the early detection of dementia. *Br J Psychiat* 1986; **149**: 698–709.
25. Robins LN, Helzer JE, Croughan J, Radcliff KS. National Institute of Mental Health Diagnostic Interview Schedule (DIS): its history, characteristics and validity. *Arch Gen Psychiat* 1981; **38**: 381–9.
26. Copeland JRM, Kellcher MJ, Kellett JM *et al*. A semi-structured clinical interview for the assessment of diagnosis and mental state in the elderly: the Geriatric Mental State Schedule I, Development and Reliability. *Psychol Med* 1976; **6**: 439–49.
27. Lawton MP, Moss M, Fulcomer M, Kleban MH. A research and service-oriented multilevel assessment instrument. *J Gerontol* 1982; **37**: 91–9.
28. Zielstorff RD, Jette AM, Gillick MR *et al*. Functional assessment in an automated medical record system for coordination of long-term care. *Topics Geriat Rehab* 1986; **1**(3): 43–57.
29. Derogatis LR, Spencer PM. *The Brief Symptom Inventory (BSI)—Administration, Scoring and Procedures Manual*, Vol. I. Baltimore, MD: Clinical Psychiatric Research, 1982.
30. Gotestam JG. A geriatric scale empirically derived from three rating scales for geriatric behavior. *Acta Psychiat Scand* 1981; **294**(suppl): 54–63.
31. Helmes E, Csapo KG, Short JA. Standardization and validation of the Multidimensional Observation Scale for Elderly Subjects (MOSES). *J Gerontol* 1987; **42**: 395–405.
32. Levin HS, High WM, Goethe KE *et al*. The Neurobehavioral Rating Scale: assessment of behavioral sequelae of head injury by the clinician. *J Neurol Neurosurg Psychiat* 1986; **50**: 183–93.
33. Katona CLE. Editorial: the dexamethasone suppression test in geriatric psychiatry. *Int J Geriat Psychiat* 1988; **3**: 1–3.
34. Branconnier RJ. A computerized battery for behavioral assessment in Alzheimer's Disease. In Poon L, Crook T, Davis KL *et al*., eds, *Handbook for Clinical Memory Assessment of Older Adults*. Washington, DC: American Psychological Association, 1986; 189–96.
35. Escobar JI, Burnham A, Karno M *et al*. Use of the Mini-Mental State Examination (MMSE) in a community population of mixed ethnicity:

cultural and linguistic artifacts. *J Nerv Ment Dis* 1986; **174**(10): 607–14.

36. Golden RR, Teresis JA, Gurland BJ. Development of indicator scales for the comprehensive assessment and referral evaluation (CARE) interview schedule. *J Gerontol* 1984; **39**: 138–46.

37. Teresi JA. Golden RR, Gurland BJ *et al.* Construct validity of indicator-scales developed for the Comprehensive Assessment and Referral Evaluation interview schedule. *J Gerontol* 1984; **39**(2): 147–57.

38. Raskin A. Validation of a battery of tests designed to assess psychopathology in the elderly. In Burrows GD, Norman TR, Dennerstein L, eds, *Clinical and Pharmacological Studies in Psychiatric Disorders*. London: John Libbey, 1985; 337–43.

39. Blessed G, Tomlinson BE, Roth M. The association between qualitative measures of dementia and senile change with cerebral matter of elderly subjects. *Br J Psychiat* 1968; **114**: 792–811.

40. Fillenbaum G. Comparison of two brief tests of organic brain impairment, MSQ and the Short Portable MSQ. *J Am Geriat Soc* 1980; **28**(8): 381.

41. Folstein MF, Folstein SE, McHugh PR. Mini-Mental State Examination: a practical method for grading the cognitive state of patients for the clinician. *J Psychiat Res* 1975; **12**: 189–98.

42. Haglund R, Shuckit M. A clinical comparison of tests of organicity in elderly patients. *J Gerontol* 1976; **6**: 654–9.

43. Kahn RI, Goldfarb AI, Pollock M *et al.* Brief objective measures for the determination of mental status in the aged. *Am J Psychiat* 1960; **117**: 326–8.

44. Katzman R, Brown T, Fuld P *et al.* Validation of a short orientation–memory–concentration test of cognitive impairment. *Am J Psychiat* 1983; **140**: 734–8.

45. McCartney JR, Palmateer L. Assessment of cognitive deficit in geriatric patients. *J Am Geriat Soc* 1985; **33**: 467–71.

46. Nelson A, Fogel B, Faust D. Bedside cognitive screening instruments. *J Nerv Ment Dis* 1986; **174**: 73–83.

47. Reisberg B, Ferris SH, de Leon MJ, Crook T. The Global Deterioration Scale (GDS): an instrument for the assessment of Primary Degenerative Dementia (PDD). *Am J Psychiat* 1982; **139**: 1136–9.

48. Beck AT. Measuring depression—the Depression Inventory. In Williams T, Katy MM, Shield JA, eds, *Recent Advances in the Psychobiology of the Depressive Illness*. Washington, DC: US Government Printing Office, 1972.

49. Beck AT, Ward CH, Mendelson *et al.* An inventory for measuring depression. *Arch Gen Psychiat* 1961; **4**: 561–71.

50. Gallagher D. Assessing affect in the elderly. *Clin Geriat Med* 1987; **3**(1): 65–86.

51. Hamilton M. Standardized assessment and recording of depressive symptoms. *Psychiat Neurol Neurochir* 1969; **72**(2): 201–5.

52. Hathaway SR, McKinley JC. *Minnesota Multiphasic Personality Inventory Manual (MMPI)*. New York: Psychological Corporation, 1951.

53. Lubin B. *Depression Adjective Checklists (DACL Manual)*. San Diego: Educational and Industrial Testing Service, 1971.

54. McNair D, Lorr M, Droppleman LF. *Profile of Mood States, Bipor Form (POMS Manual)*. San Diego, CA: Educational and Industrial Testing Service, 1971.

55. Radloff IS. The CES-D scale: a self-report depression scale for research in the general population. *Appl Psychol Meas* 1977; **1**: 385–401.

56. Zung WWK. A self-rating depression scale. *Arch Gen Psychiat* 1965; **12**: 63–70.

57. Bradburn NM. *The Structure of Psychological Well-being*. Chicago, IL: University of Chicago Press, 1969.

58. Greene JG, Smith R, Gardiner M, Timbury GC. Measuring behavioral disturbances of elderly demented patients in the community and its effects on relatives: a factor analytic study. *Age Ageing* 1982; **11**: 121–6.

59. Zarit SH, Zarit JM. Families under stress: intervention for caregivers of senile dementia patients. *Psychother Theor Res Practice* 1982; **19**: 461–71.

27

Non-computerized Assessment Procedures: Fundamental Assessment Issues

P. Logue

Duke University Medical Center, Durham, NC, USA

BASIC ASSESSMENT ISSUES

Just as individuals age, so do populations. The "graying of America" is a cliché that carries with it the inevitability of the normal aging process combining with the advancement of medical science. The average age of all industrialized countries is going up steadily. While, to some extent, these changes in basic demographics relate to improved infant mortality, there is also an increasing ability and willingness on the part of the medical profession to treat the ailments that may come with aging and extend the lifespan of individuals within the society. Control of ischemia risk factors, dialysis and organ transplant are all commonplace now but were much less advanced 30 years ago.

In many ways this demographic change is a very positive trend. Individuals at 50 now are no longer considered to be as old as they once were. There are many physically vigorous and cognitively intact individuals who function effectively well into their 70s, 80s and 90s. However, extension of life is not necessarily the extension of quality of life. With increasing age there is an increasing probability of dementing processes. Dementia is not the inevitable outcome of aging, but the diagnosis of dementing conditions increases significantly with each decade of life.

There are multiple potential dementing conditions. Some of these conditions are the by-products of physical disease and others of lifestyle choices made years earlier (*see* Table 27.1 for a partial listing of the more common dementing processes from the familiar DSM). The clear majority of dementing processes, however, fall into three general categories, Alzheimer's dementia, vascular disease-related dementia, and mixed dementias. While each has a progressive course, the potential for treatment and the speed and uniformity of the progression varies significantly. Precision of diagnosis is critical in the appropriate treatment and management in a geriatric dementia work-up.

Depression in the old, in combination with the normal aging process, can produce a condition that is treatable but that mimics the effects of central nervous system-based dementias. Depression in some cases may be the earlier preclinical precursor of dementia, but nevertheless, the accurate differential diagnosis of dementia and depression is of extraordinary importance. The consequences of a false-positive or false-negative diagnosis in dementia can be devastating. If a patient is labeled as having early-stage Alzheimer's syndrome, multiple negative consequences occur very quickly. Driving privileges, financial and medical decision-making and the independence that is critical to any person are all restricted and sometimes taken away. If the patient diagnosed with dementia is not demented but is depressed, unnecessary and

Table 27.1 DSM-IV: common dementing processes

Dementia of the Alzheimer's type
Vascular dementia
Dementia due to HIV disease
Dementia due to head trauma
Dementia due to Parkinson's disease
Dementia due to Huntington's disease
Dementia due to Pick's disease
Dementia due to Creutzfeldt–Jakob disease
Dementia due to other general medical conditions
Substance-induced persisting dementia
Dementia due to multiple etiologies
Dementia not otherwise specified

Diagnostic and Statistical Manual of Mental Disorders, 4th edn, p. 133.

potentially irreversible changes occur in the quality of the patient's life, even if the diagnosis is later changed. Similarly, if the patient does have a progressive dementia and proceeds to make decisions about finances, about health, or even about day-to-day instrumental activities of daily living, the consequences can be equally negative.

In summary, the geriatric population is growing. As people age, they become more susceptible to potentially treatable conditions. These conditions can radically alter the quality of life and the ultimate prognosis and disposition for the successful management of the case.

ASSESSMENT PROCEDURES

The assessment of geriatric patients for dementing conditions demands considerable focus in assessment and knowledge of the scientific literature. These areas would include, at minimum, an understanding of the characteristics of the normal aging process and the salient behavioral/cognitive characteristics of the dementias. Necessary and desirable parameters of geriatric evaluations are as follows.

Necessary Characteristics of Any Assessment Procedure

Norms

Test results are significantly influenced by the age of the subject and premorbid functioning levels; therefore, any assessment procedure utilized should have reasonably adequate norms that take age and educational level into consideration.

Validity and Reliability

Validity and reliability of the assessment procedure must be established and the relationship between the given dementing process and test scores well established within the scientific literature.

Depression and Cognition

Cognitive and affective diagnostic procedure should be utilized within the same battery, whether formally or informally, since the two interact so powerfully. The diagnosis of dementia vs. depression often resolves itself down to the proportion of each.

Depth/Breadth of Assessment

Sufficient breadth and depth of assessment is required so that patients can be followed over time, in improving and deteriorating conditions, so that unsuspected conditions are not easily missed in a routine assessment.

Desirable Characteristics

Short

Relative brevity, even in a multi-factorial assessment, is highly desirable. Geriatric patients become impatient, threatened and exhausted when test batteries become too lengthy. The procedure at the end of the assessment process may be less valid than that at the beginning of the assessment process.

Practical

Ideally, along with reliability and validity, the assessment encompasses those variables that are clinically important. While reaction time may be highly sensitive at the bedside, in day-to-day clinical practice memory assessment or assessment of attention is much more likely to be broadly useful. The geriatric patient is more likely to be uncooperative and sometimes appropriately contemptuous of "kid" games. If a patient can perceive the relevance of the procedure, whether or not he/she feels threatened by it, the test results are more likely to be valid and reliable.

Numbers

Quantification of the test result is very desirable, since multiple successive assessments may be done that trace the course of the syndrome or the effects of medication.

Models

It is highly desirable that the tests, in aggregate, fit together into a relatively coherent model of cognitive assessment and include formal and informal assessment of at least the following:

- General abilities.
- Speech and language.
- Constructional abilities.
- Motor functions.
- Memory and learning.
- Attention and concentration.
- Judgment and problem-solving abilities.
- Speed of processing.

At times, these assessments may be as informal as just listening to the patient, but are necessary descriptive parameters of the assessment.

NON-COMPUTERIZED ASSESSMENT OF COGNITIVE FUNCTION

Selection of Assessment Tools

As in all patient populations, neuropsychological assessment of older individuals begins with a thorough understanding of the referral question and a clear goal as to the purposes of the evaluation. The specific functional areas of cognition to be tested, and therefore the format and comprehensiveness of the entire evaluation, should be based on the initial referral question and targeted at achieving the specific goals of the referring healthcare provider. Nowhere is it more important to tailor the assessment battery to the specific diagnostic concerns, while considering the unique abilities and limitations of the patient population, than with a geriatric population. Test selection must optimally allow for an in-depth evaluation of the cognitive areas of concern, while keeping battery length and difficulty level manageable for the aging patient. Ultimately, the battery "should discriminate maximally between normal aging and CNS disorders such as the different dementias"[1]. As these authors state further, a successful test battery should also allow differentiation among the various common subtypes of dementia, as well as between dementia and affective disturbance.

Screening Evaluations vs. Full Batteries

Even when the referral question implies a broad assessment of overall cognitive abilities for the purpose of identifying the presence or absence of neuropsychological deficits, the use of a brief but well-rounded neuropsychological screening measure can be prudent. Such tools typically allow the examiner to quantify gross deficits against normative data in order to classify the tested individual as "normal" or "abnormal" in particular cognitive areas of functioning. Cut-off scores and the number of abnormal scores necessary for rating an individual's performance on such measures against target normative populations usually allow for qualitative classifications ranging from superior to severely impaired. Depending upon the psychometric soundness of the screening instrument, the examiner may be able to draw conclusions with respect to specific cognitive abilities, or may be limited to a judgment of impaired or not impaired.

The benefits of using a brief screening measure for cognitive evaluation are obvious; they tend to require less administration time for both the patient and the examiner, and they are typically less labor-intensive and intimidating for the patient. Most commercially available cognitive screens are easily scored and provide feedback for recommendations quickly, which is an asset in inpatient settings or other situations when the patient's treatment plan and disposition considerations may be urgent. As with most things in life, however, time-saving procedures may sacrifice quality. Even the most widely accepted brief cognitive screens lack the diagnostic sensitivity and specificity of the more comprehensive neuropsychological battery, particularly when they generate only a single score or are limited to largely verbal measures. When choosing to use a cognitive screen for neuropsychological evaluation of a geriatric patient, it is important to balance our desire to spare the patient a lengthy assessment time with a genuine quest to garner the most reliable diagnostic data available. This goal may best be achieved by augmenting a brief cognitive screen, with individual neuropsychological measures aimed at the more detailed evaluation of specific cognitive abilities or affective characteristics.

One neuropsychological screening assessment that has achieved wide acceptance with use in a geriatric population is the Dementia Rating Scale (DRS)[2]. This scale yields scores for attention, initiation/perseveration, construction, conceptualization and memory, and compares individuals' performances to a normative base of subjects with known Alzheimer's disease. In providing such a comparison population, the instrument controls for normal aging variation. In this way, the measure offers easily referenced cut-off scores for quick classification of outcomes as being consistent with dementia or not.

A more recent tool available to clinicians is the Repeatable Battery for the Assessment of Neuropsychological Status (RBANS)[3]. While supportive literature for its use in diagnosing dementia in the geriatric population is only now being gathered, the RBANS has the advantage of being available in parallel forms, thus allowing serial assessment. Repeatability is a valuable feature for a cognitive screen to have, especially in documenting recovery of function after a reversible neurological injury and in demonstrating progressive decline in the degenerative dementias. The authors refer readers to published review articles and commercial catalogs for the clinical findings and availability of these and other neuropsychological screening measures.

In many cases, the discrimination between dementia and pseudodementia, or the differential diagnosis between types of dementing illnesses, cannot be achieved through use of a brief cognitive screen. In these cases, a more comprehensive test battery may be the only method by which to quantify and qualify specific areas of deficits into a pattern consistent with a diagnostic picture. In selecting tests for such a battery, one may focus on specific symptomatic cognitive areas or may seek to assess global cognitive functioning with a combination of neuropsychological measures. There are numerous individual neuropsychological tests developed to assess specific cognitive functional areas (Table 27.2). The combination of these tests into a clinical battery may be based on theoretical concepts or assessment approaches; some clinicians prescribe to use of standard batteries, such as the Halstead–Reitan and the Luria–Nebraska, while others combine individual neuropsychological measures into a more flexible or "process approach" battery. Whatever one's theoretical basis, consistency and rigor in assessment procedures remains the most effective way for a clinician to develop his/her own personal bank of base rates and characteristic result profiles.

Specific Cognitive Functional Areas

Intellectual functioning is one of the broader functional areas assessed and may include assessment of fluid and crystallized knowledge. It is not a unitary entity but instead consists of multiple functions, including the ability to acquire, process, categorize and integrate information. Intellectual functioning intimately involves use of memory and learning, visuospatial skills, attentional abilities, expressive and receptive language, and aspects of adaptive reasoning and organizational structure. Assessment may involve evaluation of verbal intellect, non-verbal (performance) intellect, or overall intellectual abilities.

Attention and concentration abilities are critical for neuropsychological functioning. More complex processing depends on

Table 27.2 Examples of neuropsychological tests for specific cognitive functions

Cognitive functional area	Example neuropsychological tests
Intellectual functioning	WAIS-R or WAIS-III
	Ravens Progressive Matrices (non-verbal)
	Peabody Picture Vocabulary Test (verbal)
	Mini-Mental State Examination (MMSE)
Attention/concentration functioning	Verbal Series Attention Test
	Continuous Performance (2 and 7) Test
	Stroop Test
	Digit Span
	PASAT
Executive functioning	Wisconsin Card Sorting Test
	Short Category Test
	Trail Making Test
	Verbal Fluency/Figural Fluency
Memory and learning functioning	WMS-R or WMS-III (logical memory and visual reproduction)
	CVLT, RAVLT-R, HLVT-R
	Selective Reminding (Buschke or Levin)
	Warrington Facial Recognition Memory
	Benton Visual Retention Test
Language functioning	Western Aphasia Battery
	Wepman Aphasia Screening
	Multilingual Aphasia Examination
	Boston Naming Test
	Controlled Verbal Fluency
	Animal Fluency
Visuospatial/visuomotor functioning	Benton Facial Recognition
Judgment of line orientation	Rey-O Complex Figure
	Trail Making Test
Motor functioning	Finger Tapping
	Grooved Pegboard
	Grip Strength
	Boston Apraxia Examination
Emotional/personality functioning	Geriatric Depression Scale
	Beck Depression Inventory
	Multiscore Depression Inventory
	MMPI-2

these primary functions. Their scope involves speed of information processing, accuracy of discrimination, selectivity and use of a heightened state of awareness. Successful evaluation of attention/concentration skills is necessary for proper interpretation of other neuropsychological findings, including memory and learning.

Executive functioning is a complex phenomenon, which answers the question of how or whether one will do something. It involves the capacity to initiate activity and the process of self-monitoring and interpreting feedback. Executive functions include the planning and sequencing strategies that facilitate goal-directed behaviors. Assessment of executive functioning should include testing at varying levels of complexity to obtain an adequate picture of the patient's mental flexibility.

Memory and learning assessment is at the core of most neuropsychological evaluations of the elderly. A complete evaluation should examine verbal memory (contextual and non-contextual) and visual memory (independent of constructional ability), and should address acquisition, retention and recognition through somewhat independent means. The distinction between deficits in encoding and deficits in retrieval of newly-learned information can be crucial in differential diagnosis of the various dementias.

Expressive and receptive language abilities should be assessed directly, including auditory and reading comprehension, repetition skills and the ability to follow simple commands (praxis). Specific language characteristics, including visual confrontation naming and word fluency, may be evaluated with multiple or overlapping measures to increase the reliability of findings. Whenever possible it may be helpful to assess language abilities in both the oral and written modalities to determine the generalizability of language deficits.

Visuospatial functioning assessment should include the evaluation of near visual acuity, processing of visual stimuli, recognition of shapes, colors and forms, and overall spatial orientation of objects in space and during motor tasks. The copying and drawing of geometric or figural designs can directly assess visual perception.

Assessment of motor functioning should include both gross and fine motor abilities. Manual dexterity and gross manual strength are both important and may yield clues to hemispheric differences. Motor planning can best be evaluated through completion of complex, repetitive motor movements and with traditional go–no go motor tasks.

Emotional/personality functioning is one of the most important areas to be assessed in the elderly population. Affective disturbance can contribute to multiple cognitive deficits; therefore, the differentiation between emotional dysfunction and true CNS abnormality is essential in creating an accurate diagnostic profile. Generational differences must be considered when assessing elderly patients for signs and symptoms of depression and anxiety, and stereotypical views of expected emotional functioning of older individuals must be avoided.

ADDITIONAL RESOURCES

What has been offered in this chapter represents a brief introduction and overview of the basic concepts of non-computerized neuropsychological assessment in geriatric patients. The field of geriatric neuropsychology, while still relatively new in comparison with other disciplines, is growing exponentially as the world population continues to include more people at older ages. There exist a good number of valuable references and resources for both professionals working with older individuals, and for caregivers who must consider whether referral of their loved one for neuropsychological evaluation is indicated. The authors encourage healthcare professionals and caregivers alike to access their local centers on aging, the national Alzheimer's Association, and the various clinical neuropsychological associations (e.g. National Academy of Neuropsychology) to obtain further information on cognitive assessment and intervention in older individuals. An extensive list of reading references is also being included to encourage further exploration of related topics.

REFERENCES

1. Hestad, K, Ellersten B, Klove H. Neuropsychological assessment in old age. In Nordhus IH, VanderBos GR *et al.* (eds) *Clinical Geropsychology*. Washington, DC: American Psychological Association, 1998; 259–88.
2. Mattis S. *Dementia Rating Scale Professional Manual*. Odessa, FL: Psychological Assessment Resources, 1973, 1988.
3. Randolph C. *Repeatable Battery for the Assessment of Neuropsychological Status Manual*. San Antonio, TX: The Psychological Corporation, 1998.

RECOMMENDED READINGS

Grant I, Adams K. *Neuropsychology Assessment of Neuropsychiatric Disorders*, 2nd edn. New York: Oxford University Press, 1996.
Hunt T, Lindley CJ (eds). *Testing Older Adults: A Reference Guide for Geropsychological Assessments*. Austin, TX: Pro-Ed, 1989.
Lezak M. *Neuropsychological Assessment*, 3rd edn. New York: Oxford University Press, 1995.
Parks W, Zec R, Wilson R. *Neuropsychology of Alzheimer's Disease and Other Dementias*. New York: Oxford University Press, 1993.
Poon L (Ed.). *Clinical Memory Assessment of Older Adults*. Washington, DC: American Psychological Association, 1986.

Mini-Mental State Examination

Joseph R. Cockrell and Marshal F. Folstein*

*Department of Psychiatry, Medical University of South Carolina, Charleston, SC, USA, and
New England Medical Center, Boston, MA, USA

The Mini-Mental State Examination (MMSE) is a 10-minute bedside measure of impaired thinking in undeveloped, uneducated, diseased, or very old populations. The summed score of the individual items indicates the current severity of cognitive impairment. Deterioration in cognition is indicated by decreasing scores of repeated tests. Scores are reliable between tests and between raters[1] and correlate with other mental tests, electroencephalography[2], computerized tomography[3], magnetic resonance imaging[4], single photon emission computed tomography (SPECT) scan[5], CSF proteins and enzymes[6,7] and brain biopsy synapse numbers[8].

To administer the MMSE, gain the patient's cooperation by asking him if there is a memory problem and then asking permission to test his memory. During testing, praise successes and ignore failures so as to avoid emotional reactions that will compromise cooperation and performance.

The items of the MMSE include tests of orientation, registration, recall, calculation and attention, naming, repetition, comprehension, reading, writing and drawing. Level of consciousness is rated on a scale from coma to fully alert, but the consciousness rating is not summed with the other items. If all items are answered correctly, the score is 30. The mean score for a community-dwelling population over 65 years of age is 27, with a standard deviation of 1.7[1]. The score is lower in those who completed comparatively fewer years of education and who have diagnosable diseases[9–11]. Patients with dementia, delirium, mental retardation, Parkinson's disease, stroke and some cases of depression score lower than normal controls[1,12]. Alzheimer's disease patients lose 3–4 points per year of illness after the onset of memory disturbance, although there is wide variability in this phenomenon[13,14].

Misinterpretations of scores result from several misconceptions about the test. The MMSE is not a complete mental status examination or a complete neuropsychological examination. The MMSE does not define a clinical or pathological diagnostic category, such as dementia or brain tumor or organicity. The score does not measure decline from a previous level unless tests are repeated over time. The score does not tell the whole story. Individual items are useful for understanding the situation of the patient, since they indicate whether the patient can follow instructions, read and write. Finally, the MMSE is a weak measure of competence or disability. Competence, handicap and disability must be assessed by procedures designed for that purpose.

REFERENCES

1. Folstein MF, Folstein SE, McHugh PR. Mini-Mental State: a practical method for grading the cognitive state of patients for the clinician. *J Psychiatr Res* 1975; **12**: 189–98.
2. Tune L, Folstein MF. Post-operative delirium. *Adv Psychosom Med* 1986 **15**: 51–68.
3. Tsai L, Tsuang MT. The Mini-Mental State test and computerized tomography. *Am J Psychiat* 1979; **136**(4A): 436–8.
4. Bondareff W, Raval J, Woo B *et al*. Magnetic resonance imaging and the severity of dementia in older adults. *Arch Gen Psychiatry* 1990; **47**(1): 47–51.
5. DeKosky ST, Shih WJ, Schmitt FA *et al*. Assessing utility of single photon emission computed tomography (SPECT) scan in Alzheimer disease: correlation with cognitive severity. *Alz Dis Assoc Disord* 1990; **4**(1): 14–23.
6. Koponen H, Stenback U, Mattila E *et al*. CSF β-endorphin-like immunoreactivity in delirium. *Biol Psychiat* 1989; **25**(7): 938–44.
7. Martignoni E, Petraglia F, Costa A *et al*. Dementia of the Alzheimer type and hypothalamus–pituitary–adrenocortical factor and plasma cortisol levels. *Acta Neurol Scand* 1990; **8**(5): 452–6.
8. DeKosky ST, Scheff SW. Synapse loss in frontal cortex biopsies in Alzheimer's disease: correlation with cognitive severity. *Ann Neurol* 1990; **27**(5): 457–84.
9. Anthony JC, Leflesche L, Niaz U *et al*. Limits of the "Mini-Mental State" as a screening test for dementia and delirium among hospital patients. *Psychol Med* 1982; **12**: 397–408.
10. Folstein M, Anthony JC, Parhad I *et al*. The meaning of cognitive impairment in the elderly. *J Am Geriat Soc* 1985; **38**: 228–35.
11. Crum R, Anthony J, Bassett S, Folstein M. Population-based norms for the Mini-Mental State examination by age and educational level. *J Am Med Assoc* 1993; **269**: 2386–91.
12. DePaulo JR, Folstein MF. Psychiatric disturbances in neurologic patients: detection, recognition and hospital course. *Ann Neurol* 1978; **4**: 225–8.
13. Rebok G, Brandt J, Folstein M. Longitudinal cognitive decline in patients with Alzheimer's disease. *J Geriat Psychiat Neurol* 1990; **3**: 91–7.
14. McHugh PR, Folstein MF. Organic mental disorders. In Michels R, Cooper AM, Guze SB *et al*., eds. *Psychiatry*. Philadelphia: JB Lippincott, 1988, 1–24.

IQCODE: Informant Interviews

A. F. Jorm

Centre for Mental Health Research, The Australian National University, Canberra, Australia

In assessing patients for dementia, informants are a valuable source of information, complementing other sources such as cognitive testing. The strengths of informant data include:

- *Everyday relevance*. Informants can report on how the patient is functioning in everyday cognitive tasks. Cognitive tests, by contrast, generally involve artificial tasks removed from daily life.
- *Acceptability to patients*. Formal cognitive testing can be distressing to some people because of the limitations it reveals. However, informant interviews do not directly confront the patient's limitations.
- *Longitudinal perspective*. It is often useful to know how a patient is functioning compared to earlier in life. An interview with an informant who has known the patient for many years can provide this.
- *Ease of administration*. If necessary, informant data can be collected by telephone or mail. In some research situations, it has even been used to assess deceased subjects.
- *Cross-cultural portability*. Informant data may have greater validity than cognitive testing for patients who are from culturally different backgrounds[1].

While informant interviews are widely used in clinical practice, there is now a range of standardized informant interviews and questionnaires available for quantifying this information. Probably the most widely used and researched is the Informant Questionnaire on Cognitive Decline in the Elderly (IQCODE)[2]. The IQCODE is a 26-item questionnaire that asks the informant about cognitive changes over the previous 10 years. Items cover memory and intellectual functioning and are rated on a five-point scale from "1. Much improved" to "5. Much worse". Originally, the IQCODE was designed as an interview but it is more commonly used as a self-administered questionnaire. There is now a short 16-item IQCODE which performs as well as the original. Translations of the IQCODE are available in a range of languages. The various versions are available on the Web at http://www.anu.edu.au/iqcode/.

Principal component analysis of the IQCODE items have shown that it measures a general factor of cognitive decline. Validity studies have found that the IQCODE correlates moderately with cognitive screening tests such as the Mini-Mental State Examination (MMSE) (mean $r = 0.59$ over seven samples). Correlations with indicators of premorbid ability, such as the National Adult Reading Test (NART) and years of education are repeatedly found to be near zero.

A meta-analysis of seven studies directly comparing the IQCODE with the MMSE as a screening test for dementia found that the IQCODE performed at least as well as the

MMSE[3]. However, in clinical practice informant questionnaires and cognitive screening tests are complementary rather than competitors. A simple graphical way of combining the IQCODE and the MMSE for screening purposes is provided by the Demegraph[4]. This can be downloaded from the Web at http://www.mhri.edu.au/biostats/demegraph/.

One weakness of the IQCODE and other informant scales is that they can be biased by the affective state of the informant and the quality of the relationship between the informant and the patient. Cognitive decline is perceived to be greater where the informant is anxious or depressed or where there is a poor relationship.

REFERENCES

1. Jorm AF. Assessment of cognitive impairment and dementia using informant reports. *Clin Psychol Rev* 1996; **16**: 51–73.
2. Jorm AF, Jacomb PA. The Informant Questionnnaire on Cognitive Decline in the Elderly (IQCODE): socio-demographic correlates, reliability, validity and some norms. *Psychol Med* 1989; **19**: 1015–22.
3. Jorm A. Methods of screening for dementia: a meta-analysis of studies comparing an informant questionnaire with a brief cognitive test. *Alzheimer Dis Assoc Dis* 1997; **11**: 158–62.
4. Mackinnon A, Mulligan R. Combining cognitive testing and informant report to increase accuracy in screening for dementia. *Am J Psychiat* 1998; **155**: 1529–35.

Staging Dementia

Barry Reisberg, Gaurav Gandotra, Arshad Zaidi and Steven H Ferris

Aging and Dementia Research Center, New York University School of Medicine, USA

Dementia is a progressive pathologic process extending over a period of many years. Clinicians and scientists have long endeavored to describe the nature of this progression. Such descriptions have generally been encompassed within two broad categories, viz. global staging and more specific staging, sometimes referred to as axial or multi-axial staging. A comparison of the major current dementia staging systems with the most widespread mental status assessments in Alzheimer's disease, the major cause of dementia, is shown in Table 1, which illustrates some of the major potential advantages of staging. These advantages include: (a) staging can identify premorbid but potentially manifest conditions that may be associated with dementia, such as age-associated memory impairment, a condition which is not differentiated with mental status or psychometric tests; (b) staging can be very useful in identifying subtle, identifiable, predementia states, such as mild cognitive impairment (MCI), wherein mental status assessments and psychometric tests, while frequently altered, are generally within the normal range and consequently are not reliable markers; and (c) staging

can track the latter 50% of the potential time course of dementias such as AD, when mental status assessments are virtually invariably at bottom (zero) scores. Furthermore, apart from its utility in portions of dementia where mental status and psychometric assessments are out of range or clearly insensitive, there is evidence that staging procedures can more accurately and sensitively identify the course of dementia in the portion of the condition that is conventionally charted with mental status assessments. This latter evidence comes from longitudinal investigation of the course of AD[1], pharmacologic treatment investigation of AD[2] and study of independent psychometric assessments of AD[3]. Another seeming advantage of staging procedures in comparison with mental status or psychometric assessment of AD and other dementias is in identifying the management concomitants of severity assessments[4]. Staging procedures have also been successfully applied post mortem to assess retrospectively the diagnoses of a diverse assortment of dementia-related cases available for "brain banking" but on which no ante mortem clinical data were available[5]. Similarly,

Table SA27iii.1 Typical time course of normal brain aging and Alzheimer's disease

Clinical Diagnosis	Normal Adult	Age Associated Memory Impairment	Mild Cognitive Impairment	Mild AD	Moderate AD	Moderately Severe AD	Severe AD
CDR Stage *		0	0.5	1	2 3	4	5
GDS and FAST Stage *	1	2	3	4	5	6	7
FAST Substage						a b c d e	a b c d e f
Years [a]	Many decades	Generally many years 0		7 9 10.5		13	19
MMS-E	29	29 29	25	19 14		5 0	
Blessed IMC	35	35 35	29	23 16		0 0	

Typical Psychometric Tests = 0   Usual Point of Death

*Stage range comparisons shown between the CDR and GDS/FAST stages are based upon published functioning and self-care descriptors.
[a]Numerical values represent time from the earliest clinically manifest symptoms of Alzheimer's disease.
Adapted by permission from Reisberg *et al.*[52]

post mortem retrospective staging procedures have been successful in establishing remarkably robust clinicopathologic correlations in longitudinally-studied AD cohorts[6,7].

GLOBAL STAGING

Efforts to stage progressive dementia globally can be traced back at least to the early nineteenth century, when the English psychiatrist, James Prichard, described four stages in the progression of dementia: "(1) impairment of recent memory, (2) loss of reason, (3) incomprehension, (4) loss of instinctive action"[8]. More recently, the American Psychiatric Association's 1980 *Diagnostic and Statistical Manual of Mental Disorders*, 3rd edn (DSM-III)[9] recognized three broad stages in its definition of primary degenerative dementia. Subsequently, in 1982, two more detailed global descriptions of the progression of dementia were published. One of these, the Clinical Dementia Rating (CDR) scale[10] described five broad stages from normality to severe dementia. The other, the Global Deterioration Scale (GDS)[11], identified seven clinically recognizable stages, from normality to most severe dementia of the Alzheimer type. These two global staging instruments, the GDS and the CDR, are generally compatible except that the GDS is more detailed and specific and identifies two stages that the original CDR staging does not. One of these is a stage in which subjective complaints of cognitive deficit occur (GDS stage 2). These subjective complaints are now recognized as occurring very commonly in aged persons[12–14] and consensus workgroups have called attention to the importance of these symptoms and the need for more detailed study of their nature and treatment[15–17]. Although this stage of subjective complaints continues to be identified only by the GDS staging system, recent studies have indicated that persons with these complaints are at increased risk for subsequent overt dementia[18,19]. Also, at the other end of the pathologic spectrum, the CDR did not identify any stage beyond that in which dementia patients "require much help with personal care" and are "often incontinent", whereas the GDS identifies a final seventh GDS stage in which patients are already incontinent and over the course of which language and motor capacities are progressively lost. Subsequently, two further stages were suggested for the CDR, corresponding to the GDS stage 7 range[20–22].

Staging procedures have been shown to be valid and reliable methods for assessing the magnitude of pathology in AD and related dementing conditions. This validity and reliability is illustrated in this brief review for the GDS, probably the most detailed and explicit staging procedure.

The validity of the GDS has been demonstrated in several ways. Cross-sectional studies have confirmed the consistency of the ordinal sequence and the optimal weighting of the hierarchically sequenced items embodied in the GDS stages in aging and progressive Alzheimer's disease (AD)[22–24]. Thus, the specific impairments characteristic of each stage almost always follow the impairments described for the previous stage. Also, the grouping of impairment characteristics within stages appears to be optimal.

For example, naturalistic study has supported the identification of staging phenomena, largely identical to the GDS stages, by independent lay-person observers. In this study[23], a 30-item questionnaire derived from the GDS was completed by a relative or caregiver for each of 115 patients with varying degrees of dementia. Principal components analysis was used to combine the items into a single composite scale which more reliably represents distances between the 30 clinical manifestations along the continuum of cognitive decline. The study found that "the scale scores for the clinical manifestations were observed to cluster into relatively discrete groups, suggesting naturally occurring stages or

phases. Objective cluster analysis methods further confirmed the presence of distinct transitions along the cognitive decline continuum". It concluded that the "utility of empirically derived scale values in staging the course of primary degenerative dementia is suggested".

The relationship between the GDS stages and mental status assessments, other dementia assessments, scores on cognitive tests and other objective tests and *in vivo* assessments of brain change in aging and progressive dementia have been studied in considerable detail[11,24]. These studies have indicated significant correlations between all of these measures of dementia severity and the GDS stages. However, the strongest relationships have been observed between comprehensive dementia assessments, such as the Mini-Mental State Examination (MMSE)[25], and the progression of dementia on the GDS[24]. The GDS also correlates well with evaluations of actual functioning and activities of daily living in AD[26] and with independent physical markers of AD progression, such as changes in neurologic reflexes[27]. Thus, the construct validity of the GDS has been well substantiated.

At least six separate studies have examined the reliability of the GDS[28–33]. Reliability coefficients have ranged from 0.82 to 0.97 in these studies, using disparate procedures in diverse settings. These studies have indicated that the GDS is at least as reliable as any other instrument upon which clinicians rely, such as the MMSE. In a reliability study in a nursing home setting[32], the GDS was found to be somewhat more reliable than the MMSE. Importantly, GDS staging has also been shown to be a reliable procedure when assessed using a telephone format[33].

Global staging scales such as the GDS have certain important advantages in dementia assessment. First and foremost, these scales are strongly anchored to the clinical symptoms, behaviour and functional changes in progressive degenerative dementia and particularly that of Alzheimer's disease. Consequently, they discourage misdiagnosis. Unlike many mental status and other dementia test instruments, global stages are relatively stable over time and relatively resistant to practice effects. Equally importantly, global staging instruments are minimally influenced by educational background and socioeconomic status, whereas mental status and similar assessments are strongly influenced by such factors. Also, global staging, and in particular the GDS, covers the entire range of pathology in central nervous system (CNS) aging and progressive dementia, whereas, for example, mental status assessments and most psychometric tests entirely fail to distinguish GDS stages 1 and 2. Occasionally, patients may display GDS stage 3 symptomatology and still score a perfect 30 on the MMSE. Uncommonly, dementia patients may display GDS stage 4 symptomatology, and still score a perfect 30 on the MMSE. Much more commonly, patients may display the clear-cut dementia symptomatology characteristic of GDS stage 4 and achieve MMSE scores which are near-perfect or within the so-called "normal" range. At the other end of the pathologic spectrum, most patients at GDS stage 6 achieve only bottom scores on traditional psychometric tests. Over the entire course of the GDS 7 stage, nearly all patients attain only zero scores on the MMSE. The GDS, however, describes a final seventh stage, over the course of which patients may survive for many years.

AXIAL AND MULTI-AXIAL STAGING

The observation that the progression of dementia pathology is accompanied by progressive changes in more specifically defined processes has resulted in efforts to stage dementia in terms of those processes. Generally, axial staging has attempted to exploit progressive changes in cognition or functioning, although attempts have also been made to stage hierarchically progressive mood and behavioural changes, progressive motoric changes and progressive neurologic changes, as well as other observable concomitants of dementia. These efforts can be traced back more than 30 years to the work of de Ajuriaguerra and associates[34–36], Swiss investigators who were strongly influenced by Piaget's investigations of the stages of normal infant and childhood development. More recently, Cole and co-workers in Canada employed this approach in their Hierarchic Dementia Scale[37–39]. A similar approach was pursued, apparently independently, by Haycox[40] in the USA and Gottfries et al.[41] in Sweden.

The CDR staging has a "sum of boxes" approach that employs a hierarchical, multi-axial-like procedure[21]. Based upon their seven-stage GDS, Reisberg and associates also described axial and multi-axial concomitants of progressive dementia[42,43]. Ultimately, these latter descriptions resulted in the most detailed hierarchic staging of progressive dementia proposed to date, a 16-stage measure of progressive functional change. This latter assessment, termed Functional Assessment Staging or FAST[44], has been enumerated to be optimally concordant in dementia of the Alzheimer type, with the corresponding GDS stages, discussed above. The developers of the FAST note several advantages of this measure, including: (a) the FAST is capable of describing the entire course of dementia of the Alzheimer type, ordinally (i.e. hierarchically), in unprecedented detail; (b) the scale can assist in differentiating dementia of the Alzheimer type from other dementia processes[22,45,46]; (c) the scale can assist in identifying premature and potentially remediable functional changes in AD patients (e.g. premature loss of ambulation due, for example, to the side effects of medication)[22,45,46]; (d) the scale permits the retrospective as well as prospective examination of the temporal course of AD[6,7]; and (e) the scale is the only current measure that permits the detailed staging of severe AD[3,26,47]. A strong relationship between this FAST procedure and comprehensive cognitive assessments such as the MMSE has long been noted[48,49]. However, because the MMSE and other cognitive modalities bottom out prior to the final five to eight FAST substages, complete concurrent validation and examination of the FAST had to await the development of cognitive measures useful in most severe dementia. Such measures were developed towards the end of the twentieth century and do, in fact, evidence strong relationships with the final FAST stages[3]. Subsequent work showed equally strong relationships between this latter portion of the FAST and ostensibly cognition-independent neurologic reflex changes[27] as well as hippocampal neuropathologic changes in volume[6], cell number[7], and neurofibrillary changes[7] with the advance of AD as per the FAST stages and substages. The correlation between the advance of AD as measured with the FAST in the latter portion of the course of AD, generally after the MMSE bottom (zero) point, and cognitive, neurologic reflex and neuropathologic hippocampal measures are generally approximately 0.8–0.9, comparable to the correlation between the FAST and the MMSE in the MMSE sensitive portion of the FAST staging assessment. Because of these properties and others, the FAST, as well as the GDS staging more generally, has proved of widespread utility. For example, in the USA, the FAST staging procedure is currently utilized as the Medicare mandated "gold standard" for hospice admission (Health Care Finance Administration, 1998) and the FAST and GDS have been utilized to survey the severity mix in the US National Institute on Aging Special Care Units consortium[50]. Importantly, because of the sensitivity of the FAST staging procedure to the course of AD, not only over the final seventh stage when the MMSE is zero, but also over the course of FAST stage 6, when patients still score on measures such as the MMSE, the FAST measure has shown a significant neuroprotective effect on course in a multicenter drug trial, whereas the MMSE was not sensitive to change in this study[2].

SUMMARY

Staging can be useful in identifying potential treatments for AD and other dementias, as well as in assessing the course and the management needs of the dementia patient, and also in the diagnosis and differential diagnosis of dementing disorders. In providing an overview of the course of dementias such as AD, from the initial to final clinical symptoms, staging is uniquely useful. Staging is also uniquely useful in assessment at various specific points in the evolution of dementing processes. Very importantly, staging can uniquely relate to management needs and the general management import of dementing processes.

ACKNOWLEDGEMENTS

This work was supported in part by US DHHS Grants AG03051 and AG08051 from the National Institute on Aging of the US National Institutes of Health, by Grant 90 AR2160 from the US Department of Health and Human Services Administration on Aging, and by the Zachary and Elizabeth M. Fisher Alzheimer's Disease Education and Resources Program of the New York University School of Medicine.

REFERENCES

1. Reisberg B, Ferris SH, Franssen E et al. Mortality and temporal course of probable Alzheimer's disease: a five-year prospective study. Int Psychogeriat 1996; 8: 291–31.
2. Reisberg B, Windscheif U, Ferris SH et al. Memantine in moderately severe to severe Alzheimer's disease (AD): results of a placebo-controlled 6-month trial. Neurobiol Aging 2000; 21(1S): S275.
3. Auer SR, Sclan SG, Yaffee RA, Reisberg B. The neglected half of Alzheimer disease: cognitive and functional concomitants of severe dementia. J Am Geriat Soc 1994; 42: 1266–72.
4. Reisberg B, Kenowsky S, Franssen EH et al. President's Report: towards a science of Alzheimer's disease management: a model based upon current knowledge of retrogenesis. Int Psychogeriat 1999; 11: 7–23.
5. Rockwood K, Howard K, Thomas VS et al. Retrospective diagnosis of dementia using an informant interview based on the Brief Cognitive Rating Scale. Int Psychogeriat 1998; 10: 53–60.
6. Bobinski M, Wegiel J, Wisniewski HM et al. Atrophy of hippocampal formation subdivisions correlates with stage and duration of Alzheimer disease. Dementia 1995; 6: 205–10.
7. Bobinski M, Wegiel J, Tarnawski M et al. Relationships between regional neuronal loss and neurofibrillary changes in the hippocampal formation and duration and severity of Alzheimer disease. J Neuropathol Exp Neurol 1997; 56: 414–20.
8. Cohen GD. Historical views and evolution of concepts. In Reisberg B (ed.), Alzheimer's Disease. New York: Free Press/Macmillan, 1983, 29–33.
9. American Psychiatric Association. Diagnostic and Statistical Manual of Mental Disorders, 3rd edn. Washington, DC: American Psychiatric Association, 1980.
10. Hughes CP, Berg L, Danziger WL et al. A new clinical scale for the staging of dementia. Br J Psychiat 1982; 140: 566–72.
11. Reisberg B, Ferris SH, de Leon MJ, Crook T. The global deterioration scale for the assessment of primary degenerative dementia. Am J Psychiat 1982; 139: 1136–9.
12. Lowenthal MF, Berkman PL, and associates (eds). Aging and mental disorder in San Francisco: A Social Psychiatric Study. San Francisco, CA: Jossey-Bass, 1967.
13. Sluss TK, Rabins P, Gruenberg EM. Memory complaints in community residing men. Gerontologist (Part II) 1980; 20: 201 (abstr).
14. Wang P-N, Wang S-J, Fuh J-L et al. Subjective memory complaint in relation to cognitive performance and depression: a longitudinal study of a rural Chinese population. J Am Geriat Soc 2000; 48: 295–9.
15. Crook T, Bartus RT, Ferris SH et al. Age-associated memory impairment: proposed diagnostic criteria and measures of clinical

change—report of a National Institute of Mental Health Work group. *Dev Neuropsychol* 1986; **2**: 261–76.

16. American Psychiatric Association. *Diagnostic and Statistical Manual of Mental Disorders*, 4th edn. Washington, DC: American Psychiatric Association, 1994; 684.

17. Levy R. (Chairman), Working Party of the International Psychogeriatric Association in collaboration with the World Health Organization. Aging-associated cognitive decline. *Int Psychogeriat* 1994; **6**: 63–8.

18. Tobiansky R, Blizard R, Livingston G, Mann A. The Gospel Oak Study, stage IV: the clinical relevance of subjective memory impairment in older people. *Psychol Med* 1995; **25**: 779–86.

19. Geerlings MI, Jonker C, Bouter LM *et al*. Association between memory complaints and incident Alzheimer's disease in elderly people with normal baseline cognition. *Am J Psychiat* 1999; **156**: 531–7.

20. Heyman A, Wilkinson WE, Hurwitz BJ *et al*. Early-onset Alzheimer disease: clinical predictors of institutionalization and death. *Neurology* 1987; **37**: 980–4.

21. Hughes CP, Berg L, Danziger WL *et al*. Clinical dementia rating (CDR) scale. In *Task Force for the Handbook of Psychiatric Measures*. Washington, DC: American Psychiatric Association, 2000; 446–50.

22. Reisberg B, Ferris SH. Global deterioration scale (GDS), brief cognitive rating scale (BCRS), and functional assessment staging (FAST) measures: the GDS staging system. In *Task Force for the Handbook of Psychiatric Measures*. Washington, DC: American Psychiatric Association, 2000; 450–5.

23. Overall JE, Scott J, Rhoades HM, Lesser J. Empirical scaling of the dementia stages of cognitive decline in senile dementia. *J Geriat Psychiat Neurol* 1990; **3**: 212–20.

24. Reisberg B, Ferris SH, de Leon MJ *et al*. Stage-specific behavioural, cognitive, and *in vivo* changes in age-associated memory impairment (AAMI) and primary degenerative dementia of the Alzheimer type. *Drug Dev Res* 1988; **15**: 101–14.

25. Folstein MF, Folstein SE, McHugh PR. Mini-mental state: a practical method for grading the cognitive state of patients for the clinician. *J Psychiat Res* 1975; **12**: 189–98.

26. Reisberg B, Franssen E, Bobinski M *et al*. Overview of methodologic issues for pharmacologic trials in mild, moderate, and severe Alzheimer's disease. *Int Psychogeriat* 1996; **8**: 159–93.

27. Franssen EH, Reisberg B. Neurologic markers of the progression of Alzheimer disease. *Int Psychogeriat* 1997; **9**(suppl. 1): 297–306.

28. Foster JR, Sclan S, Welkowitz J, Boksay I, Seeland I. Psychiatric assessment in medical long-term care facilities: reliability of commonly used rating scales. *Int J Geriat Psychiat* **3**: 229–33.

29. Gottlieb GL, Gur RE, Gur RC. Reliability of psychiatric scales in patients with dementia of the Alzheimer type. *Am J Psychiat* **145**: 857–60.

30. Reisberg B, Ferris SH, Steinberg G *et al*. Longitudinal study of dementia patients and aged controls: an approach to methodological issues. In Lawton MP, Herzog AR (eds), *Special Research Methods for Gerontology*. Amityville, NY: Baywood Publishers, 1989; 198–231.

31. Dura JR, Haywood-Niler E, Kiecolt-Glaser JK. Spousal caregivers of persons with Alzheimer's and Parkinson's Disease dementia: A preliminary comparison. *Gerontologist* 1990; **30**: 332–6.

32. Hartmaier SL, Sloan PD, Guess, HA, Koch GG. The MDS Cognition Scale: a valid instrument for identifying and staging nursing home residents with dementia using the Minimum Data Set. *J Am Geriat Soc* 1994; **42**: 1173–9.

33. Monteiro IM, Boksay I, Auer SR *et al*. The reliability of routine clinical instruments for the assessment of Alzheimer's disease administered by telephone. *J Geriat Psychiat Neurol* 1998; **11**: 18–24.

34. de Ajuriaguérra J, Rey M, Bellet-Muller M, Tissot R. A propos de quelques problèmes posees par le déficit opératoire de viellards arreints de démence dégénérative en début d'évolution. *Cortex* 1964; **1**: 103–32.

35. de Ajuriaguerra J, Tissot R. Some aspects of psychoneurologic disintegration in senile dementia. In Mueller CH, Ciompi L (eds), *Senile Dementia*. Switzerland: Huber, 1968.

36. de Ajuriaguerra J, Tissot R. Some aspects of language in various forms of senile dementia: comparisons with language in childhood. In Lennenberg EH, Lennenberg E (eds), *Foundations of Language Development*, vol 1. New York: Academic Press, 1975.

37. Cole MG, Dastoor D. Development of a dementia rating scale: preliminary communication. *J Clin Exp Gerontol* 1980; **2**: 46–63.

38. Cole MG, Dastoor D. A new hierarchic approach to the measurement of dementia. *Psychosomatics* 1987; **28**: 298–304.

39. Cole MG, Dastoor DP, Koszycki D. The Hierarchic Dementia Scale. *J Clin Exp Gerontol* 1983; **5**: 219–34.

40. Haycox JA. A behavioral scale for dementia. In Shamoian CA (ed.), *Biology and Treatment of Dementia in the Elderly*. Washington, DC: American Psychiatric Press, 1984; 1–13.

41. Gottfries CG, Brane G, Steen B. A new rating scale for dementia syndromes. *Gerontology* 1982; **28**(suppl): 20–31.

42. Reisberg B, London E, Ferris SH *et al*. The Brief Cognitive Rating Scale: language, motoric, and mood concomitants in primary degenerative dementia. *Psychopharmacol Bull* 1983; **19**: 702–8.

43. Reisberg B, Schneck MK, Ferris SH *et al*. The brief cognitive rating scale (BCRS): *Psychopharmacol Bull* 1983; **19**: 47–50.

44. Reisberg B. Functional assessment staging (FAST). *Psychopharmacol Bull* 1988; **24**: 653–9.

45. Reisberg B. Dementia: a systematic approach to identifying reversible causes. *Geriatrics* 1986; **41**: 30–46.

46. Reisberg B, Ferris SH, de Leon MJ. Senile dementia of the Alzheimer type: diagnostic and differential diagnostic features with special reference to functional assessment staging. In Traber J, Gispen WH (eds), *Senile Dementia of the Alzheimer Type*, vol 2. Berlin: Springer-Verlag, 1985; 18–37.

47. Reisberg B, Kluger A. Assessing the progression of dementia: diagnostic considerations. In Salaman C (ed.), *Clinical Geriatric Psychopharmacology*, 3rd edn. Baltimore: Williams & Wilkins, 1998; 432–62.

48. Reisberg B, Ferris SH, Anand R *et al*. Functional staging of dementia of the Alzheimer type. *Ann N York Acad Sci* 1984; **435**: 481–3.

49. Franssen EH, Monteiro I, Boksay I *et al*. Retrogenesis in Alzheimer's disease: Functional and cognition relationships. *Neurobiol Aging* 2000; **21**: S27.

50. Teresi JA, Morris JN, Matlis S, Reisberg B. Cognitive impairment among SCU and non-SCU residents in the United States. Prevalence estimates from the National Institute on Aging Collaborative Studies of Special Care Units for Alzheimer's Disease. *Research and Practice in Alzheimer's Disease* 2000; **4**: 117–38.

51. Reisberg B, Sclan SG, Franssen E *et al*. Dementia staging in chronic care populations. *Alzheimer's Dis Assoc Dis* 1994; **8**(suppl): 188–205.

Psychogeriatric Assessment Scales

A. F. Jorm

Centre for Mental Health Research, The Australian National University, Canberra, Australia

The Psychogeriatric Assessment Scales (PAS) aim to assess the clinical changes of dementia and depression using a set of continuous scales[1]. The PAS consists of two parts, an interview with the patient and an interview with an informant who knows the patient well. The purpose of interviewing both the patient and an informant is to acquire different perspectives on the patient's impairments. The PAS consists of six scales, three derived from the interview with the patient and three from the interview with the informant. The content of these scales is as follows:

Patient Interview:

- *Cognitive impairment*. This consists of brief tests of cognitive functioning and is sensitive to dementia. It correlates highly with the Mini-Mental State Examination.
- *Depression*. This asks about common symptoms of depression. It correlates highly with the Goldberg Anxiety and Depression Scales.
- *Stroke*. This scale asks about symptoms of cerebrovascular disease and is useful in differentiating Alzheimer's dementia from vascular dementia. It correlates highly with the Hachinski Ischemic Score.

Informant Interview:

- *Cognitive decline*. This scale asks questions about everyday cognitive functioning and is sensitive to dementia. It correlates highly with the Informant Questionnaire on Cognitive Decline in the Elderly (IQCODE).
- *Behaviour change*. The questions in this scale cover aspects of behaviour that could cause interpersonal difficulties and are sensitive to both depression and dementia.
- *Stroke*. The scale involves the same questions as asked of the patient, but provides an independent source of information.

Each scale yields a score along a continuum, and norms are available to show how rare a given score is in the population. The scores can be plotted as a graph to give a readily interpretable summary of the patient's pattern of impairments.

The PAS scales were derived from a principal component and latent trait analysis of items that were designed to cover the ICD-10 and DSM-III-R diagnostic criteria for dementia and depression[1]. Items for the PAS scales were selected to have steep slopes (i.e. to be highly discriminating items) and to have a range of thresholds (i.e. to cover a range of severity).

Validity has been assessed against clinical diagnoses of dementia and depression using receiver operating characteristic (ROC) analysis[1,2]. The Cognitive Impairment and Cognitive Decline scales perform well as screening tests for dementia, while the Depression scale performs well as a screening test for depression. The Behaviour Change scale is non-specific, being affected by both dementia and depression. The Stroke scales perform well at discriminating vascular from non-vascular (mainly Alzheimer's) types of dementia.

The PAS materials and User's Guide[3] can be downloaded free from the Web at http://www.mhri.edu.au/pas/. For people who do not have Internet access, printed copies are available by writing to: PAS Project, Centre for Mental Health Research, Australian National University, Canberra 0200, Australia. The PAS is available in a number of other languages, including French, German, Italian, Chinese and Korean. For details on their availability, write to the above address.

REFERENCES

1. Jorm AF, Mackinnon AJ, Henderson AS *et al.* The Psychogeriatric Assessment Scales: a multi-dimensional alternative to categorical diagnoses of dementia and depression in the elderly. *Psychol Med* 1995; **25**: 447–60.
2. Jorm AF, Mackinnon AJ, Christensen H *et al.* The Psychogeriatric Assessment Scales (PAS): further data on psychometric properties and validity from a longitudinal study of the elderly. *Int J Geriat Psychiat* 1997; **12**: 93–100.
3. Jorm A, Mackinnon A. *Psychogeriatric Assessment Scales: User's Guide and Materials*, 2nd edn., Canberra: ANUTECH, 1995.

28

Computer Methods of Assessment of Cognitive Function

T. W. Robbins and Barbara J. Sahakian

Departments of Experimental Psychology and Psychiatry, University of Cambridge, UK

Almost 20 years ago, the Royal College of Physicians recommended the use of automated testing procedures in assessing the deficits of patients with dementia, particularly in the context of clinical trials, because of their greater reliability and objectivity[1]. Since then, there have been several developments that have capitalized on the explosion of computer technology and its general availability over the past decade, which have been the subject of earlier reviews[2-5].

The advantages and disadvantages of computerized testing can readily be summarized. Apart from the obvious objectivity and accuracy of the measures and the standardization of the administration of the tests themselves, there are potential gains in patient compliance. Paper and pencil tests and clinical assessment interviews are generally admitted not to be popular with patients, perhaps because of their confrontational and formal nature. In our experience, computerized tests are also preferred by clinical assessors, who find that they have more time to focus on the patient during testing, rather than upon the presentation of the test material and data recording. Well-designed computerized tests that provide adequate feedback may provide some incentive for patients to do well, thereby avoiding the difficult problems of interpretation provided by lack of motivation. On the other hand, there is often little to be gained from the mere administration of standard tests in a computerized format, except in terms of the logging and storage of the data. Certainly it is infeasible to dispense with the human assessor during computerized testing; indeed, it is vital that a trained individual is present during such testing. And requesting patients to interact with certain novel and complex forms of interface, such as keyboards and other complex manipulanda, may serve only to confuse assessment by providing the patients with an extra set of problems to master. In recent developments, these problems have been circumvented, at least in part, by the use of touch-sensitive screens, which require the patient only to respond directly to the test stimuli themselves without imposing further demands by requiring them to divide their attention between a screen and a keyboard. It can also be argued that computerized assessment removes some of the creative flexibility that an experienced clinical neuropsychologist can bring to patient testing; however, this, too, can largely be avoided by the use of sufficiently flexible computerized contingencies.

In this brief review, we will concentrate on some prominent batteries that have been used for assessing cognitive functioning in the elderly. These batteries share some common principles, but also emphasize different aspects of design and administration.

EARLY ATTEMPTS: A COMPUTERIZED EVERYDAY MEMORY BATTERY

Crook and his colleagues took into account clinical, theoretical and psychometric considerations in designing their battery which, however, no longer appears to be generally available. However, their design historically represented a methodological advance in several respects and so we describe its main features below. In particular, they addressed the problem of ecological validity by simulating everyday memory situations, such as memory for faces, the locations of objects, telephone numbers and shopping lists, narrative memory for a simulated news broadcast and topographical memory for routes[6-8]. This required at that time quite advanced computer technology, including the use of the touch-sensitive screen, laser disk and video recordings. Thus, for example, one test involves viewing a live colour video recording of people introducing themselves. The subject has to learn the names that go with the faces and retain them over a 40 min delay. Tests of immediate memory for telephone numbers are administered with the subject actually dialling numbers on a telephone linked to the computer, having read a seven- (or 10-) digit number from the monitor screen. A reaction time task is configured to resemble the familiar situation of having to stop and start a car in relation to the colour of the prevailing traffic lights. The effects of certain theoretically interesting variables, such as degree of interference, can also be simulated, for example, by having the subjects hear an "engaged" signal and then asking them to redial the number.

As well as achieving a clear face validity, the battery developed by Crook and his colleagues had a degree of theoretical or construct validity. Recognizing that many of the classical memory batteries, such as the Wechsler Memory Scale[9], in fact have a complex factorial structure including dimensions that can be labelled Attention/Concentration and Orientation, as well as Immediate and General Memory, the battery contains a more comprehensive examination of information-processing capacity that includes, for example, explicit measures of speed of reaction. In addition, evidence for dissociable forms of memory process[10-11] led to the inclusion of tests that probed different aspects of memory.

Although unfortunately this battery no longer appears to be in general use, it was potentially useful in the diagnosis of various age-related memory impairments, including those resulting from Alzheimer's disease, and in the evaluation of candidate pharmacological treatments. It was mainly used to study the relationship between ageing and memory loss in a sample of over 3000 healthy normal subjects in the USA[6]. This study revealed some interesting differences among the tests. For example, the name–face association task administered to 1547 individuals showed a decade-by-decade decline in performance beginning in mid-life, whereas a facial recognition paradigm revealed decline only in the 70+ group in another survey of 326 subjects. Moreover, in the latter study, performance was most impaired at a delay interval of 0 seconds, suggesting attentional rather than mnemonic dysfunction.

The most important theme of the Everyday Memory Battery, which still makes it of contemporary interest, is its adherence to the principle of ecological validity—cognitive functions are tested in the context of everyday functions, which makes them relevant to patient and clinician alike. This is clearly an important element of assessment, but it should also be pointed out that it may be at the expense of test sensitivity, inasmuch that patients can resort to a greater extent on well-learned routines, to overcome deficits that would be exposed by more abstract or unfamiliar test material. In this sense the following two batteries to be considered place less weight on ecological validity and more on theoretical issues, such as the nature of the brain systems damaged in dementia, as well as on practical considerations that enhance the sensitivity and stability of the results obtained.

CANTAB (CAMBRIDGE NEUROPSYCHOLOGICAL TEST AUTOMATED BATTERY)

CANTAB was developed by a group including Dr T. W. Robbins at the University of Cambridge and Dr B. J. Sahakian (Section of Old Age Psychiatry, Institute of Psychiatry) from a research programme funded by the Wellcome Trust to improve the comparative assessment of cognition from animals to humans. CANTAB is a set of computerized neuropsychological test batteries with three main components[4,13]:

1. *Visual memory.* Consists of short pattern and spatial recognition memory tests, a simultaneous and delayed-matching-to-sample test, and a test of paired-associate, conditional learning of pattern–location associations[14].
2. *Attention.* Consists of tests of intradimensional and extra-dimensional set-shifting (analogous to the Wisconsin Card Sorting Test), a reaction time-based visual search task for conjunctive features, according to the Sternberg paradigms[15], and a test of sustained attention, termed rapid visual information processing.
3. *Spatial working memory and planning.* Consists of tests of spatial span, spatial working memory and a computerized version of the Tower of London task, which includes separate measures of thinking and movement time[16].

Each battery employs a touch-sensitive screen and begins with preliminary tests of sensorimotor function, which enable subjects with marked visual or motor deficits to be screened out from subsequent testing. The theoretical rationale for the tests is based on two major themes: first, those animal tests of cognitive function (e.g. delayed matching to sample, spatial working memory and the attentional shifting task, which is based on animal learning theory) that have proved useful in establishing the neural substrates of certain types of cognitive function and can be adapted appropriately for human subjects; and second, a componential analysis of cognitive function, allowing the characterization of elementary processes contributing to cognition. This is exemplified in each battery, e.g. visual memory, where there are separate tests of spatial and pattern recognition memory, as well as a test in which patterned information has to be remembered in specific spatial contexts. In the attentional battery, the attentional shifts are preceded by stages establishing

the subject's capacities for simple rule use, acquisition of a simple rule (simple discrimination), its reversal, and its application to more complicated stimuli with additional perceptual dimensions. In the planning battery, some of the componential cognitive requirements for the Tower of London planning task itself, such as the capacities of subjects to remember and use a short spatial sequence, and to employ working memory in a strategic spatial search task, are separately measured. In addition, a "yoked motor control" is employed, which allows the computation of thinking time, corrected for any problems of movement that inevitably confound the interpretation of latency measures in brain-damaged and elderly subjects[16–17]. This yoked control is available to capitalize on some of the advantages conferred by computerized testing; the exact sequence of moves that a patient uses in attempting to solve a problem is stored on-line, and played back to him/her one at a time, in the yoked control test.

The "componential" approach also has some more practical benefits. For example, each test, in addition to containing internal controls, begins at a simple level, so that virtually all subjects achieve a score above floor levels. Moreover, if successful, a subject proceeds to difficult versions of the same test, which avoids ceiling effects. In addition, as the tests are non-verbal in nature, they avoid problems posed by specific language disorders and by illiteracy, and this also makes the tests suitable for cross-national studies. Finally, the tests are available for the IBM machines or similar clones running under WINDOWS '95 or later, which are relatively inexpensive as well as portable (in fact, CANTAB can be implemented on a portable computer equipped with a touchscreen) and so can be used by moderately equipped clinical neuropsychology departments of hospitals, as well as for testing in subjects' or patients' homes[4,13]. The tests are both comprehensive, in terms of the range of cognitive functions they cover, and also sensitive to deficits in patients with dementia of the Alzheimer type (DAT), Parkinson's disease (PD), Huntington's disease and dementia of the Lewy body type[14–20]. Some of the deficits have shown double dissociations across these groups. For example, PD patients show deficits on matching-to-sample, independently of delay, whereas patients with DAT exhibit a delay-dependent decline in performances. In addition, DAT patients early in the course of the disease can perform better than non-medicated, early-in-the course patients with Parkinson's or Huntington's diseases in tests of attentional shifting[15,18,19]. These results are important in showing different profiles of deficits in different forms of neurodegenerative cognitive disorders, which may prove important in the early detection and diagnosis of neurodegenerative diseases and for establishing the neural substrates of the early forms of dementia. For example, it seems likely that the impairments in visual recognition memory that occur early in the course of DAT may reflect temporal lobe deficits, whereas the impairments in attention shifting in unmedicated Parkinson's disease[15] and Huntington's disease[19] may depend upon fronto-striatal forms of dysfunction. Other studies have confirmed that the spatial working memory and planning tests, as well as that of attentional shifting, are sensitive to frontal (but not temporal) lobe damage in humans[16,21].

In the assessment of dementia the results are important because the computerized tests may prove to be more sensitive to cognitive decline than many of the existing instruments, e.g. Mini-Mental State Examination (MMSE)[22] and clinical stagings of dementia[23]. Follow-up testing in populations of DAT and elderly depressed patients with the visual memory battery has shown that many of the tests are sensitive to the effects of progressive intellectual decline in the DAT patients and to the effects of recovery in the depressed group[24]. Some studies have provided evidence that one of the CANTAB tests (paired associate learning) is capable of discriminating between those patients with questionable dementia that go on to be diagnosed with DAT, and those that do not[25,26]. There is evidence that some of the tests are sensitive to drug treatments in DAT patients[27], as well as to the effects of a variety of drugs in normal subjects, including those that may provide models of different aspects of dementia[28,29].

CANTAB has also been subject to several forms of validation-testing. There are, for example, data on test–retest reliability showing that most of the tests fall into categories described as "good" or "fair"[30–32], even though many tap "fronto-executive" functions that are notoriously unreliable in terms of measurement in this context. Most of the elements of the CANTAB battery have been administered to a large sample of normal subjects (>800) from the North East Age Research Panel. This has resulted in two major publications, which have provided a standardization of the test scores across a wide range of ages and several levels of intelligence[33,34]. There are also burgeoning data on developmental norms[35]. CANTAB is also validated in theoretical terms, partly from the studies of so many patient groups, including those with specific damage to different regions of the neocortex[16,21,36]. There is also a parallel CANTAB battery for testing monkeys, which potentially provides one way of achieving a vertical integration of findings across species[37]. Further data on the underlying neural substrates of the tests is provided via the availability of functional imaging data (mainly derived from positron emission tomography) that confirm which neural networks are activated by different tests[38–42].

COGDRAS: A COGNITIVE PERFORMANCE BATTERY

The Cognitive Drug Research Computerized Assessment System (COGDRAS) is rather complementary to the other two batteries described, in that it is based more on pragmatic considerations of assessing such functions as reaction time and elementary aspects of memory than on theoretical preoccupations with the ecological validity or the relationship of task performance to functional brain circuitry. COGDRAS was originally designed by Dr Keith Wesnes[43] to evaluate the cognitive effects of drugs in normal volunteers and patients. A further version of the battery (COGDRAS-D) was developed to examine cognitive performance in people with dementia[43,44]. In COGDRAS-D eight cognitive tests are presented to the subject, the system originally having been installed on a BBC microcomputer[43]. The subject faces the screen with two index fingers resting on two response buttons. All material is presented visually on the screen in large bold type. The tests comprise immediate and delayed verbal and picture recognition, a test of sustained attention similar to that used in CANTAB, simple and choice reaction time tests, and a memory scanning task. The battery deliberately sets out to avoid problem-solving tasks or the provision of negative feedback. In various extensions of the battery, tests of motor control are also incorporated. Like CANTAB, it has been employed in a wide variety of applications, especially for testing effects of drugs[45] or potential environmental toxins in normal subjects.

One validation study[44] for the dementia version of the battery has assessed 98 unselected patients from a memory clinic, who were divided into five groups on clinical assessment, including demented, depressed, "worried well", minimally cognitively impaired, and other brain disorders. The battery discriminated between some of these groups. In the key comparison of dementia and minimally impaired patients, 6/14 measures were significantly worse than for the demented group, although the level of significance obtained for these individual measures was less than

that achieved by the MMSE. It has also been used to compare patients with DAT and Huntington's disease[46]. An earlier study[43] showed good test–retest reliability coefficients for demented patients, particularly on the reaction time measures and significant correlations with other commonly-used instruments in dementia research. More recent applications of the battery have also shown that it is possible to test DAT patients over as long as a 4 h period, in the context of studying the effects of the benzodiazepine antagonist flumazenil[47].

CONCLUSIONS

The batteries reviewed above, as well as others, will ultimately have to be compared with one another, as well as with more conventional assessment procedures, and this will require large and dedicated studies, some of which are under way. A clinician anxious merely to diagnose DAT and other conditions will understandably enquire why such complex tests should supplant the use of such simple and easy-to-use instruments as the Mini-Mental State Examination[22]. The answer is that they are not intended to supplant, but rather to augment, their use. In our own experience, for example, the Mini-Mental State Examination often fails to detect the early onset of dementia, especially in individuals of high IQ. To understand the relationship between such clinical rating scales and the specific computerized tests is to consider the scale as providing a gross measure on a relatively undifferentiated range of functions, whereas the computerized tests provide more specific and precise information about particular capacities, thus providing important information for patient management.

Crook et al.[6] pointed out that they found it useful to develop in parallel their own self-rating scales for memory, although the relationships with direct performance measures are typically low. Of course, such low correlations may reflect the measurement of subtly different components of memory, all of which should be taken into account. They view self-rating data as important in assessing age-related memory disorders and family ratings and clinical scales as useful in the assessment of dementia. Certainly, it is important to relate what may be a statistically significant and consistent effect of a treatment on computerized tests of cognitive performance to the clinical improvement manifest to the patient's family in their everyday activities. However, it should be noted that such assessments of everyday activities have not so far proved to be especially discriminating for patients with mild DAT. It is particularly important to add some assessments of everyday activities to the assessments provided by CANTAB and the COGDRAS battery, as these are not specifically designed to simulate such situations. The rationale is that the use of rather visual abstract material tends to be more sensitive in detecting deficits than the use of concrete examples, as there is every indication that many well-established skills (e.g. reading) or types of knowledge (skills) may remain largely intact in early dementia. Moreover, obvious differences in life experience, e.g. produced by different occupations, will tend to be minimized. Finally, we should point out that it is important that batteries such as CANTAB, and to a lesser extent CDR, can provide means for differentiating cognitive disorders in the elderly arising from a variety of conditions, preferably on a qualitative basis. Providing a profile of which functions are spared as well as which are impaired may have implications for strategies based on rehabilitation, as well as pharmacological treatments, which will increasingly motivate attempts at cognitive remediation for the elderly.

REFERENCES

1. Royal College of Physicians. Organic mental impairment in the elderly, implications for research, education and the provision of services. *J R Coll Phys Lond* 1981; **15**: 3–38.

2. Maulucci RA, Eckhouse RH. The use of computers in the assessment and treatment of cognitive disabilities in the elderly: a survey. *Psychopharmacol Bull* 1988; **24**; 557–64.

3. Morris RG. Automated clinical assessment. In Watts F (ed.), *New Directions in Clinical Psychology*. Chichester: Wiley, 1985; 121–38.

4. Morris RG, Evenden JL, Sahakian BJ, Robbins TW. Computer aided assessment of dementia: comparative studies of Alzheimer-type dementia and Parkinson's disease. In Stahl S, Iversen SD, Goodman E (eds), *Cognitive Neurochemistry*. Oxford: Oxford University Press, 1987; 21–36.

5. Skilbeck C. Computer assistance in the management of memory and cognitive impairments. In Wilson B, Moffatt N (eds), *Clinical Management of Memory Problems*. Edinburgh: Churchill Livingstone, 1984; 112–31.

6. Crook TH, Johnson BA, Larrabee GJ. Evaluation of drugs in Alzheimer's disease and age-associated memory impairment. In Benkert O, Maier W, Rickels K (eds), *Methodology of the Evaluation of Psychotropic Drugs*. Heidelberg: Springer-Verlag, 1990; 37–55.

7. Larrabee GJ, Crook T. A computerised everyday memory battery for assessing treatment effects. *Psychopharmacol Bull* 1988; **24**: 695–7.

8. Larrabee GJ, Crook T. Assessment of drug effects in age-related memory disorders: clinical, theoretical and psychometric considerations. *Psychopharmacol Bull* 1988; **24**: 515–22.

9. Prigatano GP. Wechsler Memory Scale: a selective review of the literature. *J Clin Psychol* (Special Monograph Suppl) 1978; **34**: 816–32.

10. Baddeley AD. *Working Memory*. Oxford: Oxford University Press, 1986.

11. Tulving E. *Elements of Episodic Memory*. Oxford: Clarendon Press, 1983.

12. Mishkin M, Appenzeller T. The Anatomy of Memory. *Sci Amer* 1987; **256**: 80–9.

13. Sahakian BJ. Computerized assessment of neuro-psychological function in Alzheimer's disease and Parkinson's disease. *Int J Geriat Psychiat* 1990; **5**: 211–13.

14. Sahakian BJ, Morris RG, Evenden JL et al. A comparative study of visuospatial memory and learning in Alzheimer-type dementia and Parkinson's disease. *Brain* 1988; **111**: 695–718.

15. Downes JJ, Roberts AC, Sahakian BJ et al. Impaired extra-dimensional set-shifting performance in medicated and unmedicated Parkinson's disease: Evidence for a specific attentional dysfunction. *Neuropsychologia* 1989; **27**: 1329–43.

16. Owen A, Downes JJ, Sahakian BJ et al. Planning and spatial working memory following frontal lobe lesions in man. *Neuropsychologia* 1990; **28**: 1021–34.

17. Morris RG, Downes JJ, Sahakian BJ et al. Planning and spatial working memory in Parkinson's disease. *J Neurol Neurosurg Psychiat* 1988; **51**: 757–66.

18. Sahakian BJ, Downes JJ, Eagger S et al. Sparing of attentional relative to mnemonic function in a subgroup of patients with dementia of the Alzheimer type. *Neuropsychologia* 1990; **28**: 1197–213.

19. Lawrence AD, Sahakian BJ, Hodges JR et al. Executive and mnemonic functions in early Huntington's disease. *Brain* 1996; **119**: 1633–45.

20. Sahgal A, Galloway PH, McKeith IG et al. A comparative study of attentional deficits in senile dementias of the Alzheimer type and Lewy body types. *Dementia* 1991; **3**: 350–4.

21. Owen AM, Roberts AC, Polkey CE et al. Extra-dimensional vs. intradimensional set-shifting performance following frontal lobe excisions, temporal lobe excisions or amygdala-hippocampectomy in man. *Neuropsychologia* 1991; **29**: 993–1006.

22. Folstein MF, Folstein SE, McHugh PR. 'Mini-Mental State': a practical method for grading the cognitive state of patients for the clinician. *J Psychiatr Res* 1975; **12**: 189–98.

23. Hughes CP, Berg L, Danziger WL et al. A new clinical scale for the staging of dementia. *Br J Psychiat* 1982; **140**: 566–72.

24. Abas M, Sahakian BJ, Levy R. Neuropsychological deficits and CT scan changes in elderly depressives. *Psychol Med* 1990; **20**: 507–20.

25. Fowler K, Saling M, Conway E et al. Computerized delayed matching to sample and paired associate performance in the early detection of dementia. *App Neuropsychol* 1995; **2**: 72–8.

26. Fowler K, Saling M, Conway E et al. Computerized neuropsychological tests in the early detection of dementia: prospective findings. *J Int Neuropsychol Soc* 1997; **3**: 139–46.

27. Sahakian BJ, Owen AM, Morant NJ et al. Further analysis of the cognitive effects of tetrahydroaminoacridine (THA) in Alzheimer's disease: assessment of attentional and mnemonic function using CANTAB. *Psychopharmacology* 1993; **110**: 395–401.

28. Rusted J, Warburton DM. Effects of scopolamine on working memory in healthy young volunteers. *Psychopharmacology* 1988; **96**: 145–52.

29. Robbins TW, Semple J, Kumar R et al. Effects of scopolamine on delayed matching-to-sample and paired associates tests of visual memory and learning in human subjects: comparison with diazepam and implications for dementia. *Psychopharmacology* 1997; **134**: 95–106.

30. Paolo AM. Psychometric issues in the clinical assessment of memory in aging and neurodegenerative disease. In Troster AI (ed.), *Memory and Neurodegenerative Disease: Biological, Cognitive and Clinical Perspectives*. Cambridge: Cambridge University Press, 1998; 262–77.

31. Lowe C, Rabbitt PM. Test/retest reliability of the CANTAB and ISPOCD neuropsychological batteries. Theoretical and practical issues. *Neuropsychologia* 1998; **36**: 915–23.

32. Harrison JE, Iddon JL, Stow I et al. Cambridge Neuropsychological Test Automated Battery (CANTAB): test–retest reliability characteristics www.cambridgecognition.com

33. Robbins TW, James M, Owen AM et al. The Cambridge Neuropsychological Test Automated Battery (CANTAB): a factor analytic study in large number of elderly volunteers. *Dementia* 1994; **5**: 266–81.

34. Robbins TW, James M, Owen AM et al. A study of performance on tests from the CANTAB battery sensitive to frontal lobe dysfunction in a large number of normal volunteers: implications for theories of executive functioning and cognitive aging. *J Int Neuropsychol Soc* 1998; **4**: 474–90.

35. Luciana M, Nelson CA. The functional emergence of prefrontally-guided working memory systems in four- to eight-year-old children. *Neuropsychologia* 1998; **36**: 273–93.

36. Owen AM, Sahakian BJ, Semple J et al. Visuospatial short-term recognition memory and learning after temporal lobe excision, frontal lobe excision or amygdalo-hippocampectomy. *Neuropsychologia* 1995; **33**: 1–24.

37. Weed MR, Taffe MA, Polis I et al. Performance norms for a rhesus monkey neuropsychological testing battery: acquisition and long term performance. *Cogn Brain Res* 1999; **8**: 185–201.

38. Baker SC, Rogers RD, Owen AM et al. Neural systems engaged by planning: a PET study of the Tower of London task. *Neuropsychologia* 1996; **34**: 515–26.

39. Owen AM, Evans AC, Petrides M. Evidence for a two-stage model of spatial working memory processing within the lateral frontal cortex: a positron emission tomography study. *Cerebral Cortex* 1996; **6**: 31–8.

40. Owen AM, Doyon J, Petrides M, Evans AC. Planning and spatial working memory: a positron emission tomography study in humans. *Eur J Neurosci* 1996; **8**: 353–64.

41. Elliott R, Dolan RJ. Differential neural responses during performance of matching and non-matching to sample tasks at two delay intervals. *J Neurosci* 1999; **19**: 5066–73.

42. Rogers RD, Andrews T, Grasby P et al. Contrasting cortical and sub-cortical PET activations produced by reversal learning and attentional set-shifting in humans. *J Cogn Neurosci* 2000 (in press).

43. Simpson PM, Surmont DJ, Wesnes KA, Wilcock GK. The cognitive drug research computerized assessment system for demented patients: a validation study. *Int J Geriat Psychiat* 1991; **6**: 95–102.

44. Nicholl CG, Lynch S, Kelly CA et al. The cognitive drug research computerised assessment system in the evaluation of early

dementia—is speed the essence? *Int J Geriat Psychiat* 1995; **10**: 199–206.

45. Ebert U, Oerteal R, Wesnes K, Kirch W. Effects of physostigmine on scopolamine-induced changes in quantitative electroencephalogram and cognitive performance. *Hum Psychopharmacol* 1998; **13**: 199–210.

46. Mohr E, Walker D, Randolph C *et al*. Utility of clinical trial batteries in the measurement of Alzheimer's and Huntington's dementia. *Int J Psychogeriat* 1996; **8**: 397–411.

47. Templeton A, Barker A, Wesnes K, Wilkinson D. A double-blind, placebo-controlled single dose trial of intravenous flumazenil in Alzheimer's disease. *Hum Psychopharmacol Clin Exp* 1999; **14**: 239–45.

29

The Assessment of Depressive States

Thomas R. Thompson and William M. McDonald

Emory University School of Medicine, Atlanta, GA, USA

The diagnosis of depressive states in the elderly requires a multi-dimensional approach and should not be undertaken without a clear understanding of the normal aging process and the psychosocial factors that are unique to the elderly. The accurate assessment of depressive disorders in the elderly is essential, since this population is often subject to more adverse side effects from pharmacotherapy, and concurrent depression can limit compliance with medical treatments and worsen the cognitive decline associated with dementia. Further, depression can adversely affect the clinical course of other medical illnesses and increase morbidity and mortality[1,2]. Depression in late life is not a normal part of aging and is not necessarily more difficult to treat or chronic when compared to depression in younger people[3,4].

A number of authors have drawn attention to the psychosocial stressors that must be taken into account in the diagnosis of depression in the older population and to the high levels of depressive symptoms in the elderly living in the community[5]. Although the prevalence of individuals with major depression may not be as high as for younger subjects in such settings[6,7], the prevalence increases in elderly patients in long-term care facilities and the medically ill[8,9]. Depressive symptoms can lead to accelerated cognitive decline, physical impairment and increased health care costs. The elderly population maintains the highest suicide rate[10,11] so that the social and economic consequences of this disorder are severe.

THE SYNDROME OF LATE-LIFE DEPRESSION

To accurately assess the depressed older adult, the clinician must be aware of the major syndrome encountered in older adults. The major categories of mood disorders outlined in the *Diagnostic and Statistical Manual of Mental Disorders*, 4th edn[12], are major depression, dysthymic disorder (dysthymia) and adjustment disorder (bipolar disorder is discussed elsewhere), which correspond roughly with the International Classification of Diseases 9 (ICD-9)[13] for diagnoses of manic–depressive psychosis, neurotic depression and brief depressive reaction, respectively. The revision of the ICD (ICD-10)[14] has diagnoses of depressive episode and persistent affective state (with a subclassification of dysthymia) that closely approximate the corresponding DSM-IV classifications.

Major depression is distinguished by the severity of symptoms, which may include significant weight loss or weight gain, insomnia or hypersomnia, psychomotor agitation or retardation, diminished ability to think or concentrate, feelings of worthlessness or excessive inappropriate guilt and recurrent thoughts of death or suicide[12]. A melancholic depression (DSM-IV) or severe depression (ICD-10) represents a subtype of major depression that is felt to be preferentially responsive to somatic therapy (i.e. antidepressants and electroconvulsive therapy) and includes symptoms such as a lack of reactivity to pleasurable stimuli, diurnal variation in mood with depression worse in the morning, early morning awakening, psychomotor retardation or agitation, significant weight loss and other factors that may have a bearing on response, including no significant personality disturbance before the onset of a major depressive episode and a previous history of a major depressive episode that may have responded to somatic treatment. In the DSM-IV, depression is sub-typed according to whether the mood disturbance is associated with a seasonal variation (e.g. a temporal relationship between a distinct 60-day period of the year) or psychotic symptoms that are more likely to be mood-congruent (i.e. delusions or hallucinations of a depressive nature). Psychotic depressions may be more common in late life[15].

The DSM-IV now includes a research diagnosis of minor depression. The duration of the episode and the symptoms are the same as major depression. However, in minor depression the number of symptoms required for diagnosis is less compared to major depression. Minor depression is important in the elderly as there is evidence that these individuals have levels of cognitive and functional impairment similar to those who met full criteria for major depression[16].

Dysthymic disorder (dysthymia) is defined as a chronic low-grade depression, which lasts at least 2 years (DSM-IV), or "several" years (ICD-10). Primary dysthymia may occur in older adults due to changing roles and life conditions. Personality styles and the individual's ability to cope with changing life situations may predispose the individual to develop a dysthymic disorder (see Chapters 71, 74). Although certain severe personality disorders are less common in the elderly, long-standing patterns of perfectionism and the need for external gratification can lead to chronic low self-esteem and dysphoria. Dysthymic disorder may also develop secondary to a medical disorder, which leads to chronic debilitation or other psychiatric disorders, such as substance abuse, anxiety disorder or somatization disorder.

The elderly patient may also have to adjust to severe changes in lifestyle and the loss of loved ones. In the DSM-IV, the patient is not classified with an adjustment disorder unless his/her reaction is considered maladaptive and the level of impairment is significantly severe, so as to be greater than what would be normally expected. The ICD-10 outlines similar symptoms under the heading of mild depressive episodes. Several common life events that prove to be stressors in the elderly

Principles and Practice of Geriatric Psychiatry, 2nd edn. Edited by J. R. M. Copeland, M. T. Abou-Saleh and D. G. Blazer

include retirement, financial problems, crime rates, physical illness, the death of a spouse and moving to an institutional setting. Whether the elderly subject's reaction to these stressors is classified as a disorder is a clinical judgement. Regardless, the clinician should watch carefully for the development of symptoms of a major depression if the individual's reaction to stress is persistent or severe.

The symptom profile of older patients with depression has also been posited to differ from that of younger adults, and these subjects are more likely to demonstrate hypochondriacal or somatic symptoms. However, Blazer asserts that this issue is confounded by the significant co-morbidity with other physical illnesses, and these factors must be controlled when making such comparisons[3]. Hypochondriasis, or the belief that one has a serious physical illness, is quite different from an older patient's complaints of physical symptoms such as constipation and nausea. In the hypochondriacal patient these complaints are more likely to be long-standing and to fluctuate over time. In the depressed patient, somatic complaints may become severe and delusional. Somatic delusions can be bizarre and unshakeable. Whereas the patient with hypochondriasis is willing to consider a physical cause for the symptoms, the depressed patient is more likely to have a bizarre rationalization for his symptoms that defy logical explanation. The depressed patient is also apt to show a history of neurovegetative symptoms that have become progressively worse over time.

THE PROBLEM OF CO-MORBIDITY

The diagnosis and treatment of major depression in older adults is more often complicated by concomitant medical illness and/or cognitive decline than in their younger counterparts. For example, over 10% of patients who are initially diagnosed with dementia were found to have an affective disorder when seen in follow-up[17–19]. This misdiagnosis is due to the fact that the symptoms seen in dementia, such as withdrawal, diminished ability to think and concentrate and psychomotor retardation, occur in both dementia and depression. In fact, over 50% of patients with dementing illnesses such as Alzheimer's disease may also have depressive symptoms, with 20% meeting criteria for a major depressive episode[20].

Alexopoulos et al.[21] demonstrated that a significant minority of individuals with depression and reversible cognitive deficits eventually progress to true dementia within 3 years. Krishnan et al.[24] found an association between apolipoprotein E-e3/e4 (which has been linked to Alzheimer's disease[22,23]) and major depression in later life, further supporting the association of dementia and late-onset depression[24].

Various clinical studies have shown that depressed older subjects are less likely to demonstrate depressed mood[25] or guilt[26] and more prone to complain of fatigue[27]. Other researchers emphasize that these differing presentations are the result of accompanying dementia and medical illness that are more likely to occur in older depressed patients, and that depressed elderly patients without concomitant medical illnesses have presentations similar to younger subjects[28].

Support for this latter view has been provided by Blazer and his colleagues[29], who compared depressive symptoms in a group of middle-aged (35–50 year-old) and older (>60 years) inpatients with melancholic depression. The symptom profiles of these patients were markedly similar to the elderly, differing only in their more frequent reporting of weight loss and less frequent suicidal thoughts. Finally, Blazer discusses some of the misconceptions of depression in the elderly, pointing out that as discussed above, symptomatically there is little difference when compared to adult early-onset depression.

TAKING A HISTORY FROM THE DEPRESSED OLDER ADULT AND FAMILY

The key elements in the patient's history include evidence of a previous psychiatric illness especially a major depressive or manic episode, particularly if that episode responded to somatic therapy (e.g. lithium, antidepressants or electroconvulsive therapies). Obtaining pharmacy and other medical records regarding the symptoms, dose and the duration of medication trials can further aid in the assessment of depressed individuals. Major depression is a recurrent illness, with about half of the patients experiencing two or more episodes in their lifetime. In order to distinguish dementia from depression, researchers have relied upon the findings in the family and individual histories, mental status and laboratory examinations. Determining the time of onset of the depressive symptoms may also be useful, since most dementias are slowly developing, with early evidence of cognitive decline (e.g. the inability to balance a checkbook) being present months to years before the typical form of the disease becomes apparent. In contrast, the course of depressive illness may seem more abrupt.

An accurate family history may also provide valuable diagnostic information, since dementing illnesses (e.g. Huntington's chorea and Alzheimer's disease, particularly the early-onset form) and major depression (especially the early-onset form) have both been demonstrated to have a genetic diathesis. The family history should also include questions about neurological and medical disease, alcohol/drug abuse, anxiety, suicide and psychosis, since these conditions are often associated with concomitant depression.

THE MENTAL STATUS EXAMINATION

The mental status examination and standardized depression rating scales may also aid in determining whether the patient has depression, dementia or (as is often the case) both.

The depressed patient approaches the mental status examination with the same lack of interest that is also apparent in other areas of his/her life. The depressed patient may attempt to prematurely terminate the interview or consistently refuse to try and answer questions. On the other hand, the demented patient may be quite concerned about his/her declining cognitive skills and, at the same time, make attempts to cover their deficits with confabulation[30]. He/she may use notes and other reminders to keep up with facts and uncovering his/her deficits might be quite distressing. This is in marked contrast to the apathetic attitude of the depressed patient. The depressed inpatient is also more likely to be able to find his/her way around the ward and to keep track of the ward routine and personnel. In contrast, the demented patient will forget mealtimes and confuse familiar faces. This confusion may often get worse as evening approaches and is incorporated in the well-known clinical syndrome of "sundowning".

The mental status examination of patients with physical illnesses may show primarily problems with concentration and attention. In more severe cases, evidence of delirium may be present. Delirium is diagnosed when the level of consciousness becomes impaired. In this condition, disorientation and memory impairment may be present along with illusions (which are misinterpretations of environmental stimuli), hallucinations and disturbances in psychomotor activity and the sleep–wake cycle. As opposed to dementia, these symptoms usually evolve over hours and days rather than months and may show a waxing and waning course along with autonomic instability.

A common clinical dilemma occurs in patients who are known to be demented, but in whom the clinician seeks to make an accurate diagnosis of depression. In these patients, the clinician may need to assign more weight to neurovegetative signs, such as weight loss and insomnia, although these same symptoms may occur in non-depresssed demented patients if they are too disorganized to prepare a meal or have night-time confusion. Some researchers have pointed to the presence of cognitive symptoms of depression (i.e. depressed mood, anxiety, helplessness, hopelessness and worthlessness) as being more prominent in demented patients, whereas neurovegetative signs are notably absent[31].

Monitoring the patient over time, observing for some overall consistent pattern of depressed mood and affect, is also helpful. Although there is little or no data to support empiric trials of antidepressants, given the relatively low side-effect profile of the newer antidepressants[32] (SSRIs: see Chapter 78), many clinicians will often attempt a trial of an antidepressant in these difficult situations in hopes the treatment may improve cognition and function.

PSYCHOLOGICAL TESTS

Standardized assessments of cognitive performance (e.g. Wechsler Adult Intelligence Scale and Clinical Dementia Rating Scale[33]) may also be useful in distinguishing depression and dementia. The depressed patient will more likely show results that are inconsistent over time and are effort-dependent. The demented patient will demonstrate a more global decline, with relatively lower scores on aspects of the testing requiring adaptability and processing of information (e.g. performance IQ) as opposed to rote skills and long-term memory tasks (e.g. verbal IQ).

Standardized depression scales may yield false-positive results in demented patients, particularly if they are heavily weighted for difficulties symptoms, such as with attention and concentration, which overlap with symptoms of depression. Depression scales that have been specifically designed to grade levels of depression in patients known to be demented include the Cornell Depression Scale[34] and the Dementia Mood Assessment Scale[35]. The Geriatric Depression Scale (GDS), Beck Depression Inventory (BDI) and the Montgomery–Asberg Depression Rating Scale (MADRS) are other useful tests that can help aid in evaluation of a depressed patient[36-38].

LABORATORY TESTS

The common laboratory tests for depression may lose much of their specificity in demented patients. The Dexamet has one suppression test that is frequently abnormal in dementia[39,40].

The sleep electroencephalogram, however, does maintain its specificity and is able to distinguish a group of elderly depressed patients from those with dementia[41,42].

Any physical illness that can potentially affect the central nervous system can present with depressive and dementing symptoms; these illnesses include encephalitis, chronic subdural hematoma and normal pressure hydrocephalus. Depressive symptoms such as fatigue, insomnia, weight loss and concentration problems can occur in other illnesses that do not directly affect the central nervous system (CNS). These illnesses include infectious diseases (e.g. tuberculosis, influenza), cardiovascular disease (e.g. congestive heart failure), endocrine abnormalities (e.g. thyroid disease, diabetes), electrolyte disturbances (e.g. hyponatremia, hypocalcemia), renal and hepatic disease.

Recent evidence has indicated that both cerebral vascular accidents and periventricular[42] white matter disease are related to depressive symptoms in the elderly[44,45].

MEDICAL WORK-UP

Medical conditions also present with depressive symptoms in the elderly. Many of these medical conditions are reversible with

Table 29.1 Laboratory work-up in the depressed elderly patient

Laboratory test	Underlying condition
Complete blood count	Infectious disease
	Encephalitis
	Meningitis
	Sub-acute bacterial endocarditis
	Anemia
Electrolytes	Hypokalemia
	Hyponatremia
	Diabetes
	Uremia
B$_{12}$/Folate	Pernicious anemia
Thyroid panel	Hypo/hyperthyroidism
Liver enzymes	Hepatitis
	Liver cancer
Calcium/phosphorus	Hyperparathyroidism
Guiaic stool	Colon disease
Urinalysis	Infection
	Renal disease
Consider additional test including:	Particularly patients who complain of fatigue, edema, shortness of breath or who are being considered for antidepressant therapy
Electrocardiogram	
Electroencephalogram	When delirium may be a concern or to screen for a mass lesion
Urine drug screen	For lead (exposure to paint), mercury (textile manufacturing), organophosphates and arsenic (insecticides). Also drugs of abuse (e.g. opiates, marijuana, etc.)
Human immune deficiency virus (HIV)	Exposure to potentially contaminated blood products (surgery, drug use) or a history of promiscuity or homosexuality
Brain computed tomography	Neoplasia, stroke
Brain magnetic resonance imaging	Particularly to view the posterior brain stem

proper treatment, and estimates of the number of patients with reversible conditions presenting as dementia have been as high as 15%[17]. The work-up of medical conditions that present with depressive symptoms in the elderly includes a personal history of medical illness, mental status examination and laboratory tests[46].

The physical examination and laboratory diagnosis is crucial in the diagnosis of medical disorders. The typical laboratory screening for elderly patients with depressive symptoms is outlined in Table 29.1. Clearly, the medical history and physical examination would influence the laboratory testing that was actually done. The neurologic examination should be particularly thorough and include an examination of both subtle (e.g. frontal reflex signs) and prominent (e.g. reflex changes) signs of neurologic dysfunction.

MEDICATION HISTORY

Medication, including the antihypertensive medications such as propranolol and centrally acting α-methyldopa and reserpine, has been shown to cause depressive symptoms. Drugs such as alcohol are also frequent causes of depression in the elderly, as are the barbiturates that are used as sedatives. Patients at risk should be screened for heavy metals, including lead, arsenic and the organophosphates.

SUMMARY

Depressive symptoms are common in the elderly, whereas the syndrome of a major depressive episode is relatively rare[6,45].

Symptoms of depression can be manifestations of either dementing or medical illnesses, both of which are common in the elderly. Psychosocial factors that are unique to the elderly may be etiologic in the genesis of depressive symptoms, but nevertheless require the clinician to assess each patient fully and treat as appropriate. Accurate treatment mandates as detailed history, often with collaboration with the family, and a thorough medical evaluation for other co-morbid illnesses that may contribute to the patient's current presentation. The treatment of depressive symptoms in the elderly requires an understanding of both the origin of these symptoms and the proper treatment of the underlying disorder, whether it be due to medical, dementing, psychosocial or melancholic factors.

REFERENCES

1. Ford DE, Mead LA, Chang PP *et al*. Depression is a risk factor for coronary artery disease in men: the precursors study. *Arch Intern Med* 1998; **158**: 1422–6.
2. Marsh C. Psychiatric presentation of medical illness. *Psychiat Clin N Am* 1997; **20**(1): 181–90.
3. Blazer DG. Depression in the elderly: myths and misconceptions. *Psychiat Clin N Am* 1997; **20**(1): 111–19.
4. Blazer DG, Burchette B, Service C, George LK. The association of age and depression among the elderly. An epidemiologic exploration. *J Gerontol* 1991; **46**: M210–15.
5. Blazer DG, Williams CD. Epidemiology of dysphoria and depression in elderly population. *Am J Psychiat* 1980; **137**: 439–44.
6. Myers JK, Weissmann MM, Tischler GL *et al*. Six-month prevalence of psychiatric disorders in three communities, 1980–1982. *Arch Gen Psychiat* 1984; **41**: 959–67.
7. Blazer D, Hughes DC, George LK. The epidemiology of depression in an elderly community population. *Gerontologist* 1987; **27**: 28.
8. Parmelee PA, Katz IR, Lawton MP. Depression among institutionalized aging: assessment and prevalence estimation. *J Gerontol* 1989; **44**: M22–9.
9. Koenig HG, Meador KG, Cohen HJ *et al*. Depression in elderly hospitalized medically ill patients. *Arch Intern Med* 1988; **148**: 1929–36.
10. Meechan PJ, Saltman LE, Sattin RW. Suicides among older United States residents: epidemiologic characteristics and trends. *Am J Publ Health* 1991; **81**: 1198–2000.
11. *Suicide in the United States, 1980–1992*. Reported by the Division of Violence Prevention, National Center for Injury Prevention and Control, Center for Disease Control, Atlanta, GA, January 1996.
12. APA. *Diagnostic and Statistical Manual of Mental Disorders*, 4th edn. Washington, DC: American Psychiatric Association Press, 1994.
13. World Health Organization. *Mental Disorders: Glossary and Guide to their Classification in Accordance with the Ninth Revision of the International Classification of Diseases*. Geneva: WHO, 1978.
14. *International Classification of Diseases, 10* (ICD-10). Draft of Chapter V, Categories FOO, F99 (Mental, Behavioural and Development Disorders). Clinical descriptions and diagnostic guidelines. Geneva: WHO, 1986.
15. Kiloh LG, Garside RF. The independence of neurotic depression and endogenous depression. *Br J Psychiat* 1963; **109**: 451–63.
16. Lyness JM, King DA, Cox C *et al*. The importance of subsyndromal depression in older primary care patients: Prevalence and associated functional disability. *J Am Geriat Soc* 1999; **47**: 647–52.
17. Marsden CD, Harrison MJ. Outcome of investigation of patients with presenile dementia. *Br Med J* 1972; **ii**: 249–52.
18. Nott PN, Fleminger JJ. Presenile dementia: the difficulties of early diagnosis. *Acta Psychiat Scand* 1975; **51**: 210–17.
19. Ron MA, Toone BK, Garralda ME *et al*. Diagnostic accuracy in presenile dementia. *Br J Psychiat* 1979; **134**: 161–8.
20. Wragg RE, Jeste DV. Overview of depression and psychosis in Alzheimer's disease. *Am J Psychiat* 1989; **146**: 577–87.
21. Alexopoulous GS, Meyers BS, Young RC *et al*. The course of geriatric.
22. Saunders AM, Strittmatter WJ, Schmechel D *et al*. Association of apolipoprotein E allele epsilon 4 with late-onset familial and sporadic Alzheimer's disease. *Neurology* 1993; **43**: 1467–72.
23. Strittmatter WJ, Saunders AM, Schmechel D *et al*. Apolipoprotein E: high-avidity binding to beta-amyloid and increased frequency of type 4 allele in late-onset familial Alzheimer disease. *Proc Natl Acad Sci USA* 1993; **90**: 1977–81.
24. Krishnan KR, Tupler LA, Ritchie JC *et al*. Apolipoprotein E-epsilon 4 frequency in geriatric depression. *Biol Psychiat* 1996; **40**(1): 69–71.
25. Salzman C, Shader RI. Depression in the elderly: I. Relationship between depression, psychological defence mechanisms, and physical illness. *J Am Geriat Soc* 1978; **26**: 253–60.
26. Winokur G, Behan D, Schlesser M. Clinical and biological aspects of depression in the elderly. In Cole JO, Barrett JE (eds), *Psychopathology in the Aged*. New York: Raven, 1980; 145–55.
27. Gaitz C, Scott J. Age and measurement of mental health. *J Health Soc Behav* 1972; **13**: 55–67.
28. Himmelhock JM, Auchenbach R, Fuchs CS. The dilemma of depression in the elderly. *J Clin Psychiat* 1982; **43**: 26.
29. Blazer D, Bachar JR, Hughes DC. Major depression with melancholia: a comparison of middle-aged and elderly adults. *J Am Geriat Soc* 1987; **35**: 927–32.
30. Wells CE. Pseudodementia. *Am J Psychiat* 1979; **136**: 895–900.
31. Lazarus LW, Newton N, Cohler B. Frequency and presentation of depressive symptoms in patients with primary degenerative dementia. *Am J Psychiat* 1987; **144**: 41–45.
32. Goldberg RJ. Selective serotonin reuptake inhibitors: infrequent medical adverse effects. *Arch Fam Med* 1998; **7**: 78–84.
33. Hughes CP, Berg L, Danziger WL *et al*. A new clinical scale for the staging of dementia. *Br J Psychiat* 1982; **140**: 566–72.
34. Alexopoulos GS, Abrams RC, Young RC *et al*. Diagnosis and Assessment Cornell scale for depression in dementia. *Biol Psychiat* 1988; **23**: 271–84.
35. Sunderland T, Alterman IS, Yount D *et al*. A new scale for the assessment of depressed mood in demented patients. *Am J Psychiat* 1988; **145**: 955–9.
36. Montgomery SA, Asberg MA. A new depression scale designed to be sensitive to change. *Br J Psychiat* 1979; **134**: 382–9.
37. Beck AT, Ward CH, Mendelson M *et al*. An inventory for measuring depression. *Arch Gen Psychiat* 1961; **4**: 541–51.
38. Yesavage J, Brink TL. Development and validation of a geriatric depression screening scale: a preliminary report. *J Psychiat Res* 1983; **7**: 37–49.
39. The APA Task Force on Laboratory Tests in Psychiatry. The dexamethasone suppression test: an overview of its current status in psychiatry. *Am J Psychiat* 1987; **144**: 1253–62.
40. Krishnan KE, Heyman A, Ritchie JX *et al*. Depression in early-onset Alzheimer's disease: clinical and neuroendocrine correlates. *Biol Psychiat* 1988; **24**: 937–40.
41. Buysee DJ, Reynolds CF, Kupfer DJ *et al*. Electroencephalographic sleep in depressive pseudodementia. *Arch Gen Psychiat* 1988; **45**: 568–75.
42. Reynolds CF, Kupfer DJ, Houck PR *et al*. Reliable discrimination of elderly depressed and demented patients by electroencephalographic sleep data. *Arch Gen Psychiat* 1988; **45**: 258–64.
43. McDonald WM, Krishnan KRR, Doraiswamy PM, Blazer DG. Occurrence of subcortical hyperintensities in elderly subjects with mania. *Psychiat Res Neuroimag* 1991; **40**: 211–20.
44. Krishnan KRR, Goli V, Ellinwood EH *et al*. Leukoencephalopathy in patients diagnosed as major depressive. *Biol Psychiat* 1988; **23**: 529.
45. McDonald WM, Krishnan KRR, Doraiswamy PM *et al*. Magnetic resonance findings in patients with early-onset Alzheimer's disease. *Biol Psychiat* 1990; **27**: 162A.
46. Blazer DG. Depression and the older man. *Med Clin N Am* 1999; **83**(5): 1305–16.

The Geriatric Depression Scale: Its Development and Recent Application

Ruth O'Hara[1] and Jerome A. Yesavage[2]

[1]Department of Psychiatry and Behavioral Sciences, Stanford University School of Medicine, CA, and [2]Veterans Administration, Palo Alto Health Care System, CA, USA

Developed in 1983, the Geriatric Depression Scale (GDS) is a 30-item self-report measure for rating depression in elderly adults[1]. The identification of depression in older adults is of particular importance to clinicians, since depression is the most common psychiatric disorder in this population and can be associated with morbidity and mortality[2].

The GDS was designed to address the unique characteristics of geriatric depression and the subsequent difficulties in rating depression in older adults using scales developed for younger populations. Somatic complaints are less useful indicators of depression in the elderly than in young adults, since such symptoms often accompany the normal aging process. Depression in older adults is more often accompanied by subjective complaints regarding decline in memory and cognition than is depression in younger adults. Questions pertaining to suicidal intent or one's hopefulness regarding the future can be interpreted differently by elderly adults, who are in the latter stages of their lifespans. To address these issues, the GDS excludes questions pertaining to somatic complaints, registers a cognitive dimension of depression and focuses dominantly on the worries of the individual and how that person interprets his/her quality of life. Additionally, the GDS employs a yes–no format for both economy of time and ease of self-administration in this population.

The scale was developed and validated in two phases. First, 100 widely varied yes–no questions were selected and tested for their potential to distinguish depressed elderly adults from normal controls. The 30 questions correlating most highly with depression were chosen for inclusion in the final version of the GDS. Second, validity of the scale was established by comparing the mean GDS scores for subjects classified as normal, mildly depressed or severely depressed, using the Research Diagnostic Criteria (RDC) for depression. The mean GDS scores for these three groups were reliably different and were ordered in accordance with the differing RDC scores[1]. The scale has been found to have high internal consistency and high test–retest reliability. A score of 11 or higher has been found to indicate the presence of depression, yielding 84% sensitivity and 95% specificity[3].

The GDS has been utilized widely in clinical practice and research and has been shown to be a reliable and valid measure of depression in outpatient, nursing home and hospital settings[4-6].

Additionally, the GDS is sensitive to depression among elderly adults suffering from mild to moderate dementia and elderly adults with physical illnesses[7].

To date, the GDS has been translated into 21 languages, including Spanish and Chinese. It is in the public domain, and available on the Web (http://www.stanford.edu/~yesavage/GDS.html). A 15-item, short form of the GDS has been developed and validated[7]. Additionally, administrations of the GDS by telephone and by requiring caregivers to answer the questions have been validated[8,9].

Overall, the GDS provides a sensitive measure of depression in older adults that is time-efficient, easy to administer and reliable and valid in a broad range of clinical and research settings.

REFERENCES

1. Yesavage JA, Brink TL, Rose TL et al. Development and validation of a geriatric depression screening scale: a preliminary report. J Psychiat Res 17: 37–49.
2. McGuire MH, Rabins PV. Mood disorders. In Coffey CE, Cummings JL (eds), Textbook of Geriatric Neuropsychiatry. American Psychiatric Press: Washington, DC, 1994; 243–60.
3. Brink TL, Yesavage JA, Lum O et al. Screening tests for geriatric depression. Clin Gerontol 1982; 1: 37–44.
4. McGivney SA, Mulvihill M, Taylor B. Validating the GDS depression screen in the nursing home. J Am Geriat Soc 42: 490–2.
5. Lyons JS, Strain JJ, Hammer JS et al. Reliability, validity, and temporal stability of the Geriatric Depression Scale in hospitalized elderly. Int J Psychiat Med 1989; 192: 203–9.
6. Burke WJ, Nitcher RL, Roccaforte WH, Wengel SP. A prospective evaluation of the Geriatric Depression Scale in an outpatient geriatric assessment center. J Am Geriat Soc 1992; 40: 1227–30.
7. Sheik JL, Yesavage JA. Geriatric Depression Scale (GDS): recent evidence and development of a shorter version. In Brink TL (ed.), Clinical Gerontology: A Guide to Assessment and Intervention. New York: Hawthorn, 1986; 165–73.
8. Burke WJ, Roccaforte WH, Wengel SP. The reliability and validity of the Geriatric Depression Rating Scale administered by telephone. J Am Geriat Soc 1985; 43: 674–9.
9. Logsdon RG, Teri L. Depression in Alzheimer's disease patients: caregivers as surrogate reporters. J Am Geriat Soc 1995; 43: 150–5.

Center for Epidemiologic Studies Depression Scale: Use among Older Adults

Dan G. Blazer

Duke University Medical Center, Durham, NC, USA

The Center for Epidemiologic Studies Depression Scale (CES-D) is a depression screening instrument which has been applied widely in epidemiologic studies including many community-based studies of older adults[1–3]. The scale consists of 20 items which on factor analysis among older adults fall into four different factors. The first factor is depressed affect, and items that load on this factor include: "bothered by things that usually don't bother me", "I could not shake the blues", "I felt depressed", "I felt lonely", "I had crying spells" and "I felt sad". The second factor is positive affect and includes the items: "I felt as good as other people", "I felt hopeful about the future", "I thought my life had been a failure", "I was happy" and "I enjoyed life". The third factor is somatic complaints and includes the items: "I did not feel like eating", "I had trouble keeping my mind on what I was doing", "My sleep was restless", "I felt like everything was an effort", "I talked less than usual" and "I could not get going". The final factor is interpersonal relations and includes the items: "People were unfriendly" and "I felt that people disliked me". Each item is rated on a 1–4 scale, depending on the frequency of symptoms the week prior to the administration of the scale. Therefore, the range of answers is 0–60. A score of 16 or greater is considered indicative of clinically significant depression[1].

Murrell *et al.*[4] found, when using the CES-D in a community of over 2000 community-dwelling adults, 55 years of age and older in Kentucky, that the mean score was 8.9 for African-Americans and 9.2 for Whites. When they applied the cut-off noted above for clinically significant depressive symptoms, 12.8% of African-Americans and 13.7% of Whites had clinically significant depression[4]. Berkman *et al.*[5] found that 16% of both African-Americans and Whites in an urban community scored above the threshold for clinically significant symptoms. When control variables are taken into account, such as gender, socioeconomic status and functional health, the association of age and depression disappears (whereas in uncontrolled analysis there is a positive association between age and depression) using the CES-D[6].

When using the CES-D in older adults, there is little difference by gender and little difference by race/ethnicity[2]. In a cross-sectional analysis, age is negatively associated with somatic complaints, lower education is associated with more complaints of depressed affect and interpersonal problems, African-American race is associated with increased interpersonal complaints and cognitive impairment associated with somatic complaints and interpersonal complaints. Of all control factors, however, disability is most closely associated with all four of the factors noted above.

In summary, the CES-D is a useful screening scale for depressive symptoms in community (and clinical) samples of older adults. The one drawback to this scale is that it requires responding along a spectrum of four responses (little or none, some of the time, most of the time, or all the time) over the previous week compared to a simple yes–no format, as is found in other symptom screening scales. The scale has been used extensively in older adults and therein lies its greatest value for future epidemiologic studies as well as clinical screening efforts.

REFERENCES

1. Radloff LS. The CES-D Scale: a self-report depression scale for research in general populations. *Appl Psychol Meas* 1977; **1**: 385–401.
2. Blazer DG, Landerman LR, Hays JC *et al*. Symptoms of depression among community-dwelling elderly African-American and White older adults. *Psychol Med* 1998; **28**: 1311–20.
3. Kohout FJ, Berkman LF, Evans DA, Cornoni-Huntley J. Two shorter forms of the CES-D depression symptoms index. *J Aging Health* 1993; **5**: 179–93.
4. Murrell SA, Himmelfarb S, Wright K. Prevalence of depression and its correlates in older adults. *Am J Epidemiol* 1983; **117**: 173–85.
5. Berkman LF, Berkman CS, Casl S *et al*. Depressive symptoms in relation to physical health and functioning in the elderly. *Am J Epidemiol* 1986; **12**: 372–88.
6. Blazer D, Burchette B, Service CS, George LK. The association of age and depression among the elderly: an epidemiologic exploration. *J Gerontol Med Sci* 1991; **46**: M210–15.

30

The Development of the EURO-D Scale

Martin Prince

Institute of Psychiatry, London, UK

BACKGROUND

The 11 country EURODEP consortium, assembled an unprecedented body of data; 14 population-based surveys of mental health in late life, including 21 724 older Europeans aged 65 years and over. Most centres had used either GMS/AGECAT[1] or the very similar SHORT-CARE[2] as their index of clinical case-level depression. However, three centres had used the Centre for Epidemiological Studies Depression scale (CES-D)[3], one the Zung Self-rating Depression Scale (ZSDS)[4] and one the Comprehensive Psychopathological Rating Scale (CPRS)[5]. Our challenge, therefore, was to derive from these instruments a common depression symptom scale, allowing risk factor profiles to be compared between centres[6].

METHOD[6]

The instruments were scrutinized for common items. Algorithms for fitting items from other instruments to GMS were derived by either: (a) empirical observation of the nature of the relationship between items in different scales where they had been administered together; or (b) expert opinion. The resulting 12-item scale (see Table 30.1) was checked in each centre for internal consistency, criterion validity and uniformity of factor analytic profile.

RESULTS[6,7]

The EURO-D, however derived, is an internally consistent scale. Cronbach alphas for the 14 centres ranged from 0.58 to 0.80. It seemed also to capture the essence of its parent instrument. Correlations with the CES-D in all four centres using that measure exceeded 0.90, and the correlation with the Zung was 0.84. A cut-point of 3/4 on the EURO-D scale predicted a GMS/AGECAT computerized diagnosis of depression with 70–80% sensitivity at 80–95% specificity. Principal components factor analysis demonstrated that a very similar two-factor solution seemed appropriate in all centres, however the scale had been derived; depression, tearfulness and wishing to die loaded on the first factor (affective suffering) and loss of interest, poor concentration and lack of enjoyment on the second (motivation).

In general, EURO-D scores increased with age, women scored higher than men, and widowed and separated subjects higher than others. The gender effect was negligible among the never-married but was not modified by age. In most centres EURO-D could be reduced into two well-characterized factors; affective suffering, responsible for the gender difference, and motivation, accounting for the positive association with age.

CONCLUSIONS

Large between-centre differences in depression symptoms as assessed by EURO-D were explained neither by demography nor by the depression measure used in the survey. Consistent, small effects of age, gender and marital status were observed across Europe. Depression may be overdiagnosed in older persons

Table 30.1 EURO-D Scale.
The Geriatric Mental State (from which EURO-D is derived) is a semi-structured clinical interview. The following instructions apply:
1. Each question should be asked as it is written. The sections in parentheses are additional prompts to clarify the question if it has not been understood.
2. Sections in *italic* script provide the criteria by which the interviewer judges from the response whether the symptom is present or absent.

	EURO-D item	Corresponding GMS question
1.	Depression	Have you been sad (depressed, miserable in low spirits, blue) recently?
2.	Pessimism	How do you see your future? *Pessimistic, empty expectations or bleak future*
3.	Wishing death	Have you ever felt that you would rather be dead? *Has ever felt suicidal or wished to be dead*
4.	Guilt	Do you tend to blame yourself or feel guilty about anything? *Obvious guilt or self blame*
5.	Sleep	Have you had trouble sleeping recently? *Trouble with sleep or recent change in pattern*
6.	Interest	What is your interest in things? *Less interest than is usual*
7.	Irritability	Have you been irritable recently?
8.	Appetite	What has your appetite been like? *Diminution in the desire for food*
9.	Fatigue	Have you had too little energy (to do the things you want to do)? *Listlessness or subjective energy restriction*
10.	Concentration	How is your concentration? *Difficulty in concentrating on entertainment or reading*
11.	Enjoyment	What have you enjoyed doing recently? *Almost nothing enjoyed*
12.	Tearfulness	Have you cried at all?

Principles and Practice of Geriatric Psychiatry, 2nd edn. Edited by J. R. M. Copeland, M. T. Abou-Saleh and D. G. Blazer
©2002 John Wiley & Sons, Ltd

because of an increase in lack of motivation that may be affectively neutral, and is possibly related to cognitive decline.

The EURO-D scale shows promise as a means of harmonizing data from studies and perhaps trials that have used similar depression outcome measures. In the EURODEP datasets the EURO-D has been used informatively in three ways[7]:

1. To compare EURO-D item prevalence between centres.
2. To compare EURO-D scale distribution between centres.
3. To compare effect sizes for associations between risk factors and EURO-D score between centres.

Researchers might consider using the EURO-D in epidemiological or health services research, either on its own or as a component part of the GMS. Its principal advantage at present is the large amount of normative data available from the many population-based studies in different parts of the world to have used the GMS. A limitation of the scale is its current format, which relies upon interviewer administration and rating. A future priority will be to develop self-report forms and test their equivalence against the current version.

REFERENCES

1. Copeland JRM, Dewey ME, Griffith-Jones HM. A computerized psychiatric diagnostic system and case nomenclature for elderly subjects: GMS and AGECAT. *Psychol Med* 1986; **16**: 89–99.
2. Gurland B, Golden RR, Teresi JA *et al*. The SHORT-CARE: an efficient instrument for the assessment of depression, dementia and disability. *J Gerontol* 1984; **39**: 166–9.
3. Radloff LS. The CES-D scale: a self-report depression scale for research in the general population. *Appl Psychol Meas* 1977; **1**: 385–401.
4. Zung WWK. A self-rating depression scale. *Arch Gen Psychiat* 1965; **12**: 62–70.
5. Asberg M, Perris C, Schalling D *et al*. CPRS: development and applications of a psychiatric rating scale. *Acta Psychiat Scand* 1978; **271**(suppl): 1–69.
6. Prince M, Beekman A, Fuhrer R *et al*. Depression symptoms in late-life assessed using the EURO-D scale. Effect of age, gender and marital status in 14 European centres. *Br J Psychiat* 1999; **174**: 339–45.
7. Prince M, Reischies F, Beekman ATF *et al*. The development of the EURO-D scale—a European Union initiative to compare symptoms of depression in 14 European centres. *Br J Psychiat* 1999; **174**: 330–8.

31

Interviews Aimed at Differential Psychiatric Diagnosis

GMS–HAS–AGECAT Package

John R. M. Copeland

Department of Psychiatry, Royal Liverpool University Hospital, UK

For epidemiological and other studies of mental illness and morbidity in older age it is important to ensure as far as possible that the differences in the levels of cases of illness found between geographical areas and between studies at different points in time are not due to methodological differences and, in particular, the way the diagnoses themselves are made. To overcome this problem, standardized interviews were introduced. The GMS–HAS–AGECAT Package consists of a series of interviews designed to be given to a subject and his/her informant for assessing the dementias and depression, with optional sections for minor mental illness[1,2]. The Geriatric Mental State (GMS) was derived originally from the Present State Examination[3] and the Mental Status Schedule[4]. Substantial modifications and additions were incorporated to make it more applicable to older populations and to increase emphasis on organic states. The Package now provides, in addition to the GMS, which is an interview with the subject, the History and Aetiology Schedule (HAS) for an informant, which allows the assessment of onset and course of illness, past history, family history and certain risk factors for dementia, depression and other mental illness. The Secondary Dementia Schedule provides a semi-structured framework to aid in collecting information required for the NINCDS–ADRDA (National Institute of Neurology and Communicative Disorders and Stroke–Alzheimer's Disease and Related Disorders Association) criteria[5] and the assessment of daily living.

Standardization of diagnosis is achieved by the AGECAT (Automated Geriatric Examination for Computer Assisted Taxonomy) computer-assisted differential diagnosis[6–8]. Based on an extensive decision tree method, the system aggregates the data into scores and allots each subject to levels of diagnostic confidence on each of eight diagnostic syndrome clusters, organic, schizophrenia/paranoid, mania, depression (psychotic and neurotic type) (levels 0–5), obsessional, hypochondriacal, phobic and anxiety neurosis (levels 0–4). Levels 3 and above are what would usually be recognized by psychiatrists as cases of illness. The computer then compares these levels with one another to derive a final differential diagnosis and flags cases where the decision has been difficult. The validity of the AGECAT diagnosis has been assessed against psychiatrists' diagnoses on the same patients. The range of kappa values for the agreement between AGECAT and psychiatrists' diagnoses for organic states is 0.80–0.88 and for depressive states 0.76–0.80[6]. Outcome studies are now providing additional validation. After 3 years' follow-up, over 83% of AGECAT cases of organic disorder identified in a community study were either dead or still dementing. One-third of depressed cases were also depressed 3 years later[9]. Post mortem validation studies are in progress.

In the second stage AGECAT uses the data from the HAS to take the diagnosis to a further stage, dividing organic states into acute or chronic, and the latter into the different types of dementia using a standardized form of the Hachinski score[10]. It also identifies bereavements and flags coexistent immobility, pain, life-long intellectual function and physical illness.

The GMS can be used by trained lay workers and provides a diagnosis by AGECAT. When used in epidemiological studies it is possible to derive prevalence figures for the full range of psychiatric morbidity using a one-stage design[11]. The measures are therefore economical as well as reliable and valid. The Package does not rely on special psychological tests as these are not applicable across cultures or socioeconomic groups or with populations of varying literacy. The interviews have also been transferred for presentation on laptop computer, which improves accuracy and communication, avoids delays and costs in inputting data, and provides rapid access to results and easy quality control of interviewing techniques[12].

These measures have been used in a number of projects, including the Medical Research Council (UK) ALPHA[13,14] study of the incidence of the dementias and the multicentre Cognitive Function and Ageing Study, the EURODEP EC-funded Concerted Action[16], the ongoing ASIADEP studies in 12 Asian centres and the 10/66 Club studies on the prevalence of dementia in India, Latin America and Africa, as well as forming part of the minimum data set required by the EURODEM (EC Concerted Action on Epidemiology and Prevention of Dementia)[17,18]. The GMS has been translated and used in a wide range of languages. Recently, algorithms have been developed for ICD-10, DSM-III-R and DSM-IV and compared favourably with psychiatrists' diagnoses using these international criteria. The HAS has been shortened and modified to provide for the criteria of Lewy body dementia and other recognized dementia classifications.

REFERENCES

1. Copeland JRM, Kelleher MJ, Kellett JM *et al.* A semi-structured clinical interview for the assessment of diagnosis and mental state in

the elderly. The Geriatric Mental State 1. Development and reliability. *Psychol Med* 1976; **6**: 439–49.

2. Gurland BJ, Fleiss JL, Goldberg K *et al.* A semi-structured clinical interview for the assessment of diagnosis and mental state in the elderly. The Geriatric Mental State Schedule 2. A factor analysis. *Psychol Med* 1976; **6**: 451–9.

3. Wing JK, Cooper JE, Sartorius N. *The Description and Classification of Psychiatric Symptoms: An Instruction Manual for the PSE and Catego System.* London: Cambridge University Press, 1974.

4. Spitzer RL, Endicott J, Fleiss JL, Cohen J. Psychiatric Status Schedule: a technique for evaluating psychopathology and impairment in role functioning. *Arch Gen Psychiat* 1970; **23**: 41–55.

5. McKhann G, Drachman D, Folstein M *et al.* Clinical diagnosis of Alzheimer's disease: Report of the NINCDS–ADRDA Work Group under the auspices of Department of Health and Human Services Task Force on Alzheimer's Disease. *Neurology* 1984; **34**: 939–44.

6. Copeland JRM, Dewey ME, Griffiths-Jones HM. Computerised psychiatric diagnostic system and case nomenclature for elderly subjects: GMS and AGECAT. *Psychol Med* 1986; **16**: 89–99.

7. Copeland JRM, Dewey ME, Henderson AS *et al.* The Geriatric Mental State (GMS) used in the community. Replication studies of the computerised diagnosis AGECAT. *Psychol Med* 1988; **18**: 219–23.

8. Dewey ME, Copeland JRM. Computerised psychiatric diagnosis in the elderly: AGECAT. *J Microcomp Appl* 1986; **9**: 135–40.

9. Copeland JRM, Davidson IA, Dewey ME *et al.* Alzheimer's Disease, other dementias, depression and pseudodementia prevalence, incidence and three year outcome in Liverpool. *Br J Psychiat* 1992; **161**: 230–9.

10. Hachinski VC, Illiff LD, Zihka E *et al.* Cerebral flow in dementia. *Arch Neurol* 1975; **32**: 632–7.

11. Copeland JRM, Dewey ME, Wood N *et al.* The range of mental illness amongst the elderly in the community: prevalence in Liverpool. *Br J Psychiat* 1987; **150**: 815–23.

12. Saunders PA, Glover GR. Field use of portable computers in epidemiological surveys: computerised administration of the GMS–HAS–AGECAT package. In Dewey ME, Copeland JRM, Hofmann A, (eds), *Case-finding for Dementia in Epidemiological Studies.* Liverpool: Institute of Human Ageing, 1990: 89–94.

13. Copeland JRM, Dewey ME, Saunders PA. The epidemiology of dementia: GMS–AGECAT studies of prevalence and incidence, including studies in progress. *Eur Arch Psychiat Clin Neurosci* 1991; **240**: 212–17.

14. Copeland JRM, McCracken CFM, Dewey ME *et al.* Undifferentiated dementia, Alzheimer's disease and vascular dementia: age- and gender-related incidence in Liverpool. *Br J Psychiat* 1999; **175**: 433–8.

15. MRC–CFAS. Cognitive function and dementia in six areas of England and Wales: the distribution of MMSE and prevalence of GMS organicity level in the MRC–CFAS. *Psychol Med* 1998; **28**: 319–35.

16. Copeland JRM, Beekman ATF, Dewey ME *et al.* Depression in Europe. Geographical distribution among older people. *Br J Psychiat* 1999; **174**: 312–21.

17. Lobo A, Launer LJ, Fratiglioni L *et al.* Prevalence of dementia and major subtypes in Europe: a collaborative study of population-based cohorts. *Neurology* 2000; **54** (suppl 5): S4–9.

18. Fratiglioni L, Launer LJ, Andersen K *et al.* Incidence of dementia and major subtypes in Europe: a collaborative study of population-based cohorts. *Neurology* 2000; **54** (suppl 5): S10–15.

CAMDEX

Daniel W. O'Connor

Monash University, Melbourne, Australia

The Cambridge Examination for Mental Disorders of the Elderly (CAMDEX) was devised to assist clinicians and epidemiologists to diagnose dementia, and mild dementia in particular, as reliably and validly as possible[1]. It was developed with the following aims in mind: it addresses all elements of current diagnostic criteria; it incorporates historical material so that persons with cognitive deficits due to intellectual disability, sensory handicap or functional mental disorder are classified correctly; and its neuropsychological battery is sensitive to mild dementia.

The schedule is fully structured and incorporates: a mental status examination; a comprehensive neuropsychological battery (CAMCOG); a medical and psychiatric history; a brief physical examination; and an interview with an informant that enquires into changes in memory, intellect, personality, behaviour and self-care. Medications, laboratory investigations and imaging are all recorded. There is a clear focus on dementia but conditions such as delirium, anxiety, depression, bipolar disorder, delusional disorder and schizophrenia are considered as differential diagnoses. The respondent interview takes 30–60 minutes to complete. Informants are questioned for another 20–30 minutes, by telephone if necessary. Diagnoses are based on all available data using criteria virtually identical to those in ICD-10. Since judgement is required, interviewers should have a clinical background and have received training in formulating complex data, applying diagnostic criteria and rating dementia severity.

CAMDEX, which is available in English, Dutch, French, German, Italian, Spanish and Swedish versions, is practicable and acceptable and can be administered with high inter-observer reliability[1]. It includes the Mini-Mental State Examination[2], Hachinski Ischaemia Scale[3] and other commonly-used rating scales. When applied in community surveys, prevalence rates of dementia based on CAMDEX assessments are close to those reported in other recent Western European studies[4]. CAMDEX diagnoses are also stable over time. In a British study in which community residents rated as having mild dementia were followed for 2 years, diagnoses were maintained for 51 of the surviving 56 persons. Two were re-classified as having minimal dementia and only three were rated as having no significant impairment, mostly as the result of better-controlled diabetes mellitus[5,6]. CAMCOG has been used as a stand-alone assessment package in many clinical and community studies. Further details about its psychometric properties can be found on the website listed below.

An updated version of CAMDEX includes both DSM-IV and ICD-10 diagnostic criteria and provides better coverage of more recently described conditions, such as frontotemporal dementia and dementia of the Lewy body type. A floppy disk permits computer-assisted administration, data entry, scoring and analysis. CAMDEX is copyright but packs including the interview schedule, test materials and scoring sheets can be purchased in most countries. Consult this website (http://www.iph.cam.ac.uk/camdex-r) for further updates, access to a dedicated bulletin board, references to published reports based on CAMDEX and CAMCOG, and other relevant information.

REFERENCES

1. Roth M, Tym E, Mountjoy CQ *et al*. CAMDEX: a standardised instrument for the diagnosis of mental disorder in the elderly with special reference to the early detection of dementia. *Br J Psychiat* 1986; **149**: 698–709.
2. Folstein MF, Folstein SE, McHugh PR. Mini-Mental State: a practical method for grading the cognitive state of patients for the clinician. *J Psychiat Res* 1975; **12**: 189–98.
3. Hachinski VC, Iliff LD, Zihlka E *et al*. Cerebral blood flow in dementia. *Arch Neurol* 1975; **32**: 632–7.
4. Rocca WA, Hofman A, Brayne C *et al*. Frequency and distribution of Alzheimer's disease in Europe: a collaborative study of 1980–1990 prevalence findings. *Ann Neurol* 1991; **30**: 381–90.
5. O'Connor DW, Pollitt PA, Hyde JB *et al*. A follow-up study of dementia diagnosed in the community using the Cambridge Mental Disorders of the Elderly Examination. *Acta Psychiat Scand* 1990; **81**: 78–82.
6. O'Connor DW, Pollitt PA, Jones BJ *et al*. Continued clinical validation of dementia diagnoses in the community using the Cambridge Mental Disorders of the Elderly Examination. *Acta Psychiat Scand* 1991; **83**: 41–5.

32

Assessment of Daily Living

Kerstin Hulter Asberg

University of Uppsala, Sweden

The need for assessing activities of daily living[1] (ADL) has increased during the last few decades for several reasons. First, the number of disabled persons in the population is higher today than ever before, since more people survive longer and have to live with the consequences of diseases and other[2] disorders. Second, the costs for ADL-related services to disabled persons have surged ahead, both for sheltered living and for assistance given by people paid to provide services in the homes. Relatives and neighbours will often give voluntary help but they, too, may need professional support. Third, there is a need for outcome measures, other than mortality and morbidity, which can describe levels of function among elderly people. This is required for the evaluation of pharmacological treatments and rehabilitation programmes. Many people in different professions are involved in the care of the elderly, e.g. physicians, nurses, occupational therapists, physiotherapists and social workers. In clinical practice, they need a common language to communicate their knowledge about the individual's functional level. Although much work has already been done to develop new ADL instruments and make existing ADL assessments representative, reliable and valid, much remains to be done to reach a consensus in this field. Even a definition of the concept of ADL can still be a matter for discussion: "ADL" means "activities which are common to all human beings and which must be performed regularly in order to live an independent life". This is a very broad definition, which permits a variety of activities to be included. These activities are usually divided into several categories:

1. *Personal ADL*: activities concerning self-care, care of one's own body, e.g. feeding, dressing, bathing.
2. *Instrumental ADL*: activities concerning home management, e.g. cooking, cleaning, shopping.
   (*Communication by talking and writing may be referred to as personal ADL, while transportation and managing money may be referred to as instrumental ADL.*)
3. *Professional work*.
4. *Leisure activities*.

Ambulation or walking is not an ADL item, although it is often assessed in this context. It is rather a level of mobility on a scale from bed-ridden, through unsteady gait such as creeping, to walking and running. A certain level of mobility is usually required for independent living as is a certain level of intellectual capacity, motivation and a suitable environment.

"ADL-capacity" means that a subject can perform ADL independently of another person. Even if a person can do things, it may not be certain that he/she actually does them in practice! In the WHO Classification of Impairments, Disabilities and Handicaps, ADL-dependence is classified as a disability. "Disability" has been defined as "any restriction or lack (resulting from impairment) of ability to perform an activity in the manner or within the range considered normal for the human being"[2].

"ADL-ability" means that a subject does perform ADL. It may take time, it may hurt, or there may be other difficulties, but the person is nevertheless able to perform ADL and independently of another person. If a person does not perform ADL, it may be due to physical or intellectual capacity deficits (he/she can not or does not understand) but it may also be due to lack of motivation (he/she does not want to do it), or to environment problems (he/she is not allowed to do it or is prevented).

When assessing ADL-performance in clinical practice, it is recommended that the interviewer starts with the question: "Does the patient perform the activity or not?" If he/she does not or has difficulties, the interviewer may proceed by asking "Why should this be?" There may be physical, mental and/or social reasons, which then must be analysed in more detail to form the basis for decisions on rehabilitation.

"ADL assessment" is part of the broader concept of "functional assessment", which implies assessment not only of disability but also of impairments and handicaps. "Functional assessment" is to be found in DSM-III-R and in DSM-IV[19] in Axis V. The Global Assessment of Functioning (GAF) scale is a hierarchical assessment scale not only of psychic symptoms but also of social and professional functioning.

The ADL instruments can be constructed as check lists, a summed index or hierarchical scales.

WHAT IS AVAILABLE TO ASSESS ACTIVITIES OF DAILY LIVING?

Many structured ADL assessment instruments have been developed but rather few have been used by persons other than their inventors. Most instruments include the same types of personal items, but they often have divergent operational definitions, if indeed they are defined at all. Some instruments combine personal and instrumental items. There are also multidimensional instruments with ADL items mixed up with those for other assessments, such as mobility, physical status, mental capacity and social conditions.

An overview of such instruments, mainly from Anglo-Saxon countries, is given in Kane and Kane[4]. This field of study is also undergoing continuous and rapid development in other countries, so readers are recommended to check up on the key-word "Activities of Daily Living" in *Index Medicus*.

Principles and Practice of Geriatric Psychiatry, 2nd edn. Edited by J. R. M. Copeland, M. T. Abou-Saleh and D. G. Blazer
©2002 John Wiley & Sons, Ltd

DIAGNOSIS AND ASSESSMENT

When choosing an ADL instrument, three questions need to be asked:

Question 1: for what purpose is it to be used?
   Possible uses could be:
(a) To describe and document any need for assistance in performing ADL.
(b) To differentiate among different levels of disability.
(c) To follow and record changes in ADL performance over time.
(d) To predict outcome, survival, length of hospital care, type and quality of living, etc.
(e) To evaluate rehabilitation programmes, hospital, home and day care, etc.

Question 2: for whom is it intended?

(a) For individuals, for groups with certain medical diagnoses or receiving different types of care or for populations?
(b) For mainly healthy persons or for the mildly or severely disabled?
(c) For patients living in institutions or in their own homes or for patients with or without cognitive impairment?

Most published instruments are shown to be reliable and valid for particular purposes and for particular patient categories. The same instruments may be unsuitable for use in other circumstances, e.g. instruments that include personal items only are often adequate for the more seriously disabled patients living in institutions, whereas instruments including instrumental items are necessary for use with more healthy populations living in their own homes. For patients with serious cognitive impairment, the ADL instrument has to depend on observation or test situations. The assessment has to take into consideration the patient's own dependence on active assistance as well as the patient's dependence on supervision, and whether or not activity is initiated by another person. The quality of ADL performance has also to be assessed; for example, if the patient dresses him/herself independently, does he/she dress him/herself adequately and appropriately for the situation?

Question 3: are the results of ADL assessment expected to be compared with other ADL assessments?

If so, it is necessary to choose an ADL instrument that has been tested and documented as to its reliability and validity for the chosen purpose and the specified patient category. If a group of patients is to be compared with normal subjects, data on nationally representative samples must also be available for comparison.

It may be difficult, if not impossible, to find one ADL instrument to fit all purposes. In any case, it is usually better to choose one of the well-known instruments and then supplement it with items that seem important in that specific situation, than to start the immense work of creating a new instrument. It is also better to use a plain ADL instrument instead of a multi-dimensional one, if the purpose is simply to study ADL ability.

Time and staff resources are also limiting factors when choosing an ADL-instrument. Self-administered questionnaires are less expensive to administer, but require patients who understand the questions and can respond adequately. The number of subjects who drop out may be high, so some validation of the answers is necessary. This type of instrument is mainly used in studies of elderly general populations, who are expected to be reasonably healthy.

Observations of the patient's actual ADL performance can be carried out during a nurse's daily work, when documentation will take only a few minutes. Training of the observers is usually required, along with tests of inter-observer reliability.

Test situations that use professional observers are the most expensive measures. Even if the test situation does not correspond exactly to real life, it can still be of value for specific purposes, e.g. when occupational therapists analyse the kind of impairment that is hindering performance or how rehabilitation should be undertaken; or in methodological studies, such as in a study of the relationship between severity of dementia and ADL performance[5].

In clinical practice, occupational therapists usually combine self-report information concerning the disabled patient's own values, personal causation, interests, roles, habits and skills with observations and test situations[6].

HOW GOOD ARE THE ADL ASSESSMENTS?

The quality of an ADL instrument depends on the following factors:

1. *Its representativeness*: i.e. whether the items reflect the activities of a person's normal daily life.
2. *Its reliability*: viz. its reproducibility and stability, so that the results can be reproduced by other observers or by the same observer at different times, so that changing results reflect changes in the patient's ADL status.
3. *Its validity*: i.e. whether the results are meaningful to others; whether they can be understood and used to compare with other data reflecting different levels of disability; and whether they may predict outcome.

These aspects of instrument quality are generally easy to test, but the problem is the lack of a norm or gold standard for comparison. The closest approximation to such a norm is the Katz Index of ADL[7], which is based on a cumulative scale of personal items reflecting improvement and deterioration among disabled patients, and designed to correspond with ADL development in the small child.

Other instruments may include more or less the same items as in Katz Index, such as Barthel's Index[8], but problems arise when the authors put arbitrary nominal values on different levels of ADL ability, which are ordinal in character, and then summarize the assessments. The results may be affected by systematic statistical errors, but more importantly they may obscure the understanding of actual ADL status and undermine the possibility for interstudy comparisons using different instruments. For example, if a patient scores 75 out of 100 possible points, this will not reveal in which items the patient is dependent. Furthermore, one patient with 75 points may not be as disabled as another person with an equal number.

Quite another way of handling ordinal data is shown by the development of Katz's Index of ADL. In the 1950s, a multi-disciplinary team in Cleveland, Ohio, followed patients who were recovering from a hip fracture by assessing in which order they regained the ability to perform ADL. They found six items that usually followed in sequence: first the patients regained independence in feeding, followed by continence, movement of the body (e.g. getting out of bed), going to the toilet, dressing and bathing. A patient who was independent in bathing could be expected to be independent in the other five items, too, and a person who was dependent in feeding was also dependent in the other items. The authors defined each item carefully, and found that dependence on another person, either by active assistance or supervision, decided whether or not the subject was dependent.

The authors had discovered a hierarchical or cumulative order between these six personal activities of daily life, which formed the beginning of an ADL "staircase" where each step upwards corresponded to an improvement in the patient's condition. Later, it was shown that patients with other diagnoses, such as stroke and rheumatoid arthritis, and mentally impaired people improved and deteriorated in the same way[9]. The instrument has been used for a number of purposes among elderly and disabled people in many countries[10]. In Sweden, it is used in clinical practice by medical and geriatric departments and in home care to communicate information about the patients' ADL ability. The level of ADL performance has been shown to predict survival and death, length of hospital stay and type of hospital discharge in acute medical care[11,12].

The cumulative order of items was found to correspond to the observations made by Gesell of the ADL development in small children during their first 7 years. This sociobiological origin may explain the good predictive validity of the instrument. The limitation of the scale is primarily a ceiling effect. It does not differentiate among less disabled persons, who are independent in bathing. But the small child does not stop developing at age 7, and the very existence of a cumulative scale evoked the question of what comes after bathing.

From population studies, it was possible to derive scales of percentages of the population with activity limitations. Lawton and Brody[13] formed hierarchical scales of personal and instrumental items. These cumulative ADL items were incorporated in a comprehensive multidimensional scale, the Older American Research and Service Center (OARS) instrument[14]. In order to provide shortened measures, Fillenbaum formed a five-item cumulative instrumental ADL scale out of the OARS instrument[15]. Spector and Katz[16] reported that the instrumental items of cooking and shopping were ranked higher than personal items. From the Gothenburg population study[17], ADL reduction was found in about 30% of 70 year-old people, mostly due to dependence in the personal items of the ADL.

To understand further the cause of disability in old age, it was necessary to formulate exact definitions for instrumental activities, which could be ordered into an extended cumulative scale. Sonn and Hulter Asberg[18] found that the items of cooking, transportation, shopping and cleaning could be defined and ordered next to bathing in Katz's Index of ADL. The ADL "staircase" now consists of 10 items: feeding, continence, movement of the body (e.g. getting out of bed), going to the toilet, dressing, bathing, cooking, transportation, shopping, cleaning. This ADL staircase can be used for observation and documentation of the different levels of disability for individuals, groups of patients and for population studies. For individuals, it can be supplemented by test situations according to the occupational therapists' assessment of the need for rehabilitation. For groups of patients, it can be supplemented by disease- or symptom-specific scales, and populations can be assessed by interviews, where the interviewer also assesses whether or not the answer seems a reasonable one.

There may be special reasons for choosing other ADL instruments than the one described above, such as historical reasons, instruments that include more items and are more sensitive to small changes in disability and that offer the possibility of comparison with earlier studies. Furthermore, important research work by occupational therapists is now in progress, attempting to develop special ADL instruments for patients with psychiatric problems. The field is, as it were, "preadolescent". In order to achieve a general standard for ADL assessments, it would be valuable to use the ADL staircase alongside other instruments. This would facilitate comparisons between different studies and help promote knowledge about, and understanding of, the ADL status of elderly patients.

REFERENCES

1. World Health Organization. *International Classification of Impairments, Disabilities, and Handicaps: A Manual of Classification Relating to the Consequences of Disease*. Geneva: World Health Organization, 1980.
2. Wood PHN, Badley EM. Setting disablement in perspective. *Int Rehab Med* 1978; **1**: 32–7.
3. Eakin P. Problems with assessments of activities of daily living. *Br J Occup Therapy* 1989; **52**(2): 50–4.
4. Kane RA, Kane RL. *Assessing the Elderly*. Lexington, MA: DC Heath, 1981.
5. Skurla E, Rogers JC, Sunderland T. Direct assessment of activities of daily living in Alzheimer's disease. *J Am Geriat Soc* 1988; **36**: 97–103.
6. Hawkins Watts J, Keilhofner G, Bauer DF *et al*. The assessment of occupational functioning: a screening tool for use in long-term care. *Am J Occup Therapy* 1986; **4**: 231–40.
7. Katz S, Ford AB, Moskowitz RW *et al*. Studies of illness in the aged. The index of ADL: a standardized measure of biological and psychosocial function. *J Am Med Assoc* 1963; **185**: 914–19.
8. Mahoney Fl, Barthel DW. Functional evaluation, the Barthel index. *Maryland State Med J* 1965; **14**: 61–5.
9. Katz S, Akpom CA. A measure of primary sociobiological functions. *Int J Health Services* 1976; **6**: 493–507.
10. Hulter Asberg K. The common language of Katz Index of ADL in six studies of aged and disabled patients. *Scand J Caring Sci* 1988; **4**: 171–8.
11. Brorsson B, Hulter Asberg K. Katz index of independence in ADL. Reliability and validity in short-term care. *Scand J Rehab Med* 1984; **16**: 125–32.
12. Hulter Asberg K, Nydevik I. Early prognosis of stroke outcome by means of Katz Index of Activities of Daily Living. *Scand J Rehab Med* 1991; **23**: 187–91.
13. Lawton MP, Brody EM. Assessment of older people: self-maintaining and instrumental activities of daily living. *Gerontologist* 1969; **9**: 179–86.
14. Duke University Center for Study of Aging. *Multidimensional Functional Assessment: the OARS Methodology*, 2nd edn. Durham, NC: Duke University, 1978.
15. Fillenbaum GG. Screening the elderly: A brief instrumental activities of daily living measure. *J Am Geriatr Soc* 1985; **33**: 698–706.
16. Spector WD, Katz S, Murphy JB, Fulton JP. The hierarchical relationship between activities of daily living and instrumental activities of daily living. *J Chron Dis* 1987; **40**: 481–90.
17. Gosman-Hedstrom G, Anianson A, Persson GB. ADL-reduction and need for technical aids among 70 year-olds. From the population study of 70 year-olds in Gothenburg. *Comp Gerontol B* 1988; **2**: 16–23.
18. Sonn U, Hulter Asberg K. Assessment of activities of daily living in the elderly. A study of a population of 76 year-olds in Gothenburg, Sweden. *Scand J Rehab Med* 1991; **23**: 193–202.
19. American Psychiatric Association. *Diagnostic and Statistical Manual of Mental Disorders*, 4th edn. Washington, DC: American Psychiatric Association, 1994.

33

Rating Scales Designed for Nurses and Other Workers

Kenneth C. M. Wilson, Ben Green and P. Mottram

Department of Psychiatry, University of Liverpool, UK

The changing role of nurses and other workers in the context of clinical audit and community care has provided a fertile backdrop for the development of brief and easy-to-use clinical rating instruments. Few of these are of diagnostic validity and they require little or no training. The are usually employed to rate clusters of signs, symptoms, syndromes, behaviours or needs. They have often been developed from other instruments or through clinical observation. The majority have been exposed to validation and inter-rater reliability and some are furnished with "cut-off" scores corresponding to external diagnostic criteria. Nurses and other professionals have been successfully trained in the delivery of more complex diagnostic and assessment instruments, including CAMDEX and GMS. However, this chapter will focus on relatively brief clinical instruments requiring little or no training, primarily designed for nurses and carers. This chapter is by no means exhaustive but is designed to provide an overview in a rapidly developing field.

ORGANIC STATES INCLUDING DEMENTIA

Some of the specialized neuropsychological instruments, including the Kendrick Battery, are usually carried out by psychologists and have been extensively validated[1]. However, there now exists a wide range of brief cognitive assessments that have gained both scientific and clinical credibility, readily available to clinicians of all professions. The Mini-Mental State Examination[2] is pre-eminent in this field. It is easily administered and requires no training. The test consists of verbal and performance components. The verbal subtests evaluate orientation in time, memory and attention. The performance subtests involve the naming of objects, execution of written and spoken orders, writing, and copying a complex polygon. It takes a relatively short time to administer, and can be carried out by medical and paramedical staff. It has been extensively validated and has high inter-rater and test–retest reliability. Culture and social status significantly affect the scores[3] but it has been employed in the context of transcultural epidemiological studies in which modifications have been made[4]. The Standardized Mini-Mental State Examination is a derivative designed to promote standardization and inter-rater reliability[5].

The Blessed Dementia Rating Scale[6] has been a source scale for the development of further rating instruments. Cognitive assessment includes memory and information items. The second part consists of items of behaviour. The scale has been validated through correlation with mean brain cortical plaque counts. It "ceilinged" with the correlation declining sharply in clinically severe dementia sufferers. The 10 most useful questions differentiating between normal and abnormal cognitive functioning have been extracted[7] and are used as the Abbreviated Mental Test Score, giving comparable results to the full Blessed scale. The latter has been used in a simple test of mental impairment in functionally and mildly organically ill patients attending a day hospital[8] and has been used in screening for organic disorder and predicting change over a 2-year period[9]. The study evaluated the degree of disability and was used in the planning of social support.

The Clifton Assessment Procedures for the Elderly (CAPE) consists of two sub-scales, the Cognitive Assessment Scale and the Behaviour Rating Scale, derived from the Stockton Geriatric Rating Scale, designed to be used by nurses[10]. It was devised as a brief measure of psychological functioning for chronic psychiatric patient groups and has been validated against the outcome of day hospital and day centre care[13]. There is poor inter-rater reliability of the Gibson Maze component, which has to be completed by the patient. Despite these problems, the CAPE provides a well-validated, useful instrument that does not take too long to complete. Other common instruments include the Mental Status Questionnaire[14] (MSQ), requiring some training, as questions are asked in a standardized fashion. The Short Orientation–Memory–Concentration Test was developed from the MSQ and consists of six items concerning orientation and memory[15]. One of the more recent developments has been the Clock Drawing Test, which assesses frontal and temporoparietal functions, providing a useful bedside assessment[16].

SCALES FOR RATING BEHAVIOUR AND SELF-CARE

The Stockton Rating Scale (from which items of the CAPE were derived) is pre-dated by the Crichton Behavioural Rating Scale (CBRS)[17]. The CBRS rates 10 aspects of behaviour, including the functions of orientation, communication and mood. The addition of a memory item allows the generation of a "confusion" score that is sensitive to change in mentally ill patients. A modified version has been used in the context of nursing home residents.

The Performance Test for Activities of Daily Living (PADL)[18] was developed for the US/UK Cross-National Project. It assesses the degree of autonomy of elderly psychiatric subjects in activities of daily living. It is presented as a test of praxis containing 16 sub-tests. Lawton and Brodie developed the Instrumental Activities of Daily Living Scale (IADL) and the Physical Self-maintenance Scale[19]. The IADL is widely used to evaluate the degree of

Principles and Practice of Geriatric Psychiatry, 2nd edn. Edited by J. R. M. Copeland, M. T. Abou-Saleh and D. G. Blazer

physical and instrumental autonomy of elderly subjects. It takes 5 min to deliver and has been used as a base instrument for more recent developments in this field. Both the IADL and the PADL are task-based scales using simple scoring systems.

The Stockton and other scales[20] inspired the Physical and Mental Impairment of Function Evaluation in the Elderly (PAMIE). The assessment is completed with the aid of simply formulated items not requiring rater interpretation. It measures behavioural characteristics in patients suffering from chronic diseases, with particular reference to the elderly. Two other scales, the Psychogeriatric Dependency Rating Scale (PGDRS)[21] and the Geriatric Behavioural Scale[22], have been developed by nurses, psychologists and psychiatrists. Both scales have been used for the assessment of dementia and physical incapacity. They have been well validated in the context of prognostic ability over a period of 1–2 years. The only scale designed to examine behaviour in elderly schizophrenic subjects is the Nurses' Observation Scale for Inpatient Evaluation (NOSIE)[23]. The scale consists of 30 items and takes about 20 min to complete. It is based on 3-day consecutive observation of the patient and has a frequency scale of 0–4 for each item.

A number of scales designed to be completed by nurses and carers address disruptive, antisocial and aggressive behaviour in dementia sufferers. These include the Overt Aggression Scale[24], The Disruptive Behaviour Rating Scale[25], The Nursing Home Behaviour Problem Scale[26] and the Brief Agitation Rating Scale[27]. The Caretaker Obstreperous-Behaviour Rating Assessment (COBRA)[28] and the Ryden Aggression Scale[29] are slightly longer, taking up to 30 min to complete.

SCALES ASSESSING CARERS AND ENVIRONMENT

The Multiphasic Environment Assessment Procedure[30] is a relatively well-validated questionnaire for the assessment of the environment in which dementia sufferers are nursed. It enables the assessment of the complex relationships existing between physical environment, the policies and the characteristics of the staff and residents. Adaptations have to be made for its use in the UK, as it was designed and validated in North America[31]. The Social Network Assessment Scale[32] has been used in typing social networks of older dementia sufferers.

SCALES ASSESSING CARERS

Gilleard[33] developed the Problem Checklist and Strain Scale, designed to assess problems experienced by carers. Other less well-known instruments include those designed to assess psychological problems facing the carer: the Ways of Coping Check List[34] and the Burden Interview[35]. The Relatives' Stress Scale[36] enables the relatives to make a standard assessment of stress they are experiencing as a result of having to care for an elderly demented person living at home. The Caregiver Activity Survey[37] quantifies the time a caregiver devotes to the patient, and the Marital Intimacy Scale[38] specifically examines the psychological and emotional consequences of caring for an ill spouse.

RATING SCALES FOR MORALE AND MOOD

The Measurement of Morale in the Elderly Scale consists of items extracted from empirical observations[39]. It is a long, structured interview lasting 2–4 h. A degree of training and knowledge of the instrument is required before it is used, in order to achieve satisfactory levels of reliability. A shorter morale scale, The Philadelphia Geriatric Centre Morale Scale[40], takes 10 min and

requires no training. The questions are of a forced-choice type and are read to the respondent. There is an internal consistency of factors and the scale has had fairly wide use. It is a multidimensional instrument for use in the very old and was particularly designed not to provoke fatigue or excessive inattention.

Depression rating scales should only be employed in rating depression in older people if validation studies have been reported. Some rating scales have been specifically designed for this age group, accommodating the issues of concomitant physical illness and cognitive change. The Self Care (D)[41] is a self-administered scale. It has been used in the community for the screening and rating of severity of depression in the elderly. It was found to be a sensitive indicator of depression. It may have potential use in the monitoring of change as a consequence of antidepressant medication. The scale has been validated in a pilot study in elderly, continuing-care patients[42]. The Geriatric Depression Scale (GDS)[43] was devised by compiling 100 questions used by professionals in the diagnosis of depression. O'Riordan et al.[44] recently used the scale in a large survey of patients admitted to an acute medical geriatric assessment unit, where there was a high prevalence of physical illness and cognitive impairment. They found that the GDS appeared to be a sensitive test for depression in this group, but was sufficiently non-specific to require psychiatric evaluation of patients with high scores to establish the accurate prevalence of depressive illness. The instrument exists in 15-item[45], 10-item and four-item versions[46]. Other scales that are used by clinicians include the Cornell Scale for depression in dementia[47], the Brief Assessment Schedule Depression Cards[48] and the ELDRS[49] designed to be used with an informant as well as the patient. The Centre for Epidemiological Studies Depression Scale (CES-D)[50] is a self-rating scale that has been found to be of value in screening community samples.

CONCLUDING REMARKS

This chapter does not provide a comprehensive account of the wide variety of instruments that are available for the assessment of the elderly mentally ill. Attention has been given to those instruments that have been relatively well validated, with evidence of reliability, that are easy to use with little or no training. They have been loosely categorized by function and use. Care must be taken in their application, with appropriate supervision and standardization in view of frequent problems of inter-rater reliability. In isolation, these instruments are of limited clinical value, but in the context of a multi-professional team they do have important potential in screening, clinical audit, examining issues of service need and rating change.

REFERENCES

1. Kendrick DC, Gibson AJ, Moyes ICA. The Kendrick Battery; clinical studies. *Br J Soc Clin Psychol* 1978; **18**: 329–39.
2. Folstein MF, Folstein SE, McHugh PR. Mini-Mental State; a practical method for grading the cognitive state of patients for the clinician. *J Psychiatr Res* 1975; **12**: 189–98.
3. Dick JPR. The Mini-Mental State Examination in neurological patients. *J Neurol Neurosurg Psychiat* 1984; **471**: 491–8.
4. Li G, Shen YC, Chen CH et al. An epidemiological survey of age related dementia in an urban area of Beijing. *Acta Psychiat Scand* 1989; **79**: 557–63.
5. Molley DW, Alemayehu E, Roberts R. Reliability of a standardised Mini-Mental State Examination compared with the traditional Mini-Mental State Examination. *Am J Psychiat* 1991; **148**: 102–5.

6. Blessed G, Tomlinson B, Roth M. The association between qualitative measures of dementia and senile change in the cerebral grey matter of elderly subjects. *Br J Psychiat* 1968; **114**: 797–811.

7. Hodgkinson HM. Evaluation of a Mental Test Score for the Assessment of mental impairment in the 26 elderly. *Age Ageing* 1972; **i**: 233–8.

8. Bell JS, Gilleard CJ. Psychiatric day centre outcome. *Br J Clin Psychol* 1986; **25**: 195 200.

9. Little A, Hemsley D, Bergman K *et al.* Comparison of the sensitivity of three instruments for the detection of cognitive decline in the elderly living at home. *Br J Psychiat* 1987; **150**: 808–14.

10. Meer B, Baker JA. The Stockton Geriatric Rating Scale. *J Gerontol* 1966; **21**: 392–403.

11. Erkinjuntti T, Hokkanen L, Sulkava R, Palo J. The Blessed Dementia Scale is a screening test for Dementia. *Int J Geriat Psychiat* 1988; **3**: 267–73.

12. Pattie AH, Gilleard CJ. A brief psychogeriatric assessment schedule evaluation against psychiatric diagnoses and discharge from hospital. *Br J Psychiat* 1975; **127**: 489–93.

13. Bell JS, Gilleard CJ. Psychiatric day centre outcome. *Br J Clin Psychol* 1986; **25**: 195–200.

14. Kahn RL, Goldfarb A, Pollack M, Peck A. Brief objective measures for the determination of mental state in the aged. *Am J Psychiat* 1960; **117**: 326–8.

15. Katzman R, Bown T, Fuld P *et al.* Validation of a short orientation-memory-concentration test of cognitive impairment. *Am J Psychiat* 1983; **140**: 734–9.

16. Brodaty H, Moore CM. The clock drawing test for dementia of the Alzheimer's type: a comparison of three scoring methods in a memory disorders clinic. *Int J Geriat Psychiat* 1997; **12**: 619–27.

17. Robinson RA. Some problems of clinical trials in elderly people. *Gerontol Clin* 1961; **3**: 247–57.

18. Kuriansky J, Gurland B. The Performance Test of Activities of Daily Living. *Int J Ageing Hum Dev* 1976; **7**(4): 343–52.

19. Lawton MP, Brodie EM. Assessment of older people, self-maintaining and instrumental activities of daily living. *Gerontologist* 1969; **9**: 179–86.

20. Gurel L, Linn MW, Linn BS. Physical and mental impairment of function evaluation in the aged: the PAMIE scale. *J Gerontol* 1972; **27**(1): 83–90.

21. Wilkinson IM, Graham-White J. Psychogeriatric Dependency Rating Scales (PGDRS). A method of assessment for use by nurses. *Br J Psychiat* 1980; **137**: 558–65.

22. Gottfries CG, Brane G, Gullberg B, Steen G. A new rating scale for dementia syndromes. *Arch Gerontol Geriat* 1982; **1**: 311–30.

23. Honigfield G, Klett CJ. The Nurses' Observation Scale for Inpatient Evaluation. *J Clin Psychol* 1965; **21**: 65–71.

24. Yudofsky SC, Silver JM, Jackson W *et al.* The Overt Aggression Scale for objective rating of verbal and physical aggression. *Am J Psychiat* 1986; **143**: 35–9.

25. Mungas D, Weller P, Franzi C, Henry R. Assessment of disruptive behaviour associated with dementia: the Disruptive Behaviour Rating Scales. *J Geriat Psychiat Neurol* 1989; **2**: 196–202.

26. Ray WA, Taylor JOA, Lichtenstein MJ, Meador KG. The Nursing Home Behaviour Problem Scale. *J Gerontol* 1992; **47**: M9–16.

27. Finkel SI, Lyons JS, Anderson RL. A Brief Agitation Rating Scale (BARS) for nursing elderly. *J Am Geriat Soc* 1993; **41**: 50–2.

28. Drachman DA, Swearer JA, O'Donnell BF *et al.* The Caretaker Obstreperous-Behaviour Rating Assessment (COBRA) Scale. *J Am Geriat Soc* 1992; **40**: 463–70.

29. Ryden MB. Aggressive behaviour in persons with dementia who live in the community. *Alzheimer's Dis Assoc Dis* 1988; **2**: 342–55.

30. Moos RH, Lenke S. *Multiphasic Environmental Assessment Procedure (MEAP).* Stanford University Medical Centre: Stanford, CT, 1984.

31. Benjamin L, Spector J. Environments for the dementing. *Int J Geriat Psychiat* 1990; **5**: 15–24.

32. Wenger GC. Support networks in old age: constructing a typology. In Jefferys M (ed.) *Growing Old In the Twentieth Century.* London Routledge, 1989, 166–85.

33. Gilleard C. *Living with Dementia: Community Care of the Elderly Mental Infirm.* Beckenham: Croom Helm.

34. Vitaliano PP, Russo J, Maiuro RD, Becker J. The Ways of Coping Checklist: revision and psychometric properties. *Multivar Behav Res* 1995; **20**: 3–26.

35. Zarit SH, Reever KE, Bach-Peterson J. Relatives of the impaired elderly: correlates of feeling of burden. *Gerontologist* 1980; **20**: 649–55.

36. Greene JG, Smith R, Gardiner M, Turnbury GC. Measuring behavioural disturbance of elderly demented patients in the community and its effect on relatives; a factor analytic study. *Age Ageing* 1982; **11**: 121–6.

37. Davies KL, Kane R, Patrick D *et al.* The Caregiver Activity Survey (CAS): the development and validation of a new measure for caregivers of persons with Alzheimer's disease. *Int J Geriat Psychiat* 1997; **12**: 978–88.

38. Morris LW, Morris RG, Britton PG. The relationship between marital intimacy, perceived strain and depression in spouse caregivers of dementia sufferers. *Br J Med Psychol* 1988; **61**: 231–6.

39. Pierce RC, Clarke MM. Measurement of morale in the elderly. *Int J Ageing Hum Dev* 1973; **4**(2): 83–101.

40. Lawton MP. The Philadelphia Geriatric Centre Morale Scale; a revision. *J Gerontol* 1975; **30**: 85–9.

41. Bird AS, MacDonald AJD, Philpott MP. Preliminary experience with the Self-Care D. *Int J Geriat Psychiat* 1987; **2**: 31–8.

42. Black J, Knight P, Belford H. The use of the Self-Care D Rating Scale for depression in elderly continuing care patients—a pilot study. *Care Elderly* 1990; **2**(2): 119–21.

43. Yesavage JA, Brink TL, Rose TL *et al.* Development and evaluation of a geriatric depression screening scale: a preliminary report. *J Psychiat Res* 1983; **17**: 37–9.

44. O'Riordan T, Hayes J, O'Neill D *et al.* The effect of mild to moderate dementia on the Geriatric Depression Scale and on the General Health Questionnaire in the hospitalised elderly. *Age Ageing* 1990; **19**: 57–61.

45. Shiekh J, Yesavage J. Geriatric Depression Scale: recent findings and development of a short version. In Brink T (ed.), *Clinical Gerontology: A Guide to Assessment and Intervention.* New York: Howarth.

46. Shah A, Herbert R, Lewis S *et al.* Screening for depression among acutely ill geriatric inpatients with a short geriatric depression scale. *Age Ageing* 1997; **26**: 217–21.

47. Alexopoulos GS, Abrams RC, Young RC, Shmoian CA. Cornell Scale for Depression in Dementia. *Biol Psychiat* 1988; **23**: 271–84.

48. Adshead F, Day Cody D, Pitt B. BASDEC: a novel screening instrument for depression in elderly medical inpatients. *Br Medical J* 1992; **305**: 397.

49. Evans ME. Development and validation of a screening test for depression in the elderly physically ill. *Int Clin Psychopharmacol* 1993; **8**(4): 329–31.

50. Radloff LS, Teri L. Use of the Centre for Epidemiological Studies Depression Scale with older adults. *Clin Gerontol* 1986; **5**: 119–37.

34

Comprehensive Interviews

OARS Methodology

Gerda G. Fillenbaum

Duke University Medical Center, Durham, NC, USA

The OARS (Older Americans Resources and Services) methodology was developed over two decades ago in response to a request "to assess alternative strategies to institutionalizing frail older adults"[1]. To address this issue, a three-element model was developed, which allows one to: (a) assess adults at all levels of functioning from excellent to totally impaired, using a multidimensional perspective; (b) determine the extent of use of and perceived need for each of 24 broadly encompassing but non-overlapping generically-defined services, which can be aggregated into costable packages; and consequently (c) to examine the impact of the identified service packages on persons defined in terms of their multidimensional functional profiles.

The questionnaire developed to operationalize the first two elements of the model is not restricted to it, but has enjoyed more varied use. The questionnaire is in two parts (*see* summary in Table 1). Part A assesses the level of functioning in five areas. Three areas reflect personal functioning—mental health, physical health, and activities of daily living; two reflect environmental conditions—social resources and economic resources. In each area the information obtained (from the subject or an informant) can be summarized on a six-point scale, ranging from excellent to totally impaired functioning. Review across all five areas provides a profile, making it possible to identify where functional strengths and weaknesses lie. Each area is itself multidimensional, so allowing users to examine specific aspects of particular areas of functioning and permitting more accurate identification of service impact.

Part B focuses on services assessment. To ensure accurate identification, each service is defined in terms of its purpose, the activity involved, the personnel who may provide the service, and the units in which it is to be measured (to facilitate costing). So, a resident of a nursing home would not be rated as receiving "nursing home services", rather, the precise services received there (e.g. nursing care, meal preparation, occupational therapy), the amount, and the type of provider (formal or informal) would be recorded. Need for services is self-assessed.

On average, the OARS questionnaire takes 40 min to administer (training in this is provided). Validity and reliability have been determined. It is available, and has been validated, in a number of languages. The questionnaire has been used for purposes as varied as teaching, clinical and population assessment, agency evaluation, staffing determination, service impact, prediction of service needs, determination of preferred service aggregation, and estimating service cost in different settings. An archive of OARS-based data sets is maintained at the Duke Aging Center.

Table 1. Overview of OARS multidimensional functional assessment questionnaire

Part A, Assessment of functional status	Part B, Services assessment
Demographic	Transportation
	Social/recreational services
Social resources	Employment services
Interaction	Sheltered employment
Affect	Educational services,
Extent of availability of help	employment-related
	Remedial training
Economic resources	Mental health services
Occupation	Psychotropic drugs
Income (by source)	Personal care services
Housing	Nursing care
Self-assessed adequacy of income	Medical services
	Supportive devices and
Mental health	prostheses
Short Portable Mental Status	Physical therapy
Questionnaire (to assess level of	Continuous supervision
cognitive functioning)	Checking services
Short Psychiatric Evaluation	Relocation and placement
Schedule (to assess presence of	services
psychiatric problems)	Homemaker–household
Self-assessed mental health	services
	Meal preparation
Physical health	Administrative, legal and
Prescribed medications	protective services
Current illnesses and conditions and	Systematic multidimensional
their impact	evaluation
Alcohol use	Financial assistance
Level of activity	Food, groceries
Self-assessed physical health	Living quarters (housing)
	Coordination, information
Activities of daily living (ADL)	and referral services
Instrumental ADL	
Physical ADL	

REFERENCE

1. Maddox GL. Foreword. In Fillenbaum GG, *Multidimensional Functional Assessment of Older Adults: The Duke Older Americans Resources and Services Procedures.* Hillsdale, NJ: Erlbaum, 1988.

Principles and Practice of Geriatric Psychiatry, 2nd edn. Edited by J. R. M. Copeland, M. T. Abou-Saleh and D. G. Blazer

The Comprehensive Assessment and Referral Evaluation (CARE): An Approach to Evaluating Potential for Achieving Quality of Life

Barry Gurland and Sidney Katz

Columbia University Stroud Center, New York, USA

PURPOSES

The CARE covers a wide range of indicators of a person's potential for achieving a preferred quality of life. Its bounded focus is on health and social problems associated with aging, including psychiatric disorders. Originally developed for intensive studies of community-dwelling elders[1], the rater-administered CARE has given rise to versions that have been made briefer by concentrating on key scales (the CORE-CARE[2] and the SHORT-CARE)[3], suitable for residents of institutions (the IN-CARE)[4], clinically focused (the CLIN-CARE)[5], and capable of self-administration (the SELF-CARE). There is also an INFORMANT version[6] of the CARE.

THEORETICAL BASE[7]

The phrase "quality of life" is invoked to direct attention to processes of striving to achieve or preserve a preferred manner of living. The processes involve strategies that allow relevant choices to be made and implemented. The strategies can be impeded by certain health and social problems that may occasion help-seeking contacts with informal or formal care-givers or services. The CARE seeks to assess the person's ability to deal with the strategies necessary for choosing and attaining a preferred manner of living. It does not attempt to define the latter. Information on processes can come from many sources, touching on many aspects of living, reaching beyond the person's immediate status into the present and historical context, modified by expectations of the future, and qualified by personal and cultural preferences. It is recognized that the gathering of such information is very constrained by its complexity, openness to change and inherent uncertainties, as well as by the necessary rigidities of the systematic assessment procedures.

STYLE

The general style of the CARE relies on scripted questions with pre-coded answers. The questioning is tactful and with an organization that is understandable to the interviewee, Header questions allow sections to be skipped if unlikely to be productive. Computer-assisted programs guide interview administration, so as to avoid missed or conflicting ratings. Information can be analyzed at the level of discrete items, global ratings, scales, hierarchically-arranged classes of severity, and threshold scores relating to diagnosis and need for investigation and possible treatment.

DOMAINS

Each domain targets the capacity to meet a distinctive challenge to achieving a preferred quality of life. Nineteen quality of life domains[8] have been identified and matched to items in the CARE: moving purposefully (mobility); maintaining self routinely (basic activities of daily living); using the immediate environment (instrumental activities of daily living); manipulating household appliances (technological activities of daily living); finding one's way around (navigational orientation); keeping track of time and space (continuity orientation); gathering information (receptive communication); expressing needs (expressive communication); preserving health (health and safety practices); protecting physical and mental comfort (emotional and physical status); engaging in social relations; exercising choice; managing material resources; finding the best environment; obtaining meaningful gratifications; recognizing one's own state of health (self-perceived health); taking account of the future (pessimism, optimism. realism); balancing competing qualities of life; setting and achieving goals. The domain content and labels are keyed to adaptive behaviors in pursuit of quality of life (more conventional captions are shown in parentheses).

SUBJECTIVITY AND OBJECTIVITY

The CARE does not beg the issue of whether quality of life is primarily subjective or objective, preferring to regard both as important strategies in the pursuit of quality of life. Subjective (e.g. feelings, attitudes), quasi-objective (self-reports of objective status) and mainly objective (tests and observations) aspects of quality of life are represented, thus allowing their interrelationships and their respective effects and outcomes to be examined. For example, questions on activities of daily living probe self-reported task performance, views on the extent to which health limits desired activities, informant views on the elder's functioning, tests of range of movement and observations on mobility. A supplement tests a simulation of various basic and instrumental tasks (the Performance of Activities of Daily Living, or PADL)[2]. Similarly, inquiries on cognitive status range from self-reported difficulties with memory to formal tests of memory and orientation, and a supplement (the Medication Management Test, or MMT)[10,11] tests higher-order cognitively-driven performance.

SEVERITY LEVELS

Threats to quality of life are graded in terms of the degree to which they overshadow living at a critical point in time (intensity) and over time, experiences, and situations (extensity). This approach has been more completely modeled within the CARE domain of emotional comfort, as expressed in the seven levels of the index of affective suffering (IAS)[12,13]. Each level is operationalized by symptom criteria that convey the severity meanings of suffering in a way not equaled by symptom scores or diagnosis. This model of severity is also worked out for the CARE domains dealing with functioning in the activities of daily living. Current development is concerned with deriving a measure of the continuities underlying the progression of functional decline.

MECHANISMS

Threats to quality of life, such as those measured by the CARE, may arise from health and social conditions; the presence of the latter can be suggested by certain syndromes. The CARE items include syndromes of cardiac failure or angina, arthritic pain, respiratory problems, effort intolerance, cognitive deficits, Parkinson's disease, stroke, perceptual deficits, vertigo, falls, experience of crime, and social isolation and desolation. Conversely, there are characteristics of the threatened qualities of life that suggest certain mechanisms: one scale of functioning in the CARE is composed of higher-order tasks that are principally affected by cognitive mechanisms; similarly, certain somatic items are phrased to suggest a mood disorder and others to suggest a physical disorder. More directly, there are items to record what the individual blames as the cause of his/her threatened quality of life.

BIOMETRICS

Satisfactory reliability, validity and operational characteristics for discriminating diagnoses of the CARE scales have been established[14–18]. Transition tables show a range of incidence, chronicity and recovery from threats to quality of life[19]; these also reflect a power to predict specific quality-of-life outcomes. Cross-tabulations reveal that the various domains are sufficiently independent to be usefully measured separately but that there is substantial interaction between them.[20,21]

CULTURE-FAIR INDICATORS

Ethno-racial and educational variation in qualities of life have been found with CARE indicators[22,23], as with comparable instruments[24]. In order to minimize the confound of bias entering into such comparisons, item response theory has been applied to construct culture-fair CARE scales of mood, cognition and functioning in the activities of daily living[25].

MODULAR USES

Although the full CARE is more than the sum of its parts, the scales can be, and have been, used alone and in various combinations. This has enabled the assembly of its different versions.

WHOLE-PERSON VIEW[26]

Profiles of CARE indicator severity scales are generated by computer algorithms, giving an overview of the person's strengths and vulnerabilities for preserving and improving quality of life. Global concepts are also embodied in items on self-perceived general health and in visual analog scales on physical and psychological distress and task and social functioning: a supplementary single-page rapidly completed set of visual analog scales (the QoL-100) has proved useful for a snap-shot of the quality of life potentials of seriously ill patients or where frequent follow-up assessments are needed. Psychiatric diagnoses have been generated using a computerized decision tree[27,28].

APPLICATIONS

Taken together with its versions and supplements, the CARE has been applied to epidemiological[29] surveys[30–33], public health policy[34–39] and clinical management in primary medical care[40], home care[41] and occupational therapy. A Training Manual is available.

FURTHER DEVELOPMENT

The Stroud Center's program is designed to contribute to understanding the nature of the parts and the connected whole of a person's quality of life. Experience with applications, modifications and analyses of the CARE is leading to new and better ways of assessing quality of life.

REFERENCES

1. Gurland BJ, Kuriansky JB, Sharpe L *et al*. The Comprehensive Assessment and Referral Evaluation (CARE)—rationale, development and reliability. *Int J Aging Hum Dev* 1977; **8**: 9–42.
2. Gurland BJ, Wilder DE. The CARE interview revisited: development of an efficient, systematic, clinical assessment. *J Gerontol* 1984; **39**: 129–37.
3. Gurland B, Golden R, Teresi J, Challop J. The SHORT-CARE: an efficient instrument for the assessment of depression, dementia and disability. *J Gerontol* 1984; **39**: 166–9.
4. Mann A, Gurland B, Cross P. A comparison of the long-term care of the elderly in New York and London and implications of the differences. In Radebaugh TS, Gruenberg EM, Kramer M, Cooper B (eds), *The Chronically Mentally Ill: An International Perspective*. Baltimore, MD: Johns Hopkins School of Hygiene and Public Health, 1985, 117–29.
5. Gurland B, Lantigua R, Teressi J *et al*. The CLIN-CARE: a technique for comprehensive assessment: preliminary report of biometric properties. In Wykle ML (ed.), *Elderly Rehabilitation as Art and Science*. New York: Springer, 1990, 78.
6. Wilder DE, Gurland BJ, Chen J. Interpreting subject and informant reports of function in screening for dementia. *Int J Geriat Psychiat* 1994; **9**: 887–96.
7. Katz S, Gurland BJ. Science of quality of life of elders: challenges and opportunity. In Birren J, Lubben JE, Rowe JC, Deutchman DE (eds), *The Concept and Measurement of Quality of Life in the Frail Elderly*. New York: Academic Press, 1991, 335–43.
8. Gurland BJ, Katz S. Quality of life and mental disorders of elders. In Katschnig H, Freeman H, Sartorius N (eds), *Quality of Life in Mental Disorders*. Chichester: Wiley (in press).
9. Kuriansky J, Gurland B. The Performance Test of Activities of Daily Living. *Int J Aging Hum Dev* 1976; **7**: 343–52.
10. Fulmer T, Gurland B. Restriction as elder mistreatment: differences between caregiver and elder perceptions. *J Ment Health Aging* 1996; **2**(2): 89–99.
11. Gurland BJ, Cross P, Chen J *et al*. A new performance test of adaptive cognitive functioning: the Medication Management (MM) Test. *Int J Geriat Psychiat* 1994; **9**: 875–85.
12. Gurland BJ, Katz S, Chen J. Index of Affective Suffering: linking a classification of depressed mood to impairment in quality of life. *Am J Geriat Psychiat* 1997; **5**(3): 192–210.
13. Gurland BJ, Katz SI. Subjective burden of depression. *Am J Geriat Psychiat* 1997; **5**(3): 188–91.
14. Golden RR, Teresi JA, Gurland BJ. Development of indicator-scales for the Comprehensive Assessment and Referral Evaluation Interview schedule. *J Gerontol* 1984; **39**: 138–46.
15. Gurland BJ, Wilder DE. The CARE interview revisited: development of an efficient, systematic, clinical assessment. *J Gerontol* 1984; **39**: 129–37.
16. Teresi JA, Golden RR, Gurland BJ. Concurrent and predictive validity of indicator-scales developed for the Comprehensive Assessment and Referral Evaluation interview schedule. *J Gerontol* 1984; **39**: 158–65.

17. Teresi JA, Golden RR, Gurland BJ *et al*. Construct validity of indicator-scales developed for the Comprehensive Assessment and Referral Evaluation interview schedule. *J Gerontol* 1984; **39**: 147–57.

18. Golden RR, Teresi JA, Gurland BJ. Detection of dementia and depression cases with the Comprehensive Assessment Referral Evaluation interview schedule. *Int J Aging Hum Dev* 1983; **16**: 242–54.

19. Wilder D, Gurland BJ, Bennett R. The chronicity of depression among the elderly. In Erlemeyer-Kimling L, Miller N (eds), *Life Span Research on the Prediction of Psychopathology*. Hillsdale, NJ: Erlbaum, 1986, 205–22.

20. Gurland B, Wilder D, Berkman C. Depression and disability in the elderly: reciprocal relations and changes with age. *Int J Geriat Psychiat* 1988; **3**: 163–79.

21. Gurland B, Wilder D, Golden R *et al*. The relationship between depression and disability in the elderly—data from the Comprehensive Assessment and Referral Evaluation (CARE). In Wattis JP, Hindmarch I (eds), *Psychological Assessment of the Elderly*. London: Churchill Livingstone, 1988, 114–37.

22. Gurland BJ, Wilder DE, Lantigua R *et al*. Differences in rates of dementia between ethnoracial groups. In *Racial and Ethnic Differences in Health of Older Americans*. Proceedings of the National Academy of Sciences/National Research Council's Workshop on Racial and Ethnic Differences in Health in Late Life in the United States, held December 12–13, 1994, Washington, DC, National Academy of Sciences (in press).

23. Teresi JA, Golden RR, Cross P *et al*. Item bias in cognitive screening measures: comparisons of elderly White, Afro-American, Hispanic and high and low education subgroups. *J Clin Epidemiol* 1995; **48**(4): 473–83.

24. Wilder DE, Cross P, Chen J *et al*. Operating characteristics of brief screens for dementia in a multicultural population. *Am J Geriat Psychiat* 1995; **3**(12): 96–107.

25. Teresi J, Golden R, Cross P *et al*. Item bias in mental health screening measures: comparisons of elderly white and minority subgroups. In Padgett D (ed.), *Handbook on Ethnicity, Aging and Mental Health* (in press).

26. Katz S, Gurland BJ. Science of quality of life of elders: challenges and opportunity. In Birren J, Lubben JE, Rowe JC, Deutchman DE (eds), *The Concept and Measurement of Quality of Life in the Frail Elderly*. Los Angeles, CA: Academic Press, 1991, 335–43.

27. Copeland JRM, Gurland BJ, Dewey ME *et al*. Is there more dementia, depression and neurosis in New York? A comparative community study of the elderly in New York and London using the computer diagnosis, AGECAT. *Br J Psychiat* 1987; **151**: 466–73.

28. Copeland JRM, Gurland BJ, Dewey ME *et al*. The distribution of dementia, depression and neurosis in elderly men and women in an urban community: assessed using the GMS–AGECAT package. *Int J Geriat Psychiat* 1987; **2**(3): 177–84.

29. Gurland BJ. Methods of screening for survey research on Alzheimer's disease and related dementias. In Khachaturian ZS, Radebaugh TS (eds), *Alzheimer's Disease: Causes, Diagnosis, Treatment and Care*. Boca Raton, FL: CRC Press, 1996, 61–72.

30. Gurland BJ, Wilder DE, Chen J *et al*. A flexible system of detection for Alzheimer's disease and related dementias. *Aging Clin Exp Res* 1995; **7**(3): 165–72.

31. Gurland BJ, Wilder DE, Cross P *et al*. Relative rates of dementia by multiple case definitions, over two prevalence periods, in three cultural groups. *Am J Geriat Psychiat* 1995; **3**: 6–20.

32. Wilder D, Gurland B. Cross-cultural comparisons of disability and depression among older persons in four community-based probability samples. In Adler L (ed.), *Cross-Cultural Research in Human Development: Focus on Life Span*. Praeger-Greenwood, 1989; 223–33.
    Gurland B, Toner J. The epidemiology of the concurrence of depression and dementia. In Altman H (ed.), *Alzheimer's Disease. Problems, Prospects and Perspectives*. New York: Plenum, 1988.

33. Gurland BJ, Cross PS, Mann A, Macdonald A. Comparisons of the care of the demented elderly in New York and London. In Wertheimer J, Marois M (eds), *Senile Dementia: Outlook for the Future*. New York: Alan R. Liss, 1984, 327–37.

34. Gurland BJ. The range of quality of life: relevance to the treatment of depression in elderly patients. In Schneider LS, Reynolds CF III, Lebowitz BD, Friedhoff AJ (eds), *Diagnosis and Treatment of Depression in Late Life*. Results of the NIH Consensus Development Conference. Washington, DC: American Psychiatric Press, 1994, 61–79.

35. Gurland BJ, Toner JA, Wilder DE *et al*. Impairment of communication and adaptive functioning in community-residing elders with advanced dementia: assessment methods. *Alzheimer's Dis Assoc Disord* 1994; **8**(suppl 1): S230–41.

36. Berkman C, Gurland B. *Growing Older in New York City in the 1990s: a Study of Changing Lifestyles, Quality of Life, and Quality of Care, Vol 3, The Impact of Health Problems on the Quality of Life of Older New Yorkers*. The New York Center for Policy on Aging of the New York Community Trust, September, 1993.

37. Gurland B. The impact of depression on quality of life of the elderly. *Clinics in Geriatric Medicine*. Philadelphia, PA: W. B. Saunders, 1992, 377–86.

38. Gurland BJ, Golden R, Lantigua R, Dean L. The overlap between physical conditions and depression in the elderly: a key to improvement in service delivery. In Aronwitz E, Bromberg EM (eds), *Mental Health Aspects of Long Term Physical Illness*. Canton, MA: Watson, 1984, 23–36.

39. Mann AH, Wood K, Cross P *et al*. Institutional care of the elderly: a comparison of the cities of New York, London and Mannheim. *Soc Psychiat* 1984; **19**: 97–102.

40. Gurland BJ, Wilder D. Detection and assessment of cognitive impairment and depressed mood in primary care of older adults: a systems approach to the uses of brief scales. In Rubenstein LZ, Wieland D, Bernabei R (eds), *Geriatric Assessment Technology: The State of the Art*. Milan: Editrice Kurtis, 1995, 111–34.

41. Barrett VW, Gurland BJ, Chen J, Ratau A. The QoL-100: a new visual analog technique for quality of life assessment: a preliminary report of measurement utilities. *J Nursing Res* 2000 (in press).

Part E

Organic Disorders

EI   Delirium

EII   Dementia

EIII   Alzheimer's Disease

EIV   Vascular Dementia

EV   Other Dementias

EVI   Clinical Diagnosis of the Dementias

EVII   Outcome of the Dementias and Subtypes

EVIII   Treatment and Management of Dementias

EIX   Conditions Associated with, or Sometimes
        Mistaken for, Primary Psychiatric Conditions

EX   Investigation of Organic States and Dementia

35

Delirium—An Overview

Andrew F. Fairbairn

Centre for Health Care of the Elderly, Newcastle upon Tyne, UK

Delirium is a state of acute confusion due to an underlying physical cause. Associated with the disorder of cognition and attention, there is frequently disturbed psychomotor behaviour and disturbance to the sleep–wake cycle. It is a common feature in those, particularly older patients, who present as acute medical emergencies. As a common, potentially highly treatable condition, it is associated with major health care costs. It is also under-recognized and associated with longer periods of inpatient stay. It is a recognized mental disorder under the English Mental Health Act, which has significance in relation to compulsory treatment.

Formal diagnostic criteria for delirium were only first introduced in DSM-III. These criteria were further revised for DSM-IV and the criteria for general medical conditions are shown in Table 35.1. DSM-IV critera are also described as more specific for delirium in relation to substance abuse. The main changes in the criteria are a general simplification with less emphasis on deficits of attention and more emphasis on the syndrome developing over a short period of time.

Confusion, or cognitive impairment, commonly only occurs in three conditions, namely delirium, dementia and depression. Two of the "3Ds" are eminently treatable, therefore it is to be regretted that cognitive impairment is primarily associated with dementia and hence only belatedly recognized as a potentially treatable condition in the case of this particular chapter's subject, delirium.

The rest of the chapter will discuss incidence and risk factors. There is an expanded section on clinical features and discussion of assessment scales, neuropathogenesis, appropriate investigations and treatment.

INCIDENCE

Delirium occurs in 14–56% of older hospitalized patients[1]. It is lower after elective surgery and higher in acute medical admissions. Patients who have suffered delirium during a hospital admission tend to stay in hospital for longer and have greater requirements for rehabilitation and require increased home care services[2].

RISK FACTORS

Inouye *et al.*[1] propose a multifactorial model for delirium, including predisposing factors and precipitating factors. The study identifies four predisposing factors for delirium, visual impairment, severe physical illness, cognitive impairment and blood urea nitrogen (BUN):creatinine ratio i.e. an indicator of dehydration. Using complex methodology, they identified a hierarchy of precipitating factors, the most significant of which were major surgery, stay in intensive care, multiple medication and sleep deprivation. Their conclusion was that the aetiology of delirium is multifactorial, but that certain predisposing factors, combined with a weighting of precipitating factors can make the likelihood of delirium much more predictable. Elie *et al.*[3] similarly identified risk factors that included dementia, advanced age and medical illness. Robertsson *et al.*[4] looked at the likelihood that a pre-existing dementia could predispose to the onset of delirium and showed that late-onset Alzheimer's disease was more likely to do so than early-onset Alzheimer's disease and that vascular dementia was more likely to do so than early-onset Alzheimer's disease.

CLINICAL FEATURES

Whilst DSM-IV attempts to define the clinical features, it is worth remembering that Lipowski[5] has regularly warned about the subtle "prodromal, non-specific" features that can even precede the more formal syndrome. This can be as simple as increased anxiety or subtle levels of agitation. The cardinal feature is probably a relatively sudden change in cognition but there can also be perceptual disturbances. Patients can latterly describe great difficulties in differentiating between reality and hallucination. Visual hallucinations are classically more common than auditory hallucinations and are generally unpleasant and frightening. Thinking is disorganized, slowed and impoverished. Memory is impaired across the entire spectrum of registration, retention and recall. Short-term memory may well be impaired, secondary to poor attention, and patients may be inclined to confabulate.

The impact of delirium on psychomotor behaviour is variable. Some delirious patients will become agitated, restless and hypervigilant. In contrast, some patients will become withdrawn, with slowed physical responses. Finally, the picture of psychomotor activity can be mixed with oscillation between hyper- and hypo-activity.

Having described the classic clinical features above, it should be remembered that Treloar and McDonald[6] have placed emphasis on the "quiet syndrome". They argue that one of the reasons that delirium is under-recognized is because of the frequency of the hypo-active type of syndrome. There is evidence that nurses are better than doctors at identifying the syndrome of delirium and there is tentative evidence that different aetiologies may possibly account for differentiation in the clinical picture. Zou *et al.*[7] showed that diagnosis by a nurse clinician using a standardized rating scale (the Confusion Assessment method) and multiple

Table 35.1 Diagnostic criteria for 293.0 Delirium, due to... (indicate the general medical condition)

A. Disturbance of consciousness (i.e. reduced clarity of awareness of the environment) with reduced ability to focus, sustain, or shift attention
B. A change in cognition (such as memory deficit, disorientation, language disturbance) or the development of a perceptual disturbance that is not better accounted for by a pre-existing, established or evolving dementia
C. The disturbance develops over a short period of time (usually hours to days) and tends to fluctuate during the course of the day
D. There is evidence from the history, physical examination or laboratory findings that the disturbance is caused by the direct physiological consequences of a general medical condition

Coding note: If delirium is superimposed on a pre-existing Dementia of the Alzheimer's Type or Vascular Dementia, indicate the delirium by coding the appropriate subtype of the dementia, e.g. 290.3 Dementia of the Alzheimer's Type, with Late Onset, with Delirium.
Coding note: Include the name of the general medical condition on Axis I, e.g. 293.0 Delirium Due to Hepatic Encephalopathy; also code the general medical condition on Axis III (see Appendix G for codes)

observation points was better than a one-off assessment by a psychiatrist. This study reinforces the importance of repeated observations and the value of a structured approach to the diagnosis.

ASSESSMENT SCALES

Because of the problem clinicians have in recognizing delirium, there have been a number of attempts to create assessment scales to assist in diagnosis. In the development of these scales, one of the major problems has been that cognitive impairment is, of course, a common symptom but that it is not specific to delirium. A number of instruments to evaluate delirium have been developed, mainly using DSM-III-R criteria. Many of them are multi-item scales, which probably have limited value in the clinical setting, but one, the Confusion Assessment Method (CAM), is intended to be used by physicians and has two versions with only nine and four items, respectively. Non-specific cognitive tests, such as the well known Folstein Mini-Mental State Examination, cannot specifically address the differentiation between delirium and dementia. However, it would seem that the introduction of appropriately clinically friendly scales for delirium, used by skilled nurse clinicians, might well increase the recognition of delirium in acute medical settings[7].

NEUROPATHOGENESIS

Whilst delirium is regarded as a syndrome with global dysfunction of cognition, attempts have been made to address whether there are disorders of specific brain pathways that can account for specific symptomatology, the analogy being that certain specific strokes can be associated with syndromes, for example, left frontal strokes being associated with depression. Trzepacz[8] has reviewed a number of brain scan studies which, although they are limited to studies with only a small series or even single case reports, tend to show that frontal cortex, anteromedial thalamus, right basal ganglia, right posterior parietal cortex and medial basal temporal and occipital cortex may be areas particularly associated with delirium.

The neurochemistry of delirium is believed to mainly involve under-activity of the cholinergic system. That said, on the basis that most neurochemical systems in the brain are in dynamic relationships with others, it is highly likely that this acetylcholine hypothesis also relates to a balance with the dopamine system. It can be speculated that, in the future, there may be scope to manipulate the balance of the acetylcholine and dopamine systems in such a way as to treat the symptoms of delirium, very possibly with the new cholinesterase inhibitors.

INVESTIGATIONS

Delirium, particularly in the elderly, tends to have a multifactorial aetiology. As it can be due to almost any underlying physical problems, the old adage that "common things occur commonly" must be relevant when investigating the causes. These are likely to be infections, cardiac problems, iatrogenic medication, dehydration, stroke disease, diabetes and cancer. Naughton et al.[9] reported a study of head CT scans in delirium. 15% were positive for an acute condition (haemorrhage, haematoma, space-occupying lesion or infarct) and 95% of these positive scans were found in patients with impaired consciousness or a new focal neurological finding detected during the episode of delirium. Their main conclusion was that there was considerable variation in brain CT scanning of older people with delirium.

TREATMENT

First, the aetiological factors must be identified and treated or corrected if at all possible. Whilst these are being identified, symptomatic and supportive therapies will be required. Over the years, Lipowski[5] in particular has recommended an appropriate environment for managing patients with delirium. He has described a well-lit room with familiar items and clearly visible clock and calendar. Inouye et al.[10] have systematically studied this in a paper describing a multi-component intervention to prevent delirium in hospitalized older patients. Their risk factors and intervention protocols are detailed in Table 35.2. The study provides important evidence that a multicomponent, targeted intervention to prevent delirium in hospitalized older patients can work, particularly targeting those at high risk from previously identified precipitating and predisposing factors. Wahlund and Björlin[11] report on a specialized delirium ward and argue that such a specific ward is best placed to clinically manage, investigate and treat patients with delirium. Despite the importance of primary prevention and the probable value of special delirium wards, there may be a need for antipsychotic medication. Haloperidol probably remains the antipsychotic of choice[12], although little is currently known about the efficacy of the new atypical antipsychotics in delirium. Benzodiazepines probably remain the preferred medical treatment in delirium due to alcohol.

As noted above, delirium per se makes a longer hospital stay likely, with consequent increased health care costs. That said, the mean duration of delirium is shorter in post-operative patients compared to acute medical patients[13]. The long-term prognosis of delirium used to be felt to be simply that of the underlying condition. However, a recent publication[14] flags up the possibility that the long-term prognosis after delirium is poor and, indeed, delirium might be a marker for decline. Also in contrast to traditional views, there is now a view that delirium is not always entirely reversible.

Table 35.2 Risk factors for delirium and intervention protocols

Targeted risk factor and eligible patients	Standardized intervention protocols	Targeted outcome for reassessment
Cognitive impairment* All patients, protocol once daily; patients with base-line MMSE score of <20 or orientation score of <8, protocol three times daily	Orientation protocol: board with names of care-team members and day's schedule; communication to reorientate to surroundings Therapeutic activities protocol: cognitively stimulating activities three times daily (e.g. discussion or current events, structured reminiscence or word games)	Change in orientation score
Sleep deprivation All patients; need for protocol assessed once daily	Non-pharmacologic sleep protocol: at bedtime, warm drink (milk or herbal tea), relaxation tapes or music, and back massage Sleep enhancement protocol: unit-wide noise reduction strategies (e.g. silent pill crushers, vibrating beepers and quiet hallways) and schedule adjustments to allow sleep (e.g. rescheduling of medications and procedures)	Change in rate of use of sedative drug for sleep[†]
Immobility All patients; ambulation whenever possible, and range-of-motion exercises when patients chronically non-ambulatory, bed- or wheelchair-bound, immobilized (e.g. because of extremity fracture or deep venous thrombosis), or when prescribed bed rest	Early mobilization protocol: ambulation or active range of motion exercises three times daily; minimal use of immobilizing equipment (e.g. bladder catheters or physical restraints)	Change in Activities of Daily Living score
Visual impairment Patients with <20/70 visual acuity on binocular near-vision testing	Vision protocol: visual aids (e.g. glasses or magnifying lenses) and adaptive equipment (e.g. large illuminated telephone keypads, large-print books and fluorescent tape on call bell), with daily reinforcement of their use	Early correction of vision, ≤48 hours after admission
Hearing impairment Patients hearing ≤6 of 12 whispers on Whisper Test	Hearing protocol: portable amplifying devices, earwax disimpaction, and special communication techniques, with daily reinforcement of these adaptations	Change in Whisper Test score
Dehydration Patients with BUN:creatinine ratio ≤18, screened for protocol by geriatric nurse-specialist	Dehydration protocol: early recognition of dehydration and volume repletion (i.e. encouragement of oral intake of fluids)	Change in BUN:creatinine ratio

*The orientation score consisted of results on the first 10 items on the Mini-Mental State Examination (MMSE).
[†] Sedative drugs included standard hypnotic agents, benzodiazepine and antihistamines, used as needed for sleep.

Finally, delirium is a mental disorder and as such comes under the English Mental Health Act. Very occasionally, therefore, it may be legitimate to use the Mental Health Act to facilitate the treatment of delirium.

SUMMARY

Delirium remains a common, under-diagnosed symptom of underlying physical illness in older people. This alone makes it an important health economic issue. Primary prevention of delirium is now of proved efficacy and, generally, the prognosis of delirium is that of the underlying physical disorder.

REFERENCES

1. Inouye SK, Viscoli CM, Horwitz RI *et al.* A predictive model for delirium in hospitalised elderly medical patients based upon admission characteristics. *Ann Intern Med* 1993; **119**: 474–81.
2. Stevens LE, de Moore GM, Simpson JM. Delirium in hospital: does it increase length of stay? *Aust NZ J Psychiat* 1998; **32**(6): 805–8.
3. Elie M, Cole MG, Primeau FJ, Bellavance F. Delirium risk factors in elderly hospitalised patients. *J Gen Int Med* 1998; **13**(3): 204–12.
4. Robertsson B, Blennow K, Gottfris CG, Walkin A. Delirium in dementia. *Int J Geriat Psychiat* 1998; **13**(1): 49–56.
5. Lipowski ZJ. *Delirium (Acute Confusional State)*. New York: Oxford University Press, 1990.
6. Treloar AJ, McDonald AJ. Outcome of delirium: part 2. Clinical features of reversible cognitive dysfunction—are they the same as accepted definitions of delirium? *Int J Geriat Psychiat* 1997; **12**(6): 614–18.
7. Zou Y, Cole MG, Primeau FJ *et al.* Detection and diagnosis of delirium in the elderly: psychiatrists' diagnosis, confusion assessment method, or consensus diagnosis? *Int Psychogeriat* 1998; **10**(3): 303–8.
8. Trzepacz PT. Update on the neuropathogenesis of delirium. *Dementia* 1999; **10**: 330–4.
9. Naughton BJ, Moran M, Ghaly Y, Michalaks C. Computed tomography scanning and delirium in elderly patients. *Acad Emerg Med* 1997; **4**(12): 1107–10.
10. Inouye SK, Bogardus ST, Charpentier MPH *et al.* A multicomponent intervention to prevent delirium in hospitalised older patients. *N Engl J Med* 1999; **340**(9): 669–76.
11. Wahlund LO, Bjorlin GA. Delirium in clinical practice: experiences from a specialised delirium ward. *Dementia* 1999; **10**: 389–92.
12. Jacobson S, Schriebiman B. Behavioural and pharmacological treatment of delirium. *Am Family Physician* 1997; **56**(8): 2005–12.
13. Manos PJ, Wu R. The duration of delirium in medical and postoperative patients referred for psychiatric consultation. *Ann Clin Psychiat* 1997; **9**(4): 219–26.

14. George J, Bleasdale S, Singleton SJ. Causes and prognosis of delirium in elderly patients admitted to a district general hospital. *Age Ageing* 1997; **26**(6): 423–7.

15. Inouye SK, Van Dyck C, Alessi CA *et al*. Clarifying confusion: the confusion assessment method. A new method for detection of delirium. *Ann Intern Med* 1990; **113**: 941–8.

Delirium in Institutions

Barbara Kamholz and Christopher Colenda

Michigan State University, East Lansing, MI, USA

The prevalence of delirium is approximately 10–40% of patients on acute medical and surgical units. The incidence for newly admitted patients ranges from 25% to 60%[1]. Delirium is commonly misdiagnosed as depression; up to 41.8% of inpatient psychiatry consultations for depression actually result in a diagnosis of delirium[2,3]. Delirium has a number of adverse outcomes, and may itself be looked upon as a "symptom" of problems in the delivery of hospital services[8]. It is the single most important factor contributing to in-hospital complications, such as falls and pressure sores[4]. It has a significant impact on increasing hospital length of stay[4,5] and upon the need for discharge to long-term care institutions[6]. It is the single strongest predictor of impaired daily function (AFL) at 6 months[7], although most studies have found surprising little impact on mortality[4,7]. Delirium may not be as reversible as previously thought; Levkoff found that only 17.6% of all new symptoms of delirium had cleared fully at 6 month follow-up[5]. Delirium is the most frequent complication of hospitalization in older patients.

DIAGNOSIS

Careful diagnosis of delirium is essential, as up to 66% of cases are missed[1]. Delirium can be systematically diagnosed using the Folstein Mini-Mental State Examination (MMSE)[9] in combination with the Confusion Assessment Method[1], with the optimal technique using several observation points[10]. Inattention is a critical criterion of delirium and is essential in differentiating it from depression and dementia. A recent model developed by Inouye and colleagues[1] at the Yale University Elder Life Program demonstrates that the probability of developing delirium is somewhat predictable among a population of vulnerable patients characterized by older age, high medical co-morbidity, sensory (visual/hearing) impairment and baseline cognitive impairment. Among this vulnerable group, the introduction of specific precipitating causes of delirium (such as indwelling catheter, use of restraints, and new medical complications) has been shown to increase the probability of delirium in proportion to the number of precipitating factors present.

TREATMENT

As yet, despite promising evidence that neuroleptics may improve the course of delirium itself[11] and that cholinesterase inhibitors may be effective[12], there are as yet no specific recommended pharmacological treatments for delirium. However, there is more

hopeful evidence that delirium may be prevented. An intervention based on Inouye's approach provides: sensory correction aids (e.g. glasses and hearing aids); reorientation; therapeutic cognitive activities; a non-pharmacological sleep protocol; a dehydration protocol; and an early-mobilization protocol. This resulted in a significant reduction in new cases of delirium among patients at intermediate baseline risk for delirium. It is notable that this strategy had no impact on "delirium in progress'; its primary clinical impact lay in prevention[13]. Further work on interventions for delirium will clearly be of vital importance to the reduction of the risks for delirium in institutions and for its treatment. The costs incurred by early detection may well be more than offset by savings in decreased length of stay, decreased rates of institutionalization and decreased rates of in-hospital complications[8].

REFERENCES

1. Inouye S. Delirium in hospitalized older patients: recognition and risk factors. *J Geriat Psychiat Neurol* 1998; **11**: 118–25.
2. Farrell KE, Ganzini L. Misdiagnosing delirium as depression in medically ill elderly patients. *Arch Intern Med* 1995; **155**: 2459–64.
3. Boland RJ, Diaz S, Lamdan R *et al*. Overdiagnosis of depression in the general hospital. *Gen Hosp Psychiat* 1996; **18**: 28–35.
4. O'Keeffe S, Lavan J. The prognostic significance of delirium in older hospitalized patients. *J Am Geriat Soc* 1997; **45**: 174–8.
5. Levkoff SE, Evans DA, Liptzin B *et al*. Delirium: the occurrence and persistence of symptoms among elderly hospitalized patients. *Arch Intern Med* 1992; **152**: 334–40.
6. Inouye SK, Rushing JT, Foreman MD *et al*. Does delirium contribute to poor hospital outcomes? A three-site epidemiological study. *J Gen Intern Med* 1998; **13**: 234–42.
7. Francis J, Kapoor WN. Prognosis after hospital discharge of older medical patients with delirium. *J Am Geriat Soc* 1992; **40**: 601–6.
8. Inouye SK, Schlesinger MJ, Lydon TJ. Delirium: a symptom of how hospital care is failing older persons and a window to improve quality of hospital care. *Am J Med* 1999; **106**: 565–73.
9. Folstein MF *et al*. The Mini-Mental State Examination. *Arch Gen Psychiat* 1983; **40**(7): 812.
10. Zou Y, Cole MG, Primeau FJ *et al*. Detection and diagnosis of delirium in the elderly: psychiatrist diagnosis, confusion assessment method, or consensus diagnosis? *Int Psychogeriat* 1998; **10**(3): 303–8.
11. Breitbart W *et al*. A double-blind trial of haloperidol, chlorpromazine, and lorazepam in the treament of delirium in hospitalized AIDS patients. *Am J Psychiat* 1996; **2**: 231–7.
12. Wengel SP, Roccaforte WH, Burke WJ. Donepezil improves symptoms of delirium in dementia: implications for future research. *J Gen Psychiat Neurol* 1998; **11**(3): 159–61.
13. Inouye SK, Bogardus ST, Charpentier PA *et al*. A multicomponent intervention to prevent delirium in hospitalized older patients. *N Engl J Med* 1999; **340**(9): 669–76.

Prognosis of Delirium

A. Treloar

Memorial Hospital, London, UK

Studies of outcome have started to challenge the assumption that delirium is a truly reversible disorder with a good prognosis. Prospective outcome studies of delirium are required to describe its prognosis. Using change in MMSE[1] score as the outcome measure, Fields *et al.*[2] found that by no means all patients improve, and some get worse. Treloar and Macdonald[3] found that although many acute patients had reversible cognitive dysfunction, few regained normal cognition. Some patients took the full 3 month time-course of the study to start their recoveries. Studies based upon standard diagnoses of delirium have also reported poor recovery at follow-up[4]. Kolbeinsson and Jonsson[5] found that elderly patients with DSM-III-R[6] delirium but not dementia at outset, had dementia at follow-up in 70% of cases. Cole *et al.*[7] found that less than 50% recovered mentally at follow-up. Rudberg *et al.*[8] showed delirium lasting over periods of several weeks (even though patients did not meet Delirium Rating Scale[9] criteria for delirium continuously). Cognitive deficits and behavioural abnormalities persisted in the majority of patients for at least 6 months[10] Kaponen *et al.*[11] found infrequent good cognitive outcome following delirium at one year.

Delirious patients stay longer in hospital than those without delirium. Diagnosis-related group length of stay of 13 days for patients with delirium compares with 3.3 days for those with dementia[12]. Physical morbidity may be exacerbated by psychiatric co-morbidity. Delirium is associated with death in up to 33%[13]. It is frequently asserted that mortality is purely the result of the physical illness, but this is a difficult hypothesis to test. It would be very surprising if the stupor, retardation and poor compliance with treatments seen in delirious patients did not contribute to mortality from physical illness. Patients with delirium after hip fracture surgery are at greater risk of incontinence, urinary tract infections and pressure sores[14]. Delirium in patients with hip fractures also predicts higher long-term mortality and poor functional recovery[14-16]. Francis and Kapoor[17] found that delirium predicted a doubling of mortality attributable to functional impairment, and in survivors predicted loss of ability to live independently. Levkoff *et al.*[10] found that new symptoms of delirium resolve at 6 months in only 17.7%.

The prognosis of delirium is almost certainly not, therefore, one of early full recovery. Rather, delirium is a condition with a slow recovery and one which often fails to resolve completely.

REFERENCES

1. Folstein M, Folstein S, McHugh P. Mini-Mental State, a practical method for grading the cognitive state of patients for the clinician. *J Psychiat Res* 1975; **12**: 189–98.
2. Fields S, Mackensie R, Charlson M, Perry S. Reversibility of cognitive impairment in medical inpatients. *Arch Intern Med* 1986; **146**: 1593–6.
3. Treloar A, Macdonald AJ. Outcome of delirium diagnosed by DSM-III-R, ICD-10 and CAMDEX and derivation of the reversible cognitive dysfunction scale among acute geriatric inpatients. *Int J Geriat Psychiat* 1997; **12**: 609–13.
4. Jacobson SA. Delirium in the elderly. *Psychiat Clin N Am* 1997; **20**(1): 91–110.
5. Kolbeinsson H, Jonsson A. Delirium and dementia in acute medical admissions of elderly patients in Iceland. *Acta Psychiat Scand* 1993; **87**: 123–7.
6. American Psychiatric Association. Diagnostic and Statistical Manual of Mental Disorders, 3rd edn, revised (DSM-III-R). Washington, DC: American Psychiatric Association.
7. Cole MG, Primeau FJ. Prognosis of delirium in elderly hospital patients. *Can Med Assoc J* 1993; **149**(1): 41–6.
8. Rudberg MA, Pompei P, Foreman M *et al.* The natural history of delirium in older hospitalised patients: a syndrome of heterogeneity. *Age Ageing* 1997; **26**: 169–17.
9. Trzepacz PT, Baker RW, Greenhouse J. A symptom rating sale for delirium. *Psychiat Res* 1988; **23**: 89–97.
10. Levkoff SE, Evans DA, Liptzin B *et al.* Delirium: the occurrence and persistence of symptoms among elderly hospitalised patients. *Arch Intern Med* 1992; **152**: 334–40.
11. Kaponen H, Stenbeck U, Mattila *et al.* Delirium among elderly patients admitted to a psychiatric hospital: clinical course and one year follow-up. *Acta Psychiat Scand* 1989; **79**: 579–85.
12. Thomas R, Cameron D, Fahs M. A prospective study of delirium and prolonged hospital stay. *Arch Gen Psychiat* 1988; **45**: 937–40.
13. Rabins P, Folstein M. Delirium and dementia: diagnostic criteria and fatality rates. *Br J Psychiat* 1982; **140**: 149–53.
14. Gustafson Y, Berggren D, Brannstrom B *et al.* Acute confusional states in elderly patients treated for femoral neck fracture. *J Am Geriat Soc* 1988; **36**: 525–30.
15. Magaziner J, Simonsick EM, Kashner TM *et al.* Survival experience of aged hip fracture patients. *Am J Publ Health* 1989; **79**: 274–8.
16. Magaziner J, Simonsick EM, Kashner TM *et al.* Predictors of functional recovery one year following hospital discharge for hip fracture: a prospective study. *J Gerontol* 1990; **5**: M101–7.
17. Francis J, Kapoor W. Prognosis after hospital discharge of older medical patients with delirium. *J Am Geriat Soc* 1992; **40**: 601–6.

36

Nosology of Dementia

Ingmar Skoog[1] and **John R. M. Copeland**[2]

[1]*Institute of Clinical Neuroscience, University of Göteborg, Sweden, and*
[2]*Royal Liverpool University Hospital, Liverpool, UK*

In the early 1950s, Sir Martin Roth defined dementia as "severe decline in memory accompanied by disorientation for time and place". The modern criteria emphasize that dementia is a global decline of intellectual functions that affects more areas than just memory. However, memory impairment is mandatory for the diagnosis in the *Diagnostic and Statistical Manual of Mental Disorders*, Version III—Revised (DSM-III-R) and IV (DSM-IV) (see Tables 36.1 and 36.2), issued by the American Psychiatric Association[1,2] and in the *International Classification of Disease—Edition 10 criteria for research (ICD-10)*, issued by the World Health Organization[3] (see Table 36.3). In these criteria, dementia is a syndrome characterized by a decline in memory and other intellectual functions (e.g. orientation, visuospatial abilities, language, thinking, executive function, problem solving, apraxia, agnosia). It is often accompanied by changes in behaviour or personality (e.g. loss of initiative, emotional lability, irritability, apathy, coarsening of social behaviour, change in mood). These latter symptoms are mandatory for a diagnosis in ICD-10, diagnostic in the presence of memory dysfunction in DSM-III-R and not included in DSM-IV.

An interesting difference between DSM-III-R and DSM-IV is that DSM-III-R requires impairment in short *and* long-term memory, while DSM-IV states that the impairment should include impairment in either short *or* long-term memory. In DSM-IV, in contrast to DSM-III-R and ICD-10, the criteria for dementia are integrated with the criteria for different types of dementia (such as Alzheimer's disease and vascular dementia). It is thus not permitted to diagnose the dementia syndrome *per se*, but the subcriteria for dementia are identical for all types.

The symptoms of dementia are on a continuum with normal behaviour, which often makes it difficult to know where the line should be drawn between normal function and mild dementia. This dimensional rather than categorical character makes mild dementia difficult to separate from normal ageing[4]. Fairly small differences in criteria may have large effects on the prevalence rates. Mowry and Burvill[5] found a variation in the prevalence of mild dementia ranging from 3% to 64% when different criteria were used on the same population. Different criteria also diagnosed different individuals. If a decline from a previously higher level can be shown (by obtaining information from key informants or by following the patients over time), the validity may be higher[6]. The DSM-III-R, DSM-IV and ICD-10 use the degree of social consequences of the disorder ["sufficient to interfere with everyday activities" (ICD-10) and "significant impairment in social or occupational functioning representing a significant decline from a previous level of functioning" (DSM-IV)] as the criterion for demarcating normal from abnormal behaviour.

The modern concept of dementia does not imply anything about prognosis, i.e. the course may be progressive, static, fluctuating or even reversible.

DIFFERENT TYPES OF DEMENTIA

A dementia syndrome may be caused by more than 70 diseases, the most common being Alzheimer's disease and vascular dementias.

Alzheimer's Disease

The neuropathology of Alzheimer's disease (AD) is characterized by a marked degeneration of the neurons and their synapses and the presence of extensive amounts of extracellular senile plaques and intracellular neurofibrillary tangles in certain areas of the brain. The typical insidious onset and gradually progressive course is emphasized in the National Institute of Neurological and Communicative Disorders and Stroke and the Alzheimer's Disease and Related Disorders Association (NINCDS–ADRDA) criteria (Table 36.4), in DSM-III-R and in DSM-IV but not in ICD-10. Memory disturbance is the most prominent early symptom, but slight impairment of visuospatial functioning, language and concentration may occur. In the later stages, the symptomatology is more widespread. The NINCDS–ADRDA criteria, DSM-III-R, DSM-IV and ICD-10 require that the diagnosis of AD should be made in the absence of diseases that, in and of themselves, could account for the progressive deficits in memory and cognition. Possible AD, according to the NINCDS–ADRDA criteria, may be diagnosed in the presence of other diseases if they are not judged to have caused the dementia.

Alzheimer's disease is categorized into an early- and a late-onset form in DSM-IV and ICD-10, based on whether onset occurred before or after age 65 years. ICD-10 also specifies that the early-onset type should have a relatively rapid onset and progression or aphasia, agraphia, alexia, acalculia or apraxia, while the late-onset type should have a very slow, gradual onset and progression or predominance of memory impairment. Another subdivision is between familial AD (FAD) and sporadic AD. FAD has an autosomal dominant inheritance. Almost all cases with FAD have an early onset, while most cases of sporadic AD occur late in life. Familial clustering may occur also in sporadic AD[8].

Table 36.1 Dementia (DSM-IV) (adapted)

A1   Memory impairment (impaired ability to learn new information *or* to recall previously learned information)
      and
A2   One (or more) of the following cognitive disturbances:
      (a) Aphasia
      (b) Apraxia
      (c) Agnosia
      (d) Disturbance in executive functioning
B   The cognitive deficit in A1 and A2 *each* cause significant impairment in social *or* occupational functioning *and* represent a significant decline from
      a previous level of functioning

American Psychiatric Association[2].

Table 36.2 Dementia (DSM-III-R) (adapted)

A   Demonstrable evidence of impairment in short *and* long-term memory
      and
B   At least one of the following:
       (i) Impairment in abstract thinking
       (ii) Impaired judgement
       (iii) Other disturbances of higher cortical function, such as:
            aphasia, apraxia, agnosia, constructional difficulty
       (iv) Personality change
C   The disturbance in A + B significantly interferes with work *or* usual social activities *or* relationships with others
D   Not occurring exclusively during the course of delirium
E   Either (1) there is evidence from the history, physical examination, or laboratory tests of a specific organic factor (or factors) judged to be etiologically
      related to the disturbance, or (2) in the absence of such evidence, an etiologic organic factor can be presumed if the disturbance cannot be
      accounted for by any non-organic mental disorder

American Psychiatric Association[1].

Table 36.3 ICD-10 Criteria for dementia. Definition of dementia in the ICD-10 (adapted)

G1   There is evidence of each of the following:
(1) A decline in memory (at least) sufficient to interfere with everyday activities, though not so severe as to be incompatible with independent living
(2) A decline in other cognitive abilities characterized by deterioration in judgement and thinking, such as planning and organizing, and in the general
      processing of information (at least) sufficient to cause impaired performance in daily living, but not to a degree that makes the individual
      dependent on others
G2   Awareness of the environment (i.e. absence of clouding of consciousness)
G3   There is a decline in emotional control or motivation, or a change in social behaviour manifest as at least one of emotional lability, irritability, apathy
      or coarsening of social behaviour
G4   The symptoms in criterion G1 should have been present for at least 6 months

World Health Organization[3].

Table 36.4 NINCDS–ADRDA Criteria for Alzheimer's disease

1. Probable Alzheimer's disease:
    Dementia
    Deficits in two or more areas of cognition
    Progressive worsening of memory and other cognitive functions
    No disturbance of consciousness
    Onset between ages 40 and 90
    Absence of systemic disorders or other diseases that in and of themselves could account for the progressive deficits in memory and cognition

2. Possible Alzheimer's disease:
    Dementia
    Variations in the onset, in the presentation, or in the clinical course
    May be made in the presence of a second systemic or brain disorder sufficient to produce dementia, which is not considered to be the cause of the
    dementia
    Should be used in research studies when a single, gradually progressive severe cognitive deficit is identified in the absence of other identifiable cause

McKhann *et al.*[29].

Vascular Dementia

Vascular dementia is a dementia caused by different forms of cerebrovascular disorder (CVD)[9,10], most often stroke and ischaemic white matter lesions (WMLs). The Hachinski Ischemic Score[11] was the most widely used instrument for the diagnosis of vascular dementia, or rather multi-infarct dementia (MID), from the 1970s to the early 1990s. It consists of a symptom checklist that incorporates some of the symptoms that are believed to be essential in MID, such as abrupt onset, stepwise deterioration, fluctuating course, a history of stroke, and focal neurological symptoms and signs. The assumption was that MID was caused by embolic phenomena, so that the onset of the clinical condition would be sudden and acute. Subsequent further emboli would produce other sudden deteriorations, perhaps followed by some improvement as areas of brain oedema resolved and some function was restored.

WMLs refer to the histopathological picture of diffuse demyelination with incomplete infarction in subcortical structures of both hemispheres, and arteriosclerotic changes with hyalinization or fibrosis of the small penetrating arteries and arterioles in the white matter[9]. These lesions may appear as low-density areas on computed tomography (CT) scans and as hyperdense areas on magnetic resonance imaging (MRI). The cognitive decline in subjects with WMLs has been suggested to be caused by a disconnection of subcortical–cortical pathways, producing a decline in abilities related to subcortical or frontal lobe structures.

Memory impairment is mandatory for the diagnosis of vascular dementia in ICD-10, DSM-III-R and DSM-IV. This is not ideal to describe the cognitive dysfunction in vascular dementia, where intellectual impairment may be substantial while memory dysfunction is mild[12]. The ICD-10 requires that "deficits in higher cognitive functions are unevenly distributed" and DSM-III-R that there is "a patchy distribution of deficits (i.e. affecting some functions, but not others) early in the course". The latter was, however, no longer included in the DSM-IV.

Although stroke increases the risk of developing dementia several-fold[13,14] the contributions of a stroke or an infarct to the clinical symptoms of dementia are not always easy to elucidate. Stroke may be the main cause of dementia in an individual, it may be the event that finally overcomes the brain's compensatory capacity in a subject whose brain is already compromised by Alzheimer pathology, albeit not yet clinically manifest, and in many instances minor manifestations of both disorders which individually would not be enough to produce dementia may produce it together[15]. Sometimes the presence of stroke in a patient with AD may be coincidental. Most criteria leave it to the clinician to make the decision whether the cerebrovascular disease "may be judged to be aetiologically related to the dementia" (ICD-10, DSM-III-R, DSM IV).

In most criteria the definition of CVD is based on history or findings of focal neurological upper motor neuron symptoms/ signs, or brain imaging findings of CVD. DSM-IV (Table 36.5) gives examples of signs, while the ICD-10 (Table 36.6) specifically requires that at least one should be: (1) unilateral spastic weakness of the limbs; (2) unilateral increased tendon reflexes; (3) extensor plantar response; or (4) pseudobulbar palsy.

The DSM-IV specifies that there should be signs *and* symptoms *or* laboratory evidence indicative of CVD (e.g. multiple infarctions involving the cortex and underlying white matter) that are judged to be aetiologically related to the disturbance, while ICD-10 requires that there should be evidence from history,

Table 36.5 DSM-IV Vascular dementia

A/B General criteria for dementia
C Focal neurological signs and symptoms, e.g:
    Exaggeration of deep tendon reflexes
    Extensor plantar response
    Pseudobulbar palsy
    Gait abnormalities
    Weakness of an extremity
    or
    Laboratory evidence of cerebrovascular disease, e.g.
      Multiple infarctions involving cortex and underlying white matter
      that are judged to be etiologically related to the disturbance
D Do not occur exclusively during delirium

American Psychiatric Association[2].

Table 36.6 ICD-10 Criteria for vascular dementia (adapted)

G1 The general criteria for dementia (G1–G4) must be met
G2 Deficits in higher cognitive function are unevenly distributed, with some findings affected and others relatively spared
G3 There is clinical evidence of focal brain damage, manifest as *at least* one of the following:
    (1) Unilateral spastic weakness of the limbs
    (2) Unilaterally increased tendon reflexes
    (3) An extensor plantar response
    (4) Pseudobulbar palsy
G4 There is evidence from the history, examination, *or* tests of a significant cerebrovascular disease, which may reasonably be judged to be etiologically related to the dementia

World Health Organization[3].

examination *or* tests of a significant CVD, which may be reasonably judged to be aetiologically related to the dementia (e.g. history of stroke or evidence of cerebral infarction). In the National Institute of Neurological Disorders and Stroke and the Association Internationale pour la Recherche et l'Enseignement en Neurosciences (NINDS–AIREN) criteria[10] (Table 36.7), a diagnosis of probably vascular dementia requires that focal signs consistent with stroke *and* relevant CVD by brain imaging should be present. Tatemichi, one of the authors of the NINDS–AIREN criteria, and his colleagues published a modified version[16], in which this criterion was changed to focal signs consistent with stroke *or* relevant CVD by brain imaging. The first criterion is probably too strict and underestimates the occurrence of VaD; the latter criterion may be too broad. The NINDS–AIREN criteria recommend that a diagnosis of "possible" vascular dementia may be made in the presence of dementia with focal neurological signs in patients in whom brain imaging studies are missing; or in the absence of a clear temporal relationship between dementia and stroke; or in patients with subtle onset and variable course. This means that if CVD is present in a patient with dementia, VAD is likely to be diagnosed, which might overestimate the occurrence of this type of dementia. Furthermore, the interpretation of a single stroke leading to dementia probably differs between centres, and may be one reason for the disparate results regarding the prevalence of vascular dementia.

Table 36.7 The NINDS–AIREN criteria

Probable Vascular Dementia
  1. Dementia
  2. Cerebrovascular disease
    (a) Focal signs consistent with stroke
    and
    (b) Relevant CVD by brain imaging:
      Multiple large-vessel infarcts
      Single strategically placed infarct
      Multiple lacunes (basal ganglia, white matter)
      Extensive periventricular white matter lesions
  3. Relationship between (1) and (2):
    (a) Dementia onset within 3 months following stroke
    (b) Abrupt deterioration in cognitive functions
    (c) Fluctuating stepwise progression

Possible Vascular Dementia
  1. Dementia
  2. Cerebrovascular disease
    Focal signs consistent with stroke
  3. Absence of relationship between (1) and (2)
    (a) Dementia onset more than 3 months following stroke
    (b) Subtle onset or variable course

The temporal relationship between stroke and onset of dementia is often thought to strengthen the possibility that the two disorders are aetiologically related. The NINDS–AIREN criteria suggest an arbitrary limit of 3 months for onset of dementia after stroke. However, a stroke which occurred years before may still indicate the presence of CVD.

VAD may be underdiagnosed, as sometimes the onset is insidious, the course gradual, the infarctions clinically silent and the infarcts not detectable by CT of the brain[17,18]. VAD may be overdiagnosed, as the presence of stroke, WMLs or other CVD does not necessarily mean that they are the cause of the dementia[17]. Often AD becomes a diagnosis by exclusion, and the diagnosis of VAD will be assigned if the patient has a history of CVD. This leads to a situation where the dementias will not infrequently be divided into one group with stroke and one without, giving negative associations between risk factors for stroke and AD, and positive associations with VAD[17].

Even the histopathological diagnoses of AD and VaD are uncertain. Extensive histopathological signs of AD[19,20] and VAD[19,21] have been found in persons who show no clinical signs of dementia during life. A considerable proportion of subjects fulfilling the diagnosis of probable NINCDS–ADRDA criteria for AD or probable NINDS–AIREN for VAD have mixed pathologies[22,23]. CVD may increase the possibility that individuals with AD lesions in their brains will express a dementia syndrome[24], but some workers have suggested that there may be a causal link between AD and VAD[25].

Frontotemporal Dementia

Frontotemporal dementia is a neurodegenerative disease characterized by neuronal loss in the frontal and temporal lobes. Criteria for frontotemporal dementia was proposed by the Lund and Manchester Groups in 1994[26], and revised in 1998[27]. The latter describes five core diagnostic features that must be present: (a) insidious onset and gradual progression; (b) early decline in social interpersonal conduct; (c) early impairment in regulation of personal conduct (e.g. social disinhibition); (d) early emotional blunting (such as inertia and loss of volition); and (e) early loss of insight. It also includes supportive diagnostic features, which are not present in all patients: (a) behavioural disorder; (b) speech and language alterations (economical output, reduced number of words, aspontaneity, press of speech, stereotypy, echolalia, mutism, perseveration); (c) physical signs (primitive reflexes, incontinence, akinesia, rigidity, tremor, low or labile blood pressure); (d) investigations showing impairment in frontal lobe tests in the absence of severe amnesia, aphasia or perceptual disorder, normal EEG, and frontal or anterior temporal abnormality on CBF. Other common symptoms are stereotyped behaviour and motor perseverations. Cognitive deficits occur mainly in attention, abstraction, planning and problem solving, while memory is relatively well-preserved in the early phase[27]. In DSM-IV and ICD-10, this type of dementia is classified under the heading Dementia due to Pick's disease, while Pick's disease is a subtype of frontotemporal dementia in the criteria from Neary et al[27]. According to the ICD-10, the general criteria for dementia should be met, onset should be slow with steady deterioration, memory and parietal lobe functions should be relatively preserved in the early stages, and at least two symptoms should be either emotional blunting, coarsening of social behaviour, disinhibition, apathy or restlessness, and aphasia. The problem with the emphasis on memory impairment in the general criteria for dementia in this disorder is evident.

Two other clinical syndromes of frontotemporal degeneration are progressive nonfluent aphasia and semantic dementia, which are disorders of language. Patients with Alzheimer's disease, vascular dementia, and some other brain disorders may also exhibit symptoms of the frontal lobe type during the course of their disorders.

Lewy Body Dementia

Lewy body disease is a neurodegenerative dementia characterized by Lewy body formation in the brain stem and cerebral cortex. It has been reported that as much as 20% of demented patients coming to autopsy exhibit these changes. Criteria for Lewy body dementia are lacking in DSM-IV and ICD-10, but were proposed by McKeith et al[28] in 1992. These include: (a) fluctuating cognitive impairment affecting both memory and higher cortical functions; (b) at least one of (i) visual and/or auditory hallucinations, (ii) mild spontaneous extrapyramidal features (mainly rigidity and hypokinesia) or a neuroleptic sensitivity syndrome (i.e. exaggerated adverse response to standard doses of neuroleptic medications), or (iii) repeated unexplained falls and/or transient clouding or loss of consciousness; (c) despite the fluctuating pattern the clinical features persist over a long period of time; (d) exclusion of any underlying physical illness adequate to explain the fluctuating cognitive state, and of past history of stroke or ischaemic brain damage on brain imaging. The clinical presentation often also includes paranoid ideations and depression.

Subcortical Dementia

A special subtype of dementia is subcortical dementia. This type of dementia is seen in subcortical disorders, such as Parkinson's disease with dementia, Huntington's disease, supranuclear palsy, Lewy body disease and subcortical ischaemic WMLs. The dominating symptoms are psychomotor retardation, emotional bluntness, akinesia and slight memory disturbance, which may be helped by cues.

Secondary Dementias

Secondary dementias are caused by conditions with a known aetiology where dementia is generally not a core symptom, but may occur in some patients. Traditionally, vascular dementia is not classified among the secondary dementias, while subdural haematomas, normal pressure hydrocephalus, Creutzfeldt–Jakob disease, brain tumours, metabolic disorders and deficiency states are treated as secondary dementias.

REFERENCES

1. American Psychiatric Association. *Diagnostic and Statistical Manual of Mental Disorders*, 3rd edn, revised. Washington, DC: American Psychiatric Association, 1987.
2. American Psychiatric Association. *Diagnostic and Statistical Manual of Mental Disorders*, 4th edn. Washington, DC: American Psychiatric Association, 1994.
3. World Health Organization. *The ICD-10 Classification of Mental and Behavioural Disorders. Diagnostic Criteria for Research*. Geneva: World Health Organization, 1993.
4. Henderson AS, Huppert FA. The problem of mild dementia. *Psychol Med* 1984; **14**: 5–11.
5. Mowry B, Burvill P. A study of mild dementia in the community using a wide range of diagnostic criteria. *Br J Psychiat*, 1988; **153**: 328–34.
6. Aevarsson O, Skoog I. Dementia disorders in a birth cohort followed from age 85 to 88. The influence of mortality, non-response and diagnostic change on prevalence. *Int Psychogeriat* 1997; **9**: 11–23.

8. Blennow K, Skoog I. Genetic testing for Alzheimer's disease: how close is reality? *Curr Opin Psychiat*, 1999; **12**: 487–93.

9. Skoog I. Blood pressure and dementia. In Hansson L, Birkenhäger WH (eds), *Handbook of hypertension. Vol 18, Assessment of Hypertensive Organ Damage.* Amsterdam: Elsevier Science, 1997.

10. Román GC, Tatemichi TK, Erkinjuntti T *et al.* Vascular dementia: diagnostic criteria for research studies. Report of the NINDS–AIREN international workshop. *Neurology* 1993; **43**: 250–60.

11. Hachinski VC, Illif LD, Zihka E *et al.* Cerebral flow in dementia. *Arch Neurol* 1975; **32**, 632–7.

12. Bowler JV, Hachinski V. Vascular cognitive impairment: a new approach to vascular dementia. In *Baillière's Clinical Neurology.* London: Baillière Tindall, 1995; 357–76.

13. Tatemichi TK, Desmond DW, Mayeux R *et al.* Dementia after stroke: baseline frequency, risks, and clinical features in a hospitalised cohort. *Neurology* 1992; **42**: 1185–93.

14. Pohjasvaara T, Erkinjuntti T, Vataja R, Kaste M. Dementia three months after stroke. Baseline frequency and effect of different definitions of dementia in the Helsinki Stroke Aging Memory (SAM) cohort. *Stroke* 1997; **28**: 785–92.

15. Erkinjuntti T, Hachinski V. Dementia post stroke. In *Physical Medicine and Rehabilitation: State of the Art Reviews*, vol 7. Philadelphia, PA: Hanley & Belfus, 1993.

16. Tatemichi TK, Sacktor N, Mayeux R. Dementia associated with cerebrovascular disease, other degenerative diseases, and metabolic disorders. In Terry RD, Katzman R, Bick KL (eds), *Alzheimer Disease.* 1994; New York: Raven.

17. Skoog I. Risk factors for vascular dementia. A review. *Dementia* 1994; **5**: 137–44.

18. Fischer P, Gatterer G, Marterer A *et al.* Course characteristics in the differentiation of dementia of the Alzheimer type and multi-infarct dementia. *Acta Psychiat Scand* 1990; **81**: 551–3.

19. Tomlinson BE, Blessed G, Roth M. Observations on the brains of demented old people. *J Neurol Sci* 1970; **11**: 205–42.

20. Arriagada P, Marzloff K, Hyman B. Distribution of Alzheimer-type pathologic changes in non-demented elderly individuals matches the pattern in Alzheimer's disease. *Neurology*, 1992; **42**: 1681–8.

21. Del Ser T, Bermejo F, Portera A *et al.* Vascular dementia. A clinicopathological study. *J Neurol Sci* 1990; **96**: 1–17.

22. Holmes C, Cairns N, Lantos P, Mann A. Validity of current clinical criteria for Alzheimer's disease, vascular dementia and dementia with Lewy bodies. *Br J Psychiat* 1999; **174**: 45–50.

23. Lim A, Tsuang D, Kukull W *et al.* Clinico-neuropathological correlation of Alzheimer's disease in a community-based case series. *J Am Geriat Soc* 1999; **47**: 564–9.

24. Snowdon DA, Greiner LH, Mortimer JA *et al.* Brain infarction and the clinical expression of Alzheimer disease. The Nun Study. *J Am Med Assoc* 1997; **277**: 813–17.

25. Skoog I, Kalaria RN, Breteler MM. Vascular factors and Alzheimer disease. *Alzheimer's Dis Assoc Disord* 1999; **13**(suppl 3): S106–14.

26. Brun A, Englund E, Gustafson L *et al.* Clinical and neuropathological criteria for frontotemporal dementia. *J Neurol Neurosurg Psychiat* 1994; **57**: 416–18.

27. Neary D, Snowden JS, Gustafson L *et al.* Frontotemporal lobar degeneration: a consensus on clinical diagnostic criteria. *Neurology*, 1998; **51**: 1546–54.

28. McKeith IG, Perry RH, Fairbairn AF *et al.* Operational criteria for senile dementia of Lewy body type (SDLT). *Psychol Med* 1992; **22**: 911–22.

29. McKhann G, Drachman D, Folstein M *et al.* Clinical diagnosis of Alzheimer's disease: report of the NINCDS–ADRDA work group under the auspices of Department of Health and Human Services Task Force on Alzheimer's disease. *Neurology*, 1984; **34**: 939–44.

Cross-national Inter-rater Reliability of Dementia Diagnosis

Daniel W. O'Connor

Monash University, Melbourne, Australia

DSM-IV[1], ICD-10[2] and other glossaries have proved successful in promoting a common approach to psychiatric diagnosis. In field trials of DSM-III-R, for example, psychiatrists achieved concordance rates for diagnosing dementia of 0.91, where 1.0 represents complete agreement[3].

It cannot be assumed, however, that similar performances will be achieved in "real world" practice. Most studies of diagnostic reliability involve assessments by experienced clinicians of cooperative, physically healthy old people who are either "normal" controls or "pure cases" of dementia. In reality, cognitive function lies on a spectrum and assessment is often complicated by limited education, deafness, poor vision, physical illness, anxiety or depression.

In a study of five research teams in Australia, Germany, The Netherlands, the UK and the USA, each centre contributed 20 written vignettes of elderly persons encountered in clinics or community surveys[4]. No exclusions were made because of medical, neurological or psychiatric complications. The vignettes were brief and highly structured. The contents included subjects' demographic details, medical and psychiatric history, abbreviated cognitive test results and an informant's report of cognitive, personal and social performance.

When 13 researchers applied DSM-III-R criteria to the 100 vignettes, within-team levels of diagnostic agreement were high, ranging from kappa 0.72 in the centre with the least joint training to 0.86 in the centre with most. Between-team agreement was lower but still acceptable, with kappas ranging from 0.74 to 0.83. Some elements of DSM-III-R were easier to apply consistently than others. Mean percentage agreement was highest for social and occupational dysfunction (94%) and lowest for impairment of higher cortical function (87%). Concordance was also significantly higher for cognitively intact (98%) and severely impaired (96%) persons than for those with minimal (80%) and mild (82%) degrees of dementia.

Agreement was higher for "yes–no" DSM-III-R diagnoses than for the multilevel Clinical Dementia Rating (CDR) scale, in which six domains (memory, orientation, judgement, community affairs, home and hobbies, and personal care) are each rated on a five-point scale[5]. Kappa levels ranged from 0.61 to 0.76 within teams and from 0.50 to 0.69 between teams. Personal care was rated most consistently (85% mean agreement) and community affairs least so (74%). As with DSM-III-R, concordance was higher for cognitively intact (95%) and severely impaired (84%) persons than for those with minimal (78%) and mild (68%) dementias.

Univariate analyses of CDR ratings pointed to lower agreement levels for persons described as physically ill, deaf, partially sighted, anxious or depressed. However, multivariate analysis detected only two main effects: dementia severity and physical illness. Other variables made no significant independent contribution.

These findings suggest that dementia can be diagnosed with acceptable reliability in community surveys. Agreement is likely to be higher, though, when teams train intensively and use instruments that require simple "yes–no" choices. The reduction in agreement associated with physical illness is important given the high co-morbidity of physical and mental illness in representative elderly populations.

REFERENCES

1. American Psychiatric Association. *Diagnostic and Statistical Manual of Mental Disorders*, 4th edn. Washington, DC: American Psychiatric Association, 1994.
2. World Health Organization. *The ICD-10 Classification of Mental and Behavioural Disorders. Clinical Descriptions and Diagnostic Guidelines*. Geneva: World Health Organization, 1992.
3. American Psychiatric Association. *Diagnostic and Statistical Manual of Mental Disorders*. 3rd edn, revised. Washington, DC: American Psychiatric Association, 1987; 470.
4. O'Connor DW, Blessed G, Cooper B *et al*. Cross-national interrater reliability of dementia diagnosis in the elderly and factors associated with disagreement. *Neurology* 1996; **47**: 1194–9.
5. Hughes CP, Berg L, Danziger WL, Coben LA *et al*. A new clinical scale for the staging of dementia. *Br J Psychiat* 1982; **140**: 566–72.

37

Early Detection

Scott Henderson

Centre for Mental Health Research, The Australian National University,
Canberra ACT 0200, Australia

IS EARLY DETECTION IMPORTANT?

Why try to detect dementia early in its course? Since the advent of technologies for the early detection of disease, it has become important to ask whether early recognition is worthwhile, and for whom. Can it be shown that a lower level of morbidity is achieved in a population that has been screened, compared to others that were not screened? Is the quality of life of cases improved by their early diagnosis; or could early detection of dementia "seriously damage your health", as has been found for other disorders[1]? For a start, evaluation of the early detection of dementia would have to take note of the 10 principles of screening, as listed by Wilson and Jungner[2]. These include the requirement that there be an accepted form of treatment for persons once detected, that facilities for diagnosis and treatment be available to the population being screened, and that a suitable test be available for detecting the disease in its early stages. Clearly, screening for early dementia is a procedure where none of these requirements has yet been met.

Cooper and Bickel[3] have nevertheless indicated some of the advantages that screening or early detection could bring. They point out, first, that the biggest gap between those receiving specialist psychiatric care and the total volume of morbidity in a general population is amongst its elderly; and that mental disorders in this age group are probably under-recognized by general physicians. Second, a proportion of cases detected as dementia have reversible conditions such as depressive disorder, normal pressure hydrocephalus, metabolic disorders or brain tumours. Third, early detection can be a preliminary not to curative treatment but "to intervention aimed at reducing disability and postponing the need for institutional care". Such intervention is well placed with the general practitioner and the person's family. It can then be added that, for the general practitioner, the advantages of early detection are appreciable: the possible causes of the cognitive or behavioural deterioration may need to be pursued. Where co-morbidity emerges, as it commonly will, the physician's awareness that dementia is present will prove useful in assessment and continuing management; and the presence of dementia may influence the choice of medication.

There is one further reason for early detection, although this is not to the individual patient's immediate benefit. For research on dementia, it is of great importance to know about the earliest symptoms and signs before these become buried by the dementia itself. Without this information, and without knowing the clinical course of mild cases, it may not be possible to improve the specificity of screening, and to distinguish between mild cognitive decline and normal ageing[4]. For population-based research, where some early cases will inevitably be identified, Brayne *et al.*[5] recommend that a two-stage design should ideally be used, along with a third assessment that serves as a gold standard: evidence of progression of the dementia; or neuropathology at post mortem.

HOW IS EARLY DETECTION ACHIEVED?

Early detection will usually mean the dementia is of only mild severity. It is an advantage, therefore, that the diagnostic criteria for mild dementia have been specified in both ICD-10[6] and DSM-IV[7]. In ICD-10, the declining memory and information processing causes impaired performance in daily living, but not to a degree that is incompatible with independent living. Explicit criteria are given for the diagnosis of mild dementia.

Early detection can be carried out at three levels: in the community, in primary care settings, and in hospitals. In the community, screening is conducted only as part of research studies, and has not yet been used in a way similar to other routine screening for disease. In primary care, early detection is at present conducted informally and is based largely on the initiative and clinical skill of the practitioner. It is not clear what most commonly prompts the physician into considering a diagnosis of early dementia. Rarely it would be, say, all persons aged 70 years and over consulting in a given period, but rather those who prompt the physician's concern. Commonly, it is the patient's family who have first detected a deterioration in cognition or behaviour. The present consensus is that, in the absence of some indication, efforts to detect early dementia in general practice are unwarranted. But there may be a place for routinely obtaining a base-line measure of cognitive performance against which subsequent assessments can be placed. There is as yet no place for annual repetition of the assessment.

Tests for Early Detection of Dementia

In hospitals and clinics, the realities of clinical practice are that early detection of dementia is achieved in one of two ways. In the more common style, the clinician obtains a history from others that a *decline* in cognitive performance and/or behaviour has taken place. To this is added some non-systematic cognitive assessment of the patient, leading to a conclusion on whether or not early dementia is present. Clearly, other clinical features,

Principles and Practice of Geriatric Psychiatry, 2nd edn. Edited by J. R. M. Copeland, M. T. Abou-Saleh and D. G. Blazer
©2002 John Wiley & Sons, Ltd

such as cerebrovascular disease, would commonly play a part in this.

In the second situation, the assessment is formal and partly quantitative. A large number of standardized clinical instruments and neuropsychological tests for this are now available. They are described in Section DIII of this volume. For the purpose of *early* detection, two points need to be emphasized. Firstly, some of the tests are open to educational or cultural bias, so that they can generate false-positive results in some sociodemographic contexts, possibly to the patient's detriment. Secondly, in this writer's opinion, many tests are focused on cognitive function, ignoring changes in behaviour—yet the latter are an important clue to early dementia. The Psychogeriatric Assessment Scales developed by Jorm *et al.*[8] have gone some way to redress this imbalance (*see* Chapter 27).

Limitations

To detect dementia early in its course, and to do so with a high level of accuracy in different social and educational groups, is not a straightforward task. The only means currently available are those clinical instruments described in Section DIII. There is no biomedical test with both portability and greater accuracy than these instruments. The clinical instruments all have a number of limitations. First, the mental status questionnaires are brief, and can act only as screening instruments that sort individuals into different levels of probability of being a case of dementia. A questionnaire cannot be expected to do more than this. Second, the instrument must be acceptable; yet elderly people may dislike extensive cognitive testing, particularly if it shows them up as defective in performance. Third, whether it is a brief questionnaire or a clinical examination, the reliability and validity have to be high. The latter means achieving good levels of sensitivity and specificity. Fourth, and closely related to validity, there is the problem of bias against low intelligence or poor education. It is highly likely that this causes some false-positives to appear in the course of screening.

Whatever the method used for early detection, there are three further issues to consider. Not all the cases detected will progress[9,10] and it is hard to predict to whom this will happen.

ORGANIC DISORDERS

Rosenman[11] found very poor predictive validity for five well-established methods for making this diagnosis. Cooper and Bickel[3] argue that there are no good grounds for asking elderly persons to subject themselves to extensive investigations when some will undergo no further deterioration. A further impediment is the cost and service burden from investigating all the possible cases of dementia generated from a national screening programme. Eastwood and Corbin[12] have argued that the cost would be prohibitive. This is likely to be the case even for the older section of the community, where the frequency of secondary dementias is known to be lower than in younger adults. Lastly, there may be unexpected adverse consequences of screening. The belief may be false that early detection can contribute to prevention. O'Connor *et al.*[13] found, unexpectedly, that screening for early or mild dementia increased the likelihood of entry into residential care.

WHAT POSSIBLE SOLUTIONS ARE THERE?

Routine screening for dementia at the community level cannot yet be defended. What is required instead is work to evaluate

its impact in the manner advocated by Cooper and Bickel[3]. These authors have emphasized the need for research into the feasibility and effectiveness of early detection as a first step towards preventive action. They also argue that programmes for early detection will be successful only if they are incorporated into the work of general practitioners, community nurses and other health professionals. It is there, and not the total community of elderly, where early detection needs first to be attempted and evaluated to see what benefits, if any, it brings.

At a technical level, it has to be accepted that early detection of cognitive decline or dementia by brief screening methods has at least two unavoidable imperfections: first, there will be some error, whereby the screening test misclassifies a proportion of individuals; second, some of this error will be attributable to low intelligence in the respondent, or educational bias in the test. Since both of these are likely to produce false-positives rather than negatives, the problem can usually be overcome by more detailed clinical assessment and history in a two-phase design. In research settings, another desirable strategy in early detection is to have a second assessment after an appropriate lapse of time. This is the most certain way to ensure that deterioration has indeed taken place, and that it has progressed. Early detection of dementia is currently dependent on clinical information and on cognitive performance related to daily life. Assessment of this is now remarkably satisfactory, although the validity of the main clinical instruments has yet to be demonstrated in community instead of hospital samples. Because dementia has very explicit clinical manifestations and associated impairments, its early detection is likely to be by clinical means for some time to come. For the present, early detection brings no benefit to the elderly in the general population. But the situation may soon change in the face of current advances in the molecular biology of Alzheimer's disease, where it is conceivable that early detection may become justified for genetically high-risk individuals for whom a pharmacological intervention could be beneficial[14]. It is from these advances that far-reaching consequences for clinical practice are now imminent.

REFERENCES

1. Stewart-Brown S, Farmer A. Screening could seriously damage your health. *Br Med J* 1997; **314**: 533.
2. Wilson JMO, Jungner G. Principles and practice of screening. *Public Health Papers No. 34*. Geneva: World Health Organization, 1968.
3. Cooper B, Bickel H. Population screening and the early detection of dementing disorders in old age: a review. *Psychol Med* 1984; **14**: 81–95.
4. Henderson AS, Huppert F. The problem of mild dementia. *Psychol Med* 1984; **14**: 5–11.
5. Brayne C, Day N, Gill C. Methodological Issues in Screening for Dementia. *Neuroepidemiology* 1992; **11**: 88–93.
6. World Health Organization. *The ICD-10 Classification of Mental and Behavioural Disorders. Clinical Descriptions and Diagnostic Guidelines*. Geneva: World Health Organization, 1992.
7. American Psychiatric Association. *Diagnostic and Statistical Manual*, 4th edn (DSM-IV). Washington, DC: 1994.
8. Jorm AF, Mackinnon AJ, Christensen H *et al*. The Psychogeriatric Assessment Scales (PAS): further data on psychometric properties and validity from a longitudinal study of the elderly. *Int J Geriatr Psychiatry* 1997; **12**: 93–100.
9. Bergmann K, Kay DWK, Foster MM. A follow-up study of randomly selected community residents to assess the effects of chronic brain syndrome and cerebrovascular disease. *Psychiatry*, Part II. Excerpta Medica Congress Series 1971; **274**: 856–65.

10. Korten AE, Henderson AS, Christensen H *et al*. A prospective study of cognitive function in the elderly. *Psychol Med* 1997; **27**: 919–30.

11. Rosenman SJ. The validity of the diagnosis of mild dementia. *Psychol Med* 1991; **21**: 923–34.

12. Eastwood MR, Corbin S. Investigation of suspect dementia. *Lancet* 1981; **i**: 1261.

13. O'Connor DW, Pollitt PA, Brook CP *et al*. Does early intervention reduce the number of elderly people with dementia admitted to institutions for long-term care? *Br Med J* 1991; **302**: 871–5.

14. Breitner JCS. Inflammatory processes and anti-inflammatory drugs in Alzheimer's disease: a current appraisal. *Neurobiol Aging* 1996; **17**: 789–94.

38

Dementia Epidemiology: Prevalence and Incidence

A. F. Jorm

Centre for Mental Health Research, The Australian National University, Canberra, Australia

Prevalence is the proportion of cases of a disease present in a population at any one time, while incidence is the rate of occurrence of new cases over a given period of time, usually 1 year. Prevalence is a function of both the incidence of disease and its duration: the prevalence of a disease will rise if the rate of new cases increases or if the average case survives longer. Prevalence is useful for assessing the likely need for service provision. However, for purely scientific purposes, such as assessing risk factors, incidence is preferred over prevalence. The reason is that any differences between groups in prevalence may be due to differences in either incidence or disease duration.

The notions of prevalence and incidence are based on the assumption that a population can be neatly divided into cases and non-cases. However, for dementia this division is not straightforward. There is a gradation from normal cognitive ageing through to severe dementia, without clear breaks to define where normality ends and dementia begins. The threshold for dementia is usually defined in terms of interference with daily living, but even this is a fuzzy boundary. Furthermore, prevalence and incidence studies typically examine different levels of severity, described as "mild", "moderate" or "severe", but these descriptors are not always used consistently to divide up the continuum of severity. Various diagnostic criteria for dementia are known to divide the continuum in different ways, which can result in very different prevalence and incidence rates. For example, Erkinjuntti et al.[1] examined the rates of dementia in the same sample using six different sets of diagnostic criteria. They found that the percentage with dementia varied from 3.1% using the ICD-10 criteria to 29.1% using DSM-III. Thus, there are no "true" prevalence or incidence rates for dementia, but rather various rates dependent on the definition of dementia used.

PREVALENCE OF DEMENTIA

The number of prevalence studies is now very large and several meta-analyses have been carried out to pool the data for those that give rates for specific age groups (e.g. 65–69 years). The first meta-analysis, by Jorm et al.[2], involved fitting a statistical model to data from 22 studies published between 1945 and 1985. They found that methodological differences between studies contributed to variation in prevalence rates. For example, studies that used a broad definition of dementia (to include all cognitive impairment) had rates 64% higher than those using a more narrow definition. They fitted an exponential statistical model to the data[2]. The essence of this model is that prevalence rises

exponentially with age, doubling every 5.1 years, but the actual rates differ from study to study. Although there were differences between studies, it is possible to derive average rates across studies. These are shown in column 1 of Table 38.1. The exponential model is an adequate description up to age 90 but should not be applied above that age. If prevalence continued to double every 5.1 years above age 90, it would soon be greater than 100%, which is impossible. This limitation of the exponential model has led some researchers to use the logistic model, in which prevalence at first rises steeply, but then levels out to a maximum of 100%[3]. For prevalence rates of 0–50% the exponential and logistic curves are difficult to distinguish, and the exponential curve may be preferred because of its simplicity.

The second meta-analysis involved a pooling of data from 12 European studies dating 1980–1990, which used DSM-III or equivalent criteria[4]. This meta-analysis did not involve fitting a statistical model to the data or testing for the effects of methodological differences. Rather, the researchers simply divided the data from each study into 5 year age groups and pooled them. The results are shown in column 2 of Table 38.1. Despite the differences in approach, the results are remarkably close to those of Jorm et al.[2].

A third meta-analysis was carried out by Ritchie and Kildea[5] (this superseded an earlier meta-analysis by Ritchie et al.[6], which will not be described here). They were particularly interested in what happens to prevalence in extreme old age, in particular whether dementia is inevitable if a person lives long enough. Ritchie and Kildea[5] pooled data from nine studies that included samples of elderly people aged over 80. These data are shown in column 3 of Table 38.1 and are very similar to the earlier meta-analyses up to age 90. Ritchie and Kildea[5] fitted various curves to

Table 38.1 Prevalence rates (%) for dementia from three meta-analyses

Age group	Meta-analysis		
	Jorm et al.[2]	Hofman et al.[4]	Ritchie and Kildea[5]
60–64	0.7	1.0	—
65–69	1.4	1.4	1.5
70–74	2.8	4.1	3.5
75–79	5.6	5.7	6.8
80–84	11.1	13.0	13.6
85–89	23.6*	24.5*	22.3
90–94	—	—	33.0
95–99			44.8

* Rates for ages 85+.

Principles and Practice of Geriatric Psychiatry, 2nd edn. Edited by J. R. M. Copeland, M. T. Abou-Saleh and D. G. Blazer
©2002 John Wiley & Sons, Ltd

the data, including exponential and logistic models. The best fit was by a modified logistic curve in which prevalence levelled off at around 40% at age 95. The authors concluded that dementia is not inevitable in extreme old age. However, this conclusion has been criticized by McGee and Brayne[7] because it was based on prevalence rather than incidence data. A decrease in survival with dementia in very old age could explain the flattening of the age-curve that was observed.

PREVALENCE OF ALZHEIMER'S DISEASE AND VASCULAR DEMENTIA

The clinical diagnosis of Alzheimer's disease and vascular dementia in community surveys involves additional problems beyond those in diagnosing global dementia, so such studies have been fewer. Nevertheless, several meta-analyses have attempted to integrate data on the issue.

The original meta-analysis of Jorm et al.[2] also examined seven studies that gave age-specific data on Alzheimer's disease and vascular dementia. One study could not be fitted well by the exponential model, but the remaining six could. The prevalence of Alzheimer's was found to double every 4.5 years of age, while vascular dementia doubled every 5.3 years. In other words, the rise with age was steeper for Alzheimer's disease.

The pooling of data from European studies also examined specific dementing diseases[8]. The pooled prevalence rates for Alzheimer's disease from six studies were: 30–59 years, 0.02%; 60–69 years, 0.3%; 70–79 years, 3.2%; and 80–89 years, 10.8%. It was not possible to arrive at pooled rates for vascular dementia because of the variation across studies.

Later, Corrada et al.[9] fitted a logistic model to data from 15 studies giving age-specific data on prevalence of Alzheimer's disease. They found considerable variation in rates between studies depending on the methodology used. However, the underlying trend was for an 18% increase in the odds for Alzheimer's disease with every year of age.

The most recent meta-analysis was carried out by the US General Accounting Office[10] in response to controversy in that country about the number of people with Alzheimer's disease. A logistic curve was fitted to data from 18 studies with predominantly White populations. The data were grouped by sex and severity level of the dementia and are shown in Table 38.2. It can be seen that the results vary, depending on severity, and that females have a higher prevalence than males.

INCIDENCE STUDIES

Incidence studies are much rarer than prevalence studies because they require longitudinal data and large sample sizes to arrive at age-specific rates. It is only fairly recently that sufficient studies have become available to permit meta-analysis.

Two meta-analyses have been published at around the same time. The first of these, by Jorm and Jolley[11], used data from 23 published studies. The incidence of both dementia and Alzheimer's disease was found to increase exponentially with age up to

Table 38.2 Prevalence rates (%) for Alzheimer's disease according to a meta-analysis by the US General Accounting Office[10]

Age	All severity levels		Moderate–severe cases	
	Men	Women	Men	Women
65	0.6	0.8	0.3	0.6
70	1.3	1.7	0.6	1.1
75	2.7	3.5	1.1	2.3
80	5.6	7.1	2.3	4.4
85	11.1	13.8	4.4	8.6
90	20.8	25.2	8.5	15.8
95	35.6	41.5	15.8	27.4

Table 38.3. Incidence rates (%) for dementia from meta-analyses by Jorm and Jolley[11] and Gao et al.[12]

Age group	Jorm and Jolley[11]				Gao et al.[12] 12 studies
	Europe (mild+)	Europe (moderate+)	USA (moderate+)	East Asia (mild+)	
60–64	—	—	—	—	0.11
65–69	0.91	0.36	0.24	0.35	0.33
70–74	1.76	0.64	0.50	0.71	0.84
75–79	3.33	1.17	1.05	1.47	1.82
80–84	5.99	2.15	1.77	3.26	3.36
85–89	10.41	3.77	2.75	7.21	5.33
90–94	17.98	6.61	—	—	7.29
95+	—	—	—	—	8.68

Mild+ results from USA and Moderate+ results from East Asia are missing from the table because insufficient data were found in the literature.

Table 38.4 Incidence rates (%) for Alzheimer's disease from meta-analyses by Jorm and Jolley[11] and Gao et al.[12]

Age group	Jorm and Jolley[11]					Gao et al. 8 studies
	Europe (mild+)	Europe (moderate+)	USA (mild+)	USA (moderate+)	East Asia (mild+)	
60–64	—	—	—	—	—	0.06
65–69	0.25	0.10	0.61	0.16	0.07	0.19
70–74	0.52	0.22	1.11	0.35	0.21	0.51
75–79	1.07	0.48	2.01	0.78	0.58	1.17
80–84	2.21	1.06	3.84	1.48	1.49	2.31
85–89	4.61	2.26	7.45	2.60	3.97	3.86
90–94	9.66	4.77	-	-	-	5.49
95+	-	-	-	-	-	6.68

Moderate+ results from East Asia are missing from the table because insufficient data were found in the literature.

90 years, with no sign of levelling off. The incidence of vascular dementia showed similar trends, but the actual rates varied greatly from study to study. There was no sex difference in dementia, but women tended to have a higher incidence of Alzheimer's disease in very old age, and men a higher incidence of vascular dementia at younger ages. There were also regional differences, with East Asian countries having a significantly lower incidence of dementia than Europe, and also tending to have a lower incidence of Alzheimer's disease. Tables 38.3 and 38.4 summarize the results for different regions and levels of severity.

The second meta-analysis, by Gao et al.[12], involved only the subset of 12 studies that used DSM-III criteria for dementia and NINCDS–ADRDA criteria for Alzheimer's disease. The data were fitted with a logistic model and a levelling of the rate of increase with age was found. Women were found to have a higher incidence of Alzheimer's disease than men. The estimated incidence rates are also shown in Tables 38.3 and 38.4. It can be seen that the rates of Gao et al.[12] are different from those of Jorm and Jolley[11] and the two meta-analyses came to different conclusions about whether there is a levelling in the rise with age. The difference arises because Gao et al.[12] pooled data from different regions and different levels of severity. Their rates fall in between those of Jorm and Jolley[11] for Mild + and Moderate + dementia. Deviations from an exponential rise can result if the studies contributing cases at the upper ages are examining milder dementia or are from regions with a lower incidence.

CONCLUSIONS

The prevalence and incidence of dementia rise exponentially with age up to age 90. There is no consensus about what happens at extreme ages, because of the limited data available, but some levelling in the rise is a possibility. Women probably have a higher prevalence and incidence of Alzheimer's disease. Conversely, men may be at greater risk of vascular dementia. There appear to be important regional differences, although the proper investigation

of these requires studies with identical methodologies in the various sites.

REFERENCES

1. Erkinjuntti, T, Østbye T, Steenhuis R, Hachinski V. The effect of different diagnostic criteria on the prevalence of dementia. *N Engl J Med* 1997; **337**: 1667–74.
2. Jorm AF, Korten AE, Henderson AS. The prevalence of dementia: a quantitative integration of the literature. *Acta Psychiat Scand* 1987; **76**: 465–79.
3. Dewey ME. How should prevalence be modelled? *Acta Psychiat Scand* 1991; **84**: 246–9.
4. Hofman A, Rocca WA, Brayne C et al. The prevalence of dementia in Europe: a collaborative study of 1980–1990 findings. *Int J Epidemiol* 1991; **20**: 736–48.
5. Ritchie K, Kildea D. Is senile dementia "age-related" or "ageing-related"?—evidence from meta-analysis of dementia prevalence in the oldest old. *Lancet* 1995; **346**: 931–4.
6. Ritchie K, Kildea D, Robine J-M. The relationship between age and the prevalence of senile dementia: a meta-analysis of recent data. *Int J Epidemiol* 1992; **21**: 763–9.
7. McGee MA, Brayne C. The impact on prevalence of dementia in the oldest age groups of differential mortality patterns: a deterministic approach. *Int J Epidemiol* 1998; **27**: 87–90.
8. Rocca WA, Hofman A, Brayne C et al. Frequency and distribution of Alzheimer's disease in Europe: a collaborative study of 1980–1990 prevalence findings. *Ann Neurol* 1991; **30**: 381–90.
9. Corrada M, Brookmeyer R, Kawas C. Sources of variability in prevalence rates of Alzheimer's disease. *Int J Epidemiol* 1995; **24**: 1000–1005.
10. US General Accounting Office. *Alzheimer's Disease: Estimates of Prevalence in the United States*. Washington, DC: United States General Accounting Office.
11. Jorm AF, Jolley D. The incidence of dementia: a meta-analysis. *Neurology* 1998; **51**: 728–33.
12. Gao S, Hendrie HC, Hall KS, Hui S. The relationships between age, sex, and the incidence of dementia: a meta-analysis. *Arch Gen Psychiat* 1998; **55**: 809–15.

39

Case-control Studies

Scott Henderson

NHMRC Psychiatric Epidemiology Research Centre, Australian National University, Canberra, ACT 0200, Australia

The case-control study is aimed at aetiology. Schlesselman[1] says that it has two distinctive features: it proceeds backwards from effect to cause by trying to identify exposures or other factors that led to a given disorder; and it uses a control or comparison group without the disorder, so that a causal effect for a given exposure can be supported or refuted. The first of these features is really what a clinician does in daily practice when taking a history, but as a rule, the clinician does not go on to determine how many *normal* persons have had the same exposure. The strength of the case-control method lies in these two features. It is on the basis of them that the fundamental comparison in the case-control study lies: the frequency of an exposure in the cases, and the frequency in the controls. Such a comparison is disarmingly simple, mainly because of the biases that can bring about misleading results. Some readable accounts can be found in Cole[2], Lilienfeld and Lilienfeld[3], Feinstein[4] and Anthony[5]. A non-technical overview has been set out by Henderson[6]. An entire issue of *Epidemiologic Reviews* devoted to the case-control method has provided an excellent conspectus of this powerful tool, including the diverse applications now being made of case-control designs for problem-solving in the health field, including evaluation of service interventions[7].

In case-control parlance, "exposure" refers not only to environmental exposures, but to other properties of the individual, such as a family history of a particular disease or some other personal attribute. To identify an exposure that may contribute to the onset of a disorder, the investigator has firstly to choose a number of candidate exposures. This may be based on theory, on speculation, or on a mindless search. The first of these is particularly desirable, because it means that from the start there is some plausible biological or psychosocial basis for the putative effect. Speculation can be the vehicle for a gifted insight. The atheoretical examination of a large array of factors is undesirable and carries the risk of capitalization on chance.

CONDUCTING A CASE-CONTROL STUDY

There are five issues that deserve close attention:

1. The cases should be newly diagnosed, not ones which have been known for some time; and they should be representative of all incident cases in the population. If longer-established cases were used, the findings might be related more to factors influencing survival or chronicity than to aetiology (see below).
2. The cases should include no errors in diagnosis, which would lead to misclassification and therefore errors in estimating the relative risk for exposures.
3. The controls should either be matched demographically or be similar in overall attributes. Much thought needs to be accorded to the source of the controls if misleading biases are to be avoided.
4. In obtaining information on exposures from cases and controls, as well as from their informants, it is likely that selection effects will operate, causing information bias. That is, people may selectively recall certain experiences, or selectively report what they do recall. A likely example is a history of past head injury in Alzheimer's disease, or any other situation where "effort after meaning" may operate. Ideally, the interviewers should themselves be blind to the purpose of the study, lest they unwittingly influence the information that they elicit.
5. A case-control study that has too few cases to provide a satisfactory estimate of risk is of little value. The sample size needed can be determined beforehand by establishing the minimum size of the effect to be demonstrated, and the frequency of exposure in the controls. The more the frequency of the exposure departs from 50% of the subjects, the more cases will be needed for an association to be shown.

The assessment of risk for an exposure is obtained by calculating its odds ratio as an approximation of the relative risk, and the 95% confidence intervals for that estimate (Schlesselman[1], p. 32 *et seq.*) (Henderson[6], p. 16 *et seq.*). An odds ratio of 1.0 means that the exposure occurs as often in cases as in controls. The confidence interval should keep the estimate above unity if the exposure is to be accorded attention. It is misleading to report odds ratios without also giving their confidence intervals. For example, an odds ratio of 1.7 with a 95% confidence interval of 0.9–2.5 should be seen as a negative finding, because the lower limit is below unity.

RESULTS OF CASE-CONTROL STUDIES OF DEMENTIA

Nearly all the case-control studies of dementia have been focused on Alzheimer's disease (AD). Within this diagnostic group, the studies have covered several categories, although not always making this explicit. The cases have often been heterogeneous in age of onset and, indeed, in age *since* onset. The latter introduces the problem of Neyman's bias[5] and factors related to survival after the onset of the dementia. In looking critically at case-control studies of dementia, their strengths and deficiencies can be seen by using the above points as a checklist, to assess the value that can be attached to each observation. Most studies have had only modest sample sizes. In case-control studies of AD, the

Principles and Practice of Geriatric Psychiatry, 2nd edn. Edited by J. R. M. Copeland, M. T. Abou-Saleh and D. G. Blazer
©2002 John Wiley & Sons, Ltd

scientific significance of a result should rest on its replication by other workers on other samples; and on the development of biological evidence to support it as a risk factor in AD.

Risk and Protective Factors for Alzheimer's Disease

A comprehensive review of the evidence for a wide range of proposed risk factors, but also protective factors for AD, have been given by Jorm[8] and Henderson and Jorm[9].

Summarized, these are as follows:

Definite
  Age.
  Family history.
  Specific genetic mutations (for familial cases only).
  Apolipoprotein E ε4 allele on chromosome 19.
  Down's syndrome.
Awaiting confirmation
  Regional or ethnic differences.
  α-2 Macroglobulin gene.
  Head injury (interaction with apoE?).
  Previous depressive disorder.
  Herpes simplex virus.
  Cerebrovascular disease.
Unlikely
  Aluminium in drinking water.
  Diet.
  Industrial solvents.
  Life stress.
  Electromagnetic fields.
Possible protective factors
  Education, high premorbid intelligence or both.
  Anti-inflammatory drugs (NSAIDS).
  Oestrogen.
  Smoking.
  Moderate wine drinking.

For vascular dementia, the review by Skoog[10] lists the same risk factors as for stroke, namely hypertension, diabetes mellitus, advanced age, being male, smoking and cardiac disease. A number of recent case-control studies have suggested that vascular factors may have a part to play in AD. There are as yet no case-control studies of Lewy body or other less common dementias, although there is no impediment other than ensuring accuracy of ascertainment and recruitment of sufficient cases. The same applies to other under-researched areas of geriatric psychiatry, such as the psychoses of late onset, where case-control studies could throw much-needed light on pathogenesis.

It does seem justifiable to continue to search for environmental exposures and other risk factors for AD, for vascular dementia and possibly the rarer dementias. Case-control research may in this way contribute not only to understanding their aetiology, but to finding preventive measures—the ultimate purpose of epidemiology. With the great expansion of the world's elderly, the social significance of this would be inestimable.

REFERENCES

1. Schlesselman JL. *Case-control Studies: Design, Conduct, Analysis*. New York: Oxford University Press, 1982.
2. Cole P. The evolving case-control study. *J Chronic Dis* 1979; **32**: 15–27.
3. Lilienfeld AM, Lilienfeld DE. *Foundations of Epidemiology*, 2nd edn. New York: Oxford University Press, 1980.
4. Feinstein AR. Experimental requirements and scientific principles in case-control studies. *J Chronic Dis* 1985; **38**: 127–33.
5. Anthony JC. Case-control studies. In Henderson AS, Burrows GD (eds), *Handbook of Social Psychiatry*. Amsterdam: Elsevier, 1988; 157–71.
6. Henderson AS. *An Introduction to Social Psychiatry*. Oxford: Oxford University Press, 1988.
7. Armenian HK, Gordis L. Future perspectives on the case-control method. *Epidemiol Rev* 1994; **16**: 163–4.
8. Jorm AF. Risk factors for Alzheimer's disease. In O'Brien J, Ames D, Burns A (eds), *Dementia*, 2nd Edn. London: Kluwer Academic/Lippincott-Raven (in press).
9. Henderson AS, Jorm AF. Disease definition, natural history and epidemiology. In Maj M, Sartorius N (eds), *Evidence and Experience in Psychiatry, vol 3, Dementia*. Chichester: Wiley, 2000.
10. Skoog I. Risk factors for vascular dementia: a review. *Dementia* 1994; **5**: 137–44.

Results from EURODEM Collaboration on the Incidence of Dementia

LJ Launer[1], for the EURODEM Incidence Research Group*

[1]*Erasmus University Medical Centre, Rotterdam, The Netherlands, and National Institutes of Health, Bethesda, MD, USA*

In 1988, European investigators formed the EURODEM network to harmonize the protocols used in newly initiated population-based prospective studies on incident dementing diseases[1].

*Participants of the EURODEM Incidence Research Group: Department of Epidemiology and Biostatistics, Erasmus Medical School, The Netherlands (A. Hofman MD, L.J. Launer PhD, A. Ott MD, T. Stijnen PhD); Epidemiology, Demography, Biometry Program, National Institute on Aging, US (L.J. Launer PhD); Department of Psychiatry, Odense University, Denmark (K. Andersen MD, P. Kragh-Sorensen MD); Department of Psychiatry, Royal Liverpool University Hospital, UK (J.R.M. Copeland MD, M.E. Dewey PhD); INSERM Unit 330, France (J.F. Dartigues MD, L. Letenneur PhD); National Research Council Targeted Program on Ageing, Italy (L.A. Amaducci MD: now deceased); Institute of Public Health, Cambridge University, UK (C. Brayne MD); Department of Psychiatry, Zaragoza University (A. Lobo MD) and Department of Neurology, University of Navarra, Spain (J.M. Martinez-Lage MD).

Incident studies succeeded the case-control studies based on prevalent cases that were conducted in the 1980s[2]. Studies based on incident cases are preferred to those based on prevalent cases, as the latter have several biases that affect the validity of their results[3]. Here we summarize the findings from the pooled EURODEM analyses on the frequency and risk for dementing disease in the elderly.

STUDY DESIGN

The pooled analyses are based on studies from Denmark[4], France[5], The Netherlands[6] and the UK[7]. The sample includes

528 incident dementia cases and 28 768 person-years of follow-up. As a common core, each study included a population-based cohort of persons aged 65 years and older living in the community and nursing homes. Samples were drawn from defined geographic areas and either include all eligible individuals or individuals randomly selected within predefined strata. All studies contributed to the pooled analyses baseline data and one follow-up panel conducted after a fixed interval of about 3 years. The cohorts exclude the prevalent cases identified at baseline.

Dementia cases were identified in a two-stage procedure, whereby the total cohort was screened and screen-positive subjects underwent a detailed diagnostic assessment that included a clinical exam, neuropsychological testing and an informant interview. Dementia and vascular dementia were diagnosed according to DSM-III-R criteria[8], Alzheimer's disease (AD) was diagnosed according to NINCDS–ADRDA criteria[9].

RESULTS

AD comprised approximately 70% of all cases. Incident rates for dementia and AD were similar across studies. There was an increase with age in the incidence of all dementia and in particular AD. At 90 years of age and older the incidence of AD was 63.5 (95% CI, 49.7–81.0) per 1000 person-years. However, compared to men, women had significantly higher rates of AD after age 85 years. At 90 years of age, the rate of AD per 1000 person-years was 81.7 (63.8–104.7) in women and 24.0 (10.3–55.6) in men (Figure 1a,b)[10]. This translated into a cumulative risk for 65 year-old women to develop AD at the age of 95 years of 0.22 compared to 0.09 for men. These sex differences were not found in vascular dementia: at 90 years of age, the incidence of vascular dementia was 15.9 (6.6–38.5) and 9.2 (4.3–19.6) per 1000 person-years in men and women, respectively.

In addition to sex and age, we investigated the association of AD to four risk factors that had been previously investigated in case-control studies[1,2]. These risk factors were ascertained in a similar manner across studies. We found that low education increased the risk for dementia, specifically AD. However, the increased risk was detectable only in women: compared to those with high education, those with low education had a 4.3 (95% CI, 1.5–11.9) times, and those with middle education had a 2.6 (95% CI, 1.0–7.1) times increased risk for AD. There was no association of educational level to dementia among men[11]. Contrary to a previous EURODEM analysis based on case-control studies[2], we did not find an increased risk for AD associated with head trauma. Previous reports based on prevalent cases suggested an inverse association of smoking with the risk for AD[2]. In these current analyses based on incident cases, we found current smoking significantly *increased* the risk of AD. The risk associated with smoking was higher in men than women[1]. Finally, we found that the association of AD to family history in two or more family members was weaker (OR 1.59 95% CI, 0.78–3.26) than previously estimated on the basis of case-control studies[2].

SUMMARY

Because we had a large sample, we were able to investigate whether gender modified the risk for AD, the most common form of late-life dementia. We found that women not only had a higher risk for AD than men, but that the relations of education and smoking to the risk for AD were different in men and women. These findings suggest that the risk for AD is altered either by sex-related biological or behavioral factors or by differences in cumulative survival.

A

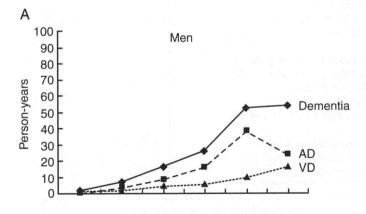

B

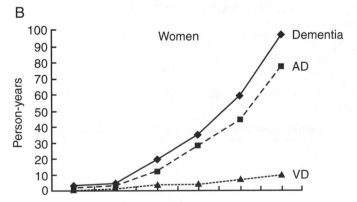

Figure 1 Incidence of dementia and major sub-types, Alzheimer's disease (AD) and vascular dementia (VD): EURODEM Studies. (A) men; (B) women

REFERENCES

1. Launer LJ, Andersen K, Dewey ME *et al*. Rates and risk for Alzheimer's disease: EURODEM collaborative analysis. *Neurology* 1999; **52**: 78–84.
2. van Duijn CM, Hofman A (eds). Risk factors for Alzheimer's disease: a collaborative re-analysis of case-control studies. *Int J Epidemiol* 1991; **20**(suppl 2): S2–73.
3. Szklo M, Nieto FJ. *Epidemiology: Beyond the Basics*. Gaithersburg, MD: Aspen, 2000.
4. Andersen K, Nielsen H, Lolk A *et al*. Incidence of very mild to severe dementia in Denmark. The Odense Study. *Neurology* 1999; **52**: 85–90.
5. Letenneur L, Commenges D, Dartigues J-F, Barberger-Gateau P. Incidence of dementia and Alzheimer's disease in elderly community residents of south-western France. *Int J Epidemiol* 1994; **23**: 1256–61.
6. Ott A, Breteler MM, van Harskamp F *et al*. Incidence and risk of dementia. The Rotterdam Study. *Am J Epidemiol* 1998; **147**: 574–80.
7. Saunders PA, Copeland JRM, Dewey ME *et al*. ALPHA: The Liverpool MRC study of the incidence of dementia and cognitive decline. *Neuroepidemiol* 1992; **11**(suppl 1): 44–7.
8. American Psychiatric Association. *Diagnostic and Statistical Manual of Mental Disorders*, 3rd edn, revised. Washington, DC: American Psychiatric Association, 1987.
9. McKhann G, Drachman D, Folstein M *et al*. Clinical diagnosis of Alzheimer's disease. Report of the NINCDS–ADRDA Work Group under the auspices of Department of Health and Human Services Task Force on Alzheimer's disease. *Neurology* 1984; **34**: 939–44.
10. Andersen K, Launer LJ, Dewey M *et al*. Sex differences in the risk for incident dementia: EURODEM pooled analyses. *Neurology* 1999; **53**: 1992–7.
11. Letenneur L, Launer LJ, Andersen K *et al*. Education and the risk for Alzheimer's disease: sex makes a difference. EURODEM pooled analyses. EURODEM Incidence Research Group. *Am J Epidemiol* 2000; **151**(11): 1064–71.

MRC/DoH Cognitive Function and Ageing Study

J. Nickson, C. F. M. McCracken and C. Brayne, on behalf of MRC CFAS

University of Cambridge, Cambridge, UK

The MRC Cognitive Function and Ageing Study (MRC CFAS) is a multi-centre prospective cohort study, set up in 1989 and funded by the MRC and Department of Health (DoH).

AIMS

CFAS aims to estimate the prevalence and incidence of cognitive decline and dementia and geographical variation; to determine the natural history of dementia, in particular the rate of progression of cognitive decline, including the distribution of the interval between identification of cognitive impairment and death; to identify factors associated with differing rates of cognitive decline and with the risk of dementia; to determine the contribution of different underlying pathologies to rates of dementia, geographical variation and burden of disability; to evaluate the degree of disability associated with cognitive decline and service needs generated; to set up a brain and blood resource; and to provide a framework to support sub-studies.

METHODOLOGY

The study has five methodologically identical centres (Cambridge, Gwynedd, Newcastle, Nottingham and Oxford) and one

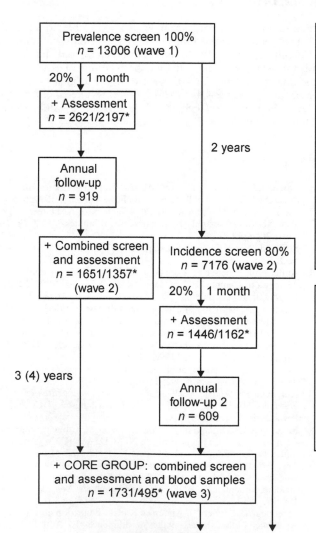

Screening interview:
Sociodemographics
Activities of daily living
Physical health
Smoking, alcohol
Cognitive function
Medication

Assessment interview:
Geriatric mental state (GMS)
allowing AGECAT
CAMCOG, MMSE
Extra items for ICD and DSM

Informant interview*:
History and aetiology schedule (HAS)
Hachinski, Blessed

Selection from screen to assessment					
Age (years)	AGECAT O3+	MMSE LE 21	MMSE 22–25	MMSE 26–30	MMSE missing
65–74					
Four centres*	1	1	2/3	1/10	1
Cambridge	1	1	1/4	1/10	1
≥ 75					
Four centres*	1	2/3	1/3	1/13	2/3
Cambridge	1/2	1/2	1/7	1/15	1/2
*Four centres: Gwynedd, Newcastle, Nottingham, Oxford					

Figure 1. MRC CFAS: methodology (five identical centres). + Declaration of intent (DoI) to donate brain at post mortem. *Informant interview

centre (Liverpool) with a different design and funded earlier. Each of the five centres obtained a stratified random sample from Family Health Service Authority lists of sufficient individuals aged 65 years and over to achieve at least 2500 interviews (*see* Figure 1 for the study design). The Liverpool study consisted of a sample of 6035 individuals aged 65 years and over, stratified by sex and 5 year age bands. 5222 received a detailed assessment interview, with a selection also receiving the same interview by a clinician 3 months later. This process was repeated at 2 and 4 years. At 7–8 years the cohort was reinterviewed using the five-centre combined screen and assessment interview.

BRAIN DONATION

At all waves of the study, selected participants and their families have been approached with a request to consider donating brain tissue after death. Procedures are in place to collect, process and examine brains from these individuals, which are stored locally. There are currently 347 brains within

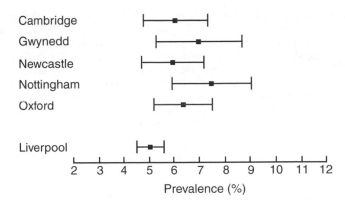

Figure 3. Prevalence estimates with 95% confidence intervals for AGECAT organicity O3+. From reference 3, with permission

Table 1. Estimated numbers of cognitively impaired or disabled elderly people in England and Wales by age group, sex and type of disability

Disability	64–74 years		75–84 years		≥85 years	
	Men	Women	Men	Women	Men	Women
Physical only	68 000	122 000	82 000	257 000	43 000	232 000
Cognitive only	32 000	29 000	45 000	57 000	20 000	61 000
Combined	14 000	11 000	26 000	57 000	27 000	99 000

From reference 1, with permission.

the Neuropathology study and 209 have been used for a first analysis. There are a further 500 people who have made a declaration of intent to donate brain tissue (DoI) and the continuing mechanism for collection will enable us to reach our target of 450.

BLOOD RESOURCE

During wave 2 in Oxford, wave 3 in Cambridge, Gwynedd, Newcastle and Nottingham and wave 4 in Liverpool, a blood sample (or saliva when blood was refused) was requested. There are 1126 blood and 193 saliva samples from the assessed groups in five sites (Cambridge, Liverpool, Gwynedd, Newcastle and Nottingham) and a further 1600 from the full wave 2 population in Oxford.

MORTALITY DATA

The full sample of 24 066 is flagged on the NHS Central Register at the Office for National Statistics (ONS); 11 104 death notifications, with causes coded to ICD-9, have been received. The death information complements and enhances data from interviews, as all eligible for entry into the study, together with those actually interviewed, were flagged. This enables tracking of all individuals from initial sampling to death.

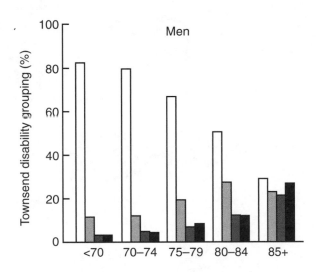

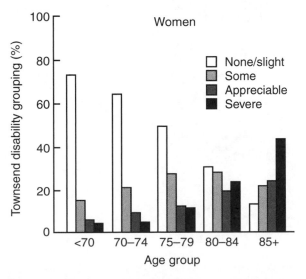

Figure 2. Percentage within Townsend disability grouping by age group and sex. From reference 2, with permission

OUTPUT FROM THE STUDY

Figures 2 and 3 and Table 1 provide some results from published papers. A full bibliography may be found on the CFAS website, http://mrc-bsu.cam.ac.uk/cfas. Work in progress includes measures of healthy life expectancy, estimation of incidence rates, medication usage, normative values for CAMCOG and its subscales, cognitive function as a marker for survival, neuropathology analysis and genetic risk for dementia.

REFERENCES

1. MRC CFAS and RIS MRC CFAS. Profile of disability in elderly people: estimates from a longitudinal population study. *Br Med J* 1999; **318**: 1108–11.
2. MRC CFAS. The description of activities of daily living in England and Wales. *Age Ageing* 1998; **27**: 605–13.
3. MRC CFA. Cognitive function and dementia in six areas of England and Wales: the distribution of MMSE and prevalence of GMS organicity level in the MRC CFA study. *Psychol Med* 1998; **28**: 319–35.

40

The Epidemiology of Alzheimer's Disease: An Update

Lenore J. Launer

*Epidemiology, Demography, Biometry Program,
National Institute on Aging, Bethesda, MD, USA*

This chapter provides a short overview on methodologic issues related to the design of epidemiologic studies of dementia, and provides an update on the epidemiology of Alzheimer's disease (AD). AD is characterized by a gradual but steady decline in cognitive and occupational function. A clinical diagnosis of AD is based on the course of the dementia and exclusion of other known causes of dementia. A definite diagnosis of AD can only be made post mortem in the presence of neuritic plaques and neurofibrillary tangles[1]. Although these lesions are considered to be pathognomonic for the disease, it is unclear as to whether they are the primary cause of the disease or are the consequence of other more fundamental processes.

METHODOLOGY

Study Design

Research into the frequency and etiology of dementia is based on studies of prevalent cases and incident cases. Prevalent cases are identified in a cross-sectional study. The probability that they are found depends on the likelihood that they developed into a case and survived until the time of the survey. Thus, there is usually over-representation of cases with long duration. Incident cases are newly developed cases identified in a prospective follow-up study of a cohort that is initially dementia-free at baseline. It is preferable to study etiologic factors related to dementia in incident cases, as there is less likelihood that factors related to survival (or severity of the disease) influence the association of the exposure to the disease.

Measurement of Risk Factors

Ascertainment and interpretation of risk factor data is also less subject to bias when collected from incident, compared to prevalent, cases. In incident cases, a risk factor can be measured at baseline before the onset of dementia. In a prevalent case, a proxy needs to be questioned because a demented person can no longer be expected to provide valid or reliable answers. In addition, some biologic markers in prevalent cases may be influenced by the dementia itself[2].

Case Identification

Most cases of dementia do not come to the attention of the health services. This is the result of many factors, including the cases themselves or their caretakers not recognizing the disease[3] and there presently being few treatment alternatives. Likewise, dementia is under-reported as cause of death. Therefore, studies relying on health care systems or records to identify cases probably only capture moderate to severe cases or cases with exceptional presentation. To fully identify the range of case presentation in the population, including mild cases, population-based studies that interview individuals in person are needed.

Diagnostic Guidelines

Strides in standardization of diagnoses used in research studies have been made in the past decade. Currently, the diagnosis of AD is made on the basis of internationally agreed guidelines for dementia (i.e. DSM-IV[4] and ICD-10[5]) and specific criteria for AD. The most widely used criteria for AD are from the NINCDS–ADRDA[6]. Although application of different guidelines for dementia can identify different individual cases[7], reasonable inter- and intra-rater reliability can be achieved[8] if the same guidelines are used.

RISK FACTORS

Much progress has been made in the past decade in testing hypotheses based on case-control studies[9], and also in identifying new hypotheses.

Age and Sex

All epidemiologic studies show an increase in the frequency of dementia with age, with an almost doubling of prevalence and incidence from age 65–85 years[10,11]. Approximately 65% of cases are attributed to AD, although the proportion of AD cases out of the total might depend on ethnic group[12]. Furthermore, as more neuroimaging is used in diagnosis, more cases of dementia associated with cerebrovascular disease may be identified[13]. The slope of the increase with age depends on the sub-type of dementia. The incidence of dementia and AD increases steeply with age. The absolute incidence and the age-related increase in vascular dementia is lower. Studies differ concerning the sex-specific risk for AD. After 85 years of age a large difference in incidence was found in European studies[14]; the incidence in women increased steadily with age (up to 82/1000 person-years at 90 years and older), but flattened out in men (at 25/1000 person-years at 90 years and older). In contrast, in USA-based cohorts[15,16], the incidence of dementia, or AD, increased in old age with no apparent differences by sex. Sex differences in the risk for AD may be due to differences in biology, cumulative survival, or behaviour and exposures. Further investigations are needed to clarify the contribution of sex to the risk for AD.

Education

The contribution of education to the risk for AD is still controversial. Some argue that an association reflects confounding by socioeconomic factors, or diagnostic bias due to poorer performance on neuropsychological tests by individuals with low education[17]. Others argue that education is a marker for biological capacity that modulates when a person reaches the threshold of clinical dementia[18]. Several studies based on prevalent cases show that low education is associated with an increased risk for AD[19]. Studies based on incident cases are inconsistent, with some showing no relation[20] and others showing a relationship[21] of low education to increased risk for AD. In one study the increased risk associated with AD was confined to women[22].

Head Trauma

Reports on the relation of AD to head trauma with unconsciousness are inconsistent. Most studies are based on prevalent cases, where a proxy has had to be asked about the case's history of head trauma. These studies have either shown no effect[23], an increased risk for AD only in men[24], or only in women with head trauma[25]. In a study based on US war veterans with independently documented history of head trauma during the war, there was a two-fold increased risk for AD[26]. One report suggested that head trauma is a risk factor in the presence of the apolipoprotein E*4 allele[27] but two other studies have failed to confirm this[24,28].

Cardiovascular Risk Factors

One new area that is being investigated is the relation to AD of cardiovascular disease and risk factors. Several direct and indirect mechanisms may explain such associations, including ischemia, hypoxia, hemodynamic factors and neurotransmitter metabolism[29]. Studies have reported an increased risk for AD associated with subclinical measures of atherosclerosis[30] and elevated levels of blood pressure[2]. Indicators of glucose metabolism, including glucose and insulin levels[3] and diabetes[32] have also been associated with an increased risk for AD, although not consistently[33]. In addition, cardiovascular risk factors have also been shown to increase the risk for AD, including smoking[34,35] and diet[36]. Since this is a relatively new area of investigation, confirmation of these findings in other studies is needed.

Steroidal Hormones

Estrogen may be linked to AD through several direct mechanisms related to amyloid processing, neurotransmitter metabolism, cerebral blood flow or through cardioprotective pathways[37]. Epidemiologic studies based on prevalent cases are inconsistent, some show a positive effect[38], others not[39,40]. Prospective studies suggest that estrogen replacement therapy is protective[41–44]. However, these observational studies may be detecting an association of AD to healthy behaviour, as hormone replacement therapy users tend to be healthier[45]. Studies examining estrogen effects in men, as well as clinical trials, are needed to confirm the association of increased estrogen levels to a reduced risk for AD.

NSAIDs

Based on finding remnants of inflammatory processes in neuropathologic material of AD brains, it has been hypothesized that anti-inflammatory medications may reduce the risk for AD[46]. There have been many case-control studies based on prevalent cases[47]. Although some of these studies show no effect, those that do provide estimates of as much as an 80% reduced risk[48]. More recently, several prospective studies have been published, with inconsistent results. Studies with one measure at baseline and subsequent follow-up found no association[49,50], and another showed a non-significant reduced risk among those using NSAIDs for 6 months or more within 10 years prior to the diagnosis of dementia[51]. In the Baltimore Longitudinal Study of Aging, the risk of AD decreased with increasing duration of NSAID use over a 16 year follow-up[52]. As with the estrogen hypothesis, that pertaining to NSAIDs needs to be tested in controlled clinical trials.

Genetics

With time, increasingly more will be known about the genetics of AD. Currently, several specific mutations have been found in familial (early onset) cases of AD, including missense mutations in the β-amyloid precursor protein on chromosome 21[53] and mutations in the presenilin-1 (chromosome 14q)[54] and presenilin-2 (chromosome 1) genes[55]. However, these mutations do not account for the vast majority of cases, which are sporadic and of later onset. To date, apolipoprotein is the only identified polymorphism that has consistently been shown to be associated with a genetic susceptibility to sporadic and late-age onset AD. Specifically, the e*4 allele increases the risk for AD[56]. Genes involved in inflammatory, apoptotic, metabolic, cytoskeletal, and neurotransmission processes are also under investigation[57]. However, their role in modulating the risk for AD needs further elucidation. There are examples where a polymorphism is found to increase the risk for AD in one sample, but the findings cannot be replicated in others (i.e. such as the polymorphism in the gene encoding α2-macroglobulin[58,59]). Identification of genetic factors contributing to AD will not be simple. The majority of cases are probably a pool of heterogeneous conditions. It is not likely that there will be one or two major genes that are identified; rather, the genetic risk for AD will likely be the product of a number of genes that make a small contribution to risk.

SUMMARY

In the past decade many more prospective population-based studies were started and have yielded valuable data. However, besides age and the apolipoprotein gene, few risk factors have been shown consistently to reduce, or to increase, the risk for AD. With advances in our understanding of the brain and our genetic code, rapid progress should be made in identifying environmental and genetic risk factors and in studying the interaction between the two.

REFERENCES

1. The National Institute on Aging, and Reagan Institute Working Group on Diagnostic Criteria for the Neuropathological Assessment of Alzheimer's Disease. Consensus recommendations for the postmortem diagnosis of Alzheimer's disease. *Neurobiol Aging* 1997; **18**(4 Suppl): S1–2.
2. Skoog I, Lernfelt B, Landahl et al. 15-year longitudinal study of blood pressure and dementia. *Lancet* 1996; **347**: 1141–5.
3. Ross GW, Abbott RD, Petrovitch H et al. Frequency and characteristics of silent dementia among elderly Japanese-American men. The Honolulu–Asia Aging Study. *J Am Med Assoc* 1997; **12**: 800–5.
4. American Psychiatric Association. *Diagnostic and Statistical Manual of Mental Disorders*, 4th edn (DSM-IV). Washington, DC: American Psychiatric Association, 1994.
5. World Heath Organization. *International Classification of Diseases*, 10th edn (ICD-10). WHO: Geneva, 1988.
6. McKhann G, Drachman D, Folstein M et al. Clinical diagnosis of Alzheimer's disease: report of the NINCDS–ADRDA Work Group under the auspices of Department of Health and Human Services Task Force on Alzheimer's Disease. *Neurology* 1984; **34**: 939–44.
7. Erkinjuntti T, Ostbye T, Steenhuis R, Hachinski V. The effect of different diagnostic criteria on the prevalence of dementia. *N Engl J Med* 1997; **337**: 1667–74.
8. O'Connor DW, Blessed G, Cooper B et al. Cross-national interrater reliability of dementia diagnosis in the elderly and factors associated with disagreement. *Neurology* 1996; **47**: 1194–9.
9. van Duijn CM, Hofman A (eds). Risk factors for Alzheimer's disease: a collaborative re-analysis of case-control studies. *Int J Epidemiol* 1991; **20**(suppl 2): S2–73.
10. Hofman A, Rocca WA, Brayne C et al. The prevalence of dementia in Europe. A collaborative study of 1980–1990 prevalence findings. *Int J Epidemiol* 1991; **20**: 736–48.
11. Jorm AF, Jolley D. The incidence of dementia: a meta-analysis. *Neurology* 1998; **51**: 728–33.
12. White L, Petrovitch H, Ross GW et al. Prevalence of dementia in older Japanese-American men in Hawaii: the Honolulu–Asia Aging Study. *J Am Med Assoc* 1996; **226**: 955–60.
13. Skoog I, Nilsson L, Palmertz B et al. A population-based study of dementia in 85 years-olds. *N Engl J Med* 1993; **328**: 153–8.
14. Andersen K, Launer LJ, Dewey ME et al. Sex differences in the incidence of Alzheimer's and vascular dementia: the EURODEM Studies. *Neurology* (in press).
15. Rocca WA, Cha RH, Waring SC, Kokmen E. Incidence of dementia and Alzheimer's disease. A reanalysis of data from Rochester, Minnesota, 1975–1984. *Am J Epidemiol* 1998; **148**: 51–62.
16. Bachman DL, Wolf PA, Linn RT et al. Incidence of dementia and probable Alzheimer's disease in a general population: the Framingham Study. *Neurology* 1993; **43**: 515–19.
17. Mortimer JA, Graves AB. Education and other socioeconomic determinants of dementia and Alzheimer's disease. *Neurology* 1993; **43**(suppl 4): S39–44.
18. Katzman R. Education and the prevalence of dementia and Alzheimer's disease. *Neurology* 1993; **43**: 13–20.
19. Fratiglioni L, Grut M, Forsell Y et al. Prevalence of Alzheimer's disease and other dementia in an elderly urban population: relationship with age, sex and education. *Neurology* 1991; **41**: 1886–92.
20. Beard M, Kokmen E, Offord K, Kurland L. Lack of association between Alzheimer's disease and education, occupation, marital status or living arrangement. *Neurology* 1992; **42**: 2063–8.
21. Stern Y, Gurland B, Tatamichi TK et al. Influence of education and occupation on the incidence of Alzheimer's disease. *J Am Med Assoc* 1994; **271**(3): 1004–10.
22. Letenneur L, Launer LJ, Andersen K et al. Education and the risk for Alzheimer's disease: sex makes a difference. EURODEM pooled analyses. *Am J Epidemiol* 2000; **51**: 1064–71.
23. Fratiglioni L, Ahlbom A, Viitanen M et al. Risk factors for late-onset Alzheimer's disease: a population-based case-control study. *Ann Neurol* 1993; **33**: 258–66.
24. O'Meara ES, Kukull WA, Sheppard L et al. Head injury and risk of Alzheimer's disease by apolipoprotein E genotype. *Am J Epidemiol* 1997; **146**: 373–84.
25. Mayeux R, Ottman R, Tang M-X et al. Genetic susceptibility and head injury as risk factors for Alzheimer's disease among community-dwelling elderly persons and their first-degree relatives. *Ann Neurol* 1993; **33**: 494–501.
26. Plassman BL, Havlik RJ, Steffens DC et al. Documented head injury in early adulthood and risk of Alzheimer's disease and other dementias. *Neurology* 2000; **55**(8): 1158–66.
27. Mayeux R, Ottman R, Maestre G et al. Synergistic effects of traumatic head injury and apolipoprotein epsilon-4 in patients with Alzheimer's disease. *Neurology* 1995; **45**: 555–7.
28. Mehta KM, Ott A, Kalmijn S et al. Head trauma and risk of dementia and Alzheimer's disease. The Rotterdam Study. *Neurology* 1999; **53**: 1959–62.
29. Erkinjuntti T, Hachinski V. Rethinking vascular dementia. *Cerebrovasc Dis* 1993; **3**: 3–23.
30. Hofman A, Ott A, Breteler MM et al. Atherosclerosis, apolipoprotein E, and prevalence of dementia and Alzheimer's disease in the Rotterdam Study. *Lancet* 1997; **349**: 151–4.
31. Kuusisto J, Koivisto K, Mykkanen L et al. Association between features of the insulin resistance syndrome and Alzheimer's disease independently of apolipoprotein e4 phenotype: cross sectional population-based study. *Br Med J* 1997; **315**: 1045–9.
32. Leibson CL, Rocca WA, Hanson VA et al. Risk of dementia among persons with diabetes mellitus: a population-based cohort study. *Am J Epidemiol* 1997; **145**: 301–8.
33. Curb JD, Rodriguez BL, Abbott RD et al. Longitudinal association of vascular and Alzheimer's dementias, diabetes, and glucose tolerance. *Neurology* 1999; **52**: 971–5.
34. Ott A, Slooter AJ, Hofman A et al. Smoking and risk of dementia and Alzheimer's disease in a population-based cohort study: the Rotterdam Study. *Lancet* 1998; **351**: 1840–3.
35. Merchant C, Tang MX, Albert S et al. The influence of smoking on the risk of Alzheimer's disease. *Neurology* 1999; **52**: 1408–12.
36. Kalmijn S, Launer LJ, Ott A et al. Dietary fat intake and the risk for incident dementing disease: The Rotterdam Study. *Ann Neurol* 1997; **42**: 776–82.
37. Henderson VW. The epidemiology of estrogen replacement therapy and Alzheimer's disease. *Neurology* 1997; **48**(suppl 7): S27–35.
38. Brenner DE, Kukull WA, Stergachis A et al. Postmenopausal estrogen replacement therapy and the risk of Alzheimer's disease: a population-based case-control study. *Am J Epidemiol* 1994; **140**: 262–7.
39. Broe GA, Henderson AS, Creasey H et al. A case—control study of Alzheimer's disease in Australia. *Neurology* 1990; **40**: 1698–707.
40. Graves AB, White E, Koepsel et al. A case control study of Alzheimer's disease. *Ann Neurol* 1990; **28**: 766–74.
41. Paganini-Hill A, Henderson VW. Estrogen deficiency and risk of Alzheimer's disease in women. *Am J Epidemiol* 1994; **140**: 256–61.
42. Tang M-X, Jacobs D, Stern K et al. Effect of oestrogen during menopause on risk and age at onset of Alzheimer's disease. *Lancet* 1996; **348**: 429–32.
43. Kawas C, Resnick S, Morrison A et al. A prospective study of estrogen replacement therapy and the risk of developing Alzheimer's disease: the Baltimore Longitudinal Study of Aging. *Neurology* 1997; **48**: 1517–21.
44. Waring SC, Rocca WA, Petersen RC et al. Postmenopausal estrogen replacement therapy and risk of AD: a population-based study. *Neurology* 1999; **52**: 965–70.
45. Posthuma WFM, Westendorp RG, Vandenbrouchke J. Cardioprotective effect of horomone replacement therapy in postmenopausal women: is the evidence biased? *Br Med J* 1994; **308**: 1268–9.
46. McGeer PL, Rogers J. Antiinflammatory agents as theraputic approach to Alzheimer's disease. *Neurology* 1992; **42**: 447–9.

47. Launer LJ, Hoes AW. NSAIDs and the risk for Alzheimer's disease: weighing the epidemiologic evidence. *Neurogeriatrics and Neurogerontology*, 1998; 133–42.

48. Breitner JC, Gau BA, Welsh KA *et al.* Inverse association of anti-inflammatory treatments and Alzheimer's disease: initial results of a co-twin control study. *Neurology* 1994; **44**: 227–32.

49. Henderson AS, Jorm AF, Christensen H *et al.* Aspirin, anti-inflammatory drugs and risk of dementia. *Int J Geriatr Psychiatry* 1997; **12**: 926–30.

50. Fourrier A, Letenneur L, Begaud B, Dartigues JF. Non-steroidal antiinflammatory drug use and cognitive function in the elderly: inconclusive results from a population-based cohort study. *J Clin Epidemiol* 1996; **49**: 1201.

51. in't Veld BA, Launer LJ, Hoes AW *et al.* NSAIDs and incident Alzheimer's disease. The Rotterdam Study. *Neurobiol Aging* 1998; **19**: 607–11.

52. Stewart WF, Kawas C, Corrada M, Metter EJ. Risk of Alzheimer's disease and duration of NSAID use. *Neurology* 1997; **48**: 626–32.

53. Goate A, Chartier-Harlin MC, Mullan M *et al.* Segregation of a missense mutation in the amyloid precursor protein gene with familial Alzheimer's disease. *Nature* 1991; **349**: 704–6.

54. Sherrington R. Cloning of a novel gene bearing missense mutations in early onset familial Alzheimer's disease. *Nature* 1995; **375**: 754–60.

55. Rogaev E. Familial Alzheimer's disease in kindreds with missense mutations in a gene on chromosome 1 related to the Alzheimer's disease type 3 gene. *Nature* 1995; **376**: 775–8.

56. Strittmatter WJ. Apolipoprotein E: high avidity binding to β-amyloid and increased frequency of type 4 allele in late-onset familial Alzheimer's disease. PNAS 1993; 1977–81.

57. Alzheimer Research Forum/Research findings/Molecular Genetics of Alzheimer's Disease, October, 1999 (http://www.alzforum.org).

58. Blacker D, Wilcox MA, Laird NM *et al.* Alpha-2 macroglobulin is genetically associated with Alzheimer's disease. *Nature Genet* 1998; **19**: 357–60.

59. Wavrant-DeVrieze F, Rudrasingham V, Lambert JC *et al.* No association between the alpha-2 macroglobulin I1000V polymorphism and Alzheimer's disease. *Neurosci Lett* 1999; **262**: 137–9.

The Lundby Study, 1947–1997

Per Nettelbladt[1], Olle Hagnell[1], Leif Öjesjö[2], Lena Otterbeck[1], Cecilia Mattisson[1], Mats Bogren[1], Erik Hofvendahl[1], Per Toråker[1]

[1]Lund University Hospital and [2]Karolinska Institute, Stockholm, Sweden

The Lundby Study is a prospective, longitudinal investigation of all kinds of mental disorders in a total population. It started in 1947, when four psychiatrists, Essen-Möller *et al.*, interviewed and described all the 2550 inhabitants of a geographically delimited area in southern Sweden. They were interested in finding out how many people were suffering from a mental illness or deviation, and also the way normal and abnormal personality traits were distributed in a normal population. They traced and examined all but 1% of the population. Only four people refused to participate. After 10 years, in 1957, the field investigation was repeated. One psychiatrist alone (Hagnell) re-examined the original population from 1947, irrespective of domicile. For deceased persons, information was collected from hospital case notes and from relatives. Hagnell also examined the 1013 newcomers in Lundby and thus performed a new prevalence study of 2612 people, as well as a 10 year incidence study of the original 2550 subjects. In 1972 Hagnell and Öjesjö made a second follow-up study[1] including the total population of 3563, also this time irrespective of domicile, thus performing a 25 year and a 15 year incidence study. The participation rate was as high as 98% at the two follow-ups.

All the three field examinations were performed in a similar way. One part of the examination was a semi-structured interview, the other part a free conversation. The task of the psychiatrist was to collect the information to the best of his ability, observantly looking for symptoms and signs. In an investigation such as this, the data should ideally be collected by a trained psychiatrist. To facilitate his task, the psychiatrist had a structured form to fill in. Each interview turned out to be different, but the information gathered was noted in a systematic way. Supplementary information was collected from, amongst other sources, official registers, hospital case notes, autopsy reports, social insurance offices, local officials and relatives. This additional information from other sources forms a rich resource and has proved to be particularly valuable when evaluating the dementias of the elderly. All the types of information collected formed the basis for the global evaluation and classification.

The material from the three field studies has enabled us not only to estimate the rates of prevalence, incidence and probability of developing a mental illness, but also to identify possible background factors of, for example, dementia, starting with people who were healthy at one investigation but who had contracted the illness before the next. Trying to identify risk factors is a weighty enterprise in which we are still involved.

In an epidemiological, psychiatric investigation, precise clinical classification tools are hardly applicable. For dementias among the elderly we use two diagnostic groups: senile dementia of the Alzheimer type (SDAT) and vascular dementia (MID), the latter characterized by focal brain symptoms. Of course, other dementias of the elderly exist but they are fairly unusual compared with SDAT and vascular dementia and not very easily recognized in epidemiological investigations.

In order also to be able to include the hereditary aspect, we have mapped out the kinship of every proband down to the sixth generation, and for the original 2550 even down to the seventh generation.

From the Lundby Study, several reports on dementias in the elderly have been published. Figures from the 1972 prevalence study are included in the EURODEM comparative prevalence studies[2,3]. For the 10 year age groups 60, 70 and 80, the prevalence rates of SDAT in the Lundby Study were, for both sexes taken together, 0.3%, 2.5%, and 10.9%, respectively, and for vascular dementia 0.8%, 3.5%, and 6.3%.

The rates of incidence and cumulative probability of contracting SDAT or vascular dementia were also published[4,5]. The cumulative lifetime probability of contracting SDAT was reported to be 25.5% in men and 31.9% in women. If only the most severely impaired cases are counted, the figures are 15.0% and 22.2%, respectively. For vascular dementia the figures are 29.8% in men and 25.1% in women, for severe cases 16.6% and 15.2%, respectively.

Attempts have been made at finding background factors of a precipitating or protective nature in SDAT and vascular dementia in the Lundby Study. Two articles on this topic have been written[6,7].

On 1 July 1997 the Lundby Study[1,8,9] celebrated its 50th anniversary by launching a new re-examination of its population, now aged 40 + . This fourth wave of the Lundby Study gives an opportunity to study the occurrence of mental disorders and, as the population has grown 25 years older since 1972, especially mental disorders in an ageing population.

Between 1 July 1947 and 1 July 1972, 736 probands had died, and between 1 July 1972 and 1 July 1997, 1028 probands had died. On 1 July 1997, in all, 1764 probands were deceased. Thus, the number of living probands on 1 July 1997 was 1799 (3563–1764). This field investigation is now completed and the participation rate is still high (approximately 90%).

In the 1997 Lundby Study, modern diagnostic systems, such as DSM-IV[10] and ICD-10[11], are used, together with the old diagnostic Lundby classifications. When the interview is finished, the proband is given a set of self-rating questionnaires. The proband is asked to complete them and to return them to the Lundby Study. The self-rating questionnaires are: the Interview Schedule for Social Interaction about social network[12], the Nottingham Health Profile about quality of life[13], the Sense of Coherence Scale (about salutogenesis)[14], and the Hopkins Symptom Check List, a mental symptom check list[15]. Also, this time supplementary information will be collected.

Focusing on the mental health/illness and its consequences as the present prospective, longitudinal study can shed light on the incidence and course of mental disorders in the middle-aged and elderly and estimate the importance of health care and treatment. By revisiting and examining the Lundby population a fourth time, the Lundby database will be updated. No comparable study has been progressing for such a long period of time.

REFERENCES

1. Hagnell O, Essen-Möller E, Lanke J et al. The Incidence of Mental Illness over a Quarter of a Century. The Lundby Longitudinal Study of Mental Illnesses in a Total Population based on 42 000 Observation Years. Stockholm: Almqvist & Wiksell International, 1990.
2. Rocca WA, Hofman A, Brayne C et al. Frequency and distribution of Alzheimer's disease in Europe. A collaborative study of 1980 1990 prevalence findings. Ann Neurol 1991; 30(3): 381–90.
3. Rocca WA, Hofman A, Brayne C et al. The prevalence of vascular dementia in Europe. Facts and fragments from 1980–1990 studies. Ann Neurol 1991; 30(6): 817–24.
4. Hagnell O, Lanke J, Rorsman B et al. Current trends in the incidence of senile and multi-infarct dementia. A prospective study of a total population followed over 25 years; the Lundby Study. Arch Psychiat Nervenkr 1983a; 233: 423–38.
5. Hagnell O, Lanke J, Rorsman B, Öhman R. The diminishing incidence of chronic organic brain syndromes among the elderly. In Book of Proceedings from the Third European Symposium on Social Psychiatry in Hanasaari, Finland. 1983; 253–61.
6. Hagnell O, Franck A, Gräsbeck A et al. Senile dementia of the Alzheimer type in the Lundby Study. II. An attempt to identify possible risk factors. Eur Arch Psychiat Clin Neurosci 1992; 241: 231–5.
7. Hagnell O, Franck A, Gräsbeck A et al. Vascular Dementia in the Lundby Study. II. An attempt to identify possible risk factors. Neuropsychobiology 1993; 27: 210–16.
8. Essen-Möller E, Larsson H, Uddenberg CE, White G. Individual traits and morbidity in a Swedish rural population. Acta Psychiat Neurol Scand 1956; suppl 100.
9. Hagnell O. A Prospective Study of the Incidence of Mental Disorder. Lund: Svenska Bokförlaget/Bonniers, 1966.
10. American Psychiatric Association (APA). Diagnostic and Statistical Manual of Mental Disorders, 4th edn. Washington, DC: American Psychiatric Association, 1994.
11. World Health Organization (WHO). The ICD-10 Classification of Mental and Behavioural Disorders. Geneva: World Health Organization, 1992.
12. Henderson S, Duncan-Jones P, Byrne DG, Scott R. Measuring social relationships: the Interview Schedule for Social Interaction. Psychol Med 1980; 10: 723.
13. Hunt SM, Wiklund I. Cross-cultural variation in the weighting of health statements: a comparison of English and Swedish valuations. Health Policy 1987; 8: 227–35.
14. Antonovsky A. Health, Stress and Coping. San Francisco, CA: Jossey-Bass, 1979.
15. Derogatis LR, Lipman RS, Rickels K et al. The Hopkins symptom check list. A self-report symptom inventory. Behav Sci 1974; 19: 1–15.

Nutritional Factors in Dementia

D. N. Anderson[1] and M. T. Abou-Saleh[2]

[1]Mossley Hill Hospital, Liverpool, and [2]St George's Hospital Medical School, London, UK

The prevalence of nutritional disorders among the elderly is substantial, particularly among the elderly mentally ill (see Chapter 138a). Those with dementing disorders are at special risk. Dementia caused by a single nutrient deficiency is rare in the UK and USA and malnourishment will normally be the result of a dementia and deranged eating patterns, rather than its cause. The elderly in hospital or residential care are more likely to be malnourished than those living in the community[1,2].

Reduced plasma and blood levels of folate[3-6], vitamin B$_{12}$[3], vitamin C[2,5,7-10], and vitamin E[8-10] in particular, have been reported in association with dementia and cognitive impairment.

Goodwin et al.[11] reported a direct relationship between water-soluble vitamins and cognitive function in healthy subjects. Those with the lowest levels of plasma folate and vitamin B$_{12}$ scored significantly worse on the Halstead–Reitan categories test and the Wechsler memory test. As part of the Basle Longitudinal Project on Ageing, involving urban-dwelling healthy elderly people, Perrig et al.[12] found that β-carotene and vitamin C levels were independently correlated with memory function after controlling for compounding variables such as age, education and gender. High intake of monounsaturated fatty acids was found to be associated with better memory function in 300 people aged 65–84 years[13]. Unsaturated fatty acids appear important for maintaining the development and integrity of neuronal function.

Botez et al.[14] having found evidence of organic brain damage on psychometric testing in folate deficient subjects, reported improvement following 12 months' supplementation. Of five patients who underwent radionucleotide cysternography, three showed improvement of cerebral atrophy. Supplementation with vitamin E has been associated with slower development of the pathology of Alzheimer's disease[15].

It is not easy to establish, from studies of this sort, whether nutritional deficiency is a cause or effect of cognitive impairment. Supplementation studies suggest that certain additional nutrients may influence cognitive performance and, whether causative or not, nutrient deficiency may increase cognitive decline. If aetiologically significant, then the relevance of many of these findings may lie in the relationship with the oxidative stress hypothesis of Alzheimer's disease and the significance of oxidative stress for the development of ischaemic vascular disease. There is increasing evidence that reactive oxidizing species contribute to the neuronal damage and formation of the amyloid plaques seen in Alzheimer's disease[16,17]. Antioxidants could be important for preventing this damage and antioxidant constituents of diet, such as vitamins E and C and β-carotene may be of particular importance. Vitamin C is actively concentrated in the brain[18] and is considered to be the most effective antioxidant in human plasma[19].

Impaired antioxidant status[20] and low plasma vitamin C levels[21] have been suggested as risk factors for coronary artery disease and, therefore, may be relevant to dementia of vascular origin. Similar associations have been reported with vitamin B$_6$ and folate consumption[22]. Preliminary suggestions that vitamin E may reduce the risk of stroke has obvious implications for the development of vascular dementia.

The causative role of thiamine deficiency for the Wernicke–Korsakoff syndrome is established and it seems that some alcoholic dementias may result from Wernicke–Korsakoff lesions[23]. Other B vitamins are capable of producing cognitive impairment and dementia[24] but are only likely to be significant causes in industrially underdeveloped countries.

Assessment of nutritional status should be part of the general management of dementing patients and nutritional deficiency corrected whenever possible. The cause of undernutrition is multifactorial and various interventions may help to improve a patient's nutritional state[25] (see Chapter 138a). For a few patients this may lead to gratifying improvements of cognitive performance, but all are likely to benefit by a reduction of morbid risk and improvements in general health. It is likely that a clearer understanding of the relationship between dietary constituents and dementia will contribute to methods of prevention and treatment of this condition.

REFERENCES

1. Burns A, Marsh A, Bender DA. Dietary intake and clinical, anthropometric and biochemical indices of malnutrition in elderly demented patients and non-demented subjects. Psychol Med 1989; 19: 383–91.
2. Hancock MR, Hullin RP, Ayland PR et al. Nutritional state of elderly women on admission to mental hospital. Br J Psychiat 1985; 147: 404–7.
3. Sneath P, Chanarin I, Hodkinson MH et al. Folate status in a geriatric population and its relation to dementia. Age Ageing 1993; 2: 177–82.
4. Shorvon SD, Carney MWP, Chanarin I, Reynolds EH. The neuropsychiatry of megaloblastic anaemia. Br Med J 1980; 28: 1036–43.
5. Kemm JR, Alcock J. The distribution of supposed indictors of nutritional status in elderly patients. Age Ageing 1984; 13: 21–8.
6. Abou-Saleh MT, Spalding E, Kellett J. Folate deficiency in dementia. Br J Psychiat 1986; 148: 336.
7. Shaw DM, Tidmarsh SF, Thomas DE et al. Senile dementia and nutrition. Br Med J 1984; 288: 792–3.
8. Jeandel C, Nicholas MB, Dubois F et al. Lipid peroxidation and free radical scavengers in Alzheimer's disease. Gerontology 1989; 35: 275–82.
9. Riviere S, Birloyez-Aragon I, Nourhashemi F, Vellas B. Low plasma vitamin C in Alzheimer patients despite an adequate diet. Int J Geriat Psychiat 1998; 13: 749–54.
10. Sinclair AJ, Bayer AJ, Johnston J et al. Altered plasma antioxidant status in subjects with Alzheimer's disease and vascular dementia. Int J Geriat Psychiat 1998; 13: 840–5.
11. Goodwin JS, Goodwin JM, Garry PJ. Association between nutritional status and cognitive functioning in a healthy population. J Am Med Assoc 1983; 249: 2917–21.
12. Perrig WJ, Perrig P, Stahelin HB. The relation between antioxidants and memory performance in the old and very old. J Am Geriat Soc 1997; 45: 718–24.
13. Solfrizzi V, Panza F, Torres P et al. High monounsaturated fatty acid intake protects against age-related cognitive decline. Neurology 1999; 8: 1563–8.
14. Botez MI, Botez T, Maag H. The Wechsler sub-tests in mild organic brain damage associated with folate deficiency. Psychol Med 1984; 14: 431–7.

15. Sano M, Ernesto C, Thomas RG et al. A controlled trial of selegiline, α-tocopherol, or both as treatment of Alzheimer's disease. *N Engl J Med* 1997; **336**: 1216–22.

16. Richardson SJ. Free radicals in the genesis of Alzheimer's disease. *Ann NY Acad Sci* 1993; **695**: 73–6.

17. Markesbury WR. Oxidative stress hypothesis in Alzheimer's disease. *Free Rad Biol Med* 1997; **23**: 134–7.

18. Grunewald RA. Ascorbic acid in the brain. *Brain Res Rev* 1993; **18**: 123–33.

19. Frei B, Stocker R, Ames BN. Antioxidant defences and lipid peroxidation in human blood plasmas. *Proc Nat Acad Sci* 1988; **85**: 9748–52.

20. Kristenson M, Zieden B, Kucinskiene Z et al. Antioxidant state and mortality from coronary heart disease in Lithuanian and Swedish men: concomitant cross sectional study of men aged 50. *Br Med J* 1997; **314**: 629–33.

21. Nyyssonen K, Parviainen MT, Salonen R et al. Vitamin C deficiency and risk of myocardial infarction: prospective population study of men from eastern Finland. *Br Med J* 1997; **314**: 634–8.

22. Rimm E, Willett WC, Hu FB et al. Folate and vitamin B_6 from diet and supplements in relation to risk of coronary heart disease among women. *J Am Med Assoc* 1998; **279**: 359–64.

23. Lishman WA. Alcohol and the brain. *Br J Psychiat* 1990; **156**: 635–44.

24. Lishman WA. Vitamin deficiencies. In *Organic Psychiatry*, 3rd edn. London: Blackwell Scientific, 1998; 570–93.

25. Watson R. Undernutrition, weight loss and feeding difficulty in elderly patients with dementia: a nursing perspective. *Rev Clin Gerontol* 1997; **7**: 317–26.

41

The Genetics of Alzheimer's Disease

Brenda L. Plassman[1] and John C. S. Breitner[2]

[1]*Duke University Medical Center, Durham, NC, and* [2]*Johns Hopkins University, Baltimore, MD, USA*

Knowledge of the genetics of Alzheimer's disease (AD) has advanced in recent years. Like many other diseases of late life, AD exhibits a complex pattern of inheritance. It is difficult to localize genes that cause such diseases, however, partly because only recent generations are available to be genotyped and phenotyped. This chapter will provide a general overview of the current state of knowledge in the genetics of AD and related dementias, and suggest approaches to interpretation of future findings in this area.

FAMILY AND TWIN STUDIES

The striking early evidence for genetic causes of AD was based on a few multigenerational kindreds with many individuals with the disease (for review, *see* ref. 1). Most of these families had onset of disease before the age of 65, and were thus arbitrarily classified as having "early onset". These multigenerational kindreds with so-called familial AD probably represent no more than 1–2% of all AD cases, but their existence strongly suggested that genes were important in at least some cases of AD.

Other early work supporting a genetic etiology of AD was based on the presence of a positive family history of the disease in clinical and population-based AD samples. Most of these studies showed an increased risk of AD in first-degree relatives, ranging from 25% to 50%, as compared with 10% or less for non-demented controls[2]. This finding suggested an up to five-fold increase in risk of AD among relatives of individuals with the disease.

The early family studies focused on families at greater risk of developing AD. Recently, however, some researchers have taken another approach to the problem by investigating families who appear to have a *lower* risk of AD[3]. They have shown that the first-degree relatives of individuals who reached the age of 90 and were not demented had a reduced liability to AD from age 60 on, as compared with the families of younger non-demented individuals. The message here is that genes may either promote or reduce the risk of AD.

Twin studies have provided other evidence for genetic causes of AD. Members of identical (monozygotic) twin pairs share 100% of their genome, while fraternal (dizygotic) twin pairs share 50% of their genes on average. The twin design assumes that the degree of similarity in the early life environments of identical and fraternal twin pairs are the same. Based on this so-called "equal environments assumption", the twin design compares concordance rates for disease in identical (monozygotic) twin pairs with that in fraternal (dizygotic) pairs. Higher concordance in identical pairs, then, implies genetic influences. The magnitude of such influences can be estimated in complex models that simultaneously assess the proportion of disease liability attributable to shared or unique environmental causes, as well as stochastic variation[4].

Like the early family studies, twin studies of AD have generally implied genetic causation without identifying particular genes or loci. The heritability of AD (proportion of disease liability attributable to genes) has been estimated from ongoing studies of AD in three population-based twin registries: (a) the NAS–NRC Twin Registry in the USA[5]; (b) the Swedish Twin Registry[6]; and (c) the Norwegian Twin Registry[7]. Based on tetrachoric correlation analyses, current estimates of heritability for AD in these studies range from 0.33 to 0.74[5-7]. We suggest that the wide range of these estimates of heritability may reflect the differences in the age distribution of twins in the three registries. We speculate that the lowest heritability estimate (0.33) from our work may underestimate the true heritability of AD because of the atypically young age (mean onset age = 67 years) of AD cases in the NAS–NRC sample. Others have shown that the risk of developing AD, for a relative of a proband with AD, increases with age at least until the mid-80s[8]. Consistent with this, we have found that the estimates of heritability in the NAS–NRC Registry have gradually increased over the past few years. As the Registry approaches the typical age of risk for AD of the late 70s, 80s and even beyond, we anticipate that heritability in the NAS–NRC sample will approximate that of the other two studies and the consensus estimate of heritability will likely be between 0.5 and 0.65.

MOLECULAR GENETICS

Autosomal genes with dominant expression

Motivated by the findings from family and twin studies, molecular genetic techniques have now identified mutations at three genetic loci that are associated primarily with early onset AD. Initial interest in the molecular genetics of AD focused on chromosome 21, because aging Down's syndrome patients (trisomy 21) often exhibit the brain pathology seen in AD patients[9,10]. The first identified AD mutation was found in the β-amyloid precursor protein (*APP*) located on chromosome 21[11]. This mutation substitutes isoleucine for valine at codon 717 in exon 17[11]. Since the first report of this missense mutation, a number of other *APP* mutations have been identified (for review, *see* ref. 12). But, in total, the *APP* mutations appear to account for the disease in less than 20 families worldwide.

The second genetic locus to show linkage to AD was found on chromosome 14[13,14] and was termed presenilin-1 (*PS-1*)[15]. Over 40 mutations in the *PS-1* locus have now been reported in at least 82 families world-wide[16]. Like the *APP* mutations, *PS-1* mutations appear to act as autosomal (i.e. not sex-linked) dominant traits with nearly complete penetrance[16]. Early reports suggested that chromosome 14 mutations may account for the majority of early-onset familial AD cases[17,18]. More recent estimates from population-based samples[16,19] have produced conflicting estimates of the proportion of early-onset cases attributable to *PS-1* mutations, with some[16] suggesting that *PS-1* mutations account for less than 20% of such cases (*see* p. 217 for more discussion of presenilins).

A third autosomal dominant locus for AD has been localized to chromosome 1 and termed presenilin 2 (*PS-2*)[20,21]. To date, *PS-2* mutations have been identified in only a few families of different ethnicity. In fact, in a population-based sample of early-onset AD cases, it was estimated that *PS-2* mutations account for less than 1% of the cases[16]. The *PS-2* mutations usually provoke onset of AD symptoms before age 65, but later onsets occasionally occur. The variability in onset age for the *PS-1* and *PS-2* mutations suggests the complexity of these otherwise Mendelian traits.

Identification of AD mutations on chromosomes 21, 14 and 1 has led to major advances in understanding the etiology of this disease. It is important to note, however, that these mutations probably account in total for less than 2% of all AD cases[22]. Importantly, it appears that they do not account even for the majority of so-called autosomal dominant familial AD[16]. Thus, there are almost certainly other major genes remaining to be identified in early-onset AD. A separate and, from a public health perspective, far more compelling issue is the search for other genetic influences in common, late-onset AD.

Apolipoprotein E

In the search for other so-called AD genes, Pericak-Vance and colleagues[23] reported linkage of disease to a locus on chromosome 19 in pedigrees with late-onset AD. Searching through the candidate genes of the implicated region on chromosome 19, Strittmatter *et al.*[24] found that the apolipoprotein E gene (*APOE*), which encodes the lipid transporter apolipoprotein E (apoE), is located in the same region that showed linkage to familial late onset AD. Their initial studies showed an increase in amyloid deposition in elderly individuals with the ϵ4 allele at *APOE*[24,25], and an increased frequency of this allele in both familial and sporadic AD cases[25–29]. Subsequent studies showed that, as the number of ϵ4 alleles increases from 0 to 2, the age of onset of AD decreases[30]. These findings have now been confirmed in over 100 studies, including some that extend the findings to early onset AD (for review, *see* ref. 31). A recent meta-analysis of data on over 14 000 subjects from 40 research teams synthesized the findings on *APOE* through 1997[32]. That study confirmed the basic findings noted above and also replicated some findings that previously had been suggested by select studies. These findings were that the *APOE* ϵ2 allele may be associated with lower risk of AD, and that risk associated with the ϵ4 allele appears to vary by age, sex, and ethnicity. The association between AD and *APOE* ϵ4 is complex, and it is not clear why some individuals with the ϵ4 allele develop the disease while others do not. But, whatever its precise role, ϵ4 is an important player in the genetics of AD, as various groups have now estimated that *APOE* accounts for 57–70% of the genetic contribution of AD[33–35]. Further discussion of the role of *APOE* on the risk of AD is provided on pp. 218–19.

Other Putative Genes

There are many pedigrees that show intense familial aggregation of either early- or late-onset AD but have no identified mutation and no *APOE* ϵ4 allele. It seems likely, therefore, that one or more genes predisposing to AD remain to be discovered. The pursuit of these other genes has produced numerous reports of associations between specific genes and AD, but none of these has been consistently replicated. Chromosome 12 has been the focal point of much of this work, since a genomic screen showed a region on this chromosome may be associated with increased susceptibility to AD in individuals without an *APOE* ϵ4 allele[36]. Further analyses by this group has suggested that a region on chromosome 12 near the one of original interest may be associated with increased risk of the Lewy body variant of AD[37]. Other groups have now demonstrated linkage to regions near the initially implicated chromosome 12 locus, although one such study suggested that the strongest such association was in individuals *with* an ϵ4 allele[38], while the other showed the strongest association in those *without* an ϵ4 allele[39].

Two of the several candidate genes in the region under scrutiny on chromosome 12 have now been shown to be positively associated with AD in at least some studies. The first is the gene for the major apoE receptor in the brain, the low-density lipoprotein receptor-related protein (LRP) that is selectively found in neurons and reactive astrocytes[40]. This gene, *LRP*, has also been shown to mediate the endocytosis and degradation of Aβ[41]. It has two alleles, called C and T. The homozygous C genotype appears to be associated with increased risk of AD, earlier onset of AD, and significantly more neuritic plaques at post mortem, as compared to individuals with at least one T allele[42]. Several groups have confirmed these results[43–46], but at least two have not[47,48].

The other candidate locus encodes α-2 macroglobulin (*A2M*) and is located just outside the area on chromosome 12 for which others have reported linkage[36]. Previous work[41] showed that *A2M* is a major LRP ligand and is a serum pan-protease inhibitor that mediates the clearance and degradation of Aβ, the major component of brain amyloid. At least three different *A2M* polymorphisms have been implicated so far[49–51]. One of these studies reported that, in a very elderly Finnish cohort, the association with the *A2M* polymorphism was only evident in neuropathologically diagnosed AD cases, but not in the clinically diagnosed AD cases. This particular polymorphism was also associated with an increase in the neocortical β-amyloid protein load[51]. Unfortunately, a number of other studies have not confirmed these associations between *A2M* and AD in several large samples[52–56]. Together, these findings suggest that if *A2M* is associated with AD, its effect may be limited to subgroups of susceptible individuals and that different polymorphisms may be influential in each of these subgroups.

With so many purported loci and mutations associated with AD, one may wonder about a common thread in the pathogenesis of AD. The pathogenic mechanisms of the *APP*, *PS-1* and *PS-2* mutations are not completely understood, but each appears to be associated with increased production of the long form of Aβ (Aβ-42), relative to the production of the shorter forms (mostly Aβ-40) of Aβ[57]. Aβ-42 seems to be a particularly pathogenic form of Aβ in AD. Both *LRP* and *A2M* are involved in the degradation of Aβ. It has been suggested that these links to Aβ may be the underlying common pathogenic event leading to AD for these genes[58].

There are reports of numerous other genes throughout the genome contributing to AD, but none of these findings has been consistently confirmed. A partial list of the contending genes includes: α_1 antichymotrypsin (*ACT*), a gene on chromosome 14[59–67]; the K variant of butyrylcholinesterase (*BCHE-K*) on chromosome 3[68–72]; bleomycin hydrolase (*BH*) on chromosome 17[73] (cf. ref 74); the non-amyloid component precursor gene (*NACP*/α-synuclein) on chromosome 4[75] (cf. ref 76); the human leukocyte antigen *(HLA)* genes on chromosome 6[77,78]; the *FE65* gene on chromosome 11[79]; the dihydrolipoyl succinyltransferase (*DLST*) gene on chromosome 14[80,81]; the interleukin-1 (IL-1) on chromosome $2^{82,83}$; and the mitochondrial cytochrome *c*-oxidase (CO) genes *CO1* and *CO2*[84]. To make matters more complicated, many of the above-named genes have been shown to interact in varying degrees with *APOE* or other genes to alter risk of AD[85].

There are several possible reasons for the contradictory results of the association studies noted above. Other authors have proposed that they may reflect: (a) different etiologies in different ethnic populations; (b) lack of adjustment for multiple comparisons (type I statistical error, resulting from simultaneous screening of many different candidate loci); (c) linkage disequilibrium in some (or all) populations between the tested polymorphism and the functional polymorphism; or (d) inability to detect an effect due to limited statistical power or weak genetic effects[39,86]. Association studies are also more difficult to interpret when one does not know such characteristics as the mode of inheritance, age-dependent expression characteristics, interaction with other loci, misdiagnosis rate, and disease allele frequency. Finally, the inconsistent findings may reflect interactions with non-genetic factors. There is convincing evidence implicating *non-genetic* factors in the etiology of AD, either alone or in interaction with specific genes[87,88]. The most compelling indications of this effect are the numerous reports of monozygotic twin pairs who, although genetically identical, remain discordant for AD for 10 or more years[5,89–91].

Collectively, the three twin studies previously described suggest that non-genetic influences account for at least 25% of the variance in AD susceptibility. Studies of these "environmental factors" have suggested that both potentiating and protective influences may operate by primarily altering the timing of onset[92–94]. Similar to the recent reports of genetic associations, however, few non-genetic risk factors have been consistently confirmed. For further discussion on the genetic epidemiology of AD, see pages 219–21.

CONCLUSION

Given the number of AD genes already identified and the proportion of cases attributed to each of these genes, we can reasonably predict that there will be more than one other new gene implicated in AD. Based on what we know about the complexity of the relationship of AD and the genes identified to date, it is likely that any newly identified genes will also interact with other genes and with non-genetic factors. Also, the effect of any one gene may be influenced by the age, sex, and ethnicity of the at-risk individual. Therefore, any newly identified genes will need extensive evaluation and confirmation in various subpopulations before they are added to the list of AD genes.

Until the search for genetic and non-genetic causes of AD is complete, there is no way of identifying those individuals who will definitely develop AD. However, the discovery of new AD genes may have benefits beyond just identifying those at increased genetic risk for the disease. At least two lines of evidence suggest that there may be a common underlying pathological mechanism regardless of the genes involved. First, multiple predisposing genes appear to produce the same AD phenotype. Second, all of the AD genes identified to date, and some of the other candidate genes under examination, have some link to the metabolism of Aβ, a neuropathological marker of the disease. Understanding this common feature may lead to evidence of a common destructive metabolic process (i.e. final common pathway) and may be the key to identifying susceptible individuals *before* they develop the full syndrome of AD, or even preventing the disease. Because clinically normal individuals with at least one *APOE* ϵ4 allele have "AD neuropathology" as early as the fourth decade of life[95], one might postulate that other "AD genes" may also begin their destructive process early in life. If one could find the common pathological mechanism for the disease, then regardless of the genetic or non-genetic factors that initiate the process, treatment could be implemented to delay or prevent progression of the disease. The underlying premise is that it may be more feasible to identify a "marker for the disease process" and develop a test to measure a single marker present fairly early in life, rather than try to develop an algorithm to predict AD that includes all possible variations of genetic and non-genetic risk factors for disease.

REFERENCES

1. Kennedy AM, Brown J, Rossor M. The genetics of Alzheimer's disease. *Baillière's Clin Neurol* 1994; **3**: 217–40.
2. Breitner JCS. Clinical genetics and genetic counseling in Alzheimer's disease. *Ann Intern Med* 1991; **115**: 601–6.
3. Silverman JM, Smith CJ, Marin DB *et al.* Identifying families with likely genetic protective factors against Alzheimer disease. *Am J Hum Genet* 1999; **64**: 832–8.
4. Plomin R, DeFries JC, McClearn GE. Twin studies. In *Behavioral Genetics—A Primer*. New York: W.H. Freeman, 1990; 309–40.
5. Breitner JCS, Welsh KA, Gau BA *et al.* Alzheimer's disease in the National Academy of Sciences–National Research Council Registry of aging twin veterans. III. Detection of cases, longitudinal results, and observations on twin concordance. *Arch Neurol* 1995; **52**: 763–71.
6. Gatz M, Pedersen NL, Berg S *et al.* Heritability for Alzheimer's disease: the study of dementia in Swedish twins. *J Gerontol* 1997; **52A**: M117–25.
7. Bergem ALM, Engedal K, Kringlen E. The role of heredity in late-onset Alzheimer disease and vascular dementia. *Arch Gen Psychiat* 1997; **54**: 264–70.
8. Silverman JM, Li G, Zaccario ML *et al.* Patterns of risk in first-degree relatives of patients with Alzheimer's disease. *Arch Gen Psychiat* 1994; **51**: 577–86.
9. Burger PC, Vogel FS. The development of the pathologic changes of Alzheimer's disease and senile dementia in patients with Down's syndrome. *Am J Pathol* 1973; **73**: 457–68.
10. Oliver C, Holland AJ. Down's syndrome and Alzheimer's disease: a review. *Psychol Med* 1986; **16**: 307–22.
11. Goate A, Chartier-Harlin MC, Mullan M *et al.* Segregation of a missense mutation in the amyloid precursor protein gene with familial Alzheimer's disease. *Nature* 1991; **349**: 704–6.
12. Van Broeckhoven CL. Molecular genetics of Alzheimer disease: identification of genes and gene mutations. *Eur Neurol* 1995; **35**: 8–19.
13. Schellenberg GD, Bird TD, Wijsman EM *et al.* Genetic linkage evidence for a familial Alzheimer's disease locus on chromosome 14. *Science* 1992; **258**: 668–71.
14. St. George-Hyslop P, Haines J, Rogaev E *et al.* Genetic evidence for a novel familial Alzheimer's disease locus on chromosome 14. *Nature Genet* 1992; **2**: 330–34.
15. Sherrington R, Rogaev EI, Liang Y *et al.* Cloning of a gene bearing missense mutations in early-onset familial Alzheimer's disease. *Nature* 1995; **375**: 754–60.
16. Cruts M, van Duijn CM, Backhovens H *et al.* Estimation of the genetic contribution of presenilin-1 and -2 mutations in a population-based study of presenile Alzheimer disease. *Hum Mol Genet* 1998; **7**: 43–51.
17. Campion D, Flaman J-M, Brice A *et al.* Mutations of the presenilin 1 gene families with early-onset Alzheimer's disease. *Hum Mol Genet* 1995; **4**: 2373–7.
18. Hutton M, Busfield F, Wragg M *et al.* Complete analysis of the presenilin 1 gene in early onset Alzheimer's disease. *NeuroReport* 1996; **7**: 801–5.
19. Campion D, Dumanchin C, Hannequin D *et al.* Early-onset autosomal dominant Alzheimer disease: prevalence, genetic heterogeneity, and mutation spectrum. *Am J Hum Genet* 1999; **65**: 664–70.
20. Levy-Lahad E, Wasco W, Poorkaj P *et al.* Candidate gene for the chromosome 1 familial Alzheimer's disease locus. *Science* 1995; **269**: 973–7.

21. Levy-Lahad E, Wijsman EM, Nemens E *et al.* A familial Alzheimer's disease locus on chromosome 1. *Science* 1995; **269**: 970–3.

22. Farrer LA. Genetics and the dementia patient. *Neurologist* 1997; **3**: 13–30.

23. Pericak-Vance MA, Bebout JL, Gaskell PC *et al.* Linkage studies in familial Alzheimer disease: evidence for chromosome 19 linkage. *Am J Hum Genet* 1991; **48**: 1034–50.

24. Strittmatter WJ, Saunders AM, Schmechel D *et al.* Apolipoprotein E: high-avidity binding to B-amyloid and increased frequency of type 4 allele in late-onset familial Alzheimer disease. *Proc Natl Acad Sci USA* 1993; **90**: 1977–81.

25. Schmechel DE, Saunders AM, Strittmatter WJ *et al.* Increased amyloid B-peptide deposition in cerebral cortex as a consequence of apolipoprotein E genotype in late-onset Alzheimer disease. *Proc Natl Acad Sci USA* 1993; **90**: 9649–53.

26. Mayeux R, Stern Y, Ottman R *et al.* The apolipoprotein E4 allele in patients with Alzheimer's disease. *Ann Neurol* 1993; **34**: 752–4.

27. Rebeck GW, Reiter JS, Strickland DK, Hyman BT. Apolipoprotein E in sporadic Alzheimer's disease: allelic variation and receptor interactions. *Neuron* 1993; **11**: 575–80.

28. Saunders AM, Strittmatter WJ, Schmechel D *et al.* Association of apolipoprotein E allele E4 with late-onset familial and sporadic Alzheimer's disease. *Neurology* 1993; **43**: 1467–72.

29. Brousseau T, Legrain S, Berr C *et al.* Confirmation of the E4 allele of the apolipoprotein E gene as a risk factor for late-onset Alzheimer's disease. *Neurology* 1994; **44**: 342–4.

30. Corder EH, Saunders AM, Strittmatter WJ *et al.* Gene dose of apolipoprotein E type 4 allele and the risk of Alzheimer's disease in late onset families. *Science* 1993; **261**: 921–3.

31. Roses AD. Apolipoprotein E alleles as risk factors in Alzheimer disease. *Ann Rev Med* 1996; **47**: 387–400.

32. Farrer LA, Cupples LA, Haines JL *et al.* Effects of age, sex, and ethnicity on the association between apolipoprotein E genotype and Alzheimer disease. *J Am Med Assoc* 1997; **278**: 1349–55.

33. Nalbantoglu J, Gilfix BM, Bertrand P *et al.* Predictive value of apolipoprotein E genotyping in Alzheimer's disease: results of an autopsy series and an analysis of several combined studies. *Ann Neurol* 1994; **36**: 889–95.

34. Roses AD, Devlin B, Conneally PM. Measuring the genetic contribution of APOE in late-onset Alzheimer disease. *Am J Hum Genet* 1995; **57**: A202.

35. Breitner JCS, Wyse BW, Anthony JC *et al.* APOE-epsilon4 count predicts age when prevalence of AD increases, then declines: the Cache County Study. *Neurology* 1999; **53**: 321–31.

36. Pericak-Vance MA, Bass MP, Yamaoka LH *et al.* Complete genomic screen in late-onset familial Alzheimer disease. Evidence for a new locus on chromosone 12. *J Am Med Assoc* 1997; **278**: 1237–41.

37. Scott WK, Grubber JM, Conneally PM *et al.* Fine mapping of the chromosome 12 late-onset Alzheimer disease locus: potential genetic and phenotypic heterogeneity. *Am J Hum Genet* 2000; **66**: 922–32.

38. Rogaeva E, Premkumar S, Song Y *et al.* Evidence for an Alzheimer disease susceptibility locus on chromosome 12 and for further locus heterogeneity. *J Am Med Assoc* 1998; **280**: 614–18.

39. Wu W, Holmans P, Wavrant-DeVrieze F *et al.* Genetic studies on chromosome 12 in late-onset Alzheimer disease. *J Am Med Assoc* 1998; **280**: 619–22.

40. Rebeck GW, Harr SD, Strickland DK, Hyman BT. Multiple, diverse senile plaque-associated proteins are ligands of an apolipoprotein E receptor, α_2-macroglobulin receptor/low-density lipoprotein receptor-related protein. *Ann Neurol* 1995; **37**: 211–17.

41. Kounnas MZ, Moir RD, Rebeck GW *et al.* LDL receptor-related protein, a multifunctional ApoE receptor, binds secreted β-amyloid precursor protein and mediates its degradation. *Cell* 1995; **82**: 331–40.

42. Kang DE, Saitoh T, Chen X *et al.* Genetic association of the low-density lipoprotein receptor-related protein gene (LRP), an apolipoprotein E receptor, with late-onset Alzheimer's disease. *Neurology* 1997; **49**: 56–61.

43. Lendon CL, Talbot CJ, Craddock NJ *et al.* Genetic association studies between dementia of the Alzheimer's type and three receptors for apolipoprotein E in a Caucasian population. *Neurosci Lett* 1997; **222**: 187–90.

44. Wavrant-De Vrièze F, Pérez-Tur J, Lambert JC *et al.* Association between the low-density lipoprotein receptor-related protein (LRP) gene and Alzheimer's disease. *Neurosci Lett* 1997; **227**: 68–70.

45. Hollenbach E, Ackermann S, Hyman BT, Rebeck GW. Confirmation of an association between a polymorphism in exon 3 of the low-density lipoprotein receptor-related protein gene and Alzheimer's disease. *Neurology* 1998; **50**: 1905–7.

46. Lambert JC, Vrieze FW-D, Amouyel P, Chartier-Harlin M-C. Association at LRP gene locus with sporadic late-onset Alzheimer's disease. *Lancet* 1998; **351**: 1787–8.

47. Clatworthy AE, Gomez-Isla T, Rebeck W *et al.* Lack of association of a polymorphism in the low-density lipoprotein receptor-related protein gene with Alzheimer disease. *Arch Neurol* 1997; **54**: 1289–92.

48. Fallin D, Kundtz A, Town T *et al.* No association between the low density lipoprotein receptor-related protein (LRP) gene and late-onset Alzheimer's disease in a community-based sample. *Neurosci Lett* 1997; **233**: 145–7.

49. Blacker D, Wilcox MA, Laird NM *et al.* Alpha-2 macroglobulin is genetically associated with Alzheimer disease. *Nature Genet* 1998; **19**: 357–60.

50. Liao A, Nitsch RM, Greenberg SM *et al.* Genetic association of an α2-macroglobulin (Val1000lle) polymorphism and Alzheimer's disease. *Hum Mol Genet* 1998; **7**: 1953–6.

51. Myllykangas L, Polvikoski T, Sulkava R *et al.* Genetic association of α_2-macroglobulin with Alzheimer's disease in a Finnish elderly population. *Ann Neurol* 1999; **46**: 382–90.

52. Chen L, Baum L, Ng HK *et al.* Apolipoprotein E promoter and alpha2-macroglobulin polymorphisms are not genetically associated with Chinese late-onset Alzheimer's disease. *Neurosci Lett* 1999; **269**: 173–7.

53. Crawford F, Freeman M, Town T *et al.* No genetic association between polymorphisms in the Tau gene and Alzheimer's disease in clinic- or population-based samples. *Neurosci Lett* 1999; **266**: 193–6.

54. Dow DJ, Lindsey N, Cairns NJ *et al.* α-2 macroglobulin polymorphism and Alzheimer disease risk in the UK. *Nature Genet* 1999; **22**: 16–17.

55. Rogaeva EA, Premkumar S, Grubber J *et al.* An α-2-macroglobulin insertion-deletion polymorphism in Alzheimer disease. *Nature Genet* 1999; **22**: 19–21.

56. Rudrasingham V, Wavrant-De Vrièze F, Lambert J-C *et al.* α-2 Macroglobulin gene and Alzheimer disease. *Nature Genet* 1999; **22**: 17–19.

57. Hardy J. Amyloid, the presenilins and Alzheimer's disease. *Trends Neurosci* 1997; **20**: 154–9.

58. Kim W, Tanzi RE. Presenilins and Alzheimer's disease. *Curr Opin Neurobiol* 1997; **7**: 683–8.

59. Kamboh M, Sanghera D, Ferrell R, DeKosky S. APOE 4-associated Alzheimer's disease risk is modified by 1-antichymotrypsin polymorphism. *Nature Genet* 1995; **10**: 486–8.

60. Thome J, Baumer A, Kornhuber J *et al.* Alpha-1-antichymotrypsin bi-allele polymorphism, apolipoprotein-E tri-allele polymorphism and genetic risk of Alzheimer's syndrome. *J Neur Transm* 1995; **10**: 207–12.

61. Muramatsu T, Matsushita S, Arai H *et al.* Alpha 1-antichymotrypsin gene polymorphism and risk for Alzheimer's disease. *J Neur Transm Parkinson's Dis Dement* 1996; **103**: 1205–10.

62. Talbot C, Houlden H, Craddock N *et al.* Polymorphism in AACT gene may lower age of onset of Alzheimer's disease. *NeuroReport* 1996; **7**: 534–6.

63. Yoshiiwa A, Kamino K, Yamamoto H *et al.* α_1-antichymotrypsin as a risk modifier for late-onset Alzheimer's disease in Japanese apolipoprotein E ϵ4 allele carriers. *Ann Neurol* 1997; **42**: 115–17.

64. Egensperger R, Herrmann H, Kosel S, Graeber MB. Association between ACT polymorphism, and Alzheimer's disease. *Neurology* 1998; **50**: 575.

65. Ezquerra M, Blesa R, Tolosa E *et al.* α_1 Antichymotrypsin gene polymorphism and risk for Alzheimer's disease in the Spanish population. *Neurosci Lett* 1998; **240**: 107–9.

66. Lamb H, Christie J, Singleton AB *et al.* Apolipoprotein E and α-1 antichymotrypsin polymorphism genotyping in Alzheimer's disease and in dementia with Lewy bodies: distinctions between diseases. *Neurology* 1998; **50**: 388–91.

67. Nacmias B, Marcon G, Tedde A *et al.* Implication of α1-antichymotrypsin polymorphism in familial Alzheimer's disease. *Neurosci Lett* 1998; **244**: 85–8.

68. Lehmann DJ, Johnston C, Smith AD. Synergy between the genes for butyrylcholinesterase K variant and apolipoprotein E4 in late onset confirmed Alzheimer disease. *Hum Mol Genet* 1997; **6**: 1933–6.

69. Brindle N, Song Y, Rogaeva E *et al*. Analysis of the butyrylcholinesterase gene and nearby chromosome 3 markers in Alzheimer disease. *Hum Mol Genet* 1998; **7**: 933–5.

70. Russ C, Powell J, Loveston S, Holmes C. K variant of butyrylcholinesterase and late-onset Alzheimer's disease. *Lancet* 1998; **351**: 881.

71. Singleton AB, Smith G, Gibson AM *et al*. No association between the K variant of the butyrylcholinesterase gene and pathologically confirmed Alzheimer's disease. *Hum Mol Genet* 1998; **7**: 937–9.

72. Wiebusch H, Poirier J, Sévigny P, Schappert K (1999) Further evidence for a synergistic association between APOE ε4 and BCHE-K in confirmed Alzheimer's disease. *Hum Genet* 1999; **104**: 158–63.

73. Montoya SE, Aston CE, DeKosky ST *et al*. Bleomycin hydrolase is associated with risk of sporadic Alzheimer's disease. *Nature Genet* 1998; **18**: 211–12.

74. Farrer L, Abraham CR, Haines JL *et al*. Association between bleomycin hydrolase and Alzheimer's disease in caucasians. *Ann Neurol* 1998; **44**: 808–11.

75. Xia Y, Rohan DeSilva HA, Rosi BL *et al*. Genetic studies in Alzheimer's disease with an NACP/α-synuclein polymorphism. *Ann Neurol* 1996; **40**: 207–15.

76. Hellman NE, Grant EA, Goate AM. Failure to replicate a protective effect of allele 2 of NACP/α-synuclein polymorphism in Alzheimer's disease: an association study. *Ann Neurol* 1998; **44**: 278–81.

77. Curran M, Middleton D, Edwardson J *et al*. HLADR antigens associated with major genetic risk for late-onset Alzheimer's disease. *NeuroReport* 1997; **8**: 1467–9.

78. Payami H, Schellenberg GD, Zareparsi S *et al*. Evidence for association of HLA-A2 allele with onset age of Alzheimer's disease. *Neurology* 1997; **49**: 512–18.

79. Hu Q, Kukull WA, Bressler SL *et al*. The human FE65 gene: genomic structure and an intronic biallelic polymorphism associated with sporadic dementia of the Alzheimer type. *Hum Genet* 1998; **103**: 295 303.

80. Nakano K, Ohta S, Nishimaki K *et al*. Alzheimer's disease and DLST genotype. *Lancet* 1997; **350**: 1367–8.

81. Sheu KFR, Brown AM, Haroutunian V *et al*. Modulation by DLST of the genetic risk of Alzheimer's disease in a very elderly population. *Ann Neurol* 1999; **45**: 48–53.

82. Grimaldi LME, Casadei VM, Ferri C *et al*. Association of early-onset Alzheimer's disease with an interleukin-1 α gene polymorphism. *Ann Neurol* 2000; **47**: 361–5.

83. Nicoll JAR, Mrak RE, Graham DI *et al*. Association of interleukin-1 gene polymorphisms with Alzheimer's disease. *Ann Neurol* 2000; **47**: 365–8.

84. Davis RE, Miller S, Herrnstadt C *et al*. Mutations in mitochondrial cytochrome *c* oxidase genes segregate with late-onset Alzheimer disease. *Proc Natl Acad Sci USA* 1997; **94**: 4526–31.

85. Wang X, DeKosky ST, Wisniewski S *et al*. Genetic association of two chromosome 14 genes (presenilin 1 and α1-antichymotrypsin) with Alzheimer's disease. *Ann Neurol* 1998; **44**: 387–90.

86. Katzman R, Kang D, Thomas R. Interaction of apolipoprotein E epsilon 4 with other genetic and non-genetic risk factors in late onset Alzheimer disease: problems facing the investigator. *Neurochem Res* 1998; **23**: 369–76.

87. Breteler MMB, Claus JJ, van Duijn CM *et al*. Epidemiology of Alzheimer's disease. *Epidemiol Rev* 1992; **14**: 59–82.

88. Henderson AS, Jorm AF, Korten AE *et al*. Environmental risk factors for Alzheimer's disease: their relationship to age of onset and to familial or sporadic types. *Psychol Med* 1992; **22**: 429–36.

89. Creasey H, Jorm A, Longley W *et al*. Monozygotic twins discordant for Alzheimer's disease. *Neurology* 1989; **39**: 1474–6.

90. Kumar A, Schapiro MB, Grady CL *et al*. Anatomic, metabolic, neuropsychological, and molecular genetic studies of three pairs of identical twins discordant for dementia of the Alzheimer's type. *Arch Neurol* 1991; **48**: 160–8.

91. Nee LE. Twins with dementia of the Alzheimer type: a follow-up study of 22 twin pairs. *Gerontologist* 1991; **31**: 139.

92. Gedye A, Beattie BL, Tuokko H *et al*. Severe head injury hastens age of onset of Alzheimer's disease. *J Am Geriat Soc* 1989; **37**: 970–3.

93. Breitner JCS, Welsh KA, Helms MJ, Gaskell PC, Gau BA, Roses AD, Pericak-Vance MA and Saunders AM (1995b) Delayed onset of Alzheimer's disease with non-steroidal anti-inflammatory and histamine H2 blocking drugs. *Neurobiology of Aging* 1995; **16**: 523–30.

94. Nemetz PN, Leibson C, Naessens JM *et al*. Traumatic brain injury and time to onset of Alzheimer's disease: a population-based study. *Am J Epidemiol* 1999; **149**: 32–40.

95. Ghebremedhin E, Schultz C, Braak E, Braak H. High frequency of apolipoprotein E ε4 allele in young individuals with very mild Alzheimer's disease-related neurofibrillary changes. *Exp Neurol* 1998; **153**: 152–5.

The Role of Presenilins in Alzheimer's Disease

David M. A. Mann

University of Manchester, UK

It is now 5 years since the presenilins and their association with Alzheimer's disease (AD) was discovered, although homologues, *sel-12* and *spe-4*, in the animal kingdom had been known about earlier. By 1994, the AD3 locus for early onset familial AD had been mapped to chromosome 14q 24.3, where causative mutations in a gene encoding a novel protein, initially called S182 but later presenilin-1 (PS-1), were identified[1]. Over 60 different PS-1 mutations have now been found. A homologous gene on chromosome 1, presenilin-2 (PS-2), is the AD4 locus; here three AD-causing mutations have been found[1]. Both presenilin proteins span the membrane six to eight times, with C- and N-termini facing intracellularly and a large cytosolic loop region occurring between transmembrane helices 6 and 7.

Recent research has focused on understanding how changes in presenilin protein structure might facilitate disease[2]. Cell lines and transgenic mice bearing PS-1 (and PS-2) mutations produce more amyloid β protein (Aβ), particularly the highly fibrillogenic $A\beta_{42}$, than wild-type PS-1. Humans with PS-1 mutations produce more $A\beta_{42}$ in cell culture, plasma levels are elevated and brain deposition is high. Catabolism of APP along pathways favouring production of Aβ is therefore enhanced when PS-1 mutations are present, driving the pathological cascade that leads to clinical dementia[2].

PS-1 protein occurs within the perikaryon and dendrites of nerve cells, mostly within the early Golgi apparatus and smooth endoplasmic reticulum. No difference in distribution or amount of

PS-1 protein or its message are seen in PS-1 AD. The holoprotein is processed into 17 kDa, C-terminal (CTF) and 27–28 kDa, N-terminal (NTF) fragments which accumulate in 1:1 stoichiometry, in a highly regulated and saturable manner. Cleavage occurs within the hydrophilic loop, around amino acid 298[2]. PS-1 (2) mutations alter neither the site nor the manner of endoproteolysis, although the cleaved products may accumulate through increased stability.

Amyloid precursor protein (APP) trafficking from Golgi to endosome and plasma membrane—the principal sites of Aβ production—is not affected by PS-1 mutations. PS-1 knockout mice show normal α- and β-secretase activity, though Aβ production is decreased with accumulation of the C-terminal stub of APP. PS-1 therefore might regulate γ-secretase, as part of the γ-secretase complex, with mutant PS-1 fragments enhancing this activity[3,4].

CTF and NTF of PS-1 form a stable complex containing GSK-3β and β-catenin[5]. The cellular trafficking, stability and turnover of β-catenin is altered by PS-1 mutations[3] and these might interfere with the binding of GSK-3β to tau, possibly promoting hyperphosphorylation and neurofibrillary tangle formation.

PS-1, therefore, probably regulates the sorting and processing of integral membrane proteins, including APP. PS-1 mutations may alter protein topology so as to favour APP catabolism along routes which, by increasing production and tissue deposition of Aβ, facilitate the pathological cascade. Other putative roles for presenilins could include signal transduction, involving *Notch* and Wnt pathways, during development or apoptosis[4]. Whether these functions are disturbed by PS-1 mutations, with repercussions for the pathogenesis of AD, is unknown.

REFERENCES

1. Tanzi R, Kovacs D, Kim T-W *et al*. The gene defects responsible for familial Alzheimer's disease. *Neurobiol Dis* 1996; **3**: 159–68.
2. Selkoe DJ. The cell biology of β-amyloid precursor protein and presenilins in Alzheimer's disease. *Trends Cell Biol* 1998; **8**: 447–53.
3. Nishimura M, Yu G, St George-Hyslop PH. Biology of presenilins as causative molecules for Alzheimer disease. *Clin Genet* 1999; **55**: 219–25.
4. Sisodia SS, Kim SH, Thinakaran G. Function and dysfunction of the presenilins. *Am J Hum Genet* 1999; **65**: 7–12.
5. Weihl C. β-catenin and PS1. *Alzheimer's Rep* 1999; **2**: 195–8.

Apolipoprotein-E (APO-E)

Dan G. Blazer

Duke University Medical Center, Durham, NC, USA

Strittmatter *et al*.[1] found that the gene apolipoprotein-E (APO-E) for the lipid transporter apolipolipoprotein-E is located on chromosome 19 in a region that was demonstrated to have strong linkage to familial late-onset Alzheimer's disease (AD). There are three common alleles formed at the polymorphic APO-E locus, E2, E3 and E4. Each individual inherits one allele from each parent; thus a person may have an APO-E genotype of E4/E4, E4/E3, E3/E3, and so forth[2]. The E3 allele is the most common and represents approximately 78% of all alleles in European and American White populations. The E4 allele frequency is approximately 15–16% and the E2 frequency approximately 7%. The risk for AD is increased and the average age of onset is decreased with increasing numbers of APO-E E4 alleles. In addition to AD, the E4 allele has been shown to be associated with cardiovascular disease, renal disease, stroke, decreased ability to recover from physiologic challenges such as amnesia and an increase in all-cause mortality. Several case-control and incidence studies of late-onset AD have shown E4 allele frequency to be more frequent in cases; 30–50% in both sporadic and familial AD (FAD), compared to the 15% in the general population. The odds ratio for E4 allele heterozygotes developing AD are approximately 2–5, whereas the odds ratios for E4 homozygotes are 5–18. The E2 allele may actually retard the development of AD.

Other studies of AD and APOE in different ethnic groups report similar associations between the E4 allele and AD. Nevertheless, the frequency of the E4 allele among African-Americans appears to be higher than in Whites, yet the frequency of AD does not appear to be greater (thus suggesting less association, perhaps, in African-Americans compared to Whites).

Despite the association of AD and the APOE-4 allele, most persons who experience AD do not express the E4 allele. In addition, there have been reports of individuals homozygous for E4 in very late life who nevertheless remain cognitively intact. The E4 allele is therefore neither necessary nor sufficient to cause AD. For this reason, the E4 allele has been considered a susceptibility gene. This represents a change in perspective from the typical approach to genetic expression for an autosomal dominant or autosomal recessive.

Most genetic determinants of health do not derive from a one gene–one disease paradigm, but rather a paradigm in which the phenotypic expression of the genome is best conceived quantitatively. A single polymorphism at a specific locus can lead to multiple adverse outcomes, outcomes which can be investigated as changes over time as well as the onset of a specific disease at a specific point in time. In other words, these are susceptibility polymorphisms that are universally distributed in the population, rather than mutations that are uncommon and family-specific. A single allele may be sufficient to cause a specific disease, yet everyone with that allele has a measurable age-dependent risk for that disease. These susceptibility polymorphisms are therefore subject to investigation in the way epidemiologists conceive environmental stressors (such as stressful life events) or health-related behaviors (such as smoking), that is, as risk factors for disease onset and change. To date, however, few such susceptibility polymorphisms have been identified. Studies of these polymorphisms have focused almost exclusively upon the association of an allele with a specific disease or specific adverse outcome, such as mortality. Yet these polymorphisms may increase the risk for multiple diseases, and therefore for generalized morbidity, and increased the risk of mortality from multiple causes. This translates into increased burden on the health care delivery system and higher costs.

Apolipoprotein E is a major serum lipoprotein involved in cholesterol metabolism. Lipoproteins derived from E4 are cleared more efficiently from the blood than those derived from E3 and E2. Apolipoprotein E does not cross the blood–brain barrier but is synthesized in the brain by astrocytes. In the brain, APOE is thought to be involved in the mobilization and redistribution of cholesterol and phospholipid during membrane remodeling associated with the plasticity of synapses[3].

The biological basis for the association between the E4 allele and AD is unclear, however. APOE is found in senile plaques and fibrillary tangles and binds to Aβ in the cerebrospinal fluid. *In vitro* studies have indicated that APOE isoforms may differentially affect deposition of Aβ. Binding studies suggest that APOE isoforms have different affinities for Aβ. However, these results are controversial because different studies suggest different isoforms have the highest affinity for Aβ. The APOE isoforms have been shown to promote Aβ fibral formation *in vitro*. Other studies, however, show that E3 but not E4 binds to tau, preventing aggregation of tau and neurofibrillary tangle formation. Neurite extension and branching is more extensive in E3-treated cells compared with E4-treated cells. APOE E4 has also been shown to have increased antioxidant activity compared with E3[3].

Although there is a consensus that APOE E4 is strongly associated with AD, this does not mean that tests for the genotype (which are comercially available) should be used for diagnostic testing. A consensus working group has recommended that, at the present time, APOE genotyping should not be used for predictive testings. APOE genotype alone does not provide sufficient sensitivity or specificity to allow genotyping to be used as a diagnostic test. Because AD develops in the absence of E4 and because many patients with APOE E4 seem to escape the disease, genotyping is also not recommended for use as a predictive genetic test[4].

REFERENCES

1. Strittmatter WJ, Saunders AM, Schmechel D *et al.* Apolipoprotein-E: high-avidity binding to B-amyloid and increased frequency of type 4 allele in late-onset familial Alzheimer's disease. *Proc Natl Acad Sci USA* 1993; **90**: 1977–81.
2. Plassman DL, Breitner JCS. Recent advances in the genetics of Alzheimer's disease and vascular dementia with an emphasis on gene–environment interactions. *J Am Geriat Soc* 1996; **44**: 1242–50.
3. Lendon CL, Shall F, Goate AM. Exploring the etiology of Alzheimer's disease using molecular genetics. *J Am Med Assoc* 1997; **277**: 835–1.
4. American College of Medical Genetics. Statement on the use of apolipoprotein E testing for Alzheimer's disease. *J Am Med Assoc* 1995; **274**: 1627–9.

Down's Syndrome and Alzheimer's Disease: Update

David W. K. Kay and Brian Moore

University of Newcastle upon Tyne, UK

One of the unresolved questions for the dementia of Down's syndrome (DS) as a model for Alzheimer's disease (AD) is the long interval, often up to 20 years, that separates the appearance of the AD pathology in the brains of individuals dying after the age of 35 from the clinical manifestations of dementia.

EPIDEMIOLOGY OF DEMENTIA

Study of decline and dementia is important for service as well as theoretical reasons. The life expectancy of a 1 year-old DS child with mild/moderate handicap is now 55 years[2]. However, the wide variation in premorbid abilities and the presence of physical, particularly sensory impairments[1] often makes the diagnosis of dementia difficult. With ICD-10 criteria as standard, the Dementia Questionnaire for Persons with Mental Retardation[3] and the Dementia Scale for Down Syndrome[4] both perform well, but the Mini-Mental State Examination is too difficult[5]. Both caregiver information and longitudinal monitoring of cognitive performance are desirable[6]. Cortical atrophy may be demonstrated by brain imaging[7,8]. Dementia is frequently associated with late-onset epilepsy, and late-onset epilepsy is associated with clinical evidence of dementia[9–11]. Serial EEGs may reveal diffuse abnormalities and slowing of the dominant rhythm associated with the decline of cortical functions[12].

In a meta-analysis of prevalence studies, the age distribution of dementia onset in DS was unimodal, with mean age of onset 51.7 years (SD 7.1, range 31–68), and earlier onset in women[13]. Age-specific prevalence rates of dementia in population-based samples were: age 30–39, 2.0–3.4%; age 40–49, 9.4–10.3%; age 50–59, 36.1–40%; and age 60–69, 54.5%[14–16]. DS subjects aged 50 years or over were significantly impaired on memory tests compared with younger subjects[17]. Dementia rates were increased in elderly people with learning disabilities (LDs) as a whole[18] but the rates in DS were higher[19]. Persons with DS and dementia are also reported to show more non-cognitive symptoms than other persons with LDs and dementia[20]. Dementia contributed significantly to decline in adaptive behaviour and skills after age 40, independently of age, while absence of medical illness had a favourable effect[21].

Longitudinal Studies

Adaptive behaviour deteriorates more in DS than in matched controls with other LDs[22]. Treatable conditions, such as depression and medical illness, may be involved[23], but dementia is the main cause; in the absence of dementia and physical illness no decline was found[24]. However, the incidence of cognitive decline and dementia seems to be very sensitive to the criteria used. Adults aged 22–56 who were dementia-free at baseline showed little change over a period of 3–4 years in most cases[25] and even over 6 years, persons aged 50 and over showed, on average, only very slight decreases in cognitive performance, attributed to precocious ageing; only 4% satisfied the criteria for dementia[26]. However, on a sophisticated neuropsychological test battery, 28% of testable persons aged 30 + were deemed to show cognitive deterioration after 4 years, and of those aged over 50 only 30% showed no cognitive decline; as in AD, memory and learning were affected early[27]. Whether persons with DS age prematurely or whether they age normally but are at increased risk of AD remains controversial. Further national and cross-national studies of the prevalence, incidence and natural history of dementia in both DS and in other LD are required[28].

NEUROPATHOLOGY AND GENETICS

The gene coding for familial Alzheimer's disease is now known to be distinct from the amyloid precursor protein (APP) gene, which is also situated on the long arm of chromosome 21. Overexpression of the triplicated APP gene results in higher concentration of APP in DS brains than in brains of elderly controls or of patients with AD[29]. The increased amyloid deposition in AD could be due to some cases of AD being trisomy-21 mosaics, resulting from non-dysjunction during mitosis; such cases might possess other features of DS[30]. A shared susceptibility to non-dysjunction and AD could account for an increased risk of dementia reported among the mothers of persons with DS[31]. Meta-analysis of seven studies of the ApoE polymorphism in DS found a similar distribution between DS adults and non-retarded controls, and no significant difference between DS persons with and without dementia[32]. There were, however, trends for the $\epsilon 2$ allele to be associated with later onset of dementia and later age at death in non-dementing persons, and for the $\epsilon 4$ allele to be associated with earlier onset. Cognitive decline in DS may be influenced by an unidentified gene situated at D21S11[33].

Clinico-pathological Correlations

The first change is the deposition of β-amyloid peptide (β/A4) in the cerebral cortex and elsewhere, in the form of diffuse, amorphous plaques, and may be seen as early as the second or third decade; soon afterwards microglial cells and ubiquitin protein can be detected, and by the age of 35 years "cored" amyloid deposits are seen at post mortem in most subjects[34]. At this stage neurofibrillary tangles (NFT) are numerous in parts of the hippocampus and amygdala but are seen only in isolated cortical neurons. Eventually, and usually after the age of 50, the distribution and density of senile plaques and NFT and loss of neurons conform to the pattern seen in AD[34]. This is the age when clinical dementia usually appears[13]. This gradual evolution of pathological change partly explains the puzzling temporal discrepancy between the onset of pathological and clinical manifestations of dementia in DS. Whether or not a similar evolution of neuropathological change occurs in AD is still unknown.

REFERENCES

1. Van Schrojenstein Lantman-de Valk HMJ, Haveman MJ, Maaskant MA et al. The need for assessment of sensory functioning in ageing people with mental handicap. J Intellect Disabil Res 1994; **38**: 289–98.
2. Strauss D, Eyman RK. Mortality of people with mental retardation in California with and without Down's syndrome. Am J Ment Retard 1996; **100**: 643–53.
3. Evenhuis HM. Further evaluation of the Dementia Questionnaire for persons with mental retardation (DMR). J Intellect Disabil Res 1996; **40**: 369–73.
4. Gedye A. Dementia Scale for Down Syndrome. Manual. Gedye Research and Consulting: Vancouver, 1995.
5. Deb S, Braganza J. Comparison of rating scales for the diagnosis of dementia in adults with Down's syndrome. J Intellect Disabil Res 1999; **43**: 400–7.
6. Aylward EH, Burt DB, Thorpe LU, Lai F, Dalton AJ. Diagnosis of dementia in individuals with intellectual disability. J Intellect Disabil Res 1997; **41**: 152–64.
7. Kesslak JP, Nagata SF, Lott I, Nalcioglu O. Magnetic resonance imaging analysis of age-related changes in the brains of individuals with Down's syndrome. Neurology 1994; **44**: 1039–45.
8. Prasher VP, Barber PC, West R, Glenholmes P. The role of magnetic imaging analysis in the diagnosis of Alzheimer's disease in adults with Down's syndrome. Arch Neurol 1996; **53**: 1310–13.
9. McVicker RW, Shanks OEP, McClelland RJ. Prevalence and associated features of epilepsy in adults with Down's syndrome. Br J Psychiat 1994; **164**: 528–32.
10. Collacott RA. Epilepsy, dementia and adaptive behaviour in Down's syndrome. J Intellect Disabil Res 1993; **37**: 153–60.
11. Prasher VP, Corbett JA. Onset of seizures as a poor indicator of longevity in people with Down syndrome and dementia. Int J Geriat Psychiat 1993; **8**: 923–7.
12. Soininen H, Partanen J, Jousmäki V et al. Age-related cognitive decline and electroencephalogram slowing in Down's syndrome as a model of Alzheimer's disease. Neuroscience 1993; **53**: 57–63.
13. Prasher VP, Krishnan VHR. Age of onset and duration of dementia in people with Down syndrome: integration of 98 reported cases in the literature. Int J Geriat Psychiat 1993; **89**: 915–22.
14. Holland AJ, Hon J, Huppert FA, Stevens F, Watson P (1998) Population-based study of the prevalence and presentation of dementia in adults with Down's syndrome. Br J Psychiat 1998; **172**: 493–8.
15. Johanssen P, Christensen JEJ, Mai J. The prevalence of dementia in Down syndrome. Dementia 1996; **7**: 221–5.
16. Prasher VP. Age-specific prevalence, thyroid dysfunction and depressive symptomatology in adults with Down syndrome and dementia. Int J Geriat Psychiat 1995; **10**: 25–31.
17. Crayton L, Oliver C, Holland AF, Bradbury J, Hall S. The neuropsychological assessment of age-related cognitive deficits in adults with Down's syndrome. J Appl Res Intellect Disabil 1998; **11**: 255–72.
18. Cooper S-S. High prevalence of dementia among people with learning disabilities not attributable to Down's syndrome. Psychol Med 1997; **27**: 609–11.
19. Zigman WB, Schupf N, Sersen E, Silverman W. Prevalence of dementia in adults with and without Down's syndrome. Am J Ment Retard 1995; **100**: 403–12.
20. Cooper S-A, Prasher VP. Maladaptive behaviours and symptoms of dementia in adults with Down's syndrome compared with adults with intellectual disability of other aetiologies. J Intellect Disabil Res 1998; **42**: 293–300.
21. Prasher VP, Chung MC. Causes of age-related decline in adaptive behavior of adults with Down syndrome: differential diagnoses of dementia. Am J Ment Retard 1996; **101**: 175–83.
22. Rasmussen DE, Sobsey D. Age, adaptive behavior, and Alzheimer disease in Down syndrome: cross-setional and longitudinal analyses. Am J Ment Retard 1994; **99**: 151–65.
23. Burt DB, Loveland KA, Primeaux-Hart S et al. Dementia in adults with Down syndrome: diagnostic challenges. Am J Ment Retard 1998; **103**: 130–45.
24. Prasher VP, Chung MC, Haque MS. Longitudinal changes in adaptive behaviour in adults with Down's syndrome: interim findings from a longitudinal study. Am J Ment Retard 1998; **103**: 40–6.

25. Burt DB, Loveland KA, Chen Y-W *et al*. Aging in adults with Down's syndrome: report from a longitudinal study. *Am J Ment Retard* 1995; **100**: 262–70.

26. Devenny DA, Silverman WP, Hill AL *et al*. Normal ageing in adults with Down's syndrome: a longitudinal study. *J Intellect Disabil Res* 1996; **40**: 208–21.

27. Oliver C, Crayton L, Holland AJ *et al*. A four-year prospective study of age-related cognitive change in adults with Down's syndrome. *Psychol Med* 1998; **28**: 1365–77.

28. Zigman W, Schupf N, Haveman M, Silerman W. The epidemiology of Alzheimer's disease in intellectual disability: results and recommendations from an international conference. *J Intellect Disabil Res* 1997; **41**: 76–80.

29. Rumble B, Retallack R, Hilbich C *et al*. Amyloid A4 protein and its precursor in Down's syndrome and Alzheimer's disease. *N Engl J Med* 1989; **320**: 1446–52.

30. Potter H. Alzheimer's disease, Down's syndrome, and chromosome segregation. *Lancet* 1996; **348**: 66.

31. Schupf N, Kapell D, Lee JH *et al*. Increased risk of Alzheimer's disease in mothers of adults with Down's syndrome. *Lancet* 1994; **344**: 353–6.

32. Prasher VP, Chowdbury TA, Rowe BR, Bain SC. ApoE genotype and Alzheimer's disease in adults with Down syndrome: meta-analysis. *Am J Ment Retard* 1997; **102**: 103–10.

33. Farrer MJ, Crayton L, Davies GE *et al*. Allelic variability in D21S11, but not APP or APOE, is associated with cognitive decline in Down syndrome. *NeuroReport* 1997; **8**: 1645–9.

34. Mann DMA. Association between Alzheimer's disease and Down syndrome: neuropathological observations. In Berg JM, Karlinsky H, Holland AJ, eds, *Alzheimer Disease, Down Syndrome, and Their Relationship*, Oxford University Press: Oxford, 1993; 71–92.

International Criteria for Alzheimer's Disease and Their Problems— ICD-10, DSM-IV and NINCDS–ADRDA

Kenneth Rockwood

Dalhousie University, Halifax, Nova Scotia, Canada

Dementia often comes to attention when an elderly person's cognition or behaviour no longer conforms to what is expected. Given inherent variability in people and their circumstances, in their past and present performance, in how this matters, in the expectation of changes with age, it is no surprise that how dementia is described, whether it is attributed to Alzheimer's disease (AD), and what that is taken to mean will vary within and across societies[1]. Comparing three sets of commonly-used criteria for AD shows that while each conceptualizes dementia similarly, differences in their literal application can give highly variable results. Such specious variability distracts from the important task of better understanding heterogeneity in disease expression—especially in the presence of medical and psychiatric co-morbidity.

THE THREE SETS OF CRITERIA

The criteria of the National Institute of Neurological and Communicative Disorders and Stroke, and the Alzheimer's Disease and Related Disorders Association (NINCDS–ADRDA)[2] require a clinical examination to produce evidence of dementia, defined as progressive deficits in memory and other areas of cognition (notably language, motor skills and perception) that occurs without a disturbance of consciousness, and in the absence of "systemic disorders other than brain diseases that in and of themselves could account for the deficits". The criteria also require that the onset be between ages 40 and 90, the initial examination include a standardized cognitive test, and the deficits be "confirmed by neuropsychological tests". "Exclusion of causes of dementia other than Alzheimer's" allows a diagnosis of *probable* AD, with neuropathological confirmation required to make the diagnosis *definitive*. *Possible* AD exists when "atypical" features or other co-morbid illnesses exist.

The 10th International Classification of Diseases (ICD-10) has both clinical guidelines[3] and research criteria[4] for Mental and Behavioural Disorders. AD is classed as a dementia, defined as progressive impairment, in the absence of clouding of consciousness, of multiple higher cortical functions, specified as: memory, thinking, orientation, comprehension, calculation, learning capacity, language and judgement. Interestingly, the criteria also note that non-cognitive features ("deterioration in emotional control, social behaviour, or motivation") can accompany or even precede dementia. The diagnosis is one of exclusion; only insidious onset and slow deterioration are cited as characteristic of AD. Subtypes include early and late onset, and "atypical or mixed". The research criteria specify mild, moderate and severe stages, based chiefly on the extent of memory loss, although the impact on daily activities is noted.

The fourth edition of the *Diagnostic and Statistical Manual of Mental Disorders* (DSM-IV) of the American Psychiatric Association defines dementia as "multiple cognitive deficits that include memory impairment and at least one of . . . aphasia, apraxia, agnosia, or a disturbance in executive functioning", provided that such deficits cause impairment, "occupational or social functioning" and represent a decline[5]. The criteria for "Dementia of the Alzheimer's Type" emphasize the need to rule out other conditions, and to exclude the syndrome if it exists only in the setting of delirium. Subtypes include early and late onset, and each of coincident delirium, delusions, and depressed mood. The accompanying text emphasizes insidious onset and gradual decline, notes that (but does not specify how) "cultural background" should be taken into account, and, while recognizing differences in levels of disability, provides no specific criteria for staging.

PROBLEMS WITH CURRENT CRITERIA

Despite cross-national studies of their individual reliability and validity[6] variability in diagnostic criteria can have profound effects on resulting epidemiological[7] and clinical[8] estimates. This is especially true with strict exact adherence to each criterion, e.g. when patients whose dementia is too severe to sit for neuropsychological tests are said not to have fulfilled the NINCDS–ADRDA criterion that such tests be administered. Now while it might be argued that there is no point in criteria except in having strict adherence to them, we cannot ignore that most such criteria are revised periodically, and that the operationalization of some criteria (notably, functional impairment) can vary widely, again with marked impact on the resulting estimates[9]. A better approach would be to make clear how the interpretation of specific criteria may affect a study's results[7].

Each set of criteria views AD as a diagnosis of exclusion. Given that AD is common and that many of the diagnoses to be excluded are rare, this approach seems perverse, despite the absence of a biological marker for the most common disorder. Perhaps it is the lack of a detailed consideration of staging, another problem with all the criteria, that has resulted in the "diagnosis of exclusion" approach. Without some understanding of systematic variation by stage, the heterogeneity of AD would seem chaotic, so that the clinician could only feel confident in the diagnosis when everything else had been rejected. By contrast, recognizing common features in how AD presents and progresses makes the task of diagnosing it with confidence much easier—indeed, where characteristic milestones are present, such confidence can extend even to a retrospective diagnosis[10]. This notion of a usual progression is, in fact, implicit in considerations of "atypical presentations", which usually are understood as deficits (*e.g.* aphasia, apraxia) that occur at an *uncharacteristically early* stage. Also, in emphasizing insidious onset, the criteria seem to exclude patients whose dementia initially presents with delirium, despite that sequence being a common path to AD[11].

Each set of criteria emphasizes a categorical approach to diagnosis, despite patients who often show more than one problem—typically AD and cerebrovascular problems[12]. While each set of criteria allows for "mixed diagnoses", they appear to underestimate the role of cerebrovascular lesions in both the risk of AD and the degree of its expression[13].

In practice, each set of criteria sees AD chiefly in cognitive terms. Another way to think of dementia, however, is as a decline of "effective behaviour"[14]—a phenomenon seen often in clinical practice, in which cognitive and non-cognitive changes can compete for prominence as the complaints of patients and families. Perhaps it is this experience which underlies the recognition of non-cognitive features in the ICD-10 clinical description, or in the DSM-IV subtypes. Nevertheless, these non-cognitive aspects have not much informed our research understanding of disease presentation, and neither are they likely to. Given the ongoing search for clinical correlates of structural or chemical preclinical features, cognitive deficits (which are readily quantifiable) are likely to achieve even greater prominence. Both the near-continuous distribution in neuropsychological test performance scores across an unimpaired to demented range[15,16] and the preference for categories mean that we are more likely to see a renewed "cut points" debate than a debate over the meaning of cognitive vs. non-cognitive symptoms as the basis for future revisions of diagnostic criteria for AD.

REFERENCES

1. Cohen L. *No Aging in India*. Berkeley, CA: University of California Press, 1998.
2. McKhann G, Drachman D, Folstein M *et al*. Clinical diagnosis of Alzheimer's disease: Reports of the NINCDS–ADRDA work group under the auspices of the Department of Health and Human Services Task Force on Alzheimer's disease. *Neurology* 1984; **34**: 939–94.
3. World Health Organization. *The ICD-10 Classification of Mental and Behavioural Disorders. Clinical Descriptions and Diagnostic Guidelines*. WHO: Geneva, 1992.
4. World Health Organization. *The ICD-10 Classification of Mental and Behavioural Disorders. Diagnostic Criteria for Research*. WHO: Geneva, 1993.
5. American Psychiatric Association. *Diagnostic and Statistical Manual of Mental Disorders*, 4th edn. Washington, DC: APA, 1994.
6. Baldereschi M, Amato MP, Nencini P *et al*. Cross-national interrater agreement on the clinical diagnostic criteria for dementia. *Neurology* 1994; **44**: 239–42.
7. Erkinjuntti T, Ostbye T, Steenhuis R, Hachinski V. The effect of different diagnostic criteria on the prevalence of dementia. *N Engl J Med* 1997; **337**: 1667–74.
8. Chui HC, Mack W, Jackson E *et al*. Clinical criteria for the diagnosis of vascular dementia. A multicenter study of comparability and interrater reliability. *Arch Neurol* 2000; **57**: 191–6.
9. Larrea FA, Fisk JD, Graham JE, Stadnyk K. Prevalence of cognitive impairment and dementia as defined by neuropsychological test performance. *Neuroepidemiology* 2000; **19**: 121–9.
10. Rockwood K, Howard K, Thomas V *et al*. Retrospective diagnosis of dementia using an informant interview based on the brief cognitive rating scale. *Int Psychogeriat* 1998; **10**(1): 53–60.
11. Rockwood K, Cosway S, Carver D *et al*. The risk of dementia and death after delirium. *Age Aging* 1999; **28**: 551–6.
12. Rockwood K, Wentzel C, Hachinski V *et al*. Prevalence and outcomes of vascular cognitive impairment. *Neurology* 2000; **54**: 447–51.
13. Snowdon DA, Greiner LH, Mortimer JA *et al*. Brain infarction and the clinical expression of Alzheimer disease. *J Am Med Assoc* 1997; **277**: 813–17.
14. Torak RM. *The Pathologic Physiology of Dementia*. New York: Springer-Verlag, 1978.
15. Brayne C, Calloway P. Normal aging, impaired cognitive function and senile dementia of the Alzheimer's type: a continuum? *Lancet* 1988; **4**: 1265–9.
16. Ritchie K, Touchon J. Mild cognitive impairment; conceptual basis and current nosological status. *Lancet* 2000; **355**: 225–8.

42

The Neuropathology of Alzheimer's Disease

David M. A. Mann

University of Manchester, Manchester UK

Alzheimer's disease (AD) is the most common cause of dementia at any time of life and, although the brains of patients with this disorder show remarkable pathological changes, the nosological status of these and their relevance to the underlying neurodegenerative process has been the subject of vigorous debate. In this chapter the gross and microscopical changes of AD will be described.

IMAGING STUDIES

Structural imaging, by CT or MRI, fails to reveal changes in the brain specific to AD. Usually there is evidence of widespread cortical atrophy and ventricular enlargement, although not in a way that obviously discriminates AD from other neurodegenerative dementing disorders. A more severe medial temporal atrophy has been claimed to distinguish AD from normal ageing[1], although this does not differentiate between AD and other disorders, such as frontotemporal dementia, where a similar degree of hippocampal atrophy is seen[2,3]. Functional imaging, using PET or SPECT, reveals a conspicuous biparietal deficit in many patients with AD, although not all individuals show this and this pattern can also be seen in patients with Lewy body dementia[4]. Hence, definitive diagnosis still remains the province of histopathology, although this is usually made retrospectively following the death of the affected person.

THE AUTOPSY APPEARANCE OF THE BRAIN

Although the pattern of atrophy in AD may be quite distinct from that of the normal elderly[2,5] and of other dementing disorders of diverse aetiology[3,6] the diagnosis cannot be made at autopsy from visual inspection alone. Nonetheless, brain weight is usually reduced due to cortical atrophy (shrinkage of the gyri and widening of the sulci), which can be widespread but most often is severe in the medial temporal regions, particularly the parahippocampal gyrus, while the occipital lobe and the motor cortex are generally spared[2].

The cortical grey matter is reduced in thickness and the white matter, while macroscopically normal in appearance, is lost proportionately to that of the grey matter[2]. The ventricular system is dilated, most markedly in the temporal horns of the lateral ventricles. The substantia nigra usually shows normal pigmentation but frequently there is loss of pigment from the locus caeruleus. Cerebrovascular changes are often coincidentally present, but do not necessarily indicate a multi-infarct dementia.

HISTOPATHOLOGICAL CHANGES

The histopathology of AD displays several abnormalities and, although these changes can also be found in the brains of most normal elderly individuals, it is their greater extent and severity and regional pattern of distribution that is characteristic of AD.

Amyloid Plaques

These are aggregates (plaques) of an amyloid protein—amyloid β protein ($A\beta$)—typically 50–200 μm in diameter, within the cerebral cortex and other grey matter regions of the brain. The $A\beta$ may be surrounded by abnormal presynaptic nerve cell processes called dystrophic neurites. The same protein is often present within the walls of leptomeningeal and intracortical blood vessels, causing an amyloid angiopathy. Four plaque types have been identified[7]:

1. *Diffuse* plaques have even $A\beta$ deposition with ill-defined borders, not forming discrete rounded masses. They are the most common plaque type in AD and can only be defined by immunohistochemical staining with antibodies to $A\beta$; they have no dystrophic neurites.
2. *Primitive* plaques are discrete rounded $A\beta$ deposits without a dense core but having some dystrophic neurites. They can be stained using conventional amyloid stains.
3. *Classical* plaques have a dense star-shaped $A\beta$ core surrounded by a corona of radiating wisps of $A\beta$ and many dystrophic neurites.
4. *Compact* or *burnt-out* plaques have dense $A\beta$ cores without a surrounding corona, or neurites.

Primitive and classical plaques with dystrophic neurites containing PHF are termed "neuritic plaques", synonymous with what used to be known as "senile plaques". Synapse loss occurs from primitive and classical plaques, but not diffuse plaques[62].

Neuritic, but not diffuse, plaques contain reactive astrocytes and activated microglial cells[8,9]; the latter may play a role in the "processing" of $A\beta$ during plaque evolution. Although unproved, the prevailing view is that amyloid plaques undergo, during their prolonged life history, a series of evolutionary changes from diffuse to cored plaques. This involves not only compositional changes in $A\beta$, but also changes in associated glial cells. This evolutionary process has largely been deduced from studies of persons with trisomy 21 (Down's syndrome) dying at different ages[9,10], who inevitably develop the histopathology of AD if they live past 50 years of age.

Principles and Practice of Geriatric Psychiatry, 2nd edn. Edited by J. R. M. Copeland, M. T. Abou-Saleh and D. G. Blazer
©2002 John Wiley & Sons, Ltd

Although plaques are always most dense in cerebral cortex, they can also be numerous in white matter and subcortical areas, including the basal ganglia and cerebellum, where the deposits may be associated with dystrophic neurites but not PHF[11]. Plaques are common in the cerebral cortex in normal ageing, even in high density in some cognitively normal elderly patients[12,13], but are generally of the diffuse or primitive types[14,15]. The number of plaques, especially those containing $A\beta_{40}$, is increased in a gene dose-dependent way in the presence of the $\varepsilon4$ allele of the apolipoprotein gene[16,17].

$A\beta$ is derived, by proteolytic cleavage, from a large precursor, the amyloid precursor protein (APP). This is a transmembrane protein with a large extracellular amino-terminal portion and a small intracellular carboxy-terminal stub. $A\beta$ protein is present in plaque amyloid as a heterogeneous mix of cleaved APP fragments, 39–43 amino acids long[18,19].

APP is catabolized by enzymes known as "secretases". One enzyme, α-secretase (a metalloprotease)[20,21] cleaves APP across the middle of its transmembrane domain and in this way $A\beta$ formation is not possible. Another enzyme, β-secretase (a transmembrane aspartic protease), termed β-site APP-cleaving enzyme (BACE)[22], cuts APP at the amino-terminus of the $A\beta$ domain. The $A\beta$ peptide can then be released from this carboxy-terminal stub by a third enzyme, γ-secretase—which requires presenilin-1 protein for its activity, acting around amino acids 40–43 of the $A\beta$ sequence. The major catabolic product of these enzyme activities is $A\beta_{40}$, with lesser quantities of the longer peptide $A\beta_{42}$. However, because of a higher propensity to form amyloid fibrils the predominant, and indeed the sole, $A\beta$ species in diffuse plaques of the cerebral cortex, corpus striatum and cerebellum is $A\beta_{42}$: $A\beta_{40}$ is mostly present within the cored, neuritic plaques[23]. Paradoxically, the predominant peptide within blood vessel walls is $A\beta_{40}$, with variable, and usually much lesser, amounts of $A\beta_{42}$[24]. Studies on Down's syndrome[25] indicate that $A\beta_{42}$ is the earliest peptide deposited, $A\beta_{40}$ deposition occurring subsequently within that subset of diffuse plaques evolving into cored plaques[23].

Some cases of familial AD result from point mutations in the APP gene ($APP_{670/671}$ and APP_{717}) on chromosome 21[26], whereas in others mutations in genes on chromosomes 14 and 1, known as presenilin-1 and presenilin-2, respectively, are responsible[27]. Clinicopathological studies indicate that these familial AD cases have an especially high tissue deposition of $A\beta$, particularly $A\beta_{42}$, and very severe amyloid angiopathy[28,29]. Facilitation of $A\beta$ deposition, particularly $A\beta_{42}$, may be the mechanism whereby the APP and presenilin mutations operate. A different mutation in the APP gene (APP_{693}) causes hereditary cerebral haemorrhage with amyloidosis (Dutch type)[30].

Neurofibrillary Tangles (NFT)

NFT are abnormal filamentous inclusions that form inside nerve cells. They are not specific to AD and are seen in other neurodegenerative disorders, as well as being present (in lower numbers) in the brains of elderly non-demented persons, particularly in the hippocampus and temporal cortex[31,32]. Typically, NFT are found in temporal, frontal and parietal cortical areas with sparing of the paracentral (sensory and motor) and occipital cortices. They occur in subcortical areas such as the hypothalamus and nucleus basalis of Meynert, as well as in the dorsal raphe and locus coeruleus. When NFT formation in these regions is severe, NFT can be seen in the substantia nigra, thalamus and basal ganglia[18].

Traditionally, NFT are demonstrated by silver staining, but they can also be detected immunohistochemically using antibodies to their constituent proteins. The classical NFT is a flame-shaped skein of fine fibrils occupying much of the cell body. In haematoxylin and eosin-stained preparations, NFT are faint basophilic fibrillar inclusions. Certain NFT, termed "ghost tangles", appear eosinophilic and represent liberated neuropil remains following death of the affected neurone. Rounded ball-like NFT are termed "globose tangles" and are most common in neurones of the brainstem nuclei, but also in smaller cortical neurones[18].

Ultrastructurally, NFT are composed of pairs of filaments, diameter 20 nm, twisted with a periodicity of 80 nm, hence termed paired helical filaments (PHF)[33]. Evidence suggests them to be a ribbon-like double helical stack of transversely-arranged subunits[34].

NFT are composed of at least two major proteins, tau[35–37] and ubiquitin[38,39]. Tau protein stabilizes the microtubular cytoskeleton. The tau protein in PHF is abnormally phosphorylated[40,41] and abnormalities in protein phosphorylation may be fundamental to the neurodegenerative process of AD[42]. Ubiquitin labels cell proteins for degradation[70] and its presence in PHF is presumably targeting the abnormal protein for (attempted) degradation.

Like plaques, NFT undergo evolutionary changes that correlate with their morphology and immunoreactivity[43]:

Stage 0: amorphous tau immunoreactivity without aggregation into filaments (pre-tangles).
Stage 1: delicate fibrillar structures immunoreactive for tau and ubiquitin.
Stage 2: skeins and whorls of densely aggregated filaments, immunoreactive for tau and (sometimes) ubiquitin, filling the nerve cell body and displacing the nucleus.
Stage 3: extracellular NFT without tau immunoreactivity but ubiquitin-positive. The NFT is infiltrated by astrocytic processes, and $A\beta$ may be deposited upon the filaments[44].

The progress of AD can be staged by following the spread of NFT from hippocampal regions to neocortex and subcortex[45].

Neuropil threads are abnormal nerve cell processes (dystrophic neurites) in the neuropil of the cerebral cortex, not associated with plaques[46]. They are swollen, distorted structures containing PHF[47], antigenically similar (for tau and ubiquitin) to, and probably contiguous with, the NFT in neurones. These abnormal processes may interfere with neuronal communication, contributing to the cortical deficit.

The importance of neurofibrillary pathology in AD has been underscored by the discovery that similar abnormal tau aggregates occur in neurones and glia in frontotemporal dementia[48], due to mutations in the tau gene[49–51]. These mutations alter the microtubule binding capacity of tau, favouring self-assembly of the mutated protein into pathological structures, or they change the expression pattern of the tau gene, leading to intracellular accumulations of tau isoforms with four microtubule binding repeat domains. Pathological tau aggregates are also formed in a related condition, progressive supranuclear palsy[52], in the absence of $A\beta$ deposition. Neurodegenerative disease leading to dementia can therefore be caused by neurofilamentous aggregations of tau *alone*, irrespective of whether amyloid plaques are present. That is not to say, however, that $A\beta$ deposition in AD is of no importance. This may represent the route towards the formation of abnormal tau in this particular disorder, whereas in other conditions other pathways to tau pathology are invoked. Nonetheless, once pathological tau is formed and accumulated, a common mechanism of cell death may be set up in all "tauopathies" and this clearly has profound therapeutic implications for AD and other dementing disorders.

Granulovacuolar Degeneration (GVD)

GVD is an accumulation of membrane-bound vesicles, containing amorphous material, within nerve cells. In haematoxylin and eosin- or silver-stained sections GVD appears as numerous dot-like particles, each with a surrounding clear halo. These bodies may also be seen in ageing brains, but their number and tissue density are considerably greater in AD. Some granulovacuoles are immunoreactive for ubiquitin[53,54] and they may represent residual bodies from lysosomal-mediated proteolysis[55].

Hirano Bodies

These are rod-shaped bodies, $15\,\mu m$ wide and $60{-}100\,\mu m$ long, that appear in neurones with ageing but, again, with greater density in AD. They are brightly eosinophilic and immunohistochemistry suggests they are derived from the cytoskeletal protein, actin[56].

Neuronal loss in AD

There is conspicuous loss of neurones from the cerebral cortex and hippocampus in AD, particularly large pyramidal cells[57–59]. This loss is more marked in younger patients (<80 years), although it is still significant in older individuals[59]. Golgi studies show loss of dendritic arborization in surviving neocortical cells[60] and electron microscopy and immunohistochemistry indicate considerable synapse loss[61–63]. Cell loss from the nucleus basalis of Meynert, the cholinergic input into the cortex, is reflected neurochemically by reduced choline acetyltransferase, and that from the locus coeruleus can be related to a decline in cortical noradrenaline[64].

Amyloid Angiopathy

The deposition of Aβ in cerebral arteries, termed "amyloid angiopathy" or "congophilic angiopathy", is almost invariable in AD but can also exist in its own right. This amyloid angiopathy may sometimes be responsible for (lobar) cerebral haemorrhage, a cause of secondary stroke in AD[65–67].

White Matter Changes

A reduction in the amount of white matter in AD is associated with a decrease in the intensity of myelin staining. This has been described as incomplete infarction[68,69] and, although it may mimic Binswanger's disease pathologically and on imaging, it is not associated with lacunar infarcts or hypertensive arteriosclerosis. Such white matter changes may sometimes be related to ischaemia due to amyloid angiopathy, but bouts of systemic hypotension might also be causal.

REFERENCES

1. Jobst K, Smith AD, Szatmari M. Detection in life of confirmed Alzheimer's disease using a simple measurement of medial temporal lobe atrophy by computed tomography. *Lancet* 1992; **340**: 1179–83.
2. Mann DMA. The topographic distribution of brain atrophy in Alzheimer's disease. *Acta Neuropathol* 1991; **83**: 81–6.
3. Mann DMA, South PW. The topographic distribution of brain atrophy in frontal lobe dementia. *Acta Neuropathol* 1993; **85**: 334–40.
4. Varma AR, Talbot PR, Snowden JS et al. A ^{99}Tc-HMPAO single photon emission computed tomography study of Lewy body disease. *J Neurol* 1997; **244**: 349–59.
5. Hubbard BM, Anderson JN. A quantitative study of cerebral atrophy in old age and senile dementia. *J Neurol Sci* 1981; **50**: 135–45.
6. Mann DMA, Oliver R, Snowden JS. The topographic distribution of brain atrophy in Huntington's disease and progressive supranuclear palsy. *Acta Neuropathol* 1993; **85**: 553–9.
7. Wisniewski HM, Bancher C, Barcikowska M et al. Spectrum of morphological appearance of amyloid deposits in Alzheimer's disease. *Acta Neuropathol* 1989; **78**: 337–47.
8. Itagaki S, McGeer PL, Akiyama H et al. Relationship of microglia and astrocytes to amyloid deposits of Alzheimer's disease. *J Neuroimmunol* 1989; **24**: 173–82.
9. Mann DMA, Younis N, Jones D, Stoddart RW. The time course of pathological events concerned with plaque formation in Down's syndrome with particular reference to the involvement of microglial cells. *Neurodegeneration* 1992; **1**: 201–15.
10. Lemere CA, Blusztajn JK, Yamaguchi H et al. Sequence of deposition of heterogenous amyloid β-peptides and APO-E in Down syndrome: implications for initial events in amyloid plaque formation. *Neurobiol Dis* 1996; **3**: 16–32.
11. Suenaga T, Hirano A, Llena JF et al. Modified Bielschowsky and immunocytochemical studies on cerebellar plaques in Alzheimer's disease. *J Neuropathol Exp Neurol* 1990; **49**: 31–40.
12. Delaere P, Duyckaerts C, Masters C et al. Large amounts of neocortical βA4 deposits without neuritic plaques or tangles in a psychometrically assessed, non-demented person. *Neurosci Lett* 1990; **16**: 87–93.
13. Braak H, Braak E. Neurofibrillary changes confined to the entorhinal region and an abundance of cortical amyloid in cases of senile and presenile dementia. *Acta Neuropathol* 1990; **80**: 479–86.
14. Dickson DW, Farlo J, Davies P et al. Alzheimer's disease: a double-labelling immunohistochemical study of senile plaques. *Am J Pathol* 1988; **132**: 86–101.
15. Barcikowska M, Wisniewski HM, Bancher C, Grundke-lqbal I. About the presence of paired helical filaments in dystrophic neurites participating in plaque formation. *Acta Neuropathol* 1989; **78**: 225–31.
16. Gearing M, Mori H, Mirra SS. Aβ peptide length and apolipoprotein E genotype In Alzheimer's disease. *Ann Neurol* 1996; **39**: 395–9.
17. Mann DMA, Iwatsubo T, Pickering-Brown SM et al. Preferential deposition of amyloid β protein (Aβ) in the form Aβ_{40} in Alzheimer's disease is associated with a gene dosage effect of the apolipoprotein E E4 allele. *Neurosci Lett* 1997; **221**: 81–4.
18. Mann DMA. *Sense and Senility: the Neuropathology of the Aged Human Brain.* Austin, TX: RG Landes, 1997, 1–198.
19. Selkoe DJ. The cell biology of β-amyloid precursor protein and presenilins in Alzheimer's disease. *Trends Cell Biol* 1998; **8**: 447–53.
20. Buxbaum JD, Liu KN, Luo Y et al. Evidence that tumor necrosis factor alpha converting enzyme is involved in regulated alpha-secretase cleavage of the Alzheimer amyloid protein precursor. *J Biol Chem* 1998; **273**: 265–7.
21. Lammich S, Kojro E, Postina R et al. Constitutive and regulated α-secretase cleavage of Alzheimer's amyloid precursor protein by a disintegrin metalloprotease. *Proc Natl Acad Sci USA* 1999; **96**: 3922–7.
22. Vassar R, Bennett BD, Babu-Khan S et al. β-secretase cleavage of Alzheimer's amyloid protein by the transmembrane aspartic protease BACE. *Science* 1999; **286**: 735–41.
23. Iwatsubo T, Odaka N, Suzuki N et al. Visualization of Aβ42(43)-positive and Aβ40-positive senile plaques with end-specific Aβ monoclonal antibodies: evidence that an initially deposited species is Aβ1–42(43). *Neuron* 1994; **13**: 45–53.
24. Suzuki N, Iwatsubo T, Odaka N. High tissue content of soluble β1-40 is linked to cerebral amyloid angiopathy. *Am J Pathol* 1994; **145**: 452–60.
25. Iwatsubo T, Mann DMA, Odaka N et al. Amyloid β protein (Aβ) deposition: Aβ42(43) precedes Aβ40 in Down syndrome. *Ann Neurol* 1995; **37**: 294–9.
26. Goate AM, Chartier-Harlin MC, Mullan M et al. Segregation of a missense mutation in the amyloid precursor protein gene with familial Alzheimer's disease. *Nature* 1991; **349**: 704–6.
27. Tanzi R, Kovacs D, Kim T-W et al. The gene defects responsible for familial Alzheimer's disease. *Neurobiol Dis* 1996; **3**: 159–68.
28. Lemere CA, Lopera F, Kosik KS et al. The E280A presenilin 1 Alzheimer mutation produces increased Aβ42 deposition and severe cerebellar pathology. *Nature Med* 1996; **2**: 1146–50.

29. Mann DMA, Iwatsubo T, Cairns NJ et al. Amyloid (Aβ) deposition in chromosome 14-linked Alzheimer's disease: predominance of Aβ42(43). Ann Neurol 1996; **40**: 149–56.

30. Levy E, Carman MD, Fernandez-Madrid IJ et al. Mutation of the Alzheimer's disease amyloid gene in hereditary cerebral haemorrhage with amyloidosis of Dutch type. Science 1990; **248**: 1124–6.

31. Wilcock GK, Esiri MM. Plaques, tangles and dementia. A quantitative study. J Neurol Sci 1982; **56**: 353–6.

32. Mann DMA, Tucker CM, Yates PO. The topographic distribution of senile plaques and neurofibrillary tangles in the brains of non-demented persons of different ages. Neuropathol Appl Neurobiol 1987; **13**: 123–39.

33. Kidd M. Paired helical filaments in electron microscopy in Alzheimer's disease. Nature 1963; **197**: 192–3.

34. Wischik CM, Crowther RA, Stewart M, Roth M. Subunit structure of paired helical filaments in Alzheimer's disease. J Cell Biol 1985; **100**: 1905–12.

35. Brion JP, Pasareiro H, Nunez J, Flament-Durant J. Mise en evidence immunologique de la protein tau au niveau des lesions de degenerescence neurofibrillaire de la maladie d'Alzheimer. Arch Biol 1985; **95**: 229–35.

36. Wischik CM, Novak M, Thogersen HC et al. Isolation of a fragment of Tau derived from the core of paired helical filaments of Alzheimer's disease. Proc Natl Acad Sci USA 1988; **85**: 4506–10.

37. Kondo J, Honda T, Mori H et al. The carboxyl third of tau is tightly bound to paired helical filaments. Neuron 1988; **1**: 827–34.

38. Mori H, Kondo J, Ihara Y. Ubiquitin is a component of paired helical filaments in Alzheimer's disease. Science 1987; **235**: 1641–4.

39. Perry G, Friedman R, Shaw G, Chau V. Ubiquitin is detected in neurofibrillary tangles and senile plaque neurites of Alzheimer disease brains. Proc Natl Acad Sci USA 1987; **84**: 3033–6.

40. Flament S, Delacourte A, Hemon B, Defossez A. Characterisation of two pathological tau protein variants in Alzheimer brain cortices. J Neurol Sci 1989; **92**: 133–41.

41. Lee VM-Y, Balin BJ, Otvos L, Trojanowski JQ. A68: a major subunit of paired helical filaments and derivatised forms of normal tau. Science 1991; **251**: 675–8.

42. Clark EA, Leach KL, Trojanowski JQ, Lee VM-Y. Characterisation and differential distribution of the three major human protein kinase C isoenzymes (PKCa, PKCb, PKCg) of the central nervous system in normal and Alzheimer's disease brains. Lab Invest 1991; **64**: 35–44.

43. Bancher C, Brunner C, Lassman H et al. Tau and ubiquitin immunoreactivity at different stages of formation of Alzheimer neurofibrillary tangles. Progr Clin Biol Res 1989; **317**: 837–48.

44. Bondareff W, Wischik CM, Novak M et al. Molecular analysis of neurofibrillary degeneration in Alzheimer's disease: an immunochemical study. Am J Pathol 1990; **137**: 711–23.

45. Braak H, Braak E. Neuropathological staging of Alzheimer-related changes. Acta Neuropathol 1991; **82**: 239–59.

46. Braak H, Braak E, Grundke-Iqbal I, Iqbal K. Occurrence of neuropil threads in the senile human brain and in Alzheimer's disease: a third location of paired helical filaments outside of neurofibrillary tangles and neuritic plaques. Neurosci Lett 1986; **65**: 351–5.

47. Yamaguchi H, Nakazato Y, Shoji M et al. Ultrastructure of the neuropil threads in the Alzheimer brain: their dendritic origin and accumulation in senile plaques. Acta Neuropathol 1990; **80**: 368–74.

48. Foster NL, Wilhelmsen K, Sima AAF et al. and Conference Participants. Frontotemporal dementia and Parkinsonism linked to chromosome 17: a consensus conference. Ann Neurol 1997; **41**: 706–15.

49. Hutton M, Lendon CL, Rizzu P et al. Coding and 5′ splice mutations in tau associated with inherited dementia (FTDP-17). Nature 1998; **393**: 702–5.

50. Poorkaj P, Bird T, Wijsman E et al. Tau is a candidate gene for chromosome 17 frontotemporal dementia. Ann Neurol 1998; **43**: 815–25.

51. Spillantini MG, Murrell JR, Goedert M et al. Mutation in the tau gene in familial multiple system tauopathy with presenile dementia. Proc Natl Acad Sci USA 1998; **95**: 7737–41.

52. Sergeant N, Wattez A, Delacourte A. Neurofibrillary degeneration in progressive supranuclear palsy and corticobasal degeneration: tau pathologies with exclusively "exon 10" isoforms. J Neurochem 1999; **72**: 1243–9.

53. Lowe J, Blanchard A, Morrell K et al. Ubiquitin is a common factor in intermediate filament inclusion bodies of diverse type in man, including those of Parkinson's disease, Pick's disease, and Alzheimer's disease, as well as Rosenthal fibres in cerebellar astrocytomas cytoplasmic bodies in muscle, and Mallory bodies in alcoholic liver disease. J Pathol 1988; **155**: 9–15.

54. Love S, Saitoh T, Quijada S et al. Alz-50, ubiquitin and Tau immunoreactivity of neurofibrillary tangles, Pick bodies, and Lewy bodies. J Neuropathol Exp Neurol 1988; **47**: 393–405.

55. Mayer RJ, Lowe J, Landon M et al. Ubiquitin and the lysosomal system: molecular immunopathology reveals the connection. Biomed Biochim Acta 1991; **50**: 4–6.

56. Goldman JE. The association of actin with Hirano bodies. J Neuropathol Exp Neurol 1983; **42**: 146–51.

57. Terry RD, Peck A, De Teresa R et al. Some morphometric aspects of the brain in senile dementia of the Alzheimer type. Ann Neurol 1981; **10**: 184–92.

58. Hansen L, DeTeresa R, Davies P, Terry RD. Neocortical morphometry, lesion counts and choline acetyltransferase levels in the age spectrum of Alzheimer's disease. Neurology 1988; **38**: 48–54.

59. Mann DMA, Yates PO, Marcyniuk B. Some morphometric observations on the cerebral cortex and hippocampus in presenile Alzheimer's disease, senile dementia of Alzheimer type and Down's syndrome in middle age. J Neurol Sci 1985; **69**: 139–59.

60. Scheibel AB. Structural aspects of the ageing brain: spine systems and the dendritic arbor. In Katzman R, Terry RD, Bick KL, eds, Alzheimer's Disease and Senile Dementia. New York: Raven, 1987, 353–73.

61. Davies CA, Mann DMA, Sumpter PQ, Yates PO. A quantitative analysis of the neuronal and synaptic content of the frontal and temporal cortex in patients with Alzheimer's disease. J Neurol Sci 1987; **78**: 151–64.

62. Masliah E, Tery RD, Mallory M et al. Diffuse plaques do not accentuate synapse loss in Alzheimer's disease. Am J Pathol 1990; **137**: 1293–7.

63. Scheff SW, Price DA. Synapse loss in the temporal lobe in Alzheimer's disease. Ann Neurol 1993; **33**: 190–9.

64. Mann DMA, Yates PO, Marcyniuk B. A comparison of changes in the nucleus basalis and locus coeruleus in Alzheimer's disease. J Neurol Neurosurg Psychiat 1984; **47**: 201–3.

65. Ferreiro JA, Ansbacher LE, Vinters HV. Stroke related to cerebral amyloid angiopathy: the significance of systemic vascular disease. J Neurol 1989; **236**: 267–72.

66. Greene GM, Godersky JC, Biller J et al. Surgical experience with cerebral amyloid angiopathy. Stroke 1990; **21**: 1545–9.

67. McCarron MO, Nicoll JAR, Stewart J et al. The apolipoprotein E ε2 allele and the pathological features in cerebral amyloid angiopathy-related haemorrhage. J Neuropathol Exp Neurol 1999; **58**: 711–18.

68. Brun A, Englund E. A white matter disorder in dementia of Alzheimer type: a pathoanatomical study. Ann Neurol 1986; **19**: 253–62.

69. Englund E, Brun A, Gustafson L. A white matter disease in dementia of Alzheimer's type: clinical and neuropathological correlates. Int J Geriat Psychiat 1988; **3**: 1–16.

70. Rechsteiner M. Ubiquitin-mediated pathways for intracellular proteolysis. Ann Rev Cell Biol 1987; **3**: 1–30.

Oxford Project to Investigate Memory and Ageing (OPTIMA): a Longitudinal Clinicopathological Study of Dementia and Normal Ageing

A. David Smith

OPTIMA, Oxford, UK

OPTIMA was founded in 1988 by A.D. Smith, K.A. Jobst, E.M.-F. King and M.M. Esiri, with the aim of studying in parallel a cohort of patients with memory problems and age-matched controls. The total number of subjects at the end of 1999 was 666, of which 361 are patients with dementia. OPTIMA is a longitudinal clinicopathological study and its main strength lies in the very high necropsy rate (94% of the 207 who have died), which permits correlation of findings in life with those of neuropathology. Each year each subject has a full clinical examination, lumbar puncture, neuropsychology (the CAMDEX, supplemented by other tests), CT scans (axial and temporal lobe-orientated) and SPECT scans (Ceretec, for cerebral blood flow). A subset of 155 subjects have had annual volumetric MRI scans and more detailed neuropsychology.

The main findings so far are:

- Comparison of standard clinical diagnostic procedures with histopathological diagnosis, showing the poor accuracy of current clinical diagnostic procedures[1].
- Development of a more accurate diagnostic procedure for Alzheimer's disease (AD) in life by a combination of structural (CT) and functional (SPECT) brain imaging[2].
- Recognition that AD is distinct from ageing and is a true disease that follows a "catastrophic event" in the brain, leading to atrophy of the medial temporal lobe[3].
- Discovery of a biological "state" marker, the thickness of the medial temporal lobe, that can be used to follow the progression of AD[4].
- Discovery that nerve cells in AD brain express markers of the cell division cycle[5].
- Recognition of the additive effect of minor cerebrovascular disease and AD-type pathology in clinical dementia[6,7].
- Identification of a gene (K variant of butyrylcholinesterase) that markedly increases the risk of AD in those who also have the ApoE4 gene[8].
- Discovery of a risk factor (elevated blood levels of homocysteine) for AD and for vascular dementia that is potentially modifiable by diet[9].
- Finding that raised blood homocysteine levels are associated with low performance on cognitive tests in the normal elderly[10].

Projects currently under way include the search for further genetic and non-genetic risk factors for dementia, with particular emphasis on modifiable risk factors; a pilot clinical trial of high-dose folic acid and vitamin B_{12} in subjects with dementia (together with Professor G. Wilcock, Bristol); development of novel memory tests to detect pre-symptomatic AD; use of sub-voxel co-registration MRI scans to follow progression of AD over a period of a few months (with Professor G. Bydder, Hammersmith Hospital).

The current Director of OPTIMA is Professor A. David Smith, the Clinical Director is Professor Robin Jacoby and the Operational Manager and Senior Nurse is Mrs Elizabeth King. Funding is from Bristol–Myers Squibb, the Medical Research Council, National Health Service R&D and several charities.

REFERENCES

1. Nagy Z, Esiri MM, Hindley NJ et al. Accuracy of clinical operational diagnostic criteria for Alzheimer's disease in relation to different pathological diagnostic protocols. *Dement Geriat Cogn Disord* 1998; **9**: 219–26.
2. Jobst KA, Barnetson LP, Shepstone BJ. Accurate prediction of histologically confirmed Alzheimer's disease and the differential diagnosis of dementia: the use of NINCDS–ADRDA and DSM-III-R criteria, SPECT, X-ray CT, and Apo E4 in medial temporal lobe dementias. Oxford Project to Investigate Memory and Aging. *Int Psychogeriatr* 1998; **10**: 271–302.
3. Jobst KA, Smith AD, Szatmari M et al. Rapidly progressing atrophy of medial temporal lobe in Alzheimer's disease. *Lancet* 1994; **343**: 829–30.
4. Smith AD, Jobst KA. Use of structural imaging to study the progression of Alzheimer's disease. *Br Med Bull* 1996; **52**: 575–86.
5. Nagy Z, Esiri MM, Smith AD. The cell division cycle and the pathophysiology of Alzheimer's disease. *Neuroscience* 1998; **87**: 731–9.
6. Esiri MM, Nagy Z, Smith MZ et al. Cerebrovascular disease and threshold for dementia in the early stages of Alzheimer's disease. *Lancet* 1999; **354**: 919–20.
7. Nagy Z, Esiri MM, Jobst KA et al. The effects of additional pathology on the cognitive deficit in Alzheimer disease. *J Neuropathol Exp Neurol* 1997; **56**: 165–70.
8. Lehmann DJ, Johnston C, Smith AD. Synergy between the genes for butyrylcholinesterase K variant and apolipoprotein E4 in late-onset confirmed Alzheimer's disease. *Hum Mol Genet* 1997; **6**: 1933–6.
9. Clarke R, Smith AD, Jobst KA et al. Folate, vitamin B_{12}, and serum total homocysteine levels in confirmed Alzheimer disease. *Arch Neurol* 1998; **55**: 1449–55.
10. Budge M, Johnston C, Hogervorst E et al. Plasma total homocysteine and cognitive performance in a volunteer elderly population. *Ann NY Acad Sci* 2000; **903**: 407–10.

Consortium to Establish a Registry for Alzheimer's Disease (CERAD)

Gerda G. Fillenbaum and Albert Heyman

Duke University Medical Center, Durham, NC, USA

CERAD was funded by the National Institute on Aging in 1986 to develop a battery of standardized instruments for the evaluation of patients with Alzheimer's disease (AD). Until that time clinical investigation of AD and comparison of research findings was hampered by the absence of standardized assessment and uniform diagnostic criteria. The assessments developed by CERAD have been evaluated on over 1000 patients with AD and nearly 500 control subjects, seen at 24 major University medical centers across the USA. Because of their sensitivity to dementia, they have also been used in epidemiologic surveys of the elderly, to aid in identification and staging of those with dementia. The measures permit uniform identification of dementia and standardized assessment of AD.

CERAD has developed and evaluated three primary assessments. These include a clinical battery, a neuropsychological battery, and a neuropathological assessment. An overview of the contents of these assessments is given in Table 1. In addition, specialized assessments have been developed to assess family history of AD, Parkinson's disease, and Down's syndrome; extrapyramidal dysfunction in AD; neuroimaging; behavioral pathology; and assessment of service use.

Videotapes demonstrating administration of these measures are available. Educational brochures on memory loss, AD, the importance of autopsy, and an autopsy resources packet to help sites, have been prepared. Many of the CERAD assessments have been translated into various European and Asian languages, and are in use internationally.

A brief but extensive review of CERAD, including a bibliography covering the first 10 years, has been published[1]. Multiyear data on CERAD patients and control subjects as well as the CERAD measures, are available on CD-ROM. This and additional information can be obtained by writing to the Principal Investigator, Dr A. Heyman, CERAD, Box 3203, Duke University Medical Center, Durham, NC 27710, USA.

REFERENCE

1. Heyman A, Fillenbaum G, Nash F (eds). Consortium to Establish a Registry for Alzheimer's Disease: the CERAD experience. *Neurology* 1997; **49**(suppl 3).

Table 1. Overview of the contents of the primary CERAD assessments

Clinical battery
  Demographic data on subject and informant
  Clinical history, including cognitive function, systemic disorders, cerebrovascular history, parkinsonism, depression, drug effects
  Blessed Dementia Scale (ADL)
  Screen for Behavior Rating Scale for Dementia (BRSD)
  Short Blessed, Calculation, Clock, Language
  Clinical examinations, including brief physical, overall neurological assessment, extrapyramidal dysfunction
  Laboratory and imaging studies
  Clinical diagnosis, including CDR staging, diagnostic impression for:
    Possible dementia prodrome
    Probable and possible AD
    Non-AD dementias

Neuropsychological battery
  Verbal fluency
  Modified Boston Naming Test
  Mini-Mental State Examination
  Word list memory
  Constructional praxis
  Word list recall
  Word list recognition
  Constructional praxis recall
  The following are used as needed:
  Shipley Scale
  Wechsler Memory Scale, Paired Association I
  Trail Making, A and B
  Wechsler Memory Scale, Paired Association II
  Nelson Adult Reading Test
  Finger tapping
  Verbal fluency (F and P words)
Neuropathology Assessment
  Demographic information and history
  Gross examination
  Cerebrovascular disease (gross)
  Microscopic findings: vascular; major non-vascular; hippocampus and neocortex
  Neurohistologic findings
  Neuropathological diagnoses
  Final assessment

43

Neurotransmitter Changes in Alzheimer's Disease: Relationships to Symptoms and Neuropathology

Paul T Francis[1] and Elaine K. Perry[2]

[1] Centre for Neuroscience Research, King's College London, UK,
and [2]MRC Building, Newcastle upon Tyne General Hospital, UK

Cell death and histopathological changes affecting a number of neuronal systems are considered to result in the development of the typical symptomology of Alzheimer's disease (AD), characterized by gross and progressive impairments of cognitive function, which are often accompanied by behavioural disturbances such as aggression, depression, psychosis, apathy and wandering. Such non-cognitive behavioural symptoms are also considered to relate to structural and functional alterations in neurotransmission. Carers find behavioural disturbances difficult to cope with and the presence of such behaviours in AD patients often leads to the need for institutionalization[1]. The challenge has been to identify changes in specific neurotransmitter systems that underlie cognitive impairment and particular behavioural problems and to develop rational therapeutic strategies.

NEUROCHEMICAL AND HISTOPATHOLOGICAL CHANGES IN AD

The majority of biochemical studies of AD have relied on information derived from post mortem brain which typically represents the late stage of the disease (8–10 years after onset of symptoms). In these studies there is considerable evidence of gross brain atrophy, histopathological features and multiple neurotransmitter abnormalities affecting many brain regions. However, investigations of biopsy tissue taken from AD patients 3–5 years (on average) after the onset of symptoms indicate that a selective neurotransmitter pathology occurs early in the course of the disease[2].

Acetylcholine

Changes affecting many aspects of the cholinergic system in patients with AD have been reported since the initial discovery of deficits in choline acetyltransferase activity in post mortem brains[3–5]. In biopsy samples from AD patients, presynaptic markers of the cholinergic system were also uniformly reduced[2]. Thus, choline acetyltransferase activity, choline uptake and acetylcholine synthesis are all reduced to 30–60% of control values. The clinical correlate of this cholinergic deficit in AD was, until recently, considered to be cognitive dysfunction. Such a conclusion was supported by clinicopathological studies in AD and parallel experiments in non-human primates or rodents, which demonstrated disruptive effects of basal forebrain cholinergic lesions on cognitive functions. Such studies led to the "cholinergic hypothesis of geriatric memory dysfunction"[6].

Furthermore, cholinergic deficits in AD occur to the greatest extent in cortical areas primarily concerned with memory and cognition—the hippocampus, adjacent temporal lobe regions and select frontal areas. In a recent study[7] regional variations in the loss of cholinergic fibres in AD were assessed on the basis of acetylcholinesterase (AChE) histochemistry. Greatest fibre loss (>75%) was apparent in temporal association areas, with various frontal areas, including granular orbitofrontal, dysgranular orbitofrontal, prefrontal association, frontal operculum, prefrontal association and frontal pole, demonstrating fibre losses in the range 45–75%. In other cortical areas, including primary motor, premotor association, anterior and posterior cingulate, fibre loss was less than 45%.

Neuropathologically, loss of neurons from the nucleus of Meynert (Ch4 cholinergic nucleus) is well documented in AD, although the extent of the loss reported varies from moderate to severe, and it has been suggested that in AD cholinergic dysfunction exceeds degeneration[8]. Detailed analysis of subpopulations of cholinergic perikarya in the nucleus basalis have been reported by Mesulam and Geula[9], who identified selective cell loss in Ch4p (the posterior section projecting to temporal cortex). In the intermediate sector, Ch4id, which includes projections to the frontal cortex, neuron loss is not as extensive, consistent with the moderate loss of cholinergic enzyme activity.

On the basis of the above evidence, neocortical cholinergic innervation appears to be lost at an early stage of the disease and this is supported by a recent study[10] in which the cholinergic deficit (reduced ChAT activity) has been related to Braak staging. Braak stages I and II are considered to represent the earliest presentation of AD, with neurofibrillary tangles in the entorhinal cortex, and a 20–30% loss of ChAT activity was reported in brains from patients at these stages of AD[11]. However, another study using the Clinical Dementia Rating Scale (CDR) suggests that the greatest reduction in markers of the cholinergic system occurs between moderate (CDR 2.0) and severe (CDR 5.0) disease, with little change between non-demented and the mild stage (CDR 0–2)[12].

There has been a recent shift of emphasis regarding the clinical significance of cholinergic deficits. Non-cognitive or neuropsychiatric, in addition to cognitive, symptoms also appear to have a cholinergic component[13]. For example, visual hallucinations relate to neocortical cholinergic deficits[14], such deficits (e.g. loss of ChAT) being greater in Lewy body dementia (DLB), where

Principles and Practice of Geriatric Psychiatry, 2nd edn. Edited by J. R. M. Copeland, M. T. Abou-Saleh and D. G. Blazer
©2002 John Wiley & Sons, Ltd

hallucinations are common, than in AD where they are less common[15]. Reductions in cortical ChAT activity in patients with dementia, in addition to correlating with cognitive decline, are also related to overactivity and aggressive behaviour[16].

It has also been suggested that acetylcholine is centrally involved in the process of conscious awareness[17], and that the variety of clinical symptoms associated with cholinergic dysfunction in AD and related disorders reflects disturbances in the conscious processing of information. There is evidence that implicit memory, for example (which does not involve conscious awareness), is relatively intact in AD[18,19].

Glutamate

Loss of synapses and pyramidal cell perikarya (both considered to be markers of glutamatergic neurones) from the neocortex of AD patients correlate with measures of cognitive decline[2]. Although neurochemical studies of glutamate neurotransmission have failed to demonstrate extensive alterations, this may be related to the difficulty in distinguishing the transmitter pool of glutamate from the metabolic pool. Nevertheless, glutamate concentration was reduced by 14% in temporal lobe biopsy samples and by 86% in the terminal zone of the perforant pathway at autopsy of AD patients[20]. Uptake of D-aspartate, a putative marker of glutamatergic nerve endings, is also reduced in many cortical areas in AD brain[2]. Thus, additional factors other than impaired cholinergic function are likely to contribute to cognitive impairment in AD. However, it is important to remember that glutamatergic neurones of the neocortex and hippocampus are influenced by acetylcholine through nicotinic and muscarinic receptors[2]. Thus, treatment of patients with cholinomimetics is likely to increase glutamatergic function.

Other neurotransmitters

Using biopsy samples from AD patients, serotonergic and some noradrenergic markers are affected, whereas markers for dopamine, γ-aminobutyric acid (GABA) or somatostatin are not altered. When post mortem studies of AD brain are considered, many neurotransmitter systems, including GABA and somatostatin, are involved or are affected to a greater extent[2]. Based on post mortem studies, however, changes in serotonergic neurotransmission may be linked to the behavioural disturbances of AD, such as depression, rather than cognitive dysfunction. For example, patients with AD who were also depressed had lower numbers of serotonin reuptake sites in the neocortex than did patients without this symptom[21]. Furthermore, both reduced serotonergic[22,23] and increased noradrenergic activities and sensitivity[24,25] have been linked to aggressive behaviour.

Neurotransmitter receptors

Many neurotransmitter receptors appear to be unaltered in AD; however, studies have demonstrated a reduction in the number of nicotinic and muscarinic (M2) ACh receptors, most of which are considered to be located on presynaptic cholinergic terminals. Despite continuing, often unconfirmed, reports of changes in one or more of the muscarinic receptor subtypes (M–M_5), it is generally agreed, on the basis of autopsy studies, that the M1 subtype is unchanged until later in the disease when it may decline, probably in relation to cholinoceptive (postsynaptic) neurodegeneration. The status of the other subtypes is not clearly established, primarily due to the lack of specific pharmacological labels. Results using antibodies against the different receptor subtypes, while specific, are complicated by discrepancies between the distribution and density of immunoreactive proteins and localized functional receptors. With respect to muscarinic receptor coupling to G-proteins, most studies using a variety of investigative procedures have identified some degree of uncoupling, especially with respect to the M1 receptor[26].

A highly consistent receptor abnormality in AD is the loss of the nicotinic receptor[27,28], which appears to primarily reflect loss of the α4-containing subtype (generally associated with β2) as opposed to α3 or α7 subtypes[29]. Immunohistochemically, loss of α4 and β2 reactive fibres has been observed in temporal cortex, associated with reactive neuropil threads, tangles and plaques[30].

NEUROIMAGING

With respect to the cholinergic deficit, whilst measurements of CSF acetylcholine, choline and acetylcholinesterase have been reported in AD, such reports are either unconfirmed or inconsistent. More promising and potentially diagnostic findings have been obtained using in vivo functional imaging. The vesicular acetylcholine transporter and acetylcholinesterase, imaged using PET and iodobenzovesamicol and N-methylpiperidin-4-yl propionate, respectively, are both reduced in AD patients, and furthermore relate to reductions in MMSE[31,32]. Using SPECT, muscarinic QNB binding is reduced in advanced but not early cases[33], and iododexetamide, with preference for M2, is also reduced in mild/early cases[34]. Reductions in nicotine binding have also been detected using PET[35]. In vivo observations relating to non-cholinergic systems (principally noradrenaline, 5-HT and dopamine) have been equally inconsistent regarding CSF parameters and, with respect to neuroimaging markers, only dopaminergic markers have so far been investigated and there is, as expected, no consistent abnormality of the transporter or D2 receptor.

LINKS BETWEEN NEUROTRANSMISSION AND NEUROPATHOLOGY

Mismetabolism of amyloid precursor protein (APP) leading to increased production of β-amyloid has been proposed as the critical event in both familial and sporadic AD causing other changes (tangles, neurone loss, synapse loss and neurotransmission dysfunction). Cholinergic neurotransmission may be a specific target for β-amyloid, since it has been shown to reduce both choline uptake and acetylcholine release in vitro[36]. Furthermore, β-amyloid is reported to bind with high affinity to the α7 subtype of the nicotinic receptor, suggesting that cholinergic function through this receptor may be compromised because of high levels of (soluble) peptide in AD brains[37].

There is increasing evidence that various neurotransmitter systems are capable of influencing the metabolism of APP, favouring the non-amyloidogenic processing[38]. In particular, stimulation of muscarinic M1 receptors increases APP secretion, while decreasing β-amyloid production[39]. Furthermore, nicotinic receptor stimulation is associated with reduced plaque densities in human brain[40]. These results suggest that compounds being developed for symptomatic treatment may have a serendipitous effect on the continuing emergence of pathology by reducing the production of β-amyloid.

CHOLINERGIC APPROACHES TO TREATMENT

Biochemical studies of postmortem brains from AD patients showing evidence of a substantial presynaptic cholinergic deficit, which correlated with cognitive impairment[41], together with the emerging role of ACh in learning and memory[6], clearly suggested a rational approach to treatment. However, more recent studies have identified a role for the cholinergic system in attentional processing rather than memory.

A prediction of the cholinergic hypothesis is that drugs that potentiate central cholinergic function should improve cognition in AD patients. There are a number of approaches to the treatment of the cholinergic deficit; however, the use of acetylcholinesterase inhibitors is the most well-developed approach to the treatment of AD to date[42].

During the late 1980s and early 1990s, the first cholinomimetic compound, tacrine, underwent large-scale clinical studies and established clearly the benefits of ChE treatment in patients with a diagnosis of probable AD. Tacrine was subsequently approved for use in some, but not all, countries. Statistically significant, dose-related improvements on objective performance-based tests of cognition, clinician- and caregiver-rated global evaluations of patient well-being and also quality of life measures have been reported[43]. Unfortunately, potentially serious adverse side effects have limited the use of this compound.

A so-called second generation of ChE inhibitors has been developed, including donepezil, rivastigmine, metrifonate and galantamine[42]. Such compounds demonstrate a clinical effect and magnitude of benefit of at least that reported for tacrine, but with a more favourable clinical profile. Furthermore, evidence is emerging from clinical trials of cholinomimetics that such drugs may improve the abnormal non-cognitive, behavioural symptoms of AD. The cholinesterase inhibitors physostigmine, tacrine, rivastigmine and metrifonate have variously been reported in placebo-controlled trials to decrease psychoses (hallucinations and delusions), agitation, apathy, anxiety, disinhibition, pacing and aberrant motor behaviour and lack of cooperation in AD[13,44]. In a recent open-label trial of Exelon (rivastigmine), patients with DLB almost all responded positively on one or more of these measures[45].

CONCLUSIONS

In AD many different pathological manifestations, such as cortical and subcortical β-amyloidosis (plaques), abnormal tau (tangles and dystrophic neurites), neuronal and synapse loss and various transmitter deficits, provide an increasingly complex framework for clinical–neuropathological correlations. It is therefore unlikely that cholinergic deficits alone will account for the full spectrum of cognitive and non-cognitive symptoms seen in AD. In these circumstances it is perhaps surprising that cholinomimetic therapy has been a modest success in many patients, improving cognitive and non-cognitive symptoms and activities of daily living. Such therapy is all that is available at present and may well still be required as new therapies designed to slow disease progression come into the clinic.

REFERENCES

1. Esiri MM. The basis for behavioural disturbances in dementia. *J Neurol Neurosurg Psychiat* 1996; **61**: 127–30.
2. Francis PT, Sims NR, Procter AW, Bowen DM. Cortical pyramidal neurone loss may cause glutamatergic hypoactivity and cognitive impairment in Alzheimer's disease: investigative and therapeutic perspectives. *J Neurochem* 1993; **60**: 1589–604.
3. Bowen DM, Smith CB, White P, Davison AN. Neurotransmitter-related enzymes and indices of hypoxia in senile dementia and other abiotrophies. *Brain* 1976; **99**: 459–96.
4. Davies P, Maloney AJF. Selective loss of central cholinergic neurones in Alzheimer's disease. *Lancet* 1976; **ii**: 1403.
5. Perry EK, Gibson PH, Blessed G et al. Neurotransmitter abnormalities in senile dementia. *J Neurol Sci* 1977; **34**: 247–65.
6. Bartus RT, Dean RL, Beer B, Lippa AS. The cholinergic hypothesis of geriatric memory dysfunction. *Science* 1982; **217**: 408–17.
7. Geula C, Mesulam MM. Systematic regional variations in the loss of cortical cholinergic fibers in Alzheimer's disease. *Cerebr Cortex* 1996; **6**: 165–77.
8. Perry RH, Candy JM, Perry EK et al. Extensive loss of choline acetyltransferase activity is not reflected by neuronal loss in the nucleus of Meynert in Alzheimer's disease. *Neurosci Lett* 1982; **33**: 311–15.
9. Mesulam MM, Geula G. Nucleus basalis (Ch4) and cortical cholinergic innervation in the human brain—observations based on the distribution of acetylcholinesterase and choline acetyltransferase. *J Comp Neurol* 1988; **275**: 216–40.
10. Braak H, Braak E. Neuropathological staging of Alzheimer-related changes. *Acta Neuropathol* 1991; **82**: 239–59.
11. Beach TG, Kuo YM, Spiegel K et al. The cholinergic deficit coincides with Aβ deposition at the earliest histopathologic stages of Alzheimer disease. *J Neuropathol Exp Neurol* 2000; **59**: 308–13.
12. Davis KL, Mohs RC, Marin D et al. Cholinergic markers in elderly patients with early signs of Alzheimer disease. *J Am Med Assoc* 1999; **281**: 1401–6.
13. Cummings JL, Kaufer DI. Neuropsychiatric aspects of Alzheimer's disease: the cholinergic hypothesis revisited. *Neurology* 1996; **47**: 876–83.
14. Perry EK, Marshal E, Thompson P et al. Monoaminergic activities in Lewy body dementia—relation to hallucinosis and extrapyramidal features. *J Neural Transm* 1993; **6**: 167–77.
15. Perry EK, Haroutunian V, Davis KL et al. Neocortical cholinergic activities differentiate Lewy body dementia from classical Alzheimer's disease. *NeuroReport* 1994; **5**: 747–9.
16. Minger SL, Esiri MM, McDonald B et al. Cholinergic deficits contribute to behavioural disturbance in patients with dementia. *Neurology* 2000; **55**: 1460–7.
17. Woolf NJ. The critical role of cholinergic basal forebrain neurons in morphological change and memory encoding: a hypothesis. *Neurobiol Learning Memory* 1996; **66**: 258–66.
18. Postle BR, Corkin S, Growdon JH. Intact implicit memory for novel patterns in Alzheimer's disease. *Learning Memory* 1996; **3**: 305–12.
19. Hirono N, Mori E, Ikejiri Y et al. Procedural memory in patients with mild Alzheimer's disease. *Dement Geriatr Cogn Disord* 1997; **8**: 210–16.
20. Hyman BT, Van Hoesen GW, Damasio AR. Alzheimer's disease: glutamate depletion in the hippocampal perforant pathway zone. *Ann Neurol* 1987; **22**: 37–40.
21. Chen CPLH, Alder JT, Bowen DM et al. Presynaptic serotonergic markers in community-acquired cases of Alzheimer's disease: correlation with depression and neuroleptic medication. *J Neurochem* 1996; **66**: 1592–8.
22. Coccaro EF. Central serotonin and impulsive aggression. *Br J Psychiat* 1989; **155** (suppl. 8): 52–62.
23. Procter AW, Francis PT, Stratmann GC, Bowen DM. Serotonergic pathology is not widespread in Alzheimer patients without prominent aggressive symptoms. *Neurochem Res* 1992; **17**: 917–22.
24. Peskind ER, Wingerson D, Murray S et al. Effects of Alzheimer's disease and normal aging on cerebrospinal fluid norepinephrine responses to yohimbine and clonidine. *Arch Gen Psychiat* 1995; **52**: 774–82.
25. Raskind MA. Evaluation and management of aggressive behavior in the elderly demented patient. *J Clin Psychiat* 1999; **60**: 45–9.
26. Jope RS, Song L, Li X, Powers R. Impaired phosphoinositide hydrolysis in Alzheimer's disease brain. *Neurobiol Aging* 1994; **15**: 221–6.
27. Aubert I, Araujo DM, Cecyre D et al. Comparative alterations of nicotinic and muscarinic binding sites in Alzheimer's and Parkinson's diseases. *J Neurochem* 1992; **58**: 529–41.
28. Perry EK, Morris CM, Court JA et al. Alteration in nicotine binding sites in Parkinson's disease, Lewy body dementia and Alzheimer's: possible index of early neuropathology. *Neuroscience* 1995; **64**: 385–95.
29. MartinRuiz CM, Court JA, Molnar E et al. Alpha 4 but not alpha 3 and alpha 7 nicotinic acetylcholine receptor subunits are lost from

the temporal cortex in Alzheimer' s disease. *J Neurochem* 1999; **73**: 1635–40.

30. Sparks DL, Beach TG, Lukas RJ. Immunohistochemical localization of nicotinic $\beta2$ and $\alpha4$ receptor subunits in normal human brain and individuals with Lewy body and Alzheimer's disease: preliminary observations. *Neurosci Lett* 1998; **256**: 151–4.

31. Kuhl DE, Minoshima S, Fessler S *et al. In vivo* mapping of cholinergic terminals in normal aging, Alzheimer's disease and Parkinson's disease. *Ann Neurol* 1996; **40**: 399–410.

32. Kuhl DE, Koeppe RA, Minoshima S *et al. In vivo* mapping of cerebral acetylcholinesterase activity in aging and Alzheimer's disease. *Neurology* 1999; **52**: 691–9.

33. Wyper DJ, Brown D, Patterson J *et al.* Deficits in iodine-labeled 3-quinuclidinyl benzylate binding in relation to cerebral blood flow in patients with Alzheimer's disease. *Eur J Nucl Med* 1993; **20**: 379–86.

34. Claus JJ, Dubois EA, Booij J *et al.* Demonstration of a reduction in muscarinic receptor binding in early Alzheimer's disease using [^{123}I] dexetimide single emission tomography. *Eur J Nucl Med* 1997; **24**: 602–8.

35. Nordberg A, Lundqvist H, Hartvig P *et al.* Kinetic analysis of regional (s)($-$) [^{11}C] nicotine binding in normal and Alzheimer brains—*in vivo* assessment using postron emission tomography. *Alzheimer Dis Assoc Disord* 1995; **9**: 21–7.

36. Auld DS, Kar S, Quirion R. β-Amyloid peptides as direct cholinergic neuromodulators: a missing link? *Trends Neurosci* 1998; **21**: 43–9.

37. Wang HY, Lee DHS, Dandrea MR *et al.* β-Amyloid(1-42) binds to alpha 7 nicotinic acetylcholine receptor with high affinity—implications for Alzheimer's disease pathology. *J Biol Chem* 2000; **275**: 5626–32.

38. Nitsch RM. From acetylcholine to amyloid: neurotransmitters and the pathology of Alzheimer's disease. *Neurodegeneration* 1996; **5**: 477–82.

39. Nitsch RM, Slack BE, Wurtman RJ, Growdon JH. Release of Alzheimer amyloid precursor stimulated by activation of muscarinic acetylcholine receptors. *Science* 1992; **258**: 304–7.

40. Court JA, Lloyd S, Thomas N *et al.* Dopamine and nicotinic receptor binding and the levels of dopamine and homovanillic acid in human brain related to tobacco use. *Neuroscience* 1998; **87**: 63–78.

41. Francis PT, Palmer AM, Sims NR *et al.* Neurochemical studies of early-onset Alzheimer's disease. Possible influence on treatment. *N Engl J Med* 1985; **313**: 7–11.

42. Francis PT, Palmer AM, Snape M, Wilcock GK. The cholinergic hypothesis of Alzheimer's disease: a review of progress. *J Neurol Neurosurg Psychiat* 1999; **66**: 137–47.

43. Davis KL, Thal LJ, Gamzu ER *et al.* A double-blind, placebo-controlled multicenter study of tacrine for Alzheimer's disease. *N Engl J Med* 1992; **327**: 1253–9.

44. Perry EK, Walker M, Grace J, Perry RH. Acetylcholine in mind: a neurotransmitter correlate of consciousness? *Trends Neurosci* 1999; **22**: 273–80.

45. McKeith IG, Grace JB, Walker Z *et al.* Rivastigmine in the treatment of dementia with lewy bodies: preliminary findings from an open trial. *Int J Geriat Psychiat* 2000; **15**: 387–92.

44

Antemortem Markers

Susan J. Van Rensburg, Felix C. V. Potocnik and Dan J. Stein

Tygerberg Hospital and University of Stellenbosch Medical School, South Africa

INTRODUCTION

It has become increasingly clear that the disease process of Alzheimer's disease (AD) is multifaceted. It is thus difficult to single out any particular factor as the root cause of the disease, since AD appears to be a complex disorder involving several genes interacting with environmental factors. Apart from the familial forms of the disease, in which the gene mutations have been elucidated, many proteins, enzymes and other factors are involved in the process of neurodegeneration, in the formation of plaques and tangles and in the development of an inflammatory state of the brain. In all, more than 100 proteins and other factors have been found to be altered in AD patients compared with controls.

For all that, very few markers suitable for antemortem diagnostic purposes have emerged, since many of the above-mentioned alterations are not specific for AD, while others pertain only to subsets of AD[1]. While it has been argued that the most powerful antemortem marker in AD is a clinical diagnosis based on an adequate range of observations[2], such diagnosis is at present to some degree still one of exclusion. An ideal biological marker would allow for greater specificity and sensitivity than clinical diagnosis, and be readily obtainable. While neuropathological biopsy diagnosis of AD allows specificity and sensitivity, it is rarely clinically warranted or available. The neurobiological alterations present in AD may be reflected in changes in cerebrospinal fluid (CSF) neurotransmitters or neurochemicals, or in a change in systemic tissues, including blood constituents. It should be borne in mind, however, that CSF measurements are influenced by a variety of factors, including CSF gradients, age and sex, diurnal and seasonal variation, state of the blood–brain barrier, blood contamination, contributions from the spinal cord, phase of illness, psychomotor activity, stress and diet. Measurement of blood constituents may also reflect concentration differences due to diurnal rhythms and other factors.

In this chapter on antemortem markers, we will briefly review neurotransmitters and neurochemistry, systemic pathology and brain imaging.

NEUROTRANSMITTERS AND NEUROCHEMISTRY

The Cholinergic System

The most effective drugs so far for the treatment of AD are the acetylcholinesterase (AChE) inhibitors. The introduction of these agents followed the discovery that cholinergic neurons were depleted and that cholinergic function was significantly decreased in the basal forebrain of AD patients[3]. CSF markers of cholinergic function have been studied, but have not yielded consistent results. For example, measurements of AChE and pseudocholinesterase (PChE) have led to the conclusion that cholinergic basal forebrain neurons are not a major source of cholinesterases in the CSF and do not provide evidence for using CSF cholinesterases as a diagnostic marker of basal forebrain cholinergic cell loss[4].

The Noradrenergic System

Autopsy studies of AD brains demonstrate loss of cells in the locus coeruleus, the major nucleus of origin of noradrenergic fibres. Reduced noradrenaline (norepinephrine NE) in autopsy samples of AD brains has been a fairly consistent finding. In contrast, CSF and plasma NE and 3-methoxy-4-hydroxyphenylethylene glycol (MHPG) appear significantly higher in patients with advanced AD than in patients with moderate AD or controls[5,6]. Patients with advanced AD have not only biochemical indices of noradrenergic hyperactivity but also physiological pointers to this, including higher heart rate and blood pressure. AD patients with the most severe dementia have the greatest rise in CSF MHPG levels following administration of probenecid. There is also evidence for blunted growth hormone response to clonidine in AD patients, suggestive of altered α-2-adrenergic receptor sensitivity[7]. It may be hypothesized that increased activity and turnover of the noradrenergic system may compensate for cell loss and that a limited number of NE cells remain highly active in AD patients. Severe neuronal loss in advanced AD may lead to a compensatory increase in locus coeruleus firing rate, contributing to symptoms such as pacing, agitation, insomnia and weight loss.

The Serotonergic System

Numerous autopsy studies of AD brains have suggested a serotonergic deficit. Although there have been reports that the major serotonin metabolite, 5-hydroxyindoleacetic acid (5-HIAA), is unchanged in the CSF of AD patients, most studies indicate a reduction in CSF 5-HIAA. In one study that demonstrated significantly lower mean 5-HIAA levels in AD, the wide variability in values suggested that the changes were non-specific, secondary to the cerebral degeneration in AD[8]. There is also evidence of increased behavioural sensitivity to *m*-chlorophenylpiperazine in AD patients, consistent with damage to serotonin pathways[9].

Melatonin, the pineal hormone biosynthesized from serotonin, has been demonstrated to be significantly decreased in the CSF of elderly patients, and more so in AD patients. In elderly (> 80 years of age) non-demented subjects, CSF melatonin levels were half those of younger (age 41–80) control subjects, and in AD patients the CSF melatonin levels were only one-fifth of those found in control subjects ($p < 0.0001$)[10].

Other neurochemical systems have been investigated as potential antemortem markers[11]. Somatostatin is reduced in AD brains and CSF somatostatin levels have been found to be significantly lower in patients with AD compared to controls. These findings do not, however, appear specific to AD. Other CSF peptidergic findings in AD include decreased vasopressin, decreased thyrotropin-releasing hormone, and decreased delta sleep-inducing peptide. Another system that may be disordered in AD brains comprises trophic factors such as gangliosides.

SYSTEMIC PATHOLOGY

It is possible to view AD as a systemic illness. Thus, if AD were a genetic disorder, then disturbances at the molecular level may be expressed in non-neural tissue, with systemic effects.

Studies of blood cell cholinergic function have been undertaken since central cholinergic dysfunction in AD became a favoured hypothesis. Studies of red blood cell (RBC) and plasma choline and AchE do not support their validity as antemortem markers. However, studies indicate differences in the dynamics of RBC choline uptake, suggesting a vulnerability of cholinergic neurons in patients with AD[12].

Fluidity of the platelet membrane (PMF) is increased in patients with AD compared to patients with vascular dementia (VaD) and elderly controls[1,13,14]. Only about 50% of AD patients demonstrate this abnormality; however, increased PMF appears to be a familial trait, and the subgroup of AD patients in whom it manifests suffer from an earlier onset and a more rapidly progressive decline[15]. In a prospective longitudinal study to evaluate PMF as a putative risk factor for AD, nine of 330 people with increased PMF (initially asymptomatic first-degree relatives of probands with AD) developed AD after 7.5 years[16]. On a biochemical level, it was found that free radical-induced lipid peroxidation increased the fluidity of platelet membranes, providing a postulated mechanism underlying increased PMF[17].

In fibroblasts, abnormalities in enzymatic activity, glucose metabolism, abnormal calcium metabolism, impaired DNA repair and potassium channel dysfunction[18] have been observed.

Inflammation

Neuropathological findings in AD brains show an inflammatory response. CSF interleukin-1β (IL-1β) concentrations were significantly higher in AD patients than in patients with VaD, normal pressure hydrocephalus or multiple sclerosis[19]. Activated microglia may participate in the initial stages of neurodegeneration. Microglial antibodies in the CSF have been found in AD patients[20]. CSF microglial antibodies were present in at-risk descendants of familial AD patients, some of whom subsequently developed AD, and in AD patients in contrast with other types of dementia[21]. The presence of microglial antibodies may, however, be non-specific, as a similar mechanism has been implicated in the pathophysiology of VaD. Drugs aimed at diminishing inflammation and the activity of microglia are currently being investigated.

A miscellany of other research areas in AD can conveniently be mentioned in this section. These include studies of visual system dysfunctions, olfactory deficits, extrapyramidal dysfunction, atypical dermatoglyphic patterns, altered sweat response, abnormal glucose tolerance and vitamin B$_{12}$ deficiency. Such work, although interesting, has not yet led to a sensitive and specific antemortem marker.

Protein Abnormalities

Mutations of the amyloid β-protein precursor (APP) have been found in familial AD with early onset. A prominent feature of the senile plaques found in AD is the deposition of β-amyloid. The other hallmark lesion for AD is the neurofibrillary tangle, which contains tau protein. Given that the clinical phase of AD may be preceded by a 15–30 year period of deposition of amyloid and tau protein, markers to predict the development of AD should ultimately be obtainable[22]. While the concentration of tau protein in CSF was found to be significantly higher in AD patients compared to non-demented controls, reports of altered APP and β-amyloid CSF concentrations have not been consistent[22].

Environmental Factors in AD

Although AD has been linked to a genetic aetiology, studies with monozygotic twins revealed variability in age at onset of as much as 9, 15 or 20 years[23]. This led to the suspicion that some environmental factor(s) ingested from food and water, or a deficiency of some protective element, may accelerate disease expression in susceptible individuals. Several metals have been investigated in AD in the hope of finding a marker for the disease. Of these, iron, aluminium, zinc and mercury are considered to be the most important. Aluminium was found in neurofibrillary tangles[24,25], aluminium and silicon were found in cores of senile plaques[26] and aluminium levels were increased in the hippocampus and cerebral cortex of AD patients compared with non-demented controls[27]. Aluminium is not easily absorbed by the body, since the gastrointestial tract forms a major cellular barrier to its absorption. In AD this barrier may be compromised[28]. The findings of increased aluminium in AD have, however, been inconsistent.

Iron metabolism is altered and the iron transport protein transferrin decreased in the serum of AD patients. Furthermore, a genetic form of transferrin, TfC2, which is associated with diseases attributed to free radical damage, has an increased allele frequency in AD[29–31]. Serum levels of the iron binding protein p97 (melanotransferrin) were reported to be elevated in AD patients, discriminating between AD patients and controls[32], a finding which has to be confirmed. Finally, blood mercury levels are also significantly raised in AD patients[33].

BRAIN IMAGING

There has been considerable interest in the use of brain imaging in the diagnosis of AD (see Section EX). The medial temporal lobe is involved in cognitive functions of the brain and is the region reflecting the most extensive pathological changes in AD. Using temporal-lobe-orientated computed tomography (CT), it was demonstrated that decreased hippocampal width predicted AD with a detection rate of 92% when a cut-off was selected to yield a 5% false-positive rate. These cases were subsequently confirmed histopathologically[34]. CT scans also revealed that the atrophy of the medial temporal lobe in AD was related to the progression of pathology[35].

Magnetic resonance imaging (MRI) studies yielded similar results. On MRI, AD patients and controls were best told apart using left amygdala and entorhinal cortex volumes[36]. Coupled to blood flow studies using single photon emission computed tomography (SPECT) and using relative left temporoparietal cortex blood flow, the imaging studies yielded 100% discrimination between AD patients and controls[36]. In addition, in older patients with mild cognitive impairment, hippocampal atrophy determined by premorbid MRI-based volume measurements was predictive of subsequent conversion to AD[37]. In distinguishing between AD and other dementias, one study differentiated AD from normal ageing, depression, VaD and other causes of cognitive impairment[38], while in another study, no significant volumetric differences were found between patients with subcortical VaD and AD patients, apart from the volume of the cerebellum[39].

Positron emission tomography (PET) has been found to differentiate between AD and VaD: in AD the typical metabolic pattern is hypometabolism in temporoparietal and frontal association areas, while in VaD scattered areas of hypometabolism extending over cortical and subcortical structures are seen[40].

CONCLUSION

It is clear that a number of difficulties beset the researcher interested in finding an antemortem marker for AD. Some of the techniques used in this search have important limitations—in particular, CSF measurements are influenced by a variety of factors. Diagnosis of AD, even at autopsy, may not always be accurate, leading to heterogeneity of the patient sample. In addition, AD may be a heterogeneous disorder, perhaps with a presenile form, but certainly with different manifestations in the much older age group. A marker may be present in a control with the AD trait who has not yet developed AD, and if a marker is related to the severity of AD, it may not distinguish between mild cases and controls. Other dementias may overlap with AD, not only in phenomenology but also in pathogenesis, and therefore display similar markers. There are also mixed cases, where patients, for example, have both AD and VaD.

Nevertheless, the work discussed here does suggest that some combination of measures may ultimately correlate strongly with biopsy diagnosis. Work in molecular and genetic biology and in brain imaging seems particularly promising and may well tie in with our knowledge of neurochemistry and neuropathology. An interdisciplinary effort to find an antemortem marker is useful not only in leading to a better delineation of AD-related dementias and AD subtypes, but also in providing a focus on central pathogenic mechanisms and their possible reversal.

Finally, markers may be expressed differently in different populations. A genetic variant of apolipoprotein E, ApoE ε4 (Chapter 41) has been shown to be a risk factor for late-onset AD. Yet, in spite of relatively high frequencies of ApoE ε4 in African countries, the prevalence of AD is very much lower than in the Western population[41], making it extremely important for us to understand the aetiology of the disease.

ACKNOWLEDGEMENTS

The authors are supported by the Medical Research Council of South Africa and the Provincial Administration of the Western Cape.

REFERENCES

1. Zubenko GS. Biological correlates of clinical heterogeneity in primary dementia. *Neuropsychopharmacology* 1992; **6**: 77–93.
2. Roth M. Antemortem markers of Alzheimer's disease: a commentary. *Neurobiol Aging* 1986; **7**: 402–5.
3. Perry EK, Tomlinson BE, Blessed G et al. Correlation of cholinergic abnormalities with senile plaques and mental test scores in senile dementia. *Br Med J* 1978; **2**: 1457–9.
4. Rossner S, Bakinde N, Zeitschel U et al. Cerebrospinal fluid cholinesterases—markers for loss of cholinergic basal forebrain neurons? *Int J Dev Neurosci* 1998; **16**: 669–73.
5. Elrod R, Peskind ER, DiGiacomo L et al. Effects of Alzheimer's disease severity on cerebrospinal fluid norepinephrine concentration. *Am J Psychiat* 1997; **154**: 25–30.
6. Sheline YI, Miller K, Bardgett ME, Csernansky JG. Higher cerebrospinal fluid MHPG in subjects with dementia of the Alzheimer type. Relationship with cognitive dysfunction. *Am J Geriat Psychiat* 1998; **6**: 155–61.
7. Balldin J, Gottfries CG, Lindstedt G et al. The clonidine test in patients with dementia disorders: relation to clinical status and cerebrospinal fluid metabolite levels. *Int J Geriat Psychiat* 1988; **3**: 115–23.
8. Blennow K, Wallin A, Gottfries CG et al. Significance of decreased lumbar CSF levels of HVA and 5-HIAA in Alzheimer's disease. *Neurobiol Aging* 1992; **13**: 107–13.
9. Lawlor BA, Sunderland T, Mellow MA et al. Hyperresponsivity to the serotonin agonist *m*-chlorophenylpiperazine in Alzheimer's disease. A controlled study. *Arch Gen Psychiat* 1989; **46**: 542–9.
10. Liu RY, Zhou JN, van Heerikhuize J et al. Decreased melatonin levels in postmortem cerebrospinal fluid in relation to aging, Alzheimer's disease, and apolipoprotein E-ε4/4 genotype. *J Clin Endocrinol Metab* 1999; **84**: 323–7.
11. Cook LL, Nemeroff CB. Neuropeptides in Alzheimer's disease. *J Clin Psychiat (Monogr Ser)* 1989; **7**: 2–12.
12. Kanof PD, Breenwald BS, Mohs RC, Davis KL. Red cell choline II: kinetics in Alzheimer's disease. *Biol Psychiat* 1985; **20**: 375–83.
13. Hicks N, Brammer MJ, Hymas N, Levy R. Platelet membrane properties in Alzheimer's disease and multi-infarct dementias. *Alzheimer's Dis Assoc Disord* 1987; **1**: 90–7.
14. Van Rensburg SJ, Carstens ME, Potocnik FCV et al. Membrane fluidity of platelets and erythrocytes in patients with Alzheimer's disease and the effect of small amounts of aluminium on platelet and erythrocyte membranes. *Neurochem Res* 1992; **17**: 825–9.
15. Zubenko GS, Huff FJ, Beyer J et al. Familial risk of dementia associated with a biologic subtype of Alzheimer's disease. *Arch Gen Psychiat* 1988; **45**: 889–93.
16. Zubenko GS, Winwood E, Jacobs B et al. Prospective study of risk factors for Alzheimer's disease: results at 7.5 years. *Am J Psychiat* 1999; **156**: 50–7.
17. Van Rensburg SJ, Daniels WMU, Van Zyl J et al. Lipid peroxidation and platelet membrane fluidity—implications for Alzheimer's disease? *NeuroReport* 1994; **5**: 2221–4.
18. Etcheberrigaray R, Ito E, Oka K et al. Potassium channel dysfunction in fibroblasts identifies patients with Alzheimer's disease. *Proc Natl Acad Sci USA* 1993; **90**: 8209–13.
19. Cacabelos R, Barquero M, Garcia P et al. Cerebrospinal fluid interleukin-1β (IL-1β) in Alzheimer's disease and neurological disorders. *Methods Findings Exp Clin Pharmacol* 1991; **13**: 455–8.
20. Lemke MR, Glatzel M, Henneberg AE. Antimicroglia antibodies in sera of Alzheimer's disease patients. *Biol Psychiat* 1999; **45**: 508–11.
21. McRae A, Ling EA, Wigander A, Dahlstrom A. Microglial cerebrospinal fluid antibodies. Significance for Alzheimer disease. *Mol Chem Neuropathol* 1996; **28**: 89–95.
22. Hock C. Biological markers of Alzheimer's disease. *Neurobiol Aging* 1998; **19**: 149–51.
23. Breitner JCS, Murphy EA, Folstein MF, Magruder-Habib K. Twin studies of Alzheimer's disease: an approach to etiology and prevention. *Neurobiol Aging* 1990; **11**: 641–8.
24. Crapper DR, Krishnan SS, Quittkat S. Aluminium, neurofibrillary degeneration and Alzheimer's disease. *Brain* 1976; **99**: 67–80.
25. Good PF, Perl DP, Bierer LM, Schmeidler J. Selective accumulation of aluminum and iron in the neurofibrillary tangles of Alzheimer's disease: a laser microprobe (LAMMA) study. *Ann Neurol* 1992; **31**: 286–92.
26. Candy JM, Oakley AE, Klinowski J et al. Aluminosilicates and senile plaque formation in Alzheimer's disease. *Lancet* 1986; **i**: 354–7.
27. Ward NI, Mason JA. Neutron activation analysis techniques for identifying elemental status in Alzheimer's disease. *J Radioanalyt Nucl Chem Art* 1987; **113**: 515–26.
28. Taylor GA, Ferrier IN, McLoughlin IJ et al. Gastrointestinal absorption of aluminium in Alzheimer's disease: response to aluminium citrate. *Age Ageing* 1992; **21**: 81–90.
29. Van Rensburg SJ, Carstens ME, Potocnik FCV et al. Increased frequency of the transferrin C2 subtype in Alzheimer's disease. *NeuroReport* 1993; **4**: 1269–71.

30. Namekata K, Imagawa M, Terashi A *et al*. Association of transferrin C2 allele with late-onset Alzheimer's disease. *Hum Genet* 1997; **101**: 126–9.

31. Van Landeghem GF, Sikström C, Beckman LE *et al*. Transferrin C2, metal binding and Alzheimer's disease. *NeuroReport* 1998; **9**: 177–9.

32. Kennard ML, Feldman H, Yamada T, Jefferies WA. Serum levels of the iron binding protein p97 are elevated in Alzheimer's disease. *Nature Med* 1996; **2**: 1230–5.

33. Hock C, Drasch G, Golombowski S *et al*. Increased blood mercury levels in patients with Alzheimer's disease. *J Neur Transmiss* 1998; **105**: 59–68.

34. Jobst KA, Smith AD, Szatmari M *et al*. Detection in life of confirmed Alzheimer's disease using a simple measurement of medial temporal lobe atrophy by computed tomography. *Lancet* 1992; **340**(8829): 1179–83.

35. Nagy Z, Hindley NJ, Braak H *et al*. The progression of Alzheimer's disease from limbic regions to the neocortex: clinical, radiological and pathological relationships. *Dement Geriat Cogn Disord* 1999; **10**: 115–20.

36. Pearlson GD, Harris GJ, Powers RE *et al*. Quantitative changes in mesial temporal volume, regional cerebral blood flow, and cognition in Alzheimer's disease. *Arch Gen Psychiat* 1992; **49**: 402–8.

37. Jack CR Jr, Petersen RC, Xu YC *et al*. Prediction of AD with MRI-based hippocampal volume in mild cognitive impairment. *Neurology* 1999; **52**: 1397–403.

38. O'Brien JT, Desmond P, Ames D *et al*. Temporal lobe magnetic resonance imaging can differentiate Alzheimer's disease from normal ageing, depression, vascular dementia and other causes of cognitive impairment. *Psychol Med* 1997; **27**: 1267–75.

39. Pantel J, Schroder J, Essig M *et al*. *In vivo* quantification of brain volumes in subcortical vascular dementia and Alzheimer's disease. A MRI-based study. *Dement Geriat Cogn Disord* 1998; **9**: 309–16.

40. Mielke B, Heiss WD. Positron emission tomography for diagnosis of Alzheimer's disease and vascular dementia. *J Neur Transmiss* (Suppl) 1998; **53**: 237–50.

41. Kalaria RN, Ogeng'o JA, Patel NB *et al*. Evaluation of risk factors for Alzheimer's disease in elderly East Africans. *Brain Res Bull* 1997; **44**: 573–7.

45

Clinical Features of Senile Dementia and Alzheimer's Disease

Brice Pitt

St Mary's Hospital, London, UK

Not all dementias in the senium are forms of Alzheimer's disease (AD), neither does AD always arise in the senium. However, the commonest form of senile dementia and of AD is senile dementia of the Alzheimer type (SDAT). In most countries this alone is thought to account for 50–60% of the senile dementias and, in a form mixed with multi-infarct dementia (MID), for another 15–20%[1].

Alois Alzheimer originally described[2] a 51 year-old woman whose morbid jealousy was followed by a rapidly progressing amnesia. She displayed paranoid delusions and, it seemed, auditory hallucinations as well as such cognitive defects as disorientation, incomprehension, perseveration, dysphasia, dysgraphia and dyspraxia. She died only 4.5 years after the onset of her disorder, when Alzheimer was enabled to make the neuropathological observations that later caused his name to be given to the disease. Thus "psychiatric" as well as cognitive symptoms were part of the syndrome from the first. Personality change and behavioural disorder are also part of the condition, especially in those referred to psychiatrists.

Most diagnostic criteria for dementia and AD, e.g. the American Psychiatric Association's *Diagnostic and Statistical Manual*, 3rd edn, Revised[3] and those of the Royal College of Physicians[4], require some degree of disability. The operational diagnostic criteria for dementia in the Cambridge Examination for Mental Disorders of the Elderly[5] include "Progressive failure in performance at work and in the common activities of everyday life—The decline in memory is sufficiently severe to impair functioning in daily life".

Presumably there must be some period of minimal impairment before the disorder becomes disabling, but it is still unclear what are the very earliest features of AD, in its senile or presenile forms. Sufferers tend not to be brought to the notice of the medical or social services until problems arise that jeopardize self-care or strain relationships, when the disease has usually been developing for at least 2 years. Epidemiological surveys using such screening instruments as the Mini-Mental State Examination[6] have, however, identified some people with mild or borderline cognitive impairment, as have the memory clinics which have been developed in recent years[7], and some of these have been shown later to have developed dementia. The distinction between those suffering from Kral's[8] "benign senescent forgetfulness" (BSF) or Crook's[9] "age-associated memory impairment" (AAMI), both of which advance very gradually, if at all, and early AD is not very clear. In a Cambridge field study[10] about half of those with mild memory impairment later developed dementia, but it would have been hard to predict which. Among BSF subjects at the Maudsley Memory Clinic[11], however, there was a tendency for men and those whose forgetfulness was noticed by others subsequently to develop dementia.

ORGANIC DISORDERS

The start of AD is usually manifest in memory impairment:

1. Things are mislaid at home, cannot be found in their once familiar places, or are left behind at home, in shops or in cars, buses and trains.
2. There is an increasing need to check that things have been done and reliance on aides-memoires; even so, appointments and plans are forgotten.
3. The same remarks are made and the same questions asked again and again, and conversation rambles on irrelevantly.
4. Recent information and activities are forgotten and messages are not passed on.
5. The start of a story is forgotten before it is over, so it is difficult to follow plays, films, books or news.
6. New locations, as when on holiday, are not learnt easily, and the patient may get lost.
7. Some things may be done twice over, like feeding an animal or cleaning teeth, and others not at all, like paying bills or taking needed medication for, say, heart-failure or diabetes.

At a later stage:

8. Once-familiar faces and places and locations seem less familiar, and eventually the sufferer may be lost in his/her own neighbourhood or even in his/her own dwelling.
9. The nearest and dearest may not be recognized, and treated as strangers, while true strangers may be greeted warmly as old friends or family.
10. The day, and the time of the day, are forgotten, and the patient may go shopping in the middle of the night, and be unable to find his/her own home on returning.
11. Sometimes the patient no longer knows his/her age or birthday, or that his/her parents are no longer alive, and has indeed entered upon a "second childhood".

Language impairment is usually regarded as a later feature of AD[12]. The sequence of deterioration begins with tasks, such as naming, which use the semantic system, concerned with the meaning of words. There follow deviations and simplifications of syntax (grammar), and then phonemic breakdown (disordered use of sounds)[13]. One study[14] found more deficits on the Boston Naming Test than the Mini-Mental State Examination in early

Principles and Practice of Geriatric Psychiatry, 2nd edn. Edited by J. R. M. Copeland, M. T. Abou-Saleh and D. G. Blazer
©2002 John Wiley & Sons, Ltd

dementia, suggesting that naming difficulties may precede memory failure. Whether the common difficulty in finding proper names experienced by the over-50s[15] is related to the later onset of dementia, or is merely a manifestation of "AAMI", has yet to be determined. Perseveration in AD is much less common than confabulation. Difficulties in understanding, as well as in finding, some words increase during the dementia, until finally there is almost total incomprehension and incoherence. Difficulties in reading and writing may precede those affecting the spoken word.

Loss of intellect is traditionally demonstrated by psychometric tests, which show a greater impairment of "performance" than "verbal" IQ[16]. It is also exposed by difficulty in defining concepts and explaining similarities in the course of cognitive testing. In everyday life it is mainly manifest in illogical thinking and often inconsistencies, e.g. "I live with my mother". "How old is she?" "Oh, in her 80s". "But how old are you?" "I'm 82". "Then you're about the same age as your mother?" "That's right!" There is a failure to draw appropriate deductions from environmental cues: a shopping expedition is undertaken in pitch dark, or, despite the blizzard evident outside the window the season is stated to be summer. A lack of "common sense" contributes to the increasing dependency.

Judgement and creativity are early casualties of dementia, and a good sense of humour may be the first loss. Taste in music, art, reading, clothing and decor may be coarsened, so that the patient wears a garish or incongruous garment, comes back from the shops with a tatty ornament which clashes with the fastidiously appointed living-room, only reads familiar books or gives up *The Times* for a tabloid newspaper. Exploitation by unscrupulous callers, who offer a few pounds for valuable heirlooms, is all too easy. Wills are changed without due regard for those who might have expected to inherit, in favour of some *parvenu* opportunist, causing deep hurt, disappointment and disputation when the patient has died. Judges and physicians become erratic and unreliable and artistic activity ceases or becomes facile, empty and repetitive.

Agnosia contributes, with amnesia, to disorientation. A failure of recognition of faces (prosopagnosia), places and objects bewilders the patient and his/her carers. Apraxia presents as difficulties in dressing—clothes are put on, if at all, in the wrong order, back to front and upside down—and feeding: knife and fork may have to be replaced by a spoon, and the patient may then use his/her hands or lap food from the plate. Apraxia may affect walking, when there is difficulty in judging the height of steps, or a change in the covering or the colour of the floor may be perceived as a step.

A personality change is not inevitable in AD, neither is it always for the worse. Occasionally, those who recognize their limitations and the need for others' help become less dominant and assertive and more docile, mellow and biddable. Commonly, however, as the dementia progresses the range of responses narrows, animation and spontaneity are subdued into apathy and indifference; the unpleasant label "vegetable-like" can apply. Some people become uncharacteristically coarse and disinhibited, swearing and using obscenities. There may be frequent, noisy, seemingly insatiable demands. Irritability, reproaches and angry outbursts can devastate and mystify carers. Regression in dementia facilitates the crude use of mental mechanisms, notably denial and projection: problems are denied or blamed on others. "There's nothing wrong with my memory—why, I can remember years back. It's other people who muddle me up by trying to catch me out. If they'd just leave me alone I'd be all right". A loss of insight, however, is not inevitable in AD, or not until loss of language prevents its expression. Alzheimer's original patient sometimes declared that she could not understand anything, and many sufferers are similarly painfully aware that there is something terribly wrong with their health.

Disordered behaviour is often the most distressing and challenging aspect of progressive AD[17]. Behavioural and psychological symptoms of dementia (BPSD) are strong predictors of caregiver burden and psychiatric morbidity[18]. Some forms arise understandably from personality change and cognitive deficits, while others might be core features of the dementia[19]. Studies based on those patients or clients referred to health and social services are likely to find disordered behaviour more often than in those who manage or are managed without such help at home, although few epidemiological studies assess behaviour as well as cognitive deficits. O'Connor et al.[20] found that among community residents in Cambridge, UK, such disturbed behaviour as demanding attention, repeating questions, using bad language, noisiness, temper outbursts, physical aggression and nocturnal wandering increased with the severity of dementia: 7% of those with mild disorder were aggressive and 42% of the severely demented.

Withdrawal and reclusiveness can have a protective function for those who find that the complexities of their former life are now beyond them. Self-neglect and squalor may be the inevitable consequence of incompetence and lack of help, often because it is refused, although sometimes demented people who live with others are reluctant to wash themselves or to change their clothes when it is time they did. Hoarding and clutter may result because of difficulty in taking the decision to throw rubbish away. Leaving the gas on, carelessness with cookers and inadvertent fire-raising are simple, although dangerous, consequences of forgetfulness and impaired judgement. Verbal abuse and acts of aggression are consistent (although still alarming) with explosive irritability, and the "catastrophic reaction" to exposure of cognitive incompetence in those who robustly deny it makes some sense, both as a form of protest and as a defence. Disinhibition—social, being excessively outspoken, tactless, fulsome or critical, yawning and nodding off during a conversation or a meal and departing from a gathering prematurely and abruptly; minor shoplifting (although this may be partly due to dysmnesia); and, occasionally, sexual disinhibition, taking the form of stripping, exposure, open masturbation and importuning—cause carers and companions various degrees of embarrassment and shame. Noisiness may be associated with boredom, deafness, the desire for attention or depression (see below). Interfering with appliances and destructiveness may be a perverted form of "do-it-yourself"! Strange actions like talking to the reflection in the mirror as if it were another person and to photographs as if they were real people may be partly attributable to prosopagnosia.

Wandering and incontinence, two of the most troublesome behaviour disorders, are often overdetermined. Wandering may arise from utter boredom and underactivity; it is difficult to interest someone who can no longer read or enjoy television or radio and who is discouraged from going out alone for a walk or to the shops, lest they should get lost. Wanderers might have been in the habit of taking a walk with the dog or to buy cigarettes or a paper, at that time of day. They may be seeking their home even if actually at home; it may not be recognized as such, and there is a vain, vague, poorly (if at all) articulated quest for the home where they used to live. Wandering is sometimes a sign of agitated depression (see below) and occasionally a wanderer may be trying to get away from a loaded bowel! Restlessness towards nightfall ("sundowning") and nocturnal roaming[21] by patients who have no idea of the time and are bored as well as restless, are a particular strain on carers[22].

Incontinence of urine may occur for other reasons than dementia—stress incontinence, the frequency of a urinary tract infection, polyuria from diabetes or a prescribed diuretic. The foresight to urinate when the chance arises may have been lost, the location of the lavatory forgotten, or a vaguely similar place (like a cupboard or a storeroom) used in its stead. In advanced dementia the patient may not appear to care any more where he/she excretes; alternatively, cortical control of the bladder may have been lost. Incontinence of faeces may be associated with impaction, compounded by poor hygiene, resulting in soiling and smearing[23].

The psychiatric features of the disease, described first by Alzheimer[2] and reaffirmed recently by Berrios and Brook[24,25] and Burns and colleagues[26–29], include affective disorder, paranoid and other delusional states and hallucinations. The affect in the disease is often blunted or labile, but it is now apparent that, at least among those seen by psychiatrists, depressive symptoms are common—63% of the 178 patients in Burns' series[28] having at least one. Depression was associated with less cognitive impairment, suggesting that it was related to insight. As most demented patients cannot describe how they feel, the Cornell Scale for Depression in Dementia[30] combines observed and informant-based signs of such possible depressive phenomena as diurnal variation, anorexia, insomnia, agitation and retardation and lack of engagement in activities, as well as overt misery.

Paranoid delusions of theft and intruders are a not uncommon reaction to losing things and are an example of projection. Such accusations are grievous to a loyal carer, as are those arising from morbid jealousy. Capgras' syndrome[31], in which it is claimed that a stranger has adopted the appearance of someone well known to the patient, is rare but intriguing. Sixteen per cent of those in Burns' series[26], and 37% of those in Berrios and Brook's[25] were deluded.

Visual hallucinations tend to occur towards nightfall, and often take the form of little people—children, dwarfs or Lilliputians—who have to be fed. This is one reason why demented people may prepare meals for a household of people when only one or two are needed (another being because they have forgotten that their children have grown up and left home, as in Margaret Forster's moving novel *Have the Men Had Enough?*[32]. Sometimes the very small people seem to emanate from a television set, which may act as a hallucinogen[33]. Visual hallucinations are more common when the eyesight is impaired, and may be symptomatic of sub-acute delirium, superimposed on the dementia. Burns[27] found that 13% of his series of patients had visual hallucinations, and 10% auditory, but in clinical practice the latter are of little or no importance.

Finally, there are a number of neurophysical and other disorders associated with AD, including (towards the end of the illness) parkinsonism[34], gait apraxia[35], fits[36] and primitive reflexes[37,38]. Weight loss in AD is particularly interesting, and not solely explicable by inadequate diet because of reluctance or forgetting to eat or to overactivity[39].

The course of AD is one of progressive deterioration from its insidious onset until death, 1–20 years later. Although younger patients live longer, they show the highest excess mortality[40]. Measures of deterioration, like the Global Deterioration Scale[41], rely upon a more uniform progression than is always found. Plateaux, when the clinical disorder seems for a while to be stationary, are not inconsistent with the diagnosis of AD[42]. Early language deficits[43] carry a poor prognosis for survival. Bondareff[44] postulated two forms of the disease: AD1, in older subjects, with a gradual course, mainly affecting memory; and AD2, in younger people, affecting temporoparietal functions and running a relatively rapid course. The two forms are also distinguished by their neuropathology and the pattern of neurobiochemical abnormalities. Death, when sooner or later it comes, is commonly from bronchopneumonia[45], developing in a person who by now is very helpless (often requiring to be fed) and debilitated.

REFERENCES

1. Jorm A, Korten A, Henderson AS. The prevalence of dementia: a quantitative integration of the literature. *Acta Psychiatr Scand* 1987; **76**: 465–79.

2. Alzheimer A. Uber eine eigenartige Erkrankung der Hirnrinde. *Allgem Zeitschr Psychiat* 1907; **64**: 146–8.

3. American Psychiatric Association. *Diagnostic and Statistical Manual of Mental Disorders*, 3rd edn, revised (DSM-III-R). Washington, DC: Division of Public Affairs, APA, 1987.

4. Royal College of Physicians of London (Committee on Geriatrics). Organic mental impairment in the elderly. Implications for research, education and the provision of services. *JR Coll Phys Lond* 1981; **15**: 141–67.

5. Roth M, Huppert F, Tyms E, Mountjoy CQ. *CAMDEX: The Cambridge Examination for Mental Disorders in the Elderly*. Cambridge: Cambridge University Press, 1988.

6. Folstein M, Folstein SE, McHugh PR. "Mini-Mental state". A practical method for grading the cognitive state of patients for the clinician. *J Psychiat Res* 1975; **12**: 189–98.

7. Van den Cammen T, Simpson J, Fraser RM et al. The memory clinic: a new approach to the detection of dementia. *Br J Psychiat* 1987; **150**: 359–64.

8. Kral VA. Senescent forgetfulness: benign or malignant. *Can Med Assoc J* 1962; **86**: 257–60.

9. Crook T, Bartus RT, Ferris SH et al. Age-associated memory impairment: proposed diagnostic criteria and measures of clinical change—report of a National Institute of Mental Health work group. *Dev Neuropsychol* 1986; **235**: 885–90.

10. O'Connor D, Pollitt P, Hyde J et al. The progression of mild idiopathic dementia in a community population. *J Am Geriat Soc* 1991; **39**: 246–51.

11. O'Brien JT, Beats B, Hill K et al. Do subjective memory complaints precede dementia? A 3 year follow-up of patients with supposed "benign senescent forgetfulness". *Int J Geriat Psychiat* 1992; **7**: 481–6.

12. Hart S. Language and dementia—a review. *Psychol Med* 1988; **18**: 99–112.

13. Appell J, Kersetz A, Esman M. A study of language functioning in Alzheimer's patients. *Brain Language* 1982; **17**: 73–91.

14. Stevens S, Pitt B, Nicholl C et al. Language impairment in a memory clinic. *J Geriat Psychiat* 1992; **7**: 45–51.

15. Baddeley A. *Your Memory: A User's Guide*. Harmondsworth: Penguin, 1983.

16. Kendrick DC. Psychological assessment. In Pitt B, ed., *Dementia in Old Age*. Edinburgh: Churchill Livingstone, 1987.

17. Argyle N, Jestice S, Brook CPB. Psychogeriatric patients: their supporters' problems. *Age Ageing* 1985; **14**: 355–60.

18. Ballard C, Lowery K, Powell I et al. Impact of behavioural and psychological symptoms of dementia on caregivers. *Int Psychogeriat* 2000; **12**(suppl 1): 93–105.

19. Cooper JK, Mungas D, Weiler PG. Relation of cognitive status and abnormal behaviors in Alzheimer's disease. *J Am Geriat Soc* 1990; **38**: 867–70.

20. O'Connor DW, Pollitt PA, Roth M et al. Problems reported by relatives in a community study of dementia. *Br J Psychiat* 1990; **156**: 835–41.

21. Lowenstein R. Disturbances of sleep and cognitive functioning in patients with dementia. *J Neurobiol Ageing* 1982; **3**: 371–7.

22. Sanford JRA. Tolerance of debility in elderly dependants by supporters at home: its significance for hospital practice. *Br Med J* 1975; **iii**: 471–3.

23. Begg AH, McDonald C. Scatolia in elderly people with dementia. *Int J Geriat Psychiat* 1989; **4**: 53–4.

24. Berrios G, Brook P. Visual hallucinations and sensory delusions in the elderly. *Br J Psychiat* 1984; **144**: 662–4.

25. Berrios G, Brook P. Delusions and psychopathology of the elderly with cognitive failure. *Acta Psychiat Scand* 1985; **72**: 296–301.

26. Burns A, Jacoby R, Levy R. Psychiatric phenomena in Alzheimer's disease. I: Disorders of thought content. *Br J Psychiat* 1990; **157**: 72–6.

27. Burns A, Jacoby R, Levy R. Psychiatric phenomena in Alzheimer's disease. II: Disorders of perception. *Br J Psychiat* 1990; **157**: 76–81.

28. Burns A, Jacoby R, Levy R. Psychiatric phenomena in Alzheimer's disease. III: Disorders of mood. *Br J Psychiat* 1990; **157**: 81–6.

29. Burns A, Jacoby R, Levy R. Psychiatric phenomena in Alzheimer's disease. IV: Disorders of behaviour. *Br J Psychiat* 1990; **157**: 86–94.

30. Alexopoulos GS, Abrams RC, Young RC, Shamoian CA. Cornell Scale for depression in dementia. *Biol Psychiat* 1988; **23**: 271–84.

31. Enoch MD, Trethowan WH. *Uncommon Psychiatric Syndromes*, 2nd edn. Bristol: Wright, 1979.

32. Forster M. *Have the Men Had Enough?* Bristol: Chatto and Windus, 1989.

33. Rubin EH, Deverts WC, Burke WJ. The nature of psychotic symptoms in senile dementia of the Alzheimer type. *J Geriat Psychiat Neurol* 1988; **1**: 16–20.

34. Pearce J. The extrapyramidal disorder of Alzheimer's disease. *Eur Neurol* 1974; **12**: 94–103.

35. Sjogren T, Sjogren H, Lindgren A. Morbus Alzheimer and morbus Pick: a genetic, clinical and patho-anatomical study. *Acta Psychiat Neurol Scand* 1952; suppl 82.

36. Pearce J, Miller E. *Clinical Aspects of Dementia*. London: Baillière Tindall, 1973.

37. Basarvaju NJ, Silverstone FA, Libow LS, Paraskevas K. Primitive reflexes and perceptual sensory tests in the elderly—their usefulness in dementia. *J Chron Dis* 1981; **34**: 367–77.

38. Burns A, Jacoby R, Levy R. Neurological signs in Alzheimer's disease. *Age Ageing* 1990; **20**: 45–51.

39. Singh S, Mulley G, Losowsky M. Why are Alzheimer's patients thin? *Age Ageing* 1988; **17**: 21–8.

40. Wang HS. The prognosis of Alzheimer's disease. In Katzman R, Terry R, Bick K eds, *Alzheimer's Disease, Senile Dementia and Related Disorders*. New York: Raven, 1978.

41. Reisberg B, Ferris SH, de Leon MJ, Crook T. The global deterioration scale for assessment of primary degenerative dementia. *Am J Psychiat* 1982; **139**: 1136–9.

42. McKhann G, Drachman G, Folstein M *et al.* Clinical diagnosis of Alzheimer's disease: report of the NINCDS–ADRDA Work Group. *Neurology* 1984; **34**: 939–44.

43. Heyman A, Wilkinson W, Hurwitz B *et al.* Early-onset Alzheimer's disease: clinical predictors of institutionalisation and death. *Neurology* 1987; **37**: 980–4.

44. Bondareff W. Age and Alzheimer's disease. *Lancet* 1983; **i**: 1447.

45. Burns A, Jacoby R, Levy R. Cause of death in Alzheimer's disease. *Age Ageing* 1990; **19**: 341–4.

46

Assessment and Management of Behavioural and Psychological Symptoms of Dementia (BPSD)

Rupert McShane[1] and Niall Gormley[2]

[1]Warneford Hospital, Oxford, and [2]Institute of Psychiatry, London, UK

ASSESSMENT

The evaluation of BPSD should include: (a) a clear description of the target behaviour, including its antecedents and consequences ("ABC" behaviour analysis); (b) a search for external (e.g. physical environment, carer behaviour), physical (e.g. pain, delirium) and mental (e.g. psychosis) precipitating factors; and (c) an assessment of the risks posed by this behaviour to the patient, carer or other residents.

One good way to understand how to assess the range of BPSD is to use one of the many scales that have been developed[1,2]. These tend to have a number of features in common. First, the principal carer should be the main source of information about the patient's behaviour. Second, the frequency of the phenomenon in question may be a more useful question than "how severe is the problem?", since the latter is more subjective. Third, the time frame should be specified—usually a month or a week.

The term "agitation" is widely used in research and clinical practice but has been used to denote restlessness or aggression or mood changes, each of which should be individually described when analysing the "agitated" patient. "Psychosis" should similarly be dissected into component phenomena: visual and auditory hallucinations, delusions and misidentifications of various types. The issue of which symptoms tend to co-occur is controversial but important, since such clusters may reflect distinct underlying aetiologies[3].

MANAGEMENT

Until recently, there were few good quality trials of treatments for BPSD. This is in part because such trials are difficult to do. Patients are by definition most unlikely to be able to give consent to participate, "BPSD" are heterogeneous and staff are often reluctant to risk stopping medication, believing that they may be making patients easier to manage[4]. In trials of pharmacological interventions, "escape" or "rescue" medication (usually chloral or lorazepam) is needed. Nevertheless, the recognition of the burden these symptoms place on carers and of their tendency to result in the breakdown of caregiving in the home, coupled with the increasing evidence of harmful effects of conventional neuroleptics, has driven a fast-moving field.

Non-pharmacological Management

I consider the direct treatment by mere medicinal applications to be very limited. A kind and soothing reception, immediate removal of restraints, a warm bath, clean clothing, comfortable food, encouraging words, a medical treatment first directed to any manifest disease... A liberal diet, moderate use of malt liquor, exercise out of doors, employment, recreation, mental occupation, friendly intercourse and judicious religious attentions, are all important auxiliaries to amendment.

John Conolly, who was Medical Superintendent at Hanwell Asylum when he wrote this in 1847, was not writing specifically about dementia. However, there is no doubt that, overall, the management of BPSD requires more attention to psychosocial factors and to physical illness than to psychiatric factors. A variety of general supportive measures and specific behavioural interventions have been used.

General Measures

Dementia therapies. Reality orientation, reminiscence therapy and validation therapy are the best-known examples of therapies developed for use with elderly people. Although these interventions may provide valuable stimulation and foster therapeutic optimism, there is little evidence to suggest that they produce significant or sustained improvements in behaviour problems.

Stimulation-orientated therapies. Inadequate stimulation appears to have a negative impact on cognitively impaired elderly people. Training carers to identify and increase the number of pleasant activities for their dependants improves depressive symptoms[5]. Musical stimulation reduces disruptive vocalization in some patients[6]. For nursing-home residents, therapeutic activity programmes, as well as the physical environment, are important sources of stimulation. Rovner *et al.*[7] found that a programme which included music, exercise and crafts, combined with guidelines on the use of psychotropic medication, reduced the prevalence of behavioural disorders and antipsychotic drug use. In one of the few environmental studies, Cohen-Mansfield and Werner[8] found that simulating a home or natural outdoor environment within a nursing home using visual, auditory and

Principles and Practice of Geriatric Psychiatry, 2nd edn. Edited by J. R. M. Copeland, M. T. Abou-Saleh and D. G. Blazer

olfactory stimuli resulted in a modest reduction in pacing and other agitated behaviours.

Behavioural Interventions

Behavioural models, most commonly based on operant learning theory, have been used to design interventions for specific behavioural problems in dementia. An "ABC" analysis may suggest the implementation of specific behavioural techniques, including: (a) antecedent control—modification of events which trigger disruptive behaviour; (b) extinction—target behaviour is discouraged when it is not rewarded; (c) differential reinforcement of other behaviour (DRO)—the provision of positive reinforcement only for behaviours incompatible with the problem behaviour.

Personal care, for example, is a common antecedent to aggressive behaviour. This may occur because an intrusion into a patient's personal space is misinterpreted as a threat. In such circumstances, careful prompting by the carer, an adequate explanation of the procedure and simple one-step instructions may reduce the perception of threat, and subsequently eliminate or reduce the defensive response. Similarly, if a nursing home resident's only input from staff occurred following verbal outbursts, the staff response might serve to reinforce the behavioural problem. A behavioural analysis would allow staff to modify the antecedent (inactivity), or their own responses, through the use of extinction or DRO.

What is the evidence for the efficacy of behavioural interventions in dementia? Teri *et al.*[9] have found that family carers can learn behavioural management strategies and that these interventions can reduce a wide variety of behavioural problems. In a controlled trial of a comprehensive carer training programme, which focused on behaviour management training and family support, carers' negative reactions to behavioural problems were reduced, even though there was no reduction in the incidence of disruptive behaviours[10]. The majority of studies evaluating behavioural interventions in agitated nursing home residents have reported favourable results, mainly through the use of antecedent control and reinforcement of positive behaviours[11].

However, two larger recent studies failed to find a significant effect of behaviour management programmes[12,13].

Conclusion

Although psychosical interventions have been shown to reduce behavioural disturbances, significant obstacles exist to their widespread implementation. There has been insufficient evaluation of clearly defined strategies targeted at specific behavioural problems. Therapeutic gains, in many cases, persist only for the duration of the intervention. In addition, staff compliance with behavioural strategies is often poor, perhaps unsurprising when their inadequate training and poor working conditions are taken into consideration. The successful implementation of psychosocial interventions in dementia requires the continuing support and training of professional and family caregivers.

Pharmacological Interventions

In this chapter, recent randomized studies are summarized and the effect of different drugs on clinically important measures is compared using "numbers needed to treat" [NNT = 1/(difference in proportion responding to each treatment)]. The lack of a consistently applied definition of "clinically important measures" can limit the validity of such comparisons, particularly when using data from meta-analyses[14]. Nevertheless, NNTs and NNHs (numbers needed to harm) are powerful and simple ways of expressing clinically meaningful information, and are the best statistics available for making comparisons[15]. An NNT of less than 5 on a clinically important variable would usually indicate a drug that clinicians would find very useful.

"Typical" neuroleptics

Three meta-analyses have considered the efficacy of typical neuroleptics. In the first, Schneider[16] showed an 18% difference between placebo and active drug in the proportion of patients responding to drug and placebo, equivalent to an NNT of 5.6. A more detailed presentation of 16 randomized trials since 1966 found an overall NNT for "improvement" on neuroleptics of 3.8 and an NNH of 4.0[17].

Thioridazone. The Cochrane meta-analysis of the effect of thioridazine in dementia[18] found only one large placebo-controlled study that reached inclusion criteria[19]. This was a multicentre study of 610 institutionalized patients in which 4 weeks of thioridazine was compared to placebo and diazepam. Thioridazine improved the "anxiety/tension/fears/insomnia" factor of the Hamilton Anxiety Scale with an NNT of 2.6, and the "cognitive impairment/agitation/depressed mood/behavioural change" factor with an NNT of 3.1. However, the overall conclusion of the Cochrane authors was that, because of the poor quality of reporting of trials: "If thioridazine were not currently in widespread clinical use, there would be inadequate evidence to support its introduction... [It] has minimal or no effect on global ratings, while other drugs such as chlormethiazole are superior to it on behavioural ratings".

Haloperidol. Devanand and colleagues[20] (1999) addressed the question of optimal dosing of haloperidol. This was a study of 71 outpatients with Alzheimer's disease with a mean Mini Mental State Examination (MMSE) of 10. The majority of patients showed both psychosis and disruptive behaviours, so it was not possible to tease out any differential effect on the two classes of disorder. Response rates according to three sets of criteria were greater with the standard dose of 2–3 mg daily (NNT 3.3–4.0) than with low dose (0.5–0.75 mg). A subgroup (20%) of those on 2–3 mg daily developed moderate to severe extrapyramidal signs (NNH = 5), but did not meet consensus criteria for dementia with Lewy bodies. The authors recommend a starting dose of 1 mg/day with upward titration.

Atypical Neuroleptics

Risperidone. The largest good quality trial to date of drug treatment for BPSD has been that of Katz *et al.*[21]. Nursing home residents with dementia were treated for 12 weeks with either 0.5 mg, 1 mg or 2 mg risperidone daily, or placebo (approximately 150 in each arm of the study). Most had severe dementia: the mean MMSE was 6.6. The primary outcome measure was a 50% reduction in the BEHAVE-AD, which occurred in 33% taking placebo, 45% on 1 mg (NNT = 8.3) and 50% on 2 mg (NNT = 5.9). Interestingly, risperidone appeared to have an anti-aggression effect (NNT = 3.4–3.9) that was independent of its effect on psychosis (NNT for delusions 7.1 at 1 mg, 10.0 at 2 mg) or its tendency to cause somnolence. The dropout rate varied from 27% in the placebo group to 42% in the 2 mg group. The NNH for sedation was 11.2 for the 1 mg dose and 5.0 for the 2 mg dose. Extrapyramidalism was more common at 2 mg (NNH = 7.2) than at 1 mg (NNH = 18.5). The optimal dose of risperidone is therefore 1 mg daily.

Olanzapine. Street et al.[22] studied 206 nursing home patients with a mean MMSE of 7.3 in a trial of six weeks of olanzapine or placebo. The main outcome measure was a 50% reduction in the Neuropsychiatric Inventory (NPI) score for a newly defined cluster of symptoms (hallucinations, delusions, agitation). The optimal dose (5 mg) was as effective as typical neuroleptic (NNT = 3.3) but seemed to be associated with relatively high rates of adverse reactions. The response rates (66% on 5 mg, 52% on 10 mg, 43% on 15 mg and 36% on placebo) suggest that doses higher than 5 mg are likely to be suboptimal. Somnolence and gait abnormality were the commonest side effects (NNH = 5.4 and 5.7, respectively) This study illustrates the difficulties that occur in comparing adverse drug reactions (ADRs) across studies, since it is very likely that ADRs were more assiduously sought in this study than earlier studies of typical neuroleptics. The lower dose of 2.5 mg, which is now available—and which one would expect to be associated with fewer ADRs than 5 mg—was not tested.

Carbamazepine. Few trials have published significant differences in responder rates on measures of Global Clinical Impression (CGI). One exception is the study of Tariot et al.[23]. At least minimal improvement on the CGI was apparent in 77% of those taking carbamazepine compared to 22% on placebo (NNT = 1.8). Furthermore, the reduction in the number of cases requiring "a great deal" or "almost constant" extra nursing time to deal with the agitation was 37% in those taking carbamazepine and 8% in those taking placebo (NNT = 3.4). This was a relatively small (ca. 25 subjects in each arm) 6 week study of predominantly female nursing home residents with severe dementia (mean MMSE 6.0), 92% of whom were aggressive. Carbamazepine was started at 100 mg/day. The modal dose reached was 300 mg/day. The NNH for any ADR was 3.3, although these were considered clinically significant in only 2 of 16 cases. The large effect size may have been at least partly attributable to the fact that a non-blind physician adjusted the dose of carbamazepine—a strategy which, of course, parallels the clinical situation, but is not commonly employed in more recent studies.

Trazodone. Trazodone is widely used for BPSD, although there has only been a single small randomized trial of its effectiveness, in which it was shown to be comparable in effect to haloperidol[24]. The CGI was "much improved" or "very much improved" at week 9 in 57% of cases on haloperidol and 71% on trazodone. However, trazodone was associated with fewer side effects (14%, mean dose 218 mg) than haloperidol (50%, mean dose 2.5 mg). Interestingly, post hoc analyses suggested that those who were verbally aggressive or had repeated behaviours or mannerisms were more likely to respond to trazodone. Those who paced, were generally restless or made unwarranted accusations were more likely to respond to haloperidol. This raises the possibility of two syndromes of behavioural change in dementia, one associated with abnormalities of dopaminergic function and one associated with serotonergic dysfunction. The replicated finding that those with depression early in dementia are more likely to go on to be physically aggressive is also consistent with the possibility that there is a distinct serotonergic syndrome of behavioural change in dementia[25,26]. It is not necessary for other signs of depression to be present to justify a trial of an antidepressant for aggressive behaviour.

Xanomeline. Xanomeline is a cholinomimetic with agonist activity at postsynaptic muscarinic M1 and M4 receptors. Bodick et al.[27] presented data from a large (87 in each arm), 6 month study of patients with mild to moderate AD. Three doses of xanomeline were compared with placebo. The dropout rate was high, ranging from 35% in the placebo group to 59% at the highest dose of active drug (NNH = 4.2), precluding its further use in the formulation used. However, there was a dose-related response to xanomeline of hallucinations (NNT = 2.1 at the highest dose) and a variety of other behaviours (e.g. vocal outbursts, delusions and mood swings; NNT = 2.7–6.4).

Rivastigmine. The cholinergic nucleus basalis of Meynert is in double jeopardy in patients with dementia with Lewy bodies (DLB) because it is likely to degenerate as a result of both Lewy body and neurofibrillary change. Cortical cholinergic parameters show even more marked depletion in DLB than in AD. There is now evidence showing that patients with DLB are preferential responders to cholinesterase inhibitors. McKeith et al.[28] conducted a 20 week placebo-controlled study of 3–12 mg rivastigmine in 120 patients with probable or possible DLB of mild to moderate severity. The main outcome measure was a 30% reduction on a newly defined cluster of symptoms derived from the NPI: hallucinations, delusions, depression and apathy. A 30% reduction was chosen because it was comparable to the effect size seen with neuroleptics. The main result was based on the observed case analysis: 63% of those on rivastigmine responded, compared to 30% on placebo (NNT = 3.0). Although there was no overall difference in the number of ADRs (59 vs. 61%), those taking rivastigmine were significantly more likely to drop out (31% vs. 16%; NNH = 7.1). As well as improvements in the pre-defined cluster, there were also marked improvements in a computer test of attention in those on rivastigmine.

These two studies provide good evidence that hallucinations in particular, and possibly other BPSD, respond well to cholinergic agonism.

When to Consider a Trial without Medication

Neuroleptics have unpleasant side effects. Sedation, falls, hip fractures and tardive dyskinesia are common sequelae. Indeed, the prescription of typical, rather than atypical, neuroleptics is likely to be a false economy, particularly if there is any risk that the drug will be taken for more than a brief period. Trials without neuroleptics are a legal requirement in nursing homes in the USA, following the OBRA-1987 regulations. What is the optimal duration of treatment before a trial without medication is indicated?

Since evanescent symptoms do not require long periods of treatment, an important related question is "How often would the symptom normally be expected to resolve without drug treatment within a given time?" Levy et al.[29] assessed 181 outpatients and found that 60–70% of those with agitation or psychosis still had the symptom 3 months later. Persistence was more common amongst those with low MMSE scores (12–17). Devanand et al.[30] in an outpatient study of 235 patients with early AD, found that 74% of those with wandering or agitation had the symptom 6 months later. Comparable figures for other behaviours were: physical aggression 53%, hallucinations 52%, paranoid ideas 45%, misidentification 56%. In a group of 48 patients with autopsy-confirmed AD, Hope et al.[31] found that aggression and hyperactivity were both still present in 75% of cases after 8 months, and hallucinations were still present in 75% of cases at 11 months. All these studies were potentially directly or indirectly confounded by the effect of psychotropics on the natural history of behaviour. Nevertheless, these data suggest that BPSD may endure for up to 8 months in approximately 75% of cases and be evanescent in 25%.

How often will trials without treatment succeed and how often will they fail? Cohen-Mansfield et al.[4] studied the effect of withdrawal of drugs from nursing home residents, many of whom will have had dementia. The doses of haloperidol (mean = 0.9–1.3 mg), thioridazine (25–27 mg) and lorazepam (0.7–0.9 mg) that were being used were within current standards of care. The design was a cross-over study with 6 weeks in the drug or placebo arm. Of 194 residents who were taking regular medication at the start of the study, only 58 (30%) participated, but only 16 (8%) cases were excluded for reasons that potentially related to their behaviour. Thirty-five (60%) completed the study. Dropouts due to emergence of BPSD were not more significantly likely to occur in the withdrawal phase (six cases) than the continuation phase (three cases). After correction for multiple comparisons, BPSD were not more likely to re-emerge following drug withdrawal than with continuation. There was also a slight improvement in cognitive function. At face value, this study suggests that a trial without medication at 6 weeks is indicated. However, the difficulty of sustaining non-pharmacological approaches to the management of BPSD in nursing homes was shown by the fact that, during the 22 weeks following discontinuation of the original drug, less than one-third of cases remained free of psychotropic medication. The mean time until receiving another psychotropic drug was 21 days.

SUMMARY

Old age psychiatrists are often called for advice when psychosocial interventions have been tried and have failed, or the resources of the staff to try such interventions are limited. Careful judgement is needed in these circumstances, since a decision not to prescribe can make a precarious situation worse. Drug treatment can provide a breathing space during which "something" has been seen to be done, as well as having a useful "real" impact in the 75% of cases in which the behaviour persists. The relatively high placebo effect (often 30–40%) can be useful, as long as the maxim 'primum non nocere" is borne in mind. It is important not to leave patients on medication without having a trial of drug withdrawal. Recent demonstrations of the efficacy of atypicals, carbamazepine, antidepressants and cholinomimetics are important evidence that this most neglected area of psychiatry need not be dominated by therapeutic nihilism. Brief programmes of behavioural management are probably only effective briefly, if at all. Continuing support and training are required for successful psychosocial interventions.

REFERENCES

1. Finkel SI. Behavioral and psychological signs and symptoms of dementia: implications for research and treatment. *Int Psychogeriat* 1996; **8**(suppl 3): 501–52.
2. De Deyn PP, Wirshing WC. Scales to assess efficacy and safety of pharmacologic agents in the treatment of behavioral and psychological symptoms of dementia. *J Clin Psychiat* 2001; **62** (suppl 21): 19–22.
3. McShane RH. What are the syndromes of BPSD? *Int Psychogeriat* 2000; **12** (suppl 1): 147–53.
4. Cohen-Mansfield J, Lipson S, Werner P et al. Withdrawal of haloperidol, thioridazine and lorazepam in the nursing home. A controlled, double-blind study. *Arch Int Med* 1999; **159**: 1733–40.
5. Teri L, Logsdon RG, Uomoto J et al. Behavioral treatment of depression in dementia patients: a controlled clinical trial. *J Gerontol* 1997; **52B**: P159–66.
6. Allen-Burge R, Stevens AB, Burgio LD. Effective behavioural interventions for decreasing dementia-related challenging behaviours in nursing homes. *Int J Geriat Psychiat* 1999; **14**: 213–32.
7. Rovner BW, Steele CD, Shmuely Y, Folstein MF. A randomised trial of dementia care in nursing homes. *J Am Geriat Soc* 1996; **44**: 7–13.
8. Cohen-Mansfield J, Werner P. The effects of an enhanced environment on nursing home residents who pace. *Gerontologist* 1998a; **38**: 199–208.

9. Teri L, Logsdon RG, Whall AL et al. Treatment for agitation in dementia patients: a behavioural management approach. *Psychotherapy* 1998; **35**: 436–43.
10. Ostwald SK, Hepburn KW, Caron W et al. Reducing caregiver burden: a randomized psychoeducational intervention for caregivers of persons with dementia. *Gerontologist* 1999; **39**: 299–309.
11. Landreville P, Bordes M, Dicaire L, Verreault R. Behavioural approaches for reducing agitation in residents of long-term care facilities. *Int Psychogeriat* 1998; **10**: 397–419.
12. Gormley N, Lyons D, Howard R. Behavioral management of aggression in dementia: a randomized controlled trial. *Age and Ageing* 2001; **30**: 141–145.
13. Teri L, Logsdon RG, Peskind E et al. Treatment of agitation in AD. A randomized placebo-controlled clinical trial. *Neurology* 2000; **55**: 1271–8.
14. Smeeth L, Haines A, Ebrahim S. Numbers needed to treat derived from meta-analyses—sometimes informative, usually misleading. *Br Med J* 1999; **318**: 1548–51.
15. Moore A, McQuay H. NNT is a tool, to be used appropriately (letter). *Br Med J* 1999; **319**: 1200.
16. Schneider L, Pollock VE, Lyness SA. A meta analysis of controlled trials of neuroleptic treatment in dementia. *J Am Geri Soc* 1990; **38**: 553–63.
17. Lanctot KL, Best TS, Mittmann N et al. Efficacy and safety of neuroleptics in behavioral disorders associated with dementia. *J Clin Psychiat* 1998; **59**: 550–61.
18. Kirchner V, Kelly CA, Harvey RJ. Thioridazine for dementia (Cochrane Review). In *The Cochrane Library*, Issue 4. Oxford; Update Software, 1999.
19. Stotsky B. Multicenter study comparing thioridazine with diazepam and placebo in elderly, non-psychotic patients with emotional and behavioral disorders. *Clin Therapeut* 1984; **6**: 546–59.
20. Devanand DP, Marder K, Michaels KS et al. A randomised, placebo-controlled dose-comparison trial of haloperidol for psychosis and disruptive behaviors in Alzheimer's disease. *Am J Psychiat* 1998; **155**: 1512–20.
21. Katz IR, Jeste DV, Mintzer JE et al. Comparison of risperidone and placebo for psychosis and behavioral disturbances associated with dementia: a randomised, double-blind trial. *J Clin Psychiat* 1999; **60**: 107–15.
22. Street JS, Clark S, Gannon KS et al. Olanzapine treatment of psychotic and behavioral symptoms in patients with Alzheimer's disease in Nursing Care Facilities *Arch Gen Psychiat* 2000; **57**: 968–76.
23. Tariot PN, Erb R, Podgorski CA et al. Efficacy and tolerability of carbamazepine for agitation and aggression in dementia. *Am J Psychiat* 1998; **155**: 54–61.
24. Sultzer DL, Gray KF, Gunay T et al. A double blind comparison of tazodone and haloperidol for the treatment of agitation in patients with dementia. *Am J Geriatr Psychiat* 1997; **5**: 60–9.
25. McShane RH, Keene J, Fairburn C et al. Psychiatric symptoms in patients with dementia predict the later development of behavioural abnormalities. *Psychol Med* 1998; **28**: 1119–27.
26. Cohen-Mansfield J, Werner P. Predictors of aggressive behaviors: a longitudinal study in senior day care centers. *J Gerontol Psychol Sci* 1998b; **53B**(5): P300–10.
27. Bodick NC, Offen WW, Levey A et al. Effects of Xanomeline, selective muscarinic receptor agonist, on cognitive function and behavioral symptoms in Alzheimer's disease. *Arch Neurol* 1997; **54**: 465–73.
28. McKeith I, Del Ser T, Spano P et al. Efficacy of Rinastigmine in dementia with Lewy bodies: a randomised, double blind, placebo-controlled international study. *Lancet* 2000; **356**: 2031–6.
29. Levy ML, Cummings JL, Fairbanks LA. Longitudinal assessmennt of symptoms of depression, agitation and psychosis in 181 patients with Alzheimer's disease. *Am J Psychiat* 1996; **153**: 1438–43.
30. Davanand DP, Jacobs DM, Tang MX et al. The course of psychopathologic features in mild to moderate Alzheimer's disease. *Arch Gen Psychiat* 1997; **54**: 257–63.
31. Hope T, Keene J, Fairburn et al. Natural history of behavioral changes and psychiatric symptoms in Alzheimer's disease. *Br J Psychiat* 1999; **194**: 39–44.

Eating Disorders in Alzheimer's Disease

Paul E. Cullen[1] and Clive Ballard[2]

[1]*Bushey Fields Hospital, Dudley, and* [2]*Newcastle upon Tyne General Hospital, UK*

Eating disorders are a recognized feature of dementia, which include a preference for sweet foods (11%), increased (21%) or decreased (22%) consumption and eating non-food substances (3%) and are particularly common in Alzheimer's disease (AD)[1]. Clinical[1] and subclinical[3] swallowing problems, general dental health and oropharyngooesophageal function are all important. The basic necessity of eating to maintain health, the frustration that disordered eating causes to caregivers and the increased risk of institutionalization and death all make this an important topic[4].

A number of rating scales to evaluate psychopathology in dementia now include an eating disorder subcategory (e.g. Neuropsychiatric Inventory), whilst other scales have been developed specifically to assess eating disorders in AD[5].

Several neurotransmitters have been linked to eating disorders in AD. Reduced neuropetide Y and norepinephrine are associated with anorexia, whilst the action of galanin in the hypothalamus is thought to increase fat intake and impact upon cholinergic hippocampal systems.

Studies have shown associations between specific brain changes and eating disorders in AD, e.g. hyperorality with widening of the third ventricle and frontal and occipital lobe atrophy, Klüver–Bucy syndrome features with temporal lobe atrophy[14] and low body weight with temporal cortical atrophy[6]. Hyperphagia may be associated with increased calorific need in patients with motor restlessness, whilst younger people with more severe dementia who are not restless may over-eat because they respond to any food stimulus, possibly as a manifestation of frontal lobe pathology[7]. The European Commission has focused upon weight loss in AD[4].

In practice there is little evidence to inform the management of these problems. The best approaches generally involve common sense and clinical judgement. The most frequent clinically significant problems relate to poor appetite and weight loss. A first step is to assess and treat underlying disorders. This may vary from assessment of oral health to the pharmacological treatment of a concurrent depression. Educating care staff and informal carers about some of the changes in food preference and encouraging flexibility with the content and timing of an individual's diet is often an effective remedy[8–10].

Giving a diet with a higher proportion of sweet foods, such as desserts, chocolate, cakes and biscuits, is a pragmatic approach. This is helpful as it takes pressure off carers to produce a strictly balanced diet of cooked dinners, which eases the stress of mealtimes. Other types of difficulty are less frequent, and are probably best treated after a detailed individual evaluation, using techniques such as an Antecedent–Behaviour–Consequence ("ABC") diary. Work pertaining to ideational apraxia[11] and attribution theory[12] has contributed to the management of these problems. The management of eating disorders in AD raises important ethical issues[13].

REFERENCES

1. Cullen P, Abid F, Patel A *et al*. Eating disorders in dementia. *Int J Geriat Psychiat* **12**, 559–62.
2. Horner J, Alberts MJ, Dawson DV, Cook GM. Swallowing in Alzheimer's disease. *Alzheimer Dis Assoc Disord* 1994; **8**, 177–89.
3. Feinberg MJ, Ekberg O, Segall L, Tully J. Deglutition in elderly patients with dementia: findings of videofluorographic evaluation and impact on staging and management. *Radiology* **183**, 811–14.
4. Riviere S, Lauque S, Micas M *et al*. European Programme: Nutrition, Alzheimer's Disease and Health Promotion. *Rev Geriat* 1999; **24**, 121–6.
5. Tully MW, Matrakas KL, Muir J, Musallam K. The Eating Behaviour Scale. A simple method of assessing functional ability in patients with Alzheimer's disease. *J Gerontol Nursing* 1997; **23**, 9–15
6. Grundman M, Corey-Bloom J, Jernigan T *et al*. Low body weight in Alzheimer's disease is associated with mesial temporal cortex atrophy. *Neurology* 1996; **46**: 1585–91.
7. Smith G, Vigen V, Evans J *et al*. Patterns and associates of hyperphagia in patients with dementia. *Neuropsychiat Neuropsychol Behav Neurol* 1998; **11**: 97–102.
8. Boylston E, Ryan C, Brown C and Westfall B. Preventing precipitous weight loss in demented patients by altering food texture. *J Nut Elderly* **15**, 43–8.
9. Soltesz KS, Dayton JH. Finger foods help those with Alzheimer's maintain weight. *J Am Dietet Assoc* 1993; **93**, 1106–8.
10. Suski NS, Nielsen CC. Factors affecting food intake of women with Alzheimer's type dementia in long-term care. *J Am Dietet Assoc* 1989; **89**, 1770–3.
11. LeClerc CM, Wells DL. Use of content methodology process to enhance feeding abilities threatened by ideational apraxia in people with Alzheimer's-type dementia. *Geriat Nursing* 1998; **19**: 261–7.
12. Fopma-Loy J, Austin JK. Application of an attribution–affect–action model of care-giving behaviour. *Arch Psychiat Nursing* **11**, 210–17.
13. Clibbens R. Eating, ethics and Alzheimer's. *Nursing Times* 1996; **92**, 29–30.
14. Burns A, Jacoby R, Levy R. Psychiatric phenomena in Alzheimer's disease. *Br J Psychiat* 1990; **157**, 86–94.

47

Pathology of Vascular Dementia

J. M. MacKenzie

Grampian University Hospitals NHS Trust, Aberdeen, UK

Cerebrovascular disease is usually considered to be the second commonest cause of dementia, although the precise prevalence and the frequency of combination with Alzheimer's disease (AD) is very variable. In the West, approximately 15% of autopsy-studied cases of dementia have been attributed to vascular disease alone and 8–18% to a combination of vascular disease and AD[1,2]. However, this has been challenged in a recent autopsy study of patients in a dementia clinic, where dementia could not be attributed in any case to vascular disease alone[3]. Vascular dementia is commoner in the Far East than in the West and still remains the commonest form of dementia in Japan[4]. In the West, it may also be commoner than AD in the very elderly[5]. Estimates based on death certification and clinical diagnosis without pathological confirmation are liable to be significantly inaccurate[6,7].

If it is difficult to determine how frequent vascular dementia is, it is also difficult to define what it is. For example, the terms "arteriosclerotic" and "multi-infarct" dementia are often used synonymously and these, together with a lacunar state and Binswanger's disease, have been grouped together[8]. In practice, three separate forms of vascular dementia can be identified, although there is often overlap between these: multi-infarct dementia; dementia due to single strategically-placed infarcts; and dementia due to diffuse white matter damage[9].

MULTI-INFARCT DEMENTIA

Multiple areas of infarction involving both cortical and sub-cortical locations, separated in both time and space, may be associated with dementia, although in its pure form this is probably uncommon[10]. The location of the infarcts is probably more important than the volume of tissue lost (100 ml is the oft-quoted figure)[1,11]. Dementia may occur with relatively little tissue loss, particularly if infarcts are strategically located (see below) and the effect of subsequent infarcts may be synergistic rather than additive[12].

Multiple small infarcts of deep white matter or grey structures ("lacunar state") may also be associated with dementia, although this often overlaps with dementia due to diffuse white matter damage[13]. Patients with a pure lacunar syndrome show features of a subcortical dementia—psychomotor slowing, poor concentration, indecision and apathy—without features of cortical dysfunction[9]. Hypertension is the most important risk factor for dementia of this kind and that is particularly true for dementia due to multiple lacunar infarcts[13,14].

DEMENTIA DUE TO SINGLE STRATEGICALLY PLACED INFARCTS

Dementia may result from single infarcts involving certain areas of the brain, such as the angular gyrus of the dominant parietal lobe, the medial thalamic nuclei and head of the caudate nucleus, especially if bilateral, the globus pallidus, basal forebrain and hippocampus[9,15]. The cognitive effects of infarction of the angular gyrus may closely resemble AD, although the sudden onset of the cognitive deficit may point to the correct diagnosis[16].

DEMENTIA DUE TO DIFFUSE WHITE MATTER DAMAGE

Whilst white matter damage due to multiple infarcts may be the substrate of dementia, there are also forms of more diffuse white matter damage due to small-vessel disease which result in dementia, and these are probably commoner than dementia due to single or multiple infarcts[17].

Binswanger's disease is considered to be a well-established clinicopathological entity: ischaemic periventricular leuko-encephalopathy manifested clinically by subcortical frontal executive dysfunction, parkinsonism, urinary incontinence, mood changes and pseudobulbar palsy[18]. However, it is still the subject of considerable controversy regarding both its frequency[19] and its relationship with the radiological entity of "leuko-araiosis"—the appearance of low attenuation areas in the white matter on CT scanning[20]. CT abnormalities are common in the elderly and may not be associated with dementia[21,22] and the clinical significance of leukoaraiosis remains incompletely defined[23]. It certainly does not equate to Binswanger's disease, despite suggestions to the contrary[24].

A review of the pathological features of all the reported cases of Binswanger's disease in the world literature, 1912–1986, together with Fisher's review, reveals that the vast majority of cases designated as Binswanger's disease show consistent pathological changes[25,26]. The general autopsy shows evidence of prolonged systemic hypertension. The brain is of average weight but there is diffuse dilatation of the lateral and third ventricles, with rarefaction, discoloration and a rubbery texture of the peri-ventricular white matter, particularly in the occipital regions. The arteries of the Circle of Willis are affected by atheroma, which in 60% of cases is severe. Lacunar infarcts are usually present but one-third of brains also contain large infarcts. Microscopically, there is incomplete diffuse demyelination, with gliosis and microinfarcts affecting the periventricular white matter but sparing the subcortical fibres, corpus callosum, anterior commissure and internal capsules. The walls of white matter penetrating arteries are hyalinized but the vessels are patent. This condition is probably caused by hypoxic–ischaemic damage to the distal watershed periventricular white matter, secondary to narrowing of arterioles[23,27,28].

A closely related cause of dementia due to diffuse white matter damage is CADASIL (cerebral autosomal dominant arteriopathy with subcortical infarcts and leukoencephalopathy)[29]. This is a disease that usually presents in the fifth decade with strokes or dementia, and is an inherited vascular disorder due to mutation affecting the *Notch3* gene on chromosome 19. Pathologically, the disease is very similar to Binswanger's disease, with widespread lacunar infarcts and diffuse cerebral white matter degeneration. The distinguishing feature is the presence of non-hypertensive arteriolosclerosis, characterized by deposition of granular osmiophilic material in relation to vascular smooth muscle cells, with degeneration of these cells and thickening of the vessel walls. This is a systemic vascular disorder, although other tissues are less severely affected than the brain, and the diagnosis is therefore possible on skin or muscle biopsy, although genetic analysis is required for confirmation[30].

In the experience of the author, vascular dementia is much less common than AD. However, it is given a significance disproportionate to its incidence by the fact that some causes of vascular dementia—such as giant-cell arteritis[31] and thromboangiitis obliterans[32]—are potentially treatable, and that vascular dementia as a whole is theoretically preventable by addressing risk factors for cerebrovascular disease[33].

REFERENCES

1. Tomlinson BE, Blessed G, Roth M. Observations on the brains of demented old people. *J Neurol Sci* 1970; **11**: 205–42.
2. Jellinger K, Danielczyk W, Fischer P, Gabriel E. Clinicopathological analysis of dementia disorders in the elderly. *J Neurol Sci* 1990; **95**: 239–58.
3. Nolan KA, Lino MM, Seligmann AW, Blass JP. Absence of vascular dementia in an autopsy series from a dementia clinic. *J Am Geriat Soc* 1998; **46**: 597–604.
4. Seno H, Ishino H, Inagaki T et al. A neuropathological study of dementia in nursing homes over a 17 year period in Shimane Prefecture, Japan. *Gerontology* 1999; **45**: 44–8.
5. Skoog I, Nilsson L, Palmertz B. A population-based study of dementia in 85 year-olds. *N Engl J Med* 1993; **328**: 153–8.
6. Alafuzoff I. The pathology of dementias: an overview. *Acta Neurol Scand* 1992; (suppl 139): 8–15.
7. Thomas BM, Starr JM, Whalley LJ. Death certification in treated cases of presenile Alzheimer's disease and vascular dementia in Scotland. *Age Ageing* 1997; **26**: 401–6.
8. Hershey LA. Dementia associated with stroke. *Stroke* 1990; **21** (suppl II): 9–11.
9. Amar K, Wilcock G. Vascular dementia. *Br Med J* 1996; **312**: 227–31.
10. Hulette C, Nochlin D, McKeel D et al. Clinical–neuropathologic findings in multi-infarct dementia: a report of six autopsied cases. *Neurology* 1997; **48**: 668–72.
11. del Ser T, Bermejo F, Portera A et al. Vascular dementia. A clinicopathological study. *J Neurol Sci* 1990; **96**: 1–17.
12. Wolfe N, Babikian VL, Linn RT. Are multiple cerebral infarcts synergistic? *Arch Neurol* 1994; **51**: 211–15.
13. Loeb C. Dementia due to lacunar infarctions: a misnomer or a clinical entity? *Eur Neurol* 1995; **35**: 187–92.
14. Forette F, Boller F. Hypertension and the risk of dementia in the elderly. *Am J Med* 1991; **90**: 14–19S.
15. Garcia JH, Brown GG. Vascular dementia: neuropathologic alterations and metabolic brain changes. *J Neurol Sci* 1992; **109**: 121–31.
16. Benson FD, Cummings JL, Tsai SY. Angular gyrus syndrome simulating Alzheimer's disease. *Arch Neurol* 1982; **39**: 616–20.
17. Esiri MM, Wilcock GK, Morris JH. Neuropathological assessment of the lesions of significance in vascular dementia. *J Neurol Neurosurg Psychiat* 1997; **63**: 749–53.
18. Roman GC. New insight into Binswanger's disease. *Arch Neurol* 1999; **56**: 1061–2.
19. Bogousslavsky J. Binswanger's disease: does it exist? *Cerebrovasc Dis* 1996; **6**: 255–63.
20. Hachinski VC, Potter P, Merskey H. Leukoaraiosis. *Arch Neurol* 1987; **44**: 21–3.
21. Ferrer I, Bella R, Serrano MT et al. Arteriosclerotic leucoencephalopathy in the elderly and its relation to white matter lesions in Binswanger's disease, multi-infarct encephalopathy and Alzheimer's disease. *J Neurol Sci* 1990; **98**: 37–50.
22. Meyer JS, Kawamura J, Terayama Y. White matter lesions in the elderly. *J Neurol Sci* 1992; **110**: 1–7.
23. Pantoni L, Garcia JH. The significance of cerebral white matter abnormalities 100 years after Binswanger's report. A review. *Stroke* 1995; **26**: 1293–301.
24. van Gijn J. Leukoaraiosis and vascular dementia. *Neurology* 1998; **51** (suppl 3): S3–8.
25. Babikian V, Ropper AH. Binswanger's disease: a review. *Stroke* 1987; **18**: 2–12.
26. Fisher CM. Binswanger's encephalopathy: a review. *J Neurol* 1989; **236**: 65–79.
27. Pantoni L, Garcia JH. Cognitive impairment and cellular/vascular changes in the cerebral white matter. *Ann N Y Acad Sci* 1997; **826**: 92–102.
28. van Swieten JC, van den Hout JHW, van Ketel BA et al. Periventricular lesions in the white matter on magnetic resonance imaging in the elderly: a morphometric correlation with arteriosclerosis and dilated perivascular spaces. *Brain* 1991; **114**: 761–71.
29. Ruchoix M-M, Maurage C-A. CADASIL: cerebral autosomal dominant arteriopathy with subcortical infarcts and leukoencephalopathy. *J Neuropathol Exp Neurol* 1997; **56**: 947–64.
30. Schultz A, Santoianni R, Hewan-Lowe K. Vasculopathic changes of CADASIL can be focal in skin biopsies. *Ultrastruct Pathol* 1999; **23**: 241–7.
31. Caselli RJ. Giant cell (temporal) arteritis. A treatable cause of multi-infarct dementia. *Neurology* 1990; **40**: 753–5.
32. Larner AJ, Kidd D, Elkington P et al. Spatz–Lindenberg disease: a rare cause of vascular dementia. *Stroke* 1999; **30**: 687–9.
33. Hachinski V. Preventable senility: a call for action against the vascular dementias. *Lancet* 1992; **340**: 645–8.

International Criteria for Vascular Dementia and Their Problems: ICD-10, DSM-IV, ADDTC and NINDS-AIREN

John V. Bowler[1] and V. Hachinski[2]

[1]Royal Free Hospital, London, UK and [2]University of Western Ontario, London, Canada

There are two sets of criteria currently available for the diagnosis of vascular dementia. The *Diagnostic and Statistical Manual of Mental Disorders*, 4th edn (DSM-IV)[1] and the *Classification of Mental and Behavioural Disorders*, 10th Revision (ICD-10)[2] are general diagnostic tools and outline the criteria but do not operationalize them. The second set, the State of California Alzheimer's Disease Diagnostic and Treatment Centers[3] and the National Institute of Neurological Disorders and Stroke and the Association Internationale pour la Recherche at L'Enseignement en Neurosciences (NINDS–AIREN)[4] criteria, are developments of the first two and offer operational criteria.

There are three fundamental flaws and several lesser errors lying in the details of these criteria. All the criteria are fundamentally similar in that they first require the presence of dementia, which is based on Alzheimer's disease (AD)-type features, and subsequently identify vascular dementia as a subset of all dementia, using vascular features that are often operationalized using the ischaemic score[5].

Unfortunately, the use of Alzheimer-based criteria for the diagnosis of dementia has now been clearly shown to be wrong. Vascular dementia does not closely resemble AD, even when Alzheimer-based criteria have been used for case identification[6]. Thus, cases selected using current criteria represent only a subset of all vascular dementia. This is the first major flaw in the current criteria.

The second problem is the increasing recognition of mixed dementia. Originally, vascular dementia and AD were separated by the presence of large infarct volumes[7]. In the nun study, in which 47% of demented patients had mixed disease, very small amounts of cerebrovascular disease profoundly altered the age of presentation and speed of progression of what otherwise appeared to be AD[8]. Reclassification of autopsy data to allow small infarct volumes to convert a diagnosis of AD to mixed dementia increased the proportion of cases with mixed dementia from 2% to 18%[9]. Thus, mixed dementia is far more important than was realized when the current criteria, which scarcely recognize mixed disease, were prepared. No good method yet exists for separating mixed dementia. Criteria that first select cases that appear like AD and then subselect those with vascular features might form an excellent basis for doing so; unfortunately, this is what the current criteria for vascular dementia do and it is very likely that much of the reported data about vascular dementia is in fact about mixed disease.

The next fault is the level of severity. The criteria define dementia as the level of cognitive impairment at which normal daily functions are impaired, and therefore will identify only late cases, underestimating the prevalence of cognitive impairment due to vascular disease. More importantly, they prevent identification of early cases that would benefit most from preventative treatment[14]. This important early stage has been termed "vascular cognitive impairment" (VCI)[10]. VCI is important because vascular disease is the largest single identifiable risk factor for dementia apart from age, and the only one currently treatable.

The above features constitute the fundamental faults of the current criteria. There are a number of additional problems that lie in their details. Differences in the details lead to great differences in the proportion of cases identified as having vascular dementia[3].

Correction of these faults requires wholesale revision of the criteria with the development of new criteria based on data rather than supposition[11–13].

REFERENCES

1. American Psychiatric Association. *Diagnostic and Statistical Manual of Mental Disorders*, 4th edn. Washington, DC: American Psychiatric Association, 1994.
2. World Health Organization. *The ICD-10 Classification of Mental and Behavioural Disorders. Diagnostic Criteria for Research*. Geneva: World Health Organization, 1993.
3. Chui HC, Victoroff JI, Margolin D *et al*. Criteria for the diagnosis of ischemic vascular dementia proposed by the State of California Alzheimer's Disease Diagnostic and Treatment Centers. *Neurology* 1992; **42**: 473–80.
4. Roman GC, Tatemichi TK, Erkinjuntti T *et al*. Vascular dementia: diagnostic criteria for research studies. Report of the NINDS–AIREN international workshop. *Neurology* 1993; **43**: 250–60.
5. Hachinski VC, Iliff LD, Zilkha E *et al*. Cerebral blood flow in dementia. *Arch Neurol* 1975; **32**: 632–7.
6. Bowler JV, Hachinski VC. Vascular dementia. In Feinberg TE, Farah M, eds, *Behavioral Neurology and Neuropsychology*. New York: McGraw-Hill, 1997, 589–603.
7. Tomlinson BE, Blessed G, Roth M. Observations on the brains of demented old people. *J Neurol Sci* 1970; **11**: 205–42.
8. Snowdon DA, Greiner LH, Mortimer JA *et al*. Brain infarction and the clinical expression of Alzheimer disease. The nun study. *J Am Med Assoc* 1997; **227**: 813–17.
9. Bowler JV, Munoz DG, Merskey H, Hachinski VC. Fallacies in the pathological confirmation of the diagnosis of Alzheimer's disease. *J Neurol Neurosurg Psychiat* 1998; **64**: 18–24.
10. Hachinski VC, Bowler J. Vascular dementia. *Neurology* 1993; **43**: 2159–60.
11. Bowler JV, Hachinski V. Criteria for vascular dementia: replacing dogma with data. *Arch Neurol* (2000b, in press).
12. Bowler JV. Vascular dementia: changing concepts and criteria. *Stroke Rev* (2000a, in press).
13. Chui HC, Mack W, Jackson JE *et al*. Clinical criteria for the diagnosis of vascular dementia: a multicenter study of comparability and inter-rater reliability. *Arch Neurol* 2000; **57**: 191–6.
14. Hachinski VC. Preventable senility: a call for action against the vascular dementias. *Lancet* 1992; **340**: 645–7.

48

Vascular Dementia

Peter Humphrey

Walton Centre for Neurology and Neurosurgery, Liverpool UK

EPIDEMIOLOGY

For many years, dementia was thought to be due to vascular disease. This seemed logical, largely on the basis that atherosclerosis and dementia are common in the elderly. In the 1970s and 1980s, many papers appeared stressing that vascular dementia was over-diagnosed[1], and most came to the conclusion that Alzheimer's disease (AD) was the commonest cause of dementia, even in patients who had had a stroke. In recent years the pendulum has swung a little back towards vascular disease being a more significant cause. Furthermore, the clear margins between some types of vascular dementia and AD have become blurred. Indeed, brain infarction may play an important part in determining the expression of the clinical symptoms of AD[2].

The epidemiology of vascular dementia is fraught with difficulties because of the lack of a reliable definition to act as a gold standard. Many groups have come to a different consensus about the criteria for the diagnosis (e.g. DSM-IV, ADDTC, NINDS–AIREN, ICD-10 and Hachinski score) Not only is the clinical diagnosis ambiguous, partly because many patients have mixed dementia (i.e. both AD and vascular disease), but the pathological differentiation of the varying types of dementia is also blurred. Does one then use clinical series, preferably community-based, or autopsy series? Reliable data are very sparse. Referral bias remains a major problem in hospital based series. In a community-based study in those aged over 85 from the USA, dementia was found in 30%[3]. In Europe and the USA, vascular disease accounts for 10–40% of all cases of dementia, whereas in Japan vascular disease is more common than AD; the lifetime risk of developing vascular dementia is approximately 25%[4-6]. Pathological studies suggest that cases of mixed AD and vascular dementia may be as common as those with just vascular dementia.

Equally good reasons can be made for thinking that vascular dementia remains both underdiagnosed and overdiagnosed[7,8]. Dementia is common following stroke occurring in approximately 16% after the first stroke[9].

RISK FACTORS

The risk factors for vascular dementia have rarely been studied in isolation to stroke. The major risk factors are age, race, hypertension, diabetes mellitus, hyperlipidaemia, smoking, transient ischaemic attack and heart disease, especially ischaemic heart disease and atrial fibrillation[10]. The level of education, volume of cerebral loss, degree of cerebral atrophy and presence of periventricular white matter lesions are important in the development of dementia[11]. Other possible risk factors include polycythaemia, homocysteinuria, hyperfibrinogenaemia, alcohol excess and lack of physical exercise.

Most of these risk factors predispose to the atherosclerotic process in all its many guises (e.g. large vessel atherosclerosis, small vessel lacunae and white matter leukoaraiosis). However, there are a number of other causes for vascular dementia which are worthy of separate mention. In the last 10 years our understanding that genetic factors can predispose to vascular disease have gained increasing importance, with the detailed understanding of the families with cerebral autosomal dominant arteriopathy with subcortical infarcts and leukoencephalopathy (CADASIL), mitochondrial diseases and hereditary cerebral haemorrhage with amyloid[12-14]. CADASIL has been shown to be linked to chromosome 19: individuals are predisposed to migraine, vascular events and dementia[12]. The genetics of mitochondrial encephalomyopathy with lactic acid and stroke-like episodes (MELAS) is of interest; only men are affected, with the disease being transmitted only by the maternal line. The clinical features include stroke-like episodes, lactic acidosis, short stature and deafness[13]. The diagnosis is confirmed by DNA analysis to look for point mutations in the RNA gene. Other rare causes of multi-infarct dementia and stroke include the antiphospholipid syndrome[15,16], arteritis[17] and late effects of cranial radiotherapy, amongst others[18-20].

CLINICAL TYPES

The pathological findings in vascular dementia are diverse. Findings range from large cortical infarctions (Figure 48.1) to small discrete deep infarcts (Figure 48.2) and to diffuse areas of white matter low-attenuation changes as seen on CT scan (Figure 48.3). Several of these changes may co-exist in the same patient (Figure 48.4).

Cortical Infarcts

Multiple cortical thrombo-embolic infarcts are a common cause of multi-infarct dementia. This will follow embolic occlusions from either the heart or the great vessels, primarily in the neck, e.g. carotid stenosis, or primary thrombosis in the major cortical arteries of the cerebral hemispheres, e.g. antiphospholipid syndrome[15,16] and arteritis[17]. Dementia may rarely result from multiple watershed infarcts in the territories between the middle and posterior cerebral arteries in the cortex: hypotension is the usual cause secondary to prolonged cardiac arrest.

Principles and Practice of Geriatric Psychiatry, 2nd edn. Edited by J. R. M. Copeland, M. T. Abou-Saleh and D. G. Blazer

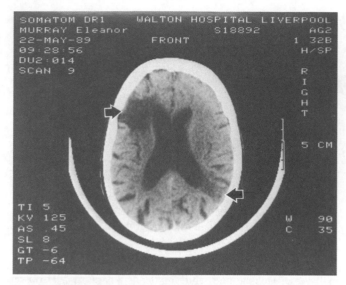

Figure 48.1 Multiple cortical infarcts

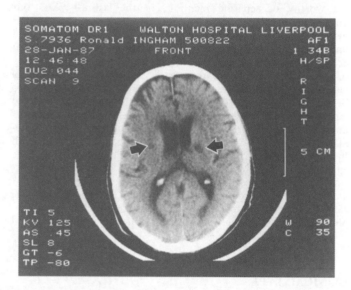

Figure 48.2 Multiple lacunae

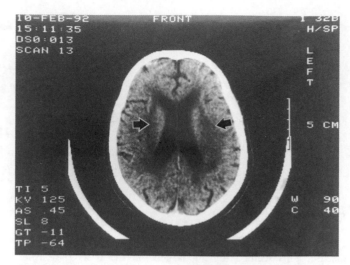

Figure 48.3 Leukoaraiosis

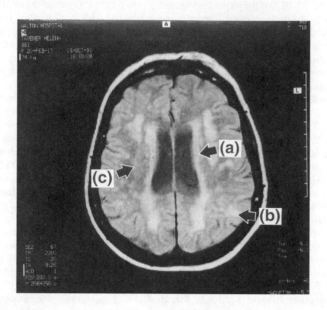

Figure 48.4 Cortical infarcts, lacunae and leukoaraiosis coexisting in the same patient

A strategic single cortical infarct in the dominant angular gyrus can also cause a picture similar to AD with dysphasia, visuospatial disorientation, agoraphobia and memory loss. Multiple cerebral haemorrhage, which particularly occurs in cerebral amyloid, may cause dementia.

Lacunar Infarction

Lacunae are small deep sub-cortical infarcts or haemorrhages. A single lacunar stroke commonly presents with pure motor hemiplegia, pure hemisensory loss or ataxic hemiparesis[21]. Multiple lacunae (état lacunaire) was described by Marie to produce dementia, dysarthria, small-stepping gait, incontinence and emotional lability. Fisher doubted the existence of a multi-lacunar dementia, although there is now no doubt that vascular dementia does occur after multiple lacunar infarcts[22,23]. Lacunar infarcts are common in hypertension and rarely follow embolic occlusion from the heart or major arteries.

While multi-infarct dementia is nearly always secondary to multiple lesions, it is possible to see memory loss after a single infarct. Discrete thalamic infarction especially in the paramedian region, may present as memory loss, often associated with somnolence and eye movement disorders[24,25].

Leukoaraiosis

This is largely a radiological diagnosis describing the diffuse or patchy low-attenuation changes seen on CT or MRI scans in the deep white matter[26]. Binswanger (1894) described eight patients with slowly progressive dementia who, at post mortem, were found to have softening and loss of deep white matter with compensatory ventricular enlargement. There is also gliosis, thickening of the arteries, within the abnormal white matter; many also show discrete lacunar infarction, although these are often too small to be seen on CT and MRI scanning. The diagnosis of Binswanger's disease (subcortical arteriosclerotic encephalopathy; SAE) has become increasingly popular.

It was initially thought that these CT findings were specific for Binswanger's disease. However, similar CT findings can occasionally be seen in normal people or even those with AD. Because of this, the term "leukoaraiosis" (Greek, for white matter of loose texture) was used to describe the CT appearances[27].

Clinically there is a stepwise or progressive course, characterized by pseudo-bulbar palsy, cognitive, behavioural and gait disturbances, with focal neurological deficits in approximately 30%. The dementia tends to be subcortical in type. Many patients are hypertensive and the pathological changes are thought to be secondary to chronic ischaemia in the deep end arteries.

Although many patients are hypertensive, the final insult is probably due to hypoperfusion. Indeed, Sulkara and Erkinjunti have reported acute dementia after periods of hypotension and cardiac arrhythmia; CT showed leukoaraiosis[28]. Although hypertension needs to be treated, episodes of hypotension need to be carefully avoided, as vasodilatory reserve is impaired[29].

Inzitari et al. noted leukoaraiosis to be present in 100% of patients with multi-infarct dementia (MID) and 33% with AD compared with 11% in the control population, although even in this control population there was evidence of intellectual fall-off, but not severe enough to be labelled dementia[30]. A history of stroke was four times more likely in those with leukoaraiosis than in those without; most, however, die from cardiac causes[31]. Overall there appears to be considerable overlap between leukoaraiosis, subcortical atherosclerotic encephalopathy and multiple lacunar states.

In CADASIL, the MRI usually shows a combination of leukoaraiosis and multiple lacunar infarction.

Cerebral Amyloid Angiopathy

Although cerebral amyloid angiopathy has been known about for many years, its role in the aetiology of dementia has attracted much attention[32]. Amyloid deposition in the small and medium-sized arteries and arterioles may present with spontaneous haemorrhage or thrombosis. More interestingly, there have now been many reports of cerebral amyloid angiopathy (CAA) presenting as dementia without any preceding history of stroke-like episodes. CAA is associated with areas of small subcortical infarction and histological changes similar to Binswanger's SAE.

Senile plaques in AD contain an amyloid core which appears to be identical to CAA. Amyloid plaque cores are often found immediately adjacent to amyloid-laden capillaries. CAA is present in more than 80% of cases of AD[33].

The association of AD with leukoaraiosis and cerebral amyloid angiopathy has renewed speculation that vascular risk factors may play a role in the pathogenesis of AD[34].

MANAGEMENT

Clinical Assessment

The following criteria point towards a diagnosis of vascular dementia:

1. Symptoms and signs of stepwise stroke-like episodes.
2. Vascular risk factors.
3. Evidence of vascular disease on CT and MRI.

The validity of the different scoring systems is discussed elsewhere (q.v.). Factors suggesting that the dementia is not vascular include:

1. Absence of the above.
2. Early presence of extrapyramidal and autonomic features.
3. Early hallucinations.
4. Cerebellar signs.

It should be noted that it is sometimes difficult in those who present with gait problems to distinguish leukoaraiosis/multiple lacunar strokes from normal pressure hydrocephalus and progressive supranuclear palsy: it is important, then, to look for poor upgaze, axial rigidity and perform CT or MRI scanning.

There is no single illness making up vascular dementia. The clinical management of any patient with vascular dementia should include a summary of the clinical presentation, the probable pathogenesis, risk factors and site of damage. This will allow a rational approach to investigation and medical treatment to minimize the risk of further recurrence/progression. An attempt should be made to decide whether the dementia is primarily a thrombotic or an embolic process from the heart or great vessels, a hypertensive deep white matter disease, a hypoperfusion process or even one of the rarer causes of stroke.

Investigation

Investigation should include a routine vascular screen and then further investigations, depending on the proposed pathophysiology. It is important to assess the routine vascular risk factors, especially as Meyer et al. have suggested that improved cognition may occur after the control of risk factors in MID[35]. A careful assessment of the cardiovascular system is necessary, particularly paying attention to blood pressure and possible sites of emboli from the cerebral arteries (i.e. carotid stenosis) and heart, (especially valvular heart disease, atrial fibrillation or tumour and left ventricular thrombus) in those with cortical infarctions. The CT/MRI scan appearances in vascular dementia have already been discussed in some detail.

All patients should have a full blood count (for polycythaemia or thrombocythaemia), ESR (for arteritis), blood sugar, chest X-ray and ECG. I also check fasting lipids, as cholesterol is an important risk factor for ischaemic heart disease and most vascular patients die a cardiac death. Neurosyphilis remains treatable. Evidence of arteritis and the antiphospholipid syndrome should be looked for, both clinically and by checking various blood tests, such as CRP, complement levels, antinuclear factor, DNA binding, lupus anticoagulant and anticardiolipin antibodies. If the ESR is raised or the patient is over 50 it is important to consider the arteritides, such as granulomatous angiitis and temporal arteritis[17,36].

The diagnosis of granulomatous angiitis can be very difficult and may require both angiography and brain/meningeal biopsy. It is often difficult to know how often one should pursue these investigations, but a stuttering onset of recent vascular dementia with a raised ESR and abnormal lymphocytic cerebrospinal fluid (CSF) should alert the physician. Unfortunately, in some cases the ESR and CSF may be normal. A high index of suspicion is needed because with steroids and cyclophosphamide these patients can do very well[17,20]. In spite of this, a raised ESR in stroke frequently remains unexplained.

Ultrasound scanning of the carotid arteries to detect carotid stenosis or occlusion may be appropriate, although these usually cause transitory ischaemic attacks or strokes, rather than a dementia[37].

Echocardiography is important if a cardiac source of emboli is considered possible and should be performed in all patients with more than one cortical infarct[18].

Skin biopsy, chromosome and DNA analysis may be helpful in the diagnosis of CADASIL and MELAS. Measuring cerebral blood flow and metabolism has become increasingly more sophisticated with the advent of positron emission tomography (PET) which uses radioactive tracers to measure metabolism and blood flow. Frackowiak et al. showed that cerebral blood flow (CBF) and metabolism fell with increasing dementia in both MID and degenerative dementia[38]. Normal CBF is 50–70 ml/100 g/min: ischaemia only occurs once the CBF falls below 10–20 ml/100 g/min. Focal abnormalities are found in both MID and degenerative dementia, although in the vascular group the individual focally deranged areas are patchy and match the unique patterns of ischaemic damage, whereas in AD the focal abnormalities are mainly temporoparietal. PET largely remains a research tool.

Single photon emission CT (SPECT) is becoming a more widely available tool, as most X-ray departments have the necessary equipment. Radioactive tracers are used to measure blood flow. Similar temporoparietal abnormalities in AD and patchy irregularities in MD have been reported[39]. However, all these studies have used a clinical scoring system with/without CT to differentiate MID and AD. None have had pathological confirmation. Because only 10–20% of dementias are multi-infarct, and because an approximate equal percentage have mixed disease (stroke with coincidental AD), it will not be possible to know the true value of PET and SPECT until serial studies are performed with pathological confirmation.

Treatment

As with all vascular disease treatment initially involves dealing with the risk factors—hypertension, hyperlipidaemia, diabetes mellitus and smoking. The Syst-Eur Hypertension trial has demonstrated that treating hypertension prevents dementia[40]. This is combined with specific treatment for the underlying disease process. Aspirin is of proven value in preventing stroke[41]. Whether adding dipyridamole to aspirin confers any greater benefit than aspirin alone remains debatable[42,43]. There is no doubt that clopidogrel is a new effective antiplatelet agent at least as good as aspirin; it should be considered in those intolerant of aspirin[44].

Warfarin is the treatment of choice in those with atrial fibrillation, but the risk of haemorrhage secondary to warfarin is higher in those with leukoaraiosis[45,46]. It must be used with caution if poor compliance and falls are a problem. Anticoagulation should also be considered in the antiphospholipid syndrome[16].

In spite of the many claims, no vasodilator, calcium antagonist or neuroprotective agent has been shown to help vascular dementia. Steroids and immunosuppression may be indicated if an arteritis is proven.

Tatemichi[37] has published a case of dementia with bilateral internal carotid occlusions which improved after extracranial–intracranial bypass surgery to improve the blood flow to the brain.

This section has dealt with the specific treatments for vascular disease: it is crucial, of course, to provide symptomatic treatment and a full care package for the many other problems the unfortunate patient with vascular dementia may experience.

REFERENCES

1. Brust JCM. Vascular dementia—still overdiagnosed. *Stroke*, 1983; **14**: 298–300.
2. Snowdon DA, Greiner LH, Mortimer JA *et al*. Brain infarction and the clinical expression of Alzheimer disease. The nun study. *J Am Med Assoc* 1997; **277**: 813–17.
3. Skoog I, Nilsson L, Palmertz B. A population-based study of dementia in 85 year-olds. *N Eng J Med* 1993; **328**: 153–8.
4. Wade JPH, Mirsen TR, Hachinski VC *et al*. The clinical diagnosis of Alzheimer's disease. *Arch Neurol* 1987; **44**: 24–9.
5. Hagnell O, Ojesjo L, Rorsman B. Incidence of dementia in the Lundby Study. *Neuroepidemiology*, 1992; **1**: 61–6.
6. Gilleard CJ, Kellett JM, Coles JA *et al*. The St. George's dementia bed investigation study: a comparison of clinical and pathological diagnosis. *Acta Psychiat Scand* 1992; **85**: 264–9.
7. O'Brien MD. Vascular dementia is underdiagnosed. *Arch Neurol* 1988; **45**: 797–8.
8. Brust JCM. Vascular dementia is overdiagnosed. *Arch Neurol* 1988; **45**: 799–801.
9. Tatemichi TK, Foulkes MA, Mohr JP *et al*. Dementia in stroke survivors in the Stroke Data Bank Cohort: prevalence, incidence, risk factors and computed tomographic findings. *Stroke* 1990; **21**: 858–66.
10. Sacco RL, Benjamin EJ, Broderick JP *et al*. Risk factors. *Stroke* 1997; **28**: 1507–17.
11. Gorelick PB. Status of risk factors for dementia associated with stroke. *Stroke* 1997; **28**: 459–63.
12. Desmond DW, Moroney JT, Lynch T *et al*. The natural history of CADASIL. *Stroke* 1999; **30**: 1230–3.
13. Hanna MG, Nelson IP, Morgan-Hughes JA, Wood NW. MELAS: a new disease-associated mitrochondrial DNA mutation and evidence for further genetic heterogeneity. *J Neurol Neurosurg Psychiat*, 1998; **65**: 512–17.
14. Haan J, Lanser JBK, Zijderveld I *et al*. Dementia in hereditary cerebral haemorrhage with amyloidosis—Dutch type. *Arch Neurol* 1990; **47**: 965–7.
15. Harle JR, Disdier P, Ali C. Antiphospholipid syndrome revealed by memory disorders. *Rev Neurol* 1992; **148**: 635–7.
16. Kerro P, Levine SR, Tietjen GE. Cerebrovascular ischaemic events with high positive anticardiolipin antibodies. *Stroke* 1998; **29**: 2245–53.
17. Hankey, GJ. Isolated angiitis/angiopathy of the central nervous system. *Cerebrovasc Dis* 1991; **1**: 2–15.
18. Martin PJ, Enevoldson TP, Humphrey PRD. Causes of ischaemic stroke in the young. *Postgrad Med J* 1997; **73**: 8–16.
19. McIlraith DM, Bahary J-P, Côte R. Delayed intracranial vasculopathy and encephalopathy following cranial radiotherapy. *Cerebrovasc Dis* 1993; **3**: 125–7.
20. Barnett HJM, Mohr JP, Stein BM, Yatsu FM. Unusual causes of stroke. *Stroke*, 3rd Edn. Edinburgh: Churchill Livingstone, 1998: 767–1013.
21. Fisher CM. Lacunar strokes and infarcts. A review. *Neurology* 1982; **32**: 871–6.
22. del Ser, T, Bermejo F, Portera A *et al*. Vascular dementia. A clinicopathological study. *J Neurol Sci* 1990; **96**: 1–17.
23. Wolfe N, Linn R, Babikian VL *et al*. Frontal systems impairment following multiple lacunar infarcts. *Arch Neurol* 1990; **47**: 129–32.
24. Bogousslavsky J, Regli F, Uske A. Thalamic infarcts: clinical syndromes, etiology and prognosis. *Neurology* 1988; **38**: 837–48.
25. Tatemichi TK, Desmond DW, Prohovnik I. Strategic infarcts in vascular dementia: a clinical and brain imaging experience. *Drug Res* 1995; **45**: 371–85.
26. Babikian V, Ropper AH. Binswanger's disease: a review. *Stroke* 1987; **18**: 2–12.
27. Hachinski VC, Potter P, Merskey H. Leuko-araiosis. *Arch Neurol* 1987; **44**: 21–3.
28. Sulkava R, Erkinjuntti T. Vascular dementia due to cardiac arrhythmias and systemic hypotension. *Acta Neurol Scand* 1987; **76** 123–8.
29. Brown MM, Pelz DM, Hachinski VC. White matter vasodilatory reserve is impaired in patients with cerebrovascular disease and diffuse periventricular lacunes. *J Neurol* 1990; **2**: 87–92.
30. Inzitari D, Diaz F, Fox A *et al*. Vascular risk factors and leuko-araiosis. *Arch Neurol* 1987; **44**: 42–27.
31. Inzitari D, Di Carlo, A, Mascalchi M *et al*. The cardiovascular outcome of patients with motor impairment and extensive leukoaraiosis. *Arch Neurol* 1995; **52**: 687–91.
32. Vinters HV. Cerebral amyloid angiography. A critical review. *Stroke* 1987; **18**: 311–24.
33. Esiri M, Wilcock GK. Cerebral amyloid angiography in dementia and old age. *J Neurol Neurosurg Psychiat* 1986; **49** 1221–6.

34. Scheinberg P. Dementia due to vascular disease—a multifactorial disorder. *Stroke* 1988; **19**: 1291–9.

35. Meyer JS, Judd BW, Tawakina T *et al.* Improved cognition after control of risk factors for multi-infarct dementia. *J Am Med Assoc* 1986; **256**: 2203–9.

36. Caselli RJ. Giant cell (temporal) arteritis: a treatable cause for multi-infarct dementia. *Neurology* 1990; **40**: 753–5.

37. Tatemichi TK, Desmond DW, Prohovnik I *et al.* Dementia associated with bilateral carotid occlusions: neuropsychological and haemodynamic course after extracranial to intracranial bypass surgery. *J Neurol Neurosurg Psychiat* 1995; **58**: 633–6.

38. Frackowiak RSJ, Pozzilli C, Legg NJ *et al.* Regional cerebral oxygen supply and utilization in dementia. *Brain* 1981; **104**: 753–78.

39. Fazekas F. Neuroimaging of dementia. *Curr Opin Neurol Neurosurg* 1990; **3**: 103–7.

40. Forette F, Seux M-L, Staessen JA *et al.* Prevention of dementia in randomised double-blind placebo-controlled systolic hypertension in Europe (Syst-Eur) trial. *Lancet* 1998; **352**: 1347–51.

41. Antiplatelet Trialists' Collaboration. Collaborative overview of randomised trials of antiplatelet therapy. *Br Med J* 1994; **308**: 81–106.

42. Davis SM, Donnan GA. Secondary prevention for stroke after CAPRIE and ESPS-2. *Cerebrovasc Dis* 1998; **8**: 73–7.

43. Diener H, Cunha L, Forbes C *et al.* European Stroke Prevention Study (ESPS)2. Dipyridamole and acetylsalicylic acid in secondary prevention of stroke. *J Neurol Sci* 1996; **143**: 1 13.

44. Caprie Steering Committee. A randomised blinded trial of clopidogrel versus aspirin in patients at risk of ischaemic events (CAPRIE). *Lancet* 1996; **348**: 1329–39.

45. European Atrial Fibrillation Study Group. Secondary prevention of non-rheumatic atrial fibrillation after transient ischaemic attack or minor stroke. *Lancet* 1993; **342**: 1255–62.

46. Gorter, J.W., Algra, A., Van Gijn *et al.* SPIRIT: predictors of anticoagulant-related bleeding complications in patients after cerebral ischaemia. *Cerebrovasc Dis* 1997; **7**(suppl. 4): 3.

Vascular Dementia Subgroups: Multi-infarct Dementia and Subcortical White Matter Dementia

Ingmar Skoog

Sahlgrenska University Hospital, Göteborg, Sweden

Until the 1960s, almost all dementias of old age were considered secondary to "hardening of the arteries" and chronic ischaemia. In the next decades, vascular causes of dementia came to be considered rare, and multi-infarct dementia (MID) almost its only cause. The term "vascular dementia" (VaD) was introduced in the 1990s to emphasize that several cerebrovascular disorders might cause dementia.

An ischaemic stroke increases the risk for dementia several-fold[1]. The dementias related to stroke are MID and strategic infarct dementia. MID is related to multiple small or large brain infarcts, often too small individually to produce a major clinical incident. The typical patient has a history of stroke or transitory ischaemic attacks with acute focal neurological symptoms and signs. The clinical picture includes sudden onset, stepwise deterioration and a fluctuating course of the dementia. In the early stages, the cognitive impairment may have a large variability, depending on the site of the lesions. However, in a large minority of cases the dementia may have a gradual onset, with a slowly progressive course[2] and without focal signs or infarcts on brain imaging (especially when computed tomography has been used), which makes it difficult to differentiate from AD. It has been suggested that the dementia may be related to the location or the volume of the infarcts. The risk factors suggested for MID are similar to those in stroke, including advanced age, male sex, hypertension, diabetes mellitus, smoking and cardiac diseases[3].

Ischaemic white matter lesions (WMLs) were first described in cases of dementia by Durand-Fardel in 1854, followed by Binswanger in 1894, and by Alzheimer in 1898. Fewer than 50 autopsied cases were described up to 1980[4]. In the 1980s, when WMLs became possible to discern on brain imaging, they were suddenly reported in thousands of patients. Before the advent of brain imaging, the level of interest in white matter disorders among pathologists was low and the white matter was not routinely evaluated in most patients. The pathologic description includes marked or diffuse demyelination and moderate loss of axons, with astrogliosis and incomplete infarction in subcortical structures of both hemispheres, and arteriosclerotic changes, with *hyalinization or fibrosis and thickening of the vessel walls and narrowing of the lumen of the small penetrating arteries and arterioles in the white matter*. The main hypothesis regarding the cause of WMLs is that long-standing hypertension causes *lipohyalinosis and thickening of the vessel walls, with narrowing of the lumen of the small perforating arteries and arterioles which nourish the deep white matter*[4]. The dementia is probably caused by subcortical–cortical or cortico–cortical disconnection, and is generally of a subcortical type with extrapyramidal signs, especially psychomotor retardation. A frontal lobe syndrome with apathy, loss of drive and emotional blunting is common.

Regarding the subtypes of VaD, there is a discussion between lumpers and splitters. In the NINDS–AIREN criteria[6], MID and WMLs are lumped together and it has been questioned whether present scientific knowledge permits anything more than a broad definition of VaD. Focal neurological deficits and brain infarcts are common in subjects with WMLs, and the presence of WMLs are reported to increase the risk for dementia in subjects with stroke. The reason for the common co-occurrence of stroke and WMLs may be that they share similar risk factors, mainly hypertension. However, not all demented subjects with WMLs have cortical infarcts in their brains, and not all individuals with MID have WMLs. Therefore, it may be better to adopt the splitting view to better categorize these entities, with the understanding that there is a large overlap.

There is also an overlap between VaD and AD. WMLs have been described in a high proportion of cases with AD on both brain imaging and at autopsy, and they seem to be more common in late-onset than in early-onset AD[4]. It has even been suggested that white matter degeneration precedes and causes the cortical atrophy in AD[5]. A considerable proportion of subjects from the general population fulfilling the research criteria for AD or VaD have mixed pathologies[7,8]. Cerebrovascular diseases may increase the possibility that individuals with AD lesions in their brains will express a dementia syndrome[9], and "post-stroke dementia" is often a mixture of the direct consequences of stroke, pre-existing AD pathology and the additive effects of these lesions and ageing[10]. The coincidence of AD and VaD may even be the most common form of dementia.

REFERENCES

1. Tatemichi TK, Desmond DW, Mayeux R et al. Dementia after stroke: baseline frequency, risks, and clinical features in a hospitalized cohort. Neurology 1992; 42: 1185–93.
2. Fischer P, Gatterer G, Marterer A et al. Course characteristics in the differentiation of dementia of the Alzheimer type and multi-infarct dementia. Acta Psychiat Scand 1990; 81: 551–3.
3. Skoog I. Guest editorial. Status of risk factors for vascular dementia. Neuroepidemiology 1998; 17: 2–9.
4. Skoog I. Blood pressure and dementia. In Hansson L, Birkenhäger WH, eds, Handbook of Hypertension, vol 18: Assessment of Hypertensive Organ Damage. Elsevier Science: Amsterdam 1997: 303–31.
5. Román GC, Tatemichi TK, Erkinjuntti T et al. Vascular dementia: diagnostic criteria for research studies. Report of the NINDS–AIREN international workshop. Neurology 1993; 43: 250–60.
6. De la Monte SM. Quantitation of cerebral atrophy in preclinical and end-stage Alzheimer's disease. Annals of Neurology, 1989; 25: 450–9.
7. Holmes C, Cairns N, Lantos P, Mann A. Validity of current clinical criteria for Alzheimer's disease, vascular dementia and dementia with Lewy bodies. Br J Psychiat 1999; 174: 45–50
8. Lim A, Tsuang D, Kukull W. Clinico-neuropathological correlation of Alzheimer's disease in a community-based case series. J Am Geriat Soc, 1999; 47: 564–9.
9. Snowdon DA, Greiner LH, Mortimer JA et al. Brain infarction and the clinical expression of Alzheimer disease. The nun study. J Am Med Assoc, 1997; 277: 813–17.
10. Pasquier F, Leys D. Why are stroke patients prone to develop dementia? J Neurol, 1997; 244: 135–42.

The Role of Blood Pressure in Dementia

Ingmar Skoog

Sahlgrenska University Hospital, Göteborg, Sweden

The association between hypertension and dementia/cognitive impairment has received increased interest recently. Both the Honolulu–Asia Aging Study[1] and the Framingham Study[2] report that low performance in psychometric tests in the population is related to a higher systolic blood pressure decades before the measurement of cognitive function. We found that systolic and diastolic blood pressure was increased 10–15 years before the onset of both Alzheimer's disease (AD) and vascular dementia, as well as in individuals with white matter lesions[3]. Furthermore, middle-aged non-demented hypertensive individuals have an increased amount of senile plaques and neurofibrillary tangles, the histopathological hallmarks of AD, in their brains[4]. In cross-sectional studies, blood pressure is generally negatively correlated to cognitive performance before age 75, while there is a positive correlation above that age. Furthermore, elderly subjects with already manifested AD and vascular dementia have lower blood pressure than the non-demented[5]. Thus, although previously high blood pressure seems to be related to cognitive decline and dementia, low blood pressure is often related to already manifested dementia.

Several mechanisms may be involved in the association between hypertension and dementia/cognitive decline. First, the risk of stroke increases with inceasing blood pressure, and stroke is a strong risk factor for dementia. It is thus reasonable to believe that high blood pressure is a risk factor for stroke-related dementia. Hypertension is also a risk factor for ischaemic subcortical white-matter lesions (WMLs)[6], which are often found in subjects with late-onset AD and multi-infarct dementia (MID). The main hypothesis regarding the cause of WMLs is that longstanding hypertension causes lipohyalinosis and thickening of the vessel walls, with narrowing of the lumen of the small perforating arteries and arterioles that nourish the deep white matter. Episodes of hypotension may lead to hypoperfusion and hypoxia–ischaemia, leading to loss of myelin in the white matter. It has been suggested that the arterial changes are due to exposure of vessel walls to increased pressure over time. The greater the pressure and/or lifespan, the more likely are these changes to be present.

A third explanation is that chronic hypertension may lead to a dysfunction of the the blood–brain barrier (BBB), with increased permeability of the endothelial cell layer and extravasation of serum proteins[7]. The CSF:serum albumin ratio is a generally accepted method of assessing the BBB function in living subjects. We recently found that AD, MID and severe forms of WMLs were all associated with an increased CSF:serum albumin ratio in a population-based study of 85 year-olds[8]. A breakdown in the BBB may cause brain lesions by cerebral oedema, activation of astrocytes, or destructive enzymes or other poisons that pass through the damaged vessel walls. Fourth, the renin–angiotensin system is an example of a system that may be involved in the pathogenesis of both hypertension and dementia[9]. Its effector peptide, angiotensin II, has several blood pressure increasing effects, promotes hyperplasia and hypertrophy in vascular smooth muscle cells, and affects memory and behaviour. Fifth, psychological stress has been suggested to be a risk factor for both hypertension and dementia[10].

The association between low blood pressure and dementia has several explanations. First, systemic hypotension associated with reduced cerebral blood flow may give rise to a spectrum of ischaemic neuronal lesions in the brain and may also lead to ischaemic loss of myelin in the white matter. Second, several of the blood pressure-regulating areas in the central nervous system are affected in dementia disorders. Therefore, dementia disorders and their associated brain changes may *per se* influence the blood pressure[5]. A correlation between the number of C-1 neurons in the medulla oblongata and blood pressure has been reported in AD[11]. Blood pressure decline during the course of AD, and low blood pressure was related to cerebral atrophy in non-demented 85 year-olds[5]. It thus seems likely that low blood pressure in demented individuals is secondary to the brain lesions. If cerebral disorder causes low blood pressure, the question arises whether cerebral changes may induce high blood pressure. Recently, it was shown that infusion of $A\beta_{42}$ (a protein deposited in the brains and cerebral vessels of AD victims) increased blood pressure in anaesthetized rats, suggesting that circulating levels of this protein may exert vasopressor actions *in vivo*[12].

Treatment of hypertension may thus have a preventive effect on cognitive decline and dementia. The recent finding from the Syst-Eur trial[13], that treatment of isolated systolic hypertension reduces the incidence of dementia by 50%, supports this hypothesis, but the number of demented in that study was small. It has been suggested that overtreatment with antihypertensive drugs may increase the risk of dementia in the very old by causing cerebral hypoperfusion. No studies so far provide support for this opinion. We recently reported[14] that subjects who became demented during a 15-year follow-up used antihypertensive drugs less often than those who did not become demented. Although these findings do not preclude the possibility that overtreatment of hypertension may cause ischaemia in the brain in a subset of individuals, they do not support the hypothesis that antihypertensive treatment may cause cognitive impairment in the elderly.

REFERENCES

1. Launer LJ, Masaki K, Petrovitch H *et al*. The association between midlife blood pressure levels and late-life cognitive function. The Honolulu–Asia Aging Study. *J Am Med Assoc*, 1995; **274**: 1846–51.
2. Elias MF, Wolf PA, D'Agostino RB *et al*. Untreated blood pressure level is inversely related to cognitive functioning: the Framingham Study. *Am J Epidemiol*, 1993; **138**, 353–64.
3. Skoog I, Lernfelt B, Landahl S *et al*. A 15-year longitudinal study on blood pressure and dementia. *Lancet* 1996a; **347**, 1141–5.
4. Sparks DL, Scheff SW, Liu H *et al*. Increased incidence of neurofibrillary tangles (NFT) in non-demented individuals with hypertension. *J Neurol Sci*, 1995; **131**: 162–9.
5. Skoog I, Andresson L-A, Palmertz B *et al*. A population-based study on blood pressure and brain atrophy in 85 year-olds. *Hypertension* 1998a; **32**: 404–9.
6. Skoog I. A review on blood pressure and ischaemic white matter lesions. *Dement Geriat Cogn Disord* 1998b; **9**(suppl 1): 13–19.
7. Johansson BB. Pathogenesis of vascular dementia: the possible role of hypertension. *Dementia* 1994; **5**: 174–6.
8. Skoog I, Wallin A, Fredman P *et al*. A population-study on blood–brain barrier function in 85 year-olds. Relation to Alzheimer's disease and vascular dementia. *Neurology* 1998c; **50**: 966–71.
9. Skoog I. Arterial hypertension and Alzheimer's disease. In Leys D, Pasquier F, Scheltens P, eds, *Stroke and Alzheimer's Disease*. The Hague: Holland Academic Graphics 1998d; 89–100.
10. Persson G, Skoog I. A prospective population study of psychosocial risk factors for late-onset dementia. *Int Geriat Psychiat* 1996; **11**: 15–22.
11. Burke WJ, Coronado PG, Schmitt CA *et al*. Blood pressure regulation in Alzheimer's disease. *J Autonom Nerv Syst*, 1994; **48**: 65–71.
12. Arendash GW, Su GC, Crawford FC *et al*. Intravascular β-amyloid infusion increases blood pressure: implications for a vasoactive role of β-amyloid in the pathogenesis of Alzheimer's disease. *Neurosci Lett*, 1999; **268**: 17–20.
13. Forette F, Seux ML, Staessen JA *et al*. Prevention of dementia in randomised double-blind placebo-controlled Systolic Hypertension in Europe (Syst-Eur) trial. *Lancet* 1998; **352**: 1347–51.
14. Skoog I, Lernfelt B, Landahl S. High blood pressure and dementia. *Lancet* 1966b; **348**: 65–6.

Neuropathology: Other Dementias

J. M. MacKenzie

Grampian University Hospitals NHS Trust, Aberdeen, UK

There are many causes of dementia in addition to Alzheimer's disease (AD) and vascular dementia, and the commonest of these seems to be dementia with Lewy bodies (DLB), which perhaps accounts for 10% of all cases of dementia, although the precise incidence depends on the population studied and the pathological criteria used for diagnosis[1,2]. In a hospital series, it may be second only to AD as a cause of dementia[3]. After DLB, other causes are distinctly rare and include Creutzfeldt–Jakob disease, Huntington's disease and the frontotemporal dementias.

DEMENTIA IN PARKINSON'S DISEASE AND DEMENTIA WITH LEWY BODIES

Parkinson's disease is a disorder characterized by rigidity, tremor and bradykinesia, usually with an onset in the sixth decade. Neuronal loss and gliosis are typically evident in the substantia nigra and loci coerulei, but also in the dorsal vagal nuclei, dorsal raphe nuclei and nucleus basalis of Meynert. Lewy bodies, spherical intracytoplasmic inclusions composed of granular and filamentous elements, immunoreactive with antibodies against neurofilament protein, paired helical filaments, ubiquitin and, in aminergic neurones, tyrosine hydroxylase protein[4–7], are found not only in pigmented brainstem neurones but also in over 20 different nuclei, pigmented and non-pigmented[8]. Changes in aminergic pathways, particularly dopaminergic, are well documented[4].

Dementia has been reported to affect 34.6% of patients with parkinsonism in one large autopsy series and it seems likely that a number of different mechanisms are responsible[9].

Concurrent AD

It has been claimed that AD is six times more common in patients with Parkinson's disease than in age-matched controls[10] and 12–25% of demented parkinsonian patients in one series had AD[4].

In Jellinger's study[9], most of the demented parkinsonians also had the pathological changes of AD. Other studies have shown that cortical senile plaques and neurofibrillary tangles are more numerous in demented patients with Parkinson's disease than non-demented Parkinson's disease sufferers or controls[11–13]. The wide spectrum of dementia in Parkinson's disease has been attributed to the overlap of clinical and subclinical pathological changes in both diseases[14].

Innominato-cortical Dysfunction

Neuronal loss from the basal nucleus of Meynert (BNM) is greater in demented than in non-demented parkinsonian patients[11] and this depletion may be 40–80% in the former as opposed to 20–50% in the latter[15,16].

Furthermore, there is also evidence of an accompanying reduction in choline acetyltransferase (CAT) and acetylcholinesterase in the BNM and all areas of the cerebral cortex. Decreased CAT activity in the temporal cortex correlates with BNM neuronal loss in Parkinson's disease, unlike AD, and also correlates with memory impairment, although not with the numbers of cortical plaques and tangles[17].

Neuronal Loss in Pigmented Brainstem Nuclei

It is generally stated that there is no correlation between neuronal loss in the substantia nigra and mental impairment[11], but it has been found that neuronal loss in the medial substantia nigra correlates with the severity of dementia, presumably due to loss of projections to the caudate nuclei, limbic system and cerebral cortex[18]. In addition, severe neuronal loss and subnormal noradrenaline metabolism in the loci coerulei are commoner in demented than non-demented parkinsonian patients[11,19]. Medial substantia nigra loss, together with cortical AD changes, seemed to underlie dementia in one study, whereas depression in Parkinson's disease was associated with more severe loss of neurones from the dorsal raphe nuclei[13].

Dementia with Lewy Bodies

Small numbers of Lewy bodies may be present in the cerebral cortex in patients without neurological impairment, or with Parkinson's disease. However, a disorder characterized by early neuropsychiatric features, dementia, visual hallucinations, fluctuating conscious level and relatively mild Parkinson's disease justifies separate identification as DLB[20] because of different therapeutic implications. Many cases also have large numbers of brainstem Lewy bodies and it seems likely that DLB, with a predominantly cortical distribution of Lewy bodies, lies at one end of a spectrum of Lewy body disorders, in which idiopathic Parkinson's disease, with Lewy bodies predominantly localized in the brainstem, is the opposite end[21].

In many reported cases, cortical Lewy bodies have been associated with AD-type changes, leading to the conclusion that the cause of dementia in diffuse LBD is cortical[22,23]. However, the distribution of neuritic plaques and neurofibrillary tangles does not necessarily parallel the distribution of Lewy bodies[24] and, in some cases with Lewy bodies in the cerebral cortex and brainstem nuclei, AD-type changes are not present[25].

The precise nosological relationship between DLB and AD, and between DLB and patients with Parkinson's disease who subsequently become demented, requires elucidation[3].

CREUTZFELDT–JAKOB DISEASE

Creutzfeldt–Jakob disease (CJD) belongs to the family of transmissible spongiform encephalopathies affecting humans and animals[26]. In humans the main forms are sporadic CJD, iatrogenic CJD (associated mostly with pituitary hormones prepared from cadaver pituitaries), familial forms, including Gerstmann–Straussler–Scheinker (GSS) syndrome and variant CJD (vCJD).

Sporadic CJD is typically a rapidly progressive dementia with associated myoclonus, but a number of different clinical and pathological variants have been described[27,28]. The worldwide incidence is approximately 1–2/million/year[29], although the average annual incidence in England and Wales was 0.3 in 1970–1979[30], and 0.49 in 1980–1984[31]. The highest reported incidence of 75 is amongst Libyan Jews[32]. Although often a presenile dementia, the peak age-specific mortality rate in England and Wales is in the seventh decade, with a mean of 63.2 years and a range of 33–82[31].

Approximately 10–15% of cases of CJD are familial and seem to follow an autosomal dominant pattern of inheritance[33]. GSS is also familial, but clinically and pathologically more closely resembles kuru than CJD, although caused by the same transmissible agent[34,35].

To date, there has been only one reported case of vCJD in the elderly[36a]. All of the other cases have been younger (mean age at death 29 years). The presenting features in both age groups are behavioural change and sensory symptoms with later development of cerebellar ataxia, dementia and mycoclonus[36].

Although pathological variants of CJD have been described, the principal features are fluctuating spongiform change of the grey matter, with neuronal loss, and astrocytic hypertrophy and hyperplasia[37]. Amyloid plaques, particularly in the cerebellum, are present in 5–10% of cases of CJD and the majority of cases of kuru and GSS[34]. Florid amyloid plaques of prion protein are also characteristic of vCJD.

The transmissible nature of CJD has been known for many years[37,38]. Prions[39,40] as proteinaceous infectious particles consisting of one protein (PrP 27-30), which is encoded by a cellular gene and derived from a larger protein. PrP 27-30 is inseparable from the infectivity of the scrapie agent and constitutes the amyloid of cerebral plaques in "prion" diseases. The PrP or a closely-related gene clearly controls the clinical expression of the disease.

The causal relationship of PrP with the disease is strengthened by the presence of disease-specific mutations linked to, or tracking with, inherited "prion" diseases, such as the substitution of leucine for proline at PrP codon 102 in ataxic forms of GSS[41] and the substitution of lysine for glutamate at codon 200 in Libyan Jews[42]. Similarly, the valine 129 homozygous genotype is associated with susceptibility to iatrogenic CJD[43] and methionine 129 homozygosity with vCJD[36].

The continued unravelling of the molecular biology of the prion diseases is likely to reveal as many surprises in the future as have already been provided by this fascinating group of

disorders. However, it seems improbable that "prion dementias" constitute a large group of as yet unrecognized neurodegenerative disorders and, for all practical purposes, transmissible spongiform encephalopathies in humans and "prion dementias", are the same[44].

HUNTINGTON'S DISEASE

Huntington's disease (HD) is a disorder of midlife onset (mean age 41 years) characterized by progressive chorea, psychological changes and dementia, although not necessarily in that order. The disease is encountered in the senium, sometimes because of prolonged survival of presenile cases, but also because chorea only appears in 28% of HD patients after the age of 50 and, occasionally, not until the seventh or eighth decade[45]. HD is inherited as an autosomal dominant trait with 100% penetrance and the HD gene has been localized near the telomere on the short arm of chromosome 4[46].

The principal neuropathological features are neuronal loss and gliosis in the corpus striatum, and a five-grade system has been devised for pathologically classifying HD[47], which closely correlates with the degree of clinical disability[48]. Most of the neuropathologically studied cases fall into Grades 2 and 3 (79%)[49]; 50% of neurones have been lost from the caudate nucleus by the time grade 1 pathological changes are recognizable and 95% by grade 4. There is an accompanying increase in astrocytes and oligodendrocytes, reaching a maximum that is significantly different from control material in grade 4 for the former and grades 0–2 for the latter[47].

The distribution of neuronal loss within the corpus striatum is non-uniform. In Grades 1 and 2 the medial caudate nucleus is more severely affected than the lateral, although this distinction is lost when the pathological changes become more severe[47]. The anteroventral part of the putamen is also spared[50]. Not only is the disease process in the corpus striatum anatomically variable, but also not all neuronal populations are equally affected. The small to medium-sized spiny neurones (which have a large synaptic surface and distant connections) are most affected in HD, and these neurones contain γ-aminobutyric acid (GABA) enkephalins and substance P[51,52]. On the other hand, medium aspiny neurones, containing NADPH-diaphorase, somatostatin and neuropeptide Y, and large cholinergic neurones, are relatively spared[53,54]. The decreased concentration of GABA and enzymes involved in its metabolism, which has been known for many years[55], together with the decreased concentrations of substance P and the enkephalins, can be explained on the basis of selective loss of striatal neuronal populations.

The disease is caused by expansion of a trinucleotide CAG repeat beyond 35 repeats in the first exon of the huntingtin gene on chromosome 4[56]. The CAG repeats are translated to polyglutamine repeats in huntingtin and, although the normal function of huntingtin is incompletely understood, it appears to be associated with the cytoskeleton and necessary for neurogenesis, and expression of mutant huntingtin is necessary for disease development. The ability of huntingtin to interact with other proteins is influenced by CAG length and it is possible that neuronal apoptosis may be triggered by abnormal interaction with caspase 3[57,58]. Furthermore, there is also evidence of abnormal metabolism in HD brain tissue, resulting in the generation of free radicals, so that more than one mechanism may be operating to produce cell death in HD[59].

Although corpus striatum changes dominate the pathological picture in HD, other areas of the brain are involved. The cerebral cortex showed 21–29% loss of substance, the cerebral white matter 29–34% and the thalamus 28% in one study[60], but cortical abnormalities may be very difficult to identify[49]. Neuronal loss has been identified in the superior frontal and cingulate cortices, particularly of laminae III and V pyramidal neurones, but this does not seem to correlate with severity of striatal pathology, suggesting that it is a primary part of the disease process[61].

However, another study[62] found evidence of loss of large pyramidal neurones from laminae III, V and VI of the prefrontal cortex, which was most severe in pathological grade 4 HD, and suggested that this represented retrograde degeneration of cortical glutamatergic neurones. Nerve cell loss from specific regions of the entorhinal cortex and subiculum has also been reported[63].

There is controversy over whether neuronal loss in the substantia nigra does[64] or does not[65] occur in HD. Preservation of neuronal populations in the nucleus basalis of Meynert, locus coeruleus and dorsal raphe nuclei has also been reported, leading to the suggestion that dementia in HD may be due not to damage to subcortical nuclei, as in the other "subcortical" dementias, but to failure of ascending systems within the basal ganglia or neuronal loss in the cerebral cortex[65].

FRONTOTEMPORAL DEMENTIA

The frontotemporal dementias (FTD) are non-Alzheimer forms of dementia characterized clinically by behavioural and personality change leading to apathy and mutism, and by progressive atrophy of the frontal, anterior parietal and anterior temporal lobes. The histology is variable and defines three separate subgroups[66]:

- *Frontal lobe degeneration*. This is characterized by microvacuolar degeneration, gliosis and neuronal loss, principally affecting laminae II and III.
- *Pick's disease* (FTD with Pick-type histology) is represented by transcortical neuronal loss, gliosis and cavitation, together with the presence of tau and ubiquitin-positive intraneuronal inclusions (Pick bodies) and αB crystallin-positive ballooned neurones (Pick cells). Although there is overlap between Pick's disease and other forms of FTD, as well as with corticobasal degeneration, the distinctive distribution of the pathological changes—such as the involvement of the dentate fascia by Pick bodies—has led some authors to regard Pick's disease as a unique disease rather than a histological variant within the FTD spectrum[67]. However, both of these different histologies can have a variable topographical distribution in the brain, producing progressive language disorder when both temporal lobes are involved or the disease primarily affects the left hemisphere, or progressive apraxia when parietal and motor areas are involved[66].
- *Motor neurone disease inclusion dementia*. Either of these histologies can overlap with classical motor neurone disease, either as a dementing disorder occurring in patients known to have MND, or also as an identical histology occurring in patients without motor dysfunction[66,68].

Fifty-eight percent of cases of FTD show a previous family history of a similar disorder, and linkage to chromosome 17 has been established in some families. Following the current trend for "molecular" classification of the dementias, the various forms of FTD have sometimes been described as "tauopathies" but 64% cases of FTD in one study showed no intracellular tau-positive inclusions[69]. This is an area where further study and clarification is required.

OTHER DISORDERS

Many other disorders may be associated with dementia in the elderly, including progressive supranuclear palsy[70] and, occasionally, multiple sclerosis[71]. There are also a number of rare dementing disorders of uncertain nosological status, such as the tangle-predominant form of dementia[72] and argyrophilic grain disease[73].

This section of the book would not be complete without the reader being reminded of the estimated 13.2%[72] of causes of dementia in the elderly—including intracranial space-occupying lesions, particularly chronic subdural haematoma; metabolic disorders, such as hypothyroidism and hypopituitarism[75]; and "normal-pressure" hydrocephalus—that are potentially treatable[76].

REFERENCES

1. Esiri MM, Hyman BT, Bayreuther K, Masters CL. Ageing and dementia. In Graham DI, Lantos PL, eds, *Greenfield's Neuropathology* 6th edn, vol II. London: Arnold, 1997; 172–3.
2. Jellinger K, Danielczyk W, Fischer P, Gabriel E. Clinicopathological analysis of dementia disorders in the elderly. *J Neurol Sci* 1990; **95**: 239–58.
3. McKeith IG, Galasko D, Kosaka K et al. Consensus guidelines for the clinical and pathologic diagnosis of dementia with Lewy bodies (DLB): report of the consortium on DLB international workshop. *Neurology* 1996; **47**: 1113–24.
4. Jellinger K. Pathology of Parkinsonism. In Fahn S et al., eds, *Recent Developments in Parkinson's Disease*. New York: Raven, 1986; 33–66.
5. Bancher C, Lassmann H, Budka H et al. An antigenic profile of Lewy bodies: immunocytochemical indication for protein phosphorylation and ubiquitination. *J Neuropathol Exp Neurol* 1989; **48**: 81–93.
6. Galloway PG, Grundke-Iqbal I, Iqbal K, Perry G. Lewy bodies contain epitopes both shared and distinct from Alzheimer's neurofibrillary tangles. *J Neuropathol Exp Neurol* 1988; **47**: 654–63.
7. Nakashima S, Ikuta F. Tyrosine hybroxylase protein in Lewy bodies of Parkinsonian and senile brains. *J Neurol Sci* 1984; **66**: 91–6.
8. Ohama E, Ikuta F. Parkinson's disease: distribution of Lewy bodies and monoamine neuron system. *Acta Neuropathol* 1976; **34**: 311–19.
9. Jellinger KA. Morphological substrates of dementia in parkinsonism. A critical update. *J Neurol Transm Suppl* 1977; **51**: 57–82.
10. Boller F, Mizutani T, Roessmann U, Gambetti P. Parkinson's disease, dementia and Alzheimer disease: clinicopathological correlations. *Ann Neurol* 1980; **7**: 329–35.
11. Gaspar P, Gray F. Dementia in idiopathic Parkinson's disease. A neuropathological study of 32 cases. *Acta Neuropathol* 1984; **64**: 43–52.
12. Hakim AM, Mathieson G. Dementia in Parkinson's disease: a neuropathologic study. *Neurology* 1979; **29**: 1209–14.
13. Paulus W, Jellinger K. The neuropathologic basis of different clinical subtypes of Parkinson's disease. *J Neuropathol Exp Neurol* 1991; **50**: 743–55.
14. Quinn NP, Rossor MN, Marsden CD. Dementia and Parkinson's disease—pathological and neurochemical considerations. *Br Med Bull* 1986; **42**: 86–90.
15. Editorial. Diffuse Lewy body disease. *Lancet* 1989; **ii**: 310–11.
16. Gibb WRG. Dementia in Parkinson's disease. *Br J Psychiat* 1989; **154**: 596–614.
17. Perry EK, Curtis M, Dick DJ et al. Cholinergic correlates of cognitive impairment in Parkinson's disease: comparisons with Alzheimer's disease. *J Neurol Neurosurg Psychiatr* 1985; **48**: 413–21.
18. Rinne JO, Rummukainen J, Paljarvi L, Rinne UK. Dementia in Parkinson's disease is related to neuronal loss in the medial substantia nigra. *Ann Neurol* 1989; **26**: 47–50.

19. Cash R, Dennis T, L'Heureux Y et al. Parkinson's disease and dementia: norepinephrine and dopamine in locus coeruleus. Neurology 1987; 37: 42–6.

20. Ince PG, Perry EK, Morris CM. Dementia with Lewy bodies. A distinct non-Alzheimer dementia syndrome? Brain Pathol 1998; 8: 299–324.

21. Kosaka K, Yoshimura M, Ikeda K, Budka H. Diffuse type of Lewy body disease: progressive dementia with abundant cortical Lewy bodies and senile changes of varying degree—a new disease? Clin Neuropathol 1984; 3: 185–92.

22. Dickson DW, Davies P, Mayeux R et al. Diffuse Lewy body disease. Neuropathological and biochemical studies of six patients. Acta Neuropathol 1987; 75: 8–15.

23. Kosaka K, Tsuchiya K, Yoshimura M. Lewy body disease with and without dementia: a clinicopathological study of 35 cases. Clin Neuropathol 1988; 7: 299–305.

24. Gibb WRG, Esiri MM, Lees AJ. Clinical and pathological features of diffuse cortical Lewy body disease (Lewy body dementia). Brain 1987; 110: 1131–53.

25. Gibb WRG, Luthert PJ, Janota I, Lantos PL. Cortical Lewy body dementia: clinical features and classification. J Neurol Neurosurg Psychiat 1989; 52: 185–92.

26. Bradley R. Bovine spongiform encephalopathy: the need for knowledge, balance, patience and action. J Pathol 1990; 160: 283–5.

27. Roos R, Gajdusek DC, Gibbs CJ Jr. The clinical characteristics of transmissible Creutzfeldt–Jakob disease. Brain 1973; 96: 1–20.

28. Traub R, Gajdusek DC, Gibbs CJ Jr. Transmissible virus dementia: the relation of transmissible spongiform encephalopathy of Creutzfeldt–Jakob disease. In Smith WL, Kinsbourne M, eds, Aging and Dementia. New York: Spectrum, 1977; 91–146.

29. Brown P, Cathala F, Raubertas RF et al. The epidemiology of Creutzfeldt–Jakob disease: conclusion of a 15 year investigation in France and review of the world literature. Neurology 1987; 37: 895–904.

30. Will RG, Matthews WB, Smith PG, Hudson C. A retrospective study of Creutzfeldt–Jakob disease in England and Wales, 1970–1979. II: Epidemiology. J Neurol Neurosurg Psychiat 1986; 49: 749–55.

31. Harries-Jones R, Knight R, Will RG et al. Creutzfeldt–Jakob disease in England and Wales, 1980–1984: a case-control study of potential risk factors. J Neurol Neurosurg Psychiat 1988; 57: 1113–19.

32. Kahana E, Alter M, Braham J, Sofer D. Creutzfeldt–Jakob disease: focus among Libyan Jews in Israel. Science 1974; 183: 90–1.

33. Masters CL, Harris JO, Gajdusek DC et al. Creutzfeldt–Jakob disease: patterns of worldwide occurrence and the significance of familial and sporadic clustering. Ann Neurol 1979; 5: 177–88.

34. Masters CL, Gajdusek DC, Gibbs CJ Jr. Creutzfeldt–Jakob disease: virus isolation from the Gerstmann–Straussler syndrome. Brain 1981; 104: 559–88.

35. Baker HF, Ridley RM, Crow TJ. Experimental transmission of an autosomal dominant spongiform encephalopathy: does the infective agent originate in the human genome? Br Med J 1985; 291: 299–302.

36. Will RG, Ironside JW, Zeidler M et al. A new variant of Creutzfeldt–Jakob disease in the UK. Lancet 1996; 347: 921–5.

36a. Lorains JW, Henry C, Agbamu DA et al. Variant Creutzfeldt–Jakob disease in an elderly patient. Lancet 2001; 357: 1339–40.

37. Manuelidis EE. Creutzfeldt–Jakob disease. J Neuropathol Exp Neurol 1985; 44: 1–17.

38. Corsellis JAN. The transmissibility of dementia. Br Med Bull 1986; 42: 111–14.

39. Prusiner SB. Novel proteinaceous infectious particles cause scrapie. Science 1982; 216: 136–44.

40. Prusiner SB, Gabizon R, McKinley MP. On the biology of prions. Acta Neuropathol 1987; 72: 299–314.

41. Hsiao K, Prusiner SB. Inherited human prion diseases. Neurology 1990; 40: 1820–7.

42. Hsiao K, Meiner Z, Khana E et al. Mutation of the prion protein in Libyan Jews with Creutzfeldt–Jakob disease. N Engl J Med 1991; 324: 1091–7.

43. Collinge J, Palmer MS, Dryden AJ. Genetic predisposition to iatrogenic Creutzfeldt–Jakob disease. Lancet 1991; 337: 1441–2.

44. Brown P, Kaur P, Sulima MP et al. Real and imagined clinicopathological limits of "prion dementia". Lancet 1993; 341: 127–9.

45. Martin JB. Huntington's disease: new approaches to an old problem. Neurology 1984; 34: 1059–72.

46. Gusella JF, Wexler NS, Conneally PM et al. A polymorphic DNA marker genetically linked to Huntington's disease. Nature 1983; 306: 234–8.

47. Vonsattel J-P, Myers RH, Stevens TJ et al. Neuropathological classification of Huntington's disease. J Neuropathol Exp Neurol 1985; 44: 559–77.

48. Myers RH, Vonsattel J-P, Stevens TJ et al. Clinical and neuropathologic assessment of severity in Huntington's disease. Neurology 1988; 38: 341–7.

49. Richardson EP. Huntington's disease: some recent neuropathological studies. Neuropathol Appl Neurobiol 1990; 16: 451–60.

50. Roos RAC, Pruyt JFM, de Vries J, Bots GTAM. Neuronal distribution in the putamen in Huntington's disease. J Neurol Neurosurg Psychiatr 1985; 48: 422–5.

51. Graveland GA, Williams RS, DiFiglia M. Evidence for degenerative and regenerative changes in neostriatal spiny neurons in Huntington's disease. Science 1985; 227: 770–3.

52. Graveland GA, Williams RS, DiFiglia M. A Golgi study of the human neostriatum: neurons and afferent fibres. J Comp Neurol 1985; 234: 317–33.

53. Ferrante RJ, Beal MF, Kowall NW et al. Sparing of acetylcholinesterase-containing striatal neurons in Huntington's disease. Brain Res 1987; 411: 162–6.

54. Ferrante RJ, Kowall NW, Beal MF et al. Morphologic and histochemical characteristics of a spared subset of striatal neurons in Huntington's disease. J Neuropathol Exp Neurol 1987; 46: 12–27.

55. Bird ED, Iversen LL. Huntington's chorea: post-mortem measurements of glutamic acid decarboxylase, choline acetyltransferase and dopamine in basal ganglia. Brain 1974; 97: 457–72.

56. Walling HW, Baldassare JJ, Westfall TC. Molecular aspects of Huntington's disease. J Neurosci Res 1998; 54: 301–8.

57. Nasir J, Goldberg YP, Hayden MR. Huntington disease: new insights into the relationship between CAG expansion and disease. Hum Mol Gen 1996; 5: 1431–5.

58. Wellington CL, Brinkman RR, O'Kusky JR, Hayden MR. Towards understanding the molecular pathology of Huntington's disease. Brain Pathol 1997; 7: 979–1002.

59. Tabrizi SJ, Cleeter MW, Xuereb J et al. Biochemical abnormalities and excitotoxicity in Huntington's disease brain. Ann Neurol 1999; 45: 25–32.

60. de la Monte SM, Vonsattel J-P, Richardson EP Jr. Morphometric demonstration of atrophic changes in the cerebral cortex, white matter and neostriatum in Huntington's disease. J Neuropathol Exp Neurol 1988; 47: 516–25.

61. Cudkowicz M, Kowall NW. Degeneration of pyramidal projection neurons in Huntington's disease cortex. Ann Neurol 1990; 27: 200–4.

62. Sotrel A, Myers RH. Morphometric analysis of prefrontal cortex in Huntington's disease (HD). J Neuropathol Exp Neurol 1990; 49: 346.

63. Braak H, Braak E. Allocrotical involvement in Huntington's disease. Neuropathol Appl Neurobiol 1992; 18: 539–47.

64. Ferrante RJ, Kowall NW, Richardson EP Jr. Neuronal and neuropil loss in the substantia nigra in Huntington's disease. J Neuropathol Exp Neurol 1989; 48: 380.

65. Mann DMA. Subcortical afferent projection systems in Huntington's chorea. Acta Neuropathol 1989; 78: 551–4.

66. Mann DM. Dementia of frontal type and dementias with subcortical gliosis. Brain Pathol 1998; 8: 325–38.

67. Bergeron C, Davis A, Pollanen MS. Pick's disease is a unique and distinct disease. Brain Pathol 2000; 10: 495–6.

68. Jackson M, Lennox G, Lowe J. Motor neurone disease-inclusion dementia. Neurodegeneration 1996; 5: 339–50.

69. Mann DMA, McDonagh AM, Snowden J et al. Molecular classification of the dementias. Lancet 2000; 355: 626.

70. Verny M, Jellinger KA, Hauw JJ et al. Progressive supranuclear palsy: a clinicopathological study of 21 cases. Acta Neuropathol 1996; 91: 427–31.

71. Mendez MF, Frey WH. Multiple sclerosis dementia. *Neurology* 1992; **42**: 696.

72. Jellinger KA, Bancher C. Senile dementia with tangles (tangle predominant form of senile dementia). *Brain Pathol* 1998; **8**: 367–76.

73. Jellinger KA. Dementia with grains (argyrophilic grain disease). *Brain Pathol* 1998; **8**: 377–86.

74. Clarfield AM. The reversible dementias: do they reverse? *Ann Intern Med* 1988; **109**: 476–86.

75. Kiloh LG. The secondary dementias of middle and later life. *Br Med Bull* 1986; **42**: 106–10.

76. Friedland RP. "Normal"-pressure hydrocephalus and the saga of the treatable dementias. *J Am Med Assoc* 1989; **262**: 2577–81.

Dementia and Parkinson's Disease

Richard B. Godwin-Austen

Queen's Medical Centre, Nottingham, UK

Although James Parkinson, in his 1817 monograph, believed that this disease left "the senses and intellects...uninjured", there has been increasing realization that Parkinson's disease (PD) is associated in many cases with dementia. The dementia has specific clinical and psychological characteristics and is now believed to be associated in the majority with specific neuropathological changes. Certainly, dementia in elderly patients with PD complicates their management, limits treatment and survival and leads to a heavy burden on medical and welfare services and family alike. The dementia of PD is therefore a subject of great importance, in which substantial advances in understanding have taken place in recent years.

In cases where parkinsonism and dementia coexist, the differential diagnosis must include Lewy body dementia (LBD), progressive supranuclear palsy, corticobasal degeneration, meso-limbo-cortical dementia and severe Azheimer's disease. In life, LBD is characterized by the association of parkinsonism and a dementia with deficits in attention, executive functions and visuospatial abilities. There are often fluctuations in alertness, sometimes amounting to transient unresponsiveness. And recurrent formed hallucinations with little or no affective component are common. In spite of these typical features, the distinction of LBD in the elderly may be very uncertain.

About 20% of all patients with PD develop dementia. The prevalence of diagnosed PD is overall about 1/1000, but the prevalence increases with age and reaches nearly 2% in the ninth decade. An undiagnosed pre-symptomatic PD is very much more common, so that pathological findings indicative of the disease are present in about 10% of the healthy population in the ninth decade[3]. Dementia in PD is more common in the elderly patient, and patients with dementia tend to be significantly older at the onset of their PD[4]. By contrast, early-onset PD tends to have a low incidence of dementia[5].

Patients who present with dementia and later develop typical PD are probably suffering from LBD, now categorized as one of the "Lewy body disorders".

Dementia associated with PD is therefore a common occurrence in clinical practice. A number of important and interesting questions arise from these facts. Has the dementia any specific clinical features that distinguish it from "senile" dementia of the Alzheimer type? Has the type of PD that is associated (perhaps at a late stage) with dementia any specific clinical features compared with the type of disease where dementia is uncommon? What is the relationship, if any, between treatment for PD and the development of dementia? What are the neuropathological correlates between PD and dementia? Are both phenomena caused by the same process?

CLINICAL FEATURES OF THE DEMENTIA ASSOCIATED WITH PARKINSON'S DISEASE

Cognitive testing in PD may be affected by a number of extraneous factors, including impaired motor function, medication or mood disturbance. In people with no associated disease, cognitive function can be compared with premorbid intelligence and the decline estimated. However, no validated method for estimating premorbid intelligence in PD has been developed. Depression is common in PD and may give a pseudodementia, relieved by antidepressant treatment. For these and other reasons, no generally accepted pattern of cognitive function has emerged as characteristic of PD and longitudinal studies are needed.

ORGANIC DISORDERS

The concept of subcortical dementia was originally introduced by Albert with reference to the dementia in the rare form of parkinsonism seen in progressive supranuclear palsy[7]. Subcortical dementia is characterized by forgetfulness, slowing of thought processes (bradyphrenia), apathy and impaired ability to manipulate acquired knowledge. This pattern of deficit is contrasted with diseases such as Alzheimer's disease, characterized by global memory impairment, aphasia, agnosia and apraxia. While much overlap seems to exist between these types of cognitive impairment, bradyphrenia, apathy and depression seem to characterize the dementia of PD. Thought-block is an early characteristic of the dementia and fluctuation of the cognitive impairment has been noted[8]. Visual hallucinations, often with little or no affective component, are common. Less common are paranoid delusional states.

Patients with PD and dementia show a treatment response for their parkinsonism that is inversely related to the severity of the cognitive changes[9].

DO SPECIFIC CLINICAL FEATURES OF PARKINSON'S DISEASE INDICATE THE LIKELIHOOD OF DEMENTIA?

Lieberman et al.[10] demonstrated that the dementia of PD was associated with a later age of onset, a poorer response to L-dopa and less abnormal involuntary movements and dose fluctuations in response to L-dopa. These findings have been confirmed[4,5,9] in later studies.

Tremor is less common as a presenting symptom in patients with PD associated with dementia, whereas dyspraxia of gait and

Principles and Practice of Geriatric Psychiatry, 2nd edn. Edited by J. R. M. Copeland, M. T. Abou-Saleh and D. G. Blazer
©2002 John Wiley & Sons, Ltd

dyspraxias for hand movements are more common. Thus, a patient who has difficulty in performing the discrete finger movements used to test for bradykinesia may commonly show early cognitive changes.

The rate of progression of the PD is significantly greater in cases where dementia further affects management and survival. Patients with dementia tolerate drug treatment less well and tend to develop more persistent and severe toxic confusional states.

Thus, many authors accept that PD may exist in a late-onset form with certain characteristic clinical features and a relatively poor response to L-dopa where dementia is common. By contrast, there is a type of PD in which dementia is rare. The disease has an earlier onset and response to L-dopa is initially very good[12,13].

All drugs used in the treatment of PD carry a risk of provoking toxic confusional states and this reaction is more likely and more severe in patients with cognitive changes. Where therapeutic benefit from a drug is likely to be modest, there is a relative contraindication to the use of that drug in an elderly patient, particularly if they are showing cognitive changes. For this reason, the anticholinergic drugs are seldom recommended in geriatric practice[14].

Conversely, in patients with classical PD in middle life, where the prospect of cognitive impairment is small (but the risks of permanent response fluctuations to L-dopa are high) anticholinergic drugs are indicated in preference to L-dopa if disability can be satisfactorily controlled.

The fluctuation of the dementia already noted may suggest that the cognitive changes are related to drug therapy. This possibility should usually be investigated by dose reduction or withdrawal, but if no improvement occurs the patient need not be deprived of the physical benefits of the drug. Many elderly patients with mild cognitive changes tolerate L-dopa therapy with benefit and without any significant exacerbation of their mental impairment. Occasionally the administration of L-dopa in patients with dementia may provoke states of excitement with impulsive behaviour and aggravation of the dementia[15].

The synthetic dopamine agonists (bromocriptine, lisuride, pergolide, ropinirole) and the anticholinergics should be used only with great caution in the parkinsonian patient with dementia.

WHAT IS THE RELATIONSHIP, IF ANY, BETWEEN TREATMENT FOR PARKINSON'S DISEASE AND THE DEVELOPMENT OF DEMENTIA?

The two drugs in most widespread use for the treatment of PD are benzhexol and L-dopa (with decarboxylase inhibitor). We must examine the evidence concerning whether either of these drugs could be causing or accelerating dementia in PD.

Alzheimer's disease is known to be associated with a reduction in brain choline acetyltransferase, and anticholinergic drugs exacerbate the neural changes in this condition, but there is no evidence of permanent effects on higher mental function from these drugs in PD. Confusional states provoked by benzhexol recover with a timescale of usually less than 4 weeks. It is noteworthy that the use of a high-dose anticholinergic drug in the treatment of dystonias over many years is not associated with any cognitive changes.

However, studies of the prevalence of dementia in PD before the L-dopa era gave figures of 3.2–10%[16] or 8<1%[17], whereas since the introduction of L-dopa, the prevalence of dementia has risen to above 20%.

Like anticholinergics, L-dopa may provoke acute confusional states that recover when the drug is withdrawn. But withdrawal of L-dopa rarely alters the decline of mental faculties in parkinsonian patients with dementia. The duration of L-dopa treatment does not appear to correlate with the likelihood of mental impairment[18]. At the present time, the evidence is against L-dopa treatment causing or accelerating the dementia of PD.

WHAT ARE THE NEUROPATHOLOGICAL CORRELATES BETWEEN PARKINSON'S DISEASE AND DEMENTIA?

With the advent of staining techniques based on anti-ubiquitin immunocytochemistry[19] neuropathological correlates between PD and dementia showed that by far the commonest cause of dementia in this condition was diffuse LBD[20]. Previously parkinsonian dementia had been attributed to a supposed association between PD and Alzheimer's disease, but the new staining techniques showed that in PD without dementia the Lewy body was substantially confined to the brainstem, whereas in PD with dementia, diffuse cortical Lewy body formation was demonstrable.

By contrast, in Alzheimer's disease, neuronal loss in the nucleus basalis is associated with neurofibrillary tangles in this region and in the dorsal raphe nucleus. In cases of PD with dementia, scanty tangle formation may be seen in the hippocampus or neocortex, but with profuse cortical Lewy bodies not seen in Alzheimer's disease.

Senile plaques have been recommended as an important neuropathological criterion for the diagnosis of Alzheimer's disease[23]. But senile plaques are commonly seen in similar density to cortical Lewy bodies in cases with dementia[20], and thus fail to distinguish between the two conditions.

The dementia seen in some cases of PD is attributable to neuronal cell loss in the cortex associated with diffuse cortical Lewy body formation.

ARE BOTH PHENOMENA CAUSED BY THE SAME PROCESS?

Lewy body disease, in which parkinsonism is associated with dementia, is probably the second commonest cause of dementia after Alzheimer's disease[24]. The Lewy body is an intra-neuronal eosinophilic inclusion body that shows ubiquitin immuno-reactivity, and is the pathological hallmark of PD.

Thus, PD is characterized by Lewy body formation in the brainstem and particularly in the substantia nigra[25]. In demented cases of PD there is cortical Lewy body formation as well and the severity of the dementia correlates with cortical Lewy body density[20]. It is therefore reasonable to conclude that the dementia and the parkinsonism are due to the same pathological process. The nature of this process is currently the subject of intense research.

LBD studied post mortem may show a variety of patterns. In the typical case, Lewy bodies may be distributed in the brainstem, diencephalon, limbic system and cortex, but in some cases Lewy bodies are confined to the brainstem and are few or absent in the cortex or limbic system. In these cases there are also no senile plaques, whereas where Lewy bodies are present in the cortex, senile plaques may also be seen.

Probably the most specific marker for the Lewy body is α-synuclein, and this protein has been associated in some families with autosomal dominant PD. The pathological process of Lewy body diseases may be partly genetic and seems to be independent from, but sometimes co-existent with, the pathological process of Alzheimer's disease. There is increasing interest in the genetic markers of PD and dementia, but it remains likely that there is an environmental trigger in genetically susceptible cases.

It has already been noted that parkinsonism with dementia is a form of PD that tends to have later onset than classical PD without dementia. This suggests that the elderly cerebral cortex is vulnerable to the same pathological processes as the substantia nigra (and which lead to parkinsonism), whereas the younger cerebral cortex is relatively resistant, so that early-onset PD tends to be unassociated with dementia. The nature of this age-related vulnerability of the cortex is unknown, but it is of interest that age-related differential vulnerability to 1-methyl-4-phenyl-1,2,3,6-tetrahydropyridine (MPTP) has been demonstrated in primates[26].

CONCLUSIONS

The dementia of PD is entirely distinct from the dementia of Alzheimer's disease. In PD dementia is associated with Lewy body formation in the cerebral cortex as well as in the substantia nigra; whereas in Alzheimer's disease neuronal loss and neurofibrillary tangle formation is characteristically in the dorsal raphe nuclei and nucleus basalis of Meynert.

The clinical features of the two forms of dementia are usually distinguishable. More difficult to distinguish clinically, especially in the earlier stages, are the two types of PD. In one the disease presents typically in middle life, progresses slowly, responds well to dopamine agonists and is not associated with dementia; whereas the other (diffuse Lewy body type) presents in late life, progresses more rapidly, responds less well to dopamine agonists and is associated with dementia. The clinical significance of making this distinction is to define prognosis and also to affect management, in particular the use of dopamine agonists and the management of dementia.

The cause of PD and of Alzheimer's disease remains unknown but there are promising lines of investigation related to the genetics and molecular biology of the Lewy body and the neurofibrillary tangle, respectively.

REFERENCES

1. Brown RG, Marsden CD. How common is dementia in Parkinson's disease? *Lancet* 1984; **ii**: 1262–5.
2. Mutch WJ, Dingwall-Fordyce I, Downie AW *et al*. Parkinson's disease in a Scottish city. *Br Med J* 1986; **292**: 534–6.
3. Gibb WR, Lees AJ. The relevance of the Lewy body to the pathogenesis of idiopathic Parkinson's disease. *J Neurol Neurosurg Psychiat* 1988; **51**: 745–52.
4. Elzan TS, Sroka H, Maker H *et al*. Dementia in idiopathic Parkinson's disease: variables associated with its occurrence in 203 patients. *J Neurol Transmiss* 1986; **65**: 285–302.
5. Godwin-Austen RB, Lowe J. The two types of Parkinson's disease. In Clifford Rose F, ed., *Current Problems in Neurology, vol. 6. Parkinson's Disease*. London: Libbey, 1987.
6. Byrne EJ, Lowe J, Godwin-Austen RB *et al*. Dementia and Parkinson's disease associated with diffuse cortical Lewy bodies. *Lancet* 1987; **i**: 501.
7. Albert ML, Feldman RG, Willis AL. The "subcortical dementia" of progressive supranuclear palsy. *J Neurol Neurosurg Psychiat* 1974; **37**: 121–30.
8. Byrne EJ, Lennox G, Lowe J, Godwin-Austen RB. Diffuse Lewy Body disease; clinical features in 15 cases. *J Neurol Neurosurg Psychiat* 1989; **52**: 709–17.
9. Taylor AE, Saint Ayr JA, Lang AR. Parkinson's disease cognitive changes in relation to treatment response. *Brain* 1987; **110**: 35–51.
10. Lieberman A, Dziatolowski M, Kupersmith M *et al*. Dementia in Parkinson's disease. *Ann Neurol* 1979; **6**: 355–9.
11. Wilson JA, Smith RG. Dementia in Parkinson's disease. *Lancet* 1987; **i**: 861.
12. Quinn NP, Critchley P, Marsden CD. Young onset Parkinson's disease. *Movem Disord* 1987; **2**.
13. Lima B, Neves G, Nora M. Juvenile Parkinsonism: clinical and metabolic characteristics. *J Neurol Neurosurg Psychiat* 1987; **50**: 345–8.
14. Maclennan WJ, Shephard AN, Stevenson IH. Disorders of the nervous system. In *The Elderly*. Berlin: Springer-Verlag, 1984; 132–3.
15. Sacks OW, Kohl MS, Messeloff CR, Schwartz WF. Effect of levodopa in Parkinsonian patients with dementia. *Neurolog* 1972; **22**: 516–19.
16. Mjones H. Paralysis agitans, a clinical and genetic study. *Acta Psychiat Neurol Scand* 1949; **54**(suppl): 1–195.
17. Pollock M, Hornabrook RW. The prevalence, natural history and dementia of Parkinson's disease. *Brain* 1966; **89**: 429–48.
18. Elizan TS, Sroka H, Maker H *et al*. Dementia in idiopathic Parkinson's disease: variables associated with its occurrence in 203 patients. *J Neurol Transmiss* 1986; **65**: 285–302.
19. Lennox G, Lowe J, Morrell K *et al*. Anti-ubiquitin immunocytochemistry is more sensitive than conventional techniques in the detection of diffuse Lewy body disease. *J Neurol Neurosurg Psychiat* 1989; **52**: 67–71.
20. Lennox G, Lowe J, Landon M *et al*. Diffuse Lewy body disease: correlative neuropathology using antiubiquitin immunocytochemistry. *J Neurol Neurosurg Psychiat* 1989; **52**: 1236–47.
21. Hakim AM, Mathieson G. Dementia in Parkinson's disease: a neuropathological study. *Neurology* 1979; **29**: 1209–14.
22. Boller F, Mizutani T, Roessmann U *et al*. Parkinson's disease, dementia and Alzheimer's disease: clinicopathological correlations. *Ann Neurol* 1980; **7**; 329–35.
23. Khachaturian ZS. Diagnosis of Alzheimer's disease. *Arch Neurol* 1985; **42**: 1097–105.
24. Mayer RJ, Landon M, Doherty F *et al*. Ubiquitin and dementia. *Nature* 1989; **340**: 193.
25. Gibb WRG, Lees AJ. The significance of the Lewy body in the diagnosis of idiopathic Parkinson's disease. *Neuropathol Appl Neurobiol* 1989; **115**: 27–44.
26. Forno LS, Langston JW, De Lanney LE *et al*. Locus coeruleus lesions and eosinophilic inclusions in MPTP-treated monkeys. *Ann Neurol* 1986; **20**: 449–55.

Clinical Criteria for Dementia with Lewy Bodies

I. G. McKeith

Newcastle upon Tyne General Hospital, UK

Why are diagnostic criteria for dementia with Lewy body (DLB) important? There are many reasons, but the most significant are to properly advise patients and carers, to minimize neuroleptic prescribing and possibly to effectively target cholinesterase inhibitor use. Also, since DLB is relatively common, it needs to be routinely excluded in the differential diagnosis of other dementia subtypes, particularly when a diagnosis of Alzheimer's disease (AD) is being considered. Several studies have now reported on either the sensitivity (proportion of cases positively identified) or specificity (proportion of negative cases correctly identified) of the International Consensus criteria for DLB, against neuropathological diagnosis. Most find "probable DLB" criteria to have a specificity >0.8, a figure comparable with the best clinical criteria for AD and Parkinson's disease (PD). High specificity means that when a diagnosis of probable DLB is made, it is likely to be correct. The more lenient "possible DLB" category should be useful as a screening tool for identifying cases in the clinic, although many false-positive diagnoses will be made.

Sensitivity rates for probable DLB are more variable and generally lower. This may in part be due to *retrospective* application of the criteria to case records in most of these studies. Spontaneous documentation of fluctuation and detailed psychiatric phenomenology in case notes is notoriously incomplete, leading some to conclude that inter-rater reliability for individual diagnostic items, especially "fluctuation", is unsatisfactory. Although a tighter operational definition, or a biological measure, of fluctuation would undoubtedly be useful, studies *prospectively* applying the DLB diagnostic criteria generally find inter-rater reliability for individual items (including fluctuation) and for a final diagnosis of DLB, to be acceptable ($\kappa > 0.6$), allowing for diagnostic sensitivities >0.8 to be achieved.

Ancillary investigations will have an important future role in improving the accuracy of clinical diagnosis of DLB. FP-CIT SPECT brain imaging demonstrates a large reduction in dopamine transport to the striatum in DLB, and this may be apparent before extrapyramidal signs are manifest. Nigrostriatal dopaminergic depletion is only rarely seen in AD or vascular dementia. Relative lack of medial temporal lobe atrophy on CT/MRI is also characteristic of DLB compared to AD.

The Second International Workshop on DLB recommended that the Consensus criteria should continue to be used in their current format for recruiting cohorts of DLB patients for research studies and clinical trials. Depression and REM sleep behaviour disorder were suggested as two additional features supporting the diagnosis.

Accurate case detection will ultimately be best achieved by increasing the index of suspicion for a diagnosis of DLB, not only in dementia assessment clinics but also in any setting where elderly patients may present with delirium, movement disorder, falls or syncope. Perhaps we might do better to frame the next revision of the diagnostic criteria within a broader spectrum of Lewy body-related disorders or α-synucleinopathies, thereby acknowledging the links between PD, DLB and primary autonomic failure, and breaking down some currently unhelpful boundaries between psychiatry, neurology and geriatric medicine.

Subcortical Dementia

J. R. Burke

Duke University Medical Center, Durham, NC, USA

Health-care workers who evaluate older patients are frequently confronted with individuals who they suspect have dementia. Although it is often straightforward to determine whether an individual is demented, determining the etiology of the dementia can be difficult. Dementia is not a single disease, but a heterogeneous complex of disorders with the common finding of impairment in multiple cognitive domains. Fortunately, clues leading to a correct diagnosis can be obtained in the physical and mental status examination.

A heuristic device that can aid in the evaluation of patients with dementia is to divide diseases into two categories, based on whether the pathology is primarily cortical or subcortical[1]. Although the cortical/subcortical dichotomy has been questioned on pathologic grounds, there are clinical features that distinguish one group from the other. The prototypical cortical dementia is Alzheimer's disease (AD). Diseases that cause subcortical dementia include small vessel cerebrovascular disease, Parkinson's disease and Huntington's disease (Table 50b.1)[2].

CLINICAL FEATURES OF SUBCORTICAL DEMENTIA

The cardinal clinical features of subcortical dementia are apathy, inattention and psychomotor slowing[1,3]. Patients with subcortical dementia typically appear apathetic. They have a blunted affect, poor personal hygiene and sloppy appearance. The patients are often aware of their cognitive deficit but appear unconcerned. In contrast, patients in the early stages of AD typically have normal affect, grooming and dress. Patients with AD who are aware of their deficit are typically quite concerned.

It is easy to become frustrated when interviewing a patient with subcortical dementia because the patient's inattention leads to frequent repetition of questions by the examiner. Surprisingly, sometimes minutes after a question is asked, patients with a subcortical dementia will respond with the correct answer. Patients with AD have normal attention.

Slowing is a key feature of subcortical dementia and one of the most obvious signs during the examination. Slowing occurs in multiple areas, including cognition (thought formulation, language generation and processing), sensation (processing of stimuli) and motor performance (bradykinesia). While forcing a patient to respond quickly impairs performance in both cortical and subcortical dementia, individuals with subcortical dementia benefit from being given more time to complete a task. Additional response time does not have a similar beneficial effect for patients with AD. The apathy, inattention and psychomotor slowing due to subcortical dementia can be difficult to distinguish from depression. Patients with AD do not demonstrate psychomotor slowing, unless they are also depressed.

The type of memory dysfunction differs between subcortical and cortical dementia. Impaired registration and retrieval characterize the memory deficit in subcortical dementia, while intact registration and rapid forgetting are seen in AD. To test registration and retrieval, a patient is asked to repeat a short list of words immediately after presentation (registration) and after a delay (retrieval). In subcortical dementia, the list may have to be presented several times before all items are registered. Registration is intact in AD patients. Patients with subcortical dementia and AD may retrieve a similar number of items, but if presented with a choice, the patient with subcortical dementia can distinguish between items that were presented and items that were not (recognition). AD patients are unable to distinguish between list and non-list items. Patients with subcortical dementia also benefit from hints to recall items (cueing), while AD patients do not.

Patients with subcortical dementia also frequently display deficits in multi-step tasks. They may perform each step of a task individually, but be unable to incorporate steps to solve the problem. For example, a patient may be able to calculate the number of nickels in $1.00 and the number of nickels in $0.35, but not the number of nickels in $1.35.

Behavioral disturbance can occur with either cortical or subcortical dementia, but apathy and depression are more common in the early stages of a subcortical dementia and may predate other cognitive problems. The cortical signs, aphasia, apraxia and agnosia, are lacking in subcortical dementia and suggest either AD or a focal process such as stroke, mass lesion or focal degeneration (e.g. primary progressive aphasia).

Motor signs, such as increased tone and bradykinesia, are common in subcortical dementia. Abnormal movements, such as tremor, chorea or dystonia, may also occur. Posture is often abnormal and patients may appear stooped or extended when standing. Gait problems include poor initiation, small step length and difficulty turning. AD patients do not demonstrate motor signs, abnormal movements or posture and gait abnormalities until the latter stages of dementia.

Table 50b.1. Causes of subcortical dementia

Parkinson's disease	Small vessel cerebrovascular disease
Progressive supranuclear palsy	Spinocerebellar ataxias
Huntington's disease	Hydrocephalus
Multiple systems atrophy	Multiple sclerosis
Wilson's disease	HIV dementia
Frontal lobe dementia	Vasculitis

Principles and Practice of Geriatric Psychiatry, 2nd edn. Edited by J. R. M. Copeland, M. T. Abou-Saleh and D. G. Blazer
©2002 John Wiley & Sons, Ltd

DISEASES CAUSING SUBCORTICAL DEMENTIA

Extrapyramidal Disorders

Parkinson's Disease (PD)

PD is a common cause of subcortical dementia and is diagnosed by the clinical findings of bradykinesia, tone abnormalities (rigidity and cogwheeling) and rest tremor. Almost all patients with PD can be shown to display cognitive slowing and other features of subcortical dementia, but only a subset progress to frank dementia[4]. Further complicating matters, some demented patients with PD develop a mixed cortical and subcortical dementia. At autopsy, patients with mixed dementia may exhibit pathologic signs of AD and PD or diffuse, intraneuronal Lewy bodies. The exact relationship between Parkinson's dementia, Lewy body dementia and AD is poorly understood[5].

Other parkinsonian syndromes are also associated with subcortical dementia. Progressive supranuclear palsy (PSP) can be distinguished from PD by limited voluntary vertical eye movements, absence of rest tremor, extended (rather than stooped) posture and lack of response to dopamine replacement[6]. Clinically significant dementia is more common in PSP than PD. Multiple systems atrophy (MSA) is another parkinsonian syndrome that can be associated with subcortical dementia. Patients with MSA have a variable combination of parkinsonism, cerebellar ataxia, corticospinal tract abnormalities and/or autonomic dysfunction[7].

Huntington's Disease (HD)

HD is an autosomal dominant inherited neurodegenerative disease characterized by psychiatric abnormalities, chorea and subcortical dementia[8]. The earliest symptoms of HD are often psychiatric and demented HD patients display the classic features of subcortical dementia. HD is caused by pathologic expansion of a CAG repeat in the huntingtin gene. A blood test is commercially available to detect the causative mutation.

Cerebrovascular Disease

The location of infarcted brain tissue in a stroke determines its clinical features. Strokes involving the cerebral cortical gray matter will cause cortical signs such as aphasia and apraxia. Subcortical dementia occurs when infarction involves the deep gray matter nuclei (e.g. basal ganglia and thalamus) and/or the periventricular white matter[9]. For dementia to develop, damage must be bilateral and multifocal. Small vessel strokes can be caused by lacunar infarction or Binswanger's disease. Lacunar strokes occur when small intracerebral penetrating blood vessels are occluded and Binswanger's disease is the result of chronic white matter ischemia. Risk factors for small vessel cerebrovascular disease include cigarette smoking, hypertension and diabetes mellitus. Patients with small vessel cerebral infarction may not experience any traditional stroke-like episodes and deny a step-wise decline in cognitive function. The physical examination will, however, demonstrate focal neurologic signs, including pseudobulbar palsy, hyper-reflexia and pathologic reflexes, such as the Babinski sign. CT or MRI is useful in demonstrating small vessel strokes in patients with suspected subcortical dementia.

Miscellaneous Causes

Multiple sclerosis (MS) and HIV infection can cause subcortical dementia. These diseases are often suspected when confronted by a young person with dementia, but should also be considered in older patients. Dementia is usually a late finding in MS and is typically associated with other neurologic signs, including eye movement abnormalities, motor findings, sensory symptoms and/or cerebellar deficits. The presence of cerebellar ataxia and subcortical dementia is also seen in patients with spinocerebellar ataxias (SCA). There are a large number of different diseases that present as SCA and the diseases may be sporadic or inherited[10]. Magnetic resonance brain imaging of patients with advanced SCA will show cerebellar and/or brainstem atrophy. Genetic testing is available for many of the inherited forms of disease.

Hydrocephalus can cause subcortical dementia. Hydrocephalus may occur in the elderly without obvious lesions obstructing cerebrospinal fluid (CSF) flow and with normal CSF pressure [normal pressure hydrocephalus (NPH)]. Brain imaging of patients with NPH shows enlarged ventricles and widely patent intraventricular foramina. The clinical signs of NPH include the well-known triad of subcortical dementia, urinary incontinence and gait apraxia. CSF shunting of patients with NPH can result in significant improvement, but is typically unsuccessful if the dementia is long-standing or far-advanced. Other potentially treatable causes of dementia can also present, with a subcortical pattern including chronic infection and vasculitis.

Frontal lobe dementia presents as a classic subcortical dementia, despite the fact that the pathology is located in frontal cortical neurons. The subcortical–frontal neuronal pathways mediate many of the features of subcortical dementia, including apathy, inattention, bradykinesia and problems with planning[3,11]. It is not surprising that damage to the subcortical nuclei, connecting white matter tracts or frontal neurons, present with a similar clinical phenotype. Other causes of frontal lobe damage can also cause a "subcortical" dementia, such as trauma, infarction, tumor or psychiatric disease.

CONCLUSION

Dividing the clinical presentation of patients with dementia into cortical and subcortical groups can be useful as a first attempt to identify the etiology of dementia, but this approach has limitations. Dementing diseases rarely cause purely cortical or subcortical pathology. Strokes can involve both white and gray matter. AD can cause degeneration in subcortical nuclei or frontal cortex and clinically resembles a subcortical dementia. Analogously, the pathology of frontal lobe dementia causes cortical neurons to degenerate, but the clinical profile is subcortical. Depression can further confuse the clinical picture by making a cortical dementia have subcortical features, leading to inaccurate diagnosis. The classical distinction between subcortical and cortical dementia is also less clear in patients with advanced dementia, because the clinical patterns tend to merge. Despite these problems, recognition of subcortical features can increase one's suspicion of unusual causes of dementia and lead to increased accuracy of diagnosis and, potentially, treatment.

REFERENCES

1. Savage CR. Neuropsychology of subcortical dementias. *Psychiat Clin N Am* 1997; **20**: 911–31.
2. Cummings JL, Benson DF. Dementia: definition, prevalence, classification, and approach to diagnosis. In Cummings JL, Benson

DF, eds, *Dementia: A Clinical Approach*. Boston, MA: Butterworth-Heinemann, 1992; 1–17.

3. Cummings JL. Subcortical dementia. Neuropsychology, neuropsychiatry, and pathophysiology. *Br J Psychiat* 1986; **149**: 682–97.

4. Cummings JL. The dementias of Parkinson's disease: prevalence, characteristics, neurobiology, and comparison with dementia of the Alzheimer type. *Eur Neurol* 1998; **28**(Suppl 1): 15–23.

5. Lowe J, Dickson D. Pathological diagnostic criteria for dementia associated with cortical Lewy bodies: review and proposal for a descriptive approach. *J Neur Transm Suppl* 1997; **51**: 111–20.

6. Litvan I, Campbell G, Mangone CA *et al*. Which clinical features differentiate progressive supranuclear palsy (Steele–Richardson–Olszewski syndrome) from related disorders? A clinicopathological study. *Brain* 1997; **120**: 65–74.

7. Kaufmann H. Multiple system atrophy. *Curr Opin Neurol* 1998; **11**: 351–5.

8. Haddad MS, Cummings JL. Huntington's disease. *Psychiat Clin N Am* 1997; **20**: 791–807.

9. McPherson SE, Cummings JL. Neuropsychological aspects of vascular dementia. *Brain Cogn* 1996; **31**: 269–82.

10. Moseley ML, Benzow KA, Schut LJ *et al*. Incidence of dominant spinocerebellar and Friedreich triplet repeats among 361 ataxia families. *Neurology* 1998; **51**: 1666–71.

11. Darvesh S, Freedman M. Subcortical dementia: a neurobehavioral approach. *Brain Cogn* 1996; **31**: 230–49.

Early-onset Dementias

Gandis Mazeika

Duke University Medical Center, Durham, NC, USA

The early-onset dementias are a heterogeneous group of neurodegenerative diseases with onset generally defined as prior to age 65. Research into these diseases has suffered from ascertainment bias, inconsistency in definitions, small numbers and inaccuracies associated with retrospective review of charts and death records. However, clinically useful information has gradually emerged over more than 60 years of study.

Liston reviewed the topic in 1979 and contributed a series of 50 cases[1,2]. Despite several significant advances in the field since that time, most notably the discovery of the presenilin genes, his review continues to be an excellent starting point in understanding this group of diseases.

EPIDEMIOLOGY

Early-onset dementia represents approximately 5–10% of all dementias seen by health caregivers.

The relative frequency of common dementia subtypes in early-onset dementia roughly parallels that for senile dementia. The most prevalent form of dementia is Alzheimer's disease (AD), followed by vascular dementia (VaD). In countries with a high rate of alcohol use, alcoholic dementia has a frequency roughly equal to vascular dementia. The frequency of less common dementing illnesses, such as inborn errors of metabolism and chronic CNS infection, is expected to be higher than in older age groups; however, epidemiological studies are lacking.

Estimates of annual incidence for early-onset AD (EOAD) vary from 2.4 to 22.6/100 000[3–7]. One study found a point prevalence of 34.6/100 000 with a 5 year survival of 68%. Median survival was estimated as 8.1 years in another study. These estimates suggest a more aggressive course for EOAD compared with the senile variant. Most studies support increased risk among females for PSAD, with a relative risk of 1.0–1.7.

Only a few epidemiological studies have attempted to include other etiologies of dementia. Two studies from Scotland varied widely with respect to relative frequencies of PSAD and vascular dementia[3,6]. One study found comparable frequencies, while another found the frequency of vascular dementia to be about 20% that of PSAD. In the latter study, of 114 patients, 60 had PSAD, 13 had vascular dementia, 14 had alcohol-related dementia, 25 had overlapping diagnoses and two had other diseases.

EARLY-ONSET ALZHEIMER'S DISEASE

EOAD differs from senile onset AD in several respects, including patterns of inheritance and disease course[8]. While

Table 50c.1 Genes linked to familial EOAD

Gene	Chromosome	Known mutation as of 1999
Amyloid precursor protein (APP)	21	5
Presenilin 1	14	45
Presenilin 2	1	2

the majority of cases of EOAD are sporadic, there is a significantly increased frequency of familial clusters in comparison to senile AD[9]. These clusters have facilitated linkage analysis, leading to the identification of a number of mutations in several genes. So far, three genes have been linked to familial EOAD (Table 50c.1). It is estimated that approximately 50% of familial cases of EOAD can be attributed to known mutations, suggesting that other genes yet to be identified are involved as well.

The mutations listed in Table 50c.1 all result in increased abnormal cleavage of APP, ultimately leading to production of amyloid plaques. The inheritance pattern for mutations in all three genes is autosomal dominant with high penetrance. No practical screening tests are currently available.

The apolipoprotein E (ApoE) gene on chromosome 19 has been identified as an important susceptibility gene for EOAD. Three naturally occurring allotypes of ApoE are known, ApoE 2, 3 and 4. Individuals homozygous for ApoE 4 have approximately twice the relative risk of developing AD as individuals homozygous for ApoE 3. Conversely, individuals with one or two copies of ApoE 2 have approximately half the risk for EOAD as individuals homozygous for ApoE 3. Risk appears to be greatest in individuals developing cognitive impairment between 60 and 65 years of age and declines in older age groups.

The role of ApoE in AD is poorly understood and is the topic of intensive research. In addition to its role in AD, homozygosity for ApoE 4 has been found to be a risk factor for poor outcome following stroke. Thus, ApoE is thought to possibly play a role in mediating inflammatory responses in the brain.

Age at onset of AD has been shown to be an important determinant of disease course and clinical presentation, with more rapid cognitive and functional decline observed in EOAD. On neuropsychological testing, individuals with EOAD score significantly worse on attentional items compared with senile AD. These observations have suggested the possibility that EOAD may be a different clinical entity than senile AD.

Principles and Practice of Geriatric Psychiatry, 2nd edn. Edited by J. R. M. Copeland, M. T. Abou-Saleh and D. G. Blazer

VASCULAR DEMENTIA

Little information exists regarding early-onset vascular dementia (EOVD), although the relative frequency in some areas, notably Japan, appears to be equal to EOAD. Risk factors are similar to senile vascular dementia and include hypertension, diabetes mellitus, smoking and hypercholesterolemia. As with EOAD, there is an increased prevalence of familial clusters in EOVD, most of which can be attributed to homocysteinuria, although other inherited coagulopathies may play a significant role. There is probably a considerable overlap between cases of EOAD and EOVD. Readers interested in additional information about the diagnosis of AD or VaD are referred to reviews by Gersing et al.[12] and by Doraiswamy et al.[13]

APPROACH TO DIAGNOSIS

There are perhaps several hundred disorders with dementia as a clinical feature. Most of these disorders are quite rare. This diversity in etiology poses a significant challenge to the clinician. For example, a case report of two patients with clinically similar features found one to have EOAD and the other to have adult onset metachromatic leukodystrophy[10].

The following general guidelines, although not exhaustive, are intended as an aid in the work-up of patients presenting with cognitive impairment at age 65 and younger:

1. History of present illness:
   (a) A gradual insidious course is suggestive of EOAD.
   (b) Cognitive decline in association with a stroke or "spells" raises the index of suspicion for EOVD.
   (c) A lifelong history of underachievement, childhood delay in milestones or difficult pregnancy or delivery is suspicious for an inherited disorder affecting cognition.
2. Ask about risk factors for less common dementias:
   (a) Exposure to toxins, including carbon monoxide, solvents, pesticides, heavy metals.
   (b) History of childhood encephalitis or meningitis.
   (c) History of multiple concussions.
   (d) History of malabsorption, diarrhea or significant change in diet.
   (e) Parental age at birth.
   (f) Detailed history of alcohol and drug use.
   (g) AIDS risk factors.
3. Past medical history:
   (a) Search for potentially reversible causes of dementia:
      (i) Thyroid disease.
      (ii) Epilepsy.
      (iii) Syphilis.
      (iv) Pernicious anemia.
      (v) Lupus, sarcoidosis, other CNS inflammatory diseases.
      (vi) Cancer.
      (vii) Hepatitis.
4. Search for illnesses that may mimic dementia:

Table 50c.2 Checklist for neurological examination in dementia diagnosis

Dementia associated with neuropathy
1. Hypothyroidism
2. Nutritional disorders, especially B_{12} deficiency
3. Vasculitis, especially Sjogren's syndrome, SLE
4. Exposure to solvents and alcohol
5. Multi-infarct dementia associated with diabetes
6. HIV
7. Neurosyphilis
8. Lyme disease
9. Metachromatic leukodystrophy
10. Adrenoleukodystrophy

Dementia associated with hemiparesis
1. Multi-infarct dementia
2. Mitochondrial encephalomyelopathy with stroke-like episodes (MELAS)
3. Vasculitis from various causes
4. Masses in the brain, including tumors, vascular malformations, hematomas, abscesses, etc.
5. Complex partial epilepsy
6. Amyotrophic lateral sclerosis

Dementia associated with tremor or rigidity
1. Early-onset Parkinson's disease
2. Multisystem atrophy
3. Spino-cerebellar degeneration
4. Multi-infarct dementia, especially with involvement of the basal ganglia
5. Huntington's disease
6. Wilson's disease
7. Progressive supranuclear palsy
8. Hallevorden–Spatz disease
9. Manganese poisoning
10. Post-encephalitic dementia
11. Multiple sclerosis
12. Carbon monoxide poisoning
13. Cryptococcal meningitis
14. Dementia pugilistica

Dementia associated with nystagmus and/or ataxia
1. Wernicke's encephalopathy
2. Spino-cerebellar degeneration

3. Alcoholic dementia
4. Paraneoplastic encephalopathy
5. Hydrocephalus

Dementia associated with dysautonomia
1. Multisystem atrophy
2. Multi-infarct dementia with diabetes
3. Parkinson's disease

Dementia associated with myoclonus
1. Early-onset fronto-temporal dementia
2. Creutzfeldt–Jakob disease
3. Post-anoxic encephalopathy
4. Autoimmune thyroiditis
5. Whipple's disease

Dementia associated with epilepsy
1. Metastatic brain lesions
2. Cryptococcal meningitis
3. Dentato-pallido-luysian atrophy
4. Anti-epileptic drug-related encephalopathy

Dementia associated with eye movement abnormalities
1. Multiple sclerosis (intranuclear ophthalmoplegia)
2. Progressive supranuclear palsy (impaired vertical gaze)

Dementia associated with myopathy
1. Myotonic dystrophy
2. Hypothyroidism
3. Diabetes mellitus

Dementia with variable physical findings
1. Primary HIV dementia
2. PML
3. ADEM
4. Metabolic causes, e.g. hypothyroidism, hypercalcemia, Addison's disease
5. Dementia with Lewy bodies

Dementia with a positive family history
1. Familial AD (Presenilin 1 and 2 mutations)
2. Inborn errors of metabolism
3. Huntington's disease
4. Mytotonic dystrophy

(a) Sleep disorders, including sleep apnea and narcolepsy.

(b) Depression, PTSD, anxiety disorders.

(c) Ongoing occult substance abuse.

(d) Subacute delirium.

5. Review medications:

(a) Long-term anticholinergic, neuroleptic and/or anti-convulsant use is associated with cognitive impairment.

(b) Overaggressive treatment of hypertension can result in hypoxic/ischemic encephalopathy.

6. Family history:

(a) Strokes or MI at an early age suggests coagulopathy or familial hypercholesterolemia.

(b) Strong family history of diabetes mellitus should prompt search for occult diabetes.

(c) Early-onset dementia without other neurological findings suggests familial EOAD.

(d) Amyotrophic lateral sclerosis has a familial association with frontotemporal dementia.

7. Mental status examination is intended to reveal the pattern of cognitive impairment and should minimally include:

(a) Mini-Mental Status Examination.

(b) Additional tests for retrieval, such as list generation.

(c) Additional tests for attention, such as asking to recite months in reverse.

(d) Additional tests for visuospatial function, such as drawing a transparent cube.

(e) Tests of motor praxis, such as demonstrating untying and tying a shoelace.

(f) Tests of frontal lobe function, such as Luria sequencing, visual go–no go testing and general assessment of judgment.

8. Thorough neurological examination:

(a) See Table 50c.2.

9. Head imaging:

(a) Some form of head imaging should probably be performed in all cases of early-onset dementia, especially if focal neurological findings are present.

(i) While CT is readily available and inexpensive, MRI is superior in imaging the posterior fossa and in distinguishing between demyelination and edema in white matter lesions.

10. Laboratory studies:

(a) Should be tailored to the findings on history, mental status and physical examinations.

(i) The interested reader is referred to an excellent and exhaustive review of rare dementia syndromes by Reichmann and Cummings[11].

(b) All patients should be tested for blood count, electrolytes, liver panel, albumin, B_{12}, folate, VDRL, sedimentation rate.

(i) While the yield of these investagations is low, their cost is low as well, and they screen for reversible causes of dementia.

(c) ApoE genotype is reasonable in cases suspicious for EOAD, especially if there is no significant family history.

REFERENCES

1. Liston E. The clinical epidemiology of presenile dementia. *J Nerv Ment Dis* 1979; **167**: 329–36.

2. Liston E. Clinical findings in presenile dementia. *J Nerv Ment Dis* 1979; **167**: 337–42.

3. McGonigal G, Thomas B, McQuade C *et al*. Epidemiology of Alzheimer's presenile dementia in Scotland, 1974–88. *Br Med J* 1993; **306**: 680–3.

4. Newens AJ, Forster DP, Kay DW *et al*. Clinically diagnosed presenile dementia of the Alzheimer type in the Northern Health Region: ascertainment, prevalence incidence and survival. *Psychol Med* 1993; **23**: 631–44.

5. Treves T, Dorczyn AD, Zilber N *et al*. Presenile dementia in Israel. *Arch Neurol* 1986; **43**: 26–9.

6. Woodburn K, Johnstone E. Measuring the decline of a population of people with early-onset dementia in Lothian, Scotland. *Int J Geriat Psychiat* 1999; **14**: 355–61.

7. Woodburn K, Johnstone E. Ascertainment of a population of people with early-onset dementia in Lothian, Scotland. *Int J Geriat Psychiat* 1999; **14**: 362–7.

8. Jacobs D, Sano M, Marder K *et al*. Age at onset of Alzheimer's disease: relation to pattern of cognitive dysfunction and rate of decline. *Neurology* 1994; **44**: 1215–20.

9. Martin J, ed. *Scientific American Molecular Neurology*. New York, NY: Scientific American, 1998.

10. Sadovnick AD, Tuokko DA, Applegarth JR *et al*. The differential diagnosis of adult-onset metachromatic leukodystrophy and early-onset familial Alzheimer disease in an Alzheimer clinic population. *Can J Neurol Sci* 1993; **20**: 312–18.

11. Reichman W, Cummings JL. Diagnosis of rare dementia syndromes: an algorithmic approach. *J Geriat Psychiat Neurol* 1990; **3**: 73–83.

12. Gersing K, Doraiswamy PM, Krishnan KR *et al*. Vascular dementia. *Curr Opin Psychiat* 1998; **11**: 425–9.

13. Doraiswamy PM, Steffens DS, Tabrizi S, Pitchumoni S. Early recognition of Alzheimer's disease. *J Clin Psychiat* 1998; **59**(s13): 6–18.

Creutzfeldt–Jakob Disease and Other Degenerative Causes of Dementia

T. F. G. Esmonde

Royal Victoria Hospital, Belfast, UK

The following disorders may have dementia as a prominent part of the illness, but overall they are not common in clinical practice. Rarely is it possible to differentiate them on the basis of the form that the dementia takes, but other features can make them sufficiently distinctive to be worthy of description.

CREUTZFELDT–JAKOB DISEASE (CJD)

This disorder was first described in 1921[1,2], when an unusual fatal neurological illness in six cases was associated with a microscopic spongy appearance of the brain at post mortem. It is a rare, rapidly progressive dementing illness, affecting both sexes, with an onset usually after the age of 55, the exceptions being those cases associated with transmission from human-derived products or tissues, or new variant CJD. The presenting features include myoclonus, cortical blindness, pyramidal/extrapyramidal/cerebellar features and akinetic mutism. It is universally fatal, with an illness duration that rarely exceeds 6 months. No cause has been found, but the existence of similar neurological illnesses in other mammals also with spongy appearances of the brain has led to much research.

In the 1950s, a disease known as kuru was discovered in a tribe that practised cannibalism in the New Guinea highlands. This had many clinical and pathological similarities to CJD, and in 1968 the disease was transmitted to monkeys by intracerebral inoculation of extracts of kuru brain[3]. Kuru was felt to have been transmitted to other members of the the tribe through their practice of eating part of the remains of a previous kuru victim, especially the brain.

Scrapie is a spongiform encephalopathy of sheep that has been recognized for over 250 years and has been known to be transmissible to other sheep by natural means, both vertically and horizontally, since the 1930s. In 1986, cattle were also found to have developed a bovine spongiform encephalopathy (BSE)[4]. The theory advanced to account for this was that they had been exposed to scrapie through the consumption of rendered sheep remains as part of their diet.

An altered form of a normal brain protein has been found in cases of spongiform encephalopathy in both man and animals, which shows resistance to protease digestion and is known as protease-resistant protein (PrP) or "prion" protein[5]. The normal variant is encoded for by a gene on chromosome 20 in humans[6]. Already a number of mutations of this gene in cases of CJD have been discovered[7], and familial cases are invariably associated with abnormalities of the gene. Homozygosity for methionine at the site of a common polymorphism at codon 129 on the PrP gene is found with twice the normal incidence in cases of sporadic CJD[8], whereas valine homozygosity incidence is higher in cases associated with human growth hormone administration.

The possibilities of the disease being due to a viral or immunological process has largely been discounted, and current opinion is focusing on somatic mutation in the PrP gene as a possible cause.

The incidence of CJD, with few exceptions, is remarkably constant worldwide, at approximately 0.5–1/million population/ year. Clustering of cases has been recognized[9] and this is thought to represent genetic susceptibility, rather than the presence of an environmental factor. Sporadic CJD is not felt to be due to transmission from consumption of or contact with animal products[10]. Cases have occurred in recipients of human-derived products such as growth hormone, gonadotrophin, corneal grafts and dura mater grafts, and following neurosurgical procedures[11–14]. Notable amongst these have been cases in patients who received human pituitary extracts, in whom pathologically confirmed CJD was manifest 10–20 years later, suggesting a prolonged "incubation period" before the disease occurs.

Diagnosis of CJD can only be made with certainty at post mortem or by brain biopsy. However, the diagnosis has been confirmed by tonsillar biopsy in suspected cases[15], although this technique is not widely recommended in view of the possible risk to operators[16]. The finding of elevated levels of cerebrospinal fluid levels of S100 and 14-3-3 proteins is relatively specific for suspected CJD, although raised levels are also found in encephalitis[17].

The rapidity with which the dementia develops, with global cortical and subcortical components as well as the specific signs mentioned earlier, should avoid confusion with other causes of dementia. The electroencephalogram (EEG) often shows a typical appearance of generalized repetitive triphasic complexes, with virtual abolition of background rhythms, but this feature is not invariable, often occurring late in the course of the illness. Its absence in no way excludes the disorder. There is almost always a slowing of cortical rhythms into the delta range. Computed tomography (CT) scan is usually normal, but is useful to exclude other conditions. Magnetic resonance imaging (MRI) can show non-specific high signal on T2-weighted images in the basal ganglia in some cases.

There is no treatment available, although there have been isolated case reports of slowing of the rate of progression of the disorder with amantadine[18].

Principles and Practice of Geriatric Psychiatry, 2nd edn. Edited by J. R. M. Copeland, M. T. Abou-Saleh and D. G. Blazer
©2002 John Wiley & Sons, Ltd

NEW VARIANT CJD

The first cases of new variant CJD appeared in 1995, when individuals under the age of 40 years developed a rapidly progressive dementing illness, and pathological analysis at post mortem confirmed the typical features of spongiform encephalopathy[19]. There were a number of important differences to typical sporadic CJD, however:

1. Many of the cases presented with features of a psychiatric disorder, such as anxiety, depression or hysteria.
2. The development of the dementia was more slowly progressive than in typical cases of CJD.
3. The typical changes of triphasic complexes on the EEG were lacking.
4. Brain microscopy revealed far more extensive PrP-positive plaques.

The evidence that these cases may be directly linked to BSE in cattle is compelling in that the PrP protein in these cases is biochemically very similar to that found in cases of BSE, and the incubation time of transmitted cases in transgenic mice expressing the human PrP gene is identical to that of transmitted BSE cases[20]. Up to September 2001, 107 cases had been described, one of which was in an elderly man aged 74.

MULTISYSTEM ATROPHY (SHY–DRAGER SYNDROME), PROGRESSIVE SUPRANUCLEAR PALSY (PSP) (STEELE–RICHARDSON–OLSZEWSKI SYNDROME), DENTATOPALLIDO–LUYSIAN ATROPHY AND OLIVOPONTOCEREBELLAR ATROPHY (OPCA)

Dementia is not an invariable accompaniment of any of the above, but thorough cognitive testing will often reveal deficits, especially in late cases. The dementia may be of frontal lobe type or sub-cortical but not severe, and may be masked by other clinical features that are more prominent[21].

Nomenclature of the above conditions is subject to debate. Extrapyramidal features are seen in most, although a clinical presentation with prominent cerebellar features tends to result in a patient being labelled as OPCA and pronounced autonomic failure as Shy–Drager syndrome, but the pathological changes of cell loss and gliosis in all are similar and may also be present in the same sites, although to varying degrees. Only in PSP is there a clearly distinct clinical presentation and histological appearance.

The early signs in all the above conditions are usually rigidity in muscle tone, bradykinesia of movement and postural instability. The signs are usually bilateral and progress over months and years.

In PSP, first described in 1964[22], there is characteristically a loss of conjugate voluntary eye movements, beginning with vertical gaze. The range of eye movement is improved if the patient is made to fixate on a target and the head moved. Upper motor neurone limb signs are common, and dystonic posturing of neck muscles resulting in extension is often seen. Reduction in verbal fluency is a prominent feature of the condition, and it has been postulated that this is due to interruption of fronto-basal circuitry[23]. The condition is confirmed pathologically by the finding of neuronal loss, neurofibrillary tangles and gliosis primarily affecting the subthalamic nucleus, globus pallidus, dentate, substantia nigra, locus coeruleus, periaqueductal grey matter and other brainstem nuclei.

Multisystem atrophy (MSA) results in a degenerative process affecting neurones throughout the central nervous system (CNS) and thus the signs may be widespread, with involvement of corticospinal tracts and especially the autonomic system. Diag-

nosis is usually clinical and may be strongly suspected when there are additional signs, such as laryngeal stridor or denervation of the urethral sphincter on electromyography.

Dentatorubral-pallido-luysian atrophy is an autosomal dominant disorder that has been found to be linked with a trinucleotide repeated on the B37 gene of chromosome 12. The clinical features include seizures, chorea, dementia, ataxia, mental retardation and psychiatric disease. Abnormalities are seen in the subcortical white matter.

Other investigations in this group of conditions are usually normal, although evidence of cortical atrophy may be present in late cases on the CT scan, and a case has been made for the differentiation of PSP from other causes of extrapyramidal syndromes and dementia by subtle findings on CT[24].

The parkinsonian features in these disorders are often resistant to treatment with conventional anti-parkinsonian drugs. In the case of MSA, L-dopa therapy can exacerbate symptoms of postural hypotension due to the coexistent autonomic neuropathy. The disorders are therefore treated along supportive lines, although MSA may require more specific drug therapy, directed at features such as postural hypotension.

In all the above disorders, depression can be a common accompanying symptom, as patients are aware of the restriction in activity caused by the disease. This may require separate treatment.

As mentioned earlier, a dementing illness may also occur, especially in the later stages. However, this may be overlooked if poor performance on a task is attributed to slowness of response or the effects of drug therapy.

MOTOR NEURONE DISEASE

This disorder, which primarily causes loss of both upper and lower motor neurones, can also be associated with a dementia. Dementia is detectable in approximately 5% of cases, although its existence may be obscured if the patient is rendered anarthric and paralysed. It may preceded the onset of the typical signs of motor neurone disease in about 50% of cases, and is more common in those with a bulbar onset or in familial cases. Myoclonus has been noted in up to 15% of cases and this is probably what has been responsible for the confusion with Creutzfeldt–Jakob disease—with many of these cases being previously labelled as the "amyotrophic form of CJD", although the other clinical features of CJD, the typical EEG findings and laboratory transmission to animals, were lacking[25]. The dementia is typically "frontal" in type, with deficits in attention, learning, naming, insight and judgement[26].

ALS may also occur in association with both parkinsonism and dementia, with the dementia being indistinguishable from that occurring in Alzheimer's disease. The age of onset was almost the same for the parkinsonism, ALS and dementia, indicating that they are probably of the same aetiology.

The studies in Guam[27] have shown the development of a parkinsonism–dementia–ALS disease on exposure of individuals to the toxins from the cycad plant. In the review by Hudson[28], it is proposed that this link between the three modes of presentation may indicate that the disorders may be variants of the same disease and not unique to Guam.

NORMAL PRESSURE HYDROCEPHALUS

The title of this condition is a misnomer, as the cerebrospinal fluid (CSF) pressure is raised, but only intermittently, to produce what are known as "B" waves on continuous CSF pressure recordings. However, classic symptoms of raised intracranial pressure are absent, the patient presenting with a triad of symptoms comprising dementia, gait dyspraxia and urinary incontinence. Cerebral atrophy is seen on CT scan, but the condition may be suspected when the ventricles are disproportionately large in comparison with the degree of sulcal widening. Unfortunately there is no reliable diagnostic test, as evidenced by recent reports in the literature[29]. Some claims have been made for isotope cisternography, which shows delayed passage of radioactivity from the ventricles to the area surrounding the cerebral convexities. Treatment is by the insertion of a CSF shunt, and in some cases this has even been used as the definitive diagnostic test. No cause has been found to account for the condition, although in some cases a "secondary" form is recognized as being due to previous meningeal inflammation or head injury and subsequent impairment of CSF uptake.

POST-TRAUMATIC DEMENTIA

Dementia pugilistica in boxers presents as a progressive neurological disease with involvement of pyramidal, extrapyramidal and cerebellar systems, in addition to memory loss and personality change. The onset may be many years after the cessation of a boxing career. The pathological appearances resemble those of Alzheimer's disease, but neurofibrillary tangles predominate, with an absence of plaques[30].

HUNTINGTON'S DISEASE

This autosomal dominant inherited condition, with an onset usually after the age of 30 and rarely after the age of 70, has choreiform movements and dementia as its most common presenting features. Diagnosis can now be confirmed by analysing the huntingtin gene on chromosome 5 for CAG triplet repeats in excess of 35. Atrophy of the caudate nucleus may be seen in typical cases on CT or MRI scan. The dementia does differ from that of Alzheimer's disease by virtue of the fact that there is more difficulty with tests of letter fluency and the copying of geometric features[31], indicating that the dementia is of the subcortical type.

FAMILIAL SPASTIC PARAPARESIS, OR SPINOCEREBELLAR ATROPHY ASSOCIATED WITH DEMENTIA

These conditions are considered together as both may produce a dementing-type illness which is in itself indistinguishable from other forms of dementia, but is set apart by the presence of other signs, such as a spastic paraparesis or a cerebellar syndrome. In both, the dementia advances only slowly, and may only be a minor feature of the illness, although recent work has shown that the cognitive impairment may be subclinical in some kindreds and overlooked with routine clinical screening tests[32].

PROGRESSIVE SUBCORTICAL GLIOSIS

This condition, described in 1967, presents as a dementing process with subcortical features and may mimic Alzheimer's disease. Infrequent findings are signs of extrapyramidal involvement, and cases with supranuclear gaze palsy have been described[33]. The clinical course extends over years, often with a final akinetic mute stage. The cardinal pathological feature is intense gliosis and astrocytic hyperplasia affecting the subcortical structures of the thalamus, basal ganglia, brainstem grey matter and ventral horns of the spinal cord.

CORTICO-BASAL DEGENERATION

The more prominent signs of extrapyramidal dystonias, cortical sensory loss, dyspraxia, myoclonus (often focal) and the "alien hand" sign, tend to obscure a slowly developing dementia which is usually cortical in nature. The presence of ideomotor dyspraxia may help to distinguish this extrapyramidal syndrome from disorders such as PSP[34]. The mean age of onset in a series of 15 patients was 60 years[35]. No investigation is diagnostic, and confirmation of the diagnosis is by finding nerve cell loss and gliosis in the frontoparietal cortex and extrapyramidal system.

DEMENTIA LACKING SPECIFIC HISTOLOGICAL FEATURES

As well as being without specific histology, the pattern of dementia is unremarkable, being of a frontal lobe type more closely resembling Pick's disease, with many cases also showing extrapyramidal features. The pathological features are cortical vacuolation and astrocytosis in the deeper layers, without neurofibrillary tangles, plaques or Pick or Lewy bodies.

REFERENCES

1. Creutzfeldt HG. Uber eine eigenartige herdformige Ekrankung des Zentralnervensystems. *Z Ces Neurol Psychiat* 1920; **57**: 1–18.
2. Jakob A. Uber eigenartige Erkrankungen des Zentralnervensystems mit bemerkenswertem anatomischen Befunde (spastiche Pseudosclerose-Encephalomyelopathie mit disseminierten Degenerationsherden) *Z Ces Neurol Psychiat* 1921; **64**; 147.
3. Gajdusek DC, Gibbs CJ Jr, Alpers M. Transmission and passage of experimental "kuru" to chimpanzees. *Nature* 1966; **209**: 794–6.
4. Wells GAH, Scott AC, Johnson CT *et al*. A novel progressive spongiform encephalopathy in cattle. *Vet Rec* 1987; **121**: 419–20.
5. Oesch B, Westaway D, Walchli M *et al*. A cellular gene encodes scrapie PrP2730 protein. *Cell* 1985; **40**: 735–46.
6. Sparkes RS, Simon M, Cohn VH *et al*. Assignment of the human and mouse prion genes to homologous chromosomes. *Proc Natl Acad Sci USA* 1986; **83**: 7358–62.
7. Goldfarb LG, Mitrova E, Brown P *et al*. Mutation in codon 200 of scrapie amyloid protein gene in two clusters of Creutzfeldt–Jakob disease in Slovakia. *Lancet* 1990; **336**: 514–15.
8. Windl O, Dempster M, Estibeiro JP *et al*. Genetic basis of Creutzfeldt–Jakob disease in the United Kingdom: a systematic analysis of predisposing mutations and allelic variation in the PRNP gene. *Hum Genet* 1996; **98**: 259–64.
9. Mayer V, Orolin D, Mitrova E, Lehotsky T. Transmissible virus dementia. An unusual space and time clustering of Creutzfeldt–Jakob disease and of other organic presenile dementia cases. *Acta Virol* 1978; **22**: 146–53.
10. Cousens SN, Zeidler M, Esmonde TF *et al*. Sporadic Creutzfeldt–Jakob disease in the United Kingdom: analysis of epidemiological surveillance data for 1970–96. *Br Med J* 1997; **315**(7105): 389–95.
11. Cochius JI, Mack K, Burns RJ *et al*. Creutzfeldt–Jakob disease in a recipient of human pituitary-derived gonadotrophin. *Aust NZ J Med* 1990; **20**: 592–3.
12. Rappaport EB, Graham DJ. Pituitary growth hormone from human cadavers: neurologic disease in ten recipients. *Neurology* 1987; **37**: 1211–15.
13. Duffy P, Wolf J, Collins G *et al*. Possible person-to-person transmission of Creutzfeldt–Jakob disease. *N Engl J Med* 1974; **290**: 692–3.
14. Will RG, Matthews WB. Evidence for case-to-case transmission of Creutzfeldt–Jakob disease. *J Neurol Neurosurg Psychiat* 1982; **45**: 235–8.
15. Hill AF, Butterworth RJ, Joiner S *et al*. Investigation of variant Creutzfeldt–Jakob disease and other human prion diseases with tonsil biopsy samples. *Lancet* 1999; **353**(9148): 183–9.

16. Zeidler M, Knight R, Stewart G *et al.* Diagnosis of Creutzfeldt–Jakob disease. Routine tonsil biopsy for new variant Creutzfeldt–Jakob disease is not justified. *Br Med J* 1999; **319**(7182): 538.

17. Hsich G, Kenney K, Gibbs CJ *et al.* The 14-3-3 brain protein in cerebrospinal fluid as a marker for transmissible spongiform encephalopathies. *N Engl J Med* 1996; **33**(13): 924–30.

18. Sanders WL. Creutzfeldt–Jakob disease treated with amantadine. *J Neurol Neurosurg Psych* 1979; **42**: 960–1.

19. Will RG, Ironside JW, Zeidler M *et al.* A new variant of Creutzfeldt–Jakob disease in the UK. *Lancet* 1996; **347**(9006): 921–5.

20. Bruce ME, Will RG, Ironside JW *et al.* Transmissions to mice indicate that "new variant" CJD is caused by the BSE agent. *Nature* 1997; **389**(6650): 498–501.

21. Berent S, Giordani B, Gilman S *et al.* Neuropsychological changes in olivopontocerebellar atrophy. *Arch Neurol* 1990; **47**: 997–1001.

22. Steele JC, Richardson JC, Olszewski J. Progressive supranuclear palsy. *Arch Neurol* 1964; **10**: 333–59.

23. Esmonde T, Giles E, Xuereb J, Hodges JR. Progressive supranuclear palsy presenting with dynamic aphasia. *J Neurol Neurosurg Psychiat* 1996; **60**: 403–10.

24. Ambrosetto P. CT in progressive supranuclear palsy. *Am J Neuroradiol* 1987; **8**: 849–51.

25. Salazar AM, Masters CL, Gajdusek DC, Gibbs CJ Jr. Syndromes of amyotrophic lateral sclerosis and dementia: relation to transmissible Creutzfeldt–Jakob disease. *Ann Neurol* 1983; **14**: 17–26.

26. Tandan R. Clinical features and differential diagnosis of classical motor neuron disease. In Williams AC, ed., *Motor Neuron Disease.* London: Chapman & Hall Medical, 1994; 3–28.

27. Tan NT, Kakulas BA, Masters CL *et al.* Neuropathology of the cortical lesions of the Parkinsonian–dementia (PD) complex of Guam. *Proc Aust Assoc Neurol* 1981; **17**: 227–34.

28. Hudson AJ. Amyotrophic lateral sclerosis and its association with dementia, Parkinsonism and other related disorders: a review. *Brain* 1981; **104**: 217–47.

29. Benzel EC, Pelletier AL, Levy PG. Communicating hydrocephalus in adults: prediction of outcome after ventricular shunting procedures. *Neurosurgery* 1990; **26**: 655–60.

30. Roberts GW, Allsop D, Bruton C. The occult aftermath of boxing. *J Neurol Neurosurg Psychiat* 1990; **53**: 373–8.

31. Hodges JR, Salmon DP, Butters N. Differential impairment of semantic and episodic memory in Alzheimer's and Huntington's diseases: a controlled prospective study. *J Neurol Neurosurg Psychiat* 1990; **53**: 1089–95.

32. Storey E, Forrest SM, Shaw JH *et al.* Spinocerebellar ataxia type 2: clinical features of a pedigree displaying prominent frontal–executive dysfunction. *Arch Neurol* 1999; **56**(1): 13–50.

33. Will RG, Lees AJ, Gibb W, Barnard RO. A case of progressive subcortical gliosis presenting clinically as Steele–Richardson–Olszewski syndrome. *J Neurol Neurosurg Psychiat* 1988; **51**: 1224–7.

34. Soliveri P, Monza D, Paridi D *et al.* Cognitive and magnetic resonance imaging aspects of corticobasal degeneration and progressive supranuclear palsy. *Neurology* 1999; **53**: 502–7.

35. Riley DE, Lang AE, Lewis A *et al.* Corticobasal ganglionic degeneration. *Neurology* 1990; **40**: 1203–12.

Frontotemporal Dementia (Pick's Disease)

John R. Hodges

MRC Cognition and Brain Sciences Unit, Cambridge, UK

"Frontotemporal dementia" is the term currently preferred to describe patients with focal cortical atrophy involving the frontal and/or temporal lobes. Pathologically, such patients show severe neuronal loss, spongiosis and gliosis, and in a minority of cases classic argyrophilic, tau-positive intraneuronal inclusions are present (Pick bodies). The hallmark changes of Alzheimer's disease are virtually always absent[1].

One of the most exciting developments in the past decade has been the discovery of mutations in the tau gene on Chromosome 17 in some families with dominantly inherited FTD[2], although it should be stressed that most cases are sporadic. Clinically, FTD patients present with one of three major syndromes, which reflect the initial locus of pathology: dementia of frontal type, semantic dementia and progressive non-fluent aphasia[3]. It should be noted that each of these syndromes can be associated with motor neurone disease and a full neurological evaluation should also be included, especially in rapidly progressive cases and if bulbar symptoms develop[4].

Patients with FTD present below the age of 65 and there is an equal sex distribution. Although rare, FTD is the second commonest cause of dementia in the presenium (after Alzheimer's disease)[5]. In Cambridge we have studied approximately 100 cases with FTD; the rarest syndrome is non-fluent progressive aphasia, the other two account for approximately 40% of cases each. The average survival from diagnosis is, on average, 10 years. In our experience, patients with the frontal form of the disease progress at the slowest rate, semantic dementia cases have a more rapid course and those with motor neurone disease-associated FTD rarely survive more than 2 years.

DEMENTIA OF FRONTAL TYPE (DFT) (FRONTAL VARIANT FTD)

The onset of symptoms is insidious and insight is lacking. Relatives complain of a change in personality and behaviour: disinhibition, poor impulse control, antisocial behaviour, stereotypical features (e.g. insisting on eating the same food at exactly the same time daily, cleaning the house in precisely the same order or the use of a repetitive catchphrase) and a change in appetite and food preference towards sweet food are the features that best discriminate FTD from Alzheimer's disease. They reflect the early involvement of the orbitobasal frontal cortex[6,7]. Apathy is also very common but non-specific. Deficits in planning, organization and other aspects of executive function are universal as the disease progresses to involve the dorsolateral prefrontal cortex. Major depression and psychosis are rare.

A major advance in the area has been the development of a semi-structured carer interview, the Neuropsychiatric Inventory, which appears to be able to differentiate patients with FTD and AD[8].

Neuropsychological Findings

Some patients show clear-cut cognitive deficits at presentation but most traditional "frontal executive" tasks are sensitive to dorso-lateral, rather than orbitobasal frontal, dysfunction; among the most useful are the Wisconsin Card Sorting Test and verbal fluency (i.e. the generation of words beginning with a given letter of the alphabet). Recently, quantifiable tasks involving decision-making and risk-taking and better able to detect orbitobasal frontal function have been developed[9].

Memory is relatively spared: orientation and recall of personal events is good but performance of anterograde memory tests is more variable, and patients tend to do poorly on recall (as opposed to recognition)-based tasks. A reduction in spontaneous conversation is common, but patients with DFT perform well on tests involving picture naming and other semantically-based tasks. Visuo-spatial abilities are strikingly preserved, particularly when the organization aspects are minimized: the Rey figure test is often copied poorly due to impulsiveness and poor strategy[10].

Simple cognitive screening tests, such as the Mini-Mental State Examination (MMSE), are unreliable for the detection and monitoring of patients with DFT, who frequently perform normally even when requiring nursing home care[11].

SEMANTIC DEMENTIA (TEMPORAL LOBE VARIANT FTD)

Patients with this variant of FTD present with a progressive fluent aphasia but the underlying cognitive deficit is a breakdown in semantic memory[3,12]. Semantic memory is the term applied to the component of long-term memory which contains the permanent representation of things in the world, including objects, words and people. It is the database which gives meaning to our sensory experiences.

Patients complain of "loss of memory for words". Although aware of their shrinking expressive vocabulary, patients are strangely oblivious to their impaired comprehension. Since the grammatical and phonological structure of language remains intact, the changes are relatively subtle, at least in the early stages. Patients with predominant right-sided atrophy may present with difficulty recognizing faces (prosopagnosia), at first affecting less commonly encountered people but with time severe prosopagnosia

Principles and Practice of Geriatric Psychiatry, 2nd edn. Edited by J. R. M. Copeland, M. T. Abou-Saleh and D. G. Blazer
©2002 John Wiley & Sons, Ltd

develops: in contrast to the true modality-specific prosopagnosia, which occasionally complicates right occipitotemporal strokes, the deficit in semantic dementia is cross-modal, so that patients are also impaired in the identification of names and voices[13].

In contrast to Alzheimer's disease, patients with semantic dementia are well orientated and have good episodic (day-to-day and autobiographical) memory, although recent studies have shown that the preservation applies only to recent memories. That is to say, they show a reversal of the temporal gradient found in amnesia and Alzheimer's disease[14].

Behavioural changes may be slight at presentation but with time features identical to those seen in DFT emerge and may be striking in patients with right-sided disease[15].

Neuropsychological Findings

The impairment of knowledge is most apparent on tasks requiring a verbal output, such as category fluency tests (in which subjects are asked to produce as many examples as possible from defined semantic categories, such as animals, within 1 minute), picture naming and the generation of verbal definitions to words and pictures. The pattern of errors reflects a loss of fine-grained knowledge, with preservation of superordinate information: on naming tasks, naming errors are initially category co-ordinates ("elephant" for hippopotamus), then with time prototype responses emerge, so that all animals are called "dog", then eventually they are simply called "animal". Single-word comprehension is also affected, as judged by tasks such as word–picture matching or synonym tasks (e.g. which of the following is the odd one out, "pond, lake or river"). Non-verbal semantic knowledge is less easy to assess, but the Pyramids and Palm Trees Test in which the subject is asked to judge the semantic relatedness of pictures, invariably reveals deficits[10,16].

In contrast to the profound semantic deficit, other aspects of language competency (phonology and syntax) are strikingly preserved. Although able to read and spell words with regular spelling-to-sound correspondence, virtually all cases have difficulty in reading and spelling irregular words (e.g. reading PINT to rhyme with hint, flint, etc.). This pattern, known as surface dyslexia (or dysgraphia), has been attributed to the loss of semantic support which is necessary for the correct pronunciation of irregular words. Patients perform normally on non-verbal problem-solving tasks, such as Raven's Matrices, and on tests of perceptual and spatial ability.

NON-FLUENT PROGRESSIVE APHASIA

The status of patients with the non-fluent form of progressive aphasia within the spectrum of FTD is less certain. Changes in behaviour are rare, but after a number of years global cognitive decline occurs. Unlike the other syndromes, a number of non-fluent cases have Alzheimer pathology[17].

Patients present with complaints of speech dysfluency and distortion or word-finding difficulty. Phonological errors are usually obvious in conversation. Comprehension is relatively well preserved, at least in the early stages, although as the disease progresses there are problems with phoneme discrimination, which the patients invariably attribute to poor hearing. In the late stages patients become mute and effectively "word deaf". Day-to-day memory is good and patients cope well in everyday life.

Neuropsychological Findings

The pattern of cognitive deficits in progressive non-fluent aphasia is the mirror image to that found in semantic dementia. They perform well on tests of semantic memory, except on those requiring a spoken output. Although conversational speech is severely disrupted, the anomia is mild and the errors are phonological (efelant for elephant). Semantic category fluency is less affected than letter fluency. Word–picture matching, synonym tasks and other semantic tests are usually performed perfectly. They perform poorly on tests of phonological competence (such as repetition of multisyllabic words and rhyming) and syntactic comprehension[16]. In common with the other syndromes, however, performance on visuo-spatial and perceptual function is well preserved.

NEURORADIOLOGICAL FINDINGS IN FTD

CT scans are of limited value in diagnosis: the temporal lobes are poorly seen due to bone artefacts but MRI with coronal images is extremely valuable, especially in cases with semantic dementia who show focal atrophy of the polar region, fusiform and infero-lateral gyri with relative sparing of the hippocampal formation. An asymmetric pattern is almost invariable, with the left temporal lobe much more often involved than the right[18]. In non-fluent cases the changes are more subtle, with widening of the left Sylvian fissure. In dementia of frontal type, atrophy of the orbitofrontal cortex can be seen, but ^{99}Tc–HMPAO–SPECT is more valuable: focal hypoperfusion is apparent before clear structural changes are obvious[11,19].

MANAGEMENT

The management of patients and their families requires a specialist multidisciplinary team approach with input from clinical psychology, genetics, psychiatry and neurology. Counselling, especially with regard to genetic implications and prognosis, are essential at an early stage. Although there are, at present, no therapies that will affect the course of the disease, many of the symptoms can be helped. The stereotypical features, disinhibition and overeating, may respond to serotonin reuptake blockers[20]. Neuroleptic drugs may be necessary to control aggressive behaviour.

REFERENCES

1. Jackson M, Lowe J. The new neuropathology of degenerative frontotemporal dementias. *Acta Neuropathol* 1996; **91**: 127–34.
2. Goedert M, Crowther RA, Spillantini MG. Tau mutations cause frontotemporal dementias. *Neuron* 1998; **21**: 955–8.
3. Snowden JS, Neary D, Mann DMA. *Frontotemporal Lobar Degeneration: Frontotemporal Dementia, Progressive Aphasia, Semantic Dementia.* New York: Churchill Livingstone, 1996.
4. Bak T, Hodges JR. Cognition, language and behaviour in motor neurone disease: evidence of frontotemporal dementia. *Dement Geriat Cogn Disord* 1999; **10**: 29–32.
5. Harvey RJ. Epidemiology of pre-senile dementia. In Hodges JR, ed., *Early Onset Dementia.* Oxford: Oxford University Press, 2001; 1–23.
6. Gregory CA, Hodges JR. Frontotemporal dementia: use of consensus criteria and prevalence of psychiatric features. *Neuropsychiat Neuropsychol Behav Neurol* 1996; **9**: 145–53.
7. Miller BL, Darby A, Benson DF, Cummings JL, Miller MH. Aggressive, socially disruptive and antisocial behaviour associated with fronto-temporal dementia. *Br J Psychiat* 1997; **170**: 150–5.
8. Levy ML, Miller BL, Cummings JL *et al.* Alzheimer disease and frontotemporal dementias: behavioral distinctions. *Arch Neurol* 1996; **53**: 687–90.
9. Rahman S, Sahakian BJ, Hodges JR *et al.* Specific cognitive deficits in early frontal variant frontotemporal dementia. *Brain* 1999; **122**: 1469–93.

10. Hodges JR, Patterson K, Ward R *et al.* The differentiation of semantic dementia and frontal lobe dementia (temporal and frontal variants of frontotemporal dementia) from early Alzheimer's disease: a comparative neuropsychological study. *Neuropsychology* 1999; **13**: 31–40.

11. Gregory CA, Serra-Mestres J, Hodges JR. The early diagnosis of the frontal variant of frontotemporal dementia: how sensitive are standard neuroimaging and neuropsychological tests? *Neuropsychiat Neuropsychol Behav Neurol* 1999; **12**: 128–35.

12. Hodges JR, Patterson K, Oxbury S, Funnell E. Semantic dementia: progressive fluent aphasia with temporal lobe atrophy. *Brain* 1992; **115**: 1783–806.

13. Evans JJ, Heggs AJ, Antoun N, Hodges JR. Progressive prosopagnosia associated with selective right temporal lobe atrophy: a new syndrome? *Brain* 1995; **118**: 1–13.

14. Graham KS, Hodges JR. Differentiating the roles of the hippocampal complex and the neocortex in long-term memory storage: evidence from the study of semantic dementia and Alzheimer's disease. *Neuropsychology* 1997; **11**: 77–89.

15. Edwards Lee T, Miller B, Benson F *et al.* The temporal variant of frontotemporal dementia. *Brain* 1997; **120**: 1027–40.

16. Hodges JR, Patterson K. Non-fluent progressive aphasia and semantic dementia: a comparative neuropsychological study. *J Int Neuropsychol Soc* 1996; **2**: 511–24.

17. Galton CJ, Patterson K, Xuereb JH, Hodges JR. Atypical and typical presentations of Alzheimer's disease: a clinical, neuropsychological, neuroimaging and pathological study of 13 cases. *Brain* 2001; **123**: 484–91.

18. Mummery CJ, Patterson K, Price CJ *et al.* A voxel-based morphometry study of semantic dementia: the relationship between temporal lobe atrophy and semantic memory. *Ann Neurol* 2000; **47**: 36–40.

19. Miller BL, Ikonte C, Ponton M *et al.* A study of the Lund–Manchester research criteria for frontotemporal dementia: clinical and single photon emission CT correlations. *Neurology* 1997; **48**: 937–42.

20. Rahman S, Sahakian BJ, Gregory CA. Drug interventions in dementia. In Hodges JR, ed., *Early Onset Dementia*. Oxford: Oxford University Press, 2001; 422–48.

52

Alcoholic and Other Toxic Dementias

E. M. Joyce

Imperial College School of Medicine, London, UK

ALCOHOLIC DEMENTIA

The concept of a dementia consequent upon the effects of long-term alcohol abuse developed from clinical observations of a gradual deterioration in personality and intellect in many alcoholics. Recent studies suggest that this is age-related, is milder in degree than the neurodegenerative dementias and can be present in 11–24% of demented patients[1-3]. Alcoholic dementia was originally considered to be distinct from the amnesia of the Wernicke–Korsakoff syndrome, which also occurs in alcoholics but is caused by thiamine malnutrition rather than alcohol neurotoxicity. Horvath[4] prospectively examined 100 chronic alcoholics presenting with a dementia syndrome and concluded that "alcoholic dementia" is not synonymous with the Wernicke–Korsakoff syndrome, and that other non-amnesic organic syndromes exist in alcoholics, characteristic of frontal, parietal or global cortical damage. Cutting[5] performed a retrospective case-note analysis of alcoholic patients with cognitive impairment and found two forms of clinical presentation. One consisted of a rapidly developing illness in younger patients with preserved intellect, akin to the traditional Wernicke–Korsakoff syndrome, whereas the other was more characteristic of dementia, being a gradual and global cognitive deterioration in older patients.

This concept was soon challenged by the results of clinicopathological studies. Torvick et al.[6] examined the clinical records of patients who, at autopsy, had diencephalic lesions characteristic of thiamine malnutrition. Of these, 75% were considered to be demented in life rather than amnesic and the majority had no additional neuropathological hallmarks of a neurodegenerative dementia. Torvick et al. concluded that the diencephalic lesions of thiamine deficiency can result in the clinical pictures of both "alcoholic dementia" and the Wernicke–Korsakoff syndrome. Victor and Adams[7] then pointed out that 10% of their pathologically-proven cases of the Wernicke–Korsakoff syndrome developed cognitive abnormalities insidiously, rather than acutely[8], and that cognitive impairments other than amnesia, and behavioural abnormalities such as inertia and apathy, can be demonstrated in these patients[9]. Thus, they argued that, depending on the severity of the non-mnemonic deficits or the mode of presentation, cases of the Wernicke–Korsakoff syndrome may be misattributed as cases of alcoholic dementia. The neuropathological studies of Harper and colleagues[10,11,62] are in agreement with this. They found that two-thirds of the alcoholics coming to post mortem in their unit had lesions of thiamine deficiency, yet only one-third of these had received a clinical diagnosis of Wernicke–Korsakoff syndrome in life. In the remainder, the most common diagnosis was dementia.

Thus far, the evidence points to the conclusion that subcortical lesions caused by thiamine malnutrition can be sufficient to explain both amnesia and dementia witnessed in alcoholics. However, Victor and Adams[7] and Torvick et al.[6] did not assume that all cases of alcoholic dementia are unrecognized cases of the Wernicke–Korsakoff syndrome. Both considered that superadded cerebral lesions may explain the dementia-like presentation of a proportion of patients with the Wernicke–Korsakoff syndrome. Because these additional lesions can be attributed to a variety of pathological processes, including chronic hepatocerebral degeneration, communicating hydrocephalus, Alzheimer's disease and ischaemic infarction, they argued that there is no need to invoke a special process of alcohol neurotoxicity. More recent research supports this contention. Kasahara et al.[2] compared young (35–45 years) and old (>60 years) alcoholics and found evidence of dementia only in the older group. Most cases had additional medical diagnoses, including hypertension, liver disease and cardiomyopathy, and no case of dementia could be accounted for by the direct effect of alcohol.

Although dementia in alcoholics is unlikely to be caused solely by alcohol neurotoxicity, there is compelling evidence to suggest that alcohol is neurotoxic. Carefully controlled neuropathological studies have frequently found whole brain atrophy, predominantly involving the white matter, in chronic alcoholics[12-16]. Neuronal death has been found in specific areas of the frontal association cortex[17-19] and neuronal shrinkage in the cingulate and motor cortex[17,20,21]. The contribution of liver failure to this neuropathology has been assessed in several studies and the bulk of evidence suggests that cirrhosis alone does not account for the brain shrinkage witnessed in alcoholics[13,15,22]. However, existing studies of the contribution of thiamine malnutrition to such findings are equivocal with evidence that thiamine deficiency both does and does not cause the cortical damage seen in alcoholics[13,15]. Medial temporal lobe limbic structures, i.e. the hippocampus and the amygdala, have been foci of interest because of their involvement in cognitive function. Reduced volumes have been reported in alcoholics but, again, it is not clear whether it is alcohol *per se* or thiamine deficiency that accounts for this[16,19,23-25].

It can be concluded from these studies that: (a) alcohol itself can cause neuronal damage; (b) liver disease *per se* is not a major factor in the aetiology of the neuropathological changes; and (c) thiamine malnutrition potentiates the neurotoxic effect of alcohol on the brain. Butterworth[26] proposes mechanisms to explain these conclusions. He argues that thiamine deficiency is common in alcoholism because of poor diet and gastrointestinal disorder. Alcohol and its metabolite acetylaldehyde are directly neurotoxic and have toxic effects on thiamine-dependent enzymes in brain and liver. In turn, liver disease disrupts thiamine homeostasis and causes astrocytic damage. The latter results in the loss of neuron–astrocyte trafficking of neuroactive amino acids and thiamine esters essential to CNS function. Thus, there are several possible routes to the production of brain damage in alcoholics. Further, these appear to be so interlinked that it may be unproductive to try and dissect the separate contribution of alcohol and thiamine deficiency to brain damage. Rather, it appears that a combination of malnutrition and alcohol intake can give rise to a range of cognitive deficits, from mild cognitive impairment to severe dementia, depending on the severity of the contributory abnormal mechanisms described by Butterworth.

Although the evidence points to alcohol being neurotoxic, the relationship between this and cognitive impairment is not clear. A major drawback of neuropathological studies is that such inferences have been either not possible or gleaned by retrospective case note analysis. In contrast, neuroimaging allows the prospective analysis of clinical features in relation to *in vivo* brain structural and functional abnormalities. Well-controlled, prospective studies using both CT and MRI have reliably confirmed the presence of cerebral shrinkage in alcoholics in life, involving both cortical grey and subcortical white matter[27-34] which are more pronounced in older patients[35] and more apparent in the frontal lobe[36,37]. The percentage of alcoholics with evidence of cerebral atrophy on brain scans is far in excess of that noted in neuropathological studies[12]. This discrepancy is probably explained by the finding that brain changes are reversible with continuing abstinence[29,33,34,38-42] indicating that neuroimaging findings do not accurately reflect the permanent neuropathological changes previously described. Some studies have found that the neuroimaging changes worsen in patients who continue to drink[41,43,44]. A recent carefully controlled study, in which alcoholic men and controls were followed over 5 years[45] found that a greater total alcohol consumption was associated with greater decrease in cortical grey matter, particularly in the frontal lobe. Thus, it is possible that prolonged alcohol ingestion leads to irreversible brain damage, which might be mirrored by irreversible cognitive deficits.

There is certainly no doubt that cognitive dysfunction can be witnessed in uncomplicated alcoholics, even though these may not reach the severity required for a diagnosis of dementia. Parsons[46], following decades of his own research, concludes that both male and female sober adult alcoholics have deficits on tests of learning, memory, abstracting, problem-solving, perceptual analysis and synthesis, and speed of information processing, which are equivalent to those found in patients with known brain dysfunction of a mild to moderate nature. Such abnormalities can also be witnessed in adolescent alcoholics[47]. Further attempts to identify factors other than alcoholism to account for these differences have been unsuccessful[46]. It is noticeable, however, that, like neuroimaging studies, these deficits are largely reversible over weeks or years of abstinence[46,48]. This may explain why studies relating cognitive and structural changes in alcoholics found weak and inconsistent correlations, the majority of which were explained mainly by age and premorbid IQ[27-30,50].

Functional imaging studies have been a bit more fruitful in this regard. One study found a reduction in overall cerebral glucose utilization[51] but all other studies found specific regional changes. For example, Samson *et al.*[52] have shown a relative decrease in glucose utilization within the medial frontal cortex of six recently detoxified neurologically intact chronic alcoholics, and Gilman *et al.*[53] have also reported the same finding in 14 alcoholics studied after at least 27 days of abstinence. In the latter study, patients made errors on the category sorting test, a test of frontal lobe function, and this correlated with glucose utilization in the medial frontal cortex. However, in a small-scale follow-up study from the same group, these deficits were partially reversible with abstinence[54] and it is not clear whether they become irreversible with continued drinking.

DISCUSSION

There are several conclusions that can be made from these studies concerning the validity of alcoholic dementia. First, diffuse cognitive impairment in alcoholic patients is common. It is an age-related phenomenon and the cognitive deficits are more mild than in patients with neurodegenerative dementias. Alcohol itself can produce irreversible brain damage, mainly of white matter and the frontal association cortex, but most studies suggest that frank dementia cannot be ascribed entirely to alcohol neurotoxicity. Other causes should therefore be sought, most notably thiamine deficiency. In younger patients, alcohol alone can also produce diffuse cognitive and cerebral abnormalities but these are largely reversible with abstinence. It remains to be determined which factors lead to the permanent alcohol-induced neuropathology seen at post mortem.

OTHER TOXIC DEMENTIAS IN THE ELDERLY

The acute and chronic psychiatric effects of ingestion of drugs of abuse, including those most relevant to the elderly—barbiturates and benzodiazepines—have been extensively reviewed by Lishman[55]. Suffice it to say that there is little evidence to suggest that these produce diffuse cognitive impairment. The neuropsychiatric effects of long-term occupational solvent exposure is also relevant to the elderly. Although there is controversy concerning whether solvents *per se* produce long-lasting effects, most studies find evidence for lasting neuropsychological abnormalities[56-59]. Of particular interest is that these studies also found that a combination of long-term solvent exposure and alcohol abuse is a particular risk factor for the development of dementia. Of final relevance to this age group is the identification of bismuth encephalopathy, which results from the over-ingestion of bismuth-containing compounds commonly taken for gastric irritation and sold without prescription. Following an acute organic reaction characterized by delirium, seizures and neurological abnormalities, persistent sequelae of diffuse cognitive impairment and cerebral atrophy have been documented[60,61].

REFERENCES

1. Carlen PL, McAndrews MP, Weiss RT *et al.* Alcohol-related dementia in the institutionalised elderly. *Alcohol Clin Exp Res* 1994; **18**: 1330–4.
2. Kasahara H, Karasawa A, Ariyasu T *et al.* Alcohol dementia and alcohol delirium in aged alcoholics. *Psychiat Clin Neurosci* 1996; **50**: 115–23.
3. Woodburn K, Johnstone E. Measuring the decline of a population of people with early-onset dementia in Lothian, Scotland. *Int J Geriat Psychiat* 1999; **14**: 355–61.
4. Horvath TB. Clinical spectrum and epidemiological features of alcoholic dementia. In Rankin JG (ed.), *Alcohol, Drugs and Brain Damage.* Toronto: Alcoholism and Drug Addiction Research Foundation of Ontario, 1975; 1–16.
5. Cutting J. The relationship between Korsakov's syndrome and "alcoholic dementia". *Br J Psychiat* 1978; **132**: 240–51.
6. Torvick A, Linboe CF, Rogde S. Brain lesions in alcoholics. *J Neurol Sci* 1982; **56**: 233–48.
7. Victor M, Adams RD. The alcoholic dementias. In Vinken PJ, Bruyn GW, Klawan HL, eds, *Handbook of Clinical Neurology*, vol. 2. Amsterdam: Elsevier Science, 1986; 335–52.
8. Victor M, Adams RD, Collins GH. *The Wernicke–Korsakoff Syndrome and Related Neurological Disorders Due to Alcoholism and Malnutrition*, 2nd edn. Philadelphia, PA: Davis, 1989.
9. Talland GA. *Deranged Memory.* New York: Academic Press, 1965.
10. Harper C. Wernicke's encephalopathy: a more common disease than realised. *J Neurol Neurosurg Psychiat* 1979; **42**: 226–31.

11. Harper CG, Giles M, Finlay-Jones R. Clinical signs in the Wernicke–Korsakoff complex: a retrospective analysis of 131 cases diagnosed at necropsy. *J Neurol Neurosurg Psychiat* 1986; **49**: 341–5.

12. Harper CG, Kril J. Brain atrophy in chronic alcoholic patients: a quantitative pathological study. *J Neurol Neurosurg Psychiat* 1985; **48**: 211–17.

13. Harper CG, Kril J. If you drink your brain will shrink. Neuropathological considerations. *Alcohol Alcoholism* 1991; **1**(suppl): 375–80.

14. Harper CG, Kril JJ, Holloway RL. Brain shrinkage in chronic alcoholics: a pathological study. *Br Med J* 1985; **290**: 501–4.

15. de la Monte SM. Disproportionate atrophy of cerebral white matter in chronic alcoholics. *Arch Neurol* 1988; **45**: 990–2.

16. Jensen G, Pakkenberg B. Do alcoholics drink their neurons away? *Lancet* 1993; **342**: 1202–4.

17. Harper CG, Kril J, Daly J. Are we drinking our neurones away? *Br Med J* 1987; **294**: 534–6.

18. Harper C, Kril J. Patterns if neuronal loss in the cerebral cortex in chronic alcoholic patients. *J Neurol Sci* 1989; **92**: 81–9.

19. Kril J, Halliday G, Svoboda M, *et al*. The cerebral cortex is damaged in chronic alcoholics. *Neuroscience* 1997; **79**: 983–98.

20. Ferrer I, Fabregues I, Rairez J *et al*. Decreased number of dendritic spines on cortical pyramidal neurons in human chronic alcoholism. *Neurosci Lett* 1986; **69**: 115–19.

21. Harper C, Corbett D. Changes in the basal dendrites of cortical pyramidal cells from alcoholic patients—a quantitative Golgi study. *J Neurol Neurosurg Psychiat* 1990; **53**: 856–61.

22. Kril J. The contribution of alcohol, thiamine deficiency and cirrhosis of the liver to cerebral cortical damage in alcoholics. *Metab Brain Dis* 1995; **10**: 9–16.

23. Alvarez I, Gonzalo L, Llor J. Effects of chronic alcoholism on the amygdaloid complex. *Histol Histopathol* 1989; **4**: 183–92.

24. Harding A, Wong A, Svoboda M *et al*. Chronic alcohol consumption does not cause hippocampal neuron loss in humans. *Hippocampus* 1997; **7**: 78–87.

25. Korbo L. Glial cell loss in the hippocampus of alcoholics. *Alcohol Clin Exp Res* 1999; **23**: 164–8.

26. Butterworth R. Pathophysiology of alcoholic brain damage: synergistic effects of ethanol, thiamine deficiency and alcoholic liver disease. *Metab Brain Dis* 1995; **10**: 1–8.

27. Bergman H, Borg S, Hindmarsh T, *et al*. Computed tomography of the brain: clinical examination and neuropsychological assessment of a random sample of men from the general population. *Acta Psychiat Scand* 1980; **62**: 47–56.

28. Cala LA, Jones B, Wiley B *et al*. A computed axial tomography (CAT) study of alcohol induced cerebral atrophy, in conjunction with other correlates. *Acta Psychiat Scand* 1980; **62**: 31–40.

29. Carlen PL, Wilkinson DA. Alcoholic brain damage and reversible deficits. *Acta Psychiat Scand* 1980; **62**: 103–18.

30. Ron M. The alcoholic brain. *Psychol Med* 1983; **13**.

31. Hayakawa K, Kumagai H, Suzuki Y *et al*. MR imaging of chronic alcoholism. *Acta Radiol* 1992; **33**: 201–6.

32. Moore JW, Dunk AA, Crawford JR *et al*. Neuropsychological deficits and morphological MRI brain scan abnormalities in apparently healthy non-encephalopathic patients with cirrhosis. A controlled study. *J Hepatol* 1989; **9**: 319–25.

33. Schroth G, Naegele T, Klose U *et al*. Reversible brain shrinkage in abstinent alcoholics, measured by MRI. *Neuroradiology* 1988; **30**: 385–9.

34. Zipursky R, Lim K, Pfefferbaum A. MRI study of brain changes with short-term abstinence from alcohol. *Alcohol Clin Exp Res* 1989; **13**: 664–6.

35. Pfefferbaum A, Sullivan E, Rosenbloom M *et al*. Increase in brain cerebrospinal fluid volume is greater in older than in younger alcoholic patients: a replication study and CT/MRI comparison. *Psychiat Res* 1993; **50**: 257–73.

36. Jernigan T, Butters N, DiTraglia G *et al*. Reduced cerebral grey matter observed in alcoholics using magnetic resonance imaging. *Alcohol Clin Exp Res* 1991; **15**: 418–27.

37. Pfefferbaum A, Sullivan E, Mathalon D *et al*. Frontal lobe volume loss observed with magnetic resonance imaging in older chronic alcoholics. *Alcohol Clin Exp Res* 1997; **21**: 521–9.

38. Artman H. Reversible enlargement of the cerebral spinal fluid spaces of chronic alcoholics as measured by computer tomographic scans. *Ann J Neuroradiol* 1981; **2**: 23–7.

39. Carlen PL, Wortzman G, Holgate RC *et al*. Reversible cerebral atrophy in recently abstinent chronic alcoholics measured by computed tomography scans. *Science* 1978; **200**: 1076–8.

40. Jacobson RR. The contribution of sex and drinking history to the CT brainscan changes in alcoholics. *Psychol Med* 1986; **16**: 547–59.

41. Muuronen A, Bergman H, Hindmarsh T *et al*. Influence of improved drinking habits on brain atrophy and cognitive performance in alcoholic patients: a 5-year follow-up study. *Alcohol Clin Exp Res* 1989; **13**: 137–41.

42. Ron M, Acker W, Shaw GK *et al*. Computed tomography of the brain in chronic alcoholism. A survey and follow-up study. *Brain* 1982; **105**: 497–514.

43. Pfefferbaum A, Sullivan E, Mathalon D *et al*. Longitudinal changes in magnetic resonance imaging brain volumes in abstinent and relapsed alcoholics. *Alcohol Clin Exp Res* 1995; **19**: 1177–91.

44. Shear P, Jernigan T, Butters N. Volumetric magnetic resonance imaging quantification of longitudinal brain changes in abstinent alcoholics. *Alcohol Clin Exp Res* 1994; **18**: 172–6.

45. Pfefferbaum A, Sullivan E, Rosenbloom M *et al*. A controlled study of cortical grey matter and ventricular change in alcoholic men over a 5-year interval. *Arch Gen Psychiat* 1998; **55**: 905–12.

46. Parsons OA. Neurocognitive deficits in alcoholics and social drinkers: a continuum? *Alcohol Clin Exp Res* 1998; **22**: 954–61.

47. Brown SA, Tapert SF, Granholm E, Delis DC. Neurocognitive functioning of adolescents: effects of protracted alcohol use. *Alcohol Clin Exp Res* 2000; **24**: 164–71.

48. Mann K, Gunther A, Stetter F *et al*. Rapid recovery from cognitive deficits in abstinent alcoholics: a controlled test-retest study. *Alcohol Alcoholism* 1999; **34**: 567–74.

49. Lee K, Moller L, Hardt F *et al* Alcohol-induced brain damage and liver damage in young males. *Lancet* 1979; **ii**: 759–61.

50. Carlen PL, Wilkinson DA, Wortzman G *et al*. Cerebral atrophy and functional deficits in alcoholics without clinically apparent liver disease. *Neurology* 1981; **31**: 377–85.

51. Sachs H, Russel J, Christman D *et al*. Alteration of regional cerebral glucose metabolic rate in non-Korsakoff chronic alcoholism. *Arch Neurol* 1987; **44**: 1242–51.

52. Samson Y, Baron J-C, Feline A *et al*. Local cerebral glucose utilisation in chronic alcoholics: a positron tomographic study. *J Neurol Neurosurg Psychiat* 1986; **49**: 1165–70.

53. Gilman S, Adams K, Koeppe R *et al*. Cerebellar and frontal hypometabolism in alcoholic cerebellar degeneration studied with positron emission tomography. *Ann Neurol* 1990; **28**: 775–85.

54. Johnson-Greene D, Adams KM, Gilman S *et al*. Effects of abstinence and relapse upon neuropsychological function and cerebral glucose metabolism in severe chronic alcoholism. *J Clin Exp Neuropsychol* 1997; **19**: 378–85.

55. Lishman WA. *Organic Psychiatry*. Oxford: Blackwell, 1997.

56. Tsai SY, Chen JD, Chao WY, Wang JD. Neurobehavioral effects of occupational exposure to low-level organic solvents among Taiwanese workers in paint factories. *Environ Res* 1997; **73**(1–2): 146–55.

57. Mikkelson S. Epidemiological update on solvent neurotoxicity. *Environmental Res* 1997; **73**: 101–12.

58. Daniell WE, Claypoole KH, Checkoway H *et al*. Neuropsychological function in retired workers with previous long-term occupational exposure to solvents. *Occup Environ Med* 1999; **56**: 93–105.

59. Albers JW, Wald JJ, Garabrant DH *et al*. Neurologic evaluation of workers previously diagnosed with solvent-induced toxic encephalopathy. *J Occup Environ Med* 2000; **42**: 410–23.

60. Collignon R, Brayer R, Rectem D *et al*. Analyse semiologique de l'encephalopathie. Confrontation avec sept cas personnels. *Acta Neurol Belg* 1979; **79**: 73–91.

61. Buge A, Supino-Viterbo V, Rancurel G, Pontes C. Epileptic phenomena in bismuth toxic encephalopathy. *J Neurol Neurosurg Psychiat* 1981; **44**: 62–7.

62. Harper C. The incidence of Wernicke's encephalopathy in Australia—a neuropathological study of 131 cases. *J Neurol Neurosurg Psychiat* 1983; **46**: 593–8.

53

Reversible Dementias

Michael Philpot and Jerson Pereira

South London and Maudsley NHS Trust, London, UK

The early literature on this subject includes numerous case series, or even single case studies, of "dementia" that seemingly resolved following treatment of the associated physical or psychiatric condition. Undoubtedly, many of the patients were actually suffering from delirium or other organic brain syndromes, an observation that is discussed in more detail by Byrne[1]. Confusion over terminology has complicated research in this area. For example, the concept of "reversible" dementia appears at odds with the European use of the term "dementia", denoting an insidiously progressive disorder[2]. In addition, the relationship between delirium and dementia is a complex one and is dealt with elsewhere in this textbook.

This chapter reviews the classification and prevalence of *potentially* reversible dementias in clinical practice, the issue of response to treatment and the cost–benefit of routine investigation. A detailed presentation of the numerous causes of reversible organic brain syndromes is provided by Lishman[2].

CLASSIFICATION

A useful scheme, which clarifies terminology, has been suggested by Maletta[3] and is shown in Table 53.1. Secondary dementias are those arising from a specific physical disorder. Drug intoxication and metabolic disorders include more acute conditions, often in association with impairment of consciousness, which clearly overlap with delirium but which have traditionally been included in studies of reversible dementia. Dementia due to psychiatric disorders includes those conditions classically referred to as the "pseudodementias"[4] mostly secondary to primary depressive illness.

PREVALENCE

The frequency with which potentially reversible dementias occur in clinical practice is an important factor in determining the rigour with which contributory physical disorders or other causes are pursued. A previous review[5] concluded that approximately 12% of patients presenting to a variety of specialist services with symptoms of dementia had treatable causes. This review was based on case series published during the 1970s and 1980s[6–11]. The prevalence of potentially reversible disorders was 18% in patients under the age of 65 years but only 5% in those over 65. Depression, drug toxicity and normal pressure hydrocephalus accounted for more than half the cases. Identification rates were higher in specialist inpatient units than in outpatient or community-based studies. Importantly, though, these studies largely failed to review patients at a later date in order to determine the true reversibility of their cognitive symptoms.

Table 53.2 shows a selection of surveys of the potentially reversible dementias published during the 1990s[12–18] grouped by specialty. Each was carried out in the setting of an outpatient memory clinic. Rates of identification of physical disorders were generally lower than in the earlier series. It has been suggested that the increasing awareness of the features of dementia and the use of internationally agreed diagnostic criteria has helped to refine clinical diagnosis[19]. This has resulted in a more rigorous exclusion of doubtful (non-dementia) cases at an early stage. Esoteric aetiologies are conspicuous by their absence, despite the comprehensive investigation carried out. This is likely to reflect the more representative nature of the patients studied. However, memory clinics specializing in the assessment of patients under the age of 65 usually still report higher rates of identification of potentially reversible conditions, particularly depression[20,21].

Table 53.1 Classification of potentially reversible dementias

Reversible dementias	Common clinical examples
1. Secondary dementias	
Associated with neurological disorders	
Structural lesions	Normal pressure hydrocephalus, brain tumour, subdural haematoma
Associated with systemic disorders	
Nutritional disorders	Vitamin B_{12} deficiency, folate deficiency
Endocrine disorders	Hypothyroidism, hyperthyroidism, hypoparathyroidism
Collagen/vascular disorders	Systemic lupus erythematosus, cerebral vasculitis
Infectious diseases	Neurosyphilis, chronic meningitis, AIDS
Alcohol related disorders	Primary alcoholic dementia
Miscellaneous	Chronic obstructive airways disease, sleep apnoea syndrome
2. Drug intoxication and metabolic disorders	Intoxication with major and minor tranquillizers, anti-hypertensives
3. Dementia due to psychiatric disorders	Depression, late-onset schizophrenia

After Maletta[3].

Principles and Practice of Geriatric Psychiatry, 2nd edn. Edited by J. R. M. Copeland, M. T. Abou-Saleh and D. G. Blazer
©2002 John Wiley & Sons, Ltd

Table 53.2 Outcome of investigation of patients presenting with clinical symptoms of dementia

Studies	Brodaty[12] Almeida et al.[13]	Ames et al.[14] Freter et al.[15]	Chui & Zhang[16] Walstra et al.[17] Hogh et al.[18]
Memory clinic specialty	Geriatric psychiatry	Geriatrics	Neurology
Total patients studied (n)	558	405	719
Clinical dementia confirmed [n (%)]	368 (100)	270 (100)	451 (100)
Mean age (range) (years)	70 (44–90)	76 (49–92)	66 (19–97)
Potentially reversible dementias			
Secondary dementias [n (%)]:	7 (1.9)	25 (9.3)	61 (13.5)
Normal pressure hydrocephalus	–	6	20
Brain tumour	–	2	1
Vitamin B_{12} deficiency	–	11	27
Folate deficiency	1		–
Hypothyroidism	1	3	8
Hyperthyroidism	–		1
Positive syphilis serology	1	3	4
Alcoholic dementia	4		–
Drug intoxication and metabolic disorders [n (%)]:	0	13 (4.8)	0
Alcohol abuse	–	2	–
Drug toxicity	–	11	–
Psychiatric disorders [n (%)]:	0	23 (8.5)	7 (1.6)
Depression	–	23	7
Follow-up period (months)	>6	>4	6[†]
'True' reversible dementia [n (%)]	0	5 (1.9)	2 (0.4)[†]

[†] Not stated in Hogh et al.[18]

RESPONSE TO TREATMENT

The degree to which reversible dementias are, in fact, reversible has long been the subject of debate. Rabins[22] reported some improvement in two-thirds of patients and complete recovery in 40%. This looks optimistic, judging by the results presented in Table 53.2 of between 0% and 2% reversibility.

A number of conditions deserve special mention. Depressive "pseudodementia" has traditionally been viewed as a treatable condition, with a distinct clinical history and symptoms that distinguish it from "true" dementia[23]. In an attempt to improve the clinical discrimination between depressive pseudodementia and progressive dementia, Yousef et al.[24] derived a rating scale from a large number of possible discriminating features. Validating the diagnosis 12–14 months later, the scale allowed correct classification of 98% of true dementia cases and 95% of depression cases. Longer-term follow-up studies tend to support the view that severe cognitive impairment in depression is a harbinger of true dementia in 25–50% of patients[24–26]. Alexopoulos et al.[26] found that, after 2–3 years, elderly depressed patients who also fulfilled DSM–III criteria for dementia were nearly five times more likely to develop dementia than those without cognitive impairment at presentation. The issue is further complicated by the high prevalence of depressive symptoms in dementia[27].

Several authors have questioned the usefulness of routine syphilis serology[28–30], while others have defended routine testing on the grounds that even one missed case would be catastrophic for the individual patient[31]. However, the erroneous diagnosis of active syphilis perhaps carries with it equally dire consequences, particularly when false positives may occur as a result of yaws and other non-venereal treponemal infection[32]. Hilton[33] has suggested that treatment should not be based solely on positive serology and that testing for syphilis should be dealt with in the same way as HIV testing and require informed consent where possible.

Normal pressure hydrocephalus is the most common neurological cause of reversible dementia[16–18]. However, the results of shunting operations indicate high rates of post-operative complications, including death, as well as a lack of evidence of effectiveness[34–35]. The best results are obtained in patients under the age of 60 years who present with dementia of less than 6 months' duration[34].

Clearly, the lack of reversibility revealed by the studies listed in Table 53.2 suggests that most of the associated disorders are really *concomitant* with true dementia, rather than of aetiological significance. They may also be secondary to the dementia, e.g. anaemia as a result of malnutrition. Hogh et al.[18] reported that 45% of those with dementia were found to have concomitant disorders. Although treatment of depressive symptoms in dementia has been shown to improve some aspects of cognition and everyday function[36,37], there is little evidence to show that the correction of other disorders, such as hypothyroidism or vitamin B_{12} deficiency, has similar benefits[17,38,39].

Table 53.3 Physical investigations for the assessment of an elderly patient presenting with cognitive impairment

Routine investigations (all cases)	Special investigations (atypical cases or clinically indicated)
Full blood count[a,b,c]	Brain CT or MRI[a,b,c]
Erythrocyte sedimentation rate[b]	EEG[a,c]
Renal function[a,b,c]	Chest X-ray[a,b,c]
Liver function[a,b,c]	Electrocardiogram[b,c]
Thyroid function[a,b,c]	Lumbar puncture[a,c]
Calcium[a,b,c]	
Vitamin B_1[c]	
Vitamin B_{12}[a,b,c]	Urine for culture[a,b]
Folate[b,c]	
Glucose[a,b,c]	HIV testing[a]
Syphilis serology[a,c]	Toxicity screen[a]
	Auto-antibody screen[b]

Recommendations for investigations: [a]American Academy of Neurology[40]; [b]Royal College of Psychiatrists[42]; [c]Dutch Consensus statement[44].

INVESTIGATION PROTOCOLS

A number of organizations have published guidelines for the investigation of dementia, largely with the aim of identifying the common reversible dementias[40–44]. Table 53.3 lists investigations suggested in three sets of consensus statements[40,42,44] and shows that there is broad agreement on the appropriate routine blood investigations. Chui and Zhang[16] examined the added value of the investigations recommended by the American Academy of Neurology[40]. After a complete clinical assessment, blood tests and neuroimaging results changed management in only 13% and 15% of cases, respectively. van Crevel et al.[44] found that the number of patients requiring investigation to find one case of reversible dementia was approximately 100, and that any financial saving on care costs was insignificant. Lastly, Foster et al.[45], in a detailed examination of the cost-effectiveness of routine computed tomography (CT), concluded that patients aged over 65 years should only be scanned if symptom duration was less than 1 year, if symptoms were rapidly progressive or if the presentation was atypical of Alzheimer's disease. Routine scanning was recommended in all patients presenting under the age of 65.

CONCLUSION

Reversible dementias are rare but their identification is important from the individual patient's perspective. The literature encompasses a polarization of views. The evidence-based view would suggest that extensive investigation is unnecessary and that, in any case, treatment of identified disorders is largely ineffective. The more traditional, patient-centred view, perhaps coloured by the early literature and the fear of litigation, would demand the continued use of routine investigations in the hope of excluding treatable aetiologies, however rare. The introduction of care protocols reached by consensus should guide clinicians and ensure that patients have equity of access to appropriate assessment.

REFERENCES

1. Byrne EJ. Reversible dementias. *Int J Geriat Psychiat* 1987; **2**: 72–81.
2. Lishman WA. *Organic Psychiatry*, 3rd edn. Oxford: Blackwell Science, 1998; 479–638.
3. Maletta GJ. The concept of reversible dementia. How non-reliable terminology may impair effective treatment. *J Am Geriat Soc* 1990; **38**: 136–40.
4. Kiloh LG. Pseudo-dementia. *Acta Psychiat Scand* 1961; **37**: 336–51.
5. Philpot MP, Burns A. Reversible dementias. In Katona C, ed., *Dementia Disorders: Advances and Prospects*. London: Chapman and Hall, 1989; 142–59.
6. Marsden CD, Harrison MJG. Outcome of investigation of patients with presenile dementia. *Br Med J* 1972; **2**: 249–52.
7. Victoratos G, Lenman JAR, Herzberg L. Neurologic investigations of dementia. *Br J Psychiat* 1977; **130**: 131–3.
8. Smith JS, Kiloh LG. The investigation of dementia: results in 200 consecutive admissions. *Lancet* 1981; **i**: 824–7.
9. Larson EB, Reifler BV, Sumi SM et al. Diagnostic evaluation of 200 elderly outpatients with suspected dementia. *J Gerontol* 1985; **5**: 536–43.
10. Renvoize EB, Gaskell RK, Klar M. Results of investigation in 150 demented patients consecutively admitted to a psychiatric hospital. *Br J Psychiat* 1985; **147**: 204–5.
11. Erkinjunntti T, Sulkava R, Kovanen J, Palo J. Suspected dementia: evaluation of 323 consecutive referrals. *Acta Psychiat Scand* 1987; **76**: 359–64.
12. Brodaty H. Low diagnostic yield in a memory disorders clinic. *Int Psychogeriat* 1990; **2**: 149–59.
13. Almeida OP, Hill K, Howard R et al. Demographic and clinical features of patients attending a memory clinic. *Int J Geriat Psychiat* 1993; **8**: 497–501.
14. Ames D, Flicker L, Helme RD. A memory clinic at a geriatric hospital: rationale, routine and results from the first 100 patients. *Med J Aust* 1992; **156**: 618–22.
15. Freter S, Bergman H, Gold S et al. Prevalence of potentially reversible dementia and actual reversibility in a memory clinic cohort. *Can Med Assoc J* 1998; **159**: 657–62.
16. Chui H, Zhang Q. Evaluation of dementia: a systematic study of the usefulness of the American Academy of Neurology's Practice Parameters. *Neurology* 1997; **49**: 925–35.
17. Walstra GJ, Teunisse S, van Gool WA, van Crevel H. Reversible dementia in elderly patients referred to a memory clinic. *J Neurol* 1997; **244**: 17–22.
18. Hogh P, Waldemar G, Knudsen GM et al. A multidisciplinary memory clinic in a neurological setting: diagnostic evaluation of 400 consecutive patients. *Eur J Neurol* 1999; **6**: 279–88.
19. Piccini C, Bracco L, Amaducci L. Treatable and reversible dementias: an update. *J Neurol Sci* 1998; **153**: 172–81.
20. Kopelman M, Crawford S. Not all memory clinics are dementia clinics. *Neuropsychol Rehab* 1996; **6**: 1871–2002.
21. Ferran J, Wilson K, Doran M et al. The early onset dementia: a study of clinical characteristics and service use. *Int J Geriat Psychiat* 1996; **11**: 863–9.
22. Rabins PV. The reversible dementias. In Arie T, ed., *Recent Advances in Psychogeriatrics*, vol 1. Edinburgh: Churchill Livingstone, 1985; 93–102.
23. Wells CE. Pseudodementia. *Am J Psychiat* 1979; **136**: 895–900.
24. Yousef G, Ryan WJ, Lambert T et al. A preliminary report: a new scale to identify the pseudodementia syndrome. *Int J Geriat Psychiat* 1998; **13**: 389–99.
25. Copeland JRM, Davidson IA, Dewey ME et al. Alzheimer's disease, other dementias, depression and pseudodementia: prevalence, incidence and three-year outcome in Liverpool. *Br J Psychiat* 1992; **161**: 230–9.
26. Alexopoulos GS, Meyers BS, Young RC et al. The course of geriatric depression with "reversible dementia": a controlled study. *Am J Psychiat* 1993; **150**: 1693–9.
27. Burns A, Jacoby R, Levy R. Psychiatric phenomena in Alzheimer's disease III. Disorders of mood. *Br J Psychiat* 1990; **157**: 81–6.
28. Boodhoo JA. Syphilis serology screening in a psychogeriatric population. Is the effort worthwhile? *Br J Psychiat* 1989; **155**: 257–62.
29. Byrne EJ, Smith CW, Arie T, Lilley J. Diagnosis of dementia 3. Use of investigations. A survey of current consultant practice, review of the literature and implications for audit. *Int J Geriat Psychiat* 1992; **7**: 647–57.
30. Powell AL, Coyne AC, Jen L. A retrospective study of syphilis seropositivity in a cohort of demented patients. *Alzheimer's Dis Assoc Disord* 1993; **7**: 33–8.
31. Cleare AJ, Jacoby R, Tovey SJ, Bergmann K. Syphilis, neither dead nor buried—a survey of psychogeriatric inpatients. *Int J Geriat Psychiat* 1993; **8**: 661–4.
32. Roman GC, Roman LN. Occurrence of congenital, cardiovascular, visceral, neurologic, and neuro-ophthalmologic complications in late yaws: a theme for future research. *Rev Infect Dis* 1986; **8**: 760–70.
33. Hilton C. General paralysis of the insane and AIDS in old age psychiatry: epidemiology, clinical diagnosis, serology and ethics—the way forward. *Int J Geriat Psychiat* 1998; **13**: 875–85.
34. Clarfield AM. Normal-pressure hydrocephalus: saga or swamp? *J Am Med Assoc* 1989; **262**: 2592–3.
35. Vanneste J, Augustijn P, Dirven C et al. Shunting normal-pressure hydrocephalus: do the benefits outweigh the risks? A multicenter study and literature review. *Neurology* 1992; **42**: 54–9.
36. Reifler BV, Teri L, Raskind M et al. Double-blind trial of imipramine in Alzheimer's disease patients with and without depression. *Am J Psychiat* 1989; **146**: 45–9.
37. Katona CL, Hunter BN, Bray J. A double-blind comparison of the efficacy and safety of paroxetine and imipramine in the treatment of depression with dementia. *Int J Geriat Psychiat* 1998; **13**: 100–8.
38. Teunissen S, Bollen AE, van Gool WA, Walstra GJ. Dementia and subnormal levels of vitamin B_{12}: effects of replacement therapy on dementia. *J Neurol* 1996; **243**: 522–9.

39. Kwok T, Tang C, Woo J *et al.* Randomised trial of the effect of supplementation on the cognitive function of older people with subnormal cobalamin levels. *Int J Geriat Psychiat* 1998; **13**: 611–16.

40. American Academy of Neurology Quality Standards Subcommittee. Practice parameter: diagnosis and evaluation of dementia. *Neurology* 1994; **44**: 2203–6.

41. Organising Committee, Canadian Consensus Conference on the assessment of dementia. Assessing dementia: the Canadian consensus. *Can Med Assoc J* 1991; **144**: 851–3.

42. Royal College of Psychiatrists. *Consensus Statement on the Assessment and Investigation of an Elderly Person with Suspected Cognitive Impairment by a Specialist Old Age Psychiatry Service.* Council Report CR49. London: Royal College of Psychiatrists, 1995.

43. Wallin A, Brun A, Gustafson L. Swedish consensus on dementia diseases. *Acta Neurol Scand* 1994; **90**(suppl 157): S1–13.

44. van Crevel H, van Gool WA, Walstra GJM. Early diagnosis of dementia: which tests are indicated? What are their costs? *J Neurol* 1999; **246**: 73–8.

45. Foster GR, Scott DA, Payne S. The use of CT scanning in dementia. *Int J Technol Assess Health Care* 1999; **15**: 406–23.

54

Differential Diagnosis of Dementia

Charlotte Busby and Alistair Burns

Withington Hospital, University of Manchester, UK

When approaching the differential diagnosis of dementia, two distinct but related issues are involved. First, the clinician has to consider whether the patient is suffering from a dementia syndrome. Differentiation has to be made from a functional psychiatric disorder, such as depression, which may be manifested as a dementing illness (so-called "pseudodementia" or the dementia syndrome of depression); from an acute organic reaction (acute or subacute confusional state); from the effects of normal ageing[1], from pre-existing handicaps; and from the deleterious effects of drugs. Second, the aetiology of the dementia, in terms of either a potentially reversible or irreversible dementia, has to be uncovered. The process is illustrated in Figure 54.1, although in practice a clinician formulates a diagnosis based on the whole presentation (see also ref. 2). This chapter will not deal with Alzheimer's disease in detail (see ref. 3) but it will be regarded as a prototype against which other disorders can be compared.

There are clinical situations in which the diagnosis of dementia is problematic. These have been well summarized[4] and include: early cases (where the effects of normal ageing need to be considered); patients with a low IQ (where intellectual symptoms may be noticed early); very old patients, especially when residents of nursing homes, without reliable informants; patients with impaired vision and hearing; patients who are mentally handicapped; patients with prominent psychiatric problems, such as paranoia, dysthymia or personality problems; and those with severe physical illness or an intercurrent delirium.

When evaluating a patient with possible dementia, the following should be performed[5–7]:

- Detailed family and personal history and history of the current illness from a reliable informant.
- Mental State Examination of the patient, with particular reference to the cognitive state (amnesia, apraxia, aphasia and agnosia); more detailed neuropsychological assessment should be considered if particular deficits are suspected).
- Physical examination, with particular emphasis on the central nervous system.
- Investigations including haematological and biochemical blood tests, serum B_{12} and folate, thyroid function tests, chest X-ray and ECG.

Some form of assessment of cerebral function/structure is desirable, the nature of the investigation being dependent on local facilities. An electroencephalogram (EEG) should be performed and is widely available. Ideally, a computed tomography (CT) scan should also be carried out, but this is not always practicable. If so, it is reasonable to limit this examination to cases in whom there is reason to suspect an intracranial lesion, i.e. clinical suspicion of such a lesion, evidence of cerebral infarction, focal neurological signs, seizure activity, a head injury thought to be contributory to the clinical picture, or a suspicion of normal pressure hydrocephalus. The main conditions in the differential diagnosis of dementia and possible causes of the dementia syndrome are discussed below.

ACUTE CONFUSIONAL STATE (DELIRIUM)

This is the most important differential diagnosis to be considered, as there is almost always a physical disorder underlying its presence. Onset is acute, disturbances often severe and the patient is usually brought to the attention of the services by worried friends, relatives or neighbours. There is a global disturbance of cognition, with marked fluctuation over the course of the day, often worse at night[8].

During affected periods, there is almost always some disorientation. Among the disturbances are disorders of perception (characterized by an inability to interpret events and to discriminate them from images and dreams), disorders of thinking (disorganized, fragmented and with disjointed thoughts and decreased ability to plan or solve problems) and disorders of memory (registration, retention and retrieval are all affected). Clouding of consciousness is the cardinal feature of delirium and has been defined in terms of a disorder of attention (decreased or increased alertness, selectiveness and directiveness) and wakefulness (diminished night sleep[9]). Psychomotor behaviour is usually disturbed, with overactivity, underactivity or a mixture of the two. The diagnosis of acute confusion is made on a characteristic history of a sudden onset of disturbance and the findings outlined above on examination of the patient. Often the physical precipitant is not obvious initially (and in a proportion of cases is never discovered). An underlying dementia may be present and is suggested by the history.

PSEUDODEMENTIA

In this condition, symptoms of disorientation and memory loss occur in a non-organic psychosis and mimic dementia. The original description of cases included patients with a number of functional psychiatric disorders[10], but in practice depression is by far the commonest cause. In contrast to dementia, the clinical course of the condition is relatively short and has a defined date of onset. There is often a previous history and/or a

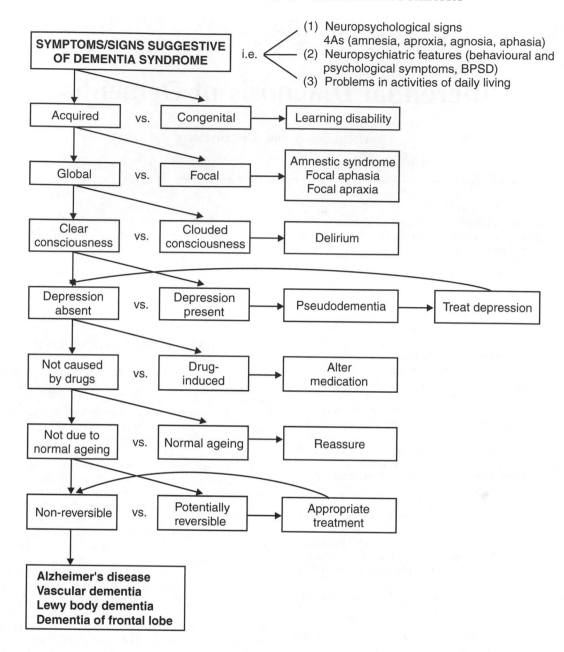

Figure 54.1 Diagnostic algorithm for dementia

family history of affective disorder. Patients tend to answer questions with "don't know" responses, there is a variability in their ability to perform tasks of similar difficulty, they communicate a sense of distress and complain of their cognitive deficits[11]. Structural brain changes have been described in this condition[12]. Pseudodementia is currently a term in disrepute and the alternative (dementia syndrome of depression) is considered to be more accurate. The diagnosis of pseudodementia is made on clinical grounds and should always be considered in a demented patient. Validation of the diagnosis is by successful treatment and return to normal of the cognitive deficit[13,14]. Some clinicians would argue that a trial of antidepressants should be given in all cases of dementia.

VASCULAR DEMENTIA

There are two main types of vascular dementia, one involving subcortical structures affecting small arteries, leading to the clinical picture of subcortical dementia (see below for cardinal features), and one involving medium-sized arteries (anterior, middle and posterior cerebral arteries), leading to a cortical dementia. The clinical features of vascular cortical dementia have been defined in the Hachinski score[15]. Physical examination will generally reveal neurological signs, such as disturbances of gait rigidity, spasticity and reflex abnormalities, and CT often reveals cerebral infarction. Diagnostic criteria have been described[16,17].

INTRACRANIAL LESIONS

Any form of intracranial mass lesion may masquerade as dementia. Cerebral tumours (primary or secondary), brain abscess or intracranial bleeds may all give rise to a dementia syndrome. Diagnosis is made through suspicion of the primary lesion and visualization on CT scan.

SUBCORTICAL DEMENTIA

This is a generic term for a particular syndrome of dementia, which has particular clinical features separating it from a cortical dementia. These include mental slowness, inertia, apathy and loss of initiative, occurring along with cognitive disturbances. The diseases associated with subcortical dementias include Parkinson's disease, Huntington's disease, progressive supranuclear palsy, Wilson's disease, spinocerebellar degeneration, hydrocephalus and the toxic/metabolic encephalopathies. The structures affected are subcortical—the basal ganglia, thalamus and the brain stem.

In Parkinson's disease, there is mental slowing, diminished problem solving, poor memory and a deterioration in abstraction, concept formation and word generation. Depression is common, as in all subcortical dementias. Cortical features (such as aphasia, apraxia and agnosia) are absent, although some authors claim there is a cortical dementia present, probably due to coexisting Alzheimer's disease. The diagnosis of Parkinson's disease is essentially a clinical one and physical manifestations of the disease will generally be present when the dementia is apparent.

Huntington's disease is characterized by choreiform movements and associated with autosomal dominant transmission. Personality changes, irritability and apathy are the first changes and predate the chorea. The dementia appears soon after the movement disorder becomes apparent, characterized by memory disturbance (impaired recall of both recent and remote memories), slowing, failure to initiate cognitions (especially those required in planning) and impaired concentration and judgement[26]. Although dementia without chorea has been described, it is very rare and the diagnosis of Huntington's disease is usually suspected prior to the onset of dementia[18].

Pseudobulbar palsy, rigidity (more pronounced in the neck and trunk) and paralysis of vertical gaze (downward gaze lost first, followed by failure of upward gaze) are hallmarks of progressive supranuclear palsy, and the associated dementia is classically subcortical (indeed, the original description of subcortical dementia was based on the dementia of progressive supranuclear palsy). Speech is disrupted (e.g. dysarthria and hypophonia) but aphasia is absent. The clinical features are such that the diagnosis will often be suspected and, although it may be confused with Parkinson's disease, the characteristic tremor of the latter is absent.

Other conditions resulting in subcortical dementias occur rarely and are of limited relevance to old age psychiatry. The amyotrophic lateral sclerosis–Parkinson–dementia complex of Guam is rare outside the Chonorro population of the Western Pacific, the dementia being profound and characterized by features of decreased memory, apathy and slowness; cerebellar degenerations are associated features of subcortical dementia but the cerebellar dysfunction is usually the prominent feature; Wilson's disease and Friedreich's ataxia are associated with dementia, but are confined to children and young adults.

NORMAL PRESSURE HYDROCEPHALUS

A potentially treatable cause for a dementia syndrome is hydrocephalus, the most widely cited being normal pressure hydrocephalus. The classical clinical triad consists of gait disturbance (ranging from mild clumsiness to akinesis), incontinence (almost always urinary incontinence, occurring late in the illness) and dementia (impaired memory, disorientation and mental slowing). The diagnosis is made by radiological examination (CT scan shows marked enlargement of the ventricles with relatively normal cortical sulci, and isotope cisternography shows obstruction to the flow over the cortex). A ventricular shunt to divert cerebrospinal fluid is the appropriate treatment but not all cases improve, even when the classical clinical picture is present.

PICK'S DISEASE

Personality changes and mood disorders (ranging from depression to elation) occur first, with coarsening of affect and antisocial behaviour. Impaired judgement occurs, with loss of insight. Aphasia and circumlocution occur early. Memory is relatively unimpaired until the later stages of the disease, as is praxic function. The Kluver–Bucy syndrome has been described early in the illness, but this also appears in Alzheimer's disease[19]. Extrapyramidal signs appear late in the illness but the clinical picture is unlikely to be confused with Parkinson's disease. Seizures are said to be less common than in Alzheimer's disease and CT scan shows frontal and temporal lobe atrophy, rather than the generalized shrinkage seen in Alzheimer's disease. The diagnosis is made on the basis of the characteristic onset of personality changes before the onset of dementia.

DEMENTIA OF THE FRONTAL LOBE TYPE

Recently, descriptions have emerged of a form of dementia that appears to affect the frontal lobes and is defined in terms of clinical presentation (personality change, speech impairment and relative preservation of visuospatial functions), neuropsychological function (frontal lobe syndrome) and blood flow studies (diminished frontal lobe blood flow on single-photon emission tomography)[20–22]. There is frontal and temporal lobe atrophy and, while the condition resembles Pick's disease, the characteristic neuronal inclusion bodies are absent. Diagnosis is made on clinical grounds but confirmation usually has to await autopsy.

DEMENTIA OF LEWY BODY TYPE

This has been described with increasing frequency and is considered to be amongst the commonest forms of primary dementia[23]. The relationship of this syndrome to Parkinson's disease is uncertain, but the clinical picture of parkinsonian features, hallucinosis and episodes of confusion should raise the diagnostic possibility.

TOXIC-METABOLIC ABNORMALITIES

Generally, these are readily identifiable by the primary cause for the syndrome (such as anoxia, renal or hepatic failure) and the symptomatology produced is more often identifiable as an encephalopathy rather than a dementia syndrome. There are a few conditions of relevance in old age psychiatry, which will be outlined briefly. Systemic carcinomas may produce effects in the brain by several mechanisms through metabolic disturbances (such as excess secretion of adrenocorticotrophic hormone or antidiuretic hormone), through structural change (cerebral secondaries or infections) or through remote effect (limbic encephalitis). This last condition is common in men, particularly with oat cell carcinomas of the lung, and has a course of up to 24 months. Affective changes dominate the picture, with amnesia the primary (and occasionally the sole) abnormality. Diagnosis of the condition is through attention to the physical condition of the individual. Vitamin deficiencies (notably B_{12} and folate) cause mental impairment, but routine testing for their levels makes the diagnosis relatively easy. The same holds true for thyroid dysfunction and hypercalcaemia. Chronic excessive alcohol intake can result in a dementia[24].

CREUTZFELDT–JAKOB DISEASE

Early features include fatigue and listlessness, elevated mood and impaired memory and concentration. Motor abnormalities occur with spasticity, ataxia and tremor. Myoclonic jerks and seizures may occur. The EEG is very abnormal, with characteristic triphasic waves superimposed on some suppression of the background rhythms. The course of the illness is very rapid and most affected individuals are dead within 2 years[25].

SUMMARY

The differential diagnosis of dementia is a two-stage process: first, the differentiation of dementia from other causes of cognitive impairment; and second, if it is found to be a form of dementia, the elucidation of the aetiology. Alzheimer's disease is the commonest form of dementia, cerebrovascular disease is probably the second commonest cause and Lewy body dementia is becoming increasingly recognized. The differential diagnosis of dementia is an excellent example of how simple logical clinical skills can be applied without the need for expensive investigations, which should be reserved for situations where there is clinical doubt about the diagnosis.

REFERENCES

1. Ritchie K, Touchon J et al. Mild cognitive impairment: conceptual basis and current nosological status. *Lancet* 2000; **355**: 225–8.
2. Corry-Bloom J, Thal L, Galasko D et al. Diagnosis and evaluation of dementia. *Neurology* 1995; **45**: 211–18.
3. McKhann G, Drachman D, Folstein M et al. Clinical diagnosis of Alzheimer's disease. *Neurology* 1984; **34**: 939–44.
4. Blessed G. Definitions and classification of the dementias. *Interdisciplinary Topics in Gerontology, vol 26: Innovative Trends in Psychogeriatrics*. Basel: Karger, 1989.
5. Clarfield AM. The reversible dementias: do they reverse? *Ann Intern Med* 1988; **109**: 476–86.
6. Walstra G, Teunisse S, van Gool W, Crevel H. Reversible dementia in elderly patients referred to a memory clinic. *J Neurol* 1998; **244**: 17–22.
7. Larson E, Reifler B, Sumi S et al. Diagnostic tests in the evaluation of dementia. *Arch Intern Med* 1986; **146**: 1917–22.
8. Lipowski Z. Transient cognitive disorders (delirium, acute confusional states) in the elderly. *Am J Psychiat* 1983; **140**: 1426–36.
9. Trzepacz PT, Mulsant BH, Dew AM et al. Is delirium different when it occurs in dementia? A study using the delirium rating scale. *J Neuropsychiat Clin Neurosci* 1998; **10**(2): 199–204.
10. Kiloh L. Pseudodementia. *Acta Psychiat Scand* 1961; **37**: 336–51.
11. Wells C. Pseudodementia. *Am J Psychiat* 1979; **136**: 895–900.
12. Pearlson G, Rabins P, Kim W et al. Structural brain CT changes in cognitive deficits in elderly depressives with and without reversible dementia. *Psychol Med* 1989; **19**: 573–84.
13. Rabins P, Merchant A, Nestadt G. Criteria for diagnosing reversible dementia caused by depression; validation by two-year follow-up. *Br J Psychiat* 1984; **144**: 488–92.
14. Alexopoulos G, Mayers B, Young R et al. The course of geriatric depression with reversible dementia. *Am J Psychiat* 1993; **150**: 1693–9.
15. Hachinski V, Iliff I, Zilhka E et al. Cerebral blood flow in dementia. *Arch Neurol* 1975; **32**: 632–7.
16. Chiu H, Victoroff J, Margolin et al. Criteria for the diagnosis of ischaemic vascular dementia. *Neurology* 1992; **42**: 473–80.
17. Roman G, Tatemechi T, Erkinjuntti T et al. Vascular dementia: diagnostic criteria for research studies. *Neurology* 1993; **43**: 250–60.
18. Chiu H. Huntington's disease. In Burns A, Levy R, eds, *Dementia*. London: Chapman & Hall, 1994; 713–62.
19. Cummings J, Duchene L. The Kluver–Bucy syndrome in Pick's disease. *Neurology* 1981; **31**: 145–52.
20. Neary D, Snowdon J, Northen B et al. Dementia of frontal lobe type. *J Neurol Neurosurg Psychiat* 1988; **51**: 353–61.
21. Neary D et al. Lund and Manchester Groups. Clinical and neuropathological criteria for frontotemporal dementia. *J Neurol Neurosurg Psychiat* 1994; **57**: 416–18.
22. Neary D et al. Frontotemporal lobar degeneration. *Neurology* 1998; **51**: 1546–54.
23. McKeith IG, Galasko D, Kosaka K, Perry E et al. Consensus guidelines for the clinical and pathologic diagnosis of dementia with Lewy bodies (DLB). *Neurology* 1996; **47**: 1113–24.
24. Kopelman MD. The Korsakoff syndrome. *Br J Psychiat* 1995; **166**: 154–73.
25. Collinge J. Human prion diseases: aetiology and clinical features. In Growdon J, Rossor M, eds, *Blue Books of Practical Neurology: The Dementias*. Oxford: Butterworth-Heinemann, 1998; 113–48.
26. McHugh P, Folstein M. Psychiatric syndromes of Huntington's chorea: a clinical and phenomenologic study. In Benson D, Blumer D, eds, *Psychiatric Aspects of Neurologic Disease*. New York: Grune and Stratton, 1975; 267–85.

Distinguishing Depression from Dementia

William E. Fox and David C. Steffens

Duke University Medical Center, Durham, NC, USA

Recent research continues to confirm the complex relationship between depression and dementia. The ability to distinguish depression from dementia is complicated by the overlap of many of their clinical manifestations. Differentiating the two illnesses is further complicated in that depression and dementia are often concurrent illnesses in the geriatric population. Depression has also become recognized as a possible prodrome, or even risk factor, for degenerative dementias. Finally, cerebrovascular disease, one of the long-established etiologies of dementia, is becoming increasingly recognized as a possible etiology of geriatric depression.

Dementia and depression are two of the most common diagnoses that clinicians encounter in geriatric psychiatry. The prevalence of dementia has been estimated to be approximately 1% at age 60, doubling every 5 years to reach 30% to 50% by age 85[1,2]. Major depression afflicts 1–2% of community-dwelling elderly, with significantly higher rates observed in hospitalized elderly and those residing in nursing homes[3]. The prevalence for minor depression or subsyndromal depression is even higher, with rates reported to be 13–27%[3].

Given the complex relationship between depression and dementia, combined with high prevalence rates, clinicians need to be familiar with the literature that addresses these issues. This chapter will begin with a review of the basic diagnostic criteria of dementia and depression. It will then explore the key points in clinically distinguishing the diagnoses. Next, it will examine the issue of concurrent depression and dementia, as well as the concept of pseudodementia of depression. It will conclude with a discussion regarding the latest research on the possibility of depression as a herald or prodrome of degenerative dementias, and the newly emerging concept of vascular depression.

CLINICAL PRESENTATIONS OF DEMENTIA AND GERIATRIC DEPRESSION

The DSM-IV diagnostic criteria for dementia include the development of multiple cognitive deficits manifested by memory impairment, and one or more of the following: aphasia, apraxia, agnosia or disturbance in executive functioning[4]. In addition to these core cognitive symptoms, numerous psychiatric symptoms are also common. In Alzheimer's disease (AD), the most common of the dementing disorders[5], significant psychiatric symptoms often occur, including personality changes, irritability, anxiety, delusions, hallucinations and depressive symptoms[5–8]. The depressive symptoms that are common in dementia include sleep disturbance, anorexia, irritability, social withdrawal, anergy and apathy[6,7].

The diagnostic criteria for major depressive disorder, as described in the DSM-IV, include depressed mood, diminished interest, weight loss, sleep disturbance, psychomotor agitation or retardation, loss of energy, feelings of worthlessness or guilt, and diminished ability to concentrate[4]. While not all studies agree, most authors report that in the elderly, compared to younger depressive counterparts, depressed mood and feelings of guilt are not as common but somatic and cognitive symptoms are more common[3,9]. The cognitive symptoms may become so severe as to lead to the development of what has been termed "pseudo-dementia".

With such significant overlap of the symptoms of dementia and depression in the elderly, the clinical or "bedside" differentiation can be quite challenging. Reynolds *et al.*[10] found that patients with pseudodementia of depression showed greater early morning awakening, higher anxiety and more severe impairment of libido. Patients with dementia showed more disorientation to time and greater difficulty with dressing and navigating through familiar surroundings.

The American Association for Geriatric Psychiatry, the Alzheimer's Association and the American Geriatric Society presented a consensus statement that included tips for differentiating dementia from depression[5]. The panel reported that patients with AD, in comparison with depressed patients, tend to minimize cognitive deficits, demonstrate impaired memory and executive function, have "indirect" symptoms of depression, such as agitation and insomnia, and demonstrate other cognitive deficits, such as aphasia and apraxia. The panel further reported that those patients with cognitive disturbance, in the context of depression, in comparison with demented patients, tended to exaggerate cognitive deficits, show impaired motivation and classic mood symptoms and have intact language and motor skills.

Abram and Alexopoulos[11] described the similarities between the clinical appearances of dementia and depression, including shared neurovegetative signs, such as weight loss, insomnia, decreased libido and fatigue. However, they also emphasized that some distinctions can be made clinically. Specifically, the authors asserted that weight loss, fatiguability and insomnia usually reflect acute changes in depression, but will be more chronic in dementia. Mood-incongruent delusions may be found in psychotic depression as well as dementia, but mood-congruent delusions are more characteristic of depression. They also reported that the agitation of dementia often manifests as "pacing", while "hand-wringing" is more characteristic of depression.

Other features of the patient's presentation, as well as personal and family history, can be helpful in distinguishing depression from dementia. Geldmacher and Whitehouse[2] suggested that, in patients with dementia, more often a relative will report decreased

Principles and Practice of Geriatric Psychiatry, 2nd edn. Edited by J. R. M. Copeland, M. T. Abou-Saleh and D. G. Blazer

memory in the patient. In contrast, in patients with depression, if cognitive symptoms are reported, it is usually by the patient. They also stated that the duration of the presentation could be helpful in clarifying the diagnosis. Depression is typically of shorter duration than dementia and usually with a more well-defined onset. The authors also recommend a review of personal or family history for depression, and a review of family history for dementia.

SCREENING INSTRUMENTS

The use of various "bedside" screening instruments has been proposed as a way to clarify the diagnoses of dementia and depression. Common instruments used in the diagnosis of depression include the Hamilton Rating Scale for Depression (HAM-D), the Beck Depression Inventory (BDI), and the Montgomery–Asberg Depression Rating Scale (MADRS). In general, many authors have found that general depression screening instruments are less helpful in the diagnosis of depression in the elderly than in the general adult population. Reasons for this age disparity include decreased specificity, due to overlap of many depression symptoms with other common geriatric presentations, including dementia and general medical illnesses. It is also believed that the sensitivity is decreased, as not all of the classic symptoms of depression are as common in the geriatric population as in the general adult population.

A number of depression screening tools specifically designed to be used in geriatric or demented patients have been developed. Among the more commonly used instruments are the Geriatric Depression Scale (GDS), Alzheimer's Disease Assessment Scale (ADAS) and the Cornell Scale for Depression in Dementia (CS). The ADAS relies on observation of the patients and thus avoids many of the difficulties inherent in interviewing a cognitively impaired individual[11]. The CS combines interviews with the patient and caregivers, focusing on behavior during the week preceding the interview, thus taking advantage of available collateral information that many other scales ignore[11,12].

The most commonly used dementia screening tool is the Mini-Mental State Examination (MMSE). The MMSE was developed by Folstein et al. in 1975[13]. Since that time, it has become the most widely used examination for rapidly assessing the cognitive status of the elderly[14]. This short test covers a broad range of cognitive domains, including orientation, registration, attention and recall, calculation, language, and constructional ability[15]. Age- and education-specific reference values have been developed to help guide the clinician in the use of the MMSE in various populations[14].

Other tests that have been developed to screen for cognitive impairment in the elderly include the Blessed Dementia Rating Scale and the Short Portable Mental Status Questionnaire (SPMSQ). A quick and simple-to-administer test, the clock-drawing test, has been shown in numerous studies to be a good screening test for dementia[16]. Numerous methods have been developed to score the clock-drawing test, ranging from complex 20-point scales to more simple ordinal scales.

Watson et al.[17], developed a scoring system that is based on a seven-point scale. With this method, the patient is instructed to draw numbers within a pre-drawn circle to make the face of a clock. After completion, the clock face is divided into quadrants and the number of digits in each quadrant is counted. An error score of one is assigned for each of the first three quadrants containing any erroneous number of digits and an error score of four is assigned for the fourth quadrant if it contains an erroneous number of digits. A score of 4 or greater has been shown to have a sensitivity of 87% and a specificity of 82% in screening for dementia[16].

Kafonek et al.[18] conducted a study to determine the sensitivity and specificity of the MMSE in detecting dementia and the Geriatric Depression Scale (GDS) for detecting depression in an academic center-affiliated nursing home population. They found that, in screening for dementia, the sensitivity of the MMSE was 81% and the specificity was 83% when using a cut-off score of 24/30. The GDS was found to be less sensitive and less specific in screening for depression, with a sensitivity of 47% and a specificity of 75%. Thus, while such screening tools can provide useful additional information, they should be taken into consideration as part of the overall clinical picture and not used as the sole basis for making or excluding a diagnosis.

NEUROPSYCHOLOGICAL ASSESSMENT

Formal neuropsychological testing is often employed to help diagnose dementia and depression in the geriatric population. Neuropsychologists are able to administer a full battery of tests that have at least three distinct functions in the assessment of geriatric patients[19]. The first goal of neuropsychological testing is to aid with differential diagnoses between normal aging, psychiatric disorders and neurodegenerative/dementing disorders. A second common use of formal testing is to establish a baseline from which changes can be tracked over time. This can help in determining the response to treatment for depression or dementia, as well as to systematically follow the progression of dementing disorders. The final common use of neuropsychological testing is to delineate the strengths and weaknesses of a particular patient, to help make clinical recommendations for treatment, daily activities and planning for the future.

In an exhaustive review of the neuropsychological testing literature dealing with the differential diagnosis of major progressive dementias and depression, Rosenstein[20] summarized the major test variables that neuropsychologists have found helpful in distinguishing depression from various dementing disorders. In general, she reports that depressed patients tend to demonstrate normal to slightly reduced attention, memory, visuospatial functions, language, executive function, reasoning and sensory-motor function, with a negative or empty response style and inconsistent performances (even within the same domain). In contrast, patients with AD tend to demonstrate more significant impairment in memory, verbal fluency and executive function (in particular, poor awareness of deficits), with a higher prevalence of false-positive responses and intrusions.

Obviously, the milder the dementia at the time of testing, the milder will be the above-mentioned deficits. However, even mild deficits will be more accurately detected on formal neuropsychological testing than with the usual clinical assessment, or with screening tests such as the MMSE. This increased sensitivity is one of the strengths of formal neuropsychological testing. As part of a prospective epidemiological study of dementia, Jacobs et al.[21] administered a comprehensive neuropsychological test battery to a group of initially non-demented older adults, in order to examine the association between baseline scores and subsequent development of dementia. The results of the study indicate that, even in the preclinical phase of AD, deficits can be found in areas of word-finding ability, abstract reasoning and memory.

MacKnight et al.[22], in their paper examining the factors associated with inconsistent diagnosis of dementia between physicians and neuropsychologists, concluded that the two disciplines have complementary strengths. The neuropsychologist has superior skills in identifying early cognitive loss, while the physician's expertise arises from a greater ability to assess the impact of the impairment on the patient's ability to function. Thus, if available to the clinician, formal neuropsychological testing can provide very helpful and complementary information.

This is particularly true in those cases where diagnostic uncertainty is high.

LABORATORY EVALUATION

For many years attempts have been made to find a reliable biological marker for depression that could be used to develop a sensitive and specific laboratory test. Early on, investigators examined the use of the dexamethasone suppression test (DST), a neuroendocrine measure of the functioning of the hypothalamic–pituitary–adrenal axis, to distinguish depression from dementia. Although the test appeared to have some discriminatory ability in some of the very early studies[23,24], subsequent research failed to demonstrate its usefulness[25–29]. Presently, the DST is not a routine part of a depression or dementia work-up.

Laboratory studies that should be a routine part of the assessment of dementia include a complete blood count (CBC), urinalysis, serum chemistry panel, liver function tests, thyroid function, serum vitamin B_{12} and folate levels, and syphilis serology[8,30]. A number of these tests are also useful in the evaluation of depression. The most commonly cited are a CBC, serum electrolytes, serum vitamin B_{12} level, serum folate level, and thyroid function. While these laboratory studies do not necessarily help to distinguish depression from dementia, they can help to evaluate a number of possible common etiologies and contributing factors. Should any of these tests have positive results, steps should be taken to correct the abnormality and the patient should then be reassessed for depression or dementia.

Genetic testing is beginning to receive much attention as a possible aid in diagnosing various dementing disorders. Early-onset AD comprises both sporadic cases and those that are now known to represent a collection of single-gene disorders. Specific mutations in three genes have been associated with the early-onset, familial-pattern AD. The identified genes are the amyloid precursor protein (APP) gene on chromosome 21, presenilin-1 (PS1) gene on chromosome 14, and presenilin-2 (PS2) gene on chromosome 1[31]. In cases where early-onset dementia is suspected, genetic testing is indicated to help confirm the diagnosis and to provide additional information to be used in counseling the patient and family members.

In the more common late-onset form of AD, one gene, apolipoprotein E (APOE), located on chromosome 19, has been associated as a risk factor. This gene has three common isoforms, $\epsilon2$, $\epsilon3$ and $\epsilon4$. Research has shown that the isoform $\epsilon4$ is associated with the development of AD in a dose-dependent manner, and that the isoform $\epsilon2$ may be protective for AD in a dose-dependent manner[31–35]. Thus, the more copies of the $\epsilon4$ allele one carries in one's genotype, the higher the risk for developing AD. One complicating factor in using this genetic test in the differential diagnosis of dementia and depression is that the $\epsilon4$ allele has also been associated with the development of late-onset major depression in a study by Krishman et al.[33] While genetic testing for APOE isoforms can be another helpful piece in distinguishing dementia and depression, it is far from conclusive and is currently not a routine part of a work-up for depressed, cognitively-impaired patients.

ELECTROENCEPHALOGRAPHY EVALUATION

A great deal of research has been conducted examining the ability of electroencephalography (EEG) studies to aid in the diagnoses of depression and dementia. In a literature review of EEG of the elderly, Klass and Brenner[36] reported several reasons why an EEG may be helpful in the evaluation of dementia. First, it may confirm that an abnormality of cerebral function exists. Second, it may indicate that a focal process is present, rather than a diffuse process. Third, it may find that a previously unidentified seizure disorder is present. Finally, certain dementing processes, such as Creutzfeldt–Jakob disease, have pathognomonic EEG change and thus the EEG can be diagnostic in those cases. The authors concluded that, in depression, the awake EEG is usually normal and when abnormalities are found they most often are mild.

As abnormalities of sleep are part of the core symptoms of depression, sleep studies using EEG have been studied extensively for many years in an attempt to find objective variables that could aid in the diagnosis of depression. Variables that have consistently been found in depression include increased rapid eye movement (REM) activity, increased sleep latency, decreased REM latency, increased REM density and high rates of sleep onset REM as compared to normal control subjects[37,38]. Dykierek et al.[38] studied the REM sleep parameters that could be useful in differentiating AD from normal aging and depression in the geriatric population. They found that they were able to correctly classify 86% of the patients studied using REM density and REM latency measures. In their study, depressed patients tended to have increased REM density and decreased REM latency, while demented patients tended to have decreased REM density and normal to increased REM latency. While the use of EEG and sleep studies are not a standard part of a dementia and depression work-up, in selected cases they may provide additional information that could be helpful to the clinician.

NEUROIMAGING

Recent years have seen significant advances in the development of technology for imaging the central nervous system. Although the value of neuroimaging in the work-up of dementia and geriatric depression is controversial, many authors present strong arguments for its diagnostic utility. The rationale for the use of magnetic resonance imaging/computed tomography (MRI/CT) scans in the work-up of dementia includes the following: (a) neuroimaging contributes to increased diagnostic accuracy and may detect occult lesions not evident on clinical examination; (b) most physicians' clinical skills in diagnosing AD are not sufficient to abandon imaging; (c) CT or MRI may identify potentially treatable causes of dementia missed by clinical evaluation; (d) imaging protects against possible malpractice suits[39]. The arguments against the routine use of neuroimaging include: (a) lack of cost-effectiveness and low yield (prevalence of < 5% for clinically significant findings); (b) lack of influence on eventual outcome; (c) imaging may result in unwanted procedures (e.g. surgery) or cause distress to patients; (d) benign small vessel changes on MRI often result in overdiagnosis of vascular dementia (false positives)[40].

Historically, the use of neuroimaging in the work-up of depression has not been as strongly recommended as it has in the work-up of dementia. However, recent research of the possibility of vascular and degenerative etiologies of geriatric depression has raised the issue of whether neuroimaging should be part of the work-up of geriatric depression[41]. As will be discussed later in this chapter, geriatric depression is becoming increasingly recognized as a heterogeneous illness with multiple possible etiologies, including cerebrovascular disease and neurodegenerative disease, as well as the genetic and psychosocial etiologies recognized in the general adult population. As these possible etiologies become better established, the use of neuroimaging may become more helpful in the classification of geriatric depression, thus impacting treatment and prognosis.

Recent research on the diagnosis of AD using MRI estimated measurements of the temporal lobes has demonstrated impressive sensitivity and specificity. O'Brien et al.[42], in a study to determine the utility of temporal lobe MRI in distinguishing AD from depression, normal aging and other causes of cognitive impairment, found that temporal lobe atrophy provided "good separation" between those patients with AD and those with other causes of cognitive impairment. In particular, anterior hippocampal atrophy was associated with a sensitivity of 83% for detection of AD, and a specificity of 80% for controls, 87% for depressed subjects and 89% for others. Jack et al.[43] found that measurements of hippocampal atrophy provided a sensitive marker for AD, even in the early stages. However, recent studies linking smaller hippocampal volume with depression may limit the utility of this measure in distinguishing depression from dementia[44,45].

The use of functional neuroimaging technology, such as positron-emission tomography (PET) scans and single photon emission tomography (SPECT) scans in the evaluation of dementia and depression is increasingly becoming a subject of research. Although some interesting findings are beginning to emerge[46–48], functional neuroimaging remains primarily a research tool, with limited application to clinical practice. As the technology becomes less expensive and the research shows more consistent and diagnostically useful findings, functional imaging studies may prove to be very powerful tools.

Overall, the use of any form of neuroimaging as a routine part of the work-up of dementia and geriatric depression remains controversial. The utility of functional neuroimaging is uncertain and its use is limited mainly to research. The utility of structural neuroimaging, such as CT or MRI, is becoming more accepted as part of a dementia work-up, but is just beginning to be considered a part of the work-up for geriatric depression. In distinguishing dementia from depression, these studies can provide another useful piece of information to the clinician. However, as with all diagnostic tests, they are not without expense and potential risks/harms, and should be utilized only when the remainder of the clinical evaluation warrants it.

CONCURRENT DEPRESSION AND DEMENTIA

To this point, depression and dementia have been discussed as though they were mutually exclusive diagnoses. However, they commonly coexist in the geriatric population. This concurrence further complicates the task of making a clear diagnosis in the patient who presents with a combination of mood symptoms and cognitive symptoms. Clinical studies report a wide range of prevalence rates for depression in dementia patients. This variance appears to depend on the criteria used and the population studied. In patients with AD, reported rates for depressive disorders have ranged from 0% to 86%, with most studies showing 30–40%[12,49]. The reported rates of depressive symptoms that do not reach diagnostic criteria for a mood disorder are even higher. Many of the less common dementing disorders, such as Parkinson's disease, Huntington's disease and frontotemporal dementia, have rates of depression that exceed those found in AD[50,51].

In light of the significant co-morbidity of depression and the dementing disorders, a number of authors[12,49] are now arguing that the clinical approach to evaluating the elderly patient with mood symptoms and cognitive symptoms should move from the traditional either/or approach to an and/or approach. The impact of not recognizing depression in the context of dementia is significant. Concurrent depression has been reported to increase the disability of patients by lowering the ability to perform instrumental activities of daily living (IADLs) in the mildly cognitive impaired, and lowering the ability to perform activities of daily living (ADLs) in the more severely cognitively impaired[49]. Concurrent depression has even been associated with a greater than 59% mortality rate during the first year in elderly patients admitted to nursing homes[49]. Thus, the recognition and treatment

of depression in the context of dementia can have a profound effect on morbidity and mortality in elderly patients.

"PSEUDODEMENTIA" AND DEPRESSION AS A PRODROME TO DEMENTIA

A great deal has been written about depression with cognitive impairment, generally referred to as "pseudodementia". This has been classically listed as one of the most common causes of reversible dementia. The most commonly described clinical scenario would be of an elderly patient undergoing an evaluation for cognitive impairment and being found to meet diagnostic criteria for depression. With appropriate treatment and resolution of the depression, a significant proportion of such patients would no longer have identifiable cognitive impairment. Increasing evidence, however, has convincingly shown that depression with an initially reversible dementia syndrome will frequently be followed by the development of an irreversible dementia[52,53].

Recent studies have also shown that depressive symptoms in the geriatric population, even without evidence of "pseudodementia", may be a prodrome of degenerative dementias. In a large epidemiological study, Berger et al.[54], found a significantly higher number of depressive symptoms in individuals who later developed AD than in those individuals who did not go on to develop AD. Reding et al.[55] found that, in a sample of patients evaluated in a dementia clinic, 57% of the depressed, non-demented patients develop frank dementia at a 3 year follow-up. The relationship between preclinical depression and the development of dementia is complicated by the difficulty in discerning whether the depression is truly part of a prodrome phase of dementia or whether it is a risk factor for later development of dementia[35]. In either case, the former concept of pseudodementia, separate and apart from true dementia, is not as clear as it once seemed.

VASCULAR DEPRESSION

Recent research has indicated yet another factor that further complicates the relationship between dementia and geriatric depression. It has long been recognized that depression is a common complication of strokes. It is now beginning to be recognized that depression and mood symptoms can be secondary to "silent strokes" or the accumulation of microvascular lesions in the CNS[41,56–58]. Numerous studies are now reporting that significant proportions of elderly patients with depression have evidence of cerebrovascular disease found on MRI and CT studies[56,57]. In particular, lesions in the basal ganglia, periventricular white matter and deep cortical white matter have been associated with depressive symptoms and depression in the elderly[59,60].

This has led to the development of the "vascular depression" hypothesis. Like the dementia in vascular dementia, the depression in vascular depression is thought to arise from vascular insults to the central nervous system. Instead of affecting the systems involved in cognitive processes, the injuries are thought to affect the systems involved in the maintenance of a normal affective state. Thus, it is possible that cerebral vascular disease can not only result in classic stroke symptoms but can also lead to the development of dementia and/or depression.

CONCLUSION

Distinguishing depression from dementia is a difficult clinical task. The cornerstone of making an accurate diagnosis remains the clinical information gathered "at the bedside" from the patient and his/her family. Various screening instruments and routine laboratory studies can contribute useful additional information to the clinician. More advanced studies, such as formal neuro-psychological testing, EEG, neuroimaging and genetic testing, can be helpful in selected patients. In every case, the clinician must keep in mind the high concurrence rate of dementia and depression, the increasing evidence that geriatric depression may be a prodrome of dementia, as well as the research that points to shared etiologies of dementia and geriatric depression, and thus avoid taking a strict either/or approach.

REFERENCES

1. Evans DA, Funkenstein HH, Albert MS *et al*. Prevalence of Alzheimer's disease in a community population of older persons: higher than previously reported. *J Am Med Assoc* 1989; **262**: 2551–6.
2. Geldmacher DS, Whitehouse PJ. Differential diagnosis of Alzheimer's disease. *Neurology* 1997; **48** (suppl 6): S2–9.
3. Lebowitz BD, Pearson JL, Schneider LS *et al*. Diagnosis and treatment of depression in late life: consensus statement update. *J Am Med Assoc* 1997; **278** (14): 1186–90.
4. American Psychiatric Association. *Diagnostic and Statistical Manual of Mental Disorders*, 4th edn (DSM-IV). Washington, DC: American Psychiatric Association, 1994.
5. Small GW, Rabins PV, Barry PP *et al*. Diagnoses and treatment of Alzheimer's disease and related disorders. *J Am Med Assoc* 1997; **278**: 1363–71.
6. US Department of Health and Human Services, Public Health Service, Agency for Health Care Policy and Research. *Recognition and Initial Assessment of Alzheimer's Disease and Related Dementias*. Clinical Practice Guideline No. 19, 1996.
7. Patterson CJS, Gauthire S, Howard B *et al*. The recognition, assessment and management of dementing disorders: conclusions from the Canadian Consensus Conference on Dementia. *Can Med Assoc J* 1999; **160** (suppl 12): S1–15.
8. Doraiswamy PM, Steffens DC, Pitchumoni S, Tabrizi S. Early recognition of Alzheimer's disease: what is consensual? What is controversial? What is practical? *J Clin Psychiat* 1998; **59** (suppl 13): 6–18.
9. Blazer D, Bacher JR, Hughes DC. Major depression with melancholia: A comparison of middle aged and elderly adults. *J Am Geriat Soc* 1987; **35**: 927–32.
10. Renolds CF, Hoch CC, Kupfer DJ *et al*. Bedside differentiation of depressive pseudodementia from dementia. *Am J Psychiat* 1988; **145** (9): 1099–103.
11. Abrams RC, Alexopoulos GS. Assessment of depression in dementia. *Alzheimer's Dis Assoc Disord* 1994; **8** (suppl 1): S227–9.
12. Katz IR. Diagnosis and treatment of depression in patients with Alzheimer's disease and other dementias. *J Clin Psychiat* 1998; **59** (suppl 9): 38–44.
13. Folstein MF, Bassett SS, Anthony JC. Dementia: case ascertainment in a community survey. *J Gerontol* 1991; **46**: M132–8.
14. Bravo G, Hebert R. Age- and education-specific reference values for the Mini-Mental and modified Mini-Mental State Examinations derived from a non-demented elderly population. *Int J Geriat Psychiat* 1997; **12**: 1008–18.
15. Brayne C. Key papers in geriatric psychiatry Mini-Mental State: a practical method for grading the cognitive state of patients for the clinician. *Int J Geriat Psychiat* 1998; **13**: 285–94.
16. Agrell B, Dehlin O. The clock-drawing test. *Age Aging* 1998; **27**: 399–403.
17. Watson YI, Arfken CL, Birge SJ. Clock completion: an objective screening test for dementia. *J Am Geriat Soc* 1993; **41**: 1235–40.
18. Kafonek S, Ettinger WH, Roca R *et al*. Instruments for screening for depression and dementia in a long-term care facility. *J Am Geriat Soc* 1989; **37**: 29–34.
19. Ogrocki PK, Welsh-Bohmer KA. Assessment of cognitive and functional impairment in the elderly. *Neurodegenerative Dementias: Clinical Features and Pathological Mechanisms*. New York: McGraw-Hill, 2000.
20. Rosenstein LD. Differential diagnosis of the major progressive dementias and depression in middle and late adulthood: a summary of the literature of the early 1990s. *Neuropsychol Rev* 1998; **8** (3): 109–67.
21. Jacobs DM, Sano M, Dooneief G *et al*. Neuropsychological detection and characterization of preclinical Alzheimer's disease. *Neurology* 1995; **45**: 957–62.
22. Macknight C, Graham J, Rockwood K. Factors associated with inconsistent diagnosis of dementia between physicians and neuropsychologists. *J Am Geriat Soc* 1999; **47** (11): 1294–9.
23. Carnes M, Smith JC, Kalin NH, Bauwens SF. Effects of chronic medical illness and dementia on the dexamethasone suppression test. *J Am Geriat Soc* 1983; **31**: 269–71.
24. McAllister TW, Ferrell RB, Price TRP, Neville MB. The dexamethasone suppression test in two patients with severe depressive pseudodementia. *Am J Psychiat* 1982; **139**: 479–81.
25. Spar JE, Gerner R. Does the dexamethasone suppression test distinguish dementia from depression? *Am J Psychiat* 1982; **139**: 238–40.
26. Raskind M, Peskind E, Rivard MF *et al*. Dexamethasone suppression test and cortisol circadian rhythm in primary degenerative dementia. *Am J Psychiat* 1982; **139**: 1468–71.
27. Alexopoulos GS, Young RC, Haycox JA *et al*. Dexamethasone suppression test in depression with reversible dementia. *Psychiat Resid* 1985; **16**: 277–85.
28. McAllister TW, Hays LR. TRH test, DST and response to desipramine in primary degenerative dementia. *Biol Psychiat* 1987; **22**: 189–93.
29. Shrimanker J, Soni SD, McMurray J. Dexamethasone suppression test in dementia and depression. Clinical and biological correlates. *Br J Psychiat* 1989; **154**: 372–7.
30. American Academy of Neurology. Practice parameter for diagnosis and evaluation of dementia. *Neurology* 1994; **44**: 2203–6.
31. Lovestone S. Early diagnosis and the clinical genetics of Alzheimer's disease. *J Neurol* 1999; **246**: 69–72.
32. Corder EH, Saunders AM, Strittmatter WJ *et al*. Gene dose of apolipoprotein E type 4 allele and the risk of Alzheimer's disease in late-onset families. *Science* 1993; **261**: 921–3.
33. Krishnan KRR, Tupler LA, Ritchie JC *et al*. Apolipoprotein E4 frequency in geriatric depression. *Biol Psychiat* 1996; **40**: 69–71.
34. Yoshizawa T, Yamakawa-Kobayashi K, Komatsuzaki Y *et al*. Dose-dependent association of apolipoprotein E allele 4 with late-onset, sporadic Alzheimer's disease. *Ann Neurol* 1994; **36**: 656–9.
35. Steffens DC, Plassman BL, Helms MJ *et al*. A twin study of late-onset depression and apolipoprotein E E4 as risk factors for Alzheimer's disease. *Biol Psychiat* 1997; **41**: 851–6.
36. Klass DW, Brenner RP. Electroencephalography of the elderly. *J Clin Neurophysiol* 1995; **12**: 116–31.
37. Perlis ML, Giles DE, Buysse DJ *et al*. Which depressive symptoms are related to which sleep electroencephalographic variables? *Biol Psychiat* 1997; **42**: 904–13.
38. Dykierek P, Stadtmuller G, Schramm P *et al*. The value of REM sleep parameters in differentiating Alzheimer's disease from old-age depression and normal aging. *J Psychiat Res* 1998; **32**: 1–9.
39. Katzman R. Should a major imaging procedure (CT or MRI) be required in the workup of dementia? Affirmative view. *J Fam Pract* 1990; **31**: 405–10.
40. Clarfield AM, Larson EB. Should major imaging procedure (CT or MRI) be required in the workup of dementia? Opposing view. *J Fam Pract* 1990; **31**: 405–10.
41. Steffens DC, Krishnan KRR. Structural neuroimaging and mood disorders: recent finding, implications for classification and future directions. *Biol Psychiat* 1998; **43**: 705–12.
42. O'Brien JT, Desmond P, Schweitzer AI *et al*. Temporal lobe magnetic resonance imaging can differentiate Alzheimer's disease from normal ageing, depression, vascular dementia and other causes of cognitive impairment. *Psychol Med* 1997; **27**: 1267–75.
43. Jack CR, Petersen RC, Xu YC *et al*. Medial temporal atrophy on MRI in normal aging and very mild Alzheimer's disease. *Neurology* 1997; **49**: 786–94.
44. Sheline YI. Hippocampal atrophy in major depression: a result of depression-induced neurotoxicity. *Mol Psychiat* 1996; **4**: 298–9.
45. Steffens DC, Byrum CE, McQuoid DR *et al*. Hippocampal volume in geriatric depression. *Biol Psychiat* 2000; **48**: 301–9.

46. Bench CJ, Friston KJ, Brown RG *et al*. Regional cerebral blood flow in depression measured by positron emission tomography: the relationship with clinical dimensions. *Psychol Med* 1993; **23**: 579–90.

47. Kennedy SH, Javanmard M, Vaccarino FJ. A review of functional neuroimaging in mood disorders: positron emission tomography and depression. *Can J Psychiat* 1997; **42**: 467–75.

48. Bench CJ, Frackowiak DJ, Dolan RJ. Changes in regional cerebral blood flow on recovery from depression. *Psychol Med* 1995; **25**: 247–51.

49. Meyers BS. Depression and dementia: comorbidities, identification, and treatment. *J Geriat Psychiat Neurol* 1998; **11**: 201–5.

50. Swartz JR, Miller BL, Lesser IM *et al*. Behavioral phenomenology in Alzheimer's disease, frontotemporal dementia, and late life depression: a retrospective analysis. *J Geriat Psychiat Neurol* 1997; **10**: 67–74.

51. Cummings JL, Masterman DL. Depression in patients with Parkinson's disease. *Int J Geriat Psychiat* 1999; **14**: 711–18.

52. Kral VA, Emery OB. Long-term follow-up of depressive pseudodementia of the aged. *Can J Psychiat* 1989; **34**: 445–6.

53. Alexopoulos GS, Young RC, Meyers BS. Geriatric depression: age of onset and dementia. *Biol Psychiat* 1993; **34**: 141–5.

54. Berger AK, Fratiglioni L, Forsell Y *et al*. The occurrence of depressive symptoms in the preclinical phase of AD: a population-based study. *Neurology* 1999; **53** (9): 1998–2002.

55. Reding M, Haycox J, Blass J. Depression in patients referred to a dementia clinic. *Arch Neurol* 1985; **42**: 894–6.

56. Alexopoulos GS, Meyers BS, Young RC *et al*. Clinically defined vascular depression. *Am J Psychiat* 1997; **154** (4): 562–5.

57. Krishnan KRR, Hays JC, Blazer DG. MRI-defined vascular depression. *Am J Psychiat* 1997; **154** (4): 497–501.

58. Alexopoulos GS, Meyers BS, Young RC *et al*. Vascular depression hypothesis. *Arch Gen Psychiat* 1997; **54**: 915–22.

59. Fujikawa T, Yamawaki S, Touhouda Y. Incidence of silent cerebral infarction in patients with major depression. *Stroke* 1993; **24**: 1631–4.

60. Steffens DC, Helms MJ, Krishnan KRR, Burke GL. Cerebrovascular disease and depression symptoms in the cardiovascular health study. *Stroke* 1999; **30**: 2159–66.

Benign Senescent Forgetfulness, Age-associated Memory Impairment, and Age-related Cognitive Decline

Kathleen A. Welsh-Bohmer and David J. Madden

Duke University Medical Center, Durham, NC, USA

Changes in cognitive functioning are prevalent in aging. These changes are perhaps best considered as falling along a continuum, with normal aging at one end of the scale and brain diseases producing bona fide dementias at the other end. It is not clear that the continuum of cognitive changes in aging and disease is entirely linear. There may be periods of plateaux in cognitive declines or even improvements in cognition as a function of adaptive brain changes. The relationship of cognitive change in normal aging and brain disease, such as Alzheimer's disease (AD) is an area of active investigation, benefiting from the advances in behavioral methods and imaging technologies[1,2].

Normal aging is now recognized as a complex mosaic of cognitive changes in which there is decline in some areas and a substantial degree of either stability or improvement in others[3]. It has been frequently observed, for example, that *fluid* abilities, those relying primarily on the efficiency of current processing (e.g. measures of spatial and reasoning abilities), exhibit pronounced and approximately linear age-related decline, whereas *crystallized* abilities, those relying more on accumulated knowledge and expertise (e.g. vocabulary measures) exhibit greater stability as a function of age. A prominent feature of normal age-related cognitive change is a decline in the speed of information processing, a decline that is more critical to the functioning of fluid abilities than to the functioning of crystallized abilities. Salthouse[4] has developed a general theory of age-related changes in fluid cognition. The theory contains two central components: a limited time mechanism and a simultaneity mechanism. According to Salthouse, changes in these mechanisms, at an elementary level, lead to changes that are observed in a variety of cognitive tasks. For example, the time available to perform higher-order cognitive operations would be limited by an increase in the proportion of the available time occupied by initial processing stages. Similarly, if initial processing is slowed, then the products of this processing may not be available simultaneously, as required by later operations.

Between the two boundaries of normal aging and genuine cognitive impairment is a broad transition state comprising gradations of cognitive change attributable to any of a host of etiologies, including benign effects of aging to early-stage AD. Over the last three decades, a variety of nomenclatures have emerged to describe the observed transitional memory state attributed to aging. The most commonly recognized terms include "benign senescent forgetfulness", "age-associated memory impairment" and, more recently, "mile cognitive impairment".

These terms vary in subtle ways from one another. However, regardless of which terminology is used, all of these categorization schemas basically describe the same phenomenon, an admixture of mild memory problems that exceeds the range of normal cognition but falls short of being classified as dementia.

The term "benign senescent forgetfulness" (BSF) was originally coined by Kral[5] in the early 1960s to describe a form of mild memory impairment that occurred in the context of aging and did not appear to progress to dementia. In cohorts of elderly nursing home residents followed over 4 years, Kral *et al.*[6] observed that approximately 18% demonstrated a form of mild memory loss described as "subjective complaints of memory loss" and "difficulty in retrieving stored recent or remote information", such as names or other proper nouns. Frequently, these individuals were able to retrieve the "forgotten" information at a later time and they had well-maintained mental faculties otherwise. Compared to this group, another subgroup emerged with a more significant memory impairment, characterized by a prominent inability to retain recent information over even brief periods of time. These individuals typically had limited awareness of their difficulties and had tendencies to confabulate. This latter group, designated as "malignant memory loss", was associated with progression in symptoms to dementia, shorter survival times and increased mortality rates[6]. Kral believed that BSF was associated with physiological aging, whereas the more malignant form of memory decline was related to either vascular or degenerative disease.

The construct of BSF, although useful in succinctly describing the boundary conditions of aging, fell out of favor in later years, primarily due to a lack of standardization in the diagnostic criteria and the absence of clinical validation within representative elderly populations. The samples used in Kral's early work were criticized because of the inclusion of a very large proportion of chronic conditions, such as neurodegenerative diseases, cerebrovascular conditions and neuropsychiatric disorders. In more recent years, interest in aging and AD led to a re-emergence of attention on transitional memory states. In 1986, a workgroup convened under the auspices of the National Institute of Mental Health (NIMH) proposed the construct "age-associated memory impairment" (AAMI) to replace BSF. The new terminology had a firmer theoretical basis than its predecessor, with clinical and anatomical data to support its validity. The new nomenclature also improved upon BSF in that it included well-delineated standardized diagnostic criteria. The latter feature rendered the new terminology more amenable to cross-laboratory investigation and potential intervention through pharmaceutical treatment trials[7].

Briefly, the criteria for the AAMI diagnosis includes: (a) the presence of subjective memory decline in an individual over the age of 50; (b) objective evidence of memory loss on standardized testing of memory function; (c) adequate intellectual function; and (d) the absence of global cognitive decline (i.e. dementia) or other disorders that could account for the symptoms. Although similar in form to the types of criteria used in arriving at other neurological diagnoses, such as AD and vascular dementia[8], the definition of AAMI differs in its specification of strict psychometric cut-points for the demonstration of memory loss and the absence of dementia. A patient diagnosed as AAMI must: (a) perform at least one standard deviation below the mean (for young adults) on at least one standardized test of memory function (e.g. Logical Memory from the Wechsler Memory Scale); and (b) demonstrate the absence of dementia, defined by normal performance on mental status screening using another psychometric measure, the Mini-Mental State examination (MMSE; a score of 24 or higher required).

The approach to defining the memory loss of aging based on a psychometric algorithm has been challenged on several grounds[9,10]. One of the main issues raised is the potential for diagnostic unreliability, particularly the threat of high false-positive rates, because the criteria rely on the results of a single memory test rather than on a consistent pattern of memory deficit. Spuriously low scores on a memory test (such as on the proposed use of the Logical Memory subtest) can be obtained for any of a variety of reasons. Similarly, patients with bona fide disorders may score quite well on the test but manifest difficulties in everyday life and on more tasking neuropsychological procedures. Related to this point, the criteria do not take into account individual differences in performance (e.g. effects of low education opportunities) or any of a variety of conditions that may alter performance and result in the mistaken impression of memory deficits, such as test anxiety or mood disorders. Finally, the choice of psychometric cut-points in the criteria for AAMI are criticized as insensitive. Dementias, particularly in early but clinically diagnosable stages, cannot be satisfactorily ruled out with MMSE scores of 24 or higher. Beyond these criticisms there is an even more fundamental concern that relates to the validity of AAMI as a process distinct from AD and other dementias. There is still considerable debate as to whether serious memory loss in the absence of dementia is actually a prodromal form of AD. The provision of an acronym, along with diagnostic criteria, implies that AAMI is an independent process associated with normal aging. However, much like its predecessor, BSF, there is ambiguity in the relationship between AAMI and AD. In fact, the similarity between the two conditions with respect to the underlying pathophysiology and proposed mechanisms for drug action suggest that AAMI is either a risk factor for AD or a mild, prodromal form of the illness. Despite these limitations, the notion of AAMI has advanced studies of aging by providing uniform criteria which could be applied across multiple sites. In so doing, the AAMI construct has allowed useful cross-study comparisons of the memory loss seen in the later decades of life.

Recently, studies from the investigative team at the Mayo Institute Alzheimer's Disease Center have suggested an alternative nomenclature for patients with memory impairments of aging, suspected to include substantial numbers of patients with preclinical AD[11]. These investigators refer to the boundary between normal aging and dementia as "mild cognitive impairment" (MCI), and characterize its clinical characterization and outcome. Unlike the terms AAMI and BSF, MCI is not considered benign and is instead viewed as being a risk factor or transitional state between normal aging and AD. This premise has some empirical support, including incidence data suggesting that there is a significant conversion rate from MCI to AD of approximately 12–15%/year (in line with other studies suggesting 50% conversion in 5 years). Normal controls, by contrast, convert to AD on an average of 1–2%/year. Because of the care devoted towards empirically defining the borderline condition of AD and aging, the "MCI" terminology is now growing in general acceptance and is becoming the standard nomenclature used by AD investigators involved in preclinical AD studies. It is still unclear whether all patients with symptoms conforming to MCI will convert to AD. Most likely the group of patients have some heterogeneity to their symptoms, reflecting multiple physical or medical causes (e.g. cardiovascular disease, diabetes, pulmonary conditions, etc.). With continuing progress in the identification of the underlying neuronal mechanisms of cognitive decline within normal aging, more clarity will be achieved in separating the various types of age associated memory conditions. This information is critical for secondary prevention efforts in preclinical AD.

REFERENCES

1. Gabrieli JDE. Memory systems analyses of mnemonic disorders of aging and age-related diseases. *Proc Natl Acad Sci* 1996; **93**: 13 534–40.
2. Small SA, Perera GM, De La Paz R *et al*. Differential regional dysfunction of the hippocampal formation among elderly with memory decline and Alzheimer's disease. *Ann Neurol* 1999; **45**: 466–72.
3. Craik FIM, Salthouse TA (eds). *The Handbook of Aging and Cognition*, 2nd edn. Mahwah, NJ: Erlbaum, 2000.
4. Salthouse TA. The processing-speed theory of adult age differences in cognition. *Psychol Rev* 1996; **103**: 403–28.
5. Kral VA. Senescent forgetfulness: benign and malignant. *Can Med Assoc J* 1962; **86**: 257–60.
6. Kral VA, Cahn C, Mueller H. Senescent memory impairment and its relation to general health of the aging individual. *J Geriat Soc* 1964; **12**: 101–13.
7. Crook T, Bartus RT, Ferris SH *et al*. Age-associated memory impairment: proposed diagnostic criteria and measures of clinical change. Report of a National Institute of Mental Health group. *Dev Neuropsychol* 1986; **2**: 261–76.
8. McKhann G, Drachman D, Folstein MF *et al*. Clinical diagnosis of Alzheimer's disease: report of the NINCDS–ADRDA Work Group under the auspices of Department of Health and Human Services Task Force on Alzheimer's disease. *Neurology* 1984; **34**: 939–44.
9. Derouesne C, Kalafat M, Guez D *et al*. The age-associated memory impairment construct revisited: comments and recommendations of a French-speaking work group. *Int J Geriat Psychiat* 1994; **9**: 577–87.
10. Larrabee GJ, McEntree WJ. Age-associated memory impairment: sorting out the controversies. *Neurology* 1995; **45**: 611–14.
11. Petersen RC, Smith GE, Waring SC *et al*. Mild Cognitive impairment: clinical characterization and outcome. *Arch Neurol* 1999; **56**: 303–8.

56

Minor Cognitive Impairment

Karen Ritchie and Jacques Touchon

INSERM E99-30, Montpellier, France

Normal cognitive functioning in the elderly has commonly been conceptualized as the range of performance found in persons without identified pathology. Comparisons of mean performance between age cohorts show decrement with increasing age, which has been attributed in the past to normal physiological ageing processes. So-called ageing-related cognitive impairment, while being considered "normal", nonetheless has been of interest to clinicians because of the physical dependency it engenders, and as such it has been given independent nosological status. A number of concepts have been proposed to describe this tail-end of the normal cognitive range, beginning with the notion of "benign senescent forgetfulness", first proposed by Kral[1]. The publication of formal diagnostic criteria for minor cognitive impairment as "age-associated memory impairment" (AAMI) was undertaken by Crook *et al.*[2] for the National Institute of Mental Health. AAMI refers to subjective complaints of memory loss in elderly persons verified by a decrement of at least one standard deviation on a formal memory test in comparison with means established for young adults.

As memory impairment in the elderly is more commonly observed to be accompanied by deficits in other areas of cognitive performance, an alternative concept, ageing-associated cognitive decline (AACD), has been proposed by the International Psychogeriatric Association in collaboration with the World Health Organization[3]. AACD refers to a wider range of cognitive functions (attention, memory, learning, thinking, language and visuospatial function), and is diagnosed by reference to norms for elderly subjects. Application of AACD and AAMI to elderly persons within the general population suggests that they are distinct clinical entities, the latter referring to a more severe state of impairment[4].

More recently, recognition that the wide variability in cognitive functioning observed in the normal elderly may be due at least in part to the inclusion in this group of persons with prodromal dementia or other sub-clinical syndromes has led to the generation of alternative formulations, which situate minor cognitive impairment as potential pathology, for which the clinical response should be therapeutic rather than palliative. Within the 10th revision of the International Classification of Diseases (ICD-10)[5], criteria are given for "mild cognitive disorder" (MCD), which refers, like AACD, to a broader range of cognitive disorders than memory, demonstrable by formal neuropsychological testing and hypothetically attributable to cerebral disease or damage or to systemic physical disease known to cause dysfunction. MCD is thus construed as being secondary to physical illness or impairment, excluding dementia, amnesic syndrome, concussion or post-encephalitic syndrome. MCD is also applicable to all ages, not just the elderly. Early attempts to apply MCD criteria to population studies of elderly persons has so far met with limited success, which has cast doubt on the validity of MCD as a separate nosological entity[22]. On the other hand, Gutierrez *et al.*[6], arguing for the inclusion of a similar category in DSM ("mild neurocognitive disorder") have reviewed numerous studies implicating diverse forms of underlying pathology, in which such a nosological category would have been appropirate.

Early evidence that elderly persons with minor cognitive disorder may be at high risk of developing senile dementia has led to the development of the concept of "mild cognitive impairment" (MCI)[7]. MCI has provoked considerable interest amongst clinicians and the pharmaceutical industry, as it refers to a much larger potential therapeutic target group than senile dementia. As such, it is likely to become a more widely-adopted concept than its predecessors. The essential feature of MCI is that it is a pathological state that is potentially progressive. Beyond this, specific diagnostic criteria found in the current literature are inconsistent. Petersen *et al.*[7] initially refer to "complaints of defective memory" and "demonstration of abnormal memory functioning for age", with normal general cognitive functioning and conserved ability to perform activities of daily living. A later definition refers to "memory impairment beyond that expected for both age and education level"[8]. Krasuki *et al.*[9] refer to cognitive impairment with a score of 20 or more on the MMSE, and Zaudig[10] defines MCI as a score of more than 22 on MMSE or 34–47 on the SIDAM dementia scale. Others have referred to criteria based on the Clinical Dementia Rating Scale or the Global Deterioration Scale scores[11,12].

A central problem in the definition of MCI has been whether or not it should be confined exclusively to isolated memory impairment. Petersen *et al.*[8] specify that in MCI general intellectual functioning should be preserved, and that only memory should be affected, as it is the restriction of the impairment to amnesic abilities which differentiates the syndrome from AD. Isolated memory impairment was observed by the authors in a series of 76 MCI subjects; however, this appears to have been part of the diagnostic criteria for entry into the study, so that the situation is somewhat circular. Apart from the general problem of cognitive domain specificity in neuropsychometric testing (i.e. ascertaining that poor performance on a memory task is purely related to memory and does not implicate other functions, such as attention and language comprehension), other researchers have noted that subjects with MCI, although primarily having memory complaints, also commonly show deficits in other cognitive domains[11–14]. If the concept of MCI is extended to include areas of cognitive impairment other than memory, then it may be considered to be identical to that of AACD, except for the underlying assumption that it is a potentially pathological, progressive syndrome rather than a feature of normal ageing.

To what extent may MCI be considered a prodromal phase of AD? A number of studies have suggested a significantly elevated risk of dementia in MCI subjects, with estimates of 10–15%/year of MCI subjects developing dementia to 100% over 4 years[8,9,14–17]. These studies are, however, all small hospital-based series. Risk factors for progression to dementia derived from larger-scale studies are ApoE 4, higher age, fine motor deficit and lower pre-morbid IQ[8,12,18].

A number of studies have described neurological changes in CT studies of MCI that distinguish it from normal ageing and senile dementia[9,14]. The principal characteristic observed in these studies is temporal lobe atrophy. Celsis et al.[19] (1997) report reduced parietal–temporal perfusion and left/right parietal–temporal asymmetry using SPECT in MCI. The observed hypoperfusion levels were found to be intermediate between those found in normal and AD subjects. Julin[20] used aligned SPECT and MRI images to compare MCI with early AD. AD patients were found to have atrophy and cerebral blood flow (CBF) reduction in both medial temporal and temporoparietal regions, whereas MCI showed significant reduction in CBF without atrophy in the temporoparietal region only. Jelic et al.[21] have used quantified EEG to demonstrate similarities between AD and MCI that differentiate both groups from the normal elderly on temporoparietal coherence and α and θ relative power. These findings suggest that MCI and AD have similar anatomical loci, with MCI being principally differentiated by the degree of impairment, and functional rather than structural change.

In a 3 year follow-up study, McKelvey et al.[17] reported that 64% of MCI subjects had abnormal SPECT scans at baseline; 53% of this cohort developed dementia, but of those developing dementia only 67% had initially abnormal scans, giving a positive predictive value of only 50%. On the other hand, Johnson et al.[15] have demonstrated a clear progression from MCI to dementia, based on SPECT perfusion levels from four regions; the hippocampal–amygdaloid complex, the anterior and posterior cingulate and the anterior thalamus. The authors conclude that, with semi-quantitative analysis and a spatial resolution sufficient to detect perfusion in limbic structures, it is possible to differentiate MCI from AD.

In conclusion, a number of nosological entities have been proposed to describe minor cognitive disorders occurring in elderly persons without dementia. MCI will probably evolve as one of the most important concepts in this area, with its underlying assumption that cognitive disorders in elderly persons are potential pathologies for which therapeutic care should be sought, rather than inevitable features of the normal ageing process. The concept appears to be almost identical to that of AACD, apart from its supposition of underlying pathology, but presently lacks clear operational criteria for either research or clinical application.

REFERENCES

1. Kral VA. Senescent forgetfulness: benign and malignant. *Can Med Assoc J* 1962; **86**: 257–60.
2. Crook T, Bartus RT, Ferris SH *et al*. Age associated memory impairment: proposed diagnostic criteria and measures of clinical change—report of a National Institute of Mental Health Work Group. *Dev Neuropsychol* 1986; **2**: 261–76.
3. Levy R on behalf of the Aging-associated Cognitive Decline Working Party. Aging-associated cognitive decline. *Int Psychogeriat* 1994; **6**: 63–8.
4. Richards M, Touchon J, Ledésert B, Ritchie K. Cognitive decline in ageing: are AAMI and AACD distinct entities? *Int J Geriat Psychiat* (in press).
5. World Health Organization. *The ICD-10 Classification of Mental and Behavioural Disorders. Diagnostic Criteria for Research*. Geneva: World Health Organization, 1993.
6. Gutierrez *et al*. (1993).
7. Petersen RC, Smith GE, Waring SC *et al*. Aging, memory and mild cognitive impairment. *Int Psychogeriat* 1997; **9**: 65–9.
8. Petersen RC, Smith GE, Waring SC *et al*. Mild cognitive impairment: clinical characterization and outcome. *Arch Neurol* 1999; **56**: 303–8.
9. Krasuki JS, Alexander GE, Horwitz B *et al*. Volumes of medial temporal lobe structures in patients with Alzheimer's disease and mild cognitive impairment (and in healthy controls). *Biol Psychiat* 1998; **43**: 60–8.
10. Zaudig M. A new systematic method of measurement and diagnosis of "Mild Cognitive Impairment" and dementia according to ICD-10 and DSM III-R criteria. *Int Psychogeriat* 1992; **4**: 203–19.
11. Flicker C, Ferris FH, Reisberg B. Mild cognitive impairment in the elderly: predictors of dementia. *Neurology* 1991; **41**: 1006–9.
12. Kluger A, Gianutsos JG, Golomb J *et al*. Motor/psychomotor dysfunction in normal aging, mild cognitive decline, and early Alzheimer's disease: diagnostic and differential diagnostic features. *Int Psychogeriat* 1997; **9**: 307–16.
13. Flicker C *et al*. (1998).
14. Wolf H, Grunwald M, Ecke GM *et al*. The prognosis of mild cognitive impairment in the elderly. *J Neural Transm* 1998; **54**: 31–50.
15. Johnson KA, Jones K, Holman BL. Preclinical prediction of Alzheimer's disease using SPECT. *Neurology* 1998; **50**: 1563–72.
16. Black SE. Can SPECT predict the future for mild cognitive impairment? *Can J Neurol Sci* 1999; **26**: 4–6.
17. McKelvey R, Bergman H, Stern J. Lack of prognostic significance of SPECT abnormalities in elderly subjects with mild memory loss. *Can J Neurol Sci* 1999; **26**: 23–8.
18. Ritchie K, Leibovici D, Ledésert B, Touchon J. Sub-clinical cognitive impairment: epidemiology and clinical characteristics. *Comp Psychiat* (in press).
19. Celsis P, Agneil A, Cardebat D. Age related cognitive decline: a clinical entity? A longitudinal study of cerebral blood flow and memory performance. *J Neurol Neurosurg Psychiat* 1997; **62**: 601–8.
20. Julin P. MRI and SPECT neuroimaging in mild cognitive impairment and Alzheimer's disease. Doctoral dissertation, Karolinska Institute, 1997.
21. Jelic V, Shigeta M, Julin P *et al*. Quantitative electroencephalography power and coherence in Alzheimer's disease and mild cognitive impairment. *Dementia* 1996; **7**: 314–23.
22. Christensen H, Henderson AS, Jorm AF *et al*. ICD-10 mild cognitive disorder: epidemiological evidence on its validity. *Psychol Med* 1995; **25**: 105–20.

Alzheimer's Disease: One or Several?

C. Holmes and A. Mann

Institute of Psychiatry, London, UK

The current research diagnostic criteria for psychiatric illness, DSM-IV[1] and ICD-10[2] have evolved from a clinically descriptive exercise to an operationally defined procedure with a sharp demarcation between disease categories. In studies of dementia, diagnostic criteria with a hierarchical approach to diagnosis have also been widely adopted, in which the probability of a diagnostic subtype of dementia being present in a subject is also specified[3–5]. Subjects who fulfil clinical diagnostic criteria for probable disease are considered to have a purer form of the disease than those fulfilling the possible diagnostic category alone. This categorical approach aims to maximize differences between cases so that they are cleanly diagnosed. Thus, the presence of a delirium excludes the diagnosis of dementia, and the presence of cerebrovascular disease debars the diagnosis of probable Alzheimer's disease (AD). So widespread is the use of these diagnostic criteria that it is now almost impossible to practise clinical psychiatry, let alone get research findings published, without reference to them.

Clearly, this approach has its uses. It enables psychiatrists from different cultures to know, within the restraints of the diagnostic criteria, what collection of phenomenology or associated pathology they are talking about. An expertise (and associated research projects) can be developed within these diagnostic categories.

However, there are problems with such an approach and these are particularly clear in the area of dementia research. Thus, a categorical approach to diagnosis can lead to the exclusion of a large and interesting group of patients who do not fall into neat divisions. Such an approach emphasizes research into differences rather than similarities, between diagnostic categories. Finally, the assumption that clinical diagnostic categories have biological meaning is questionable.

In dementing illness, mixed pathologies are common. Indeed, the presence of vascular or Lewy body pathology, in the absence of other pathology, is relatively rare[6]. The reasons why various pathologies coexist could give important clues to the aetiology of both. However, for example, examination of patients fulfilling NINCDS–ADRDA diagnostic criteria for probable AD will lead to the exclusion of patients who have vascular risk factors, and so their importance in the development of AD pathology will be underestimated[7]. Common risk factors that are likely to be important in the development of AD and vascular disease have been recently reviewed[8], with associations found between AD and atherosclerosis, smoking, type 2 diabetes and high cholesterol. The mechanisms of such a link are not yet established. Does vascular disease play a part in the promotion of AD pathology or its presentation? Do common factors, such as insulin resistance, oxidative stress or cytokine activation, underlie both pathologies? Clearly, the examination of mixed cases in research studies would be beneficial in understanding common aetiological mechanisms.

The separation of some diagnostic categories lends an emphasis to differences where in fact greater similarities exist. Dementia and delirium, like the common subgroups of dementia, often coexist and also share many similar clinical and biological features. This finding is, ironically, emphasized by the demarcation of one subgroup of dementia, dementia with Lewy bodies, which has clinical characteristics such as prominent attentional deficits, hallucinations and fluctuating cognition that can make differentiation from delirium, particularly in initial presentation, very difficult. Rather than emphasize differences, another approach would be to accept the clinical similarities and to examine in more detail common epidemiological factors and pathological mechanisms of action, such as acetylcholine depletion and cytokine activation[9].

The adoption of clinical diagnostic criteria often presumes that a group of individuals, having reconciled a number of different opinions of varying political strength, have been able to define a single biological entity on the basis of its clinical features. Clearly, this is highly unlikely. Indeed, in dementia research (where we are fortunate in having generally agreed neuropathological hallmarks by which this hypothesis can be tested) it can be seen that the application of clinical research diagnostic criteria to a community-based sample of patients with dementia suggests that, while they are efficient in identifying pathology *per se*, they are notably less efficient when other pathologies are present[6].

In summary, whilst clinical diagnostic criteria have their uses, they also have their limitations. A broader perspective is needed, which can encompass research into the common aetiological mechanisms that explain the existence of common clinical or pathological phenomena across, and between, different clinical diagnostic categories.

REFERENCES

1. American Psychiatric Association. *Diagnostic and Statistical Manual of Mental Disorders*, 4th edn (DSM-IV). Washington, DC: APA, 1994.
2. World Health Organization. The ICD-10 *Classification of Mental and Behavioural Disorders*. Geneva: WHO, 1992.
3. McKhann G, Drachman D, Folstein M *et al*. Clinical diagnosis of Alzheimer's disease. Report of the NINCDS–ADRDA work group under the auspices of Department of Health and Human Services Task Force on Alzheimer's Disease. *Neurology*: 1984; **34**: 939–44.
4. Roman GC, Tatemichi TK, Erkinjuntti T *et al*. Vascular dementia: diagnostic criteria for research studies. Report of the NINDS–AIREN International Workshop. *Neurology* 1993; **43**: 250–60.
5. McKeith IG, Galasko D, Kosaka K *et al*. Consensus guidelines for the clinical and pathologic diagnosis of dementia with Lewy bodies (DLB): report of the consortium on DLB international workshop. *Neurology* 1996; **47**: 1113–24.
6. Holmes C, Cairns N, Lantos P, Mann A. Validity of current clinical criteria for Alzheimer's disease, vascular dementia and dementia with Lewy bodies. *Br J Psychiat* 1999; **174**: 45–50.
7. Prince MJ. Vascular risk factors and atherosclerosis as risk factors for cognitive decline and dementia. *J Psychosom Res* 1995; **39**(5): 525–30.
8. Stewart R. Cardiovascular factors in Alzheimer's Disease. *J Neurol Neurosurg Psychiat* 1998; **65**: 143–7.
9. Eikelenboom P, Hoogendijk WJ. Do delirium and Alzheimer's dementia share specific pathogenetic mechanisms? *Dement Geriat Cogn Disord* 1999; **10**(5): 319–24.

Prognosis of Dementia

Barry Reisberg, Alan Kluger and Emile Franssen

Aging and Dementia Research Center, New York, USA

Dementia occurs on a continuum with the cognitive changes of normal aging and with mild cognitive impairment (MCI)[1,2]. Also, the process of dementia proceeds for many years after mental status assessments and conventional psychometric measures have reached floor (bottom) scores. Consequently, a clinically meaningful and useful description of the prognosis of dementia requires measures that are capable of spanning this vast cognitive continuum. Two kinds of measures that have been found to be particularly useful in describing this continuum and associated prognostic features are global assessments and assessment of the progressive functional course of brain aging and dementia. Two specific measures that have been found to be particularly useful in this regard are the Global Deterioration Scale[3] and the Functional Assessment Staging (FAST) procedure[4] (*see* Tables 1 and 2).

In a recent longitudinal study of more than 200 normal aged and MCI subjects followed over a mean interval of 4 years, the overall accuracy of GDS stage assignment at baseline (i.e. GDS stage 1, 2 or 3) in predicting subsequent decline to dementia was 81%[5]. In another longitudinal study of more than 100 community-residing patients with probable Alzheimer's disease (AD), who were followed over a mean interval of nearly 5 years, the correlation between change in GDS stage and time elapsed was 0.48, the correlation between change in FAST stage and time elapsed was 0.45, and the correlation between change in MMSE score and time elapsed was 0.32[6]. Consequently, the GDS and FAST measures each individually explained approximately twice the variance in AD temporal course of that accounted for by MMSE change. Furthermore, the GDS and FAST measures to some extent accounted for independent temporal variance. Consequently, these staging procedures (the GDS and FAST measures) together explained 28% of the variance (corresponding to a multiple regression correlation of 0.53), whereas change on the MMSE accounted for only 10% of variance (corresponding to a correlation of 0.32). This latter variance in the MMSE was entirely subsumed within that of the change on the GDS and FAST assessments.

What these statistics mean is that, with the staging procedures outlined in Tables 1 and 2, we can much more accurately chart the boundaries of normal aging and progressive AD and much more accurately predict the course of AD than with mental status assessments. The staging procedures also have the advantage of being clinically meaningful. This section briefly outlines the boundaries and prognosis of normal brain aging and progressive dementia, especially the dementia of AD, in terms of global, functional and traditional mental status assessments.

NORMAL BRAIN AGING

Although many, and perhaps most, persons over the age of 65 experience at least subjective cognitive complaints, many aged individuals have neither subjectively nor objectively manifest decrements in cognitive functioning. On the GDS and FAST measures, these individuals are in Stage 1. Current data indicates that the prognosis for these persons may be better than that for equivalently aged subjects with subjective complaints[5,7]. Clearly,

the general prognosis for these persons is for continued healthy cognitive functioning.

AGE-ASSOCIATED MEMORY IMPAIRMENT

This entity is most clearly and usefully defined as one in which individuals experience subjective complaints of impairment, but in which even subtle deficits are absent upon clinical evaluation[8]. Although this condition (Stage 2 on the GDS and FAST scales), is largely benign, a recent longitudinal study found that nearly 15% of more than 100 subjects at a mean baseline age of approximately 70 years at this stage declined to a dementia diagnosis over a 4 year follow-up interval[5]. This rate of decline is higher than would be anticipated from current incidence data[9]. This rate of decline is also consistent with a recent study of Geerlings *et al.*[7], which concluded that the presence of memory complaints in an otherwise normal elderly population is associated with an increased risk of subsequent dementia.

MILD COGNITIVE IMPAIRMENT

At the present time, the precise definition of this entity remains quite fluid[10]; however, the initial definition employed by Flicker *et al.*[1] remains quite useful in understanding the nature of this condition and its associated prognosis. Flicker *et al.* defined this condition as the equivalent of GDS and FAST Stage 3. This is a stage in which subtle deficits are manifest on a careful clinical interview. These subtle deficits are generally of sufficient magnitude to interfere with complex occupational and social tasks. Studies indicate that many of these subjects develop overt dementia when followed after some years. For example, Kluger *et al.*[5] found that about two-thirds of more than 85 subjects followed at this stage manifested dementia when followed after 4 years.

DEMENTIA

The prognosis of dementia varies with the nature of the dementing disorder. The major form of dementia is Alzheimer's disease (AD). The prognosis of AD is described in Tables 1 and 2 in terms of progression of clinical global changes, mental status changes and functional changes. The progression of cerebrovascular dementia is generally quite similar to that shown for AD, with two major caveats: (a) cerebrovascular dementia has been shown to have a somewhat increased risk of death and morbidity than AD[11]; and (b) overt strokes will produce a somewhat different clinical picture and course from that shown in Tables 1 and 2. Similarly, it has been noted that AD patients who develop significant cerebrovascular disease with the progression of their condition, have a significantly more rapid illness course than AD patients who do not develop cerebrovascular dementia[6].

Lewy bodies occur in approximately 15–25% of dementia cases. However, in a great majority of these cases there is co-existing AD or cerebrovascular dementia. In these cases with Lewy bodies in addition to AD and/or cerebrovascular dementia, the clinical presentation and course appear to be those of AD or cerebro-

Table 1 Global Deterioration Scale (GDS) for age-associated memory impairment and Alzheimer's disease[3] (choose the most appropriate global stage based upon cognition and function)

GDS stage	Clinical characteristics	Diagnosis and prognosis	Approximate mean MMSE[5,25,26]
1	*No subjective complaints of memory deficit.* No memory deficit evident on clinical interview	Normal adult	29–30
2	*Subjective complaints of memory deficit*, most frequently in following areas: (a) Forgetting where one has placed familiar objects (b) Forgetting names one formerly knew well No objective evidence of memory deficit on clinical interview No objective deficit in employment or social situations Appropriate concern with respect to symptomatology	Age-associated memory impairment (sometimes termed "normal aged forgetfulness" or "age-associated cognitive decline"). 15% develop dementia within 4 years[5]	29–30
3	*Earliest clear-cut deficits.* Manifestations in more than one of the following areas: (a) Patient may have become lost when traveling to an unfamiliar location (b) Co-workers become aware of patient's relatively poor performance (c) Word- and/or name-finding deficits become evident to intimates (d) Patient may read a passage or book and retain relatively little material (e) Patient may demonstrate decreased facility in remembering names upon introduction to new people (f) Patient may have lost or misplaced an object of value (g) Concentration deficit may be evident on clinical testing Objective evidence of memory deficit obtained *only with an intensive interview* Decreased peformance in demanding employment and social settings Denial begins to become manifest in patient Mild to moderate anxiety frequently accompanies symptoms	Mild cognitive impairment. Two-thirds develop dementia within 4 years[5]	25–27
4	*Clear-cut deficit on careful clinical interview.* Deficit manifest in following areas: (a) decreased knowledge of current and recent events (b) may exhibit some deficits in memory of one's personal history (c) concentration deficit elicited on serial subtractions (d) decreased ability to travel, *handle finances*, etc Frequently no deficit in following areas: (a) orientation to time and place (b) recognition of familiar persons and faces (c) ability to travel to familiar locations Inability to perform complex tasks Denial is dominant defense mechanism Flattening of affect and withdrawal from challenging situations	Mild AD. Mean duration, 2 years	20
5	*Patient can no longer survive without some assistance. Patient is unable during interview to recall a major relevant aspect of his/her current life*, e.g.: (a) Address or telephone number of many years. (b) Names of close members of his/her family (such as grandchildren). (c) Name of the high school or college from which he/she graduated. Frequently, some disorientation to time (date, day of the week, season, etc.) or to place An educated person may have difficulty in counting back from 40 by 4s or from 20 by 2s Persons at this stage retain knowledge of many major facts regarding themselves and others They invariably know their own names and generally know their spouse's and children's names They require no assistance with toileting or eating, but may have difficulty in choosing the proper clothing to wear	Moderate AD. Mean duration, 1.5 years	14
6	*May occasionally forget the name of the spouse upon whom they are entirely dependent for survival.* Will be *largely unaware of all recent events and experiences in their lives* Retain some knowledge of their surroundings; the year, the season, etc. May have difficulty counting by 1s from 10, both backwards and sometimes forwards *Will require some assistance with activities of daily living*: (a) May become incontinent (b) Will require travel assistance but occasionally will be able to travel to familiar locations Diurnal rhythm frequently disturbed Almost always recall their own name Frequently continue to be able to distinguish familiar from unfamiliar persons in their environment Personality and emotional changes occur. These are quite variable and include: (a) Delusional behavior, e.g. patient may accuse his/her spouse of being an imposter; may talk to imaginary figures in the environment, or to his/her own reflection in the mirror (b) Obsessive symptoms, e.g. person may continually repeat simple cleaning activities (c) Anxiety symptoms, agitation, and even previously non-existent violent behavior may occur (d) Cognitive abulia, e.g. loss of willpower because an individual cannot carry a thought long enough to determine a purposeful course of action	Moderately severe AD. Mean duration, 2.5 years	5
7	*All verbal abilities are lost over the course of this stage.* Early in this stage words and phrases are spoken but speech is very circumscribed. Later there is no speech at all—only unintelligible vocalizations *Incontinent; requires assistance in toileting and feeding* *Basic psychomotor skills (e.g. ability to walk) are lost with the progression of this stage.* The brain appears to no longer be able to tell the body what to do. Generalized and cortical neurologic signs and symptoms are frequently present.	Severe AD. Mean time to demise 2–3 years; potential for survival, 7 or more years	0

Table 2 Functional assessment stages (FAST) and time course of functional loss in normal aging and AD*

FAST stage	Clinical characteristics	Clinical diagnosis	Estimated duration of FAST stage or substage in AD[†]
1	No decrement	Normal adult	
2	Subjective deficit in word finding or recalling location of objects	Age-associated memory impairment (normal aged forgetfulness)	
3	Deficits noted in demanding employment settings	Mild cognitive impairment	7 years**
4	Requires assistance in complex tasks, e.g. handling finances, planning dinner party	Mild AD	2 years
5	Requires assistance in choosing proper attire	Moderate AD	18 months
6a	Requires assistance dressing	Moderately severe AD	5 months
6b	Requires assistance in bathing properly		5 months
6c	Requires assistance with mechanics of toileting (such as flushing, wiping)		5 months
6d	Urinary incontinence		4 months
6e	Fecal incontinence		10 months
7a	Speech ability limited to about a half-dozen words	Severe AD	12 months
7b	Intelligible vocabulary limited to a single word		18 months
7c	Ambulatory ability lost		12 months
7d	Ability to sit up lost		12 months
7e	Ability to smile lost		18 months
7f	Ability to hold head up lost		12 months or longer

*Adapted from Reisberg[27]. Copyright © 1984 by Barry Reisberg, M.D.
[†]In subjects without other complicating illnesses who survive and progress to the subsequent deterioration stage.
**Although the potentially observed duration is 7 years, patients are generally past the midpoint of this stage when brought for evaluation.

vascular dementia. Only in a small minority of dementia cases, an estimated 4% of the total, do Lewy bodies appear independently of AD and/or cerebrovascular disease. In these cases, a distinctive clinical picture has been described, marked by fluctuating cognition, recurrent well-formed visual hallucinations, and parkinsonian features[12]. There is a relatively rapid progression of the dementing disorder in Lewy body dementia, in comparison with AD.

Other forms of dementia that occur earlier, as well as in later life, including frontotemporal dementia and Creutzfeldt–Jakob disease, also differ in presentation and course from the classical AD course outlined in Tables 1 and 2. This AD course, which applies to the great majority of dementia patients, is described in Tables 1 and 2 and very briefly outlined below.

Mild AD

Stage 4 on the GDS and FAST scales, this stage has a mean duration of 2 years. Although overt deficits are present on assessment, patients are still capable of independent community survival, although the ability to manage financial and similarly complex affairs becomes compromised. Patients at this stage generally endeavor to conceal their deficits, just as humans in general endeavor to appear intelligent and try to present themselves well. This concealment may also take the form of

denial, whereby the patient tries to hide his/her problems from him/herself. Another defense mechanism is a flattening of affect, in which the patient is less participatory in social situations and appears to become more quiet and withdrawn. Medications frequently prescribed for AD patients, such as the SSRI antidepressants, may mask these otherwise common symptoms of affective flattening, making these patients appear even more overtly normal, despite their cognitive deficits.

Moderate AD

Stage 5 on the GDS and FAST scales, this stage has a mean duration of 1.5 years. Patients at this stage have deficits that are sufficient to interfere with independent community survival. Patients who are left alone in the community at this stage are either assisted by neighbors, relatives or others, or they are preyed upon by less scrupulous persons in our society. Functionally, persons at this stage develop incipient deficits with basic activities of daily life. More specifically, patients begin to require assistance in choosing the proper clothing to wear for the season and/or the occasion. Without assistance, patients will, for example, wear the same clothes day after day. A variety of emotional responses develop in an attempt to cope with the deficits in this stage. These commonly include suspiciousness, anger and false beliefs[13]. The magnitude of these emotional responses is probably dependent in part on the social supports provided to the patient. Patients who perceive themselves as secure may present themselves in socially appropriate ways at this stage and may successfully conceal their deficits in social situations.

Moderately Severe AD

Stage 6 on the GDS and FAST scales, this stage has a mean duration of 2.5 years. Patients at this stage develop deficits in basic activities of daily life. First, difficulties with dressing and bathing occur. Patients will put on clothing in the improper order or backwards unless assisted. At about the same time, patients develop difficulties with independently adjusting the shower- or bath-water temperature. With the progression of this stage, problems with independent toileting and independent continence occur. Collectively, these problems are such that not only can the patient not survive independently but, additionally, spouses or other caregivers begin to require additional help to manage the patient in a community setting. Emotional problems in the patient peak in this stage and generally include aggressivity and activity disturbances[13]. The newer atypical neuroleptics can be very useful in managing the overt emotional reactions in the patient, as can psychological non-pharmacological, management approaches[14,15].

Severe AD

Stage 7 on the GDS and FAST scales, this is the final stage of AD. Patients succumb throughout the course of this stage; however, the mean time to demise is about 2–3 years. Patients who progress to the final substage of severe AD, may survive for 7 or more years in this stage. Speech ability breaks down prior to the advent of this stage in the course of AD, and patients emerge in the final seventh stage with very limited remaining speech; generally a half dozen or fewer intelligible words are discernible in the course of an intensive interview in which numerous queries are presented to the patient. With the progression of this stage, speech becomes even more circumscribed. Ambulatory ability may be lost prematurely; however, after speech is lost, the ability of the patient to walk is inevitably lost. Subsequently, the ability to sit

Table 3 Functional landmarks in normal human development and AD

Approximate age		Approximate duration in development	Acquired abilities	Lost abilities	AD stage	Approximate duration in AD (years)	Developmental age of AD
Adolescence	13–19 years	7 years	Hold a job	Hold a job	3, Incipient	7 years	19–13 years: adolescence
Late childhood	8–12 years	5 years	Handle simple finances	Handle simple finances	4, Mild	2 years	12–8 years: late childhood
Middle childhood	5–7 years	2.5 years	Select proper clothing	Select proper clothing	5, Moderate	1.5 years	7–5 years: middle childhood
Early childhood	5 years	4 years	Put on clothes unaided	Put on clothes unaided	6a, Moderately severe	2.5 years	5–2 years: Early childhood
	4 years		Shower unaided	Shower unaided	6b		
	4 years		Toilet unaided	Toilet unaided	6c		
	3–4.5 years		Control urine	Control urine	6d		
	2–3 years		Control bowels	Control bowels	6e		
Infancy	15 months	1.5 years	Speak 5–6 words	Speak 5–6 words	7a Severe	7 years	15 months–birth: infancy
	1 year		Speak 1 word	Speak 1 word	7b		
	1 year		Walk	Walk	7c		
	6–10 months		Sit up	Sit up	7d		
	2–4 months		Smile	Smile	7e		
	1–3 months		Hold up head	Hold up head	7f		

(Left margin: Normal development: approximate total duration, 20 years)
(Right margin: Alzheimer's degeneration: approximate total duration, 20 years)

up independently, to smile, and to hold up the head independently are lost. Each of the six functional substages in this final seventh stage of AD lasts a mean of a year or longer. Studies have shown continuing cognitive, neurological, and neuropathological changes over the course of this final AD stage[16–19]. Throughout this stage, patients require continuous assistance for survival. Even with assistance, patients are very susceptible to disability. For example, physical deformities known as contractures occur in about 40% of patients in the early portion of this stage and become nearly universal as this stage progresses[20]. Overt behavioral symptoms become less manifest in this stage and the need for psychotropic medications steadily declines[13]. Patients commonly succumb to conditions such as pneumonia, resulting from aspiration or stroke or infections from decubiti or other sources.

Retrogenesis

It has been noted that the progression of losses in many domains in AD, and also in select other dementing disorders, reverses the normal human developmental pattern, a phenomenon which has been termed "retrogenesis"[21,22]. This process is particularly striking with regard to the progression of functional losses in AD, which precisely reverse the order of functional acquisition from birth to the adult (Table 3). Cognitive changes also reverse the normal human developmental patterns. For example, the correlation between the MMSE and mental age has been found to 0.83[23]. Neurologic reflexes have been found to be approximately as robust markers of AD course as the same reflexes are useful as markers of normal infant and child development[24]. Other physiological and pathological phenomena in AD also appear to follow a retrogenic pattern[21]. Because of these striking retrogenic relationships, the stages of AD can be usefully understood in terms of corresponding developmental ages (DAs). The management and care needs, and many AD emotional changes can be understood on the basis of the DA model[22].

ACKNOWLEDGEMENTS

This work was supported in part by US DHHS Grants AG03051 and AG08051 from the National Institute on Aging of the US National Institutes of Health, by Grant 90 AR2160 from the US Department of Health and Human Services Administration on Aging, and by the Zachary and Elizabeth M. Fisher Alzheimer's Disease Education and Resources Program of the New York University School of Medicine.

REFERENCES

1. Flicker C, Ferris SH, Reisberg B. Mild cognitive impairment in the elderly: predictors of dementia. *Neurology* 1991; **41**: 1006–9.
2. Petersen RC, Smith GE, Waring SC et al. Mild cognitive impairment: clinical characterization and outcome. *Arch Neurol* 1999; **56**: 303–8.
3. Reisberg B, Ferris SH, de Leon MJ, Crook T. The global deterioration scale for assessment of primary degenerative dementia. *Am J Psychiat* 1982; **139**; 1136–9.
4. Reisberg B. Functional assessment staging (FAST). *Psychopharmacol Bull* 1988; **24**: 653–9.
5. Kluger A, Ferris SH, Golomb J et al. Neuropsychological prediction of decline to dementia in nondemented elderly. *J Geriat Psychiat Neurol* 1999; **12**: 168–79.
6. Reisberg B, Ferris SH, Franssen E et al. Mortality and temporal course of probable Alzheimer's disease: a five-year prospective study. *Int Psychogeriat* 1996; **8**: 291–311.
7. Geerlings MI, Jonker C, Bouter LM et al. Association between memory complaints and incident Alzheimer's disease in elderly people with normal baseline cognition. *Am J Psychiat* 1999; **156**: 531–7.
8. Reisberg B, Ferris SH, Franssen E et al. Age-associated memory impairment: the clinical syndrome. *Dev Neuropsychol* 1986; **2**: 401–12.
9. Henderson AS, Jorm AF. Definition and epidemiology of dementia: a review. In Maj M, Sartorius N, eds, *Evidence and Experience in Psychiatry, vol 3: Dementia.* Chichester: Wiley, 2000: 1–33.
10. Ritchie K, Touchon J. Mild cognitive impairment: conceptual basis and current nosological status. *Lancet* 2000; **355**: 225–8.
11. Reding MJ, Haycox J, Wigforss K et al. Follow-up of patients referred to a dementia service. *J Am Geriat Soc* 1984: **32**: 265–8.
12. McKeith IG, Galasko D, Kosaka K et al. Consensus guidelines for the clinical and pathologic diagnosis of dementia with Lewy bodies (DLB). *Neurology* 1996; **47**: 1113–24.
13. Reisberg B, Franssen E, Sclan SG et al. Stage-specific incidence of potentially remediable behavioral symptoms in aging and Alzheimer's disease: a study of 120 patients using the BEHAVE-AD. *Bull Clin Neurosci* 1989; **54**: 95–112.
14. Katz IR, Jeste D, Mintzer JE et al. Comparison of risperidone and placebo for psychosis and behavioral disturbances associated with dementia: a randomized, double-blind trial. *J Clin Psychiat* 1999; **60**: 107–15.
15. Reisberg B, Monteiro I, Boksay I et al. Do many of the behavioral and psychological symptoms of dementia constitute a distinct clinical

syndrome? Current evidence using the BEHAVE-AD. *Int Psychogeriat* 2000; **12**(suppl 1): 155–64.

16. Auer SR, Sclan SG, Yaffee RA, Reisberg B. The neglected half of Alzheimer disease: Cognitive and functional concomitants of severe dementia. *J Am Geriat Soc* 1994; **42**: 1266–72.

17. Franssen EH, Reisberg B. Neurologic markers of the progression of Alzheimer disease. *Int Psychogeriat* 1997; **9**(suppl 1): 297–306.

18. Bobinski M, Wegiel J, Wisniewski HM *et al*. Atrophy of hippocampal formation subdivisions correlates with stage and duration of Alzheimer disease. *Dementia* 1995; **6**: 205–10.

19. Bobinski M, Wegiel J, Tarnawski M *et al*. Relationships between regional neuronal loss and neurofibrillary changes in the hippocampal formation and duration and severity of Alzheimer disease. *J Neuropathol Exp Neurol* 1997: **56**: 414–20.

20. Souren LEM, Franssen EM, Reisberg B. Contractures and loss of function in patients with Alzheimer's disease. *J Am Geriat Soc* 1995: **43**: 650–5.

21. Reisberg B, Franssen EH, Hasan SM *et al*. Retrogenesis: clinical, physiologic and pathologic mechanisms in brain aging. Alzheimer's and other dementing processes. *Eur Arch Psychiat Clin Neurosci* 1999; **249**(suppl 3): 28–36.

22. Reisberg B, Kenowsky S, Franssen EH *et al*. President's report: towards a science of Alzheimer's disease management: a model based upon current knowledge of retrogenesis. *Int Psychogeriat* 1999: **11**: 7–23.

23. Ouvrier RA, Goldsmith RF, Ouvrier S, Williams IC. The value of the Mini-Mental State Examination in childhood: a preliminary study. *J Child Neurol* 1993; **8**: 145–8.

24. Franssen EH, Souren LEM, Torossian CL, Reisberg B. Utility of developmental reflexes in the differential diagnosis and prognosis of incontinence in Alzheimer's disease. *J Geriat Psychiat Neurol* 1997; **10**: 22–8.

25. Folstein MF, Folstein SE, McHugh PR. Mini-Mental state: a practical method for grading the cognitive state of patients for the clinician. *J Psychiat Res* 1975; **12**: 189–98.

26. Reisberg B, Ferris SH, de Leon MJ *et al*. Stage-specific behavioral, cognitive and *in vivo* changes in community-residing subjects with age-associated memory impairment (AAMI) and primary degenerative dementia of the Alzheimer type. *Drug Dev Res* 1988; **15**: 101–14.

27. Reisberg B. Dementia: a systematic approach to identifying reversible causes. *Geriatrics* 1986; **41**(4): 30–46.

57

Acute Management of Dementia

Brice Pitt

St Mary's Hospital, London, UK

Alzheimer's disease (AD) and senile dementia of the Alzheimer type (SDAT) have an insidious onset and a prolonged course (sometimes running for 20 years); so, on the face of it, the need for acute management should seldom arise.

Indeed, perhaps for many sufferers—the "silent majority"—it may not. Some old people become ever more forgetful and adapt gradually and graciously to their limitations, while their families and friends perceive them simply as starting to show their age rather than as demented. They give them a little more help every few months, which is accepted appreciatively as appropriate. The old person may receive a lot of care at home, or move to live near or with one of the family, or agree that it would be wise to go into sheltered housing or a home, until in due course a gentle death brings life to a dignified end.

However, the course in those referred to professional services—general practitioners, social workers, geriatricians and psychogeriatricians—is often less tranquil. Usually such patients have been dementing for a year or two and the referral has been precipitated by a crisis.

CRISES

Such a crisis could be when the family doctor is telephoned by anxious and irate relatives who have visited their parent over the weekend and found things worse than when they last visited 2 months previously, or the belated awareness that he/she is not coping very well and that a long weekend, like Christmas or Easter, is imminent and that there could be problems. Relatives are usually very caring and the culture supportive, but in the developed nations families are small and dispersed and both men and women are employed, while the elderly population is large—over the age of 65 in Britain[1]; so to take care of a dementing elder at a distance requires considerable adaptation.

Crises also arise where the demented people react to their disorder not with insight, but with robust denial. These are exemplars of the "Dylan Thomas syndrome":

> Do not go gentle into that good night;
> Rage, rage against the dying of the light!

They age disgracefully, fighting the implications of a failing memory, mind and body every step of the way, stubbornly independent unto death unless society intervenes, either by overruling their rights or by using some form of mental health legislation. These denying demented patients are a huge challenge to the health and social services.

Traditionally, the dementias may be dichotomized into the presenile and senile forms, or Alzheimer's and non-Alzheimer's.

However, for the purposes of this chapter, the most practical division is into those who live with others and those who live all alone. The prognosis for survival of the latter, even if given good domicilary support, is far worse[2].

LIVING ALONE

Demented people who live alone may do so because they are single, divorced or widowed and without children. Widowing can be an acute event, and one of the crises in dementia is when a key carer dies, leaving the dependant not only emotionally bereft but also suddenly deprived of his/her main prop. An acute grief reaction is compounded by the abrupt removal of a principal support. The work of grieving is complicated by forgetting or denying that the loss has taken place. Plans for the future may be undermined by the fitful expectation that the lost one will return.

There may be personal as well as social factors in a demented person's living alone. Some people react to the early intimations of their disorder by withdrawing and leading a very simplified, limited existence. Finding it an effort to sustain conversation with neighbours, friends and even family, they adopt an isolated, frugal life. Those who deny that they have any difficulties are unlikely to accept the help that is willingly offered. "I don't want anyone coming to my house to do my housework and shopping—poking their nose in where it's not wanted". "Are you saying I can't look after myself? I've managed very nicely for all these years?" "Why would I want to come and live with you (or in sheltered housing, or in a home)? I've got a perfectly good home of my own, thank you very much!" These denials are often made by people with a well-preserved, assertive personality, and enough retention of language to make their wishes plain (although without the hearing, comprehension, insight or will to listen to reason!).

Living alone with so devastating a disorder as dementia is evidently risky. Accidents occur easily in those who lack the foresight or the judgement to prevent them, and demented old people are consequently over-represented in general hospital wards. Drugs needed to control diabetes, heart failure, epilepsy or arthritis may be taken erratically or not at all, with serious consequences. Malnutrition is a hazard for those who cannot remember whether they have eaten or not, to draw their money or where they have put it, where and when to shop and for what, and what to do with what they may have bought if they can find it. Cold weather adds to the dangers of falls and hypothermia. Floods and conflagrations are always possible, and failings

Principles and Practice of Geriatric Psychiatry, 2nd edn. Edited by J. R. M. Copeland, M. T. Abou-Saleh and D. G. Blazer
©2002 John Wiley & Sons, Ltd

in personal hygiene may amount in due course to alarming squalor.

LIVING WITH OTHERS

Dementia may develop in those already living with their family—a spouse or a son or (most often) a daughter. Crises then arise from the dependant's growing infirmity and the increasing burden on the carer(s)[3]. Acute exacerbations of the dementia intensify the strain. These may arise from:

- The swift progression of the dementia from one stage to the next[4]. This is said to be characteristic of multi-infarct dementia[5], but may also occur in Alzheimer's disease.
- Events affecting bodily health, such as heart failure, a urinary or respiratory tract infection, a fall leading, perhaps, to head injury; even impaction of faeces may all add to the patient's confusion.
- Depression may have a similar but more prolonged effect. Dementia is no protection against depression, especially where there is some preservation of insight[6].
- The dynamics of the household may have altered because of some comings or goings or change in the attitudes or well-being of one of its members. Marital strain can cause, as well as arise from, disturbed behaviour in a demented member of the household.

The demented person may have moved to be with family because of increased infirmity and dependency. Occasionally, one of the family moves in with the demented person, as when a son returns home after being divorced. Such a move may be the result of some critical failure in self-care—getting lost, having an accident, being bereft, coming out of hospital unable to cope. By moving, the demented person gains safety and security, but dependency increases, autonomy dwindles, friends and familiar haunts are now at a distance and the activities necessary for daily living are much reduced. The carer has gained peace of mind at the cost of privacy and some disruption of the household[7]. The arrival of a confused grandparent, repeating him/herself, disapproving and getting in the way, may be less than welcome to the carer's adolescent children. Also, confusion in the demented is commonly aggravated by a move, so the earliest days are not the easiest.

Occasionally the strain on carers can erupt into "elder abuse"[8]. This may take the form of physical violence, as well as angry outbursts and verbal abuse. The commonest form is when there has been mutual dependency between the demented parent and the abusing son or daughter, now at the end of his/her tether and feeling trapped in the situation.

HOSPITAL, SHELTERED HOUSING AND HOMES

Demented people are, because of their accident-proneness and deficiencies in self-care, far more prevalent among the elderly in general hospital wards than in the population at large[9]. Here their problems may be exacerbated by sudden admission, hasty and inadequate communication, the discomfort and disability of whatever they have been admitted with and sometimes, unfortunately, the indifferent, dismissive, patronizing and even hostile attitudes of staff, wary of another "social admission" or "bed-blocker"[10]. Medication may add to confusion by lowering blood pressure, causing drowsiness, or through anticholinergic side-effects. In the setting of a busy medical or surgical ward, an apparently able-bodied but deranged older person may be perceived as a threat—disturbing sick patients by being noisy and interfering—or an undue responsibility, liable to wander off

and become lost. Consequently it is still not unknown for physical restraint—binding hands, body or feet, trapping the patient in a "geriatric" chair, using cot-sides—to be added to sedation[11].

A move into sheltered housing seems to have much to commend it for those who are now too forgetful and erratic to manage readily at home but not in need of full-time care. However, such a move is better made sooner than later. Otherwise, the strangeness of the new environment aggravates the confusion, and problems may arise in the use of the alarm cord or bell to call the warden, who is summoned frequently in error. Too often the stay in sheltered housing proves quite brief, before a further move into institutional care is necessary.

Although most demented people are in their own or relatives' homes, they are also major users of residential and nursing homes, some taking all comers, others specializing in the elderly mentally infirm ("EMI"). Even in ordinary homes, as many as 60–70% of the residents may be found to be demented[12]. Homes which were already looking after the old person before the onset of dementia usually cope very well, but where someone is admitted because of their dementia there may be clashes because the parties have not had time to get to know each other. Demented people can, of course, be difficult, demanding and highly irrational, but sometimes "it takes two to make a quarrel" and tactless, hasty, overbearing staff may provoke escalation of a minor dispute into a major row. Other problems that may arise from communal living include fights between residents, say where one accuses the other of going off with his/her belongings or of wandering into his/her room and interfering with the bedding (which may well be true!), and antisocial behaviour such as stripping, masturbation, sexual advances, noise and disgusting eating habits. Another crisis is that the money runs out for costly care and there are urgent demands to find the resident another place!

ACUTE MANAGEMENT

Acute problems may be lessened by early identification of the dementia, taking account of how it is managed at that time, who is (or may become) the key carer and designating a key worker to guide, advise and support that person. If no key carer is identifiable among family or friends one may need to be enlisted, such as a home help or a paid "good neighbour". Such arrangements are highly dependent on good, well-organized primary health care and social services, with support from voluntary agencies and a well-resourced psychogeriatric service, all working well together. A "case manager", generally someone with a background in nursing or social services may be the best person to assemble a "package of care"[13], but is more effective when the client is merely elderly and infirm[14] than significantly demented[15].

Where dementia is identified early as the result of a screening programme (e.g. for the over-75s)[16], some discretion as to how, when or, indeed, whether to impart that information. There is the possibility of an adverse reaction to the label "dementia"; the family may feel that the task of caring will prove too much—beforehand they thought they were just helping someone who was ageing normally—while demented persons may be distressed by the diagnosis. However, there is the possibility of involving them with the carers in plans for their future, to prefer one kind of management to another, make a will, give an enduring power of attorney and feel that they retain some control over their own destiny[17]. The advent of the oral anticholinesterases for Alzheimer's disease[18] demands informed consent to their use.

Key carers need respite before they feel burdened by their continuous responsibility. "Sitters-in" enable them to take a few hours out of the home alone. Meals on wheels and home helps should not be reserved solely for demented people living alone;

they ease the load on carers and help them to feel less alone with the problem. An incontinence service providing pads and collecting soiled sheets and garments for laundering is a huge help. Financial recognition of the work that has to be done in the form of an attendance allowance is often greatly appreciated, although the sum may not be great. Day hospitals and respite admissions have been demonstrated to reduce scores measuring stress and strain in carers[19]. Relatives' support groups, personal counselling by a community psychiatric nurse, social worker, psychologist or doctor and, where feelings in the household are running high, family therapy[20], may all have their place. It is important for the key worker to keep in touch with the situation, to be easily available and able to offer extra assistance, e.g. admission to hospital or a home, as and when that is needed. The credibility of the service is seriously jeopardized if the help that all recognize to be required cannot in fact be given.

An interesting field study in Cambridge[21] randomly divided demented people living alone or at home with others into those who received routine care and those who received extra home care. Extra care made no significant difference to those living with others, but those living alone were far more likely to be in a residential home 2 years into the study if they were getting extra care than if they were not! This was less a demonstration of the ineffectiveness of community care than an indication that those who received it were correctly placed where they needed to be at the appropriate time.

The demented who live alone are especially in need of close monitoring by the key worker. Those who will accept help are obviously an easier proposition than those who will not. The home help is the chief provider of "hands-on" care, and may be required from 2 h/week to 6 h/day (at which stage, of course, the cost is not negligible). Meals on wheels not only support nutrition but also provide regular human contact, as do lunch clubs, day centres and day hospitals for those who can make their way there or be taken to them. Community ("district") nurses may get patients up, bathe them, help them to bed and give their medication—but the supply of such skilled staff is not limitless. Reliable, trustworthy volunteers are useful in befriending, doing small chores and running errands. Financial arrangements need to be made with banks, post offices, lawyers, social workers and whoever either holds the power of attorney or has been nominated as the Receiver by such a body as England's Court of Protection[22].

Demented people seriously at risk who refuse help may occasionally be compelled into care or placed on a guardianship order under mental health legislation (UK)[22]. This, or the decision not to take such an action, is usually the result of a case conference, often convened by a social worker, and attended by relatives, neighbours, nurses, home helps and their organizers, the general practitioner, the psychiatrist and perhaps concerned volunteers, clergy and the police. Often the conclusion is that what cannot be achieved by persuasion cannot be achieved, so a close eye is to be kept on the subject of the conference until he/she becomes more willing to accept help, falls ill and goes into hospital or dies, or confounds expectations by living on in much the same state for years!

Staff in hospitals and homes need to be trained to give demented people proper care, by example and experience as well as by precept. The inculcation of respect is a good starting point—breezy, patronizing familiarity may give offence. It is important to learn not to take umbrage, to blame, to accuse of attention-seeking or provocation and to avoid futile arguments. A spacious, bright, cheerful environment and a full, appropriate programme, including some conversation, entertainment (a sing-song is much preferable to the ubiquitous television, but people should be free to opt out), exercise and bringing visitors into the regime help to prevent problems arising from boredom and inaction.

Alertness to health problems may prevent some of the exacerbation of confusion by physical illness. Depression afflicts not a few demented people, causing agitation and restlessness by day and night. A trial of antidepressant therapy is indicated, but the old antidepressants are too powerfully anticholinergic, sedative or hypotensive to be the first choice. Serotonin-specific reuptake inhibitors are to be preferred, and citalopram 20 mg daily has been shown to improve depressive symptoms in dementia in a placebo-controlled study[23]. Rarely, in those who appear severely depressed, are not eating and who may have a history of severe depression, there could be a place for electroconvulsive therapy.

A full day's activities reduce sleep problems (and patients can often catch up on their sleep by day) but carers need sleep, and the use of a hypnotic for a restless patient may thus be justified. None is ideal, but among those to be considered are temazepam, a very popular benzodiazepine, 20–40 mg (which may induce a hangover); zopiclone, a cyclopyrrolone, 3.75–7.5 mg; chlormethiazole, a short-acting drug which occasionally causes sneezing, 250–500 mg, at night; or chloral hydrate, in tablet form (the equivalent of 414 mg in a tablet), one or two at night.

There is no perfect neuroleptic in old age psychiatry: all can cause as much trouble from side effects, notably drowsiness, extrapyramidal symptoms and falls, as any benefit they bring. Demented people seem particularly susceptible to such side effects and to tardive dyskinesia[24]. However, where the urgent control of a very disturbed patient is necessary in a setting where alternatives are not practicable, one of the major tranquillizers may be warranted[21]. The butyrophenone haloperidol, 5–10 mg i.m. or i.v. (often with procyclidine 10 mg through the same needle to prevent acute extrapyramidal reactions) is a most useful drug, and can be repeated up to 6-hourly. Once the acute crisis is over it may be replaced by one of the newer, "atypical" antipsychotics, risperidone (0.5–2 mg, twice a day), olanzepine (5 mg once or twice a day), with fewer extrapyramidal side-effects than haloperidol[25] and shown by meta-analysis[26] effectively to ameliorate symptoms of psychosis, aggression and agitation. Very popular, and reasonably safe, although quite sedative and anticholinergic, is thioridazine, 10–100 mg, up to four times a day.

REFERENCES

1. Department of Health. *Epidemiological Overview of the Health of Elderly People.* London: Central Health Monitoring Unit, 1991.
2. Bergmann K, Foster E, Justin A et al. Management of the demented elderly in the community. *Br J Psychiatr* 1978; **132**: 441–7.
3. Gilleard C, Gilleard E, Gledhill K et al. Caring for the elderly mentally infirm at home: a survey of the supporters. *J Epidemiol Comm Health* 1984; **38**: 319–25.
4. Reisberg B, Ferris S, de Leon M, Crook T. The global deterioration scale for assessment of primary degenerative dementia. *Am J Psychiat* 1982; **139**: 1136–9.
5. Wade J, Hachinski V. Multi-infarct dementia. In Pitt B, ed., *Dementia in Old Age.* Edinburgh: Churchill Livingstone, 1987.
6. Burns A, Jacoby R, Levy R. Psychiatric phenomena in Alzheimer's disease. III: Disorders of mood. *Br J Psychiat* 1990; **157**: 81–6.
7. Norman A. *Mental Illness in Old Age: Meeting the Challenge.* London: Centre for Policy on Ageing, 1982.
8. Homer A, Gilleard C. Abuse of elderly people by the carers. *Br Med J* 1990; **301**: 1359–62.
9. Johnston M, Wakeling A, Graham N, Stokes F. Cognitive impairment, emotional disorder and length of stay of elderly patients in a district general hospital. *Br J Med Psychol* 1987; **60**: 133–9.
10. Pitt B. The mentally disordered old person in the general hospital ward. In Judd F, Burrows G, Lipsitt D, eds, *Handbook of Studies on General Hospital Psychiatry.* Oxford: Elsevier, 1991.

11. Robbins L, Boyko E, Lane J, Cooper D, Jahnigen D. Binding the elderly: a prospective study of the use of mechanical restraints in an acute care hospital. *J Am Geriat Soc* 1987; **35**: 290–6.

12. Mann A, Graham N, Ashby D. Psychiatric illness in residential homes for the elderly: a survey in one London borough. *Age Ageing* 1984; **13**: 257–65.

13. Griffiths R. *Community Care: Agenda for Action*. London: HMSO, 1988.

14. Challis D, Davies B. *Case Management in Community Care*. Aldershot: Gower, 1986.

15. Askham J, Thompson C. *Dementia and Home Care*. London: Age Concern, 1990.

16. Department of Health and the Welsh Office. *General Practice in the National Health Service. A New Contract*. London: DOH & WO, 1989.

17. Johnson H, Bouman WP, Pinner G. On telling the truth in Alzheimer's disease. *Int Psychogeriat* 2000; **12**: 221–30.

18. Kelly C, Harvey R, Cayton H. Therapies for Alzheimer's disease. *Br Med J* 1997; **314**: 693–4.

19. Gilleard C. Influence of emotional distress among supporters on the outcome of psychogeriatric day care. *Br J Psychiat* 1987; **150**: 219–23.

20. Benbow S. Family therapy in the elderly. In Murphy E, Parker S, eds, *Current Approaches to Affective Disorders in the Elderly*. Southampton: Duphar, 1988.

21. O'Connor D, Pollitt P, Brook C *et al*. Does early intervention reduce the number of elderly people with dementia admitted to institutions for long-term care? *Br Med J* 1991; **302**: 871–4.

22. Jefferys P. Law. In Butler R, Pitt B, eds, *Seminars in Old Age Psychiatry*. London: Gaskell Books, 1998: 291–312.

23. Nyth AI, Gottfries CG. The clinical efficacy of citalopram in treatment of emotional disturbances in dementia disorders. A Nordic multicentre study. *Br J Psychiat* 1990; **157**: 894–901.

24. Mehta D, Mehta S, Mathews P. Tardive dyskinesias in psychogeriatric patients. *J Am Geriat Soc* 1977; **25**: 545–7.

25. DeDeyn PP, Rabheru K, Rasmussen A *et al*. A randomized trial of risperidone placebo and haloperidol for behavioral problems of dementia. *Neurology* 1999; **53**: 946–55.

26. Davidson M, Weiser M, Soares K. Novel antipsychotics in the treatment of psychosis and aggression associated with dementia: a meta-analysis of randomized controlled trials. *Int Psychogeriat* 2000; **12**:(Suppl 1): 271–80.

27. Sunderland T, Silver M. Neuroleptics in the treatment of dementia. *Int J Geriat Psychiat* 1988; **3**: 79–88.

Present and Future Treatments of Alzheimer's Disease

Lawrence J. Whalley[1] and John M. Starr[2]
[1]*University of Aberdeen and* [2]*University of Edinburgh, UK*

Modern theories of disease predict that, when valid diagnostic criteria are available and causes can be confidently ascribed to a disease condition, then effective treatments will be developed[1]. In clinical practice, the diagnosis of late-onset Alzheimer's disease (AD) is not supported by definitive diagnostic findings and no consensus exists on its causes. Currently, diagnosis depends on a cluster of neuropsychological features combined with the absence of other pathologies, identified clinically or by investigation. In those patients who present at a later stage, neuropsychological deficits are so severe and global that differentiation from other aetiologies is difficult. Moreover, the presence of other causes of cognitive decline, such as stroke, does not exclude AD; indeed, the prevalence of AD is far more common in people with stroke than would be expected by chance alone.

Observational longitudinal studies suggest that both genetic and environmental factors are important in early-onset AD[2]. Best estimates in late-onset AD are that genetic and environmental influences are approximately equal[3]. In early-onset AD genetic factors seem more important but at present can account for fewer than 10% of cases[4]. Known mutations that contribute to the causes of late-onset AD appear so far to be relatively infrequent[2,5] but genetic contributions to functional ability in late life are also established[6]. Genetic susceptibility factors are less well established; apolipoprotein E polymorphisms are best known and may influence the timing of the onset of AD in almost 50% of cases[7]. For many commentators, these sparse facts encourage the search for environmental factors that certainly contribute to the onset of dementia and, by extension, to the possible modification of those exposures. These interventions may slow or even prevent the onset of dementia. So far, however, no single factor or group of factors has been reliably confirmed as an environmental contributor to the risk of dementia. This situation is similar to the problems faced by specialists in old age medicine about 30 years ago. At that time, there was some concern about the accumulation of disabilities in old age, so much so that population projections predicted increasing longevity and an increased burden posed by large numbers of disabled old people[8]. One of the great successes of modern geriatric medicine was the postponement of the expected accumulation of disability into the final year of life. This in turn has reduced the period of dependency in old age, especially for men[9]. Prevention of disability was the key outcome of the interdisciplinary research programme one "successful ageing" in the USA[10]. Compression of disability and morbidity has been so great that the proportion of men aged 80 years in North America and Northern Europe with at least one disability halved between 1975 and 1995[11].

These reductions were achieved by preventative measures to detect and reduce environmental exposures in old people known to be at increased risk for vascular disease. Hypertension, smoking, diabetes, obesity and hyperlipidaemia proved susceptible to such interventions. Likewise, smoking reduction and improvements in air quality reduced the burden posed by respiratory disease and cancer. Reduction of disease incidence and subsequent improvements in well-being in old age have prompted some researchers to speculate that much of what is regarded as "ageing" is made up of at least two processes[12]. One process comprises the accumulated effects of disease and the acquired handicaps and disabilities of old age. The other is made up of at least one process, usually termed "intrinsic ageing". The nature and cause of intrinsic ageing processes are currently described using terms such as "the oxidative stress model" or "accumulated DNA damage" or "inefficient DNA repair". The formation of advanced glycated end products, the consequences of membrane lipid peroxidation and failure of immune surveillance are all included in current hypotheses concerning intrinsic ageing. However, given that the brain enjoys specific privileges, e.g. in terms of immuno-surveillance and neurons being naturally in a post-mitotic state throughout most of the lifespan, whether some general "intrinsic ageing" process applies to the central nervous system or is the same as that for other organs is questionable.

From the standpoint of dementia prevention and/or treatment, brain ageing research is now of pivotal importance to future progress. The success of modern geriatric medicine has been achieved largely by translation of epidemiological data into public health-based preventative programmes. This chapter first considers what is currently available to treat or prevent dementia. Second, it examines some of the potential for neuroprotection and dementia prevention and/or treatment provided by recent research findings in brain ageing. Third, lessons learnt from general medicine in the prevention of heart disease and cerebrovascular accidents will be considered. Fourth, future strategies proposed to slow or even prevent brain ageing and the characteristic features of AD will be briefly summarized.

CURRENT TREATMENTS

Who is Eligible for Treatment?

AD is the most frequent cause of late-onset cognitive impairment in the UK and probably affects around 350 000 people. Incidence rates approximately double every 5 years (65–90), such that about 20–25% of those over 80 are affected. UK demographic studies predict that old people who are cognitively impaired will increase by 11% during 2001–2011. The prevalence of AD seems likely to double by 2050. All AD sufferers are currently regarded as potentially eligible for dementia treatment.

What Are the Benefits of Current Dementia Treatment?

Anti-dementia therapy benefits are now recognized to be wider than just the slowing or improvement of cognitive decline. Additional improvements include reduced disability, time to institutionalization and fewer acute medical or surgical emergencies. Disabilities place considerable burdens on health and social services and the incidence of disability increases with age. These burdens include needs for social support, especially in best use of available health services, problems of co-morbidity and institutionalization. In London, the Gospel Oak studies reported disability in 38% of community residents aged 65–74, 77% aged 75–84 and 96% aged 85+[13] and the overall prevalence of dementia was 9.8%. Predictions based on the MRC Cognitive Function and Ageing Study (MRC CFAS) suggest that people aged 65+ with severe disability will make up 2.2% and 3.9% of the population in 2011 and 2051, respectively[14]. In general terms, disability from whatever cause forecasts both mortality and prolongation of length of stay after admission to hospital.

The MRC CFAS provides further valuable information on the burden of health care linked to cognitive impairment. Cognitive impairment was detected in 38% of disabled people aged 65 years and in 46% of people in institutional care. Cognitive impairment also generates other health service demands, some not immediately obvious. For example, a reduction of dementia prevalence of 1–2% would reduce the number of hip fractures in the UK by 20 000/year[15,16].

The Anti-dementia Drugs

Currently available drugs are based on the established cholinergic deficits in AD and early recognition that these may be sufficient to explain "core" symptoms. There are no claims that current drugs do any more than provide symptomatic relief. Large-scale randomized placebo-controlled trial results are available for three anticholinesterase drugs: donepezil[17,18], rivastigmine[19,20] and galantamine[21,22]. These show that, in general, these drugs: (a) improve global outcome; (b) slow or arrest cognitive decline; and (c) improve activities of daily living. Carers also report that some troublesome behaviours, such as apathy and apparent responses to hallucinations or delusions, are helped by drugs of this type but as yet no satisfactory clinical trial data are available. There is a consensus to support a relatively enduring good cognitive response equivalent to an arrest of disease progression of about 9 months. This is not sustained, however, and is followed by a fairly rapid decline that reverses any earlier benefit. Primarily for this reason, most commentators agree that anticholinesterase drugs do *not* modify any underlying disease process.

The generality can obscure some quite remarkable and sustained improvements in a subset of patients. Almost half of AD patients show evidence of improvement and sustain that improvement for up to about 18 months. Within this group there is a small proportion (roughly around 1 in 12) who show very extensive improvements, sometimes sufficient to permit resumption of mentally effortful recreational pursuits. Unfortunately, there is no evidence that this group of high responders obtain long-term benefits. Such patients are highly encouraging in routine clinical practice and certainly help motivate and improve morale in dementia care teams.

This class of drugs is usually well tolerated. Common unwanted effects include cholinergic actions on the GI tract (nausea, vomiting and diarrhoea). Few data are available on the effects of these drugs on disability and institutionalization rates. Tacrine was one of the early antidementia drugs and is now discontinued. Patients receiving tacrine and remaining on doses greater than 80 mg/day may be less likely to enter a nursing home than those on lower doses or who have stopped the drug[23,24].

Cost Concerns

Although the licensing of cholinesterase inhibitors has introduced widely available drug treatment for AD for the first time, the costs of these drugs prohibits extensive use in less developed countries, where the greatest increase in numbers of people with AD is expected. Even within the UK there is considerable geographical variation in the availability of antidementia drugs. In part this remains attributable to poorly informed pessimism about dementia treatment, but the fact that much-needed pharmacoeconomic data were not collected in trials sponsored by the pharmaceutical industry must share part of the responsibility. Largely at the direction of regulatory authorities, the sponsors include clinically meaningful measures of competencies in daily living, and these have become the cornerstone of current recommendations to administer these drugs as widely as possible. At present, there is an impression that these drugs are "cost-beneficial" and reduce overall spending on services for dementia. If delay to institutional care is accepted as a valid proxy in economic analyses, the eventual conclusion seems likely to support their use[25]. Data from Canada indicate that the largest proportion of costs is attributable to institutionalization. Use of donepezil for mild-to-moderate AD was associated with lower 5 year costs and less time spent with severe AD when compared with the alternative of usual care[26]. In a retrospective cost analysis in Dutch patients with Alzheimer's disease who were being cared for at home at the start of the study period, treatment with donepezil did not increase overall direct medical costs[27].

To obtain an improvement of four points on the ADAS-COG, it is estimated that between four and six patients taking donepezil 10 mg once daily for 6 months would need to be treated. Clinical experience in the UK suggests the NNT to achieve clinically significant activities of daily living score improvement is likely to be about twice that for the cognitive end point of ADAS-COG improvement of four points.

BRAIN AGEING: NEUROPROTECTION AND PREVENTION OF DEMENTIA

Neurochemical studies support an association between brain oxidative stress and AD[28,29]. Current studies are examining whether this association is a cause or a consequence of AD, perhaps an artifact of the AD process. Therapeutic agents are currently available (and more potent compounds are under investigation) that reduce oxidative stress. These agents may prove to be potent neuroprotective agents relevant to AD.

Evidence of oxidative stress in AD is detectable throughout the brain, irrespective of the site or extent of AD neuropathology. This evidence includes increased concentrations of advanced glycation end products[30], nitration[31], increased products of lipid peroxidation[32] and carbonyl modified proteins[33,34]. The sources of oxidative stress in AD extend beyond the generation of reactive oxygen species (ROS) during aerobic metabolism. Contributions are made by activated microglia near senile plaques[35] and by interactions between the receptor for advance glycation end products and β-amyloid[36,37]. These observations have supported the hypothesis that the neurotoxic effects of β-amyloid are mediated through oxidative stress.

Therapeutic agents that reduce oxidative stress may reduce the incidence and slow AD progression. These include non-steroidal anti-inflammatory agents[38–43]; inhibitors of advanced glycation end product formation[44,45] and α-tocopherol[46]. The benefits in AD of *Ginkgo biloba* extract may also involve reduction of brain oxidative stress[47].

Neuroprotective actions of oestrogen in women were linked to reduced AD prevalence in some early studies[48] and prompted many subsequent observational and experimental longitudinal studies. As yet, no single study has overcome all the methodological problems associated with complex biopsychosocial questions of this type. A recent meta-analysis of 29 studies on the putative dementia-protective effects of oestrogen replacement therapy (HRT) suggested that HRT was linked with reduced risk of dementia (summary odds ratio, 0.66; confidence intervals 0.53–0.82). The authors cautioned that control for potential confounders may remove this association[49]. When demographic and health confounders were taken into account, HRT was not associated with cognitive benefits in a large ($n = 1907$) US study[50] of post-menopausal women. In the UK, the general practice research database identified women born before 1950, of whom 112 481 received HRT and 108 925 did not[51]. Among these subjects there were 59 newly diagnosed AD cases, of whom 15 (25%) were current HRT users. Expected HRT use was estimated at 24% and the authors concluded that this type of cross-sectional observation did not support a link between HRT and protection against AD.

Raloxifene is an oestrogen receptor modulator (mixed agonist/antagonist) that is tissue selective. Potential advantages are that it does not stimulate breast or uterine tissue but is active in bone and on lipid metabolism, the last being of specific relevance to the possible involvement of cholesterol in AD (see below). Osteoporotic postmenopausal women ($n = 7478$) were entered into a 3 year multicentre randomized placebo-controlled trial of raloxifene[52]. Mean cognitive scores were similar at baseline and there were no differences between groups over the study period. The authors concluded that, in osteoporotic women, raloxifene did not modify cognitive function over time.

As yet, it is unclear whether oestrogens are involved in AD. Although early observational studies were encouraging, recent large-scale and well-conducted studies do not provide cause for continuing optimism.

LESSONS FROM THE PREVENTION OF HEART DISEASE AND STROKE

Homocysteine and Vascular Disease

There is a rare autosomal recessive condition in which very high blood concentrations of total homocysteine are associated with increased incidence of occlusive vascular disease in adolescence— even in childhood[53]. This disease, homocysteinuria, is caused by one of several genetic defects in the enzymes that metabolize methionine; these defects occur in methylene tetrahydrofolate reductase (MTHFR) or cystathionine β-synthase (CBS). Premature vascular disease develops irrespective of the genetic defect and this indicates that homocysteine is probably responsible for the vascular damage[54,55]. Blood concentrations of homocysteine are also increased (but to a lesser extent) in individuals who are heterozygous for either of these two enzymes, MTHFR and CBS. Inadequate intake of folic acid and vitamins B_6 and B_{12} (co-factors in the metabolism of homocysteine) is also associated with increased blood concentrations of homocysteine[56–58]. Dietary

supplementation using these vitamins is an important part of the treatment of genetically determined homocysteinuria. In the general ageing population, the contributions of genetic polymorphisms and nutritional intake to the determination of plasma homocysteine concentration (and in turn the risk of vascular disease) is largely unknown[59].

Epidemiological studies indicate that there is a strong positive association between blood homocysteine concentration and the risk of vascular disease. There is now considerable interest in the possible role of increased blood homocysteine concentration in brain ageing and cognitive decline leading to AD[60,61]. Nutritional factors are important in the maintenance of cognitive function in late life and specific dietary deficiencies may be relevant to the failure to retain mental abilities and progression to dementia[62–66]. Nutritional factors of most interest have been antioxidants, marine oils and fat-soluble vitamins. Maternal and infant nutrition is critical in neurodevelopment; folic acid is involved in the closure of the neural tube, and maternal folate deficiency during pregnancy is associated with neural tube defects. The maintenance of normal nervous system functioning in adulthood depends on an adequate consumption of B vitamins, including folate, B_6 and B_{12}. Acute deficiencies of these water-soluble vitamins are linked to neuropathy and psychosis. Age-related changes in metabolic and physiological systems may result in old people obtaining insufficient dietary folate and B_{12} or, to an uncertain extent, through mechanisms linked to atrophic gastritis, to failure to absorb these vitamins. In turn, insufficient intake can result in the accumulation of homocysteine[60], which is associated with greater unexpected cognitive decline and poor quality of life in old people[67] and in AD[68]. A recent review[60] commented on reports that low blood concentration of folate and B_{12} is associated with poor memory, impaired and non-verbal abstract thinking in old people. Low folate concentration is associated with poor spatial copying skills and, in very old age (90–101 years), lower blood folate concentration is linked to impaired encoding and retrieval.

The mechanisms by which homocysteine could impair mental function are uncertain. Homocysteine can undergo auto-oxidation to various metabolites and ROS (free radicals) that are directly toxic to the endothelium and also negatively alter the ability of vascular muscles to relax[69,72]. Homocysteine metabolites, such as homocysteic acid and cysteine sulphinic acid, act as endogenous agonists of NMDA receptors, over-stimulating glutamate receptors and ultimately inducing cytotoxic damage and brain cell death. Homocysteine is also associated with elevated cycline E (a marker of cell division) in the hippocampus of AD sufferers[68]. This raises the possibility that homocysteine may be involved in neuronal stimulation and trigger proliferative mechanisms, including the induction of new amyloid formation[69].

Currently, studies are under way to determine the cognitive effects in old people of strategies to reduce blood homocysteine concentrations, and early results are encouraging[70,71]. These strategies, if effective, may prove useful in community-based interventions to prevent cognitive decline and dementia in old people.

Cholesterol Metabolism and the Risk of Dementia

There is extensive evidence to support a link between lipid metabolism and dementia. Epidemiological evidence is as follows: (a) there is an established association between apolipoprotein E allele (APOEϵ4) polymorphism and AD; and (b) raised systolic blood pressure and high serum cholesterol in mid-life will increase the risk of AD in late life[73]; and (c) use of cholesterol-lowering agents (3-hydroxy-3-methylglutaryl co-enzyme A reductase inhibitors—the statins) is connected with reduced risk of dementia[74]. These findings were supported by Wolozin *et al.*[75] when they observed a lower prevalence of probable AD in subjects prescribed two different statins (lovastatin and pravastatin). Laboratory evidence also supports an association between lipid metabolism and dementia. This includes decreased processing of amyloid precursor protein when cholesterol is removed from cell culture[6] and possible interactions between β-amyloid and low-density receptor-related protein in AD.

These observations have prompted renewed speculation along two separate lines. First, dietary manipulation of lipid metabolism may modify susceptibility to AD in subjects genetically predisposed to AD[77–81]. Second, randomized controlled trials that compare statins known to cross the blood–brain barrier with statins that do not will prove informative in the prevention of AD. Such studies are under way at several centres.

A substantial body of epidemiological data supports a proposed causal link between blood cholesterol concentrations and risk of coronary heart disease. The relationship is somewhat unusual, in that there is a steady increase of coronary heart disease risk from the lowest to the highest cholesterol concentrations observed in free-living communities. Some rural communities in China have mean cholesterol concentrations around 3 mmol/l and mean coronary heart disease death rates about 5% of those seen in England and Wales. This observation has prompted intensive strategies to lower cholesterol in the Western world to concentrations well below those typically aimed for. Individuals not previously considered to be hypercholesterolaemic now seek cholesterol-reducing regimes in order to reduce their perceived risk of myocardial infarction. It is as yet unknown whether these greater than previously sought-for reductions in cholesterol will be associated with reduced rates of coronary heart disease, as the epidemiological data suggest. Likewise, it is uncertain whether cholesterol-lowering regimes reduce the risk of cerebrovascular accidents. Nevertheless, these general principles in the modification of serum cholesterol concentrations in health and disease seem likely to inform the use of statins in the prevention and treatment of dementia[28].

FUTURE STRATEGIES

The cholinergic hypothesis provided a rational basis for drug development in AD[83]. Some symptomatic relief is consistently observed after the introduction of cholinesterase inhibitors, but subsequent attempts to improve modification of cholinergic transmission have not brought substantial improvements in rate or extent of response. There is, however, a reasonable expectation that longer-acting cholinesterase inhibitors with improved safety profiles will be available. The proposition that selective cholinergic neuronal death is a primary event in AD pathogenesis has prompted a search for therapeutic neurotrophic factors specific for cholinergic neurones.

Nerve growth factor (NGF) therapy is an example of this type of approach. It is based on extensive evidence that NGF is critical in the maturation and maintenance of cholinergic neurones and a possible modulatory role for NGF in amyloid precursor protein (APP) expression and secretion[84]. So far, problems of drug delivery have largely thwarted any chance of success. NGF shares these problems with other peptide drug delivery to brain sites. In summary, these are: (a) extra CNS peptide digestion; (b) failure to cross the blood–brain barrier and achieve therapeutic concentrations in the CNS; (c) inefficient distribution within the CNS; and (d) unwanted actions in CNS. The clinical pharmacology of neurotrophic factors is in its infancy and, once mature, seems likely to offer realistic prospects of contributing to AD treatment and prevention. Uses of neurotrophic mimetics (usually small synthetic molecules with growth factor-like activity) are likely to include the promotion of neuronal survival and differentiation

after cell-based therapy[85–88]. Antisense strategies in AD therapy face similar problems. They possess considerable potential to target specific genes but so far none have been found useful in neurodegenerative disease[89].

Current drug development is based largely on better understanding of AD molecular pathology[90]. The "amyloid cascade hypothesis" of AD postulates that amyloid deposition is critical to the development of dementia and to neuronal death. Interventions are now proposed to prevent amyloid deposition and, when it occurs, to cause amyloid to disaggregate and be scavenged from the CNS[91,92]. Relatively little attention is paid to the development of therapies to prevent neurofibrillary tangle formation. A separate strand of research (described above) seeks to protect the brain against oxidative stress, inflammatory reactions, perturbations of calcium homeostasis, apoptosis and cerebrovascular endothelial function.

Figure 58a.1 shows key steps in the processing of APP. The deposition of extracellular amyloid is postulated to be the key event in AD pathogenesis. Three enzymes are involved; α-, β- and γ-secretases. The identification of these secretases raises the possibility that therapies aimed to modify their function could be useful in AD[93]. Several modulators of secretase function have been described, but so far none appear to have therapeutic applications[94].

The prevention of β-amyloid deposition may prove critical in AD treatment. Senile plaques contain not only β-amyloid deposits but copper and zinc that can be solubilized by Cu/Zn chelators *in vitro*. Recently researchers in Australia and Germany[95] successfully reduced β-amyloid accumulation in APP2576 transgenic mice (predisposed to β-amyloid deposition). This raises the possibility that therapies designed to remove brain Cu/Zn may be valuable in AD.

An alternative approach to β-amyloid deposition in AD is based on the production of antibodies to β-amyloid[96–99]. This technique seeks to dissolve senile plaques after they have formed and has the potential to prevent their formation. In studies of transgenic mice (TgCRND8 predisposed to β-amyloid accumulation), immunization with β-amyloid antibodies produced a marked (around 50%) reduction of β-amyloid in brain and was linked to reduced cognitive impairment[100]. More detailed behavioural studies were reported at about the same time[101]. These concluded that treated mice performed

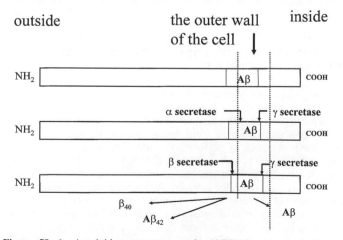

Figure 58a.1 Amyloid precursor protein (APP) is a transmembrane cellular adhesion molecule involved in synaptogenesis. It is processed by enzymatic cleavage to yield amyloid fragments (β_{50}, β_{42} and Aβ) of the original APP. Each cleavage enzyme acts at a specific point on APP. β- and γ-Secretases cleave at one or other end of the amyloid fragment. α-Secretase cleaves at a point between the two

"superbly" on the Morris water maze, whereas untreated mice did not. The authors remarked that their data did not support concerns that attempts to remove β-amyloid from brain might inadvertently cause wider dispersal and, therefore, more extensive β-amyloid neurotoxic damage. A later population-based observational study tested the hypothesis that the natural occurrence of antibodies to β-amyloid might reduce the incidence of dementia[102]. Although antibodies to β-amyloid could be detected, no reduction in AD was found.

CONCLUSION

The future for AD therapy holds much promise. As the general health of old people continues to improve and the incidence of functional disabilities is reduced, so the achievement of dementia prevention seems not only attainable but worthwhile. The huge collaborative international effort to understand the molecular pathology of AD and to design drugs to modify critical steps is certain to bring great benefit to those at risk of dementia.

REFERENCES

1. Porter R. *The Greatest Benefit to Mankind: A Medical History of Humanity from Antiquity to the Present.* Fontana, 1997; 201–44.
2. Whalley LJ. Early onset Alzheimer's disease in Scotland: environmental and familial factors. *Br J Psychiat* 2001; **178** (suppl.) s53–9.
3. Rao VS, Cupples A, van Duijn CM *et al.* Evidence for major gene inheritance of Alzheimer's disease in families of patients with and without apolipoprotein E₄. *Am J Hum Genet* 1996; **59**: 664–75.
4. Cruts M, van Duijn CM, Backhoven H *et al.* Estimation of the genetic contribution of presenilin-1 and -2 mutations in a population-based study of presenile Alzheimer disease. *Mol Genet* 1998; **7**: 43–51.
5. Liddell MB, Lovestone S, Owen MJ. Genetic risk of Alzheimer's disease: advising relatives. *Br J Psychiat* 2001; **178**: 7–11.
6. Christensen K, McGue M, Yashin A *et al.* Genetic and environmental influences on functional abilities in Danish twins aged 75 years and older. *J Gerontol Ser A Biol Sci Med Sci* 2000; **55**: 446–52.
7. Corder EH, Saunders AM, Strittmatter WJ *et al.* Gene dose of apolipoprotein E type 4 allele and the risk of Alzheimer's disease in late onset families. *Science* 1993; **261**: 921–3.
8. Tallis R. Increasing longevity: medical, social and political implications. *J R Coll Physicians* 1998; vii–ix.
9. Grimley Evans J. Implications for health services. *Phil Trans R Soc Lond Biol Sci* 1997; **352**: 1887–93.
10. Rowe JW, Kahn RL. *Successful aging.* New York: Dell, 1999.
11. Khaw K-T. Epidemiological aspects of Alzheimer's disease. *Phil Trans R Soc Lond B Biol Sci* 1997; **352**: 1829–35.
12. Whalley LJ. *The Ageing Brain.* London: Weidenfeld and Nicolson, 2001; 9–14.
13. Harwood RH, Prince MJ, Mann AH *et al.* The prevalence of diagnoses, impairments, disabilities and handicaps in a population of elderly people living in a defined geographical area: the Gospel Oak Project. *Age Ageing* 1998; **27**: 707–14.
14. MRC CFAS. Profile of disability in elderly people: estimates from a longitudinal population study. *Br Med J* 1999; **318**: 1108–11.
15. Holmes J, House A. Psychiatric illness predicts poor outcome after surgery for hip fracture: a prospective cohort study. *Psychol Med* 2000; **30**: 921–9.
16. Holmes J, House A. Psychiatric illness in hip fracture. *Age Ageing* 2000; **29**: 537–46.
17. Rogers SL, Farlow MR, Doody RS *et al.* A 24-week, double-blind, placebo-controlled trial of donepezil in patients with Alzheimer's disease. Donepezil Study Group. *Neurology* 1998; **50**: 136–45.
18. Matthews H, Korbey J. Wilkinson D, Rowden J. Donepezil in Alzheimer's disease—eighteen months results from Southampton Memory Clinic. *Int J Geriat Psychiat* (in press).
19. Corey-Bloom J, Anand R, Veach J. A randomized trial evaluating the efficacy and safety of ENA 713 (rivastigmine tartrate), a new acetylcholinesterase inhibitor, in patients with mild to moderately severe Alzheimer's disease. *Int J Geriat Psychopharmacol* 1998; **1**: 55–65.
20. Rosler M, Ananad R, Cicin-Sain A *et al.* Efficacy and safety of rivastigmine in patients with Alzheimer's disease: international randomised controlled trial. *Br Med J* 1999; **318**: 633–8.
21. Raskind MA, Peskind ER, Wessel T, Yuan W. Galantamine in AD: a 6-month randomized, placebo-controlled trial with a 6-month extension. The Galantamine USA-1 Study Group. *Neurology* 2000; **54**: 2261–8.
22. Tariot PN, Solomon PR, Morris JC *et al.* A 5-month randomized, placebo-controlled trial of galantamine in AD. The Galantamine USA-10 Study Group. *Neurology* 2000; **54**: 2269–76.
23. Winblat B, Wimo A. Assessing the societal impact of acetylcholinesterase inhibitor therapies. *Alzheim Dis Rel Dis* 1999; suppl. **2**: s9–19.
24. Smith F, Gracon S, Knopman D *et al.* Tacrine and nursing home placement: application of the Cox proportional hazards model with time-dependent covariates. *Drug Inf J* 1998; **32**: 729–35.
25. Schumock GT. Economic considerations in the treatment and management of Alzheimer's disease. *Am J Health Syst Physicians* 1998; **55**(suppl 2): s17–21.
26. O'Brien BJ, Goeree R, Hux M *et al.* Economic evaluation of donepezil for the treatment of Alzheimer's disease in Canada. *J Am Geriat Soc* 1999; **47**: 570–8.
27. McDonnell J, Redekpo WK, van der Roer *et al.* The cost of treatment of Alzheimer's disease in The Netherlands—a regression-based simulation model. *Pharmacoeconomics* 2001 **19**: 379–90.
28. Nunomura A, Perry G, Pappolla MA *et al.* Neuronal oxidative stress precedes amyloid-B deposition in Down syndrome. *J Neuropathol Exp Neurol* 2000; **59**: 1011–17.
29. Nunomura A, Perry G, Pappolla MA *et al.* RNA oxidation is a prominent feature of vulnerable neurons in Alzheimer's disease. *J Neurosci* 1999; **19**: 1959–64.
30. Vitek MP, Bhattacharya K, Glendening JM *et al.* Advanced glycation end products contribute to amyloidosis in Alzheimer disease. *Proc Natl Acad Sci USA* 1994; **91**: 4766–70.
31. Good PF, Werner P, Hsu A *et al.* Evidence of neuronal oxidative damage in Alzheimer's disease. *Am J Pathol* 1996; **149**: 21–8.
32. Sayre LM, Zelasko DA, Harris PLR *et al.* 4-Hydroxynonenal-derived advanced lipid peroxidation end products are increased in Alzheimer's disease. *J Neurochem* 1997; **68**: 2092–7.
33. Smith MA, Harris PLR, Sayre LM, Perry G. Iron accumulation in Alzheimer disease is a source of redox-generated free radicals. *Proc Natl Acad Sci USA* 1997; **94**: 9866–8.
34. Smith MA, Harris PLR, Sayre LM *et al.* Widespread peroxynitrite-mediated damage in Alzheimer's disease. *J Neurosci* 1997; **17**: 2653–7.
35. Colton CA, Gilbert DI. Production of superoxide anions by a CNS macrophage, the microglia. *Fed Exp Biol Sci (letter)* 1987, 284–8.
36. Yan S-D, Chen X, Schmidt A-M *et al.* Glycated tau protein in Alzheimer's disease: a mechanism for induction of oxidant stress. *Proc Natl Acad Sci USA* 1994; **91**: 7787–91.
37. El Khoury J, Hickman SE, Thomas CA *et al.* Scavenger receptor mediated adhesion of microglia to β-amyloid fibrils. *Nature* 1996; **382**: 716–19.
38. McGeer P, Rogers J. Anti-inflammatory agents as a therapeutic approach to Alzheimer's disease. *Neurology* 1992; **42**: 447–9.
39. Rogers J, Kirby LC, Hempelman SR *et al.* Clinical trial of indomethacin in Alzheimer's disease. *Neurology* 1993; **43**: 1609–11.
40. Breitner JCS, Gau BA, Welsh KA *et al.* Inverse association of anti-inflammatory treatments and Alzheimer's disease: initial results of a co-twin control study. *Neurology* 1994; **44**: 227–32.
41. Rich JB, Rasmusson DX, Folstein MF *et al.* Nonsteroidal antiinflammatory drugs in Alzheimer's disease. *Neurology* 1995; **45**: 51–5.
42. Smallhieser NR, Swanson DR. Indomethacin and Alzheimer's disease. *Neurology* 1996; **46**: 583.
43. Stewart WF, Kawas C, Corrada M *et al.* Risk of Alzheimer's disease and duration of NSAID use. *Neurology* 1997; **48**: 626–31.
44. Munch G, Taneli Y, Schraven E *et al.* The cognition enhancing drug tenilsetam is an inhibitor of protein crosslinking by advanced glycation. *J Neur Transm* 1994; 193–208.
45. Munch G, Mayer S, Michaelis J *et al.* Influence of advanced glycation end products and ACE-inhibitors on nucleation dependent

polymerization of β-amyloid peptide. *Biochim Biophys Acta* 1997; **1360**: 17–29.

46. Sano M, Ernesto C, Thomas RG *et al*. A controlled trial of selegiline, α-tocopherol or both as a treatment for Alzheimer's disease. *N Engl J Med* 1997; **336**: 1216–22.

47. Stoll S, Scheuer K, Pohl O *et al*. Ginkgo biloba extract (Egb761) independently improves changes in passive avoidance learning in the ageing mouse. *Pharmacopsychiatry* 1996; **29**: 144–9.

48. Henderson VW. The epidemiology of estrogen replacement therapy and Alzheimer's disease. *Neurology* 1997; suppl 7: s27–35.

49. LeBlanc ES, Janowsky J, Cha BKS *et al*. Hormone replacement therapy and cognition: systematic review and meta-analysis. *J Am Med Assoc* 2001; **285**: 1489–99.

50. Fillenbaum G, Hanlon JT, Landerman LR *et al*. Impact of estrogen use on decline in cognitive function in a representative sample of older community resident women. *Am J Epidemiol* 2001; **153**: 137–44.

51. Seshadri S, Zornberg GL, Derby LE *et al*. Postmenopausal estrogen replacement therapy and the risk of Alzheimer's disease. *Arch Neurol* 2001; **58**: 435–40.

52. Yaffe K, Krueger K, Sarkar S *et al*. Cognitive function in post menopausal women treated with raloxifene. *N Engl J Med* 2001; **344**: 1207–13.

53. Mudd SH, Levy HL, Skovby F. Disorders of trans-sulfuration. In Scriver CP, Beaudet AL, Sly WS *et al*., eds., *The Metabolic Basis of Inherited Disease*. New York: McGraw-Hill, 1989; 693–734.

54. McCully KS. Vascular pathology of homocysteinemia: implications for the pathogenesis of arteriosclerosis. *Am J Pathol* 1969; **56**: 111–28.

55. McCully KS, Wilson RB. Homocysteine theory of arteriosclerosis. *Atherosclerosis* 1975; **22**: 215–27.

56. Selhub J, Jacques PF, Bostom AG *et al*. Association between plasma homocysteine concentrations and extracranial carotid-artery stenosis. *N Engl J Med* 1995; **32**: 286–91.

57. Selhub J, Bagley LC, Miller J *et al*. B vitamins, homocysteine and neurocognitive function in the elderly. *Am J Clin Nutr* 2000; **1**: s614–20.

58. Selhub J, Jacques PF, Wilson PWF *et al*. Vitamin status and intake as primary determinants of homocysteinemia in an elderly population. *J Am Med Assoc* 1993; **270**: 2693–8.

59. Mayer EL, Jacobson DW, Robinson K. Homocysteine and coronary atherosclerosis. *J Am Coll Cardiol* 1996; **27**: 517–27.

60. Miller JW. Homocysteine, Alzheimer's disease and cognitive function. *Nutrition* 2000; **16**: 675–7.

61. Miller JW, Green R, Allen LH *et al*. Homocysteine correlates with cognitive function in Sacramento Area Latino Study of Ageing (SALSA). *Fed Am Soc Exp Biol* 1999; **13**: A374.

62. Riggs KM, Spiro A, Tucker K *et al*. Relations of vitamin B_{12}, vitamin B_6, folate and homocysteine to cognitive performance in the normative ageing study. *Am J Clin Nutr* 1996; **63**: 306–14.

63. Kalmijn S, Launer LJ, Lindemans J *et al*. Total homocysteine and cognitive decline in a community-based sample of elderly subjects. *Am J Epidemiol* 1999; **150**: 283–9.

64. Prins ND, Vermeer SE, Clarke R *et al*. Homocysteine and cognitive function in the elderly: the Rotterdam Scan Study. *Neurology* 2001; suppl. 3: A240–41.

65. Morris MS, Jaques PF, Rosenberg IH *et al*. Hyperhomocysteinemia associated with poor recall in the third National Health and Nutrition Examination Survey. *Am J Clin Nutr* 2001; **73**: 927–33.

66. Breteler MMB. Vascular risk factors for Alzheimer's disease: an epidemiological perspective. *Neurobiol Ageing* 2000; **1**: 153–60.

67. Leblhuber F, Walli J, Artner-Dworzak E *et al*. Hyperhomocysteinemia in dementia. *J Neur Transm* 2000; **107**: 1469–74.

68. Wang HX, Wahlin A, Basun H *et al*. Vitamin B_{12} and folate in relation to the development of Alzheimer's disease. *Neurology* 2001; **156**: 1188–94.

69. White AR, Huang XD, Jobling MF *et al*. Homocysteine potentiates copper and amyloid peptide-mediated toxicity in primary neuronal cultures: possible risk factors in the Alzheimer's type neurodegenerative pathway. *J Neurochem* 2001; **6**: 1509–20.

70. Nilsson K, Warkentin S, Hultberg B *et al*. Treatment of cobalamin deficiency in dementia, evaluated clinically and with cerebral blood flow measurements. *Ageing Clin Exp Res* 2000; **12**: 199–207.

71. Nilsson K, Gustafson L, Hultberg B. Improvement of cognitive functions after cobalamin/folate supplementation in elderly patients with dementia and elevated plasma homocysteine. *Int J Geriat Psychiat* 2001; **16**: 609–14.

72. Ho Pi, Collins SC, Dhitavat S *et al*. Homocysteine potentiates β-amyloid neurotoxicity: role of oxidative stress. *J Neurochem* 2001; **78**: 249–53.

73. Kivipelto M, Helkala EL, Laasko MP *et al*. Midlife vascular risk factors and Alzheimer's disease in later life: longitudinal, population-based study. *Br Med J* 2001; **322**: 1447–51.

74. Jick H, Zornberg HJ, Jick SS *et al*. Statins and the risk of dementia. *Lancet* 2000; **56**: 1627–31.

75. Wolozin BW, Ruosseau P, Celesia GG, Siegel G. Decreased prevalence of Alzheimer disease associated with 3-hydroxy-3-methyglutaryl co-enzyme A reductase inhibitors. *Arch Neurol* 2000; **57**: 439–43.

76. Simons M, Keller P, De Strooper B *et al*. Cholesterol depletion inhibits the generation of β amyloid in hippocampal neurons. *Proc Natl Acad Sci USA* 1998; **95**: 460–4.

77. Jarvik GP, Wijsman EM, Kukull WA *et al*. Interactions of apolipoprotein E genotypes, total cholesterol level, age and sex in prediction of Alzheimer's disease: a case-control study. *Neurology* 1995; **45**: 1092–6.

78. Games D, Adams D, Alessandrini R *et al*. Development of neuropathology similar to Alzheimer's disease in transgenic mice overexpressing the 717_{V-F} β-amyloid precursor protein. *Nature* 1995; **373**: 523–8.

79. Sparks DL. Coronary artery disease, hypertension, ApoE, and cholesterol: a link to Alzheimer's disease? *Ann NY Acad Sci* 1997; **826**: 128–46.

80. Notkola IL, Sulkava R, Pekkanen J *et al*. Serum total cholesterol, apolipoprotein E epsilon 4 allele, and Alzheimer's disease. *Neuroepidemiology* 1998; **17**: 14–20.

81. Refolo LM, Duff K, Malester B *et al*. Hypercholesterolemia accelerates amyloid pathology in a transgenic mouse model of Alzheimer's Disease. *J Neuropathol Neurol* 2000; **59**: 20–23.

82. Fassbender K, Simons M, Bergmann C *et al*. Simvastatin strongly reduces levels of Alzheimer's disease β-amyloid peptides Aβ42 and Aβ40 *in vitro* and *in vivo*. *Proc Natl Acad Sci USA* 2001; **98**: 5856–61.

83. Glen AIM, Whalley LJ. *Alzheimer's Disease: Early Recognition of Potentially Reversible Deficits*. Edinburgh: Churchill Livingstone, 1979.

84. Villa A, Latasa MJ, Pasual A. Nerve growth factor modulates the expression and secretion of β-amyloid precursor protein through different mechanisms in PC12 cells. *J Neurochem* 2001; **77**: 1077–84.

85. Grudnman M, Correy-Bloom J, Thal LJ. Perspectives in clinical Alzheimer's disease research and the development of antidementia drugs. *J Neur Transm* 1998; suppl. **53**: s255–75.

86. Emilien G, Beyreuther K, Masters CL, Maloteaux JM. Prospects for pharmacological intervention in Alzheimer's disease. *Arch Neurol* 2000; **57**: 454–9.

87. Cacabelos R, Alvarez A, Lombardi A *et al*. Pharmacological treatment of Alzheimer's disease: from psychotropic drugs and cholinesterase inhibitors to pharmacogenomics. *Drugs Today* 2000; **36**: 415–99s.

88. Maimone D, Dominici R, Grimaldi LME. Pharmacogenomics of neurodegenerative disorders. *Eur J Pharmacol* 2001; **413**: 11–29.

89. Stoessl AJ. Antisense strategies for the treatment of neurological disease. *Expert Opin Therapeut Patents* 2001; **11**: 547–62.

90. Wiltfang J, Esselmann H, Maler JM *et al*. Molecular biology of Alzheimer's dementia and its clinical relevance to early diagnosis and new therapeutic strategies. *Gerontology* 2001; **47**: 65–71.

91. Selkoe D. Translating cell biology into therapeutic advances in Alzheimer's disease. *Nature* 1999; **399**: A23–31.

92. Selkoe DJ. Alzheimer's disease: a central role for amyloid. *J Neuropathol Exp Neurol* 1994; **53**: 438–47.

93. Jhee S, Shiovitz T, Crawford AW, Cutler NR. β-amyloid therapies in Alzheimer's disease. *Expert Opin Invest Drugs* 2001; **10**: 593–605.

94. Creemers JWM, Dominguez DI, Plets E *et al*. Processing of β-secretase by furin and other members of the proprotein convertase family. *J Biol Chem* 2000; **276**: 4211–17.

95. Cherny RA, Atwood CS, Xilinas ME *et al*. Treatment with a copper–zinc chelator markedly and rapidly inhibits β-amyloid

accumulation in Alzheimer's disease transgenic mice. *Neuron* 2011; **30**: 665–7.

96. Esiri MM. Is an effective immune intervention for Alzheimer's disease in prospect? *Trends Pharmacol Sci* 2001; **22**: 2–3.

97. Ingram DK. Vaccine development for Alzheimer's disease: a shot of good news. *Trends Neurosci* 2001; **24**: 305–37.

98. Schenk D, Barbour R, Dunn W *et al.* Immunization with amyloid-β attenuates Alzheimer disease-like pathology in the PDAPP mouse. *Nature* 1999; **400**: 173–7.

99. Bard F, Cannon C, Barbour R *et al.* Peripherally administered antibodies against amyloid β peptide enter the central nervous system and reduce pathology in a mouse model of Alzheimer disease. *Nature Med* 2000; **6**(8): 16–19.

100. Janus C, Pearson J, McLaurin J *et al.* A β-peptide immunization reduces behavioural impairment and plaques in a model of Alzheimer's disease. *Nature* 2000; **408**: 979–82.

101. Morgan D, Diamond DM, Gottschall PE *et al.* A β-peptide vaccination prevents memory loss in a model of Alzheimer's disease. *Nature* 2000; **408**: 982–85.

102. Hyman BT, Smith C, Buldyrev I *et al.* Autoantibodies to amyloid-β and Alzheimer's disease. *Ann Neurol* 2001; **49**: 808–10.

Possible Future Treatments and Preventative Strategies for Alzheimer's Disease

Simon Lovestone

Institute of Psychiatry, London, UK

PREVENTION OR CURE?

It is a truism that prevention is better than cure, although historically both are usually preceded by palliation. Whilst this seems to be true also for Alzheimer's disease (AD), in that drugs for symptomatic treatment have preceded other approaches, the situation is complicated, both because these drugs may themselves alter the disease process and because prevention and cure (in the sense of reversing or modifying the disease pathogenesis) may be inseparable. The confusion largely results from the timing of the onset of AD. At the point of diagnosis, disease has already been established, probably for many decades. Careful pathological studies have demonstrated that a marker of neuronal damage in AD—highly phosphorylated tau—accumulates in neurons in certain cortical areas in mid-life and progresses to frank neurofibrillary tangle formation and neuronal death in these areas before the onset of clinical dementia[1]. Neuroimaging studies show that those with genetic risk factors for AD have evidence of functional damage decades before onset[2]. Truly preventative strategies, therefore, preventing even the onset of AD pathology, are probably not realistic. Rather, prevention will be secondary—preventing the disease process progressing to the point where it becomes clinically manifest. This approach (prevention) differs from approaches designed to slow the progression of disease once started (treatment) only in timing. It is best perhaps to think only of disease modification; either late, in which case it looks like slowing of disease, or early, in which case it looks like prevention. From the biological point of view, both are the same.

DISEASE MODIFICATION—DIRECTIONS FROM EPIDEMIOLOGY

Identification of risk factors for AD, such as vascular factors or diabetes, points the way towards obvious potential interventions to slow disease progression. It would be hoped that reducing hypertension and head injury, improving cardiovascular health and controlling diabetes well would all reduce the conversion of early pathology to clinical dementia. Time will tell whether this is the case. Worrying for this long-term strategy is the observation that treatment with insulin carries a higher risk than diabetes alone[3]. This may be a surrogate for disease severity but it does highlight that the route between epidemiology and public health may not always be obstacle-free.

Other population-based studies have suggested interventional possibilities for disease modification. Most promising at present is evidence suggesting that non-steroidal anti-inflammatory drugs may delay progression or prevent the appearance of symptoms[4]. Similarly, there is evidence linking oxidative damage to pathology and antioxidants to protection, and there may be an important role for vitamin E or some other antioxidant therapy in disease modification in the near to middle future[5]. The evidence linking hormone replacement and protection has a more limited potential, if only by virtue of gender. Studies are currently in progress that will determine whether any of these three approaches will have a clinical role in modifying the pathogenesis of AD.

DISEASE MODIFICATION—DIRECTIONS FROM MOLECULAR BIOLOGY

The advances in understanding the molecular biology of AD have been rapid and profound. It is clear already that this work will yield compounds designed to modify disease, although whether these compounds make the difficult passage between laboratory and clinic is a different matter. Preventing amyloid formation is the most obvious drug target and compounds designed to do this by inhibiting γ-secretase are in the late stages of development. Another, complementary approach is to increase the activity of α-secretase (thus hopefully reducing amyloidogenic metabolism). Interestingly, all cholinomimetic therapies should increase the activity of α-secretase indirectly, and this has been shown to be the case for M1 agonists[6].

The other pathology of AD, tangles, is a harder target as it is not yet clear why tau aggregates. However the importance of tau aggregation as a target is emphasized by the fact that this occurs in many neurodegenerative conditions[7], correlates with cognitive impairment and has functional consequences for neurons. Tau phosphorylation precedes aggregation and may cause aggregation in AD; certainly it inhibits tau function[8]. In neurons, tau is phosphorylated by an enzyme, glycogen synthase kinase-3β (GSK-3β), and inhibition of this would be expected to prevent tau phosphorylation[9]. Lithium inhibits GSK-3β and, as predicted, reduces tau phosphorylation[10,11]. Might lithium modify disease progression? Other GSK-3β inhibitors are in development. GSK-3β is also inhibited through the same signal transduction route as that induced by muscarinic agonists, and in line with this is the finding that muscarinic agonists reduce tau phosphorylation in cellular models[12]. It is possible that cholinomimetic therapies (including the cholinesterase inhibitors) will have some disease-modifying effect as well as a palliative effect[13].

Perhaps the most surprising and exciting development suggests that a vaccine is a therapeutic possibility for AD[14]. Amyloid peptide was used to inoculate transgenic animals overexpressing the amyloid precursor protein gene. In these animals, amyloid inoculation reduced amyloid deposition in the brain without any apparent adverse effects on the animals. It remains to be seen whether this is true in other animal models and whether cognitive deficits are also prevented. More importantly, it will be necessary to be very sure that there are no adverse consequences in man. The brain is supposedly (but probably not entirely) immunologically sacrosanct, and injecting a normal brain protein and stimulating an immune reaction has the very real potential of inducing auto-immune damage. Toxicity studies are under way that will address this concern.

TOWARDS DISEASE MODIFICATION —A TIME SCALE

The time scale of science is not linear; progress comes quicker these days and the only reliable prediction regarding the future is that predictions will continue to be usually wrong. However, disease-modifying treatments are already in clinical trials, and strategies such as HRT, anti-inflammatories and vitamin E are in use in other contexts. Another potential disease-modifying approach is to use the cholinergic therapies that are already in use for palliation. It should be known within the first few years of the new millennium whether any of these approaches have a true benefit for patients in modifying disease and, if so, given that experience in using these compounds in other contexts is extensive, then approval for use in secondary prevention may be rapid. Other approaches modifying amyloid and tau will take longer, not least because the time taken for novel drugs to travel from laboratory to clinic is best measured in decades.

REFERENCES

1. Braak E, Braak H, Mandelkow E-M. A sequence of cytoskeleton changes related to the formation of neurofibrillary tangles and neuropil threads. *Acta Neuropathol* 1994; **87**: 554–67.

2. Small GW, Mazziotta JC, Collins MT *et al.* Apolipoprotein E type 4 allele and cerebral glucose metabolism in relatives at risk for familial Alzheimer disease. *J Am Med Assoc* 1995; **273**: 942–7.

3. Ott A, Stolk RP, Hofman A *et al.* Association of diabetes mellitus and dementia: the Rotterdam Study. *Diabetologia* 1996; **39**(11): 1392–7.

4. Breitner JC, Welsh KA, Helms MJ *et al.* Delayed onset of Alzheimer's disease with nonsteroidal anti-inflammatory and histamine H_2 blocking drugs. *Neurobiol Aging* 1995; **16**: 523–30.

5. Sano M, Ernesto C, Thomas RG *et al.* A controlled trial of selegiline, α-tocopherol, or both as treatment for Alzheimer's disease. *N Engl J Med* 1997; **336**: 1216–22.

6. Nitsch RM, Slack BE, Farber SA *et al.* Regulation of proteolytic processing of the amyloid β-protein precursor of Alzheimer's disease in transfected cell lines and in brain slices. *J Neural Transm* 1994; **44** (suppl): 21–7.

7. Spillantini MG, Goedert M. Tau protein pathology in neurodegenerative diseases. *Trends Neurosci* 1998; **21**: 428–33.

8. Lovestone S, Hartley CL, Pearce J, Anderton BH. Phosphorylation of tau by glycogen synthase kinase-3β in intact mammalian cells: the effects on organisation and stability of microtubules. *Neuroscience* 1996; **73**(4): 1145–57.

9. Lovestone S, Reynolds CH. The phosphorylation of tau: a critical stage in neurodevelopmental and neurodegenerative processes. *Neuroscience* 1997; **78**(2): 309–24.

10. Lovestone S, Davis DR, Webster M-T *et al.* Lithium reduces tau phosphorylation—effects in living cells and in neurons at therapeutic concentrations. *Biol Psychiat* 1999; **45**(8): 995–1003.

11. Muñoz-Montaño JR, Moreno FJ, Avila J, Díaz-Nido J. Lithium inhibits Alzheimer's disease-like tau protein phosphorylation in neurons. *FEBS Lett* 1997; **411**: 183–8.

12. Sadot E, Gurwitz D, Barg J *et al.* Activation of m1 muscarinic acetylcholine receptor regulates tau phosphorylation in transfected PC12 cells. *J Neurochem* 1996; **66**: 877–80.

13. Lovestone S. Muscarinic therapies in Alzheimer's disease: from palliative therapies to disease modification. *Int J Psychiat Clin Pract* 1997; **1**(1): 15–20.

14. Schenk D, Barbour R, Dunn W *et al.* Immunization with amyloid-β attenuates Alzheimer-disease-like pathology in the PDAPP mouse. *Nature* 1999; **400**(6740): 173–7.

Psychological and Psychosocial Interventions

Edgar Miller

Centre for Applied Psychology, University of Leicester, UK

Psychological interventions in dementia offer attempts to ameliorate the consequences of the disorder. They do not affect the underlying pathological process but are directed at helping those afflicted to function better and more independently. Interventions of this kind are based on the implicit assumption that those with dementia remain sensitive to environmental influences, even though the extent to which this is the case may be reduced. There is now good evidence that this assumption is justified[1,2].

GENERAL METHODS

Psychosocial interventions in dementia have been dominated by a number of approaches, which are designed to be generally applicable to all sufferers. These carry with them, whether explicitly or implicitly, the assumption that attention to a key impairment or principle is the key to effective intervention.

The assumption that an important feature of those with dementia is that they lose their orientation to time, place and person, lies behind reality orientation (RO), which is the earliest of these general methods[3]. There are two facets to RO. Firstly, regular group sessions, known as "classroom" or "group RO", involve sessions in which members may be led to recall the date and time of year, where they are, and so on. Secondly, "24-hour RO" may operate continuously and involves all who come into contact with sufferers, stressing information relating to orientation. An example of this is the nurse saying, "It is now 12 o'clock and time to take your tablets, Mrs Smith". This emphasizes information relating to time and person and links the time to the activity to be undertaken.

Evaluative studies have largely concentrated on group rather than 24 hour RO. In a review of these[4], it was concluded that sessions did lead to increases in verbal orientation (e.g. group members are more likely to be able to say what day it is). When it comes to changes in a wider range of cognitive functions or in behaviour, the evidence is very much less convincing.

Another general approach is that of reminiscence. This was originally proposed for normally functioning old people and is linked to the assumption that reminiscence and life review is a major task of old age. As used with those who suffer from dementia, it also builds on an area of relative strength, that of memory for the distant past. Group sessions are organized, with participants discussing how things used to be, usually with special materials such as photographs of the local city centre as it used to be 40–50 years ago. Reminiscence about how things were can be used as a basis for turning the discussion to how things are now.

Like RO, reminiscence has been popular, but relevant research has not offered strong support. The evidence that old people are especially prone to reminisce or that it necessarily leads to beneficial effects, such as increases in well-being or mood, has proved far from overwhelming[5]. Attempts to formally evaluate effectiveness in those with dementia have produced both negative findings[6] as well as some indications of modest benefit[7].

A more recent development of relevance to this section is what has become known as "dementia care mapping" (DCM), which is based on the writings of Tom Kitwood[8,9]. Kitwood stressed the "personhood" of people with dementia, and in his view the central aspect of personhood is found in social relationships with others. Good care is that which enhances personhood and well-being in terms of such things as enhancing self-esteem, enabling individuals to influence their own personal lives, promoting social confidence in terms of being at ease with others, and a sense of hope.

DCM is built more on a set of values than psychological principles, albeit values that almost no-one who is concerned for the welfare of these people would wish to dissent from, at least in general terms. What is lacking in this general approach is any detailed analysis of how these might best be turned into caring practices for elderly people with dementia, other than by feedback from an evaluative process, or "dementia care mapping" as more narrowly defined[10], to assess quality of care. This is based, firstly, on coding activities or inactivities according to whether they are expressions of "well-being" or "ill-being". Secondly, there is recording of episodes in which the person is demeaned or diminished. The obvious problems are those of reliably defining what is "well-being", "demeaning", etc., and no data as to the reliability of the method appear to be available.

This is just a selection of the general approaches or methods that are available and others are described elsewhere[1,2]. Most of these suffer from the limitation that, explicitly or implicitly, they see the problem of dementia as a single issue (e.g. loss of orientation in RO) or, as in the case of DCM, offer a set of very general values and principles. The best evidence as to effectiveness is still for RO, although even the positive impact of that is limited in extent. However, the search for better methods of care is not necessarily futile, since there is evidence that different forms of intervention, such as altering the layout of the furniture to make interaction easier, or enhanced activity programmes, can produce improvement[11,12].

SPECIFIC METHODS

As already indicated, approaches like those described in the previous section all assume a particular key factor, whether it be lack of orientation or the minimizing of personhood, offers the key to optimal care. Against this is the argument that even such an ultimately devastating disorder as dementia does not obliterate all individuality and, in consequence, different people with dementia will have different problems and varied needs, even if there are some common elements. This does not deny that things like DCM and RO might have a general role, but it does mean there is also a need to consider individuals and their particular problems and circumstances.

A wide range of psychological interventions directed at specific problems, such as incontinence, memory failures and social behaviour, have now been described. These are based more in the kinds of psychological treatments developed for use with other clinical populations. Space does not permit an extensive description of these and more detailed information can be gained from other sources[1,2,13]. This section will merely offer a few illustrative examples.

Incontinence has always proved a difficult and almost intractable problem for psychological intervention. Nevertheless, some evidence of techniques able to produce beneficial effects has appeared. A system of checking for wetness and prompting going to the toilet has been found to produce positive effects, increasing the number of "dry checks"[14]. It is also interesting that one study has suggested that earlier failures to produce benefits with similar programmes might be at least partially attributable to staff failing to comply with the regime, rather than a failure of the method to provide positive effects when properly applied[15].

Aimless wandering can also be another feature that is difficult to manage. The adaptation of principles based on operant conditioning has shown some promise as a means to reduce this behaviour[16,17]. An interesting point in relation to this particular problem and, by implication, other problems as well, is that it is often unfortunately seen as secondary to intellectual loss and therefore only remediable if the primary problem can be tackled[13].

Finally, one possible way of ameliorating the problem of memory loss is to use external memory aids as prompts in order to lessen the load on the individual's own memory and to support retrieval. An encouraging account has described the use of this strategy with some success in the execution of daily living tasks, such as preparing a drink or snack[18].

COMMUNITY-BASED INTERVENTIONS

Most of the elderly population with dementia live in the community and are looked after by relatives, who can be under considerable strain[1]. Supporting carers therefore assumes considerable importance and extensions of the approaches described above have been made to deal with problems encountered in those resident in the community[13] (a wider discussion of community care issues is provided in Sections MI and MII).

One of the most obvious strategies is to provide support groups for carers, which may concentrate on providing information about dementia and discuss coping strategies, especially those used by group members. This strategy is described in greater detail elsewhere[1].

More formal methods, such as RO, have been adapted for use with community residents attending day hospitals. Similar effects to those obtained in applying RO in psychogeriatric wards and nursing homes were obtained. Again, the impact was most pronounced for orientation measures but with some effect on mood as well[19].

Finally, it is possible to use informal caregivers, such as spouses and children, as agents to implement more specific psychological interventions of the kind outlined in the immediately preceding section[20,21]. Problems tackled with some indication of success include the improvement of self-care skills and social interaction.

COMMENT

The most important conclusion that can be reached after surveying the evidence on psychological and psychosocial interventions for those with dementia is that people with even quite marked levels of dementia are responsive to psychological and environmental manipulation. This offers the essential foundation for the development of therapeutic or management strategies based on psychological principles.

Quite simple manoeuvres, such as rearranging chairs in groups to facilitate conversation, rather than leaving them in long regimented lines, can improve social interaction. Other relatively simple interventions can contribute to maintaining the basic skills associated with independent living. Despite being positively regarded by staff and patients, general methods like RO and reminiscence are of limited value and DCM remains to be evaluated. The best support is for RO, and indicates that small positive changes in orientation can be achieved. Since these methods are easy to apply, they can also be used as a general background on which more specific interventions can be built, and the successful addition of behavioural training to RO exploited in one investigation[22] can be seen as an example of this.

It may be that an important spin-off from general methods like RO is their popularity with direct care staff. Whilst this remains to be formally demonstrated, their use may help create and maintain a more optimistic and therapeutic attitude in staff, which can be a very worthwhile achievement in itself. In turn, this should make it easier to implement more specific interventions, more focused on individual needs.

As with psychological interventions in other contexts, the best results are likely to follow from the careful functional analysis of problem behaviour, whether this be a lack of behaviour or excessive and inappropriate behaviour, with specific interventions chosen in relation to the exact nature of the problem.

Overall, psychological and psychosocial interventions in the treatment and management of those with dementia are now capable of achieving modest but useful beneficial effects. They now must be regarded as a worthwhile part of any overall management strategy.

REFERENCES

1. Miller E, Morris R. *The Psychology of Dementia*. Chichester: Wiley, 1993.
2. Woods RT. Psychological "therapies" in dementia. In Woods RD, ed., *Handbook of the Clinical Psychology of Ageing*. Chichester: Wiley, 1996.
3. Folsom JC. Reality orientation for elderly mental patients. *J Geriat Psychiat* 1968; **1**: 291–307.
4. Holden UP, Woods RT. *Reality Orientation: Psychological Approaches to the "Confused" Elderly*. Edinburgh: Churchill Livingstone, 1988.
5. Holden UP, Woods RT. *Positive Approaches to Dementia Care*. Edinburgh: Churchill Livingstone, 1995.
6. Goldwasser AN, Auerbach SM, Harkins SW. Cognitive, affective and behavioural effects of reminiscence group therapy on demented elderly. *Int J Aging Hum Dev* 1987; **25**: 209–22.
7. Gibson S. What can reminiscence contribute to people with dementia? In Bornat J, ed., *Reminiscence Reviewed: Evaluations, Achievements, Perspectives*. Buckingham: Open University Press, 1994; 46–60.
8. Kitwood T, Bedin K. Towards a theory of dementia care: personhood and well being. *Ageing Soc* 1992; **12**: 269–87.
9. Kitwood T. *Dementia Reconsidered: The Person Comes First*. Buckingham: Open University Press, 1997.
10. Fox L. Mapping the advance of the new culture in dementia care. In Kitwood T, Benson S, eds, *The New Culture of Dementia Care*. Buckingham: Open University Press, 1995; 70–4.

11. Sommer R, Ross H. Social interaction on a geriatric ward. *Int J Soc Psychiat* 1958; **4**: 128–33.

12. Karlsson I, Brane G, Melin E *et al*. Effects of environmental stimulation on biochemical and psychological variables in dementia. *Acta Psychiat Scand* 1988; **77**: 207–13.

13. Carstensen LL. The emerging field of behavioral gerontology. *Behav Therapy* 1988; **19**: 259–81.

14. Burgio L, Engel BT, McCormick K *et al*. Behavioral treatment for urinary incontinence in elderly inpatients: initial attempts to modify prompting and toileting procedures. *Behav Ther* 1988; **19**: 345–57.

15. Schnelle JF, Traughber B, Morgan DB *et al*. Management of geriatric incontinence in nursing homes. *J Appl Behav Anal* 1983; **16**: 235–41.

16. Hussian RA. *Geriatric Psychology: A Behavioral Perspective*. New York: Van Nostrand Rheinhold, 1981.

17. Hussian RA, Brown DC. Use of two-dimensional grid patterns to limit hazardous ambulation in demented patients. *J Gerontol* 1987; **42**: 558–60.

18. Josephsson S, Backman L, Borrell L *et al*. Supporting everyday activities in dementia: an intervention study. *Int J Geriat Psychiat* 1993; **8**: 395–400.

19. Green JG, Timbury GC, Smith R, Gardiner M. Reality orientation with elderly patients in the community. *Age Ageing* 1983; **12**: 38–43.

20. Green R, Linsk NL, Pinkston EM. Modification of verbal behaviour of the mentally impaired elderly by their spouses. *J Appl Behav Anal* 1986; **19**: 329–36.

21. Pinkston E, Linsk N. Behavioral family intervention with the impaired elderly. *Gerontologist* 1984; **24**: 576–83.

22. Hanley I, McGuire RJ, Boyd WD. Reality orientation and dementia: a controlled trial of two approaches. *Br J Psychiat* 1981; **138**: 10–14.

Informal Carers and Their Support

D. Buck

University of Liverpool, UK

This chapter is concerned with the need to support informal carers of people with dementia. It will describe how the importance of informal carers has been officially recognized in the UK, albeit partially. The shortcomings of state legislation are reflected in the narrow definitions of informal care that are still prevalent. Following a discussion of "What is caring?", this text will describe the significance of the role played by informal carers for both individuals with dementia and at the wider level. Then the chapter will explain how the rewards of providing informal care are often overshadowed by the adverse effects on carers' physical and emotional well-being. Some of the economic barriers faced by carers will also be outlined. Without adequate support, the ability of informal carers to maintain their role may diminish. A brief overview of the various interventions intended to "care for carers" will follow. It will be seen that many interventions are inadequate, and the need for proper evaluation will be highlighted. The chapter will end with a summary of the key messages.

POLICY BACKGROUND

In the UK the Carers (Recognition and Services) Act 1995 (1996)[1], gave some informal carers the right to ask for an assessment of their ability to care, and gave local authorities a duty to take into account the results of this when deciding what support to provide for the care recipient. However, carers can only have an assessment if they provide "regular and substantial" care and the person they care for is receiving an assessment. Thus, although the Act was a step forward, it should be extended if the true needs of dementia carers are to be met.

WHAT IS CARING?

Informal caring has been defined in many ways[2]. On the one hand, it is often defined solely in terms of the physical activities involved, e.g.:

> Anyone who looks after or cares for a handicapped person to any extent in their own home or elsewhere[3].

More recently, the Carers Act (1996)[1] promoted this view with its restriction to those providing "regular and substantial" care. In contrast, some argue that whilst "caregiving" is best thought of as the physical and behavioural activity of an informal supporter, "caring" can be seen as the emotional/affective element. Nolan *et al.*[2] provide a very useful definition, which will set the context for the remainder of this chapter:

> . . . caring comprises emotional, social and psychological aspects, as well as a general concern for others, in addition to practical tending.

THE IMPORTANCE OF THE INFORMAL CARER'S ROLE

The majority of caring is undertaken by relatives, and there are around 7 million informal carers of older or disabled relatives at home in the UK[4]. The extent and nature of the care provided is diverse, from continual to occasional help, and from assistance with personal care to the provision of a sympathetic ear. The number of people in England and Wales living with dementia is estimated to be around 550 000[5]. Although the number of people here caring for someone with dementia is not known, most people with dementia will have an informal carer. A study with which the author was involved[6] found that out of 502 mentally frail older people, 68% identified an informal carer. In the USA, Haley[7] found that 80% of the care of people with Alzheimer's disease in 1987 was provided by relatives.

Informal caring offers enormous benefit, both to the individual (carer and care recipient) and at a wider level. Tax-payers benefit in that institutionalization of the older person is prevented or delayed where there exists a willing and able informal carer. The Carers' National Association in the UK estimated that should just 10% of informal carers feel unable to continue their caring role, the cost of alternative care would be £2 billion/year[8]. On the individual level, many people in need of care prefer to receive it from their families, rather than formal carers[9]. However, this tendency is often dependent on the quality of the relationship[10]. The decision to choose formal care, on the other hand, is associated with a desire not to inconvenience or overload family and friends. Being able to provide care can be a fulfilling experience from the perspective of the carers, who often feel satisfaction at being able to improve the well-being and maintain the dignity of the older person, experience appreciation and companionship and feel they are reciprocating past help[6,11].

ADVERSE EFFECTS OF CARING

Despite the potential rewards of caring, many carers feel their own physical health, social and working life are adversely affected[6,8,12]. One survey of a district health authority in England found that 14% of its workforce were providing informal care for older people[13]. Many people who are working at the same time as caring for an older relative are eager to fulfil both responsibilities. But trying to balance competing demands is often problematic, with

Principles and Practice of Geriatric Psychiatry, 2nd edn. Edited by J. R. M. Copeland, M. T. Abou-Saleh and D. G. Blazer

many carers having to work fewer hours, take unpaid leave or stop working completely[14]. Thus, middle-aged carers may become disadvantaged, both in the short term in terms of loss of income, and in their later years because they have relinquished pension contributions.

Moreover, psychological distress is common among informal carers[7,15]. This is of wider concern, because psychological distress in carers is considered to be a predictor of breakdown of community care, i.e. of the older person's admission to long-term care[16,17]. The likelihood of poor psychological well-being (depression, anxiety, psychological stress) is greater in the carers of people with dementia compared with relatives of older people without dementia[12,18]. Vedhara et al.[19] found that stress levels were higher in carers of people with dementia than in a control group of similar socioeconomic status.

There are inconsistencies in longitudinal research of carers of people with dementia. Several studies found no significant deterioration in psychological well-being over time in carers of people with dementia[20–22], whereas other studies found significant changes[23,24]. It could be that depression levels are determined early in the caregiving career and remain stable for the duration of caregiving[21]. Although Wright[22] found no significant changes over time in depression, carers were significantly more depressed than non-carers by two year follow-up.

TYPES OF CARE

Bowers[25] proposed a useful typology of caring, beginning with anticipatory care, then preventive, supervisory and instrumental care. Central to all of these is the notion of protective care, whereby carers attempt to maintain the self-esteem and autonomy of the care recipient. In many cases this clashes with instrumental aspects of caregiving. Given that formal services often provide instrumental care, conflict may occur between service providers and carers[26].

CARING FOR CARERS

Much of the literature has called for assessment of the needs not only of older people but also of their informal carers. The UK Carers Act (1996)[1] has answered this call, up to a point. Ideally, interventions should be "facilitative" in nature[26], that is, systematic, planned in conjunction with the informal carer and care-recipient, and complementing the type of care that the carer already provides. Such interventions should be evaluated using sound methodological techniques, perhaps by a partnership of academic institutions and service providers. However, not all interventions are successful in alleviating carer stress, and some carers feel that interventions create rather than relieve the pressure (the place of informal carers in the therapeutic team is covered in Chapter 123 of this volume). Various types of assistance have been designed for informal carers. These include the provision of in-home or institutional respite services, support groups, skills training and education. Although carers value such interventions, they tend to be less effective than more intensive psychosocial interventions[7], such as counselling and psychotherapy. For a more detailed examination of a particular intervention for carers, readers may wish to refer to a special article in this book which outlines a training programme for carers of people with dementia in Sydney: see Chapter 138b.

Graham et al.[27] found that carers with greater knowledge of dementia were less likely to be depressed and more likely to perceive themselves as competent in their caregiving role. Buckwalter et al.[28] evaluated a psychoeducational nursing intervention for carers of people with dementia. In this individual-based intervention, carers learnt how to manage behavioural problems in the care recipient, and this resulted in decreased carer depression.

However, Knight et al.[29], in a review of interventions, concluded that while the effectiveness of respite and individual psychosocial interventions is moderate, such interventions with groups of carers are weak. This can be observed in a recent study that examined the effects of a group-based, dementia carer education programme[30]. This increased carers' knowledge of dementia, but there was no significant impact on their psychological well-being. The authors proposed that more intensive or individual interventions may be more successful. In another review of interventions, Melzer et al.[31] note that the optimum type of intervention (that is, individual vs. group) may vary, depending on the needs of the individual carer. Those requiring social support may benefit more from support groups, whereas those with psychological symptoms or problems with the caring role may benefit more from individual interventions. Furthermore, a brief intervention can be of short-term benefit but may dilute over time and become ineffective. McNally et al.[32], in their review of respite provision for carers, found little support for the existence of long-term benefits.

Zarit et al.[33] note that disappointing findings such as these may be due to methodological problems and/or the fact that services are provided at an inadequate level. Interventions are frequently optimistic and carers themselves not always as prepared to incorporate change as one might expect. Moreover, it is not always possible to balance the needs of carers with those of care recipients, or with cost issues, within one intervention. Thus, interventions should be facilitative in the way described by Nolan et al.[26]. They should incorporate the experiences of carers, and qualitative research methods ought to be used to elicit their concerns early on in the caring career. This could prove invaluable in determining the best way to help carers, whether that be to continue caring for their relative at home or in long-term care. Social changes, such as the size and structure of the family, and increasing geographical mobility amongst the workforce already pose a threat to the availability and willingness of informal carers. Failure to extend current legislation and provide the resources necessary to ensure adequate implementation, may well result in the further depletion of this pool of carers. Finally, some economic barriers to informal caring could be removed with the provision of full-time national insurance and pension contributions for carers.

SUMMARY

This chapter has discussed the importance of supporting informal carers of people with dementia. These carers represent the foundation of physical and emotional support for people with dementia, yet the rights and needs of carers themselves are not fully recognized. Supporting a relative with dementia can be a rewarding experience but many carers suffer adverse effects on their own physical and mental well-being. Not only that, but wider social and demographic changes may jeopardize the informal caring network as it currently exists. Should these "invisible" carers become unwilling, or unable, to sustain their caring role, then the consequences would be bleak, not only for people with dementia but also in terms of the costs of alternative care. On the other hand, some would question the view that such care should be left to those, usually female, family members who may otherwise have pursued a very different way of life. Whilst moves have been made officially to recognize the importance of the carers' role, there is still a long way to go before legislation will safeguard not only their needs but also their rights, including the right not to care. But if willing carers are to remain able carers, then adequate and appropriate support for these individuals is crucial. The problem with this is that many interventions that are meant to support carers are inadequate or have been poorly evaluated. In particular, the effectiveness of group interventions is often weak compared with individual interventions, and there has been little evaluation of long-term benefits. Innovative approaches to caring for carers are needed, but at the same time barriers to implementation, such as lack of readiness in carers to embody change or inflexibility of the socioeconomic system, need to be removed.

REFERENCES

1. Carers (Recognition and Services) Act 1995. *Legal Exec* 1996; **7**: 42.
2. Nolan M, Grant G, Caldock K, Keady J. *A Framework for Assessing the Needs of Family Carers: A Multidisciplinary Guide*. Guildford: B.A.S.E. Publications, University of Surrey, in association with Rapport Publications, 1994.
3. Equal Opportunities Commission. *Who Cares for the Carers: Opportunities for Those Caring for the Elderly and Handicapped*. Manchester: Equal Opportunities Commission, 1982.
4. Court C. Caring for the carers. *Br Med J* 1995; **310**: 617.
5. MRC CFAS (Medical Research Council Cognitive Function and Ageing Study). Cognitive function and dementia in six areas of England and Wales: the distribution of MMSE and prevalence of GMS organicity level in the MRC CFA study. *Psychol Med* 1998; **28**: 319–35.
6. RIS MRC CFAS (Resource Implications Study Group of the MRC Cognitive Function and Ageing Study). Mental and physical frailty in older people: the costs and benefits of informal care. *Ageing Soc* 1998; **18**: 317–54.
7. Haley WE. The family caregiver's role in Alzheimer's disease. *Neurology* 1997; **48**(suppl 6): S25–9.
8. O'Reilly F, Finnan F, Allwright S *et al*. The effects of caring for a spouse with Parkinson's disease on social, psychological and physical well-being. *Br J Gen Pract* 1996; **46**: 507–12.
9. Johansson L, Thorslund M. Care needs and sources of support in a nationwide sample of elderly in Sweden. *Z Gerontol* 1992; **25**(1): 57–62.
10. Wielink G, Huijsman R. Elderly community residents' evaluative criteria and preferences for formal and informal in-home services. *Int J Aging Hum Dev* 1999; **48**(1): 17–33.
11. Grant G, Nolan MR. Informal carers: sources and concomitants of satisfaction. *J Health Soc Care Comm* 1993; **1**(3): 147–59.
12. Baumgarten M, Battista RN, Infante-Rivard C *et al*. The psychological and physical health of family members caring for an elderly person with dementia. *J Clin Epidemiol* 1992; **45**(1): 61–70.
13. Rands G. Working people who also care for the elderly. *Int J Geriat Psychiat* 1997; **12**: 39–44.
14. Stone RI, Short PF. The competing demands of employment and informal caregiving to disabled elders. *Med Care* 1990; **28**(6): 513–26.
15. RIS MRC CFAS (Resource Implications Study Group of the MRC Cognitive Function and Ageing Study). Psychological distress amongst informal supporters of frail older people at home and in institutions. *Int J Geriat Psychiat* 1997; **12**: 737–44.
16. Levin E, Moriarty J, Gorbach P. *Better for the Break*. National Institute for Social Work Research Unit. London: HMSO, 1994.
17. Jerrom B, Mian I, Rukanyake NG, Prothero D. Stress on relative caregivers of dementia sufferers, and predictors of the breakdown of community care. *Int J Geriat Psychiat* 1993; **8**: 331–7.
18. Grafstrom M, Fratiglioni L, Sandman P-O, Winblad B. Health and social consequences for relatives of demented and non-demented elderly. A population-based study. *J Clin Epidemiol* 1992; **45**(8): 861–70.
19. Vedhara K, Cox NKM, Wilcock GK *et al*. Chronic stress in elderly carers of dementia patients and antibody response to influenza vaccination. *Lancet* 1999; **35**: 627–31.
20. Baumgarten M, Hanley JA, Infante-Rivard C *et al*. Health of family members caring for elderly persons with dementia. A longitudinal study. *Ann Intern Med* 1994; **120**: 126–32.
21. Collins C, Stommel M, Wang S, Given CW. Caregiving transitions: changes in depression among family caregivers of relatives with dementia. *Nurs Res* 1994; **43**(4): 220–25.
22. Wright LK. AD spousal caregivers. Longitudinal changes in health, depression and coping. *J Gerontol Nurs* 1994; **20**: 33–48.
23. Pot AM. *Caregivers' Perspectives. A Longitudinal Study on the Psychological Distress of Informal Caregivers of Demented Elderly*. Thesis, University of Vrijel, Amsterdam, 1996.
24. Gold DP, Reis MF, Markiewicz D, Andres D. When home caregiving ends: a longitudinal study of outcomes for caregivers of relatives with dementia. *J Am Geriat Soc* 1995; **43**: 10–16.
25. Bowers BJ. Inter-generational caregiving: adult caregivers and their aging parents. *Adv Nurs Sci* 1987; **9**(2): 20–31.
26. Nolan M, Keady J, Grant G. Developing a typology of family care: implications for nurses and other service providers. *J Adv Nurs* 1995; **21**: 256–65.
27. Graham C, Ballard C, Sham P. Carers' knowledge of dementia, their coping strategies and morbidity. *Int J Geriat Psychiat* 1997; **12**(9): 931–6.
28. Buckwalter KC, Gerdner L, Kohout F *et al*. A nursing intervention to decrease depression in family caregivers of persons with dementia. *Arch Psychiat Nurs* 1999; **XIII**(2): 80–88.
29. Knight BG, Lutzky SM, Macofsky-Urban E. A meta-analytic review of interventions for caregiver distress: recommendations for future research. *Gerontologist* 1993; **33**(2): 240–48.
30. Coen RF, O'Boyle CA, Coakley D, Lawlor BA. Dementia carer education and patient behaviour disturbance. *Int J Geriat Psychiat* 1999; **14**: 302–6.
31. Melzer D, Pearce K, Cooper B, Brayne C. Epidemiologically based needs assessment: Alzheimer's disease and other dementias. London: NHS Executive, 1999 (in press).
32. McNally S, Ben-Shlomo Y, Newman S. The effects of respite care on informal carers' well-being: a systematic review. *Disability Rehabil* 1999; **21**(1): 1–14.
33. Zant SH, Gaugler JE, Jarrott SE. *Useful services for families: research findings and directions*. *Int J Geriat Psychiat* 1999; **14**: 165–81.

The Role and Influence of the Alzheimer's Society

Nori Graham

Alzheimer's Disease International, London, UK

Over the last 20 years there has been a quantum leap in awareness of the fact that carers of people with dementia are among the most stressed and underprivileged members of the community. This has led carers to seek each other out, support one another and form self-help groups. Self-help groups form the backbone of national Alzheimer's societies, whose aim is to use professional means to improve the quality of life for people with dementia and their carers.

It is well recognized that carers have needs which, if met, can go some way to alleviate the stress. Alzheimer's societies can be a mechanism through which carers can articulate these needs and provide and give guidance to others.

The Alzheimer's Society in the UK arose from a small beginning in 1979 to one of the fastest growing and respected voluntary organizations in the UK, with a current income of £20 million. It has helped to raise public awareness about dementia amongst all sections of the population. Its success is due to its role in defining core services, a successful fund-raising strategy and the involvement of people with personal, business and professional experience. Its particular strength is that members all belong to one national society and are encouraged to meet locally in self-help groups and other activities. This has led to a branch structure, with local committees and paid workers supported by the national body.

Dissemination of information is the most important task for an Alzheimer's society. Answering enquiries and the availability of good professional material is a proven route to greater awareness and recognition.

Carers need services. These include domiciliary care, day care and residential care. With government grants a rarity and many societies operating on a shoe-string, there are insufficient or no services in most countries. Voluntary organizations, such as Alzheimer's societies, because of their great flexibility, are in a better position to be innovative than are statutory bodies. Alzheimer's societies can provide models of good practice and promote these vigorously as a basis for government action.

Building a strong national society takes a number of years. One has to decide on the aims, look at fund-raising opportunities, make financial plans, computerize the office, get together a good set of publications, put into place parliamentary lobbying, collect a good team of staff and volunteers and decide on a branch structure. Funding research is only possible for those larger societies with significant resources. All national societies face this array of tasks. The challenge for Alzheimer's Disease International, the umbrella organization of currently 60 national societies, is to support the very varied needs of national societies in different stages of development and with different cultural attitudes to older people and voluntary help.

Psychiatrists and other mental health professionals will find it well worth their while to become members of their national society and involved in its work. This increases the likelihood that governments worldwide will take seriously the impact of dementia on the individual and family, and provide resources to support people with dementia and their families.

60

The Psychiatric Manifestations of CNS Malignancies

M. Glantz and E. Massey

Duke University Medical Center, Durham, NC, USA

DIAGNOSIS

A variety of signs and symptoms may lead to the diagnosis of central nervous system (CNS) cancer. One-quarter to one-third of patients will be diagnosed following a recognized seizure[4,13,14,30]. Others will come to neurologic or neurosurgical attention because of focal weakness or headache[21,43,44]. Tumor-related alterations in behavior will be demonstrated by 50–90% of patients at some time during their illness[13,14,31–33], and in as many as two-thirds of all patients, a psychiatric manifestation is the initial or only complaint[31–39]. In a majority of these patients, the diagnosis of cancer is only made once "hard" neurologic deficits appear[14,24,26,36,39] or at autopsy[21,22]. Meanwhile, treatment for the psychiatric disturbance is often initiated. This pattern is most frequent in the elderly[77] in cases where the tumor occurs in a relatively "silent" area of the brain (the frontal lobe, occipital lobe, ventricle, corpus callosum or septum pellucidum)[37,40–46] and when the tumor is relatively slow-growing (astrocytoma, oligodendroglioma, meningioma)[11,14,31,32,34,37,43,45,47,48].

THE PSYCHIATRIC MANIFESTATIONS OF BRAIN TUMORS

Many factors, including the tumor itself, increased intracranial pressure[63], a variety of treatments, the patient's response to his illness and the premorbid personality, contribute to the psychiatric symptoms of patients with neoplasms (Table 60.1). These may be difficult to separate. Moreover, the signs and symptoms (both neurologic and behavioral) of a CNS cancer may be intermittent or may fluctuate[24,41,50,51]. Behavioral disturbances may resolve with surgery or radiation therapy, even if long-standing[39,45,48,51,52]. Frequently, they improve following ECT[55–57] or conventional

Table 60.1 Causes of neurobehavioral disturbance in patients with cancer

Direct involvement of the nervous system with cancer focal lesions
Increased intracranial pressure
Seizures
Metabolic derangements
Nutritional deficiencies
Endocrinologic dysfunction
Opportunistic infections
Complications of therapy
Psychological response to the illness
Neurologic paraneoplastic syndromes

pharmacotherapy—tricyclic antidepressants, selective seratonin re-uptake inhibitors or methylphenidate for depression[58]; lithium, haloperidol or carbamazepine for mania[31,32,59,60]; neuroleptics for schizophrenic symptoms[31,32,41]. Paradoxically, successful treatment of the psychiatric symptoms may delay the correct diagnosis if treatment is initiated without an appropriate search for underlying disease.

Tumor-related Symptoms

Neurologic and psychiatric disturbances related directly to the presence of cancer in the CNS can be catalogued according to the type of symptom, or the site of the lesion (Tables 60.2 and 60.3).

Behavioral symptoms are most frequently reported (75–90% of cases) with frontal or temporal lobe tumors[33,47,61]. In about one-third of patients these are the initial manifestations

Table 60.2 Common neurologic deficits associated with focal brain lesions

Location of the lesion	Corresponding sign or symptom
Frontal lobe	Contralateral hemiparesis or hemisensory deficit; motor aphasia; Brun's ataxia; incontinence; frontal release signs (snout, grasp, etc)
Temporal lobe	Contralateral hemiparesis or hemisensory deficit; visual field abnormalities; aphasias
Parietal lobe	Contralateral neglect; visuospatial and cognitive disturbances; apraxia; contralateral visual field deficit
Occipital lobe	Contralateral visual field deficit
Basal ganglia, diencephalon, limbic structures	Contralateral hemiparesis or sensory disturbance; aphasias; visual field deficits; apraxia
Cerebellum	Limb (cerebellar hemisphere) or gait (midline) ataxia; dysarthria; eye movement disturbances
Spinal cord	Pain, weakness and sensory disturbance below the level of the lesion; sphincter dysfunction
Leptomeningeal	Cranial neuropathy; diminished (often asymmetric) deep tendon reflexes; weakness; radicular pain; sphincter dysfunction

Principles and Practice of Geriatric Psychiatry, 2nd edn. Edited by J. R. M. Copeland, M. T. Abou-Saleh and D. G. Blazer
©2002 John Wiley & Sons, Ltd

Table 60.3 Focal central nervous system lesions associated with neuropsychiatric symptoms

Location of the lesion	Corresponding sign or symptom
Right hemisphere (especially temporal lobe and central lesions)	Delusions; schizophrenia-like behavior; mania
Temporal lobe Central lesions Parietal lobe (left) Occipital lobe (left)	Hallucinations
Frontal lobe Leptomeningeal Multifocal brain metastases	Delirium; encephalopathy; abulia
Temporal lobe Occipital lobe (right)	Anxiety; irritability
Frontal lobe Temporal lobe Central lesions Parietal lobe (left)	Depression
Frontal lobe Temporal lobe Central lesions Leptomeningeal Occipital lobe (left)	Memory impairment
Frontal lobe Temporal lobe	Euphoria; facetiousness

of the tumor. Distractibility, indifference, disinhibition, euphoria or mania[43,62], facetiousness, memory impairment[52,53,55], abulia, depression[31,43,45,54,64–67,73] and confusion are common in frontal lobe tumors[24,31,42,43,68,69]. Temporal lobe lesions can produce memory dysfunction (especially in the dominant hemisphere)[70–72], depression, and intellectual impairment[31,61,73,74]. Anxiety attacks, irritability, dissociative states, altered sexual behavior, mania (in right-sided or bilateral lesions)[32,60,62,75], and schizophrenic symptoms[24,35,46,76–79] have also been noted. The delusions which occur in this setting are usually paranoid in content and less complex in nature than those seen in true schizophrenia[80]. Non-epileptic visual and auditory hallucinations develop occasionally with frontal, temporal, parietal and occipital tumors, and probably represent "release" phenomena[82,83]. They are frequently prolonged, non-stereotyped and complex, in contrast to hallucinations produced by a seizure.

Tumors involving the limbic system, thalamus, basal ganglia, and diencephalon produce the next highest frequency of psychiatric symptoms[33,46,84–92]. Memory deficits[63], including Korsakoff's syndrome[90], depression[53], apathy and psychomotor slowing, have been described. Delusions, visual hallucinations, disinhibition, childish behavior, mania[59,75,91,93,94] and violent or emotional outbursts are also common[92].

A smaller number of patients (20–30%) with tumors confined to the parietal lobe develop psychiatric symptoms[33,61]. Intellectual impairment, depression and (with right-sided lesions) mania[34,44,60,95] are typical. Tumors of the occipital lobe are occasionally accompanied by behavioral symptoms[96], including memory impairment, irritability and visual hallucinations[82,96,97]. Behavioral disturbance is a relatively unusual finding in infratentorial tumors, although irritability, apathy, poor concentration and encephalopathy have all been reported[31,46,98] and a well-characterized "cognitive affective syndrome" can occur in the setting of cerebellar tumors or tumor surgery[99].

Leptomeningeal carcinomatosis is heralded by confusion, memory loss and cognitive impairment in at least 20% of patients, and mental symptoms ultimately develop in the majority of patients[14,17,100–102]. While myelopathy, radiculopathy and pain are the hallmarks of spinal cord and epidural tumors, psychiatric symptoms have also been reported[103].

Seizures

Seizures are the presenting sign of primary and metastatic brain tumors in one-quarter to one-third of patients, and occur in half of such patients at some point[14,30,104,105]. For patients with leptomeningeal disease, the corresponding frequencies are 6–7% and 14–26%[14,16,17,30]. Tumors located in the frontal and temporal lobes are most often associated with seizures; occipital lobe foci are uncommon; lesions in the basal ganglia, brainstem and cerebellum rarely if ever produce seizures[30,104,105]. Focal or generalized motor seizures are the most frequent and easily recognized seizure type; however, seizures may have solely behavioral manifestations[105]. Confusion may be the only observed manifestation of a seizure arising from any location. Visual and olfactory hallucinations may arise from frontal, temporal or occipital lobe foci. Memory lapses[106], feelings of anxiety or fearfulness[107], aggressive, inappropriate or psychotic behavior[108] and distortions of sound, space or size occur with temporal and frontal lobe seizures[109–113]. Rarely, the sensation of fear can be so overpowering that patients will run from a vaguely perceived threat ("cursive" epilepsy)[114]. Visual, auditory and olfactory hallucinations may be poorly formed (flashes of light, hissing or buzzing, unpleasant smells) or quite elaborate[115]. Patients may describe familiar (*déjà vu*) or unfamiliar (*jamais vu*) pictures or situations, snatches of music or overpowering (but inappropriate) feelings[112]. Disinhibition and feelings of compulsion[116] can occur with frontal lobe seizures. Schizophrenic[101,116] and manic–depressive symptoms[112–117] have been reported with temporal lobe foci in the dominant and non-dominant, hemispheres, respectively. Depression, weeping or laughter ("gelastic" epilepsy) also occur[114–118]. Although controversial, interictal behavioral abnormalities probably develop in a higher percentage of epileptic than non-epileptic patients[119–124].

Paraneoplastic Disorders

Psychiatric disturbances can also be produced by a number of indirect effects of cancer on the nervous system (Table 60.1). Of these, the neurologic paraneoplastic syndromes are the most difficult to diagnose[125–129]. These are seen much more frequently in the setting of systemic cancer than with primary brain tumors, and produce identifiable syndromes resulting in profound neurologic disability, in the absence of other causes. One type of "remote effect", paraneoplastic encephalomyelitis (PEM), frequently produces behavioral symptoms[129–132]. PEM is an inflammatory disorder of grey matter that may involve any level of the CNS, including the limbic system, cerebellum and spinal cord. With limbic encephalitis, the gradual (average 10.5 months) onset of anxiety, depression, hallucinations, bizarre behavior, paranoia and marked impairment of recent memory, progressing to dementia (the "Ophelia syndrome")[132], are characteristic. In one-third of cases, behavioral symptoms precede the diagnosis of cancer. Small cell carcinoma of the lung is the most common underlying malignancy, followed by breast, ovarian, gastric, testicular, uterine and non-small cell lung cancers and Hodgkin's disease. In addition to a characteristic clinical presentation and setting, well-defined serum antibody markers (Hu, Ma/Ta, CV2) are often present[133–135] and characteristic MRI findings have also been described[136,137].

Effects of Treatment

A final very important contributor to the psychiatric morbidity of patients with brain tumors is the effect of treatment[138]. Because patients are living longer and treatments are becoming more aggressive, the psychiatric complications of treatment have become common. While these "late effects" have traditionally been blamed on cranial irradiation, concurrent chemotherapy, corticosteroids and surgery are important contributors. The best-studied late effect is cerebral radionecrosis[139]. Typically, an enhancing mass develops at the site of previous cranial irradiation several months to several years after the completion of treatment. While headache, seizures and focal neurologic defects are often present, insidiously progressive personality change, abulia and lethargy may be the only early manifestations. A second late complication of cranial irradiation, also developing months to years after the completion of treatment, has been termed "radiation-related dementia"[40]. This is a more diffuse brain process, betokened radiographically by cortical atrophy, ventricular enlargement and increased white matter signal on T2-weighted and FLAIR MRI images. Again, gradually progressive cognitive impairment, abulia, short-term memory loss and personality change occur. Focal neurologic deficits are uncommon, although gait impairment and incontinence may develop. Frequently the correct diagnosis of a treatment-related complication is delayed while the diagnoses of depression, Alzheimer's disease, Parkinson's disease or normal pressure hydrocephalus are considered.

APPROACH TO THE PATIENT

The need for integration of psychiatric, neurologic and oncologic insights arises in at least three diagnostically different settings in patients with CNS cancer. In the most common scenario, a patient with known cancer or a proven primary brain tumor develops new or progressive psychiatric deficits. Frequently the symptom is iatrogenic, and withdrawal of the offending agent or substitution of some other therapy will be of benefit. Sometimes recurrent or progressive disease (a new metastasis, regrowth of a treated brain tumor) is the cause, and antineoplastic therapy is indicated. The new onset of seizures or a paraneoplastic disorder may be at fault, the symptom may have evolved from the patient's reaction to his illness. Recognition of these possibilities and an appropriately directed evaluation will often be of diagnostic and therapeutic value and will improve both the length and quality of life.

The patient with known psychiatric disease who develops new symptoms represents a second type of challenge. If focal neurologic deficits are prominent, a vigorous evaluation usually ensues. If the earliest or most obvious signs and symptoms are behavioral, a malignant etiology may be overlooked. Because psychiatric disease and cancer are both common, the chance development of cancer in a behaviorally abnormal patient will account for some of the apparent excess of brain tumors arising in patients in psychiatric hospitals. However, because behavioral changes are a common manifestation of CNS tumors and are especially easy to overlook in patients with chronic psychiatric illness, many cases elude early diagnosis. In patients with long-standing psychiatric illness, therefore, periodic evaluations should also include a detailed neurologic assessment.

A third diagnostically difficult situation occurs when an elderly patient presents with new psychiatric symptoms and no known cancer. Submitting all such patients to periodic neuroradiographic, electroencephalographic, neurologic and laboratory evaluations would eliminate most misdiagnoses, but is impractical and costly. Most secondary psychiatric disturbances in the elderly are due to toxic-metabolic, endocrine, cerebrovascular or infectious etiologies[41]. A detailed history supplemented by a few simple laboratory tests is usually adequate for diagnosis of these disorders. In most patients with CNS cancer, at least subtle neurologic abnormalities are demonstrable at the time of psychiatric presentation, although a careful neurologic examination may be required[47,52]. If not attributable to another known etiology (e.g. stroke, trauma, multiple sclerosis), such abnormalities should prompt additional studies. The presence of seizures, evidence of increased intracranial pressure (papilledema, headaches, nausea and vomiting), a disturbed level of consciousness, gradual intellectual decline, "frontal lobe" findings (also seen with temporal lobe and deep cortical lesions; Table 60.2), or persistent, unexplained headaches should also trigger further evaluation. In such patients, neuroimaging or examination of the cerebrospinal fluid (if leptomeningeal disease is suspected) is the best diagnostic approach.

Elderly patients with the new onset of psychoses, mania or hallucinations, suggestive family histories, normal neurologic examinations and no neurologically worrisome complaints rarely harbor CNS malignancies. Nevertheless, the number of these "idiopathic" cases, after toxic and metabolic etiologies have been excluded, will be so few and so unusual that neuroimaging is probably justified. In contrast, depression is common in the elderly. A careful history and examination are obligatory.

REFERENCES

1. Eby NL, Grufferman S, Flannelly CM *et al.* Increasing incidence of primary brain lymphoma in the US. *Cancer* 1988; **62**: 2461–5.
2. Russell DS, Rubinstein LJ. *Pathology of Tumours of the Nervous System* 5th edn. Baltimore, MD: Williams & Wilkins, 1989; 1–6.
3. Greenlee RT, Murray T, Bolden S, Wingo PA. Cancer statistics, 2000. *CA Cancer J Clin* 2000; **50**: 7–33.
4. Prados MD, Berger MS, Wilson CB. Primary central nervous system tumors: advances in knowledge and treatment. *CA Cancer J Clin* 1998; **48**: 331–60.
5. Nelson JS, Tsukada Y, Schoenfeld D *et al.* Necrosis as a prognostic criterion in malignant supratentorial, astrocytic gliomas. *Cancer* 1983; **52**: 550–54.
6. Burger PC, Vogel FS, Green SB, Strike TA. Glioblastoma multiforme and anaplastic astrocytoma: pathologic criteria and prognostic implications. *Cancer* 1985; **56**: 1106–11.
7. Piepmeier JM. Observations on the current treatment of low-grade astrocytic tumors of the cerebral hemispheres. *J Neurosurg* 1987; **67**: 177–81.
8. North CA, North RB, Epstein JA *et al.* Low-grade cerebral astrocytomas. Survival and quality of life after radiation therapy. *Cancer* 1990; **66**: 6–14.
9. Schiff D, Wen PY. Uncommon brain tumors. *Neurol Clin* 1995; **13**: 953–74.
10. Black PM. Meningiomas. *Neurosurgery* 1993; **32**: 643–57.
11. Bullard DE, Rawlings CE, Phillips B *et al.* Oligodendroglioma. An analysis of the value of radiation therapy. *Cancer* 1987; **60**: 2179–88.
12. Fokes EC, Earle KM. Ependymomas: clinical and pathological aspects. *J Neurosurg* 1969; **30**: 585–94.
13. Wen PY, Loeffler JS. Management of brain metastases. *Oncology* 1999; **13**: 941–61.
14. Posner JB. *Neurologic Complications of Cancer*. Philadelphia, PA: F. A. Davis, 1995.
15. Delattre JY, Krol G, Thaler HT, Posner JB. Distribution of brain metastases. *Arch Neurol* 1988; **45**: 741–4.
16. Wasserstrom WR, Glass JP, Posner JB. Diagnosis and treatment of leptomeningeal metastases from solid tumors: experience with 90 patients. *Cancer* 1982; **49**: 759–72.
17. Grossman SA, Krabak MJ. Leptomeningeal carcinomatosis. *Cancer Treat Rev* 1999; **25**: 103–19.
18. Sorensen PS, Borgesen SE, Rohde K *et al.* Metastatic epidural spinal cord compression. Results of treatment and survival. *Cancer* 1990; **65**: 1502–8.

19. Morse ME. Brain tumours as seen in hospitals for the insane. *Arch Neurol Psychiat* 1920; **3**: 417–28.

20. Larson CP. Intracranial tumors in mental hospital patients: a statistical study. *Am J Psychiat* 1940; **97**: 49–54.

21. Waggoner RW, Bagchi BK. Initial masking of organic brain changes by psychic symptoms: clinical and electroencephalographic studies. *Am J Psychiat* 1954; **110**: 904–10.

22. Patton RB, Sheppard JA. Intracranial tumors found at autopsy in mental patients. *Am J Psychiat* 1956; **113**: 319–24.

23. Klotz M. Incidence of brain tumors in patients hospitalised for chronic mental disorders. *Psychiat Q* 1957; **31**: 669–80.

24. Selecki BR. Intracranial space-occupying lesions among patients admitted to mental hospitals. *Med J Aust* 1965; **I**: 385–90.

25. Andersson PG. Intracranial tumors in a psychiatric autopsy material. *Acta Psychiat Scand* 1970; **46**: 213–24.

26. Cole G. Intracranial space-occupying masses in mental hospital patients: necropsy study. *J Neurol Neurosurg Psychiat* 1978; **41**: 730–6.

27. Davison K. Schizophrenia-like psychoses associated with organic cerebral disorders: a review. *Psychiat Dev* 1983; **1**: 1–34.

28. Larson EB, Laurence MPH, Mack A *et al.* Computerized tomography in patients with psychiatric illness: advantage of a "rule-in" approach. *Ann Intern Med* 1981; **95**: 360–4.

29. Roberts JK, Lishman WA. The use of the CAT head scanner in clinical psychiatry. *Br J Psychiat* 1984; **145**: 152–8.

30. Glantz M, Recht L. Epilepsy in the cancer patient. In Vinken PJ, Bruyn GW, eds, *Neuro-Oncology, Part III. Neurological Disorders in Systemic Cancer. Handbook of Clinical Neurology*, vol 69. Amsterdam: Elsevier, 1997; 9–18.

31. Filley CM, Kleinschmidt-DeMasters BK. Neurobehavioral presentations of brain neoplasms. *West J Med* 1995; **163**: 19–25.

32. Cummings JL. Neuropsychiatric manifestations of right hemisphere lesions. *Brain Lang* 1997; **57**: 22–37.

33. Hecaen H, Ajuriaguerra J. *Troubles Mentaux au Cours des Tumeurs Intracrâniennes.* Paris: Masson, 1956.

34. Moersch FP, Graig W McK, Kernohan JW. Tumors of the brain in aged persons. *Arch Neurol Psychiat* 1941; **45**: 235–45.

35. Pool JL, Correll JW. Psychiatric symptoms masking brain tumor. *J Med Soc NJ* 1955; **55**: 4–9.

36. Remington FB, Rubert SL. Why patients with brain tumors come to a psychiatric hospital: a thirty-year survey. *Am J Psychiat* 1962; **119**: 256–7.

37. Gautier-Smith P. *Parasagittal and Faix Meningiomas.* London: Butterworth, 1970.

38. Tomita T, Raimond AJ. Brain tumors in the elderly. *J Am Med Assoc* 1981; **246**: 53–5.

39. Law J. Late diagnosis of frontal meningiomas. *Br Med J* 1988; **297**: 423.

40. Zeman W, King FA. Tumors of the septum pellucidum and adjacent structures with abnormal affective behavior: an anterior midline structure syndrome. *J Nerv Ment Dis* 1958; **127**: 490–502.

41. Gassel MM, Davies H. Meningiomas in the lateral ventricles. *Brain* 1961; **84**: 605–27.

42. Selecki BR. Cerebral mid-line tumours involving the corpus callosum among mental hospital patients. *Med J Aust* 1964; **2**: 954–60.

43. Hunter R, Blackwood W, Bull J. Three cases of frontal meningiomas presenting psychiatrically. *Br Med J* 1968; **3**: 9–16.

44. Binder RL. Neurologically silent brain tumors in psychiatric hospital admissions: three cases and a review. *J Clin Psychiat* 1983; **44**: 94–7.

45. Maurice-Williams RS, Dunwoody G. Late diagnosis of frontal meningiomas presenting with psychiatric symptoms. *Br Med J* 1988; **296**: 1785–6.

46. Tanaghow A, Lewis J, Jones GH. Anterior tumour of the corpus callosum with atypical depression. *Br J Psychiat* 1989; **155**: 854–6.

47. Malamud N. Psychiatric disorder with intracranial tumors of limbic system. *Arch Neurol* 1967; **17**: 113–23.

48. Chee PC, David A, Calbraith S, Giliham R. Dementia due to meningioma: outcome after surgical removal. *Surg Neurol* 1985; **23**: 414–16.

49. Rice E, Gendelman S. Psychiatric aspects of normal pressure hydrocephalus. *J Am Med Assoc* 1973; **223**: 409–12.

50. Ross RT. Transient tumor attacks. *Arch Neurol* 1983; **40**: 633–6.

51. Araga S, Fukada M, Kagimoto H *et al.* Transient global amnesia and falcotentorial meningioma—a case report. *Jap Psychiat Neurol* 1989; **43**: 201–3.

52. Riisoen H, Fossan GO. How shall we investigate dementia to exclude intracranial meningiomas as cause? An analysis of 34 patients with meningiomas. *Age Ageing* 1986; **15**: 29–34.

53. Upadhyaya AK, Sud PD. Psychiatric presentation of third ventricular colloid cyst. A case report. *Br J Psychiat* 1988; **152**: 567–9.

54. Weller R, Clague HW. Late diagnosis of frontal meningiomas. *Br Med J* 1988; **297**: 423.

55. Maltbie AA, Wingfield MS, Volow MR. Electroconvulsive therapy in the presence of brain tumor. Case reports and an evaluation of risk. *J Nerv Ment Dis* 1980; **168**: 400–405.

56. Goldstein MZ, Richardson C. Meningioma with depression: ECT risk or benefit? *Psychosomatics* 1988; **29**: 349–51.

57. Greenberg LB, Mofson R, Fink M. Prospective electroconvulsive therapy in a delusional depressed patient with a frontal meningioma. A case report. *Br J Psychiat* 1988; **153**: 105–7.

58. Meyers CA, Weitzner MA, Valentine AD, Levin VA. Methylphenidate therapy improves cognition, mood, and function of brain tumor patients. *J Clin Oncol* 1998; **16**: 2522–7.

59. Stern K, Dancey TE. Glioma of the diencephalon in a manic patient. *Am J Psychiat* 1942; **98**: 716–19.

60. Jamieson RC, Wells CE. Manic psychosis in a patient with multiple metastatic brain tumors. *J Clin Psychiat* 1979; **40**: 280–83.

61. Keschner M, Bender MB, Strauss I. Mental symptoms in cases of tumor of the temporal lobe. *Arch Neurol Psychiat* 1936; **35**: 572–96.

62. Starkstein SE, Boston JD, Robinson RG. Mechanisms of mania after brain injury: 12 case reports and review of the literature. *J Nerv Ment Dis* 1988; **176**: 87–100.

63. Busch E. Psychical symptoms in neurosurgical disease. *Acta Psychiat Neurol Scand* 1940; **15**: 257–90.

64. Smith S. Organic syndromes presenting as involutional melancholia. *Br Med J* 1954; **ii**: 274–7.

65. Abrams R, Taylor MA. Catatonia. A prospective clinical study. *Arch Gen Psychiat* 1976; **33**: 579–81.

66. Carlson RJ. Frontal lobe lesions masquerading as psychiatric disturbances. *Can Psychiat Assoc J* 1977; **22**: 315–18.

67. Feigin G. Suicide and meningioma. *Am J Forens Med Pathol* 1988; **9**: 334–5.

68. Strauss I, Keschner M. Mental symptoms in cases of tumor of the frontal lobe. *Arch Neurol Psychiat* 1935; **33**: 986–1007.

69. Avey TL. Seven cases of frontal tumor with psychiatric presentation. *Br J Psychiat* 1971; **119**: 19–23.

70. Meador KJ, Adams RJ, Flanigin HF. Transient global amnesia and meningioma. *Neurology* 1985; **35**: 769–71.

71. Mastromarino JH. Acute presentations of memory loss and emotional lability. *Ann Emerg Med* 1987; **16**: 709–11.

72. Schlesinger B. Mental changes in intracranial tumors and related problems. *Confinia Neurol* 1950; **10**: 225–63; 322–55.

73. Strobos RRJ. Tumors of the temporal lobe. *Neurology* 1953; **3**: 752–60.

74. Bingley T. Mental symptoms in temporal lobe epilepsy and temporal lobe gliomas. *Acta Psychol Neurol Scand* 1958; **33** (suppl 120): 1–143.

75. Cummings JL, Mendez MF. Secondary mania with focal cerebrovascular lesions. *Am J Psychiat* 1984; **141**: 1084–7.

76. Mulder DW, Daly D. Psychiatric symptoms associated with lesions of temoral lobe. *J Am Med Assoc* 1952; **150**: 173–6.

77. Hobbs GE. Brain tumors simulating psychiatric disease. *Can Med Assoc J* 1963; **88**: 186–8.

78. Bollati A, Galli G, Gandolfi M *et al.* Visual and auditory hallucinosis (the only symptoms of meningioma of the lesser sphenoidal wing). *J Neurosurg Sci* 1980; **24**: 41–4.

79. Cummings JC. Organic delusions. *Br J Psychiat* 1985; **146**: 184–97.

80. Kanakaratnam G, Direzke M. Aspects of primary tumors of the frontal lobe. *Br J Clin Pract* 1976; **30**: 220–1.

81. Ron MA. Psychiatric manifestations of frontal lobe tumours. *Br J Psychiat* 1989; **155**: 735–8.

82. Critchley M. Types of visual perseveration: "palinopsia" and "illusory visual spread". *Brain* 1951; **74**: 267–99.

83. Cogan DG. Visual hallucinations as release phenomena. *Albrecht Von Graefes Arch Klin Exp Ophthalmol* 1973; **188**: 139–50.

84. Smyth GE, Stern K. Tumors of the thalamus—a clinicopathological study. *Brain* 1938; **61**: 339–74.

85. Williams M, Pennybacker JB. Memory disturbances in third ventricle tumors. *J Neurol Neurosurg Psychiat* 1954; **17**: 115–23.

86. Russell RWR, Pennybacker JB. Craniopharyngioma in the elderly. *J Neurol Neurosurg Psychiat* 1961; **24**: 1–13.

87. Tovi D, Schisano G, Liljeqvist B. Primary tumors of the region of the thalamus. *J Neurosurg* 1961; **18**: 730–40.

88. Ziegler DK, Kaufman A, Marshall HE. Abrupt memory loss associated with thalamic tumor. *Arch Neurol* 1977; **34**: 545–8.

89. Gutmann DH, Grossman RI, Mollman JE. Personality changes associated with thalamic infiltration. *J Neuro-oncol* 1990; **8**: 263–67.

90. Delay J, Brion S, Derouesne C. Mémoires originaux—syndrome de Korsakoff et étiologie tumorale: étude anatomo-clinique de trois observations. *Rev Neurol* 1964; **111**: 97–133.

91. Mendez MF, Adams NL, Lewandowski KS. Neurobehavioral changes associated with caudate lesions. *Neurology* 1989; **39**: 349–54.

92. Lobosky JM, Vangilder JC, Damasio AR. Behavioural manifestations of third ventricular colloid cysts. *J Neurol Neurosurg Psychiat* 1984; **47**: 1075–80.

93. Krauthammer C, Klerman G. Secondary mania. *Arch Gen Psychiat* 1978; **35**: 1333–9.

94. Greenberg DB, Brown GL. Mania resulting from brain stem tumor. *J Nerv Ment Dis* 1985; **173**: 434–6.

95. Oppler W. Manic psychosis in a case of parasagittal meningioma. *Arch Neurol Psychiat* 1950; **64**: 417–30.

96. Allen IM. A clnical study of tumours involving the occipital lobe. *Brain* 1930; **53**: 194–243.

97. Bender MB, Feldman M, Sobin AJ. Palinopsia. *Brain* 1968; **91**: 321–38.

98. Keschner M, Bender MB, Strauss I. Mental symptoms in cases of subtentorial tumor. *Arch Neurol Psychiat* 1937; **37**: 1–18.

99. Levisohn L, Cronin-Golomb A, Schmahmann JD. Neuropsychological consequences of cerebellar tumour resection in children: cerebellar cognitive affective syndrome in a paediatric population. *Brain* 2000; **123**: (5): 1041–50.

100. Bleyer WA, Byrne TN. Leptomeningeal cancer in leukemia and solid tumors. *Curr Probl Cancer* 1988; **12**: 181–238.

101. Remington SB, Rubert SL. Why patients with brain tumors come to a psychiatric hospital. *Am J Psychiat* 1962; **119**: 256–7.

102. Byrne TN, Cascino TL, Posner JB. Brain metastases from melanoma. *J Neuro-oncol* 1983; **1**: 313–17.

103. Epstein BS, Epstein JA, Postel DM. Tumors of spinal cord simulating psychiatric disorders. *Dis Nerv Syst* 1971; **32**: 741–3.

104. Glantz MJ, Cole BF, Forsyth PA et al. Practice parameter: anticonvulsant prophylaxis in patients with newly diagnosed brain tumors. *Neurology* 2000; **54**: 1886–93.

105. Porter RJ. Epilepsy. In Walter JN, ed., *Major Problems in Neurology*, vol. 12. Philadelphia, PA: WB Saunders, 1984.

106. Glowinski H. Cognitive deficits in temporal lobe epilepsy. An investigation of memory functioning. *J Nerv Ment Dis* 1973; **157**: 129–37.

107. Gillig P, Sackellares JC, Greenberg HS. Right hemisphere partial complex seizures: mania, hallucinations, and speech disturbances during ictal events. *Epilepsia* 1988; **29**: 26–9.

108. Ghadirian AM, Gauthier S, Bertrand S. Anxiety attacks in a patient with a right temporal lobe meningioma. *J Clin Psychiat* 1986; **47**: 270–71.

109. Ervin F, Epstein RW, King HE. Behavior of epileptic and nonepileptic patients with "temporal spikes". *Arch Neurol Psychiat* 1955; **74**: 488–97.

110. Currie S, Heathfield KWG, Henson RA, Scott DF. Clinical course and prognosis of temporal lobe epilepsy. A survey of 666 patients. *Brain* 1971; **94**: 173–90.

111. Williamson PD, Spencer DD, Spencer SS et al. Complex partial seizures of frontal lobe origin. *Ann Neurol* 1985; **18**: 497–504.

112. Boone KB, Miller BL Rosenberg L et al. Neuropsychological and behavioral abnormalities in an adolescent with frontal lobe seizures. *Neurology* 1988; **38**: 583–6.

113. Kan R, Mori Y, Suzuki S et al. A case of temporal lobe astrocytoma associated with epileptic seizures and schizophrenia-like psychosis. *Jap J Psychiat Neurol* 1989; **43**: 97–103.

114. Chen R-C, Forster FM. Cursive epilepsy and gelastic epilepsy. *Neurology* 1973; **23**: 1019–29.

115. Sowa MV, Pituck S. Prolonged spontaneous complex visual hallucinations and illusions as ictal phenomena. *Epilepsia* 1989; **30**: 524–6.

116. Ward CD. Transient feelings of compulsion caused by hemispheric lesions: three cases. *J Neurol Neurosurg Psychiat* 1988; **51**: 266–8.

117. Larson EW, Richelson E. Organic causes of mania. *Mayo Clin Proc* 1988; **63**: 906–12.

118. Gumpert J, Hanisota P, Upton A. Gelastic epilepsy. *J Neurol Neurosurg Psychiat* 1970; **33**: 479–83.

119. Flor-Henry P. Schizophrenic-like reaction and affective psychoses associated with temproal lobe epilepsy: etiological factors. *Am J Psychiat* 1969; **126**: 400–403.

120. Pritchard PB, Lombroso CT, Mcintyre M. Psychological complications of temporal lobe epilepsy. *Neurology* 1980; **30**: 227–32.

121. Mendez MF. Psychopathology in epilepsy: prevalence, phenomenology and management. *Int J Psychiat Med* 1988; **18**: 193–210.

122. Stevens JR. Psychiatric aspects of epilepsy. *J Clin Psychiat* 1988; **49** (suppl): 49–57.

123. Trimble MR. The psychoses of epilepsy. In Laidlaw J, ed., *A Textbook of Epilepsy*. London: Churchill Livingstone, 1988; 393–405.

124. Kido H, Yamaguchi N. Clinical studies of schizophrenia-like state in epileptic patients. *Jap J Psychiat Neurol* 1989; **43**: 433–8.

125. Henson RA, Urich H. *Cancer and the Nervous System: the Neurological Manifestation of Systemic Malignant Disease*. Oxford: Blackwell Scientific, 1982.

126. Posner JB, Dalmau JO. Paraneoplastic syndromes of the nervous system. *Clin Chem Lab Med* 2000; **38**: 117–22.

127. Newsom-Davis J. Paraneoplastic neurological disorders. *J R Coll Physicians Lond* 1999; **33**: 225–7.

128. Dalmau JO, Posner JB. Paraneoplastic syndromes. *Arch Neurol* 1999; **56**: 405–8.

129. Henson RA, Hoffman HL, Urich H. Encephalomyelitis with carcinoma. *Brain* 1965; **88**: 449–64.

130. Gultekin SH, Rosenfeld MR, Voltz R et al. Paraneoplastic limbic encephalitis: neurological symptoms, immunologic findings and tumor association in 50 patients. *Brain* 2000; **123**(7): 1481–94.

131. Alamowitch S, Graus F, Uchuya M et al. Limbic encephalitis and small cell lung cancer. Clinical and immunologic features. *Brain* 1997; **120**(6): 923–8.

132. Carr I. The Ophelia syndrome: memory loss in Hodgkin's disease. *Lancet* 1982; **i**: 844–5.

133. Sutton I, Winer J, Rowlands J, Dalmau J. Limbic encephalitis and antibodies to Ma2: a paraneoplastic presentation of breast cancer. *J Neurol Neurosurg Psychiat* 2000; **69**: 266–8.

134. Dalmau J, Voltz RD, Posner JB et al. Paraneoplastic encephalomyelitis: an update of the effects of the anti-Hu immune response on the nervous system and tumour. *J Neurol Neurosurg Psychiat* 1997; **63**: 133–6.

135. Voltz R, Gultekin SH, Rosenfeld MR et al. *N Engl J Med* 1999; **340**: 1788–95.

136. Lacomis D, Koshbin S, Schick RM. MR imaging of paraneoplastic limbic encephalitis. *J Comput Assist Tomogr* 1990; **14**: 115–17.

137. Glantz MJ, Biran H, Myers ME et al. The radiographic features of paraneoplastic central nervous system disease. *Cancer* 1994; **1**: 168–75.

138. Glantz M. Central nervous system complications of radiation. In Gilman S, Goldstein GW, Waxman SG, eds, *Neurobase*. San Diego, CA: Arbor, 1999.

139. Sheline GE, Wara MM, Smith V. Therapeutic irradiation and brain injury. *Int J Radiat Oncol Biol Phys* 1980; **6**: 1215–28.

140. DeAngelis L, Delattre J-Y, Posner J. Radiation-induced dementia in patients cured of brain metastases. *Neurology* 1989; **39**: 789–96.

61

Peripheral Neuropathy and Peripheral Nerve Lesions

Janice M. Massey and E. Wayne Massey

Duke University Medical Center, Durham, NC, USA

Peripheral neuropathy is a diffuse process involving either sensory nerves, motor nerves or, more frequently, both. It is the most common neurologic disease of the elderly. The known causes of polyneuropathy are numerous and are frequently associated with other systemic illness (Table 61.1). Many occur in patients with psychiatric symptoms. Additionally, drugs must always be considered as possible etiologies.

In addition to diffuse peripheral neuropathy, the pattern of single peripheral nerve involvement is termed mononeuropathy. The causes include acute trauma or entrapment but often are non-traumatic in origin, presumably representing either chronic trauma or due to other factors, such as infarction of the nerve (diabetes mellitus or collagen vascular disease). Patients with many psychiatric diseases are more prone to these problems, i.e. peroneal or ulnar pressure palsies in depressed patients.

POLYNEUROPATHY

Symptoms of diffuse peripheral neuropathy include a "stocking glove" distribution of sensory loss usually involving the feet and later the hands. With sensory involvement, patients complain of numbness and tingling or pain in the feet. Early on, the hands are rarely involved to any significant degree. On examination, varying degrees of decreased perception to pain, temperature or vibratory sense and, less often, joint position sense may be seen in the distal extremities, particularly in the feet. When this sensory loss is severe in the lower extremities, there may be unsteadiness of gait, worse with the eyes closed.

When the motor nerves are involved, distal muscles of the feet and hands may be weak. The patient may walk with a "foot drop" or be unable to stand on tiptoe due to distal lower extremity weakness. Intrinsic hand muscle weakness produces decreased hand grip. Reflexes are hypoactive, initially at the ankles, but may subsequently be absent at the knees and even in the upper extremities. All symptoms and signs, including the reflexes, are usually symmetrical.

The temporal profile of the symptoms may suggest possible etiologies. Neuropathy of sudden onset is seen in inflammatory or vasculitic disease, whereas patients with familial history and long-standing neuropathy are more likely to have hereditary disease.

We will discuss only the most common diffuse neuropathies.

Landry–Guillain–Barré–Strohl Syndrome (AIDP)

Immune polyradiculoneuropathy (polyradiculoneuropathy, Guillain–Barré syndrome) may be preceded by a minor febrile illness or following immunization. Symmetrical motor weakness, often beginning in the legs and ascending, and areflexia with minimal sensory involvement, are the primary features. The cerebrospinal fluid (CSF) protein is usually increased and no cells are present. This relationship is termed cytoalbuminologic dissociation. Facial diplegia without extra-ocular muscle or pupillary involvement may occur. Respiratory weakness may develop rapidly. The severity of the illness ranges from minimal weakness to flaccid quadriparesis. Although usually idiopathic, known causes include AIDS, rabies, cytomegalic and other viruses. Porphyria may cause neuropathy along with psychiatric symptoms.

Quadriparesis may develop rapidly, requiring respiratory support within an hour. Usually the symptoms progress over 3–4 days, although occasionally it may take weeks to develop the maximum deficit. Spontaneous recovery, usually complete, occurs over weeks or months as a rule. However, some patients have serious residual deficits.

Respiratory function may deteriorate rapidly, even without obvious respiratory distress. When Guillain–Barré syndrome is suspected, serial pulmonary functions should be performed. When the forced vital capacity drops below 1–1.5 L, intubation is indicated. Autonomic dysfunction is common, with symptoms ranging from bladder dysfunction and labile blood pressures to cardiac rhythm disturbances.

Therapy is supportive. Maintenance of adequate respiration and nutrition, treatment of infection and autonomic disturbances, good nursing care and physical therapy to prevent contractures are required. Plasmapheresis, immunoglobulin therapy (IgG) and, less often, steroid therapy may shorten the course of the illness.

A chronic relapsing form of inflammatory demyelinating neuropathy (CIDP) is an increasingly important neuropathy and often responds to corticosteroid treatment. Nerve biopsy is occasionally helpful to confirm the diagnosis.

Diabetic Neuropathy

Various portions of the peripheral nervous system can be affected by diabetes mellitus. Diabetes is common in the elderly. Individuals with psychiatric disease will frequently have diabetes with neuropathy concomitantly. The most frequent pattern is a distal symmetric predominantly sensory polyneuropathy. Painful

Table 61.1 Peripheral neuropathy: etiology and classification

1. Neuropathy associated with toxic metabolic states
   A. Vitamin deficiency (B_1, B_{12}, B_6, nicotinic acid, pantothenic acid and folic acid)
   B. Diabetic
   C. Uremic
   D. Hepatic
   E. Thyroid disease
   F. Dysproteinemias and paraproteinemias
   G. Alcohol
   H. Amyloid

2. Inherited peripheral neuropathy
   A. Charcot–Marie–Tooth
   B. Dejerine–Sottas (hypertrophic)
   C. Roussy–Lévy
   D. Refsum's disease
   E. Tangier disease and $A\beta$-lipoproteinemia (Bassen–Kornzweig's)
   F. Neuropathy associated with the leukodystrophies (metachromatic leukodystrophy, Krabbe's disease, adrenoleukodystrophy)
   G. Fabry's disease
   H. Porphyric neuropathy
   I. Friedreich's disease
   J. Tomaculous neuropathy

3. Infectious, inflammatory and post-infectious neuropathy
   A. Guillain–Barré syndrome, inflammatory polyradiculoneuropathy
   B. Diphtheria
   C. Leprosy
   D. Sarcoid
   E. CIDP (chronic inflammatory)
   F. AIDS
   G. *Campylobacter*

4. Neuropathies associated with malignancy
   A. Neuropathy associated with lymphoma and Hodgkin's disease (sensory, motor, mixed)

5. Toxic neuropathies
   A. Heavy metals
      1. Lead
      2. Arsenic
      3. Mercury
      4. Thallium
   B. Toxins
      1. Acrylamide
      2. Trichloroethylene
      3. Benzene
      4. Carbon tetrachloride
      5. TOCP (triorthocresyl phosphate)
   C. Drugs
      1. Vincristine, vinblastine
      2. Chloroquine
      3. Nitrofurantoin
      4. Phenytoin
      5. Disulfiram
      6. Isoniazid
      7. Thalidomide
      8. Excessive B_6 administration
      9. Dapsone
      10. Amiodarone
      11. *cis*-platin

burning or numbness and tingling in the toes and feet, and less commonly the hands, are present. Often a "stocking glove" distribution of decreased pain, temperature and vibration perception is present, along with decreased distal reflexes.

Patients with longstanding diabetes or poor glucose control usually have more severe neuropathy, although these do not always correlate well. In addition, mononeuropathy (involvement of single motor or sensory nerves) is frequently seen in diabetes.

Femoral neuropathy produces pain in the anterior medial thigh, with weakness in the proximal muscles of the leg. Lumbosacral plexus involvement with weakness and atrophy of the thigh muscles is termed diabetic amyotrophy. Mononeuritis multiplex involves multiple sensory and motor nerves in an asymmetrical fashion, usually due to infarction of the nerves. However, multiple mononeuropathies may also occur, due to pressure or entrapment. These need recognition so that patients can be taught how to prevent further trauma or compression of their nerve. Radiculopathy in the thoracic or lumbar area without disc herniation also occurs frequently in diabetes. In the thoracic area, patients complain of chest wall or abdominal pain, usually unilaterally, and may have abdominal musculature weakness. The autonomic nervous system may also be involved, causing orthostatic hypotension, bladder and gastrointestinal disturbances, skin changes, sweating abnormalities and impotence. A penile prosthesis may be helpful in male patients with impotence.

Alcoholic Neuropathy (Nutritional/Toxic)

This neuropathy is most often sensory, with pain on the soles of the feet and loss of ankle reflexes. Minor motor involvement may occur, but is seldom severe. This is associated with vitamin B_1 deficiency, but is also likely a direct toxic effect from chronic alcohol use. A history of the amount and frequency of alcohol intake is essential in evaluating these problems. Abstinence from alcohol is necessary to result in any improvement. Psychiatric care is usually the predominant need in these patients, however.

Evaluation of Patients with Neuropathy

Evaluation for systemic disease in patients with peripheral neuropathy must include several factors: patient history, physical examination, basic laboratory studies and special laboratory analysis.

The history should include a detailed family history, but this may be difficult to obtain. Sometimes additional family members must also be examined. The social history should include occupation, types of hobbies and possible exposure to toxins. Other medical illness should be noted. A complete record of all drugs used, including prescription, non-prescription and recreational drugs, should be obtained. One should determine whether onset of symptoms correlates with initiation of a drug regimen. Recent medical history should include risk factors for possible infectious etiologies, such as tick exposure, high-risk sexual

Table 61.2 Approach to history in peripheral neuropathy

Family history: diabetes mellitus, pernicious anemia, amyloidosis, porphyria, Refsum's disease, Tangier disease
Social history: alcoholism, occupation or hobbies with possible toxic exposure (carbon tetrachloride, carbon disulfide, carbon monoxide, trichloroethylene, trinitrotoluene, benzene, *o*-dinitrophenol, lead, arsenic, bismuth, mercury, thallium, copper, silver, gold, antimony, zinc), intentional poisoning (suicide, homicide), heavy smoking (carcinoma of lung)
Medication history: sulphonamides, emetine, hydralazine, nitrofurantoin, diphenylhydantoin, glutethimide, isoniazid, allopurinol, thalidomide, insulin
Recent medical history: infections (AIDS, diphtheria, tuberculosis, infectious mononucleosis, infectious hepatitis, syphilis, typhoid, typhus, "strep throat", cat-scratch fever), malignancy (direct invasion or remote effects), gastrointestinal disturbances (seen with arsenic, lead, porphyria, thallium, vitamin deficiencies, pernicious anemia, hepatitis, Tangier disease)

Table 61.3 Physical examination in peripheral neuropathy

Hair: alopecia (thallium, arsenic), premature graying (pernicious anemia)
Skin: dry skin (myxedema), dermatitis of exposed surfaces (pellagra, porphyria), erythematous sweaty palms (alcohol, arsenic), depigmented areas (leprosy), ecchymoses (blood dyscrasias, hypercortisonism), butterfly rash or poikiloderma (lupus), ichthyosis (Refsum's disease)
Nails: Aldrich–Mees lines (arsenic), petechiae under nails (subacute bacterial endocarditis)
Gums: lead line (lead), gingival hyperplasia (diphenylhydantoin)
Tongue: glossitis (pernicious anemia, pellagra), large tongue (acromegaly, amyloid)
Sore throat: infectious mononucleosis, diphtheria, leukemia
Salivary glands: enlargement (sarcoid)
Eyes: third-nerve palsy without pupillary involvement (diabetes)
Fundi: Roth's spots (subacute bacterial endocarditis, blood dyscrasia), hypertensive changes (uremia, periarteritis), dilated veins (macroglobulinemia), retinitis pigmentosa (Refsum's disease)
Adenopathy: infection, malignancy, sarcoid
Cardiac enlargement: myxedema, beri beri
Hypertension: periarteritis, porphyria, thallium
New heart murmurs: subacute bacterial endocarditis
Hepatomegaly: alcoholism, malignancy, hepatitis
Ankle edema: uremia, beri beri, malignancy of kidney (especially if unilateral)
Wristdrop: lead
Slow relaxation of deep tendon reflexes: myxedema
Joint deformities: rheumatoid arthritis with or without vasculitis, gout
Reddish brown urine: porphyria

Table 61.4 Initial laboratory studies in evaluation of peripheral neuropathy

Urinalysis: chronic nephritis, hematuria (malignancy, proteinuria, myeloma)
Erythrocyte blood count and hemoglobin: anemia (infection, malignancy), macrocytic anemia (pernicious anemia, diphenylhydantoin), basophilic stippling (lead), acanthocytosis on fresh smear
Blood smear, fresh: acanthocytosis
Leukocytes: depressed count (lupus, toxicity), increased count (periarteritis, infection), hypersegmented neutrophilis (pernicious anemia), abnormal leukocytes (leukemia, malignancy, toxicity, infectious mononucleosis)
Sedimentation rate: elevated in collagen disease, infection, malignancy, cirrhosis
Chest X-ray: carcinoma of lung, sarcoidosis infection, enlarged heart (myxedema, beri beri, hypertension)
Serum creatinine: uremia (including lupus)
Fasting blood sugar (glucose tolerance test): diabetes mellitus
Thyroid panel: myxedema
Serum cholesterol: decreased in thyrotoxicosis and Tangier disease, increased in myxedema

Table 61.5. Additional laboratory studies (if clinically indicated)

Genetic studies: (GM1, H5MN)
Antibodies: (anti-maG, anti-Hu)
HTLV I, HIV (serum)
Hair and nail analysis: arsenic
Urine: heavy metals, porphyrins
Liver function studies: hepatitis, alcholism
Schilling's test: pernicious anemia
Cultures: infection
Serum uric acid: gout
Rheumatoid factor
Lupus erythematosus preparation (FANA)
Heterophil antibody titer
Biopsy of nodes, liver, kidney, testicle (periarteritis): malignancy, sarcoid, lupus, cirrhosis
Rectal biopsy: amyloid, Tangier disease
Nerve biopsy: vasculitis, amyloidosis, leprosy, sarcoidosis, embolic disease, Refsum's disease

Table 61.6 Genetic (DNA) tests in peripheral neuropathy

1. Hereditary
   CMT1 Evaluation (DNA) CMT 1A, 1B, 1X
   Peripheral myelin protein 22 (PMP22)
   Early growth response 2 gene (EGR2)
   Axonal HMSN, Dejerine–Sottas, congenital hypomyelination, HNPP, Refsum's
   TTR 30 Amyloidosis DNA Test
2. Acquired peripheral neuropathy:
   MAG, GM1 Triad, Sulfatide, Galop,
   Hu, MAG "Dual" Antigen
   Autoantibodies for GM1, MAG, GQ16,
   Sulfatide, Galop

activity or blood product exposure, and include a detailed review of systems (Table 61.2).

In addition to the neurologic examination, one should include attention to the general examination for evidence of systemic illness that could cause the underlying neuropathy (Table 61.3). Initial studies in the evaluation of peripheral neuropathy include many routine laboratory tests (Table 61.4). Specific laboratory studies are also useful. Nerve conduction studies reveal diffuse abnormalities in the motor and sensory nerves in patients with diffuse neuropathy. Electromyography is abnormal if axonal damage has occurred. These tests characterize the neuropathy as primarily demyelinating or axonal and recognize unusual patterns of response. Specific patterns are useful in establishing an etiology[2].

Genetic studies, analysis of hair, nails, and urine for heavy metals, liver function studies, Schilling's test, cultures, fluorescent antinuclear antibody (FANA), sedimentation rate, rheumatoid factor, evaluation for malignancy and possibly nerve biopsy, may be required in specific cases (Tables 61.5 and 61.6).

COMMON MONONEUROPATHIES

The most common mononeuropathies include involvement of the median, ulnar and radial nerves in the upper extremity and femoral, peroneal, lateral femoral cutaneous and sciatic nerves in the lower extremity. In addition, truncal neuropathies and even cranial nerve involvement may cause a localized sensory or motor deficit (Table 61.7).

Table 61.7. Common mononeuropathies

Cranial mononeuropathy
   VII Facial (Bell's palsy)
   V Trigeminal (mental nerve)
   IV, VI, II, III
Extremity mononeuropathies
   Median
   Ulnar
   Radial
   Brachial plexus
   Lateral femoral cutaneous (meralgia paresthetica)
Femoral
Peroneal
Obturator
Sciatic
Truncal neuropathy
   Intercostal (*Herpes zoster* and diabetic)
   Posterior primary rami T2–T6 (notalgia paresthetica)

Knowledge of the symptoms, signs and anatomic distribution of specific peripheral nerves is essential to recognize and diagnose the mononeuropathies. These mononeuropathies are common in the elderly. The most common chronic mononeuropathy is carpal tunnel syndrome (CTS), entrapment of the median nerve as it passes under the carpal ligament at the wrist.

Entrapment injury to the ulnar nerve is common in chronic illness, particularly in the elderly population. Psychiatric patients restricted to bed or a wheel chair use their elbows for support and often compress the ulnar nerve at the olecranon notch, producing a "tardy ulnar palsy". The supine position, with the arms in a position of mild flexion with the forearm pronated, exposes the ulnar nerve to chronic pressure.

The radial nerve innervates the extensor muscles for the fingers, wrist and elbow. The most common site of injury of the radial nerve is in the proximal portion of the nerve as it wraps around the humerus. Injury often occurs when the patient is deeply asleep or unconscious (usually due to alcohol or sedation) while the arm is held in abduction and lateral rotation. Injury results when the nerve is compressed by the head of a sleeping partner lying against the humerus ("honeymoon palsy"); or falling asleep with the arm propped over a bench, chair or bar ("Saturday night palsy").

The lateral femoral cutaneous nerve, a sensory nerve that arises from the lumbar plexus, is often entrapped at the medial border of the anterior superior iliac crest, producing an acute or subacute onset of numbness and a disagreeable prickly sensation over the lateral thigh (meralgia paresthetica). Sigmund Freud was one of three early describers of this and experienced it himself. Recognition is important, if only to avoid intervention to treat other conditions, such as lumbar radiculopathy.

Peroneal nerve injury produces footdrop or loss of sensation in the anterolateral surface of the foot. This can be subtle. The most common cause of common peroneal nerve injury is crossing the legs. Immobility is a predisposing cause, and depression, stroke or dementia is present among many patients.

Sciatica is usually caused by a protruded lumbar disc affecting the S1 root. However, the sciatic nerve is susceptible to injury at various sites in the buttocks causing identical symptoms and signs.

Idiopathic inflammation of the brachial plexus (neuralgic amyotrophy, cryptogenic brachial plexopathy, Parsonage–Turner) predominantly affects the superior trunk of the brachial plexus. A deep aching pain in the axilla or shoulder is followed within a few days by weakness of muscles supplied by the superior brachial trunk.

REFERENCES

1. Massey JM. Neurology. In Crapo J, Hamilton M, Edgman S, eds, *Medicine and Pediatrics in One Book*, Philadelphia, PA: Hanley & Belfus, 1988; 425–58.
2. Donofrio PD, Albers JW. Polyneuropathy: classification by nerve conduction studies and electromyography. AAEM Minimonograph 34. *Muscle Nerve* 1990; **13**: 889–903.

62

Electroencephalography (EEG)

The Late George W. Fenton
University of Dundee, Scotland, UK

It is 60 years since Berger[1] demonstrated electroencephalographic abnormalities in an histologically confirmed case of Alzheimer's disease. Since then, the electroencephalograph (EEG) has been widely used in the investigation of patients with suspected organic brain disease. To interpret the results in an individual patient, a number of observations relating to the nature and origin of the EEG signal and the impact of healthy ageing on its waveforms must be considered.

PRINCIPLES OF EEG INTERPRETATION

The EEG samples the electrical activity of the cerebral cortex only. Further, widespread synchronous involvement (6 cm^2 or more) of the cortex is required to significantly alter the scalp EEG waveforms. Cerebral neuronal dysfunction caused by different disease processes produces essentially similar patterns of EEG disturbance. Hence, with a few exceptions, the type of EEG change cannot predict the precise nature of the underlying pathology. Finally, acute cerebral disease or rapidly deteriorating dysfunction cause the most florid electrical disturbance, while static lesions produce little or none, unless epileptogenic activity develops with the generation of spikes, sharp waves, spike–wave complexes, etc.[2]

EFFECTS ON HEALTHY AGEING

The more important changes that accompany healthy ageing include alpha rhythm frequency slowing, changes in beta (fast) rhythm abundance, the appearance of diffuse delta activity, local anterior temporal delta wave foci and alterations in nocturnal sleep patterns[3,4].

Mean Alpha Rhythm Frequency

In young adults, this is around 10 Hz and does not change until 60 years. Subsequently there is a gradual decline, the rate of decrement varying from 0.05 to 0.75 Hz/decade across studies; 9.0–9.5 Hz at 70 and 8.5–9.0 Hz after 80 years. Indeed, in healthy subjects of any age it is rare to have a dominant (alpha) rhythm frequency of less than 8 Hz. In elderly patients, the degree of alpha frequency slowing is significantly related to the extent of cognitive impairment.

Low-voltage Beta (Fast) Activity

This is a low voltage 15–30 Hz rhythm, arising from the frontocentral areas of both hemispheres and sometimes diffuse in distribution, which increases in abundance in middle age and is more prominent in females. It persists into old age but diminishes markedly after 80 years.

Diffuse Slow Activity

This consists of background theta (4–7 Hz) and delta (1–3 Hz) waves of generalized distribution, is not seen in healthy people under 65 years and is relatively rare in early senescence (7% of people under 75 years), but occurs in up to 20% of persons over 75 years. Even in this relatively aged population the degree of diffuse slowing is mild. When moderate or severe, there is a significant association with a clinical diagnosis of dementia.

Focal Delta Waves

A substantial minority (30–40%) of healthy people over 60 years have focal delta (slow) waves strictly localized to the anterior temporal region and often lateralized to the left side. More extensive spread beyond the anterior temporal area indicates local pathology.

Paroxysmal Activity

Paroxysmal EEG events are transient, higher voltage waveforms that arise suddenly from the EEG background. The healthy brain generates some normal paroxysmal activity, namely lambda waves during wakefulness when the eyes are open and paroxysmal waveforms during sleep as part of the alerting process (lambdoid waves in light sleep and K-complexes in medium to deep sleep). Abnormal paroxysmal discharges include bifrontal delta wave episodes, spikes, and sharp waves and spike–wave complexes. Such phenomena are extremely rare in healthy elderly people.

Nocturnal Sleep Patterns

EEG sleep studies of healthy elderly individuals show decreases in sleep efficiency, greater numbers of awakenings from sleep with increases in total time awake (especially in the last 2 h of the night) as well as marked diminution in stages 3 and 4 sleep. These

Principles and Practice of Geriatric Psychiatry, 2nd edn. Edited by J. R. M. Copeland, M. T. Abou-Saleh and D. G. Blazer
©2002 John Wiley & Sons, Ltd

changes, which usually begin somewhere around 50 years of age, are age-related and generally more pronounced in men[5]. A shortened rapid eye movement (REM) latency may be helpful in separating early dementia (normal REM latency) from depression (shortened REM latency). The former show decreased amounts of sleep spindles and K-complexes with reduced REM sleep percentage and a normal REM temporal distribution.

EEG IN DEMENTIA

With important exceptions, the changes in dementia are qualitatively similar to those of healthy ageing, although the degree of change is much more marked. Since the days of Berger, there have been many studies of the routine clinical EEG in dementia (reviewed by Busse[6], Pedley and Miller[7], Fenton[4]).

Changes Common to Most Dementing Disorders

Slowing of the dominant, parieto-occipital (alpha 8–13 Hz) rhythm over both hemispheres, a moderate to marked increase in generalized theta (4–7 Hz) and delta (1–3 Hz) activity (diffuse slowing) and a bilaterally symmetrical decline in low voltage beta (fast) activity are common background activity changes. One autopsy study reports a significant correlation between alpha frequency slowing and the number of senile plaques counted in Alzheimer's disease (AD) patients' brains[8]. Paroxysmal runs of bifrontal delta activity are not uncommon in dementia patients. In one investigation these have been related to degenerative brain stem changes at autopsy[9]. The occipital responses to photic stimulation at fast flicker rates (equal to or greater than 18 flashes/s) tend to disappear in a significant minority of dementia patients (1 in 5).

Differences Between the Various Dementias

AD vs. Pick's Disease

Studies that have compared the various types of dementing illnesses indicate that less than 5% of patients with histologically confirmed AD have a normal EEG even when first referred to the psychiatric services[4,10–12]. In contrast, Pick's disease and multi-infarct dementia (MID) are not infrequently associated with normal EEGs. The number of Pick's disease patients in any study is small, but a consistent finding is that around 50% have normal records. Even when diffuse slowing is present in Pick's disease patients, the alpha rhythm is better preserved[9,12,13]. The alpha rhythm is generated by the parieto-occipital areas of the cerebral cortex modulated by thalamocortical influences. The histological changes in Pick's disease are largely confined to the frontotemporal regions, which are relatively "silent" electrically, compared to the parieto-occipital areas, where the predominant AD changes occur. Indeed, it has been recently suggested that a normal EEG is one of the characteristic features of dementia of frontal lobe type: a dementing syndrome with onset in the presenium and selective frontal lobe dysfunction. It is not clear whether it represents a form of Pick's disease[14].

Multi-infarct Dementia (MID)

The EEG in MID differs from AD in displaying significantly more asymmetry between the hemispheres, localized slow wave disturbances being particularly common, while the alpha tends to be better preserved. For example, Constantinidis et al.[15] report three

times more alpha rhythm and five times more local slow wave foci in MID. Often, the laterality of the EEG focus in MID correlates with past or present clinical evidence of an ischaemic lesion lateralized to the same side. In contrast, AD patients have a significantly higher incidence of diffuse delta activity.

Huntington's Disease

The EEG in Huntington's disease differs from the dementias already discussed. In a variable number (30–80%) depending on the series reported, a low voltage tracing with an average amplitude of 10 μV or less is a characteristic feature. This amplitude reduction correlates with caudate nucleus involvement but only becomes apparent by the time the disease is clinically well-established[16,17].

The Significance of Paroxysmal Abnormalities with Periodocity

Paroxysmal bifrontal runs of delta waves are common in dementia patients, especially those with AD. In one histological investigation, this bifrontal delta activity has been related to degenerative brain stem changes[9]. Regularly recurring (periodic) generalized biphasic or triphasic sharp wave or slow wave complexes of generalized origin with a characteristic recurrence rate of 0.5–1.0 s (intervals between successive bursts of complexes) are a characteristic feature of Creutzfeldt–Jakob disease (CJD). Early in the illness, diffuse background slowing occurs and in most cases the characteristic periodic complexes emerge. In a minority of patients (up to one-third in some series), especially the amyotrophic cases, this pattern may not be seen or may appear late. If practical, serial recordings are recommended[18]. On rare occasions, the periodic discharges may be temporarily focal, later generalizing and becoming bilaterally synchronous as the disease progresses. Their presence in a middle-aged or elderly patient with dementia is highly suggestive of CJD. Periodic triphasic waves of generalized distribution can be seen in other conditions, notably hepatic and other metabolic encephalopathies, subacute sclerosing leucoencephalitis and Unverricht's myoclonus epilepsy. Rarely they may appear in advanced AD patients and in Binswanger subcortical encephalopathy but do not show the characteristic periodicity or evolution of CJD.

EEG, COGNITIVE AND CT SCAN CHANGES

McAdam and Robinson[19] reported a correlation of +0.79 between ratings of EEG change and clinical severity in dementia patients of mixed aetiology. The association between EEG slowing and severity of dementia has been replicated by many subsequent studies[4,6,20]. However, Johannesson et al.[12] report that this electroclinical relationship held for 100% of their AD cases but almost half of their Pick's and MID patients had normal EEGs in the presence of significant cognitive decline. The correlation between the EEG slowing and extent of cortical atrophy as measured by computed tomography (CT) is weak, the link being obvious only in advanced cases. The EEG correlates better with clinical scales sensitive to early dementia, while the converse is true for the CT scan[20]. Combining the two measures improves their diagnostic power. A discriminant function analysis study of 56 AD patients and 84 normal controls correctly classified 86% using the EEG data and 84% using the CT scan information. Combining the EEG and CT scan variables improved the correct classification rate to 90%[2]. Interestingly enough, the degree of functional brain impairment as measured by the EEG predicts survival time while the extent of cortical activity does not[22].

THE APPLICATION OF QUANTITATIVE ELECTROENCEPHALOGRAPHY

Recent computerized EEG (CEEG) investigations have used frequency spectral analyses of the background activity and have generally replicated the earlier reports obtained by visual inspection of the EEG tracings. An overall slowing in mean EEG frequency is an invariable finding, with relative power increases in the slower frequencies (theta/delta) and decreases in the fast (beta) frequencies. The degree of frequency slowing correlates reasonably well with clinical ratings of dementia severity, e.g. Mini-Mental State and Clinical Dementia rating scales.

Is there a Relationship to Clinical Severity?

Alterations in the distribution of power across the various frequency bands seem to relate to the severity of the dementing process. In less severe cases, the main changes are increases in theta and reductions in beta power. When the disease is advanced, the respective amounts of delta and alpha power are also affected, the former being increased and the latter reduced. These associations have been observed during cross-sectional studies, there being a paucity of longitudinal investigations.

What About Early Cases?

Much of the work has been on populations of patients with established AD being cared for in hospital. A number of recent studies have examined mild probable AD patients (clinical dementia ratings of 1) compared to age-matched controls. These have replicated the earlier findings of frequency spectral slowing which have a specificity of virtually 100%[23]. However, the sensitivity is only 20%. This means that only one in five of early cases of AD will have CEEG findings that deviate three standard deviations from the mean and therefore fall into the AD range.

The Potential Role of Brain Mapping

A new development in EEG technology has been brain electrical activity mapping (BEAM). This involves sampling the cortical electrical activity from multiple scalp electrodes and calculating the distribution of voltage across the whole of the scalp using a mathematical interpolation method. The patterns of scalp voltage distribution are displayed as colour-coded contour maps. This technique investigates the patterns of electrical activity generated at the same time by different areas of cerebral cortex. It can be used to detect regional differences and promises to be a useful tool in the investigation of the dementias. Several investigators have used multichannel or BEAM recordings to demonstrate localized left temporal lobe delta power abnormalities, which may in AD patients be an early manifestation of the disease[24–27]. Hence, BEAM may prove especially useful in the early detection of dementia.

Does the CEEG Change as the Dementia Progresses?

The few longitudinal CEEG studies that have been carried out over several years give conflicting results. Some report significant decreases in mean frequency over time, with increases in delta/theta power and reduced alpha and beta activity[28–29], but others have found either statistically insignificant trends in the direction of frequency slowing or that only about half of AD patients show progressive EEG changes over 12 months[30–31]. It is noteworthy that the negative reports deal with relatively short time scales; 18 months or less. This may not be long enough to establish significant progression. There is also some evidence that frontal lobe quantitative changes may precede more generalized slowing[31].

Differences between AD and MID

Few CEEG investigations have investigated the question of quantitative differences between AD and MID patients. A recently completed study in my laboratory reveals significantly greater amounts of delta power and less alpha power in the temporal and parieto-occipital areas of both hemispheres in AD patients, compared to those with a clinical diagnosis of multi-infarct dementia. As well as having less alpha power, the peak alpha frequency is slower in AD patients with mean values of 7 Hz and 8 Hz in AD and MID subjects, respectively, and significant asymmetry between the hemispheres in the MID patients[31].

The degrees of synchrony between different areas of cortex within each cerebral hemisphere and between homologous areas of the right and left hemisphere can be assessed by coherence spectral analyses, which measures the similarity between pairs of EEG signals generated by different cortical areas. The coherence function is essentially a frequency correlation coefficient and measures the correlation at each frequency. It varies from 0 (signals quite different) to $+1.0$ (signals identical).

The main coherence differences between the AD and MID patient are seen in the temporal and parieto-occipital areas of both hemispheres. Compared to the MID patients, the within-hemisphere alpha and beta synchrony is lower in AD subjects. The pattern of between-hemisphere synchrony is different, being higher in AD patients for theta components between the temporal areas and lower for the alpha and beta frequencies between the parieto-occipital areas[31].

Do Elderly Patients with "Non-organic" Psychiatric Illness Deviate from Normals?

In my laboratory we have also investigated age-matched controls and elderly patients with major depressive illness. Compared to the normals, the depressive patients had significantly more theta power and less alpha power, such changes being maximal in the temporal regions. Indeed, the mean spectral values of the three patient groups could be ranked roughly according to degree of deviation from the healthy controls. The AD patients were the most deviant, then those with MID, and finally the depressed patients. The deviation of the elderly depressives from the healthy controls raises the issue of the contribution of organic brain disease to the genesis of affective disorder in old age, as suggested by current CT and single photon emission computed tomography (SPECT) scan work[32,33].

EVENT-RELATED POTENTIALS IN DEMENTIA

What is an Event-related Potential?

Event-related or evoked potentials (ERPs or EPs) consist of transient voltage changes that occur in response to a sensory stimulus. These take the form of a series of negative and positive waves, which last a number of milliseconds (ms) and measure a few microvolts (μV) in amplitude. They are "buried" amongst the "noise" of the ongoing EEG and are "extracted" by summating or averaging the response to a series of identical stimuli. This results in a waveform that lasts from a few ms up to several s.

Types of Event-related Potential

It takes about 20 ms for information to reach the cerebral cortex from a peripheral sense organ. Hence the early ERP components reflect neuronal activity in the sensory receptor itself and the afferent pathways of the brainstem. They depend on the functional integrity of the relevant sensory system, being relatively impervious to changes in psychological state. The brainstem responses consist of five positive (I–V) waves within 10 ms of the stimulus, and are especially stable and stimulus-bound, having prolonged latencies in brainstem disease. In contrast, the middle-latency (80–200 ms) and long-latency (> 200 ms) components are influenced by attention processes and how the subject perceives or processes the stimulus. The long-latency waves are termed cognitive or endogenous potentials, since their form is largely determined by the subjects' psychological state.

Healthy Ageing

The latency and waveform of sensory ERPs are critically affected by peripheral receptor changes. Hence, impaired hearing and visual acuity, common in the elderly, can cause problems in interpretation. If such sensory deficits are controlled for, the early and mid-latency potentials are little affected by healthy ageing. In contrast, the P_{300} wave, a positive going cognitive ERP that appears about 300 ms after a subject receives an important but unexpected stimulus, declines in latency and amplitude with advancing years.

Brainstem ERPs

Since there are brainstem changes, neuronal cell loss and neurofibrillary tangles in AD early ERP abnormalities can be predicted. The available brainstem auditory evoked response data are conflicting, two studies reporting delayed central conduction times (prolonged I–V intervals) with negative findings in a third[34–36].

Visual ERPs

A promising finding is the differential latency pattern of visual evoked potentials in dementia. Wright et al.[37] report completely normal pattern reversal responses with significant latency delay of the major positive component (P_2) of the flash response. The difference value between the prolonged flash P_2 latency and the normal latency value of the equivalent positive (P_{100}) wave of the pattern response is much longer in dementia patients compared to controls. It has the advantage of being little affected by drugs and only slightly lengthened by the ageing process, but does not discriminate between AD and MID[38]. These findings have been replicated twice[39,40].

Cognitive ERPs

The P_{300} wave is elicited by a task requiring discrimination between two types of stimuli, one frequent and the other rare in repetition. It develops as a response to the rare stimulus, which is used as a target and is a measure of cognitive processing time. Its latency may well reflect the time required for stimulus evaluation and categorization, while the amplitude is inversely related to probability of occurrence of the target stimuli. Healthy ageing increases the latency by around 1.36 ms/year and decreases the amplitude at a rate of about 0.18 μV/year[41]. The P_{300} latency is prolonged in many dementia patients by more than 1.5 standard deviations from the normal age-related mean and lengthens progressively over time[42,43]. Positron emission tomography (PET) scanning of early patients has shown that P_{300} latency is inversely correlated with the relative metabolic rates of the parietal and, to a lesser extent, temporal and frontal association areas, but not with the subcortical areas[44]. There is also a significant positive correlation between P_{300} amplitude and CSF 5-hydroxyindole-acetic acid (5-HIAA) concentration in AD patients[45].

Distinctions between Cortical and Subcortical Dementia

Some work suggests that auditory ERP patterns may be useful in distinguishing cortical from subcortical dementia. The P_{300} wave is abnormal in both. In contrast, the earlier waves (middle-latency components; N_1, P_2 and N_2) are intact in the former but abnormal in the latter[46]. Indeed, a recent preliminary study reports correlations with specific aspects of cognitive functioning; N_1 and P_2 with motor speed and N_2 with short-term memory[47].

OVERVIEW

The potential application of the ERP recordings to the diagnosis of dementia has yet to be clearly defined. None of the available techniques are capable of distinguishing between AD and MID. The visual flash-pattern reversal latency pattern is a robust finding in established cases of dementia of cortical origin. Further, there is some evidence that it reflects a specific cholinergic deficit. However, the abnormality rate in patients during the early stages of dementia remains to be determined. On the other hand, the P_{300} latency delay has been shown to be present in a majority of recent-onset AD patients[44]. A difficulty is that the correct classification rate for AD patients using the P_{300} data alone has varied widely across studies, from 89% to 20%, most having rates of more than 70%. This variability reflects not only differences in the clinical material and selection of controls but also the type and level of task difficulty of the experimental paradigm used to record the P_{300} wave. The paradigm has differed in the various studies. Research is required to determine the optimum paradigm for eliciting abnormality in early dementia cases, so that standardization across studies becomes possible. Further work on central brainstem conduction times and the pattern of middle latency components in subcortical dementia is also indicated.

REFERENCES

1. Berger H. Uber das elektrenkephalogramm des menschen. Funfte mitteilung. *Arch Psychiat Nervenkr* 1932; **98**: 231–54.
2. Fenton GW. EEG in neuropsychiatry. In Reynold EH, Trimble MR, eds. *The Bridge between Neurology and Psychiatry*. Edinburgh: Churchill Livingstone, 1989; 302–33.
3. Obrist WD. Problems of aging. In Laing GC, ed. *Handbook of Electroencephalography and Clinical Neurophysiology*. Amsterdam: Elsevier, 1976; 273–92.
4. Fenton GW. Electrophysiology of Alzheimer's Disease. *Br Med Bull* 1986; **42**: 29–33.
5. Reite ML, Nagel KE, Ruddy JR. *The Evaluation and Management of Sleep Disorders*. Washington, DC: American Psychiatric Press, 1990.

6. Busse EW. Electroencephalography. In Reisberg B, ed. *Alzheimer's Disease*. New York: Free Press, 1983; 231–6.

7. Pedley TA, Miller JA. Clinical neurophysiology of aging and dementia. In Mayeux R, Rosen WG, eds. *The Dementias*. New York: Raven, 1983; 31–49.

8. Deissenhammer E, Jellinger K. EEG in senile dementia. *Electroencephalogr Clin Neurophysiol* 1974; **36**: 91 (abstr).

9. Johannesson G, Brun A, Gustafson I, Ingvar DH. EEG in presenile dementia related to cerebral blood flow and autopsy findings. *Acta Neurol Scand* 1977; **56**: 89–103.

10. Soininen H, Partanen VJ, Puranen M, Riekkinen PJ. EEG findings in senile dementia and normal aging. *Acta Neurol Scand* 1982; **65**: 59–70.

11. Gordon EB, Sim M. The EEG in presenile dementia. *J Neurol Neurosurg Psychiat* 1967; **30**: 285–91.

12. Johannesson G, Hagberg B, Gustafson L, Ingvar DH. EEG and cognitive impairment in presenile dementia. *Acta Neurol Scand* 1979; **59**: 225–40.

13. Stigsby B, Johannesson G, Ingvar DM. Regional EEG analysis and regional cerebral blood flow in Alzheimer's and Pick's diseases. *Electroencephalogr Clin Neurophysiol* 1981; **51**: 537–47.

14. Neary D, Snowden JS, Northern BM, Goulding P. Dementia of frontal lobe type. *J Neurol Neurosurg Psychiat* 1988; **51**: 353–61.

15. Constantinidis J, Krassoievitch M, Tossit R. Corrélations entre les perturbations électroencéphalographiques et les lésions anatomo-histologiques dans les démences. *Encéphale* 1969; **58**: 19–52.

16. Scott DF, Heathfield WG, Toone B, Margerison JH. The EEG in Huntington's chorea: a clinical and neuropathological study. *J Neurol Neurosurg Psychiat* 1972; **35**: 97–102.

17. Sishta SK, Troupe A, Marszalek KL, Kremer LM. Huntington's chorea: an electroencephalographic and psychometric study. *Electroencephalogr Clin Neurophysiol* 1974; **36**: 387–93.

18. Knight R. Creutzfeldt–Jakob disease. *Br J Hosp Med* 1989; **41**: 165–71.

19. McAdam W, Robinson RA. Senile intellectual deterioration and the electroencephalogram: a quantitative correlation. *J Ment Soc* 1956; **102**: 819–25.

20. Merskey H, Ball MJ, Blume WT *et al*. Relationships between psychological measurements and cerebral organic changes in Alzheimer's disease. *Can J Neurol Sci* 1980; **7**: 45–59.

21. Soininen H, Partanen VJ, Puranen M, Riekkinen PJ. EEG and computed tomography in the investigation of patients with senile dementia. *J Neurol Neurosurg Psychiat* 1982; **45**: 711–14.

22. Kaszniak AW, Fox J, Gandell DL *et al*. Predictors of mortality in presenile and senile dementia. *Ann Neurol* 1978; **3**: 246–52.

23. Coben LA, Chi D, Snyder AZ, Storandt M. Replication of a study of frequency analysis of the resting awake EEG in mild probable Alzheimer's disease. *Electroencephalogr Clin Neurophysiol* 1990; **75**: 148–54.

24. Leuchter AF, Spar JE, Walter DO, Weiner H. Electro-encephalographic spectra and coherence in the diagnosis of Alzheimer's type and multi-infarct dementia. *Arch Gen Psychiat* 1987; **44**: 993–8.

25. Saletu B, Anderer P, Paulus E *et al*. EEG brain mapping in SDAT and MID patients before and during placebo and Xantinolnicotinate therapy: reference considerations. In Samson-Dollfys D, Guieu JD, Gotman J, Stevenson P, eds. *Statistics and Topography in Quantitative EEG*. Paris: Elsevier, 1988; 251–68.

26. Breslau J, Storr A, Sicotte N, Higa J, Buchsbaum MS. Topographic EEG changes with normal aging and SDAT. *Electroencephalogr Clin Neurophysiol* 1989; **72**: 281–9.

27. Rice DM, Buchsbaum MS, Storr A *et al*. Abnormal EEG slow activity in left temporal areas in senile dementia of the Alzheimer type. *J Gerontol* 1990; **45**: M145–51.

28. Coben LA, Danziger W, Storandt M. A longitudinal 40. EEG study of mild senile dementia of Alzheimer type: changes at one year and at 2.5 years. *Electroencephalogr Clin Neurophysiol* 1985; **61**: 101–12.

29. Hooizer C, Jonker C, Posthume J, Visser SL. Reliability, validity and follow-up of the EEG in senile dementia: sequelae of sequential measurement. *Electroencephalogr Clin Neurophysiol* 1990; **76**: 400–12.

30. Soininen H, Partanen J, Laulumaa V *et al*. Longitudinal EEG spectral analysis in early stage of Alzheimer's disease. *Electroencephalogr Clin Neurophysiol* 1989; **72**: 290–7.

31. Sloan EP, Fenton GW. EEG power and coherence spectra in dementia: a longitudinal study (in preparation).

32. Abas M, Sahakian B, Levy R. Neuropsychological deficits and CT scan changes in elderly depressives. *Psychol Med* 1990; **20**: 507–20.

33. Upadhyaya AK, Abou-Saleh MT, Wilson K *et al*. A study of depression in old age using single-photon emission computed tomography. In Abou-Saleh MT, ed. *Brain Imaging in Psychiatry*. *Br J Psychiat* 1990; **157** (suppl 9): 76–81.

34. Harkins SW. Effects of presenile dementia Alzheimer's type on brainstem transmission time. *Int Neurosci* 1981; **15**: 165–70.

35. Grimes AM, Grady CL, Pikus A. Auditory evoked potentials in patients with dementia of the Alzheimer's type. *Ear Hearing* 1987; **8**: 157–61.

36. Tachibana H, Takeda M, Sugita M. Brainstem auditory evoked potentials in patients with multi-infarct dementia and dementia of the Alzheimer type. *Int J Neurosci* 1989; **48**: 325–31.

37. Wright CE, Harding GF, Orwin A. Presenile dementia—the use of flash and pattern VEP in diagnosis. *Electroencephalogr Clin Neurophysiol* 1984; **57**: 405–15.

38. Wright CE, Furlong P. Visual evoked potentials in elderly patients with primary or multi-infarct dementia. *Br J Psychiatry* 1988; **152**: 679–82.

39. Philpot M, Amin D, Levy R. Visual evoked potentials in Alzheimer's disease: correlations with age and severity. *Electroencephalogr Clin Neurophysiol* 1990; **77**: 323–9.

40. Sloan EP, Fenton GW. Serial visual evoked potential recordings in geriatric psychiatry. *Electroencephalogr Clin Neurophysiol* 1992; **84**: 325–31.

41. Picton TW, Stuss DT, Champagne SC, Nelson RF. The effects of age on human event-related potentials. *Psychophysiology* 1984; **21**: 312–25.

42. Polich J. P300 and Alzheimer's disease. *Biomed Pharmacother* 1989; **43**: 493–9.

43. Ball SS, Marsh JT, Schubarth G *et al*. Longitudinal P_{300} latency changes in Alzheimer's disease. *Gerontology* 1989; **44**: M195–200.

44. Marsh JT, Schubarth G, Brown WS *et al*. PET and P_{300} relationships in Alzheimer's disease. *Neurobiol Aging* 1990; **11**: 471–4.

45. Ito J, Yamao S, Fukuda H *et al*. The P_{300} event-related potentials in dementia of the Alzheimer type. Correlations between P_{300} and monoamine metabolites. *Electroencephalogr Clin Neurophysiol* 1990; **77**: 174–8.

46. Goodin DS, Aminoff MJ. The distinction between different types of dementia using evoked potentials. In Johnson R Jr, Rohrbaugh JW, Parasuraman R, eds. *Current Trends in Event-related Potential Research*. Amsterdam: Elsevier, 1987, 695–8.

47. Verma NP, Nichols CD, Greiffenstein MF *et al*. Waves earlier than P_3 are more informative in putative subcortical dementias: a study with mapping and neuropsychological techniques. *Brain Topogr* 1989; **1**: 183–91.

63

Computed Tomography (CT)

Alistair Burns[1] and Godfrey Pearlson[2]

[1]*University of Manchester, UK, and* [2]*Johns Hopkins Hospital, Baltimore, MD, USA*

Computed tomography (CT) was introduced in the early 1970s and has become one of the standard investigations in the clinical neurosciences. In cranial CT, X-radiation is passed through the head in the form of a tightly collimated beam and is measured by a series of detectors. Radiation is absorbed by the intervening structures, which results in "attenuation" of the beam. Attenuation is maximal in high-density regions such as bone and minimal in low-density regions such as cerebrospinal fluid (CSF). The information from the detectors is processed by computer and the product is a numerical output. The brain is divided into three-dimensional volume elements (or voxels) and each is given an attenuation number, which represents the average attenuation in that area. The numerical output is transferred to a grey scale and each voxel is represented by a two-dimensional pixel. The familiar CT scan images are the result of the pictorial representation of the pixels on the grey scale. Areas of high attenuation are represented by white and areas of low attenuation by black. Areas with intermediate attenuation (such as brain substance) appear grey. The amount of radiation exposure in an average CT scan is slightly less than that in a set of conventional skull X-rays.

USE OF CT IN CLINICAL PRACTICE

CT has several advantages over magnetic resonance imaging (MRI) in the investigation of dementia. Acute haematomas can be easily distinguished from areas of infarction, the increased density of the former contrasting significantly with the hypodensity of the latter. In practice, CT is more widely available than MRI and the examination is less arduous and can be completed much faster. The presence of a cardiac pacemaker or the presence of surgical clips from previous brain surgery are not contra-indications to CT scanning in the same way that they are for MRI.

Guidelines have been published that suggest the circumstances under which a CT scan should be performed for the work-up of dementia[1,2]. Essentially, where the duration of the illness is short (<6 months and certainly <3 months), and where the features of the illness indicate that there may be cerebral pathology, then the chances of a CT scan detecting a clinically significant lesion is increased. Such features include: focal neurological signs; epileptic fits; variations in the course of the illness; and indicators of the presence of normal pressure hydrocephalus (gait disturbance, and incontinence in the presence of dementia). One study specifically examined a population sample aged 65+ and found that potentially treatable lesions (subdural haematoma, hydrocephalus, non-metastatic intracranial tumour) were present in 145 out of a possible 137 000 patient years at risk[33]. Specific features predicting the detection of such a lesion were: cognitive

impairment for 1 month or less; head trauma in the week before mental state change; rapid onset of change over 48 h; history of CVA; seizures or incontinence; focal neurological signs; papilloedema; visual field defects; gait abnormalities; postural instability; or headaches. Paris *et al.*[3] estimate that the yield of potentially treatable conditions is about 3%. Factors on CT scan that predict who will respond positively to a CSF shunt have been documented by Vanneste *et al.*[4]—cerebral atrophy and the presence of white matter disease were poor predictors of response to the insertion of a shunt.

DIFFERENTIAL DIAGNOSIS

CT scanning is helpful in confirming certain diagnoses, e.g. Alzheimer's disease (AD), but is not the definitive investigation, whereas in other disorders, e.g. 'subdural haematoma' the CT is the definitive investigation.

The CT scan has been used to differentiate vascular dementia from primary degenerative dementia. Generally speaking, good concordance between the presence of vascular lesions on CT and the presence of vascular dementia (defined purely clinically or using the Hachinski score) has been achieved[5–7].

White matter lesions on CT scan have been widely reported[8,9] and are associated with impaired cognitive function (in both AD patients and non-demented subjects) and neurological signs (gait disturbance and extensor plantar response). Scheltens *et al.*[10] described a number of rating scales used to detect white matter changes on CT and MRI brain imaging, concluding that the ideal rating scale is not yet in existence but that different rating scales serve individual purposes.

Excessive ingestion of alcohol can result in cerebral atrophy and ventricular dilatation on CT scan, particularly affecting the frontal lobe and cerebellar vermis. It is apparent that the changes occur relatively early (but do not antedate alcohol excess), are apparent before any clinical evidence of declining cognitive function and may be partially reversible with abstinence[11]. There is also evidence that third ventricular size is correlated with memory impairment in alcoholics without Korsakoff's deterioration. Patients with Korsakoff's psychosis have more cortical atrophy and lateral ventricular enlargement, but the size of the third ventricle is particularly increased.

Depression has been shown to be accompanied by both cerebral atrophy and ventricular enlargement[12,13]. CT scan appearances in depressed patients appear to be midway between those of normal controls and demented subjects, tending to be nearer the latter. More recently, it has been shown that patients with reversible dementia secondary to depression (pseudodementia, or dementia

Table 63.1 Clinical and structural correlates on CT in AD

Reference	Mean age (or range)	n	CT measure	Clinical features	Association†
36	70.0	43	Cortex	GRD	C = 0.56
			Lateral ventricles		C = 0.62
37	78.6	40	Cortex	Age, paranoid delusions	NS, C = −0.65**
			Lateral ventricles	Age, digit symbol test	NS, C = −0.31*
			Evan's ratio	Age, digit symbol test	NS, C = −0.31*
38	NS	22	Lateral ventricles	GRD, duration	C = 0.73**, NS
			Sylvian fissures	GRD, duration	C = 0.59* NS
			Surface sulci	GRD, duration	NS, C = 0.61**
(a) Presenile	59.6	10	Cortex	Age	NS
(b) Senile	77.6	7			
40	53–87	59	Cortex	GRD, age	NS, C = 0.27*
			Lateral ventricles	GRD, age	C = 0.29*, C = 0.50***, C = 0.46***
			III ventricle	GRD	NS
			IV ventricle	GRD	
41	77.0	57	Cortex	Age, duration, cognition, AD	NS, NS, NS, NS
			Lateral ventricles	Age, duration, cognition, AD	NS, C = 0.29*, C = −0.35**, C = −0.43***
			III ventricle	Age, duration, cognition, AD	NS, NS, C = −0.40***, C = −0.30**
42	72.7	35	Lateral ventricles	Age, GDS, MSQ	C = 0.55*, C = 0.37*, C = 0.42**
32	58.1	8	Lateral ventricles	Memory	C = −0.68**
			Lateral ventricles	Verbal fluency	C = −0.59**
			Lateral ventricles	Proverb interpretation	C = 0.74***
			Lateral ventricles	Clock drawing	C = 0.60**
43	78.1	47	Lateral ventricles	Digit copying test, MTS	C = 0.24* NS
			Regional density: pontine		C = −0.31***, C = 0.40**
44	60.7	60	Cortex	Aphasia, GRD	*, *
			Lateral ventricles	Aphasia, GRD	*, *
45	67.9	42	Cortex	Memory, deterioration in IQ	C + 0.30* , NS
			Lateral ventricles	Memory, deterioration in IQ	NS, NS
46	45–84	39	Total intracranial CSF	IMC, MMSE, BDS	*, *, *
47	72.2	16	Lateral ventricles	MMSE	C = −0.46*
31	63.4	30	Cortex	Age, duration, MMSE, GDS	NS, *, ***, ***
			Lateral ventricles	Age, duration, MMSE, GDS	NS, NS, NS, NS
			III ventricle	Age, duration, MMSE, GDS	**, NS, **, ***
17	79.7	138	Cortex	Age, duration, MMSE, CAMCOG	C = −0.27***, C = 0.24**, C = −0.42**, C = −0.41***
			Lateral ventricles	Age, duration, MMSE, CAMCOG	NS, NS, C = −0.25**, C = −0.31***
			III ventricle	Age, duration, MMSE, CAMCOG	NS, C = 0.22**, C = −0.31***, C = −0.34***
			R Sylvian fissure	Age, duration, MMSE, CAMCOG	C = 0.21**, NS, C = −0.25**, C = −0.27**
			L Sylvian fissure	Age, duration, CAMCOG	NS, NS, C = −0.28**, C = −0.30***
48	79.7	138	Lateral ventricles	Delusions	** (Smaller venticles)
			Basal ganglia calcification	Delusions	**
			Temporal atrophy	Aggression	*
			Frontal/occipital atrophy	Hyperorality	***
50	75.0	60	Brain quadrants	Misidentification symptoms (MS)	MS associated with larger right anterior horn of lateral ventricles and left anterior brain areas
51	75.0	60	III ventricle	Age, duration, MMSE, CAMCOG	NS, C = 0.34**, C = −0.23**, C = −0.27**
			L anterior horn	Age, duration, MMSE, CAMCOG	NS, C = 0.39***, C = −0.33***, C = −0.36***
			R anterior horn	Age, duration, MMSE, CAMCOG	NS, NS, C = −0.25**, C = −0.23**
			Subarachnoid areas:		
52	75.0	60	L frontal	Age, duration, MMSE, CAMCOG	NS, C = 0.32**, NS, NS
			R frontal	Age, duration, MMSE, CAMCOG	NS, C = 0.39**, NS, NS
			L posterior	Age, duration, MMSE, CAMCOG	NS, C = 0.36**, NS, NS
			R posterior	Age, duration, MMSE, CAMCOG	NS, NS, NS, NS
			Total intracranial density	Age, duration, MMSE, CAMCOG	NS, NS, NS, NS
			Grey matter	Age, duration, MMSE, CAMCOG	NS, NS, NS, NS
			White matter	Age, duration, MMSE, CAMCOG	NS, C = 0.32***/, NS, NS

†Associations reflect the information in the original paper: NS, not significant; C, correlation coefficient (Spearman or Pearson), given if significant followed by significance level: *$p < 0.05$; **$p < 0.01$; ***$p < 0.001$.
‡In L parietal only.
GRD, Global rating of dementia (varies from study to study): GDS, Global Deterioration Scale: MSQ, Mental Status Questionnaire: MTS, Mental Test Score; MMSE, Mini-Mental State Examination; CAMCOG, part of Camdex[53]; IMC, Information memory and Concentration Test; BDS, Blessed Dementia Scale. Table reproduced from O'Brien, J., Ames, D., and Burns, A. (eds), *Dementia*, 2nd edn, 2000, by permission of Edward Arnold.

syndrome of depression) have CT scan changes such as increased lateral ventricular size and decreased tissue density numbers[14]. In paraphrenia, there is dilatation of the lateral ventricles, preservation of cortical structures and loss of the normal ventricular size/age correlation seen in normal ageing[15].

CT IN AD

Two areas of clinical interest are important in relation to CT scanning in AD. First, what is the diagnostic ability of the CT scan? Second, what CT changes take place in AD and how are they related to the clinical features of the disorder?

DIAGNOSTIC ABILITY OF CT

The second area of clinical interest relates to the ability of CT scan changes to differentiate patients with dementia from non-demented control subjects. It is well recognized that demented subjects can have normal CT scans, whereas normal subjects can have marked atrophic changes. Discriminant analyses are able to differentiate the two groups using CT scan appearances in about 80% of cases[16], a rate that has remained virtually constant over time in spite of advances in CT technology and methods of scan analysis[49]. In a meta-analysis, De Carli et al.[18] estimated sensitivity and specificity for a variety of CT measures. Specificity was high for most measures (about 90%, i.e. few normal subjects were classified as having abnormal CT appearances). Sensitivity (i.e. the number of AD patients regarded as having abnormal CT scans) was lower.

Serial CT scans in individual patients have been performed and have the potential for greater diagnostic accuracy. Increases in ventricular size have been shown to outstrip those which take place in normal ageing. Luxenberg et al.[19] found that the rate of lateral ventricular enlargement in male AD patients over 12 months completely differentiated these patients from controls (i.e. 100% sensitivity and 100% specificity). Increase in ventricular size correlates with deterioration in cognitive function[19] and two subgroups of patients with AD have been described on this basis of one with significantly increasing ventricular size and deteriorating cognitive function and one without these chages[20].

CLINICO–RADIOLOGICAL CORRELATIONS

Early studies demonstrated correlations between the degree of intellectual impairment and both cortical and subcortical atrophy on CT[21–23] but often included normal controls in the correlations. Normal control subjects tended to be patients referred for investigations and found to have normal scans, rather than people screened first and then scanned.

With regard to clinico-radiological changes, both cortical atrophy and lateral ventricular enlargement occur with normal ageing and tend to accelerate after the age of 60. There is a significant correlation between cerebral atrophy and age in normal subjects but this has not been as consistently found in dementia. Correlations have been described between cognitive function and both cortical atrophy and ventricular size. Generally, correlations are higher in the latter relationship (ventricular size can be measured as a continuous variable, which may partly explain the greater association), although some studies have reported no association between degree of dementia (measured by both specific cognitive tests and global ratings) and either CT measure. The third ventricle has been examined in a number of studies, and was found to be larger in demented patients than in age-matched controls, correlating with degree of cognitive impairment[17,24].

In addition to measures of global cerebral atrophy and ventricular enlargement, CT scans can provide other information of clinical interest. Regional cerebral atrophy has been shown to be related to certain behavioural disturbances[49]. Basal ganglia calcification is found in a significantly greater proportion of patients with delusions and demented patients with affective symptomatology have less severe CT scan changes, including relative preservation of the interhemispheric fissure[49].

Table 63.1 summarizes the relevant studies; 88% of ventricular measures show significant correlations with cognitive tests, whereas only 41% of cortical assessments do so ($\times 2 = 11.3$, $p < 0.001$, d.f. $= 1$).

The diagnostic potential of the specific temporal lobe views of the brain has attracted some interest in AD[25]. Pathologically, the temporal lobe discriminates well between AD and normal controls[26] and coronal plane CT images can be reformated to display the temporal lobes in fine detail.

CT has been combined with SPET (single-photon emission tomography) in order to improve diagnostic accuracy in AD. Jobst and colleagues, in the OPTIMA project in Oxford[27,28], reported a series of studies demonstrating that views of the temporal lobe could be achieved during CT scan, with the plane orientated along the long axis of the medial temporal lobe (20–25° anterior to standard CT angle). In this way, 92% of patients with AD were correctly diagnosed compared to a 5% false-positive rate. Simple measurement of the narrowest thickness of the medial temporal lobe (right or left) was about 50% thinner in patients with AD compared to controls. Combining these measurements with SPET in patients with histologically proven AD compared to controls, the medial temporal lobe atrophy provides 94% sensitivity and 93% specificity, parietotemporal hypoperfusion on SPET gave 96% sensitivity and 89% specificity, and the combination of both changes gave a sensitivity of 97%. The results of Lavenu et al.[29] who carried out a similar study using CT and SPET, resulting in a diagnostic accuracy rate which was much less—68%. Stage of disease is an important influencing factor in this rate and replication of the results of these studies is needed before they can be incorporated into clinical practice. O'Brien et al.[7] found reduced temporal lobe width in AD, vascular dementia and Lewy body dementia compared to controls, suggesting a lack of specificity of the finding with a single cross-sectional measurement.

CONCLUSION

In summary, the role of the CT scan in old age psychiatry is as a relatively non-invasive and widely available neuroradiological technique to exclude intracranial mass lesions. Regional changes may be helpful in the differential diagnosis of the dementia syndrome. The concordance between the CT changes and a clinical diagnosis of dementia is not absolute and significant overlap exists between the changes seen in dementia and those seen in normal ageing. Some methods of CT scan analysis are better than others in this differentiation and serial CT scans on individual patients may be an even better indicator.

REFERENCES

1. Bradshaw J, Thomas J, Campbell M. Computed tomography in the investigation of dementia. *Br Med J* 1985; **286**: 277–80.
2. Larson E, Reifler B, Featherstone J, English D. Dementia in elderly outpatients: prospective study. *Ann Intern Med* 1984; **100**: 417–23.

3. Paris B. The utility of CT scanning in diagnosing dementia. *M Sinai J Med* 1997; **64**(6), 372–5.

4. Vanneste J, Augustijn P, Tan W, Dirven C. Shunting normal pressure hydrocephalus. *J Neurol Neurosurg Psychiat* 1993; **56**: 251–6.

5. Loeb C, Gandolfo C. Diagnostic evaluation of degenerative and vascular dementia. *Stroke* 14: 339–401.

6. Cummings J, Miller B, Hill N et al. Neuropsychiatric aspects of multi-infarct dementia and dementia of the Alzheimer type. *Arch Neurol* 1987; **44**: 389–93.

7. O'Brien J, Metcalfe S, Swann A et al. Medial temporal lobe width on CT scanning in Alzheimer's disease: a comparison with vascular dementia, depression and dementia with Lewy bodies. *Dement Geriat Cogn Disord* 1999; **648**: 1–8.

8. Hachinski V, Potter P, Mersky H. Leuko-araiosis. *Arch Neurol* 1987; **44**: 21–3.

9. Steingart A, Hachinski V, Lau C et al. Cognitive and neurologic findings in subjects with diffuse white matter lucencies on CT scan. *Arch Neurol* 1987; **44**: 32–5.

10. Scheltens P, Erkinjuntit F, Leys D et al. White matter changes on CT and MRI. *Eur Neurol* 1998; **39**: 289–9.

11. Ron M. The alcoholic brain: CT scan and psychological findings. *Psychol Med Monogr Suppl* 1983; 3.

12. Jacoby R, Levy R. Computed tomography in the elderly. III. Affective disorder. *Br J Psychiat* 1980; **136**: 270–5.

13. Pearlson GD, Rabins PV, Burns A. CT changes in centrum semiovale white matter in dementia of depression. *Psychol Med* 1991; **21**: 321–8.

14. Pearlson GD, Rabins P, Kim W et al. Structural brain CT changes and cognitive deficits in elderly depressive with and without reversible dementia. *Psychol Med* 1989; **19**: 573–84.

15. Burns A, Carrick J, Amers D et al. The cerebral cortical appearance in late paraphrenia. *Int J Geriat Psychiat* 1989; **4**: 31–4.

16. Jacoby R, Levy R. Computed tomography in the elderly. II, Senile dementia: diagnosis and functional impairment. *Br J Psychiat* 1981; **362**: 256–69.

17. Burns A, Jacoby R, Philpot M, Levy R. CT in Alzheimer's disease—methods of scan analysis, comparison with normal controls and clinical radiological correlations. *Br J Psychiat* 1991; **159**: 609–14.

18. De Carli C, Kaye J, Horwitz B, Rapoport S. Critical analysis of the use of CT to study human brain in ageing and dementia of the Alzheimer type. *Neurology* 1990; **40**: 872–83.

19. Luxenberg J, Haxby J, Creasey H et al. Rate of ventricular enlargement in dementia of the Alzheimer type correlates with the rate of psychological deterioration. *Neurology* 1987; **37**: 1135–40.

20. Naguib M, Levy R. CT scanning in senile dementia. A follow-up of survivors. *Br J Psychiat* 1982; **141**: 618–20.

21. Roberts MA, Caira FI. Computerised tomography and intellectual impairment in the elderly. *J Neurol Neurosurg Psychiat* 1976; **39**: 986–9.

22. Brinkman SD, Sarwar M, Levine HS, Morris HH III. Quantitative indexes of computed tomography in dementia and normal aging. *Radiology* 1981; **138**: 89–92.

23. Wu S, Schenkenberg T, Wing SD, Osborn AG. Cognitive correlates of diffuse cerebral atrophy determined by computed tomography. *Neurology* 1981; **3**: 80–4.

24. Leyl D, Prudo J, Pretty H et al. Maladie d'Alzheimer. *Rev Neurol (Paris)* 1989; **145**: 134–9.

25. De Leon MJ, George AE, Styulopoulos LA et al. Early marker for Alzheimer's disease: the atrophic hippocampus. *Lancet* 1989; **6**: 672–3.

26. Tomlinson B. Observations on the brains of demented old people. *Neurol Sci* 1970; **II**: 205–42.

27. Jobst K, Smith A, Barker C. Association of atrophy of the medial temporal lobe with reduced blood flow in the posteria parietotemporal cortex in patients with a clinical and pathological diagnosis of Alzheimer's disease. *J Neurol Neurosurg Psychiat* 1992; **55**: 190–4.

28. Jobst K, Smith A, Szetmari M et al. A detection in life of confirmed Alzheimer's disease using a simple measurement of medial temporal lobe atrophy by computer tomography. *Lancet* 1992; **340** 1179–83.

29. Lavenu L, Pasquier IF, Leberte F. Association between medial temporal lobe atrophy on CT and parietal temporal uptake and decrease on SPET in Alzheimer's disease. *J Neurol Neurosurg Psychiat* 1997; **63**: 441–5.

30. Jacoby R, Levy R. Computed tomography in the elderly. II. Senile dementia: diagnosis in functional impairment. *Br J Psychiat* 1980; **136**: 256–69.

31. Leys D, Prudo J, Pretty H et al. Maladie d'Alzheimer. *Rev Neurol (Paris)* 1989; **145**: 134–9.

32. Albert M, Naeser MA, Levine HL, Garvey AJ. Ventricular size in patients with presenile dementia of the Alzheimer's type. *Arch Neurol* 1984; **41**: 1258–63.

33. Alexander E, Wagner E, Buchner D et al. Do surgical brain lesions present as isolated dementia? A population-based study. *J Am Geriat Soc* 1995; **43**: 138–43.

34. Baldy R, Brindley G, Mensah I et al. A fully automated computer-assisted method of CT scan brain analysis for the measurement of CSF spaces and brain absorption density. *Neuroradiology* 1986; **28**: 108–17.

35. Philpot M, Burns A. Reversible dementias. In Katona C, ed. *Dementia Disorders: Advances and Prospects*. London: Chapman and Hall, 1989; 142–59.

36. De Leon MJ, Ferris SH, George AE et al. Computed tomography evaluations of brain–behaviour relationships in senile dementia of the Alzheimer type. *Neurobiol Aging* 1980; **1**: 69–79.

37. Jacoby R, Levy R. Computed tomography in the elderly II, Senile dementia: diagnosis in functional impairment. *Br J Psychiat* 1980; **136**: 256–69.

38. Merskey H, Ball MJ, Blume WT et al. Relationships between psychological measurements and cerebral organic changes in Alzheimer's disease. *Canadian J Neurol Sci* 1980; **7**: 45–9.

39. Naeser MA, Gebhardt C, Levine HL. Decreased computerized tomography numbers in patients with presenile dementia. *Arch Neurol* 1980; **37**: 401–9

40. Ford CV, Winter J. Computerized axial tomograms and dementia in elderly patients. *J Gerontol* 1981; **36**: 164–9.

41. Soininen H, Puranen M, Riekkinen PJ. Computed tomography findings in senile dementia and normal aging. *J Neurol Neurosurg Psychiat* 1982; **45**: 50–4.

42. George AE, De Leon MJ, Rosenbloom S et al. Ventricular volume and cognitive deficit: a computed tomographic study. *Radiology* 1983; **149**: 493–8.

43. Colgan J. Regional density and survival in dementia. *Br J Psychiat* 1985; **147**: 63–6.

44. Drayer BP, Heyman A, Wilkinson W et al. Early-onset Alzheimer's disease: an analysis of CT findings. *Ann Neurol* 1985; **17**: 407–10.

45. Bigler ED, Hubler DW, Cullum CM et al. Intellectual and memory impairment in dementia. Computerized axial tomography volume correlations. *J Nerv Ment Dis* 1985; **173**: 347–62.

46. Creasy H, Schwartz M, Frederickson H et al. Quantitative computed tomography in dementia of the Alzheimer type. *Neurology* 1986; **36**: 1563–8.

47. Pearlson GD, Tune LE. Cerebral ventricular size and cerebrospinal fluid acetylcholinesterase levels in senile dementia of the Alzheimer type. *Psychiatry Res* 1986; **17**: 23–9.

48. Burns A. Cranial computerised tomography in dementia of the Alzheimer type. *Br J Psychiat* 1990; **157**(suppl 9): 10–15.

49. Burns A, Jacoby R, Levy R. Psychiatric phenomena in Alzheimer's disease. *Br J Psychiat* 1990; **157**: 72–94.

50. Förstl H, Burns A, Jacoby R et al. Quantitative CT scan analysis in senile dementia of the Alzheimer type: 1 Computerized planimetry of cerebrospinal fluid areas. *Int J Geriatr Psychiat* 1991; **6**: 709–13.

51. Förstl H, Burns A, Jacoby R et al. Quantitative CT scan analysis in senile dementia of the Alzheimer type: 2 Radio-attenuation of grey and white matter. *Int J Geriatr Psychiat* 1991; **6**: 715–19.

52. Förstl H, Burns A, Jacoby R, Levy R. Neuro-anatomical correlates of clinical misidentification and misperception in senile dementia of the Alzheimer type. *J Clin Psychiat* 1991; **52**: 268–71.

53. Roth M, Tym E, Mountjoy CQ et al. CAMDEX, A standardised instrument for the diagnosis of mental disorder in the elderly with special reference to the early detection of dementia. *Br J Psychiat* 1986; **149**: 698–709.

64

Magnetic Resonance Imaging

K. Ranga R. Krishnan

Duke University Medical Center, Durham, NC, USA

The property that is the basis for magnetic resonance imaging is the interaction between hydrogen and a magnetic field. A hydrogen atom is a nuclear magnet which, when placed on the magnetic field, aligns itself in the direction of the field. In the process of aligning it develops a spin at a frequency which is called the Larmor frequency. If the magnetic field is varied, then the frequency of this oscillation also varies. Besides hydrogen, when a nucleus contains an odd number of either protons or neutrons, it is magnetic. As indicated earlier, the frequency of oscillation of hydrogen is proportional to the strength of the magnetic field. Resonance occurs when the applied frequency (magnetic frequency) is the same as that of the object. Magnetic nuclei in a magnetic field can be stimulated by other magnetic fields. These fields can usually be created by radio-frequency waves. When the radio-frequency waves are tuned to the Larmor frequency of the atomic nuclei, namely hydrogen, then the direction of oscillation of the atom moves towards the direction of the newly applied magnetic field. When the field is turned off, the nuclei relax, emit absorbed energy and return to the state prior to the radio frequency stimulation. This process can be repeated over and over again, provided that enough time is allowed for the relaxation of the atom. When consideration is given to an entire object composed of billions of atoms, the relaxation of these atoms will depend upon local effects, i.e. what molecule the atom is attached to, etc., the most common attachment being water for hydrogen. The signal detected when the hydrogen atom relaxes after the radio frequency and pulse has stopped can be detected by using a radio frequency antenna tuned to the Larmor frequency. The decay of this signal over time is called free induction decay. The time to recover two-thirds of the magnetization after stopping the radio-frequency stimulus is called the T1 relaxation time, or spin lattice relaxation time. This relaxation time is influenced by the environment of the hydrogen atom and can vary between gray matter, white matter, and fluid. T1 primarily refers to the longitudinal vector of relaxation, which is along the direction of the magnetic field. Another vector at right angles to the field, called the transverse vector, can also be measured, and its relaxation is called T2 relaxation. By convention, this refers to the time when it disappears, rather than the two-thirds used for measuring T1. T2 is always shorter than T1. Based on the properties of the longitudinal and transverse vector, one acquires images that are predominately T1-weighted, or those which are predominately T2-weighted, a third type that appear intermittent in appearance. In a T1-weighted image, fluid appears dark. In a T2-weighted image, fluid appears bright and white. Scanning sequences can be optimized by emphasizing one contrast vs. another. This allows a better distinction of both pathology and normal tissue.

MAGNETIC RESONANCE MORPHOMETRY

Magnetic resonance morphometry basically utilizes the acquired images to identify objects and then to quantitate their volumes. Volumes can be estimated in either two dimensions or three. The most common method of estimation is to use two-dimensional slices through a given object. A number of studies have indicated that systematic sampling is better than the randomized sampling of the particular object of interest. Segmentation of the object can be accomplished manually or by semi-automated means, and more recently in an automated fashion. Factors that effect the sensitivity and accuracy of the estimation of the volume include the number of slices that go through the object, the orientation of the slices, contrast, and any inhomogeneities in the magnetic field. Magnetic resonance morphometry methods have greatly improved over the last decade and are now widely utilized for studying a variety of neuropsychiatric disorders. The techniques, which were initially primarily manual outlining of an object, have vastly improved and now include semi-automated and automated techniques to estimate the volume of the object.

GERIATRIC PSYCHIATRY

The application of MRI in geriatric psychiatry has been extensive. There are two broad areas to which MR techniques have been applied. One is to evaluate the presence of gross pathology and the other is to evaluate morphemetric changes in a variety of disorders in the elderly. MRI is often utilized to look for tumors, infarcts, etc. when one suspects disease in a patient. MRI can detect space-occupying lesions and, given that images can be acquired in three dimensions, it can often provide better resolution than computed tomography (CT) (it must be kept in mind that newer forms of CT provide sufficiently high resolution). MRI is not useful in identifying calcifying objects, and in this particular case CT is far better. The use of contrast agents, such as gadolinium, can distinguish any breaking of the blood–brain barrier and often these agents are utilized to produce additional contrast of pathological tissue. Full-blown infarcts can be easily identified on MRI. In addition, MRI can be utilized to measure blood flow through large vessels, a technique known as called magnetic resonance angiography.

BRAIN ATROPHY

The second aspect as it relates to geropsychiatry is a measurement of brain atrophy and dementia. Patients with frontal temporal

---

Principles and Practice of Geriatric Psychiatry, 2nd edn. Edited by J. R. M. Copeland, M. T. Abou-Saleh and D. G. Blazer
©2002 John Wiley & Sons, Ltd

dementia have significant atrophy of the frontal lobes. This can be easily visualized using MRI and quantitated if need be. Patients who have significant Alzheimer's disease (AD) will demonstrate observable hippocampal atrophy. Over time this can be measured and utilized for assessing the progression of the disease. MRI can be acquired with a different contrast, as noted earlier, and in three dimensions. Utilizing this one can develop specific methods to identify objects of interest and quantitate these objects. Fluid measurements of cerebrospinal fluid in different locations can also be easily measured. The technique also seems to be of particular use in mild cognitive impairment, in which commencing atrophy, especially of the hippocampus and temporal cortex, are often seen.

SILENT INFARCTS

Another area of growing interest in geropsychiatry is the identification of silent infarct or leukoencephalopathy. These are a function of aging. The risk factors are very similar to those of stroke, including high blood pressure, diabetes, etc. These changes are usually present in the deep white matter, the periventricular region, and subcortical nuclei such as the caudate putamen and thalamus. These silent strokes occur at the ends of the perforating blood vessels of the brain. These blood vessels do not have collaterals and are therefore more susceptible to the development of occlusions and the ischaemia that results from them. These silent strokes have been characterized pathologically as areas of myelin pallor, true infarcts (dead tissue and lacuna). A lacuna is distinguished by the presence of fluid inside the area and this can be determined by a bright signal on T2 and a dark signal on the T1 images. These changes have been related to depression, bipolar disorder and dementia. They are present in both AD and vascular dementia. The contributing role of these factors in AD is controversial. Epidemiological studies indicate that the presence and extent of these changes is a good indicator of a development of dementia and it has the same odds ratio as APO-E studies.

In summary, MRI is widely utilized to study various types of neuropsychiatric disorders. It has particular application and utility for identifying pathology and atrophy in the context of dementia, and lesions such as silent strokes in late-life depression and late-life bipolar disorder.

REFERENCE

For a more thorough update, see Krishnan KR, Doraiswamy PM. *Brain Injury in Clinical Psychiatry*. New York: Marcel Dekker, 1997.

65

Functional Magnetic Resonance Imaging (fMRI)

K. Ranga R. Krishnan

Duke University Medical Center, Durham, MC, USA

Functional MRI (fMRI) is a new technique that has allowed the non-invasive assessment of physiological function of the brain in humans. The phenomena of nuclear magnetic resonance has been utilized to accomplish this. The first attempt at producing a functional image of the human brain utilized an invasive technique of evaluating blood flow changes in the brain, assessed by using a contrast agent. The non-invasive method was introduced by Ogawa, and is based on a blood oxygenation level-dependent contrast (BOLD) This contrast originates from the homogeneity induced by deoxy-haemoglobin in red blood cells. Signal intensities in MRIs are therefore acquired in a manner sensitive to this BOLD contrast, which is effected with regional deoxyhaemoglobin content. The rationale underlying the changes in deoxyhaemoglobin is that regional blood flow increases, while the oxygen consumption rate is not altered significantly, resulting in a lower deoxy-haemoglobin content per unit volume of brain tissue. The signal intensity in the image acquired sensitive to BOLD therefore increases in active regions relative to those regions which are not active.

Another technique that has been developed, called EPISTAR and FAIR, utilizes tagging of blood spins to measure cerebral blood flow changes. In a recent study, we have demonstrated that, using EPISTAR, there is a reduction in blood flow in the left frontal lobe in depressed patients. BOLD as well as FAIR can be developed and utilized in regular MRI 1.5 tesla scanners. However, many particularly exciting findings are emerging from high-field MRI, 4 tesla and greater. BOLD response is greater in a higher magnetic field, which produces an improved contrast.

APPLICATION OF fMRI

fMRI has been mostly utilized with the BOLD type of measure to evaluate brain regions involved in a task performance. Unlike positron emission tomography (PET), fMRI allows a single trial design and a single subject design and measures images that can be acquired in tenths of milliseconds, which is still much slower than the temporal response of neurons but similar to the response of the vascular system. In the design paradigms in general, the contrast is measured before and during a task and this can be done repeatedly to obtain an average within a subject on/off task. It can also be used to track the evolution of a particular task over time, that is the temporal evolution of the signal relative to the execution of this task can be obtained and averaged following repeated executions of the same task. It also allows evaluation of learning, errors, habituation, etc. The technique has had limited applicability so far to disease conditions, except as it relates to the evaluation of working memory tasks and other components of memory in patients with mild cognitive impairment, as a prelude to assessing whether they are likely to develop dementia over time. Clearly, this technique offers a significant possibility for understanding many of the neuropsychological functions that are altered in aging and acquiring the ability to assess their changes relative to particular diseases of aging.

REFERENCE

Ugurbil K, Hu X, Chen W *et al.* Functional mapping in the human brain using high magnetic fields. *Phil Trans R Soc Lond* 1999; **354**: 1195–213.

66

Positron Emission Tomography (PET)

Peter F. Liddle[1] and Cheryl L. Grady[2]

[1]*University of British Columbia, Vancouver, British Columbia*
and [2]*Rotman Research Institute, Toronto, Ontario, Canada*

Positron emission tomography (PET) provides quantitative images of the function of the brain in life. It generates an image of the distribution of a radioactively-labelled tracer substance that is distributed in the brain according to its pattern of physiological activity. By appropriate choice of tracer substances, it is possible to measure physiological variables such as blood flow, metabolism, neurotransmitter receptors, presynaptic neurotransmitter pools and aspects of amino acid metabolism.

The essence of any tomographic technique is a mathematical reconstruction of a two-dimensional image of the distribution of some physical variable (e.g. concentration of radioactivity), from a set of measurements of the value of that physical variable, averaged along a large number of intersecting straight-line paths through the brain. The feature that distinguishes PET from single photon emission computed tomography (SPECT) is the fact that a PET camera detects the paired photons generated by positron annihilation. When a positron is emitted from the tracer substance, it is annihilated by collision with an electron in the surrounding matter. This annihilation generates two γ-ray photons, which each have an energy of 511 keV and must travel in opposite directions. When two photons are detected simultaneously in different crystals arranged in a ring around the head, it can be concluded that a positron annihilation event has occurred at some point along the straight line connecting the two detectors. This use of coincidence detection of pairs of photons to determine the direction of travel of the photons is intrinsically more efficient than the use of collimators to determine the direction of travel, as is necessary in SPECT. Furthermore, correction for absorption in the brain tissue is straightforward in PET studies, because the amount of absorption along the straight-line path between a pair of detectors can be measured directly in a preliminary transmission scan, using a ring source. It is thus possible to quantify the local concentration of the positron-emitting isotope in the brain in absolute terms.

The positron-emitting isotopes used in PET are ^{15}O [half-life for radioactive decay (T/2) 2 min]; ^{13}N (T/2, 10 min); ^{11}C (T/2, 20 min); and ^{18}F (T/2, 110 min). The relatively short half-life of positron-emitting isotopes presents a logistic problem, since the PET camera must be located near to the cyclotron required to produce the isotopes. However, an advantage of short-lived isotopes is that the rapid decay of radiation minimizes unnecessary radiation exposure after the procedure is completed. In addition, in the case of ^{15}O, it is possible to carry out multiple separate PET scans within a single session of investigation, allowing the measurement of changes in brain function in response to various mental or pharmacological stimuli.

PET TRACER SUBSTANCES

In principle, virtually any substance involved in physiological processes that can be labelled with a positron-emitting isotope might be used in PET, but quantitative measurement requires an adequate mathematical model of the processes governing distribution of the substance in the brain.

An image of regional cerebral blood flow (rCBF) can be obtained from the distribution of intravenous [^{15}O]H$_2$O which is delivered to the brain at a rate depending on cerebral perfusion. Inhaled [^{15}O]oxygen provides an image of oxygen distribution in brain tissue which, when combined with an rCBF image, can be used to generate an image of regional oxygen metabolism (rCMRO$_2$). Intravenous [^{18}F]deoxyglucose (FDG) can be used to provide an image of regional glucose metabolism (rCMRGlu). This technique relies upon the fact that deoxyglucose is transported into cells by the same mechanism as is responsible for glucose uptake, but its metabolism is arrested after the first reaction in the glycolytic pathway. Hence, deoxyglucose accumulates within cells at a rate which reflects the rate of entry of glucose into the glycolytic pathway.

The development of labelled ligands that are suitable for measuring the characteristics of neurotransmitter binding sites is a difficult task, because of the difficulty in achieving a high level of specific binding at tolerable doses of the ligand. An example of a well-behaved ligand is [^{11}C]raclopride, which binds to D2 dopamine receptors[1]. It associates and dissociates rapidly from receptors, so that equilibrium is established relatively quickly, making it possible to determine an equilibrium binding curve. From such a binding curve, it is possible to determine the strength of binding (KD) and the density of receptors (B$_{max}$). Other ligands that have been used to study neurotransmitter function include [^{11}C]SCH 23390 for D1 dopamine receptors[2], [^{11}C]WAY-100635[3] to measure 5-HT$_1$ serotonin receptors, and [^{18}F]altanserin[4] and [^{18}F]setoperone[5] for measurement of 5-HT$_2$ receptors.

SOURCES OF VARIATION IN PET IMAGES

If an imaging technique is to be useful for delineating pathological processes, it is necessary that the variation in image due to the pathological process of interest should not be swamped by

Principles and Practice of Geriatric Psychiatry, 2nd edn. Edited by J. R. M. Copeland, M. T. Abou-Saleh and D. G. Blazer
©2002 John Wiley & Sons, Ltd

variation arising from other factors. The difficulties in dealing with the multiple sources of confounding variation in PET images has hitherto limited the contribution of PET to the delineation of psychiatric disorders. From the clinician's viewpoint, the biological sources of variation are the most relevant, some of which are considered below.

In the study of elderly patients, one of the potentially confounding differences between subjects is brain atrophy, which is liable to produce variation in partial volume effects. Partial volume effects are due to the limited spatial resolving power of PET cameras, resulting in the contamination of the signal from high-intensity regions by adjacent tissue with low intensity. For example, if grey matter volume is reduced, the measured functional activity of the grey matter will be lowered by an increased contribution from adjacent white matter or CSF. A number of studies have examined the effect of cerebral atrophy on metabolic measures obtained with PET in both healthy older adults and patients with Alzheimer's disease[6,7]. A recent study by Ibanez et al.[8] used measures of grey matter volume obtained from MRI scans to correct PET FDG images in a group of mildly to moderately demented AD patients. They found that metabolic values in parietotemporal and frontal cortex were reduced compared to a control group, even after correction for atrophy. These data suggest that, despite the undoubted contribution of partial volume effects, the metabolic deficits seen in these patients are not due simply to atrophy, but reflect true decreases in metabolic activity.

When evaluating images of brain function, it is necessary not only to be aware of confounding variance introduced by extraneous factors, but also to know that the functional impairments in a single disease are quite heterogeneous. For example, the clinical manifestations of AD are diverse, including not only impairments of memory but also many different aspects of cognitive function and behaviour. In accord with this behavioural heterogeneity, PET studies reveal that cases differ in the degree of laterality of the abnormalities, and also in the degree of frontal involvement[9]. On the other hand, different diseases can produce phenomenologically similar mental states, raising the possibility that different diseases might produce similar patterns of perturbation of regional blood flow and metabolism. This possibility is illustrated by the fact that hypometabolism of frontal cortex has been reported in AD[9], depression[10], Parkinson's disease[11] and in the psychomotor poverty syndrome in schizophrenia[12]. The greatest value of PET thus may lie in the sensitive measurement of particular patterns of brain malfunction, rather than the distinction between diseases differing in aetiology.

ACTIVATION STUDIES

A potentially useful approach to the measurement of brain function is within-subject comparison of brain activity during behavioural or pharmacological activation with that in an appropriate reference state. Behavioural activation has been used to identify the brain areas involved in specific mental activities in healthy young adults[13,14] and in older individuals[15]. Interestingly, older adults have been found to have greater activation in frontal areas during some types of cognitive activity, compared to younger adults[16,17]. These results have led to the suggestion that frontal cortex may play a compensatory role in the face of reduced function in other task-relevant brain areas, an idea that also is relevant to diseases of ageing.

Measurement of rCBF during pharmacological activation allows measurement of the response of the brain to drugs that alter neurotransmission. Although not yet used in psychiatric populations, the feasibility of this type of strategy has been demonstrated in normal subjects. For example, Friston et al.[18]

demonstrated that buspirone (a partial agonist at serotonergic 5-HT_{1A} receptors) caused an attenuation of the normal increase in rCBF in the parahippocampal gyrus produced by a verbal memory task, as well as a transient impairment of memory test performance. Conversely, Furey et al.[19] have shown improved performance and reduced activity in the frontal lobe during a working memory task after administration of physostigmine, a cholinesterase antagonist. These studies suggest that modulation of neurotransmitter systems has specific effects on brain function during cognitive activity, and have interesting implications for the use of pharmacologic modulation in understanding psychiatric disorders.

BLOOD FLOW AND METABOLISM IN AD

PET studies have produced a moderately consistent picture of the abnormalities of blood flow and metabolism in AD. The most common pattern is bilateral reduction in parietal and temporoparietal flow and metabolism, especially in early cases[9,20,21], but the patterns of flow and metabolism show considerable variation between patients[22]. These variations correlate with variation in behavioural and neuropsychological impairments[9]. Longitudinal studies have demonstrated that focal metabolic abnormalities are detectable before the corresponding neuropsychological impairment becomes apparent, and that the metabolic abnormalities progress as the disease progresses[23]. Recent studies have shown that metabolic abnormalities similar to those seen in the cortex of AD patients can be found in asymptomatic persons at risk for familial AD[24] and that these deficits are associated with the presence of the APOE-4 allele[25].

A few activation experiments with AD patients also have been conducted. Mildly demented AD patients have shown greater frontal activations, compared to healthy elderly, during memory tasks[26,27] and during perceptual tasks[28]. This is similar to the increased frontal activity seen in the healthy elderly, compared to young adults, and indicates that recruitment of cognitive resources mediated by frontal regions may be a common response to a decline in brain function, whether caused by normal ageing or by disease.

BASAL GANGLION FUNCTION IN HUNTINGTON'S DISEASE

The major neuropathological process in Huntington's disease (HD) is degeneration of the basal ganglia, especially the corpus striatum. Hence, it would be expected that there would be a loss of postsynaptic D1 and D2 dopamine receptors in the striatum, which has been amply demonstrated with imaging of these receptors using [^{11}C]SCH 23390 and [^{11}C]raclopride, respectively[29]. It has been shown that a striatal decrease in dopamine is detectable even in asymptomatic persons who carry the HD gene mutation[30], and further that the degree of reduction is correlated with reduced performance on cognitive tests of frontal lobe function[31]. Glucose metabolism is also reduced in the striatum of HD patients and patients at risk for HD[32]. Longitudinal studies of disease progression in HD have shown declines in both striatum and frontal lobe metabolism[33], indicating that PET could be useful in following the effects of treatment over time.

Only a few activation studies have been carried out with HD patients. Patients have been studied with [^{15}O]water during hand or finger movements and show reduced flow in the striatum, motor areas and prefrontal cortex[34,35]. Of particular interest is that activity in parietal cortex in one study[34] was increased relative to control subjects, suggesting a compensatory role of this region, similar to that postulated above for AD patients.

GERIATRIC DEPRESSION

Depression is a serious problem in older adults, and can occur as a symptom of a dementing illness or in the absence of dementia. The most common neuroimaging finding in depression is reduced glucose metabolism or flow in prefrontal cortex, although cingulate and paralimbic regions also are involved in mood disorders[36,37]. These regional patterns of reduction are seen in elderly as well as younger patients, although elderly depressed individuals are more likely to have global metabolic reductions in metabolism[38]. There is considerable evidence that the serotonergic neurotransmitter system is altered in depression[39] and ligands for measuring these receptors have recently been developed. A few studies have used PET to examine levels of serotonin receptors in depressed patients, but have reported conflicting results. In one experiment, 5-HT$_2$ binding was reduced in orbitofrontal areas in depressed patients[40], but no differences between depressed patients and controls were found in another study[41]. In older healthy adults 5-HT$_2$ receptor binding is reduced compared to young adults[42], but is not further reduced in elderly depressed patients. However, serotonin binding is reduced in AD patients[43], indicating that results from studies of geriatric depression should be viewed with caution, as they may have been influenced by co-exisiting dementia, which is difficult to rule out clinically[39]. It is clear that much work in this area remains to be done, including the assessment of brain function during serotonergic challenge in the elderly.

CONCLUSION

The accumulating evidence that detectable changes in brain function precede structural changes in neurodegenerative conditions and, in addition, that PET can provide a measure of severity of disordered brain function, indicates the potential value of PET in early detection and in monitoring the effects of treatments intended to modify the progression of these conditions. One important contribution of PET to the investigation of geriatric disorders will likely be in its use to delineate the mechanisms of disordered cerebral function. In addition, the use of pharmacological challenges and the measurement of neurotransmitter function hold promise for our understanding of neuropsychiatric disorders in the elderly.

REFERENCES

1. Sedvall G, Farde L, Persson A, Wiesel F-A. Imaging of neurotransmitter receptors in the living human brain. *Arch Gen Psychiat* 1986; **43**: 995–1005.
2. Farde L, Halldin C, Stone-Elander S, Sedvall G. PET analysis of human dopamine receptor subtypes using 11C-SCH 23390 and 11C-raclopride. *Psychopharmacology* 1987; **92**(3): 278–84.
3. Pike VW, McCarron JA, Lammerstma AA *et al.* First delineation of 5-HT$_{1A}$ receptors in human brain with PET and [11C]WAY-100635. *Eur J Pharmacol* 1995; **283**(1–3): R1–3.
4. Sadzot B, Lemaire C, Maquet P *et al.* Serotonin 5-HT$_2$ receptor imaging in the human brain using positron emission tomography and a new radioligand, [18F]altanserin: results in young normal controls. *J Cerebr Blood Flow Metab* 1995; **15**(5): 787–97.
5. Blin J, Sette G, Fiorelli M *et al.* A method for the *in vivo* investigation of the serotonergic 5-HT$_2$ receptors in the human cerebral cortex using positron emission tomography and 18F-labeled setoperone. *J Neurochem* 1990; **54**(5): 1744–54.

6. Schlageter NL, Horwitz B, Creasey H *et al.* Relation of measured brain glucose utilisation and cerebral atrophy in man. *J Neurol Neurosurg Psychiat* 1987; **50**: 779–85.
7. Alavi A, Newberg AB, Souder E, Berlin JA. Quantitative analysis of PET and MRI data in normal aging and Alzheimer's disease: atrophy weighted total brain metabolism and absolute whole brain metabolism as reliable discriminators. *J Nuc Med* 1993; **34**: 1681–87.
8. Ibanez V, Pietrini P, Alexander GE *et al.* Regional glucose metabolic abnormalities are not the result of atrophy in Alzheimer's disease. *Neurology* 1998; **50**: 1585–93.
9. Haxby JV, Grady CL, Koss E *et al.* Heterogeneous anterior–posterior metabolic patterns in Alzheimer's type dementia. *Neurology* 1988; **38**: 1853–63.
10. Baxter LR, Schwartz JM, Phelps ME *et al.* Reduction of prefrontal cortex glucose metabolism common to three types of depression. *Arch Gen Psychiat* 1989; **46**: 243–50.
11. Mayberg HS, Starkstein SE, Sadzot B *et al.* Selective hypometabolism in the inferior frontal lobe in depressed patients with Parkinson's disease. *Ann Neurol* 1990; **28**(1): 57–64.
12. Liddle PF, Friston KJ, Hirsch SR, Frackowiak RSJ. Regional cerebral metabolic activity in chronic schizophrenia. *Schizophrenia Res* 1990; **3**: 23–4.
13. Cabeza R, Nyberg L. Imaging cognition: an empirical review of PET studies with normal subjects. *J Cogn Neurosci* 1997; **9**: 1–26.
14. Grady CL. Neuroimaging and activation of the frontal lobes. In Miller BL, Cummings JL, eds *The Human Frontal Lobes: Function and Disorders*. New York: Guilford, 1999; 196–230.
15. Grady CL, Craik FIM. Changes in memory processing with age. *Curr Op Neurobiol* 2000; **10**(2): 224–31.
16. Grady CL, Maisog JM, Horwitz B *et al.* Age-related changes in cortical blood flow activation during visual processing of faces and location. *J Neurosci* 1994; **14**: 1450–62.
17. Madden DJ, Turkington TG, Provenzale JM *et al.* Adult age differences in the functional neuroanatomy of verbal recognition memory. *Hum Brain Map* 1999; **7**: 115–35.
18. Friston KJ, Grasby PM, Frith CD *et al.* The neurotransmitter basis of cognition: psychopharmacological activation studies using positron emission tomography. *Ciba Foundation Symposium* 1991; **163**: 76–87, discussion 87–92.
19. Furey ML, Pietrini P, Haxby JV *et al.* Cholinergic stimulation alters performance and task-specific regional cerebral blood flow during working memory. *Proc Natl Acad Sci USA* 1997; **94**: 6512–16.
20. Frackowiak RSJ, Pozzilli C, Legg NJ *et al.* Regional cerebral oxygen supply and utilization in dementia. A clinical and physiological study with oxygen-15 and positron tomography. *Brain* 1981; **104**: 753–78.
21. Foster NL, Chase TN, Mansi L *et al.* Cortical abnormalities in Alzheimer's disease. *Ann Neurol* 1984; **16**: 649–54.
22. Grady CL, Haxby JV, Schapiro MB *et al.* Subgroups in dementia of the Alzheimer type identified using positron emission tomography. *J Neuropsychiat Clin Neurosci* 1990; **2**: 373–84.
23. Grady CL, Haxby JV, Horwitz B *et al.* Longitudinal study of the early neuropsychological and cerebral metabolic changes in dementia of the Alzheimer type. *J Clin Exp Neuropsychol* 1988; **10**: 576–96.
24. Kennedy AM, Frackowiak RS, Newman SK, *et al.* Deficits in cerebral glucose metabolism demonstrated by positron emission tomography in individuals at risk of familial Alzheimer's disease. *Neurosci Lett* 1995; **186**: 17–20.
25. Small GW, Mazziotta JC, Collins MT *et al.* Apolipoprotein E type 4 allele and cerebral glucose metabolism in relatives at risk for familial Alzheimer disease. *J Am Med Assoc* 1995; **273**(12): 942–7.
26. Becker JT, Mintun MA, Aleva K *et al.* Compensatory reallocation of brain resources supporting verbal episodic memory in Alzheimer's disease. *Neurology* 1996; **46**: 692–700.
27. Woodard JL, Grafton ST, Votaw JR *et al.* Compensatory recruitment of neural resources during overt rehearsal of word lists in Alzheimer's disease. *Neuropsychology* 1998; **12**: 491–504.
28. Horwitz B, McIntosh AR, Haxby JV *et al.* Network analysis of PET-mapped visual pathways in Alzheimer type dementia. *NeuroReport* 1995; **6**: 2287–92.
29. Andrews TC, Brooks DJ. Advances in the understanding of early Huntington's disease using the functional imaging techniques of PET and SPET. *Mol Med Today* 1998; **4**(12): 532–9.

30. Hayden MR, Hewitt J, Stoessl AJ *et al*. The combined use of positron emission tomography and DNA polymorphisms for preclinical detection of Huntington's disease. *Neurology* 1987; **37**(9): 1441–7.

31. Lawrence AD, Weeks RA, Brooks DJ *et al*. The relationship between striatal dopamine receptor binding and cognitive performance in Huntington's disease. *Brain* 1998; **121**: 1343–55.

32. Mazziotta JC, Phelps ME, Pahl JJ *et al*. Reduced cerebral glucose metabolism in asymptomatic subjects at risk for Huntington's disease. *N Engl J Med* 1987; **316**(7): 357–62.

33. Kremer B, Clark CM, Almqvist EW *et al*. Influence of lamotrigine on progression of early Huntington disease: a randomized clinical trial. *Neurology* 1999; **53**(5): 1000–11.

34. Bartenstein P, Weindl A, Spiegel S *et al*. Central motor processing in Huntington's disease. A PET study. *Brain* 1997; **120**: 1553–67.

35. Weeks RA, Ceballos-Baumann AO, Piccini P *et al*. Cortical control of movement in Huntington's disease. A PET activation study. *Brain* 1997; **120**: 1569–78.

36. Soares JC, Mann JJ. The functional neuroanatomy of mood disorders. *J Psychiat Res* 1997; **31**(4): 393–432.

37. Mayberg HS. Limbic-cortical dysregulation: a proposed model of depression. *J Neuropsychiatr Clin Neurosci* 1997; **9**: 471–81.

38. Kumar A, Newberg A, Alavi A *et al*. Regional cerebral glucose metabolism in late-life depression and Alzheimer disease: a preliminary positron emission tomography study. *Proc Natl Acad Sci USA* 1993; **90**(15): 7019–23.

39. Nobler MS, Mann JJ, Sackeim HA. Serotonin, cerebral blood flow, and cerebral metabolic rate in geriatric major depression and normal aging. *Brain Res–Brain Res Rev* 1999; **30**(3): 250–63.

40. Biver F, Wikler D, Lotstra F *et al*. Serotonin 5-HT$_2$ receptor imaging in major depression: focal changes in orbito-insular cortex. *Br J Psychiat* 1997; **171**: 444–8.

41. Meyer JH, Kapur S, Houle S *et al*. Prefrontal cortex 5-HT$_2$ receptors in depression: an [18F]setoperone PET imaging study. *Am J Psychiat* 1999; **156**(7): 1029–34.

42. Meltzer CC, Smith G, Price JC *et al*. Reduced binding of [18F]altanserin to serotonin type 2A receptors in aging: persistence of effect after partial volume correction. *Brain Res* 1998; **813**(1): 167–71.

43. Meltzer CC, Price JC, Mathis CA *et al*. PET imaging of serotonin type 2A receptors in late-life neuropsychiatric disorders. *Am J Psychiat* 1999; **156**(12): 1871–8.

67

Single-photon Emission Computerized Tomography (SPECT)

Mohammed T. Abou-Saleh[1] and D. P. Geaney[2]

[1]*St George's Hospital Medical School, London, UK, and* [2]*Warneford Hospital, Oxford, UK*

The introduction of single-photon emission computed tomography (SPECT) has markedly enhanced the study of brain function. The development of SPECT was the culmination of a series of investigations of cerebral blood flow (CBF) pioneered by Kety and Schmidt[1] in the late 1940s, combined with the introduction of transmission computed tomography (CT) in the early 1960s, in which three-dimensional images are derived from two-dimensional data. This chapter provides a review of the principles and basic techniques of SPECT, its present utility and application to clinical practice.

PRINCIPLES AND TECHNIQUES

Kety and Schmidt[1] pioneered CBF studies in man using nitrous oxide as a diffusible agent. These early studies required inhalation of nitrous oxide and sampling of arterial and internal jugular venous blood and could only provide a measure of whole-brain blood flow. Techniques to measure regional rCBF followed and used freely diffusible radionuclides, such as [85]krypton and [133]xenon, which were injected into the carotid artery[2]. [133]Xenon emits γ-radiation, which can be detected through the intact skull, and multiple scintillation probes allow the measurement of CBF in specific regions of the brain. Further technological advances in detector sensitivity and data analysis allowed the replacement of intra-arterial injections by intravenous infusions or inhalation of gaseous ^{133}Xe, so that the measurement of rCBF became a non-invasive procedure. The rCBF data were initially presented in two dimensions and essentially reflected cortical flow, but with the development of the tomographic technology for SPECT, a three-dimensional measurement of rCBF could be obtained. The radiotracers used in SPECT emit a single γ-ray (or photon), as opposed to the dual simultaneous γ-rays of PET radiotracers, and hence the term "single-photon".

Recently, new radiotracers labelled with [123]iodine and [99m]technetium have been introduced. These lipophilic radiopharmaceuticals cross the blood–brain barrier and distribute in proportion to the rCBF shortly after intravenous injection. They are trapped in the brain and have a stable or static distribution over time, unlike freely diffusible, dynamic radiotracers such as ^{133}Xe, enabling images of higher resolution to be obtained. These agents can be used with the conventional rotating γ-cameras that are widely available in most nuclear medicine departments, whereas ^{133}Xe-labelled agents are not. The most advanced SPECT systems are now capable of a resolution of 8 mm and imaging times as short as 2–3 min for rCBF.

Unlike PET, there is no current prospect of SPECT being able to provide a direct measure of regional cerebral metabolism. However its use to measure neurotransmitter receptors is an evolving technique. The radioligand ^{123}I,3, quinuclidinyl 4-iodobenzilate (QNB) has been developed for the measurement of muscarinic acetylocholine receptors and has been applied to the study of Alzheimer's disease[3].

NORMAL SUBJECTS AND NORMAL AGEING

Dynamic tomographic studies with ^{133}Xe produce similar values for grey matter flows as found with PET, but substantially overestimate white-matter rCBF and consequently give a limited distinction between grey and white matter. Static tomographic studies with [123]I- and ^{99m}Tc-labelled radiotracers cannot, as yet, provide an absolute measure of rCBF, but the pattern of rCBF, which can be expressed semiquantitatively, is similar to that found in PET studies, and the resolution is better than with ^{133}Xe dynamic tomographic studies.

The pattern of rCBF reported in normal subjects reflects, at least in part, the conditions of the subjects at the time. For example, if subjects are studied with eyes open, the visual cortex has the highest individual rCBF, but if the eyes are closed, the rCBF is reduced[4]. At present there are no generally accepted standard conditions for the control or resting state but it is clear that these should be standardized in any individual study.

CBF is reduced in relation to both advancing age and progressive cerebrovascular disease, and hypertension is the most important predisposing factor for a significant reduction in CBF.

The reduction in rCBF with age is confined to the grey matter—the white matter is unaffected and is more marked in anterior cortical regions. Females have higher rCBF than males for subjects up to 60 years of age, but the difference lessens above this age.

In the normal individual at rest, the rCBF is closely coupled to the regional metabolism of glucose and oxygen and is felt to reflect the underlying cerebral function. PET studies have shown that during visual stimulation, the rCBF and metabolic rate of glucose have similar marked focal increases in the visual cortex, while the regional cerebral metabolic rate of oxygen has a much smaller increase[5]. This uncoupling of glucose uptake and oxygen metabolism suggests that most of the extra glucose taken up during physiological stimulation is not oxidized and presumably lactate production by glycolysis increases. The implication of

Principles and Practice of Geriatric Psychiatry, 2nd edn. Edited by J. R. M. Copeland, M. T. Abou-Saleh and D. G. Blazer

these findings is that in normal resting individuals, rCBF and the regional cerebral metabolic rate of oxygen or glucose will provide similar information about the underlying cerebral function, but when physiologically (or perhaps pharmacologically) stimulated, they may convey information about different aspects of cerebral function, with none being an index of cerebral function. Similarly, in pathological cerebral conditions, close coupling of rCBF and the cerebral metabolic rates of glucose and oxygen cannot automatically be presumed to be retained.

STUDIES IN DEMENTIA

In addition to the effects of normal ageing, functional imaging studies in dementia have three further problems: (a) the normal variation in measures of cerebral blood flow or metabolism; (b) uncertainty of diagnosis of type of dementia (e.g. Alzheimer's disease (AD) or multi-infarct dementia (MID))—AD accounts for over 50% of cases, and can only be diagnosed definitively by cerebral biopsy or at autopsy; (c) the presence of cerebral atrophy. However, some demented individuals have little atrophy, while some normal subjects show considerable atrophy. Consequently, areas of apparently reduced rCBF in patients with dementia may be due to reduced flow to a normal volume of brain, normal flow to a reduced volume of brain or reduced flow to a reduced volume of brain.

The studies by Kety and Schmidt[1] indicated lower rates of mean CBF in patients with dementia than in normal subjects, and most subsequent studies have confirmed these findings. Whole-brain studies have suggested that coupling between CBF and the cerebral metabolic rates of oxygen and glucose is present in the later stages of dementia, and although the link between CBF and the metabolic rate of oxygen is apparent in the early stages also, the metabolic rate of glucose is dissociated from these, such that it is relatively decreased in AD but increased in MID[6].

The use of SPECT to study dementia has been reported since the mid-1980s. Using the ^{133}Xe inhalation technique, Bonte et al.[7] found that out of 24 patients with probable AD, 19 had perfusion deficits, which were most commonly found in the parietotemporal flow, but instead had a patchy distribution pattern. However, ^{133}Xe SPECT involves measuring temporal variations in activity and is only possible with purpose-built equipment. The image characteristics are relatively poor because of scatter of the low-energy γ-rays and low counts obtained over the brief scanning periods.

The radiopharmaceutical ^{123}I-iodoamphetamine (IMP) does not present these technical problems and its initial cerebral uptake is proportional to rCBF. It was the first tracer to be

Table 67.1 ^{99m}Tc-HMPAO SPECT studies in dementia

Study	Patients (n)	Normal controls	Diagnosis	Assessment of images	Results
Neary et al. (1987)[11]	AD (23) FLD (9) PSP (9)	None	Clinical, NINCDS–ADRDA, CT scan	Qualitative	AD: posterior Cr Cerebral abnormalities, FLD and PSP anterior Cr abnormalities
Perani et al. (1988)[25]	AD (16) early	16	NINCDS–ADRDA, CT scan/MRI neuropsychology	Semiquantitative ratio of ratio of ROI to cerebellum	Decreased rCBF in frontal and temporo-parietal areas, hemisphere asymmetry
Burns et al. (1989)[26]	AD (20)	6	NINCDS–ADRDA, CT scan, psychometry	Semiquantitative ratio of ROI to cerebellum	Decreased rCBF in temporal and posterior parietal areas, regional rCBF correlations with memory, praxis and language functions
Gemmell et al. (1987)[10]	AD (17) MID (10)	3	DSM-III, Hachinski, MRI	Qualitative	Perfusion defects (temporoparietal occipital) more common in AD than MID, more bilateral defects in AD than MID
Battistin et al. (1989)[27]	AD (21) Mixed (9)	None	DSM-III, CT Scan	Semiquantitative ratio of ROI to cerebellum	Decreased rCBF (parietal) in AD than mixed AD and MID form, few showed right–left asymmetry
Goldenberg et al. (1989)[17]	AD (23)	None	Clinical CT scan neuropsychology tests	Semiquantitative ratio of ROI to all ROIs	Co-variation of neuropsychology test results with frontal inferior parietal and superior temporal regions
Podreka et al. (1987)[28]	Dementia (12)	None	CT scan	Semiquantitative (region/whole brain)	All patients showed perfusion defects
Upadhyaya et al. (1991)[24]	AD (15)	10	NINCDS–ADRDA Geriatric Mental State, CAMCOG	Qualitative, semi-quantitative (ROI/cerebellar)	All AD patients showed perfusion defects Significantly low ratios in parietal, frontal and occipital areas.
Jobst et al. (1998)	Dementia (200) Annual evaluation to necropsy	119	NINCDS-ADRDA DSM-IIIR	Semiquantitative	AD had medial temporal lobe atrophy (CT Scan) and parietotemporal hypo-perfusion. Both markers had better diag-nostic accuracy than NINCDS-ADRDA and DSM-IIIR.
Shih et al. (1999)	AD (18) Repeated 5–23 months	None	MMSE	Semiquantitative	All AD had decreased CBF in consecutive SPECT
Defebvre et al. (1999)	DLB (20) AD (20) PD (20)	None	MMSE	Semiquantitative	DLB: frontal CBF lower than AD
Mullet et al. (1999)	AD (116)	20	DSM-IIIR MMSE	Semiquantitative	3 regions with decreased CBF AD: 48% Controls: 10%

widely used in static SPECT studies of dementia. These have generally reported that patients with AD have deficits in flow which are maximal bilaterally in the parietotemporal cortex, while patients with MID vary from having a normal pattern to marked asymmetrical focal deficits anywhere in the cortex. Sharp et al.[8] found that, despite having characteristic regional abnormalities on SPECT, the majority of patients with AD had a normal appearance in those regions on magnetic resonance imaging (MRI). Ebmeier et al.[9] found that while MRI was not able to differentiate between AD and MID, 19 out of 21 patients showed bilateral deficits on IMP SPECT scans. Although the distribution of ^{123}I-IMP initially reflects the rCBF, redistribution of the tracer occurs approximately 1 h after injection. The use of ^{123}I-IMP is also limited by the restricted availability of ^{123}I, which has a half-life of 13 h, and is costly to produce, as this requires a cyclotron.

^{99m}Tc-HMPAO SPECT

[99m]Technetium is readily available from commercial generators in nuclear medicine departments, is inexpensive and has a shorter half-life (6 h) and better dosimetry than [123]I. Labelling with ^{99m}Tc is a much more complex procedure than with ^{123}I and the development of a ^{99m}Tc-labelled compound to provide a measure of rCBF was a major advance in SPECT technology. Technetium-labelled hexamethyl propylenaemine oxime (HMPAO) is a lipophilic tracer which, after intravenous administration, crosses the blood–brain barrier with high extraction and is retained in the brain in hydrophilic form. The brain uptake occurs over the first 2 min and has a stable distribution for many hours. This enables conventional equipment to be used to detect the radiation emitted from the brain. Comparative studies with PET in humans reveal a tendency to underestimate flow in areas of high rCBF but a good correlation with areas of low and medium rCBF. Although ^{99m}Tc-HMPAO cannot, at present, be used to quantify rCBF absolutely, the results can be expressed semi-quantitatively by comparing the counts in each brain region of interest (ROI) to a reference area, such as the whole brain or cerebellum.

A number of SPECT studies have now been performed using ^{99m}Tc-HMPAO to investigate dementia and the characteristics of these are shown in Table 67.1. The studies varied in the populations studied, diagnostic criteria used and the methods of assessment of images. Some of these studies had no data on control subjects for comparison. The majority carried out initial screening with CT or MRI to exclude structural lesions.

The early studies used qualitative assessment of the images and found that most patients with AD had bilateral parietotemporal deficits; those who did not tended to be less impaired cognitively[10].

Frontal deficits were also seen in AD. Deficits were less common in MID than AD, particularly when known infarcts on MRI were excluded, and they occurred in a more variable and asymmetrical pattern. Neary et al.[11] also investigated patients with progressive supranuclear palsy (PSP) and others with the clinical syndrome of dementia of frontal-lobe type, which is consistent with, although not necessarily diagnostic of, Pick's disease.

The later studies have generally been semi-quantitative. When a rotating γ-camera has been used, the whole brain is scanned and the cerebellum has usually been chosen as the reference area, as it is relatively unaffected by the pathology of AD[12]. Also, patients with AD have a normal cerebellar metabolic rate of glucose, compared with elderly controls, on PET study[13]. A recent study validated the use of the cerebellum as a reference region for SPECT quantification in patients with AD[14]. Studies using dedicated head scanners, which acquire their data in the form of transverse tomographic slices, have not usually obtained cerebellar data, so they have used the occipital region as a reference area because the latter also appears relatively unaffected by AD[15].

These studies have consistently found that patients with AD have a bilateral decrease in rCBF in the posterior temporal and parietal regions, adjacent to the occipital lobe, and sometimes the frontal lobes are affected, although the basal ganglia are not (Table 67.1). Several studies have demonstrated correlations in AD between rCBF and neuropsychological function, and these have tended to be more apparent for language, praxis and global function than for memory[15,19]. Recent studies of AD have also evaluated the correlates of changes in CBF in relation to psychopathology and behaviour disturbance. Reduced frontal CBF in AD is associated with negative symptoms[20], with presence of delusions[24], disinhibited behaviour, apathy and blunted affect[22].

Pharmacological activation studies of the effect of central cholinergic stimulation upon rCBF in AD have recently been reported. These require paired SPECT studies, basal (after saline infusion) and activated (after infusion of a cholinergic agent, e.g. physostigmine). In patients with AD, the reduced rCBF in the posterior parietotemporal region in the basal scan was focally increased in the scan after the cholinergic agent, which did not occur in control subjects[19]. AD is associated with striking abnormalities in the central cholinergic system, of a functional cholinergic deficit that is at least partly reversible. Also a SPECT study of nootropic drugs showed regional improvement in CBF[23]. Donepezil treatment in AD was associated with a significant increase in CBF in the frontal lobes[24].

Studies have also addressed the diagnostic value of SPECT in differentiating AD from other types of dementia. Dementia with Lewy bodies (DLB) is associated with reduced frontal CBF than AD[25]. Importantly DLB is associated with severe degeneration of the dopamine system as shown by a recent SPECT study[26]. Primary progressive aphasia is associated with reduced CBF in fronto-temporal regions[27]. Fronto-temporal dementia FTD is characteristically associated with reduced CBF in fronto-temporal regions[28]. Alzheimer's disease and FTD could be differentiated by discriminant analysis applied to 99m Tc-HMPAO SPECT data with 100% correct classification of patients with FTD and 90% correct clarification of patients with AD[29].

Moreover fronto-temporal dementia is characterized by early non-cognitive behavioural changes with relatively spared cognitive function, frontal atrophy and SPECT deficits in CBF in frontal and temporal regions whilst AD is associated with early cognitive changes and medial temporal and parietal-temporal deficits in CBF[38].

Patients with Korsakoff's psychosis, in contrast to patients with AD, have normal rCBF in the posterior temporal region.

It is well established that Parkinson's disease (PD) is characterized by degeneration of dopaminergic neurons in the substantia nigra, which project to the corpus striatum. In an HMPAO SPECT study, 36 patients with PD were found, overall, to have normal rCBF in the caudate and putamen; however, those on no therapy had lower rCBF, and those on L-dopa-replacement therapy had higher rCBF, in the caudate and putamen, than controls. Bilateral reductions in rCBF in the parietal region, similar to those found in AD, were also found in patients with PD. No patients had focal lesions on CT scans. Interestingly, the parietal reductions in rCBF were more pronounced in those PD patients with cognitive impairment and those receiving chronic anticholinergic therapy. Dopamine deficiency is the main, but not the only, neurochemical deficit in PD, and these SPECT findings are consistent with the concept that AD and PD may overlap to some extent. Patients with Huntington's Disease (HD), characterized by chorea and progressive dementia, have reduced rCBF in the caudate nucleus, matched by caudate atrophy on MRI. However, the size of the rCBF deficit in the SPECT study exceeded that predicted by the MRI findings[39].

There has been a case report of a patient with pathologically proven Creutzfeldt–Jakob disease, who had strikingly reduced rCBF throughout the cortex on HMPAO SPECT study, but a normal CT scan[40]. Patients with the AIDS dementia complex have been found, using SPECT, to have multiple or focal rCBF deficits, correlating with focal signs or symptoms, while CT scans showed diffuse cerebral atrophy[41].

DISCUSSION

Studies employing SPECT and PET can reveal cerebral abnormalities when CT and MRI do not, because the latter are measures of cerebral structure, while the former are measures of cerebral function. SPECT is, and is likely to remain, much more generally available than PET, but it is not currently capable of absolute quantification.

The characteristic SPECT findings in AD are bilaterally decreased rCBF in the parietal and temporal lobes adjacent to the occipital lobes, sometimes involving the frontal lobes, particularly in later cases. The primary motor, sensory and visual cortices and basal ganglia are relatively unaffected. This contrasts with typical CT findings of diffuse cerebral atrophy, although the CT scans have not generally been orientated along an axis that obtains optimum views of any focal atrophy in the hippocampus and temporal lobe[42]. However the Oxford Project to Investigate Memory and Aging (OPTIMA), which involved 200 patients with dementia and 119 normal controls evaluated annually till necropsy showed that medial temporal lobe atrophy (CT Scan), (80% diagnostic accuracy) and parietotemporal hypoperfusion by SPECT (83%) predicted the pathology of AD better than the established clinical criteria of NINCDS-ADRDA (66%) and DSM-IIIR (66%)[35]. On careful assessment, focal features can be seen on CT scans which correlate with individual symptoms, such as aggression or wandering[43], but the extent of the focal CT abnormalities is less than that seen on SPECT, and it appears that structural atrophy lags behind clinical deficit.

The diagnosis of dementia and its differentiation from other clinical syndromes, such as depression, is still primarily a clinical matter. If a structural lesion, such as a cerebral tumour, is suspected, then a structural scan, such as CT, is likely to be the best test for this. What, then, is the appropriate role of SPECT in current clinical practice in the assessment of dementia? The study by Upadhyaya et al.[34] suggests that it would be unwise to expect SPECT to assist in the differentiation of dementia from depression in the elderly because similar, albeit less marked, changes are seen in depression, as in AD. It would be interesting to know if those elderly individuals who present with the clinical syndrome of depression, and who have the characteristic AD abnormalities on SPECT, have a worse prognosis than those with normal SPECT scans. They might be individuals at risk of developing AD where depression has been one of the early clinical features, but much more information, including follow-up studies, is needed on this patient group to evaluate the utility of SPECT. More information is also needed on the frequency with which perfusion deficits (particularly those with a pattern similar to that in AD) are seen on visual inspection of SPECT studies in healthy, elderly controls. Patients with PD, particularly those who are cognitively impaired or receiving chronic anticholinergic treatment, also have similar SPECT abnormalities to patients with AD. Perhaps it is not surprising that there may be similarities on this measure of brain function, as there can be a degree of overlap of the clinical syndromes.

If the clinical diagnosis of dementia is made in an individual patient and it appears to be a primary degenerative dementia, the SPECT study can add weight to the clinical impression that the underlying diagnosis is that of AD, frontal lobe dementia (FLD) or progressive supranuclear palsy (PSP). AD is most characteristically associated with posterior rCBF deficits, while FLD and PSP are strongly associated with anterior rCBF deficits and

themselves have distinctive patterns when CT scans are not particularly helpful in this situation. Similarly, Korsakoff's psychosis appears to be more characteristically associated with frontal rCBF deficits than posterior temporal deficits[17]. SPECT can also assist the clinical assessment in the differentiation of AD from MID: bilateral parietotemporal deficits are strongly suggestive (but not diagnostic) of AD, although it must be remembered that AD and MID coexist in a substantial minority of cases. There is no particular single pattern of rCBF deficits seen in MID. SPECT findings vary from normal to asymmetrical deficits and theoretically MID could mimic any other pattern. However, if an asymmetrical pattern is found affecting areas other than the parietotemporal region, it is suggestive of MID. This impression is strengthened if the rCBF deficits coincide with cerebral infarcts seen on structural imaging with CT or MRI. If a patient with relatively advanced dementia has a normal SPECT, it is unlikely to be AD and may be consistent with MID.

All these conclusions, however, must be tempered by the knowledge that our present association of SPECT and PET patterns with specific conditions is based on studies where clinical diagnoses of patients are made initially and are then correlated with the SPECT findings. We need follow-up studies and pathological findings at post mortem to make more definitive assessments of the significance of specific SPECT patterns. Indeed a recent study evaluated early AD (mild cognitive impairment) using brain perfusion SPECT who were diagnosed to have AD 2 years later with a follow-up SPECT[44]. Selective reduction in CBF was observed in the left hippocampus and parahippocampal gyrus in the follow-up SPECT. We could also learn whether SPECT studies can help predict clinical outcome in individual cases. There is evidence from PET studies of patients with early AD that focal cortical reductions in glucose metabolism precede the appearance of focal neuropsychological deficits.

However, if the early whole-brain studies are correct and the metabolic rate of glucose is uncoupled from CBF in early AD, such that it is decreased relative to CBF and the rCBF is reduced later in the course of the disease, SPECT might have different predictive power in comparison with PET in early AD. It is possible that patients at risk for HD may be diagnosed in the presymptomatic phase by the SPECT finding of reduced rCBF in the caudate nucleus.

It is clear that SPECT will be used substantially in further research in AD. More significant advances in our knowledge of AD are likely to come from follow-up and activation studies. The latter would involve paired SPECT studies, basal and activated, and the activation could be cognitive or pharmacological. For paired studies, the important measure is the difference in rCBF between the two SPECT studies, which indicates the effect of activation. This avoids the problem of variation in basal values between individuals and the problem of the effect of an uncertain degree of cerebral atrophy upon rCBF. The semi-quantitative measures of SPECT are adequate, and may be preferable, for this analysis. Cognitive activation studies in controls and in patients with AD would provide a better understanding of the cerebral processes involved in cognitive function in normal individuals, and knowledge about the form of disruption of these processes in disease. Pharmacological activation studies would enable direct measures of specific neurotransmitter function to be made and hence the pharmacological characterization of disease in an individual, with implications for treatment and prognosis[19].

Another promising direction for SPECT is the study of neurotransmitter receptors. The radioligand ^{123}I-QNB has been developed for the measurement of muscarinic cholinergic receptors and it has been used in the study of AD[3]. Currently it requires a radiochemist on site to produce ^{123}I-QNB, and so it is not commercially available, but the development of radioligands for general use in receptor studies is likely to continue and may further extend the role of SPECT.

REFERENCES

1. Kety S, Schmidt C. The nitrous oxide method for quantitative determination of cerebral blood flow in man: theory, procedure, and normal values. *J Clin Invest* 1948; **27**: 475–83.

2. Lassen N, Ingvar D. Regional cerebral blood flow measurement in man: a review. *Arch Neurol* 1963; **9**: 615–22.

3. Holman B, Gibson R, Hill T *et al*. Muscarinic acetylcholine receptors in Alzheimer's disease: *in vivo* imaging with iodine 123-labelled 3-quinuclidinyl-4-iodobenzilate and emission tomography. *J Am Med Ass* 1985; **254**: 3063–6.

4. Devous M. Imaging brain function by single-photon emission computer tomography. In Andreasen N, ed., *Brain Imaging: Applications in Psychiatry*. Washington, DC: American Psychiatric Press, 147–234.

5. Fox P, Raichle M, Mintum M *et al*. Nonoxidative glucose consumption during focal physiological neural activity. *Science* 1988; **241**: 462–4.

6. Hoyer S. The abnormally aged brain. Its blood flow and oxidative metabolism. A review—part 11. *Arch Gerontol Geriatr* 1982; **1**: 195–207.

7. Bonte F, Ross E, Chehabi H *et al*. SPECT study of regional cerebral blood flow in Alzheimer's disease. *J Comp Assist Tomogr* 1986; **10**: 579–83.

8. Sharp P, Gemmell H, Cherryman G *et al*. Application of iodine-123-labelled isopropylamphetamine imaging to the study of dementia. *J Nucl Med* 1986; **27**: 761–8.

9. Ebmeier K, Besson J, Crawford J *et al*. Nuclear magnetic resonance imaging and single photon emission tomography with radio-iodine labelled compounds in the diagnosis of dementia. *Acta Psychiat Scand* 1987; **75**: 549–56.

10. Gemmell H, Sharp P, Besson J *et al*. Differential diagnosis in dementia using the cerebral blood flow agent ⁹⁹ᵐTc-HMPAO: a SPECT study. *J Cerebr Blood Flow Metab* 1987; **11**: 398–402.

11. Neary D, Snowden J, Shields R *et al*. Single photon emission tomography using ⁹⁹ᵐTc-HMPAO in the investigation of dementia. *J Neurol Neurosurg Psychiat* 1987; **50**: 1101–9.

12. Pearson R, Powell T. The neuroanatomy of Alzheimer's disease. *Rev Neurosci* 1989; **2**: 101–22.

13. Kushner M, Tobin M, Alavi A *et al*. Cerebellar glucose consumption in normal and pathologic states using fluorine-FDG and PET. *J Nucl Med* 1987; **28**: 1667–70.

14. Pickutt NA, Dierckx RA, Dobbeleir A, Audenaert K, Van Laere K, Vervaet A, De Deyn PP. Validation of the cerebellum as a reference region for SPECT quantification in patients suffering from dementia of the Alzheimer type. *Psychiatry Res* 1999; **90**: 103–12.

15. Montaldi D, Brooks D, McColl J *et al*. Measurements of regional cerebral blood flow and cognitive performance in Alzheimer's disease. *J Neurol Neurosurg Psychiat* 1990; **53**: 33–8.

16. Burns A, Philpot A, Costa D *et al*. The investigation of Alzheimer's disease with single photon emission tomography. *J Neurol Neurosurg Psychiat* 1989; **52**: 248–53.

17. Hunter R, McLuskie R, Wyper D *et al*. The pattern of function-related regional cerebral blood flow investigated by single photon emission tomography with ⁹⁹ᵐTc-HMPAO in patients with presenile Alzheimer's disease and Korsakoff's psychosis. *Psychol Med* 1989; **19**: 847–55.

18. Goldenberg G, Podreka I, Suess E *et al*. The cerebral localisation of neuropsychological impairment in Alzheimer's disease: a SPECT study. *J Neurol* 1989; **236**: 131–8.

19. Geaney D, Soper N, Shepstone B *et al*. Effect of central cholinergic stimulation on regional cerebral blood flow in Alzheimer disease. *Lancet* 1990; **335**: 1484–7.

20. Galynker II, Dutta E, Vilkas N, Ongseng F, Finestone H, Gallagjher R, Serseni D, Rosenthal RN. Hypofrontality and negative symptoms in patients with dementia of Alzheimer type. *Neuropsychiatry Neuropsychol Behav Neurol* 2000; **13**: 53–9.

21. Staff RT, Shanks MF, Macintosh L, Pestell SJ, Gemmell HG, Venneri A. Delusions in Alzheimer's disease: spet evidence of right hemispheric dysfunction. *Cortex* 1999; **35**: 549–60.

22. Sultzer DL. Behavioural Syndrome in Dementia: Neuroimaging Insights. *Semin Clin Neuropsychiatry* 1996; **1**: 261–71.

23. Dormehl IC, Jordaan B, Oliver DW, Croft S. SPECT monitoring of improved cerebral blood flow during long-term treatment of elderly patients with nootropic drugs. *Clin Nucl Med* 1999; **24**: 39–34.

24. Staff RT, Gemmell GH, Shanks MF, Murray AD, Venneri A. Changes in the Rcbf images of patients with Alzheimer's disease receiving Donepezil therapy. *Nucl Med Commun* 2000; **21**: 37–41.

25. Defebvre LJ, Leduc V, Duhamel A, Lecouffe P, Pasquier F, Lamy-Lhullier C, Steinling M, Destee A. Technetium HMPAO SPECT study in dementia with Lewy bodies, Alzheimer's disease and idiopathic Parkinson's disease. *J Nucl Med* 1999; **40**: 956–62.

26. Walker Z, Costa DC, Ince P, McKeith IG, Katona CL. In-vivo demonstration of dopaminergic degeneration in dementia with Lewy bodies. *Lancet* 1999; **354**: 646–7.

27. San Pedro EC, Deutsch G, Liu HG, Mountz JM. Frontotemporal decreases in Rcbf correlate with degree of dysnomia in primary progressive aphasia. *J Nucl Med* 2000; **41**: 228–33.

28. Miller BL, Geerhart R. Neuroimaging in the diagnosis of frontotemporal dementia. *Dement Geriaty Cogn Disord* 1999; **10** Suppl 1: 71–4.

29. Charpentier P, Laveny I, Defebvre L, Durhamel A, Lecouffe P, Pasquier F, Steinling M. Alzheimer's disease and frontotemporal dementia are differentiated by discriminant analysis applied to (99m) Tc HMPAO SPECT data. *J Neurol Neurosurg Psychiatry* 2000; **69**: 661–3.

30. Perani D, Di Piero V, Vallar G *et al*. Technetium-99m-HMPAO-SPECT study of regional cerebral perfusion in early Alzheimer's disease. *J Nucl Med* 1988; **29**: 1507–14.

31. Burns A, Tune L, Steele C *et al*. Positron emission tomography in dementia: a clinical review. *Int J Geriat Psychiat* 1989; **4**: 67–72.

32. Battistin L, Pizzolato G, Dam M *et al*. Single photon emission computed tomography studies with ⁹⁹ᵐTc-hexamethylpropylene-amine oxime in dementia: effects of acute administration of L-acetylcarnitine. *Eur Neurol* 1989; **29**: 261–5.

33. Podreka I, Suess E, Goldenberg G *et al*. Initial experience with technetium-99m HM-PAO brain SPECT. *J Nucl Med* 1987; **28**: 1657–66.

34. Upadhyaya AK, Abou-Saleh MT, Wilson K *et al*. A study of depression in old age using single-photon emission computerised tomography. *Br J Psychiat* 1990; **157**(suppl 9): 76–81.

35. Jobst KA, Barnetson LP, Shepstone BJ. Accurate prediction of histologically confirmed Alzheimer's disease and the differential diagnosis of dementia: the use of NINCDS-ADRDA and DSM-III-R criteria, SPECT, X-ray CT, and Apo E4 in medial temporal lobe dementias. Oxford Project to Investigate Memory and Ageing. *Int Psychogeriatr* 1998; **10**: 271–302.

36. Shih WJ, Ashford JW, Coupal JJ, Ryo YU, Stipp V, Magoun SL, Gross K. Consecutive brain SPECT surface three-dimensional displays show progression of cerebral cortical abnormalities in Alzheimer's disease. *Eur Arch Psychiatry Clin Neurosci* 1999; **249**: 190–6.

37. Muller H, Moller HJ, Stippel A, Fric M, Grunswald F, Laux G, Klemm E, Biersack HJ. SPECT patterns in probable Alzheimer's disease. *Eur Arch Psychiatry Clin Neurosci* 1999; **249**: 190–6.

38. Duara R, Barker W, Luis CA. Frontotemporal dementia and Alzheimer's disease: differential diagnosis. *Dement Geriatr Disord* 1999; **10** Suppl 1: 37–42.

39. Smith F, Besson J, Gemmell H *et al*. The use of technetium-99m-HMPAO in the assessment of patients with dementia and other neuropsychiatric conditions. *J Cerebr Blood Flow Metab* 1988; **8**: S116–22.

40. Hunter R, Gordon A, McLuskie R *et al*. Gross regional cerebral hypofunction with normal CT scan in Creutzfeldt–Jakob disease. *Lancet* 1989; **333**: 214–15.

41. Pohl P, Vogl G, Fill H *et al*. Single photon emission computed tomography in AIDS dementia complex. *J Nucl Med* 1988; **29**: 1382–6.

42. George A, de Leon M, Stylopoulos L *et al*. CT diagnostic features of Alzheimer disease: importance of the choroidal/hippocampal fissure complex. *Am J Neuroradiol* 1990; **11**: 101–7.

43. Burns A, Jacoby R, Levy R. Psychiatric phenomena in Alzheimer's disease. IV: Disorders of behaviour. *Br J Psychiat* 1990; **157**: 86–94.

44. Kogure D, Matusda H, Ohnishi T, Asada T, Uno M, Kunihiro T, Nakano S, Tkasaki M. Longitudinal evaluation of early Alzheimer's disease using brain perfusion SPECT. *J Nucl Med* 2000; **41**: 1155–62.

Part F

Affective Disorders

FI   Nosology and Classification

FII   Depression, Dysthymia, Bereavement
        and Suicidal Behaviour

FIII   Mania

68

Nosology and Classification of Mood Disorders

Dan G. Blazer

Duke University Medical Center, Durham, NC, USA

The mood or affective disorders are a group of disorders characterized by disturbance of mood and accompanied by a partial or complete change in mood or affect that is either manic (or hypomanic) or depressed (or mildly dysphoric). These disorders are classified in both the DSM diagnostic system and the ICD diagnostic system in the three-digit rubic of 296[1,2]. There have been recommendations for changes in the ICD system from ICD-9 to ICD-10 that would reclassify some disorders previously classified elsewhere (such as neurotic depression, 300.4) to the mood or affective disorders. Another minor change in the new ICD diagnostic system (already represented in DSM-IV) is replacing the title "affective disorder" (affective psychosis) with "mood disorder". With some exceptions noted below, the nosology of mood disorders in ICD-10 and DSM-IV is appropriate for the classification of mood disturbances in older adults. The classification of the disorders will therefore be described below, with specific comments related to older adults.

MANIC EPISODE

A manic episode is characterized by an elevated mood that is unrelated to the patient's circumstances. This elevated mood usually varies from an expansive or irritable syndrome to an almost uncontrollable excitement and psychotic agitation. Changes in mood are accompanied by increased energy, a decreased need for sleep, a decline in normal social inhibitions, as well as inflated and grandiose ideas, which frequently become delusional. Older persons can experience a typical episode of mania as well as hypomania (a less severe elevation of mood) but are more likely to suffer a so-called "irritable" or "angry" manic episode. Joviality and elation are replaced by irritability and agitation (as described elsewhere in this text). Nevertheless, older persons who suffer manic episodes usually meet both ICD-I0 and DSM-IV criteria, even when the predominant symptoms are irritability and anger, as other diagnostic criteria are met.

DEPRESSIVE (OR MAJOR DEPRESSIVE) EPISODE

A major depressive episode is characterized by a depressed, disinterested or irritable mood, associated with the loss of interest or pleasure in all or almost all activities, accompanied by a number of other symptoms. These additional symptoms include a reduced capacity for enjoyment, reduced interest in surroundings, difficulty concentrating, lethargy, sleep distur-bances, appetite disturbances, decreased self-esteem and self-confidence, and frequent ideas of guilt or worthlessness. Although older persons are somewhat less likely to report a specific decrease in their mood, they almost always describe a loss of interest in usual activities (anhedonia) in the midst of a major depressive episode. The categories of severe depressive episode in ICD-10 and major depressive episode in DSM-IV are very similar. DSM-IV criteria permit the diagnosis of a minor depressive episode, that is, a depressive episode which fulfills some of the symptom criteria for a major depressive episode and/or dysthymia and which lasts 2 weeks or longer. The more severe consequences of a depressive episode, such as a successful suicide or a retardation that progresses to stupor, would be characteristic of a severe but not a mild depressive episode in ICD-10.

Older persons who suffer a complicated, severe depression are easily diagnosed according to both ICD-10 and DSM-IV criteria. Problems do arise, however, when the episode experienced by older persons is accompanied by a severe medical illness or significant cognitive impairment. The frequency of psychobiologic symptoms in more severe depressions renders the distinction between symptoms of depression and symptoms of physical illness/functional impairment difficult in the midst of a depressed mood associated with medical illness. The current nosology is not helpful in disaggregating mood disorders from either the symptoms of physical illness or normal psychologic reactions to physical illness. Some have suggested that a unique rating for older persons for depression should include a measure of cognitive functioning (but this is yet to be included in any extant diagnostic system). The co-morbidity of depressive symptoms in organic mental disorders such as dementia, Parkinson's disease and stroke renders such an approach potentially useful in improving the current nosology. Major (or severe) depression can be specified as severe, with or without psychotic features in DSM-IV. Psychotic depression is relatively more frequent in the elderly and the recognition of psychotic features may direct the specific therapeutic intervention considered by the clinician.

BIPOLAR AND UNIPOLAR DISORDER

In both ICD-10 and DSM-IV, individuals who present with a history of recurrent mood disorder (at least two), in which mood and activity were profoundly disturbed and at least one of the episodes is manic, are classified as suffering from bipolar mood disorder. Bipolar disorder usually has an early age of onset, although it can have its onset later in life, and the categorization is useful in older as well as younger persons. Bipolar disorders are classified as manic (the individual is currently in a manic episode), depressed (the individual is currently in a depressed episode and has at least one well-authenticated manic episode in the past), or mixed (the individual's current episode involves a full symptomatic picture of both manic and depressed episode, except for the duration requirement of 2 weeks of depressed episodes). Symptoms are often intermixed or rapidly alternating within hours or days in the latter category.

Bipolar II disorder is characterized by at least one hypomanic episode and at least one episode of major depression. These disorders are probably more common among older persons than the more classic bipolar disorder described above. Older persons frequently experience depression and occasionally mania secondary to medical illness or medications, categories which are specified in DSM-IV as mood disorder due to a general medical disorder and substance-induced mood disorder. Common examples of causes of these secondary mood disorders in the elderly include hypothyroidism. Parkinson's disease, chronic obstructive pulmonary disease, various forms of cancer, alcohol, β-adrenergic blockers and L-dopa. Mood disorders with a seasonal pattern are less frequent in the elderly.

Individuals who never experience an episode of mania or hypomania but nevertheless suffer episodes of major depression are generally classified as "single-episode" or "recurrent". Most depressive disorders are recurrent, that is, if an individual (regardless of age) suffers an episode of major depression, the chances are high that he/she will suffer an additional episode at some time in his/her life. Recurrent or persistent depressive episodes are not always easily classified, that is, distinct episodes of major depression followed by distinct episodes of normal functioning may be the exception rather than the rule. For this reason, additional diagnostic categories have been instituted in the nosology to disaggregate the classification of the natural history of depressive episodes. In ICD-10, a category of "recurrent severe depressive disorder" is analogous to the DSM-IV category of "major depression, recurrent". Recurrent mild depressive disorder is categorized in ICD-10 by repeated episodes of depression, the majority of which fulfill the description given for mild depressive episode above. These recurrent mild episodes may or may not be associated with environmental stress and may be either acute or insidious in onset. Recovery is usual, although not always complete.

Cyclothymia is included in both DSM-IV and ICD-10. According to ICD-10, cyclothymia is a persistent instability of mood involving numerous periods of mild depression and mild elation. The instability usually develops early in adult life and pursues a chronic course, although at times mood may be normal and stable for months. Cyclothymia is difficult to establish without a prolonged period of observation or an unusually good account of the subject's past behavior. In DSM-IV, cyclothymia must persist for at least 2 years to be diagnosed and involve numerous hypomanic episodes.

Yet another phenomenon has emerged in the study of the natural history of depression—rapid cycling. Rapid cycling is the occurrence of four or more episodes of depression or mania per year, with either 2 weeks of normal mood between episodes, or a shift directly from mania to depression, or vice versa. Others have classified rapid cycling as involving either mixed mood states, or frequent mood fluctuation without discrete intermorbid periods, or involving 24 or 48-h cycles of mood disturbance. Rapid cycling occurs in persons regardless of age, although there may be some tendency for individuals to decrease their propensity to rapid cycling with increased age. Rapid cycling appears to be more common in individuals with bipolar disorder than unipolar disorder, but it is not limited to individuals with bipolar disorder. Rapid cycling is a specifier of bipolar mood disorder in DSM-IV.

DYSTHYMIA

Dysthymia is a category included in both ICD-10 and DSM-IV. Dysthymia is a chronic depression of mood which does not fulfill the description and guidelines of mild recurrent depressive disorders (in ICD-10) and is characterized by periods of days or weeks at a time when patients feel tired and depressed, where everything is an effort and where nothing is enjoyed. They "brood and complain", sleep badly and feel inadequate, but are usually able to cope with the basic demands of everyday life. This description is similar to the description of dysthymia in DSM-IV, where the essential feature is a chronic disturbance of mood, involving a depressed mood for most of the day and more days than not for at least 2 years (the 2 year minimum duration is not a criterion in ICD-10). In addition, individuals suffering dysthymia suffer many of the symptoms of the more severe depressions, but with less severity, such as poor appetite, insomnia, low energy and low self-esteem. Older persons often meet criteria for a dysthymic disorder when diagnosed with major depression. It is often difficult to determine, however, whether the dysthymic disorder is a separate entity or whether it is part of the same syndrome which "waxes and wanes" in severity. Recent studies have suggested that dysthymic disorder may exist most often in the elderly as an entity not associated with major depression. Dysthymic disorder has usually been equated with depressive neuroses, as described in earlier versions of both the ICD and DSM diagnostic systems, which assumes that the depressed mood results from psychoneurotic and stress-related difficulties.

Yet another category which has been suggested is minor or mild depression. Criteria for minor depression can be found in the appendix of DSM-IV and variants can be found in the Research Diagnostic Criteria and in ICD-10. There is virtually no data to substantiate a specific entity for minor depressions, except that persons who experience minor depression (that is, symptoms less severe than major depression for at least 2 weeks, according to DSM-IV) exhibit a similar risk factor profile and are at much greater risk for developing major depression over time. There have been a number of studies of minor depression (see Chapter 71) among the elderly. The renewed interest in minor depression once again brings the categorical vs. continuum controversy to the forefront in the phenomenology of depression.

ADJUSTMENT DISORDER WITH DEPRESSED MOOD

In the DSM-IV system of classification, an adjustment disorder is a reaction to an identifiable psychosocial stressor that leads to maladaptive reactions, including impairment in occupational functioning and symptoms that are in excess of normal and expected reaction to this stressor. The maladaptive reaction may take many forms and an exaggerated depressed mood is one of the forms.

Symptoms of adjustment disorder with depressed mood include tearfulness and feelings of hopelessness. By definition, the maladaptive reaction can persist no longer than 6 months, does not meet criteria for other disorders and does not represent uncomplicated bereavement. ICD-10 includes the category of adjustment disorder and the clinical form may take the characteristic of a "prolonged depressive reaction", that is, a mild depressive state occurring in response to prolonged exposure to a stressful situation but of a duration not lasting 6 months. The categories of adjustment disorder are therefore very similar for both diagnostic systems. In theory, the stressor may include physical illness and therefore this category is most relevant to depressive episodes in later life. A lack of acceptable longitudinal data on the association of depressive symptoms with physical illness renders it difficult to determine whether older persons do recover from the depressive episode, which often accompanies a physical illness within the 6 months required by the diagnostic category of adjustment disorder.

DEPRESSED MOOD ASSOCIATED WITH DEMENTIA OF THE ALZHEIMER'S TYPE AND VASCULAR DEMENTIA

DSM-IV provides for the classification of dementia of the Alzheimer's type (both early and late onset) as "with depressed mood as well as vascular dementias". The frequency of co-morbid depression and cognitive impairment renders this classification a common one among dementia patients. As the actual pathophysiological and psychopathological relations between depression and cognitive impairment are unclear, the simple recognition of the co-morbidity is sufficient. For example, the depression may be a reaction to cognitive decline or an actual symptom of the underlying disease process, which also causes the cognitive problems. Some recent studies have suggested that a separate category of vascular depression be introduced. This condition is present when individuals meet the criteria for major depression and have MRI-confirmed vascular brain changes. Persons with vascular depression appear to have more symptoms of apathy (perhaps due to disruption of prefrontal systems or their modulating pathways) and may be at increased risk of non-recovery.

CONCLUSION

In general, the current classificatory system of both DSM-IV and ICD-10 work relatively well for classifying older persons suffering from mood disorders. A number of distinct exceptions must be recognized, however. Categories such as dysthymic disorder, adjustment disorder and minor depression in DSM-IV do not appear to be adequate, and therefore more exploration of the ICD-10 construct of mild depression (but possibly not utilizing the specific diagnostic criteria of ICD-10) would appear in order. A major problem with the current classification systems is the inability to take into account co-morbidity, especially co-morbid depression and physical illness. Co-morbid depression and physical illness is a grossly unstudied area, compared to the clinical relevance of the condition. To what extent do our current classification systems accommodate individuals suffering mild or even severe depressive symptoms in the midst of physical illness? In addition, depression is often co-morbid with other psychiatric symptoms, especially anxiety disorders and somatic complaints. Neither ICD-10 nor DSM-IV adequately accommodates the co-morbid psychiatric syndromes that are frequently seen in older adults.

Finally, when classifying mood disorders, many individuals suffer a depressed mood in late life that is not disordered. Uncomplicated bereavement is an expected accompaniment of older persons who experience a significant loss in old age. In addition, other older persons may become demoralized, given the current circumstances in their lives. Such persons should not be classified in a disease-orientated classification system. Nevertheless, these human experiences are not to be ignored by the clinician working with the older adult suffering a mood disorder.

REFERENCES

1. ICD-10. 1986 Draft of Chapter 5 (Categories FOO-F99). *Mental, Behavioral and Developmental Disorders. Clinical Descriptions and Diagnostic Guidelines.* Geneva: World Health Organization, Division of Mental Health, 1987 (1986 draft for field trials).
2. *Diagnostic and Statistical Manual of Mental Disorders*, 4th edn. Washington, DC: American Psychiatric Association, 1994.
3. Akiskal HS. The clinical management of affective disorders. In Michels R, ed., *Psychiatry*, vol 1. Philadelphia, PA: Lippincott, 1989; chapter 61.
4. Dunner DL, Patrick V, Fieve RR. Rapid cycling in manic depressive patients. *Comp Psychiat* 1977; **18**: 561–6.
5. Berman E, Wolpert EA. Intractable manic-depressive psychosis with rapid cycling in an 18 year-old woman successfully treated with electroconvulsive therapy. *J Nerv Ment Dis* 1987; **175**: 236–9.
6. Wolpert EA, Goldberg JF, Harrow M. Rapid cycling in unipolar and bipolar affective disorders. *Am J Psychiat* 1990; **147**: 725–8.
7. Krishnan KR, Hays JC, George LK, Blazer DG. Six-month outcomes for MRI-related vascular depression. *Depression Anxiety* 1998; **8**: 142–6.

69

Genetics of Affective Disorders

John L. Beyer and David C. Steffens

Duke University Medical Center, Durham, NC, USA

The observation that affective disorders aggregated in families has been present from the time of Socrates, through the analysis of Sigmund Freud, the behavioral work of B. F. Skinner and in the genetic studies of the past 40 years. In each of these views, the family unit recurs as a major focal point in mood disorders. But how is one to understand this relationship? Affective disorders may be aggregated in families for a variety of reasons, such as shared genes, shared culture, shared adversity, or multiple other reasons.

In the past, research in families followed two non-overlapping tracks: genes and environment. This was known popularly as "nature vs. nurture." In recent years, researchers have become more aware that attempts to dichotomize the cause of affective disorders into "genes" and "environment" has hindered understanding of mood disorders. The emerging science of genetic epidemiology focuses on causes, distribution and control of disease in groups of relatives, and with inherited causes of disease in populations[1]. Thus, the goal of genetic research is to identify both genetic and environmental causes of illness. In fact, certain types of genetic studies (e.g. twin studies) have provided some of the strongest evidence that environment plays a significant etiologic role in the expression of mental illness.

Research findings clearly show that the etiology of mood disorders in early and middle adulthood is multifactorial. Both environmental factors (e.g. parental loss, stroke) and genetic factors are strongly implicated, although what occurs and how this happens remain as areas of intense research. In recent years, investigations in late-life affective disorders have asked the same questions regarding cause, but the answers suggest that there are etiologic differences among affective disorders at different ages. This observation only leads to new questions. Is the development of late-life affective disorders related to the genetic make-up of the individual? Are late-life affective disorders a continuation of mood disorders which developed earlier in life or do they represent unique reactions to specific challenges presented by the process of aging? If so, what are these challenges and how are they related to an individual's genetic make-up? How do genetic and environment factors contribute to the understanding of diagnostic subsets of affective disorders?

In this chapter, we will review the current state of genetic research of affective disorders, primarily studied in early and middle life. Then we will contrast that with what is known about affective disorders that have their first onset in late life. Finally, we will discuss the implications of these findings and suggest a theoretic framework to understand genetic and environmental contributions to geriatric affective disorders.

GENETIC INFLUENCES IN AFFECTIVE ILLNESS

There are four types of studies that demonstrate the influence of genetic factors on the development of disease: (a) studies of familial aggregation; (b) twin studies; (c) adoption studies; and (d) association and linkage studies of an illness with a genetic marker.

Family Studies

Family studies are the most basic research form in evaluating genetic risk. They attempt to answer the question, "Does this disorder run in families?" Logically, if genes cause a disorder, then relatives of an individual affected by that disorder (the proband) should be more likely to have that particular disorder than others in the general population, since they share common genes. However, common environmental factors may also contribute to the clustering in families. Therefore, the major goal of family studies is to understand the magnitude and patterns of a disease's aggregation, rather than identify specific genetic causes.

In affective disorders, six landmark studies[2–7] have supported the observation of familial aggregation. First-degree relatives (parents, siblings, offspring) of depressed patients are twice as likely to develop depression than those in the general population. First-degree relatives of bipolar patients are at even greater risk for developing bipolar disorder (incidence of 3.7–17.5%, depending on the study). The risk of bipolar disorder is less in second-degree relatives (grandparents, grandchildren, aunts, uncles) of bipolar patients, although still elevated over the general population.

Twin Studies

Twin and adoption studies are especially helpful in answering the next question, "What are the relative contributions of genes and environment to the development of a mental disorder?" Twins provide a natural experiment in genetics. Monozygotic (MZ) twins, known as identical twins, share 100% of their genes. Dizygotic (DZ) twins, known as fraternal twins, share approximately 50% of their genes, the same proportion as with other siblings. In the "twin experiment", it is assumed that both dizygotic and monozygotic twins share the same environment, but only monozygotic twins share the same genes. Thus, if genes are a putative cause for a disorder, then the MZ co-twin of a proband should be at higher risk to develop a disorder than the DZ co-twin of a proband. This is expressed as the concordance rate.

In affective disorders, the average concordance rate for bipolar disorders in monozygotic twins was 60%, while the concordance rate in dizygotic twins was 12%[8]. The five-fold greater rate of concordance strongly indicates the importance of genetic factors in the familial aggregation. For major depressive disorders, the role of genes is much weaker. Two recent twin studies[9,10] found that the relative risk for monozygotic twins was 1.9, while the risk for dizygotic twins was 1.2. Both findings of heritability were statistically significant.

Adoption Studies

Adoption studies provide a powerful method of evaluating genetic and environmental contributions to the familial aggregation of disease. In these cases, adopted children have a genetic relationship with their biological family, but share the primary environmental relationship with their adopted family. Thus, if genes are responsible for the familial transmission of a disorder, then the risk for the adopted child should more closely match the risk of the biological family. However, if environmental factors are more responsible, the relative risk of the adopted child would match the risk of the adoptive family.

In affective disorders, five studies have reviewed adoption and incidence of affective illnesses[11]. Two of these studies have demonstrated strong genetic influences, while the others show a more variable response. One adoption study[12] suggested certain environmental influences, especially parental loss and parental alcoholism, as predictors of depression.

Genetic Markers and Linkage Studies

The most specific studies for genetic involvement are genetic marker and linkage studies. Genetic markers are specific areas on the chromosome where laboratory procedures may differentiate individuals on the composition of DNA at that location. They are used to identify where a specific gene may be on a chromosome. Linkage refers to the nearness of two or more genes or markers on a chromosome. Linkage studies are based on the principle that as the genetic distance decreases, the probability that they will be inherited increases.

A number of gene loci for affective illness have been proposed through linkage work, but the results have been disappointingly inconsistent, and a number of the most striking findings have proven controversial[13]. One possible exception is a small subset of bipolar disorders that may be X-linked[11,14]. Recent investigations in an ethnically homogeneous American Amish population initially suggested linkage to a marker on chromosome 11[15]. Unfortunately, more recent work has cast doubt on this conclusion[16] and has prompted greater caution generally in the interpretation of the linkage results in psychiatry.

LATE-LIFE AFFECTIVE DISORDERS

Just as affective disorders in early and middle life are quite heterogeneous, late-life mood disorders are also a heterogeneous entity. However, it is unclear whether late-life affective disorders comprise the same notions of heterogeneity as those in early and middle life. In late-life mood disorders, two groups of patients are usually differentiated: those who had an early-onset of illness and continue to have symptoms or episodes in their later life, and those who had a late-onset of illness (usually defined as a first onset after the age of 60 years).

Mendlewicz[17] and other researchers have suggested that the age of onset is an important clinical variable in the genetic study of affective illness. When differentiated by age of onset, late-onset depressive disorders have qualities that suggest they may be genetically different from early-onset forms. These characteristics include the non-conformity of affective disorders to expected genetic models and clinical differences observed between late- and early-onset depression.

Most genetic models propose that strong genetic influences are most often found in the most severe forms of an illness and in the early expressions of the illness. However, late-onset affective illness syndromes are typically among the severest and most refractory to treatment[18,19]. Older patients with affective disorders who require hospitalization tend to have a slower resolution of symptoms and a longer duration of hospitalization than younger adult patients[20]. Further, patients with late-onset depression and bipolar disorders have less familial aggregation of mood disorders than those with the early-onset affective disorders. This finding has been extensively validated in many studies[21–26]. Late-onset mood disorders are also less likely to display the gender disparity[21] present in early-onset mood disorders.

Clinically, patients with late-onset mood disorders tend to have increased impairment on neuropsychological testing and higher rates of incident dementia noted at follow-up[27]. While inadequate support appears particularly difficult among middle-aged patients, stressful life events appear to pose the greater risk of poor outcomes among geriatric patients[28].

Gatz et al.[29] studied the characteristics of depression in a sample of elderly reared-apart and reared-together Swedish twins. They found evidence of only limited heritability (16%). In contrast a study[30] of a sample of Danish twins 75 years of age and older found that depression symptomatology is moderately heritable in late life (approximately 35%). However, both studies consistently implicated environmental factors as the major source of variance in depression symptoms among the elderly.

GENETICS OF LATE-LIFE AFFECTIVE DISORDERS

How can one understand the differences noted above, and how are they important for the genetic study of late-life mood disorders? Two explanations have been proposed for the age-related variation in genetic influence for affective illnesses: multifactorial inheritance and increased phenocopy expression with age. Multifactorial inheritance (also called polygenic inheritance) suggests that inheritance patterns are a result of a combination between multiple interacting genes and environmental factors. Examples of traits that have multifactorial inheritance include stature, intelligence and blood pressure[17].

According to the multifactorial theory, the onset of an affective disorder results from the additive effects of several genetic and environment factors. This concept is graphically illustrated in Figure 69.1. The horizontal axis represents the level of genetic predisposition, while the vertical axis represents the level of environmental risk. Thus, the more factors present (the number of implicated genes or environmental events that contribute to an affective illness), the more likely an individual would develop an affective illness and the more severe that illness would be. One could also assume that early-onset illnesses probably result from greater genetic loading, while late-onset illnesses may have less genetic loading but increased occurrence of environmental events with age.

The second explanation, increased phenocopies, illustrates the limited specificity of the affective disorders diagnosis. Both bipolar disorder and major depressive disorder are syndrome diagnoses, that is, the diagnosis is based on the presence of a collection of observed symptoms (phenotype) rather than an etiological cause. In this theory, late-onset affective illness is a collection of phenocopies. Phenocopies are illnesses with a

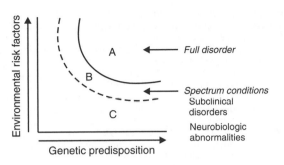

Figure 69.1 How genes and environment lead to illness. Adapted from Faraone *et al.*[31]

characteristic phenotype but different underlying causes. Hypothyroidism is an example of a phenocopy. Individuals with hypothyroidism may meet major depression criteria, but they require quite different treatment.

It should be noted that the two explanations postulated for the observed differences in age-related affective disorders are not mutually exclusive. We have already noted that affective disorders are heterogeneous. Figure 69.2 demonstrates two dimensions of heterogeneity—clinical and causal. Clinical heterogeneity occurs when more than one clinical condition can occur by the same cause. Causal heterogeneity occurs when two or more causes can independently produce the same clinical syndrome[31]. In Figure 69.2 the small circle at the top represents all patients who have the full disorder (in this case, bipolar disorder or major depressive disorder). The larger circle demonstrates three outcomes attributed to disease genes: "full disorder", "spectrum conditions" and "symptom-free". Some individuals with the disease genes will develop the full disorder. Others will not meet criteria for the full disorder, but will show abnormalities and trends toward the disorder. These are called "spectrum conditions". Finally, some individuals will remain symptom-free despite carrying the same disease genes.

The small circle at the top of Figure 69.2 also shows that not all patients who have the full disorder have the disease genes. This

subgroup represents those patients with phenocopies of the full disorder. They have an illness that looks like a genetic disorder but it is not caused by genes, at least not the same disease genes.

It has long been known that depressive syndromes are very common in neurological disorders such as Parkinson's disease, Alzheimer's disease and stroke. More recently, researchers[32,33] have proposed a subtype of depression called "vascular depression", based on the presence of white and gray matter changes observed on magnetic resonance imaging (MRI) scans. These changes are frequently seen as patients age, and both the pattern and intensity of lesions appear to have a direct relationship to major depressive episodes (and possibly bipolar disorder). This subtype is differentiated from other depressive types by demonstrating a constellation of depressive symptoms, increased incidence of apathy, psychomotor retardation, cognitive impairment, functional disability and a decreased incidence of familial affective disorders. If this is shown to be true, then the age-related variation in late-life affective disorders may be explained by increasing phenocopies in older adults who have late-onset affective disorders. Patients with early-onset affective disorders (which would include elderly patients with previous diagnosis of affective disorders) may be more likely to have a genetic cause.

As research like this sharpens our understanding of disease, the "heterogenous" group of affective disorders will be differentiated into various subtypes, each with a more specifically defined course, prognosis and treatment. Each new subtype will also suggest new ways that genes and the environment may contribute to the expression of the illness. For example, current research is examining how other "disease genes" may cause various phenocopies. One of the major complications of Alzheimer's disease is the development of a major depressive disorder. Research has suggested that the presence of one of the ApoE alleles, which has been implicated in Alzheimer's disease and is genetically determined, may predispose patients to the development of major depression[34,35]. Other researchers have not found this finding to be consistent[36–38]. However, the implication is clear. Environmental and genetic patterns in late-onset affective disorders are emerging that are different from patterns seen in early-onset disease.

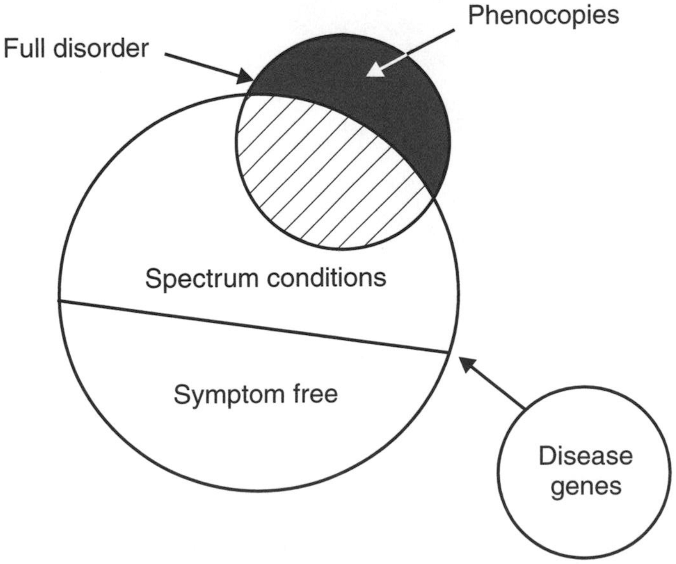

Figure 69.2 Causal and clinical heterogeneity. Adapted from Tsuang and Faraone[11]

Labels in Figure 69.2: Phenocopies; Full disorder; Spectrum conditions; Symptom free; Disease genes

REFERENCES

1. Morton NE. *Outline of Genetic Epidemiology*. Basel: S Karger, 1982.
2. Gershon ES, Mark A, Cohen N *et al*. Transmitted factors in the morbid risk of affective disorders: a controlled study. *J Psychiat Res* 1975; **12**: 283.
3. Tsuang MT, Winokur G, Crowe RR. Morbidity risks of schizophrenia and affective disorders among first-degree relatives of patients with schizophrenia, mania, depression, and surgical conditions. *Br J Psychiat* 1980; **137**: 497–504.
4. Winokur G, Crowe RR. Bipolar illness: the sex-polarity effect in affectively ill family members. *Arch Gen Psychiat* 1983; **40**(1): 57–8.
5. Gershon ES, Hamovit J, Guroff JJ *et al*. A family study of schizoaffective, bipolar I, bipolar II, unipolar and normal control probands. *Arch Gen Psychiat* 1982; **39**(10): 1157–67.
6. Maier W, Hallmayer J, Lichtermann D *et al*. Continuity and discontinuity of affective disorders and schizophrenia. Results of a controlled family study. *Arch Gen Psychiat* 1991; **50**: 871–83.
7. Weissman MM, Merikangas KR, John K *et al*. Family genetic studies of psychiatric disorders. *Arch Gen Psychiat* 1986; **43**(11): 1104–16.
8. Merikangas KR, Kupfer DJ. Mood disorders: genetic aspects. In Kaplan HI, Sadock BJ, eds, *Comprehensive Textbook of Psychiatry*, 6th edn. Baltimore, MD: Williams & Wilkins, 1995.
9. McGuffin P, Katz R, Rutherford J. Nature, nurture and depression: A twin study. *Psychol Med* 1991; **21**: 329–35.

10. Kendler KS, Neale MC, Kessler RC *et al*. A population-based twin study of major depression in women: the impact of varying definitions of illness. *Arch Gen Psychiat* 1992; **49**: 257–66.

11. Tsuang M, Faraone S. *The Genetics of Mood Disorders*. Baltimore, MD: Johns Hopkins University Press, 1990.

12. Cadoret RJ, Cunningham L, Loftus R, Edwards J. Studies of adoptees from psychiatrically disturbed biological parents. III. Medical symptoms and illnesses in childhood and adolescence. *Am J Psychiat* 1976; **133**: 1316–18.

13. Editorial. Troubles encountered in gene linkage land. *Science* 1989; **243**: 313–14.

14. Risch N, Baron M. X-linkage and genetic heterogeneity in bipolar-related major affective illness: re-analysis of linkage data. *Am J Hum Genet* 1982; **46**(2): 153–66.

15. Egeland JA, Gerhard DS, Pauls DL *et al*. Bipolar affective disorders linked to DNA markers on chromosome 11. *Nature* 1987; **325**: 782–7.

16. Kelsoe JR, Ginns EE, Egeland JA *et al*. Reevaluation of the linkage relationship between chromosome 11p loci and the gene for bipolar disorder in the Old Order Amish. *Nature* 1989; **342**(16): 238–43.

17. Mendlewicz J. Juvenile and late onset forms of depressive disorder: genetic and biological characterization of bipolar and unipolar illness—a review. *Maturitas* 1979; **1**(4): 229–34.

18. Post F. The management and nature of depressive illness in late life: a follow-through study. *Br J Psychiat* 1972; **121**: 393–404.

19. Murphy E. The prognosis of depression in old age. *Br J Psychiat* 1983; **142**: 111–19.

20. Young RC, Klerman GL. Mania in late-life: focus on age at onset. *Am J Psychiat* 1992; **152**(5): 722–30.

21. Krishnan KRR, Hays JC, Tupler LA *et al*. Clinical and phenomenological comparisons of late-onset and early-onset depression. *Am J Psychiat* 1995; **152**: 785–8.

22. Rice J, Reich T, Andreason NC *et al*. The familial transmission of bipolar illness. *Arch Gen Psychiat* 1987; **44**(5): 441–7.

23. Bland RC, Newman SC, Orn H. Recurrent and nonrecurrent depression: a family study. *Arch Gen Psychiat* 1986; **43**: 1085–9.

24. Baron M, Mendlewicz J, Klotz J. Age-of-onset and genetic transmission in affective disorders. *Acta Psychiat Scand* 1981; **64**: 373–80.

25. Mendlewicz J Baron M. Morbidity risks in subtypes of unipolar depressive illness: differences between early- and late-onset forms. *Br J Psychiat* 1991; **134**: 463–6.

26. Hopkinson G. A genetic study of affective illness in patients over 50. *Br J Psychiat* 1964; **110**: 244–54.

27. Alexopoulos GS, Young RC, Meyers BS. Geriatric depression: age of onset and dementia. *Biol Psychiat* 1993; **34**: 141–5.

28. Hays JC, Krishnan KRR, George LK, Blazer DG. Age of first onset of bipolar disorder: demographic, family history, and psychosocial correlates. *Depress Anxiety* 1998; **7**: 76–82.

29. Gatz M, Pedersen NL, Plomin R *et al*. Importance of shared genes and shared environments for symptoms of depression in older adults. *J Abnorm Psychol* 1992; **101**(4): 701–8.

30. McGue M, Christensen K. Genetic and environmental contributions to depression symptomatology: evidence from Danish twins 75 years of age and older. *J Abnorm Psychol* 1997; **106**(3): 439–48.

31. Faraone SV, Tsuang MT, Tsuang DW. *Genetics of Mental Disorders: A Guide for Students, Clinicians and Researchers*. New York: Guilford, 1999.

32. Krishnan DRR, Hays JC, Blazer DG. MRI-defined vascular depression. *Am J Psychiat* 1997; **154**: 497–501.

33. Alexopoulos GS, Meyers BS, Young RC *et al*. Clinically defined vascular depression. *Am J Psychiat* 1997; **154**: 562–5.

34. Holmes C, Russ C, Kirov G. *et al*. Apolipoprotein E: depressive illness, depressive symptoms, and Alzheimer's disease. *Biol Psychiat* 1998; **43**(3): 159–64.

35. Krishnan KR, Tupler LA, Ritchie JC Jr, McDonald WM. Knight DL, Nemeroff CB, Carroll BJ. Apolipoprotein E-epsilon of frequency in geriatric depression. *Biol Psychiatry* 1996; **40**: 69–71.

36. Zubenko GS, Henderson R, Stiffler JS *et al*. Association of the APOE epsilon 4 allele with clinical subtypes of late life depression. *Biol Psychiat* 1996; **40**(10): 1008–16.

37. Schmand B, Hooijer C, Jonker C *et al*. Apolipoprotein E phenotype is not related to late-life depression in a population-based sample. *Soc Psychiat Psychiat Epidemiol* 1998; **33**(1): 21–6.

38. Papassotirpoulos A, Bagli M, Jessen F *et al*. Early-onset and late-onset depression are independent of the genetic polymorphism of apolipoprotein E. *Dement Geriat Cogn Disord* 1999; **10**(4): 258–61.

Environmental Factors, Life Events and Coping Abilities

Toni C. Antonucci and James S. Jackson
University of Michigan, Ann Arbor, MI, USA

Understanding environmental factors, life events and coping abilities in the lives of older people is best accomplished by applying a life-span developmental perspective. Baltes *et al.*[1] emphasize that people evolve throughout their lifetime and become more heterogeneous with age. As people grow older, the experiences of a lifetime combine uniquely to shape them. This is especially important to the question of how individuals cope with the challenges of old age. The lifespan framework allows us to incorporate information about an individual's experiences, the successes or failures an individual has had in coping with these experiences, and the people who have or have not been helpful in aiding the individual to achieve those successes. Social support is not always or solely considered a coping ability or strategy. However, it has been argued that successful coping is the ability to activate the kinds of support needed to meet the needs of specific situations and to help the individual achieve a positive affective disposition.

The Convoy Model of Social Relations[2,3] suggests that individual and situational characteristics combine to explain and predict the amount, type and adequacy of support an individual is capable of garnering to cope with life events and circumstances, thus enabling the individual to adapt successfully to life's challenges. The individual moves through time and circumstance surrounded by a "convoy" of people, who either help or inhibit the individual's ability to successfully cope with the problems he/she faces, consequently affecting both his/her health and well-being. The Convoy Model incorporates both personal and situational factors to predict coping skills and success. Available evidence indicates that most convoys consist of both family and friendship relationships within a multigenerational context.

These contexts are characterized by exchanges that are perceived as either reciprocal or non-reciprocal. Since reciprocity is the norm of social relationships[4], it is useful to consider how people assess the reciprocity of their relationships. As one gets older, it is often the case that one requires more support, both emotionally and instrumentally, to cope with the challenges of life. There is some danger that older people will come to perceive their relationships as non-reciprocal, and feel that they are over-benefited, i.e. receive more support than they provide, by these exchanges. There would then be the danger that this will lead to a sense of indebtedness. However, many people are quite resourceful about maintaining relationship equity by using what has been termed a "support bank"[3] accounting system. Older people have been known to consider support provided by them to others earlier in life as contributions to a "support bank" from which they can make withdrawals, as needed, later in life. This interpretation of support exchanges can be especially useful for understanding how some older people cope with crises by accepting considerable support from others but without the disadvantage of feeling overly indebted by the receipt of more aid than they are currently able to reciprocate. Also interesting is the phenomenon whereby the older person recalibrates support received of one type to equal support provided of another type. Thus, a drive to the doctor's office can be completely reciprocated by a freshly baked loaf of bread. Some might argue that the ability to cognitively construct an equitable exchange is not necessarily a reality assessment, but rather an exercise in adaptive illusions[5].

Several recent theoretical developments should be noted. Baltes and Baltes[6] have proposed the Selective Optimization with Compensation Theory. This theory suggests that an important strategy of successful aging is to carefully select those behaviors, goals or activities that are personally most important, and to develop multiple strategies to compensate for the limitations increasingly evident with age. This theory suggests that some goals will be ignored, dropped or otherwise disregarded, while others will be achieved but only through compromise and compensation. A related theory has been proposed, the Socio-emotional Selectivity Theory[7]. This theory focuses specifically on social relations and suggests that, with age, people reduce the number of social relationships in which they invest time, energy and emotional commitment, to only those which are truly close and important to them. The argument suggested is that with fewer years left to live, older people are less interested in relationships that are troublesome or otherwise unsatisfying to them and more interested in maximizing their time and commitment to those relationships that are truly important to them. It could also be that individuals are selected who allow the elder to maintain reciprocity or those with whom the elders have had a particularly satisfying exchange relationship in the past. Empirical data are available to support both perspectives. Especially interesting, in light of the Socio-emotional Selectivity Theory, is the finding that older people report significantly fewer negative social relations and are more satisfied than younger people with the relationships they do have.

We know that people vary in their ability to cope with the problems they face and in their ability to develop supportive relationships. We can best understand these differences as indications of how older people differentially experience their environments and life events and how they cope with these experiences. Although it is clearly true that some people experience more crises than others, it is not always the case that those who experience a great many crises are the ones

Principles and Practice of Geriatric Psychiatry, 2nd edn. Edited by J. R. M. Copeland, M. T. Abou-Saleh and D. G. Blazer

overwhelmed by them. The same environmental conditions or life events that might devastate one person may have less of a negative impact on another.

The Support/Efficacy Model[8] proposes a lifespan framework to explain these differences. This model suggests that supportive interactions over time are essential to developing in the individual a sense of efficacy that instills in that person the belief that he/she can successfully meet the challenges of life. With time, exchanges and interactions accumulate which either lead the individual to feel competent and capable of coping with the problems he/she confronts (i.e. efficacious) or, under less optimal circumstances, leaves the individual feeling overwhelmed by, and personally incapable of, coping with the problems and circumstances of life.

It is also important to consider the influence of non-psychiatric factors on the experience of events in old age and how one copes with stress. Jackson et al.[9] have noted that racial, cultural and other sociodemographic factors fundamentally affect how a situation is experienced. If an individual is one of many suffering the same negative experience(s), the etiology of that experience may not be devastatingly personalized. On the other hand, if everyone else in one's reference group is significantly more successful, the relative comparison can be devastating, even if "objectively" the situation is quite positive. Similarly, there now exists empirical evidence indicating that different national groups appear to vary considerably in the degree to which they respond negatively to environmental factors and life events. Fuhrer et al.[10] have shown that normal French elderly score markedly higher on measures of depressive symptomatology than their American counterparts, despite the fact that their general environmental circumstances and their experienced life events are actually quite similar. Antonucci et al.[11], comparing Black and White Americans with French elderly on a variety of factors, have shown that the general mental health of American and French elderly are similar in some respects and different in others. All three groups are negatively affected by functional limitations. On the other hand, Black American and French elderly men are less satisfied with life than women in these groups, although there is no sex difference among White Americans. A recent study of the elderly in the Netherlands and Italy[12] is also of interest. It suggests that objective characteristics, such as living arrangements, which some might consider indicators of coping, need to be understood in terms of the individual's psychological state. Dutch elders tend to live alone, while Italians tend to live with their families. However, Italian elders reported less social integration and more loneliness than Dutch elders. Despite the appearance of family integration, these data suggest that an individual's ability to cope with environmental factors is not always directly predictable from the objective characteristics of the situation. As with the French and Americans reporting of depressive symptomology, this could simply, but importantly, be a difference in expressive style.

It has been suggested that an individual's ability to cope with specific environmental conditions and life events is best understood through a consideration of the resources and experiences available to that person. One simplistic way to consider this is that successfully coping with stresses and strains in early life is the best predictor of the individual's ability to cope with stressful situations in later life. This is likely to be true, even if the exact nature of the stressful event varies. There is also reason to believe that some individuals develop coping styles over their lifetime that can be seen to be generally successful and adaptive, while others develop coping styles that are generally unsuccessful or maladaptive. At best, these coping strategies match the environmental conditions and life events that the individual experiences. For example, Jackson[13] and Jackson et al.[14] have argued that the harsh environmental conditions faced by many racial and ethnic minorities lead to the development of novel and effective coping strategies. Over the lifecourse, however, many of these strategies actually may be deleterious to health status, e.g. alcohol use. Although the specific nature of these experiences will change with age, an individual's ability to cope with these environmental events is likely to show fairly stable lifespan continuity. At the same time, as research clearly demonstrates, individual coping and adaptation competencies can be improved through informal and professional intervention at all points in the individual lifecourse.

REFERENCES

1. Baltes PB, Reese HW, Lipsitt LP. Life-span developmental psychology. *Ann Rev Psychol* 1980; **31**: 65–110.
2. Kahn RL, Antonucci TC. Convoys over the life course: Attachment, roles, and social support. In Baltes PB, Brim O, eds, *Lifespan Development and Behavior*, vol. 3. New York: Academic Press, 1980; **3**: 253–86.
3. Antonucci TC. Personal characteristics, social support, and social behavior. In Binstock RH, Shanas E, eds, *Handbook of Aging and the Social Sciences*, 2nd edn. New York: Van Nostrand Reinhold, 1985; 94–128.
4. Gouldner AW. The norm of reciprocity: a preliminary statement. *Am Sociol Rev* 1960; **25**(2): 161–78.
5. Taylor SE, Kemeny ME, Reed GM et al. Psychological resources, positive illusions, and health. *Am Psychol* 2000; **55**(1): 99–109.
6. Baltes PB, Baltes MM, ed. *Successful Aging: Perspectives from the Behavioral Sciences*. Cambridge: Cambridge University Press, 1990.
7. Cartensen LL, Isaacowitz DM, Charles ST. Taking time seriously: a theory of socioemotional selectivity. *Am Psychol* 1999; **54**(3): 165–81.
8. Antonucci TC, Jackson JS. Social support, interpersonal efficacy, and health. In Carstensen LL, Edelstein BA, eds, *Handbook of Clinical Gerontology*. New York: Pergamon, 1987; 291–311.
9. Jackson JS, Antonucci TC, Gibson R. Cultural, racial and ethnic minority influences on aging. In Birren JE, Schaie KW, eds, *Handbook of the Psychology of Aging*, vol. 6. New York: Academic Press, 1990; **6**: 103–23.
10. Fuhrer R, Antonucci TC, Alperovitch A et al. Depressive symptomatology and cognitive functioning in later life. *Psychol Med* 1992; **22**: 159–72.
11. Antonucci TC, Fuhrer R, Jackson JS. Social support and reciprocity: a cross-ethnic and cross-national perspective. *J Soc Pers Relat* 1990; **7**(4): 519–30.
12. Tilburg T, de Jong Gierveld J, Lecchini L, Marsiglia D. Social integration and loneliness: a comparative study among older adults in the Netherlands and Tuscany, Italy. *J Soc Pers Relat* 1998; **15**(6): 740–54.
13. Jackson JS. African American experiences through the adult years. In Kastenbaum R, ed., *Encyclopedia of Adult Development*. Phoenix, AZ: Orvx Press, 1993; 18–26.
14. Jackson JS, Williams DR, Lisansky Gomberg E. Aging and alcohol use and abuse among African Americans: a life-course perspective. In Lisansky Gomberg ES, Hegedus AM, Zucker RA, eds, *Alcohol Problems and Aging* 1999; **33**: 63–87.

The Aetiology of Late-life Depression

Martin Prince and Aartjan Beekman

Institute of Psychiatry, London, UK

It is vain to speak of cures or think of remedies, until such time as we have considered of the causes (Galen)

Empirics may ease, and sometimes help, but not thoroughly root out . . . as the saying is, if the cause be removed, the effect is likewise vanquished (Burton, *The Anatomy of Melancholy*)

Late-life depression, when defined according to the broad criterion of clinical significance, is a common disorder affecting 10–15% of the 65+ population[1,2]. Prevalence rates for major depression are substantially lower, but this category excludes common forms of late-life depression, particularly those associated with bereavement and physical co-morbidity. Longitudinal population-based studies suggest that incidence and maintenance rates are both high, balanced by a high mortality ratio for those affected.

The aetiology of late-life depression remains unclear in some respects. While many population-based studies have been carried out in Europe and the USA, most of these have been cross-sectional in design, and have limited themselves to univariate analyses. The results of these investigations therefore appear as lists of cross-sectional associations, possibly confounded by other factors. While causal models can, and have been, inferred from such data, the process is fraught with difficulty and can lead to errors. More recently, good quality prospective studies have been carried out that have the potential to clarify the aetiology of these common disorders and inform primary and secondary prevention.

AGE

The data on the prevalence of major depression from the US Epidemiological Catchment Area (ECA) survey suggested a lower rate for those aged 65 (1.0%) than for those aged 45–64 (2.3%) and those aged 18–44 (3.4%)[3]. This relatively low prevalence rate among the older population was confirmed in a Canadian study using similar methodology[4]. These findings have been particularly controversial, as they could be taken to imply that the management of depression may require less resources per capita for the old than for the young[5]. They conflict with the general impression that the frequency of depressive symptoms and broader depressive syndromes either increases[6-8] or remains stable[9] with increasing age. The lay administered Diagnostic Interview Schedule (DIS) used to derive DSM-III diagnoses in the ECA excludes symptoms attributable to bereavement, physical illness or cognitive impairment. The ECA findings have been criticized on the grounds that the complex standardized symptoms, and the judgemental process required for responding to probes used in the DIS, may exceed the cognitive capacity of many older adults, leading to a systematic

response bias. This may have been a particular problem where subjects were required to attribute symptoms to physical or non-physical causes. Older subjects report as many lifetime depressive symptoms as younger subjects, but are more likely to attribute them to physical causes, meaning that they are then excluded as a basis of diagnosing depression[10]. However a re-analysis of ECA data reattributing physical symptoms to psychiatric symptoms did not lead to a disproportionate rise in major depression among the older age groups[11].

A further curiosity has been the consistent finding that the lifetime prevalence of major depression seems to be lower for elderly subjects (1.4% for those aged 65 in the ECA survey) than for younger subjects (7.5% for those aged 30–44, from the same survey). It has been suggested that this may represent a cohort effect, with successive birth cohorts carrying an increasing propensity for major depression. More plausibly, this finding may have arisen from a selective tendency for older subjects not to recall earlier undiagnosed episodes[12] and from the selective mortality of those most vulnerable to repeated severe episodes of depression[8,13]. A broad review of this area reported similar findings for most psychiatric diagnoses, including schizophrenia, and concluded that cohort trends cannot be safely extrapolated from cross-sectional data[14].

GENDER AND MARITAL STATUS

One of the clearest and most reproducible findings in psychiatric epidemiology is the apparent excess of depression among women. It has been suggested that the extent of this excess varies across the life course, increasing from menarche into mid-life, and then declining gradually into late life[15]. The EURODEP consortium[16,17] reported a clear-cut excess of depression symptoms in older women in population-based studies from 13 out of 14 European centres. Interestingly, this association was consistently modified by marital status, with marriage being protective for men but a risk factor among women. Marriage is associated with relatively low mortality and good health, although this protective effect seems to be stronger for men than for women[18,19]. In younger people, marriage also protects against depression among men but not among women[20]. In Gove's[20] study, the excess of depression in women relative to men was greatest in married people. This striking finding has been variously attributed to the mundanity of housework and the unfavourable position of women who work outside the home[20] to the differences in the number and range of role identities by gender and marital status[21] and to the burden of childcaring[22]. Brown *et al.* drew attention to the lack of satisfaction with the married state expressed by working class Camberwell women. In older people these observations are consistent with the observation from several studies that married older men cite their wife as their main confidante, whereas women more often cite a friend outside the home[24]. Also, in Finland, a prospective study showed that for men the risk of onset of depression over 5 years is increased for those having poor emotional relations with their wives, while for women the risk is greatest among those not living alone at the beginning of the follow-up period[25]. These findings led Kivels to suggest that marital counselling should be made available for older people. However, there may be external factors which, to the extent to which they affect wives and husbands and single men and single women differently, may have explained some of the observed gender/marital status interaction. One such factor may be the social integration and activity of single men and women. Never-married men reported fewer supportive friends and neighbours, less attendance at clubs or church, and more loneliness than never-married women in Gospel Oak[26,27]. Another area worthy of investigation is the relative health of male and female marital partners. A national US survey showed that 64% of all spousal carers were wives, suggesting that in older age the burden of care in marriages may generally derive from the husband and devolve on the wife[28].

DISABLEMENT

Of the world population, 7–10% are significantly affected by disablement, defined as the long-term consequences of chronic disease[29]. These estimates have varied little between world regions, and are similar for developed and developing countries[29]. There is, however, a strong positive relationship between disablement and age. The OPCS Surveys of Disability in Great Britain reported a near doubling of disability prevalence rates with each 10 year increase in age, from 7% for those aged 40–49, to 67% for those aged 80+[30]. Among older subjects, most detectable physical illness is chronic rather than acute[31].

Many studies have commented on the strength of the cross-sectional relationship between physical health variables and depression in older age. Gurland reviewed 70 years of research endeavour in this field, carried out in primary care, hospital and community settings, and concluded that there was strong accumulated evidence of a tendency for both physical illness and disability to co-exist with major and minor depression at a frequency greater than that expected by chance[32].

There have been suggestions from clinical populations of specific associations between late-life depression and diseases such as stroke[33] and Parkinson's disease[34]. Results from community surveys are less clear. However, stroke, respiratory disease and arthritis were all found to be associated by most studies which have assessed individual diagnoses[35–40], while hypertension and diabetes were less salient. This pattern of association with individual diseases would suggest that disablement, the limiting long-term consequences of disease, may be more relevant than any particular pathology. Indeed, the strongest reported associations have generally been between depression and summary measures of disablement. A systematic review of the literature, using MEDLINE for the period 1984–1996 and secondary references for earlier publications, revealed 10 cross-sectional studies which had used population samples[41]. They were consistent in reporting strong positive associations between disablement, measured in various ways, and depression[36–38,42–46]. However, the strong associations might not reflect a causal relationship. Bias (somatic contamination of the measurement of depression), confounding and, in particular, reverse causality (depression leading to disablement, rather than vice versa) were plausible alternative explanations. Later prospective population-based research has

clarified the association. At least five longitudinal studies have now shown a very strong association between disablement at baseline and the subsequent onset of depression[47–51]. In the Gospel Oak survey[26,27], after adjusting for confounders, the most restricted quarter of the Gospel Oak population (London Handicap Scale) were 20 times more likely to be depressed at baseline than the least restricted quarter. Those among them who were not depressed at baseline were five times more likely than the least restricted quarter to have experienced an onset of depression at 1 year[50]. The population attributable fraction (the proportion of new cases that might notionally be prevented if the risk factor were removed) was 0.69. Most studies agree that it is the level of disablement associated with a health condition, rather than the nature of the pathology, that determines the risk for depression[50,52,53]. Three population-based studies have suggested an interaction between disablement and social support, with the strongest effect of disablement in those with the least social support[1,50,51]. Beekman et al.[1] reported that the association between disablement and depression was only apparent for minor rather than major depression. However, this finding was based upon cross-sectional research, and requires replication. Interestingly, in community studies, disablement does not seem to influence directly the process of recovery from late-life depression[50].

Ormel et al.[54] argue in a separate publication that synchronicity of changes in depression and disability observed longitudinally in a primary care-based study support the hypothesis that there is an important pathway leading from depression to disability. In reality, as most authors have acknowledged, the situation may be more complex; the causal direction may vary between individuals, and components of each direction may co-exist within the same individual. A case can also be made for reciprocal causation, with a physical impairment leading to handicap, provoking depression which may in turn exacerbate the degree of handicap associated with the original impairment.

LIFE EVENTS

The literature on life events in older people was recently reviewed[55]. In the main, two methods have been used. The Bedford College Life Events and Difficulties Schedule (LEDS)[56] elicits events in a lengthy semi-structured recorded interview. These are then rated independently for contextual threat by a trained panel. Studies using this detailed method have shown that depressed older subjects have experienced more recent life events than non-depressed subjects[57]. However, older samples differ from younger ones in that chronic difficulties are more prevalent than life events, and events typically carry relatively low levels of threat[58,59]. Also, in contrast with Brown's work on younger adults, health difficulties are an important source of adversity[57,58]. The second and more common approach has been to use a pre-determined checklist of events. In a community survey in the USA, the onset of illness affecting a subject or relative, the onset of money problems, and becoming a victim of crime were among the most common and most undesirable life events affecting subjects aged 55+[59]. Deaths of spouses, children and siblings were rated as highly undesirable, but were individually relatively infrequent. However, 14% of females and 12% of males experienced a family bereavement of some kind over 1 year. Most checklists focus on these event categories, with a particular bias towards bereavement and personal illness events. Evidence for a relationship between depression in older age and life events measured using checklists is generally weaker than in LEDS-based studies. Linn[64] found a small significant difference in the mean number of events experienced by depressed and non-depressed community subjects. Other studies have not replicated this finding[60–63]. In this study, subjects' history of exposure to serious life events was ascertained retrospectively, at index assessment, over a period of up to 2 years prior to the time of interview. Perhaps for this reason, associations with prevalent depression at index assessment were more impressive than the prospective associations with the onset of depression 1 year later. It may be that the categories used by some life event checklists carry too little "contextual threat" to be relevant to the subsequent onset of depression. In the longitudinal Gospel Oak survey[20,27], at index assessment depressed subjects reported more life events, measured using a checklist of events likely to carry high contextual threat, than did non-depressed subjects. However, at follow-up only a weak non-significant trend towards an increased risk for the onset of depression was observed. Having something important lost or stolen was the only individual event associated with the onset of depression over 1 year.

SOCIAL SUPPORT AND THE BUFFER HYPOTHESIS

Brown demonstrated in a younger sample that negative self-esteem and lack of social support were vulnerability factors, increasing the risk of depression in the presence of a life event[23]. Murphy[57] reported a similar vulnerability for older subjects lacking a confiding relationship. Not all studies have replicated this finding. Murrell[61] found a direct protective relationship between self-esteem and depression, but noted that neither self-esteem nor health modified the association between life events and later depression scores. Social support has been infrequently investigated in older community samples, and the findings have not all been consistent. Murphy's finding of an association between a lack of confidants and depression was confirmed in New York[44]. Bowling reported a positive association between the number of confidants and well-being in a London sample, which was, however, not apparent in a sample drawn from a smaller town in Essex[65]. In both samples, health status accounted for more of the variance in well-being than did subjects' social support or social network characteristics. Bowling's finding of no association between social participation and well-being was contradicted by Palinkas' report, in a Californian study, of inverse associations between participation in church and other community organizations and depression[35,36]. Palinkas also reported an inverse relationship between social network size and depression. Both Palinkas[35,36] and Woo[66] in a study from Hong Kong[66], report inverse associations between the frequency of contacts with friends and depression. The Bowling, Woo and Palinkas studies all adjusted to some extent for subjects' physical health status, and Palinkas also controlled for age and gender. Each of these variables is a potential confounder of an association between social support and late-life depression. There are large differences between the social support networks of older men and women, women typically having more supportive and extensive networks of friends than men[35,36,67]. Palinkas hypothesized a deterioration of social network with increasing age consequent upon bereavement; he found an inverse association between age and network size in women, but not in men. Bowling[65] comments that active social engagement, such as visiting friends, is often confounded by functional ability, but unfortunately does not report her data on associations between social support or social network and health status. Palinkas found no association between physical health and social participation, or the number or frequency of social contacts[35,36], but other studies have observed disablement to be associated with smaller social networks[68,69].

One of the more consistent findings from the literature appears to be the salience to late-life depression of contact with friends, in particular intimate, confiding relationships. While older people typically receive instrumental support from spouses and relatives,

they value friends for the companionship and emotional support that they can provide[70]. A review of recent research in the area concludes that interaction with friends, rather than frequency of contact with relations, is positively associated with emotional well-being[24]. This view was borne out in the longitudinal Gospel Oak study. No contact with friends was the only social support variable prospectively associated with the onset of depression[50]. In this study, lack of social support and social participation were more evidently associated with the maintenance rather than with the onset of depression.

SOCIAL CLASS, INCOME AND EDUCATION

Brown and Harris reported that working-class women with children at home were four times more likely to have experienced a depression than middle-class women[23]. Although they were more likely to experience life events, the class difference in depression was mediated more by the higher prevalence of four vulnerability factors among the working-class women. Murphy has reported a less dramatic social class effect in an older sample[57]. In her older subjects, the excess of depression among the lower social classes was largely explained by their poorer health and greater social difficulties. Social class, as measured by best pre-retirement occupation, may retain some validity after retirement, to the extent to which it relates to retirement income, housing quality, social network, and access to and use of formal services. There have been reports from cross-sectional community surveys from a variety of cultures of associations between late-life depression and relative disadvantage in income[37,38,44,66,71,72], housing status[37,38,66] and education[37,38,44,46,66,72]. These are, of course, highly correlated variables, and it will always be difficult to determine the effect of one independent of the others. The possibility of reverse causality also needs to be considered because of the well-recognized phenomenon of social drift; people whose adult life has been scarred by depression may experience occupational and economic disadvantage.

FAMILY HISTORY, GENETIC LIABILITY AND PAST PSYCHIATRIC HISTORY

The earliest evidence of a familial tendency in depression came from family studies in which the life-time prevalence of depressive disorder was compared between relatives of probands with depression and a control sample. Many such studies have been completed, with consistent results. Higher than expected rates of major depression and minor depression are found among relatives of probands with major depression, and higher rates of bipolar disorder and major depression among relatives of probands with bipolar disorder[73]. Such studies could only identify familial aggregation, and could not distinguish between familial similarity arising from shared environment or shared genes.

Early twin studies suggested a substantial contribution from both genes and shared environment[74]. Incorporation of environmental measures in genetically sensitive designs has advanced our understanding of the interplay between genetic and environmental risk factors for major depression. Kendler et al.[75] have completed extensive quantitative genetic analyses in a large cohort of same-sex (female) twins from the population-based Virginia Twin Registry. The heritability for a life-time diagnosis of major depression was 33–45%, depending on the diagnostic criteria that were applied. This estimate varied little between more and less restrictive criteria[75]. The heritability for 1 year prevalence of major depression also lay between 41% and 46%[76]. There was some suggestion that improving the reliability of the diagnosis of major depression might increase the estimates for the heritability of the disorder, with up to half of the environmental contribution to the variance having reflected measurement error, leading to a dilution of the previous reported genetic contributions[77]. About 60% of the genetic effect contributed was indirect, mediated by past history of depression, neuroticism, life events and childhood adversity. Two coping strategies, turning to others and problem solving, which had been negatively correlated with levels of depression, were also found to have substantial heritability[78]. The relationship between genetic liability, stressful life events and depression was explored in detail, and evidence provided to support a gene–environment interaction in which genetic factors determined sensitivity to serious life events[79].

Data on older subjects is relatively lacking. Two studies from The Netherlands examined cross-sectional relationships between depression and the exposures of a family history of mental illness, and a personal past history of depression. In the Amstel study, based on a large population sample of 2540 subjects aged 65+, there was a positive association between a family history of mental problems and a diagnosis of GMS–AGECAT depression[80]. This association was modified by both cognitive status and personal past psychiatric history. The strongest association was seen in the group with a past psychiatric history and no cognitive impairment. However, only 22% of depressed subjects reported a family history of mental health problems, suggesting a modest population-attributable fraction. Van Ojen[13] also reported that, while depression was twice as common in those with a psychiatric history with an onset before the age of 65, the prevalence of this exposure decreased linearly with increasing age[13]. Only 22% of currently depressed subjects reported a previous episode of psychiatric illness with an onset before age 65. While failure of recall and "telescoping" of ages of onset might have accounted for these findings, the reduction in the prevalence of past history with increasing age was consistent with predictions based upon the known excess mortality among those so affected. The LASA study, based on a national Dutch sample of over 3000 subjects aged 65+, used two definitions of depressive disorder, major depression diagnosed using DIS, and minor depression defined as those scoring 16 or more on the Center for Epidemiological Studies Depression Scale. A family history of depression was associated with neither outcome. A past history of psychiatric disorder was strongly associated with major depression, with an odds ratio (OR) of 90.8 (39.1–211.1) and a population-attributable fraction (PAF) of 74%, but much more weakly associated with minor depression; OR 4.1 (2.3–7.3) PAF 7%.

COGNITIVE DECLINE

An inverse association between depression scores and cognitive test scores has been reported in four cross-sectional surveys[46,71,81,82] with one negative report[42]. These cross-sectional studies did not permit further analysis of direction of causality. However, at least one study has suggested that low mood may be a risk factor for subsequent decline in cognitive ability[83]. A biological basis for this association has been suggested; the failure, seen in chronically depressed subjects, of fast-feedback mechanisms to shut off the cortisol stress response may lead to high concentrations of neurotoxic metabolites, causing specific damage to hippocampal regions essential to new learning and memory recall tasks[84]. Alternatively, microvascular lesions leading to cognitive decline may also cause late-life depression through critical subcortical damage to frontotemporal cortical projections necessary for the maintenance of mood and motivation. MRI evidence suggests that first onsets of late-life depression may be associated with characteristic deep white matter lesions[85]. The finding from the Amstel study, that the associations between life events and depression and living alone and depression were not apparent in those with cognitive impairment, would be consistent with a hypothesis of an alternative pathway to late-life depression mediated through cerebral deterioration[86]. There may be a more prosaic explanation for a prospective association between cognitive decline and depression. Cognitive impairment, like other health impairments, may lead to depression to the extent to which it causes disability and handicap.

CONCLUSION

The factors most consistently implicated in these studies are similar to those observed in younger adults: constitutional or genetic vulnerability, e.g. a family history or past history of psychiatric disorder; current vulnerability, e.g. lack of social support, recent stress, as in life events, and current adversity, as in low socioeconomic class, poor housing or low income. However, some factors may be particularly salient for late-life depression, either because, as in the case of disablement or bereavement, they are a much more common exposure among the older population, or because they may impact differently upon those who are exposed, depending on their age. There is already evidence to suggest that disablement associated with declining health in older age may be a prime determinant of the prevalence, incidence and maintenance of late-life depression.

In younger adult populations, depression is a substantially heritable disorder in which both direct genetic effects and genetic effects mediated through childhood adversity, neurotic personality, coping styles, propensity for life events and sensitivity to life events can be discerned. Evidence from genetically sensitive designs in older populations is lacking, but circumstantial evidence suggests that the selective early death of those with an early first onset and multiple episodes of depression, who perhaps have a higher genetic loading for the disorder, may mean that the heritability of depression in late life is lower than in younger populations. The finding that the large majority of older depressed subjects are experiencing a first onset of the disorder raises the possibility of aetiological dissimilarity between early adult and late-life depression. There is a clear case for focusing in our investigations on those aspects of physical health status, cognition and social milieu that change most acutely in late-life and best distinguish the life experience of older and younger adults.

REFERENCES

1. Beekman AT, Penninx BW, Deeg DJ et al. Depression and physical health in later life: results from the Longitudinal Aging Study Amsterdam (LASA). J Affect Disord 1997; 46: 219–31.
2. Chen R, Copeland JR, Wei L. A meta-analysis of epidemiological studies in depression of older people in the People's Republic of China. Int J Geriatr Psychiat 1999; 14(10): F21–30.
3. Weissman MM, Leaf PJ, Tischler GL et al. Affective disorders in five United States communities [published erratum appears in Psychol Med 1988 Aug; 18(3): following 792]. Psychol Med 1988; 18: 141–53.
4. Bland RC, Newman SC, Orn H. Prevalence of psychiatric disorders in the elderly in Edmonton. Acta Psychiat Scand Suppl 1988; 338: 57–63.
5. Snowdon J. The prevalence of depression in old age. Int J Geriat Psychiat 1990; 5: 141–4.
6. Tannock C, Katona C. Minor depression in the aged. Concepts, prevalence and optimal management. Drugs Aging 1995; 6: 278–92.
7. Kanowski S. Age-dependent epidemiology of depression. Gerontology 1994; 40(suppl 1): 1–4.
8. Ernst C, Angst J. Depression in old age. Is there a real decrease in prevalence? A review. Eur Arch Psychiat Clin Neurosci 1995; 245: 272–87.
9. Henderson AS, Jorm AF, Mackinnon A et al. The prevalence of depressive disorders and the distribution of depressive symptoms in later life: a survey using draft ICD-10 and DSM-III-R. Psychol Med 1993; 23: 719–29.

10. Knauper B, Wittchen HU. Diagnosing major depression in the elderly: evidence for response bias in standardized diagnostic interviews? *J Psychiat Res* 1994; **28**: 147–64.

11. Heithoff K. Does the ECA underestimate the prevalence of late-life depression? *J Am Geriat Soc* 1995; **43**: 2–6.

12. Giuffra LA, Risch N. Diminished recall and the cohort effect of major depression: a simulation study. *Psychol Med* 1994; **24**: 375–83.

13. Van Ojen R, Hooijer C, Jonker C *et al*. Late-life depressive disorder in the community, early onset and the decrease of vulnerability with increasing age. *J Affect Disord* 1995; **33**: 159–66.

14. Simon GE, Vonkorff M. Reevaluation of secular trends in depression rates. *Am J Epidemiol* 1992; **135**: 1411–22.

15. Jorm AF. Sex and age differences in depression: a quantitative synthesis of published research. *Aust N Z J Psychiat* 1987; **21**: 46–53.

16. Prince M, Beekman A, Fuhrer R *et al*. Depression symptoms in late-life assessed using the EURO-D scale. Effect of age, gender and marital status in 14 European centres. *Br J Psychiat* 1999; **174**: 339–45.

17. Prince MJ, Reischies F, Beekman ATF *et al*. The development of the EURO-D scale—a European Union initiative to compare symptoms of depression in 14 European centres. *Br J Psychiat* 1999; **174**: 330–38.

18. Jacobs S. An epidemiological review of the mortality of bereavement. *Psychosom Med* 1977; **39**: 344–57.

19. Berkman LF, Syme SL. Social networks, host resistance, and mortality: a nine year follow-up study of Alameda county residents. *Am J Epidemiol* 1979; **109**: 186–204.

20. Gove WR. The relationship between sex roles, marital status and mental illness. *Social Forces* 1972; **51**: 34–44.

21. Thoits PA. Multiple identities: examining gender and marital status differences in distress. *Am Sociol Rev* 1986; **51**: 259–72.

22. Elliot BJ, Huppert FA. In sickness and in health: associations between physical and mental well-being, employment and parental status in a British nationwide sample of married women. *Psychol Med* 1991; **21**: 515–24.

23. Brown GW, Harris T, Alder Z, Bridge L. Social support, self-esteem and depression. *Psychol Med* 1986; **16**: 813–31.

24. Bowling A. Social networks and social support among older people and implications for emotional well-being and psychiatric morbidity. *Int Rev Psychiat* 1994; **6**: 41–58.

25. Kivela SL. Depression and physical and social functioning in old age. *Acta Psychiat Scand* 1994; **377**(suppl); 73–6.

26. Prince M, Harwood H, Blizard R *et al*. Gospel Oak VI. Social support deficits, loneliness and life events as risk factors for depression in old age. *Psychol Med* 1997; **27**: 323–32.

27. Prince M, Harwood H, Blizard R *et al*. Gospel Oak V. Impairment, disability and handicap as risk factors for depression in old age. *Psychol Med* 1997; **27**: 311–21.

28. Stone R, Cafferata GL, Sangl J. Caregivers of the frail elderly: a national profile. *Gerontologist* 1987; **27**: 616–26.

29. Thuriaux MC. Consequences of disease and their measurement: introduction. *World Health Statist Qu* 1989; **42**: 110–14.

30. Martin J, Meltzer H, Elliot D. *OPCS Surveys of Disability in Great Britain. Report 1. The Prevalence of Disability among Adults*. London: HMSO, 1988.

31. Burvill PW, Mowry B, Hall WD. Quantification of physical illness in psychiatric research in the elderly. *Int J Geriat Psychiat* 1990; **5**: 161–70.

32. Gurland BJ, Wilder DE, Berkman C. Depression and disability in the elderly: reciprocal relations and changes with age. *Int J Geriat Psychiat* 1988; **3**: 163–79.

33. Eastwood MR, Rifat SL, Nobbs H, Ruderman J. Mood disorder following cerebrovascular accident. *Br J Psychiat* 1989; **154**: 195–200.

34. Cummings JL. Depression and Parkinson's disease: a review. *Am J Psychiat* 1992; **149**: 443–54.

35. Palinkas LA, Wingard DL, Barrett-Connor E. Chronic illness and depressive symptoms in the elderly: a population-based study. *J Clin Epidemiol* 1990; **43**: 1131–41.

36. Palinkas LA, Wingard DL, Barrett Connor E. The biocultural context of social networks and depression among the elderly. *Soc Sci Med* 1990; **30**: 441–7.

37. Murrell SA, Himmelfarb S, Wright K. Prevalence of depression and its correlates in older adults. *Am J Epidemiol* 1983; **117**: 173–85.

38. Berkman LF, Berkman CS, Kasl S *et al*. Depressive symptoms in relation to physical health and functioning in the elderly. *Am J Epidemiol* 1986; **124**: 372–88.

39. Lindesay J. The Guy's/Age Concern Survey: physical health and psychiatric disorder in an urban elderly community. *Int J Geriat Psychiat* 1990; **5**: 171–8.

40. Beekman ATF. Physical health and depression in later life. In *Depression in Later Life: Studies in the Community*. Hilversum: 1996: 92–117.

41. Prince MJ. The classification and measurement of disablement, with emphasis on depression, and its applications for clinical gerontology. *Rev Clin Gerontol* 1998; **8**: 227–40.

42. Gurland BJ, Copeland J, Kuriansky J *et al. The Mind and Mood of Aging*. London: Croom Helm, 1983.

43. Turner RJ, Noh S. Physical disability and depression: a longitudinal analysis. *J Health Soc Behav* 1988; **29**: 23–7.

44. Kennedy GJ, Kelman HR, Thomas C *et al*. Hierarchy of characteristics associated with depressive symptoms in an urban elderly sample. *Am J Psychiat* 1989; **146**: 220–25.

45. Livingston *et al*. 1990.

46. Fuhrer R, Antonucci TC, Gagnon M *et al*. Depressive symptomatology and cognitive functioning: an epidemiological survey in an elderly community sample in France. *Psychol Med* 1992; **22**: 159–72.

47. Phifer JF, Murrell SA. Etiologic factors in the onset of depressive symptoms in older adults. *J Abnorm Psychol* 1986; **95**: 282–91.

48. Kennedy GJ, Kelman HR, Thomas C. The emergence of depressive symptoms in late life: the importance of declining health and increasing disability. *J Commun Health* 1990; **15**: 93–104.

49. Beekman ATF, Deeg DJH, Smit JH, Van Tilburg W. Predicting the course of depression in the older population: results from a community-based study in The Netherlands. *J Affect Disord* 1995; **34**: 41–49.

50. Prince MJ, Harwood R, Thomas A, Mann AH. A prospective population-based cohort study of the effects of disablement and social milieu on the onset and maintenance of late-life depression. Gospel Oak VII. *Psychol Med* 1998; **28**: 337–50.

51. Schoevers RA, Beekman AT, Deeg DJ *et al*. Risk factors for depression in later life; results of a prospective community based study (AMSTEL). *J Affect Disord* 2000; **59**: 127–37.

52. Ormel J, Kempen GI, Penninx BW *et al*. Chronic medical conditions and mental health in older people: disability and psychosocial resources mediate specific mental health effects. *Psychol Med* 1997; **27**: 1065–77.

53. Broe GA, Jorm AF, Creasey H *et al*. Impact of chronic systemic and neurological disorders on disability, depression and life satisfaction [published erratum appears in *Int J Geriat Psychiat* 1999 Jun; 14(6): 497–8]. *Int J Geriat Psychiat* 1998; **13**: 667–73.

54. Ormel J, Von Korff M, Van Den Brink W *et al*. Depression, anxiety, and social disability show synchrony of change in primary care patients. *Am J Publ Health* 1993; **83**: 385–90.

55. Orrell MW, Davies ADM. Life events in the elderly. *Int J Geriat Psychiat* 1994; **6**: 59–71.

56. Brown GW, Harris TO. *Social Origins of Depression: A Study of Psychiatric Disorder in Women*. London: Tavistock, 1978.

57. Murphy E. Social origins of depression in old age. *Br J Psychiat* 1982; **141**: 135–42.

58. Davies ADM. Life events in the normal elderly. In Copeland JRM, Abou-Saleh MT, Blazer DG, eds, *Principles and Practice of Geriatric Psychiatry*, 1st edn. Chichester: Wiley, 1994; 106–13.

59. Davies ADM. Life events in the rural elderly. In Copeland JRM, Abou-Saleh MT, Blazer DG, eds, *Principles and Practice of Geriatric Psychiatry*, 1st edn. Chichester: Wiley, 1994; 114–15.

59. Murrell SA, Norris FH, Hutchins GL. Distribution and desirability of life events in older adults: population and policy implications. *J Commun Psychol* 1984; **12**: 301–11.

60. Smallegan M. Level of depressive symptoms and life stresses for culturally diverse older adults. *Gerontologist* 1989; **29**: 45–50.

61. Murrell SA, Meeks S, Walker J. Protective functions of health and self-esteem against depression in older adults facing illness or bereavement. *Psychol Aging* 1991; **6**: 352–60.

62. Cutrona CE, Russell D, Rose J. Social support and adaption to stress by the elderly. *J Psychol Aging* 1986; **1**: 47–54.

63. Hurwicz M-L, Durham CG, Boyd-Davis SL *et al*. Salient life events in three generation families. *J Gerontol* 1992; **47**: 11–13.

64. Linn MW, Hunter K, Harris R. Symptoms of depression and recent life events in the community elderly. *J Clin Psychol* 1980; **36**: 675–83.

65. Bowling A, Farquhar M, Browne P. Life satisfaction and associations with social network and support variables in three samples of elderly people. *Int J Geriat Psychiat* 1991; **6**: 549–66.

66. Woo J, Ho SC, Lau J *et al*. The prevalence of depressive symptoms and predisposing factors in an elderly Chinese population. *Acta Psychiat Scand* 1994; **89**: 8–13.

67. Fischer CS, Phillips SL. Who is alone? Social characteristics of people with small networks. In Peplau LA, Perlman D, eds, *Loneliness: a Source Book of Current Theory, Research and Therapy*. New York: Wiley, 1982.

68. Fitzpatrick R, Newman S, Lamb R, Shipley M. Social relationships and psychological well-being in rheumatoid arthritis. *Soc Sci Med* 1988; **27**: 399–403.

69. Reed D, McGee D, Yano K, Feinleib M. Social networks and coronary heart disease among Japanese men in Hawaii. *Am J Epidemiol* 1983; **117**: 384–96.

70. Lee GR. Kinship and social support of the elderly: the case of the United States. *Ageing Society* 1985; **5**: 19–38.

71. Madianos MG, Gournas G, Stefanis CN. Depressive symptoms and depression among elderly people in Athens. *Acta Psychiat Scand* 1992; **86**: 320–26.

72. O'Hara MW, Kohout FJ, Wallace RB. Depression among the rural elderly. A study of prevalence and correlates. *J Nerv Ment Disord* 1985; **173**: 582–9.

73. Weissman MM, Gershon ES, Kidd KK *et al*. Psychiatric disorders in the relatives of probands with affective disorders. *Arch Gen Psychiat* 1984; **41**: 13–21.

74. McGuffin P, Katz R, Rutherford J. Nature, nurture and depression: a twin study. *Psychol Med* 1991; **21**: 329–35.

75. Kendler KS, Neale MC, Kessler RC *et al*. A population-based twin study of major depression in women. The impact of varying definitions of illness. *Arch Gen Psychiat* 1992; **49**: 257–66.

76. Kendler KS, Neale MC, Kessler RC *et al*. A longitudinal twin study of 1-year prevalence of major depression in women. *Arch Gen Psychiat* 1993; **50**: 843–52.

77. Kendler KS, Neale MC, Kessler RC *et al*. The lifetime history of major depression in women. Reliability of diagnosis and heritability. *Arch Gen Psychiat* 1993; **50**: 863–70.

78. Kendler KS, Kessler RC, Heath AC *et al*. Coping: a genetic epidemiological investigation. *Psychol Med* 1991; **21**: 337–46.

79. Kendler KS, Kessler RC, Walters EE *et al*. Stressful life events, genetic liability, and onset of an episode of major depression in women. *Am J Psychiat* 1995; **152**: 833–42.

80. Van Ojen R, Hooijer C, Bezemer D *et al*. The relationship between psychiatric history, MMSE and family history. *Br J Psychiat* 1995; **166**: 316–19.

81. Kay DW, Henderson AS, Scott R *et al*. Dementia and depression among the elderly living in the Hobart community: the effect of the diagnostic criteria on the prevalence rates. *Psychol Med* 1985; **15**: 771–88.

82. Scherr PA, Albert MS, Funkenstein HH *et al*. Correlates of cognitive function in an elderly community population. *Am J Epidemiol* 1988; **128**: 1084–101.

83. Prince M, Lewis G, Bird A *et al*. A longitudinal study of factors predicting change in cognitive test scores over time, in an older hypertensive population. *Psychol Med* 1996; **26**: 555–68.

84. Sapolsky RM, Krey LC, McEwin B. The neuroendocrinology of stress and ageing: the glucocorticoid cascade hypothesis. *Endocr Rev* 1986; **7**: 284–301.

85. O'Brien J, Desmond P, Ames D. A magnetic resonance imaging study of white matter lesions in depression and Alzheimer's disease. *Br J Psychiat* 1996; **168**: 447–85.

86. Van Ojen R. Origins of Depression: A Study in the Elderly Population. Chapter 5 Etiological Factors in Depression. PhD Thesis, Vrije Universiteit, Amsterdam, 1995; 57–76.

87. Beekman ATF, Copeland JRM, Prince MJ. Review of community prevalence of depression in later life. *Br J Psychiat* 1999; **174**: 307–11.

88. Blazer D, Burchett B, Service C, George LK. The association of age and depression among the elderly: an epidemiologic exploration. *J Gerontol* 1991; **46**: M210–15.

Risk Factors and the Incidence of Post-stroke Depression

P. W. Burvill

University of Western Australia, Australia

Post-stroke depression (PSD) is the most common psychiatric syndrome following stroke, but there is no specific PSD syndrome. It is commonly unrecognized and untreated in clinical practice. Rao[1] has reviewed the literature on the relationship between depression and cerebrovascular disease, including strokes.

PREVALENCE

Reported prevalence of PSD has varied between 30–60%, 8–30% major and 20–40% minor depression. The reasons for this wide variation include different assessment methods, diagnostic criteria, time elapsed after the stroke and patient settings, together with assessment difficulties in the presence of aphasic, cognitive and physical disabilities.

The lowest number of reported cases have come from community population-based studies. Several authors have concluded that it is unproved that depression is commoner in an unselected group of patients after strokes than it is among the elderly with other physical conditions. Most cases of PSD develop during the first 2–3 months post-stroke.

RISK FACTORS

Described pre-stroke risk factors include personal or family history of depression or other psychiatric disorder, socially impaired personality, neuroticism, high alcoholic intake, social isolation and negative life events. Post-stroke factors include perception of the effects of the stroke as a significant loss, dysphasia, significant disability, impaired cognition, living in a nursing home, isolation and poor social supports. Most, but not all, studies have reported age, gender, educational level and marital status as unimportant.

Described biological risk factors include pre-stroke subcortical atrophy, especially of periventricular white matter, site and size of the lesions, and ischaemic rather than haemorrhagic stroke.

Disruption of adrenergic and serotonergic pathways by the lesion, giving depletion of biogenic amines, has been postulated.

Robinson and Starkstein[2] considered the location of the lesion in the brain as the single most important aetiological factor in PSD, with the highest frequency of PSD associated with anterior lesions in the left hemisphere. Their method of neuroradiological lesion location has been criticized[3]. Lesions of the globus pallidus, putamen and caudate nucleus in association with PSD have been described.

A recent literature review by Singh *et al.*[4] concluded that any definitive statements about stroke lesion location and risk of depression have not yet been substantiated. Anatomical correlates of PSD change over time and may explain interstudy differences in the association of lesion location with PSD[5]. Furthermore, mood changes may be mediated through the distant effects of lesions, as shown by PET studies, or the lesions may play a facilitatory role for another primary mechanism leading to depression. Many of these risk factors may be interrelated, e.g. size of lesions, disability, impaired cognition and living in a nursing home.

REFERENCES

1. Rao R. Cerebrovascular disease and late life depression: an age-old association revisited. *Int J Geriat Psychiat* 2000; **15**: 419–33.
2. Robinson RG, Starkstein SE. Current research in affective disorders following stroke. *J Neuropsychiat Clin Neurosci* 1990; **2**: 1–14.
3. Burvill PW, Johnson GA, Chakera TMH *et al.* The place of site of lesion in the aetiology of post-stroke depression. *Cerebrovasc Dis* 1996; **6**: 208–15.
4. Singh A, Herrmann N, Black SE. The importance of lesion location in poststroke depression: a critical review. *Can J Psychiat* 1998; **43**: 921–7.
5. Shimoda K, Robinson RG. The relationship between poststroke depression and lesion location in long-term follow-up. *Biol Psychiat* 1999; **45**: 187–92.

71

Epidemiology of Depression: Prevalence and Incidence

Dan G. Blazer

Duke University Medical Center, Durham, NC, USA

Many symptom checklists have been used to estimate the burden of depressive symptoms in community populations. The results of these studies are remarkably consistent, with the range of significant depressive symptoms estimated to be 10–25% (see Table 71.1). Estimates of the prevalence of major depression and dysthymic disorder are presented in Table 71.2 from four different countries. The prevalence of major depression is much lower in community samples than is the prevalence of depressive symptoms, 1–5% in most community surveys. Lower prevalences of major depression have been found in more rural samples with an estimate of less than 1% in a North Carolina rural sample, whereas urban studies have typically estimated higher prevalence. The prevalence of dysthymic disorder is generally higher than that for major depression, approximately 2–8%, depending on the instrument used in the survey. Prevalence estimates are difficult to compare cross-nationally, as different instruments are used. Comparison is even more difficult when symptom burden is confused with diagnosed cases. For example, if the prevalences of dysthymic disorder and major depression are combined and the frequent co-morbidity of dysthymic disorder and major depression taken into account, the majority of subjects suffering significant depressive symptoms in community populations still do not qualify for diagnosis. One of the major tasks facing psychiatric epidemiologists studying depression cross-nationally in the elderly is to explain the residual depressive symptoms in community samples not easily captured by the usual diagnostic categories.

In a recent review of 34 studies of the prevalence of late-life depression by Beekman *et al.*[11] (part of the EURODEP Study),

the prevalence varied (0.4–35%). Arranged according to diagnostic category, major depression was relatively rare (weighted average prevalence of 1.8%), minor depression more common (weighted average prevalence of 9.8%) while all depressive syndromes deemed clinically relevant yield an average prevalence of 13.5%. Depression was more common among women and among older people living under adverse socioeconomic circumstances. In a cross-national comparison of nine European centers using the GMS–AGECAT package to abstract diagnoses, differences in prevalence by country were most evident, with a range from 8.8% in Iceland to 23.6% in Munich. The overall prevalence estimated by meta-analysis was 12.3%, 14.1% for women and 8.6% for men. Among the elderly, there was little variation by age across all sites.

The prevalence of depression in acute medical facilities is presented in Table 71.3. Estimates range from 5% to 10% for major depression but, of more importance, an additional 15–25% experience clinically significant symptoms not captured by the diagnosis of major depression. The same is true for estimates of prevalence in long-term care facilities (see Table 71.4). Estimates range between 5% and 15% for major depression, yet an additional 30% of the sample subjects (in one study) suffered clinically significant depressive symptoms that did not meet the criteria for major depression. Estimates of depressive symptoms and depressive diagnoses (major depression and dysthymic disorder) among the elderly should not be based solely on community samples. Older adults in hospital or residing in long-term care facilities are much more likely to

Table 71.1 Prevalence of depressive symptoms in community samples of older adults

Author	Sample	(*n*)	Screening method	Findings
Blazer and Williams, 1980[1]	Community sample in North Carolina (65+)	997	OARS Depression Scale	14.7% significant depressive symptoms. No age, gender or racial difference in prevalence
Kivela *et al.*, 1986[2]	Community sample of elderly in Finland	1529	Zung SDS	29.7% of females and 22.4% of males with significant depressive symptoms
Ben-Arie *et al.*, 1987[3]	Community sample of the elderly "coloured" in Cape Town	139	PSE symptoms	13% with significant depressive symptoms
Kennedy *et al.*, 1989[4]	Community sample in Bronx, NY	2317	CES-D	16.9% with significant depressive symptoms, more prevalent in females and the oldest-old
Ihara, 1993[5]	Rural community sample in Japan	695	CES-D	5.3% with significant depressive symptoms
Livingstone *et al.*, 1990[6]	Community sample of elderly in inner London	813	CARE	15.9% with significant depressive symptoms

OARS, Older Americans Resources and Services; SDS, Self-rating Depression Scale; PSE, Present State Examination; CES-D, Center for Epidemiologic Studies Depression Scale; CARE, Comprehensive Assessment and Referral Evaluation

Principles and Practice of Geriatric Psychiatry, 2nd edn. Edited by J. R. M. Copeland, M. T. Abou-Saleh and D. G. Blazer
©2002 John Wiley & Sons, Ltd

Table 71.2 Prevalence of dysthymia, minor depression and major depression in community samples of older adults

Author	Sample	(n)	Screening method	Findings
Blazer et al., 1987[7]	Community sample in North Carolina, USA	1304	Diagnostic Interview Schedule (DIS)	0.8% with major depression, 2% with dysthymia, 4% with minor depression
Copeland et al., 1987[8]	Community sample in Liverpool	1070	Geriatric Mental State Schedule	2.9% with major depression, 8.3% with minor depression
Beekman et al., 1995[9]	Community sample in The Netherlands	3056	CES-D/DIS	2.0% with major depression, 12.9% with minor depression
Pahkala et al., 1995[10]	Community sample in Finland	1086	DSM-III diagnosis	2.2% with major depression, 14.3% with minor depression

Table 71.3. Prevalence of depression in acute care medical facilities

Author	Sample	(n)	Diagnostic method	Findings
Koenig et al., 1986[12]	VA inpatient sample of men 70+	171	Screening plus modified DIS	11.5% with major depression; 23% with significant depressive symptoms
O'Riordan et al., 1989[13]	Acute medical geriatric assessment unit	111	Geriatric Depression Scale and Clinical Interview	4.5% with major depression; 3.6% with dysthymic disorder; 10.8% with significant depressive symptoms (most with dementia)

experience depressive symptoms and be diagnosed with major depression or dysthymic disorder than persons living in the community.

Incidence studies of depression in the elderly are extremely rare in the literature. Two studies provide some estimate of incidence, however. Rorsman et al.[18] estimated incident depression from the Lundby cohort in Sweden among 2612 individuals evaluated in 1957 and later in 1972 (i.e. 15 year incidence) until the age of 70. The cumulative probability of suffering a first episode of depression was 27% for men and 45% for women, a very high incidence figure in this cohort (especially compared to lifetime prevalence figures, reported in other studies, of less than 15%). The annual age-standardized first incidence for depression, all degrees of impairment included, was 0.43 for men and 0.76 for women. Incidence appears to decrease in the studies as individuals aged, especially for men. Eaton et al. (1997)[19] estimated the incidence of major depression over 10 years for the ECA cohort from Baltimore. They found an overall estimated annual incidence of 3.0 per 1000 per year, with a peak while subjects were in their 30s, a smaller peak when subjects were in their 50s and a definite lower incidence in the elderly. Prodromal symptoms were present many years before the full criteria for major

depression were met, further linking the minor and major depression, Foster et al. (1991)[20] estimated the incidence of depression in long-term care facilities. In a cohort of 104 new admissions followed for a year, they found an incidence of 14%. One-third of these new cases were diagnosed as major depression, two-thirds as minor depression.

HISTORICAL TRENDS OF DEPRESSIVE DISORDERS

Historical studies in epidemiology assist investigators to establish the frequency of disorders in populations at different points in time. To understand the prevalence of major depression in late life compared to earlier stages of the life cycle in modern Western societies (e.g. major depression appears to be less frequent in older adults), an historical approach is necessary. Depressive disorders, such as tuberculosis, acquired immune deficiency syndrome (AIDS) and smallpox, wax and wane in frequency through time. Unfortunately, historical studies in psychiatric epidemiology are rare. Therefore, temporal changes in mental illness are difficult to determine.

Table 71.4. Prevalence of depression in long-term care facilities

Author	Sample	(n)	Diagnostic method	Findings
Parmelee et al., 1989[14]	Nursing home and congregate apartment residence in Philadelphia	708	DSM-IIIR checklist	12.4% with major depression; 35% significant depressive symptoms
Bond et al., 1989[15]	Three British NHS nursing homes	568	Critchton Royal Behavioral Scale and the Survey Psychiatric Assessment Scale	32–42% with severe affective disorder or psychoneurosis
Phillips and Henderson, 1991[16]	24 Australian nursing homes	323	DSM-IIIR criteria	6.1% of residents suffered from a severe depressive episode, 6.7% from a moderate depressive episode and 6.7% from a mild depressive episode
Gerety et al., 1994[17]	5 Nursing homes	135	Structured Clinical Interview for DSM-III-R diagnoses	26% diagnosed with a major depressive episode

Some investigators, however, have explored historical trends via the so-called "cohort effect". Klerman[21] noted that, in contrast to the "age of anxiety" following the Second World War, modern Western society may be entering an "age of melancholy", precipitated by social factors, such as the threat of nuclear warfare, a perceived threat of environmental pollution and economic instability. Estimates of prevalence by age from the Epidemiologic Catchment Area Studies in the USA reveal a significant decrease in both current and lifetime prevalence of major depression by age cross-sectionally. In a separate study, Klerman et al.[22], analyzing family history data from subjects in the Psychobiology of Depression Study, found a progressive increase in the rates of depression in successively younger birth cohorts throughout the twentieth century, with an earlier age of onset of depression with each successive birth cohort. However, these cross-sectional studies, which suggest an "age of melancholy", must be considered in the context of historical studies.

To interpret historical trends, one must consider the cohort effect. Four findings suggest that younger birth cohorts carry a higher prevalence of depression than older cohorts. First, longitudinal studies have typically demonstrated a consistent burden of depression across the life cycle for each birth cohort[23]. That is, the prevalence of depression within a birth cohort does not change with increasing age. Second, younger birth cohorts appear to experience higher prevalences of depression than the older birth cohorts in the latter two decades of the twentieth century[24,25]. Third, suicide rates do increase with age, which in turn drives the overall rate of suicide up with age[26]. Fourth, the changes in rates of suicide and depression by age group over the past 50 years have been of such magnitude that the varying rates are best explained by psychosocial rather than biological or evolutionary factors.

Those factors that contributed to a relative protection of older birth cohorts from depression and suicide in the 1990s in Western societies, compared to younger cohorts, and that contributed to the relative increase in depression and suicide among younger cohorts in the 1990s, are unknown (but subject to much speculation). Interpreting these data, investigators and clinicians must take care to recognize that significant methodological problems in historical studies remain. Even a clear and decisive endpoint, such as suicide, can be misleading, for suicide rates are obtained from a review of death certificates, which are subject to considerable bias. Methods for estimating the prevalence of depression change through time, and therefore it is difficult to compare studies from many years in the past with current studies (due to an evolving instrumentation for measuring depression in community and clinical samples).

CONCLUSION

In summary, it appears that results from cross-sectional studies in Western societies estimate the prevalence of depression in older adults to be lower than the prevalence in young and middle-aged adults. These findings are most striking in the USA (particularly the Epidemiologic Catchment Area Studies) but also appear in other studies. Nevertheless, these findings must be interpreted with caution. Methodological problems in identifying depression across the life cycle may contribute to these difficulties. In addition, birth cohorts, with the well-known stability of function and disease that birth cohorts demonstrate, must be taken into account before cross-sectional data are translated into longitudinal interpretations.

REFERENCES

1. Blazer DG, Williams CD. The epidemiology of dysphoria and depression in an elderly population. *Am J Psychiat* 1980; **137**: 439–44.
2. Kivela SL, Pahkela K, Laippala P. Prevalence of depression in an elderly population in Finland. *Acta Psychiat Scand* 1988; **78**: 401–13.
3. Ben-Arie T, Swartz L, Bickman BJ. Depression in the elderly living in the community: its presentation and features. *Br J Psychiat* 1987; **150**: 169–74.
4. Kennedy GJ, Kelman HR, Thomas C et al. Hierarchy of characteristics associated with depressive symptoms in an urban elderly sample. *Am J Psychiat* 1989; **146**: 220–5.
5. Ihara, 1993.
6. Livingstone et al., 1990.
7. Blazer D, Hughes DC, George LK. The epidemiology of depression in an elderly community population. *Gerontologist* 1987; **27**: 281–7.
8. Copeland JRM, Dewey ME, Wood N et al. Range of mental illness among the elderly in the community: Prevalence in Liverpool using the GMS–AGECAT package. *Br J Psychiat* 1987; **150**: 815–23.
9. Beekman ATF, Deeg DJH, vanTilburg T et al. Major and minor depression in later life: a study of prevalence and associated factors. *J Affect Disord* 1995; **36**: 65–75.
10. Pahkala K, Kesti E, Kongas-Saviaro P et al. Prevalence of depression in an aged population in Finland. *Soc Psychiat Epidemiol* 1995; **30**: 99–106.
11. Beekman ATF, Copeland, JRM, Prince MJ. Review of community prevalence of depression in later life. *Br J Psychiat* 1999; **174**: 307–11.
12. Koenig HG, Meador KG, Cohen HJ, Blazer DG. Depression in elderly hospitalized patients with a medical illness. *Arch Intern Med* 1989; **148**: 1929–36.
13. O'Riordan TG, Hayes JP, Shelley R et al. The prevalence of depression in an acute geriatric medical assessment unit. *Int J Geriat Psychiat* 1989; **4**: 17–21.
14. Parmelee PA, Katz IR, Lawton MP. Depression among the institutionalized aging: Assessment and prevalence estimation. *J Gerontol* 1989; **44**: M22–9.
15. Bond J, Atkinson A, Gregson BA. The prevalence of psychiatric illness among continuing-care patients under the care of departments of geriatric medicine. *Int J Geriat Psychiat* 1989; **4**: 227–33.
16. Phillips CJ, Henderson AS. The prevalence of depression among Australian nursing home residents: results using draft ICD-10 and DSM-III-R criteria. *Psychol Med* 1991; **21**: 739–48.
17. Gerety MB, Williams JW, Mulrow CD et al. Performance of case-finding tools for depression in the nursing home: influence of clinical and functional characteristics and selection of optimal threshold scores. *J Am Geriatric Soc* 1994; **42**: 1103–9.
18. Rorsman B, Grasbeck A, Hagnell O et al. A prospective study of first-incidence depression: the Lundby Study, 1957–1972. *Br J Psychiat* 1990; **156**: 336–42.
19. Eaton WW, Anthony JC, Gallo J et al. Natural history of Diagnostic Interview Schedule/DSM-IV major depression. The Baltimore Epidemiologic Catchment Area follow-up. *Arch Gen Psychiat* 1997; **54**: 993–9.
20. Foster JR, Cataldo JK, Boksay IJE. Incidence of depression in a medical long-term facility: findings on a restricted sample of new admissions. *Int J Geriat Psychiat* 1991; **6**: 13–20.
21. Klerman GL. Affective disorders. In Nicholai A, ed., *The Harvard Guide to Modern Psychiatry*. Cambridge, MA: Belknap, 1978; 253–81.
22. Klerman GL, Lavori PW, Rice J et al. Birth-cohort trends and rates of major depressive disorders among relatives of patients with affective disorder. *Arch Gen Psychiat* 1985; **42**: 689–95.
23. Srole L, Fischer AK. The mid-town Manhattan longitudinal study vs. "the mental Paradise Lost" doctrine. *Arch Gen Psychiat* 1980; **37**: 209–21.
24. Robins LN, Helzer JE, Weissman MM et al. Life-time prevalence of specific psychiatric disorders in three sites. *Arch Gen Psychiat* 1984; **41**: 949–58.

25. Myers JK, Weissman MM, Tischler GL *et al*. Six-month prevalence of psychiatric disorders in three communities. *Arch Gen Psychiat* 1984; **41**: 959–70.
26. Blazer DG, Bachar JR, Manton KG. Suicide in late life: review and commentary. *J Am Geriat Soc* 1986; **34**: 519–25.
27. Jensen K. Psychiatric problems in four Danish old age homes. *Acta Psychiat Scand* 1966; **169** (suppl): 411–18.
28. Copeland JRM, Beekman ATF, Dewey ME *et al*. Depression in Europe: geographical distribution among older people. *Br J Psychiat* 1999; **174**: 312–29.
29. Kua EH. Depressive disorder in elderly Chinese people. *Acta Psychiat Scand* 1990; **81**: 386–8.

Epidemiological Catchment Area Studies of Mood Disorders

Dan G. Blazer

Duke University Medical Center, Durham, MC, USA

The National Institute of Mental Health Multi-site Epidemiologic Catchment Area (ECA)[1] Program consists of a combined community and institutional survey of five communities in the USA: New Haven, Connecticut; Baltimore, Maryland; Durham, North Carolina; St Louis, Missouri and Los Angeles, California. Because of the large sample drawn for this study and because oversamples of the elderly were drawn at three sites, data are available that permit the estimate of the prevalence of affective disorders from a larger sample of community-dwelling elders than from any other extant study.

The goals of the Epidemiologic Catchment Area Program were to: (a) estimate the prevalence of specific psychiatric disorders using a similar methodology across multiple geographic sampling areas; (b) determine correlates of these specific psychiatric disorders; and (c) determine the relationship between psychiatric disorders and health services utilization.

The 6-month prevalence of the affective disorders from the five ECA sites overall range from 4% to 7%[2]. All affective disorders, except for bereavement, were less prevalent in the elderly than at other stages of the life cycle. For example, the prevalence of major depression in men ranged between 1% and 4% among the 18–24 year-olds but was consistently less than 1% in the 65 age group. Among 18–24 year-old women, the prevalence of major depression was 7%, whereas in women in the 65+ age group it did not exceed 3% at any of the ECA sites. Recent incidence studies from the ECA sample suggest that the incidence for major depression peaks in the 30s with a smaller peak during the 50s. Incidence is much lower for the elderly.

Dysthymic disorder varied less by age in prevalence than major depression and was more prevalent than major depression in the elderly[3]. For example, the prevalence of dysthymic disorder was 0.5–3% in 18–24 year-old men and 0.5–2% in 65 year-old men. Among women, dysthymic disorder was 1–4% in 18–24 year-old women and between 1–4% in 65+ year-old women. Overall, current affective disorders of all types were less frequent in older persons (65+ years of age) than for any other age group. Manic disorders were extremely rare in the sample overall (0.5–1%). No cases of mania were identified in the 65+ age group across the five ECA sites.

The lifetime prevalence rates for the DSM-III specific psychiatric disorders evaluated in the ECA sample paralleled rates of current prevalence but, as would be expected, were higher[3]. Lifetime prevalence for major depression was 4–10% in the 25–44 age group but was not higher than 2% in the 65+ age group at any ECA site. Only one lifetime occurrence of manic episode was identified in this very large sample.

The ECA studies have received considerable criticism from geriatric psychiatrists who perceive that the study design significantly underestimates the prevalence of affective disorders in older adults. The dramatic differences in prevalence (both current and lifetime) by age surely calls for some explanation. Studies are emerging to suggest that the Diagnostic Interview Schedule, the instrument used to determine the prevalence of psychiatric disorders in the ECA sample, may possibly be biased toward underestimating the prevalence of affective disorders in older persons. Specifically, the threshold for a symptom being identified by the instrument may be increased for older persons. Nevertheless, the threshold effect does not appear to explain the dramatic differences in prevalence and has led a number of investigators to suspect that a cohort phenomenon is operative[5]. That is, older persons not only have lower current prevalence of depression in the 1990s, they have always experienced a lower prevalence. According to a number of studies, this is true among more modern, Western societies.

REFERENCES

1. Regier DA, Myers JK, Kramer M *et al*. The NIMH Epidemiologic Catchment Area Program. *Arch Gen Psychiat* 1984; **41**: 934–41.
2. Myers JK, Weissman MM, Tischler GL *et al*. Six-month prevalence of psychiatric disorders in three communities. *Arch Gen Psychiat* 1984; **41**: 959–70.
3. Robins LN, Helzer JE, Weissman MM. Lifetime prevalence of specific psychiatric disorders in three sites. *Arch Gen Psychiat* 1984; **41**: 949–58.
4. Klerman GL, Weissman MM. Increasing rates of depression. *J Am Med Assoc* 1989; **261**: 229–35.
5. Blazer, DG, Bachar JR, Manton KG. Suicide in late life: review and commentary. *J Am Geriat Soc* 1986; **34**: 519–25.
6. Eaton WW, Anthony JC, Gallo J *et al*. Natural history of Diagnostic Interview Schedule/DSM-IV major depression. The Baltimore Catchment Area Follow-up. *Arch Gen Psychiat* 1997; **54**: 989–99.

EURODEP—Prevalence of Depression in Europe

John R. M. Copeland

Royal Liverpool University Hospital, Liverpool, UK

The aims of the EURODEP Concerted Action were to use existing studies which had employed the GMS–AGECAT method of diagnosis to assess the prevalence of depression in nine European countries (10 centres)—Liverpool, Amsterdam (sample A), Berlin, Dublin, Iceland, London, Maastricht, Munich, Verona and Zaragoza. Later Tirana was added (not reported here), and five non-AGECAT centres joined after the study commenced— Bordeaux, Oulu, Antwerp, Amsterdam (sample B) and Göteborg.

All subjects were aged 65 or over. In Munich the subjects were aged 85 and above and in Iceland 85–87. The Amsterdam study (sample A) had an upper age limit of 84. All the studies took random samples in the community except Dublin, which sampled a general practice. Sample size varied from 202 in Verona to 5222 in Liverpool, giving a total sample of 13 803. Substantial differences in the prevalence of depression were found, with Iceland having the lowest level at 8.8%, followed by Liverpool, 10.0%; Zaragoza, 10.7%; Dublin, 11.9%; Amsterdam, 12.0%; Berlin, 16.5%; London, 17.3%; Verona, 18.3%; and Munich, 23.6%. When all five AGECAT depression levels, including both subcases of depression and cases, were added together, five high-scoring centres emerged, namely Amsterdam, Berlin, Munich, London and Verona (30.4–37.9%) and four low-scoring centres, Dublin, Iceland, Liverpool and Zaragoza (17.7–21.4%). There was no constant association between prevalence and age. A meta-analysis of the pooled data on the nine European centres yielded an overall prevalence of 12.3% (95% CI, 11.8–12.9); for women, 14.1% (95% CI, 13.5–14.8) and for men, 8.6% (95% CI, 7.9–9.3%)[1].

The proportions of depressive symptoms were found to vary between centres. In Amsterdam, for example, 40% of a general population of older people admitted to depressive mood, compared to only 26% in Zaragoza. Symptoms such as "future bleak", "hopelessness", "wish to be dead", were generally rare, but the last reached higher levels in Berlin, Munich and Verona. Sleep disturbance was admitted by only 15% of the population in Dublin, but 54% and 60% in Munich and Berlin. Large differences for some depressive symptoms were found within the very old populations, with lower levels in Iceland and higher levels in Munich. Overall, the levels of depressive symptoms among over 60% of the older general population of Europe were low, so that pejorative stereotypes of old age in Europe were not upheld[2].

In order to include non-AGECAT centres, attempts were made to harmonize the depression measures that had been used with items from the Geriatric Mental State examination. A scale was constructed, the Euro-D scale[3]. The scale appeared to work well and was applied to data from 21 724 subjects. Euro-D scores tended to increase with increasing age, unlike the levels of prevalence of depression. Women had generally higher scores than men, and widowed and separated subjects higher than those who were currently or never married[4].

Depression was confirmed as a common illness among older people in Europe. A number of other studies have shown poor treatment levels. It was concluded that opportunities for effective treatment were almost certainly being lost.

REFERENCES

1. Copeland JRM, Beekman ATF, Dewey ME *et al*. Depression in Europe. Geographical distribution among older people. *Br J Psychiat* 1999; **174**: 312–21.
2. Copeland JRM, Beekman ATF, Dewey ME *et al*. Cross-cultural comparison of depressive symptoms in Europe does not support stereotypes of ageing. *Br J Psychiat* 1999; **174**: 322–9.
3. Prince MJ, Reischies F, Beekman ATF *et al*. Development of the EURO-D Scale—A European union initiative to compare symptoms of depression in 14 European centres. *Br J Psychiat* 1999; **174**: 330–8.
4. Prince MJ, Beekman ATF, Deeg DJH *et al*. Depression symptoms in late life assessed using the EURO-D Scale. The effect of age, gender and marital status in 14 European Centres. *Br J Psychiat* 1999; **174**: 339–45.

Depression in Older Primary Care Patients: Diagnosis and Course

Jeffrey M. Lyness and Eric D. Caine

University of Rochester Medical Center, Rochester, NY, USA

Depressive symptoms and syndromes in later life are a major public health problem[1,2]. Primary care clinical settings are especially important venues to better understand depressive psychopathology among older people. Older people with psychiatric disorders utilize mental health services infrequently, especially in comparison with younger persons, yet they are *more* likely to see their primary care physicians regularly[3,4]. Elders who complete suicide have often seen their primary care providers shortly before death, and the majority of them were suffering from depressive conditions at the time of their death[4]. There are also many lines of evidence suggesting that the nature of psychopathology seen in primary care differs from that seen in psychiatric or residential care sites[3,4,6,7]. Thus, to better understand the nature of depression seen among primary care elders, we must study subjects recruited from primary care practices[8–11].

A growing number of studies have examined the prevalence of mood disorders among older primary care patients. Similar to younger and mixed-age primary care samples, major depression is common, with a point prevalence of 5–10% in the elderly[6,12,13]. An even greater number of patients have a history of major depression but are currently not fully syndromic, i.e. the point prevalence of major depression in partial or full remission is approximately 12%. Thus, one-fifth of all older persons seen in primary care settings have a depressive condition that, at the least, requires vigilance and education regarding recurrence and may require acute, continuation or maintenance therapy.

The prevalence of so-called "lesser" depressive conditions is also considerable among primary care elders. Dysthymic disorder is relatively uncommon, however, with an estimated point prevalence of 1%, of which half is co-morbid with superimposed major depression[6]. This low prevalence primarily reflects that the specific entry criterion of dysthymia seems to be less applicable to elders, where they fail to fulfill the requirement that depressed mood occurs for "most of the day, for more days than not . . . for at least two years". However, studies using any of various definitions of "minor", "subsyndromal" or "subthreshold" depression have noted point prevalences comparable to those for major depression[7,14,15]. For example, one study used the criteria set for minor depressive disorder proposed in the Appendix to DSM-IV, finding a prevalence of 5%[7]. The same group also arbitrarily defined a subsyndromal group comprising patients scoring >10 on the Hamilton Rating Scale for Depression (but *not* meeting criteria for major or minor depression) and noted a point prevalence of 10%. Some have raised concerns that classifying such "lesser" depressive symptoms as mood disorder is bringing "normal" age-related distress under the rubric of psychopathology. In fact, patients with minor and subsyndromal depression suffer both medical co-morbidity and functional disability comparable to that of major depression (and substantially greater than non-depressed controls), suggesting that these are conditions of considerable clinical importance, albeit a heterogeneous and as-yet poorly characterized group.

While studies of younger or mixed-age groups of primary care patients have demonstrated that major depression has high rates of persistence in both remitting–recurring and continuous patterns, broadly comparable to the chronicity seen in psychiatric treatment settings, much less is known about elders. So-called "lesser depressive symptoms" were powerful risk factors for subsequent new onset, or recurrent, diagnosable depression disorders in mixed-age or younger adults[16,17]. However, few investigations have focused on older persons or disentangled the findings of their older subjects from their younger subjects. Two prospective studies[18,19] of older depressed subjects found that depressive symptoms (at 33 months and 9 months, respectively) had considerable rates of persistence but also of remission and recurrence. Both studies assessed depression solely by use of self-report depressive symptom scales, and therefore were unable to determine specific depressive diagnoses. These results were also limited by the potentially reduced validity of self-report methodology regarding depressive symptoms among older persons. One recent report[12], using well-operationalized measures to establish a research diagnosis of major depression among older patients seen at university-affiliated internal medicine centers, found that at 6 month follow-up 38% of subjects with major depression continued to be fully syndromic, and only 11.5% were fully recovered. Preliminary data from our group showed that more than half of older primary care patients suffering major, minor or subsyndromal depression still suffered clinically significant depressive symptoms at 1 year (Lyness *et al.*, manuscript in preparation). In sum, the course of major and other depressions among primary care elders is largely unknown, but available evidence suggests considerable persistence, as well as variability of symptoms, over time.

Similarly, examination of specific predictors of outcome in this group is largely lacking. Medical illness burden is the most powerfully and consistently identified factor associated with the presence or course of depression in later life[1,20,21]. However, most studies of the relationship of medical illness to depression in later life have used psychiatric patient populations or mixed-community samples, rather than subjects from primary care settings. There have been cross-sectional studies demonstrating an association between medical illness burden and depression in primary care elderly[6,12,22]. Two published longitudinal investigations of older primary care patients[18,19] found that medical status (number of illnesses and self-health perception, respectively) predicted depressive symptoms at 33 and 9 month follow-up, respectively. However, these studies were limited by the use of relatively crude proxies for medical co-morbidity and by a lack of diagnostic assessments for depression. Thus, the predictive role of medical illness (measured by validated instruments) with regard to major or subsyndromal depression in primary care elderly remains to be defined. Similarly, other factors that predict depression outcome in younger adults, or in older psychiatric or nursing-home patients, include functional disability, personality trait neuroticism and social support; with few exceptions, these predictors have not been studied in primary care elders.

Little is known about treatment, too. In our above-cited study, less than half of patients with current major depression were prescribed antidepressant treatment[7], consistent with findings in younger people that depression is frequently undertreated. A wide variety of physician, patient and physician–patient interaction factors may underlie this low treatment rate, but these remain to be defined rigorously through a variety of quantitative and qualitative study methods. Also, antidepressant treatment rates were similar for major, minor and subsyndromal depression groups, despite the lack of empirical support for medication efficacy for the latter conditions. This suggests that the primary care physicians did not discriminate among these diagnostic categories. Rather, they appear to make treatment decisions based on factors that do not directly relate to the symptomatic or syndromic severity of their patients' depressive conditions.

ACKNOWLEDGEMENTS

Supported by NIMH Grants K07 MH01113 to J. M. L. and T32 MH18911 to E. D. C.

REFERENCES

1. Caine ED, Lyness JM, King DA. Reconsidering depression in the elderly. *Am J Geriat Psychiat* 1993; **1**: 4–20.
2. NIH Consensus Development Panel on Depression in Late Life. Diagnosis and treatment of depression in late life. *J Am Med Assoc* 1992; **268**: 1018–24.
3. Regier DA, Farmer ME, Rae DS *et al.* One-month prevalence of mental disorders in the United States and sociodemographic characteristics: the Epidemiologic Catchment Area study. *Acta Psychiat Scand* 1993; **88**: 35–47.
4. Shepherd M, Wilkinson G. Primary care as the middle ground for psychiatric epidemiology. *Psychol Med* 1988; **18**: 263–7.
5. Conwell Y. Suicide in elderly patients. In Schneider LS, Reynolds CF III, Lebowitz BD, Friedhoff AJ, eds, *Diagnosis and Treatment of Depression in Late Life*. Washington, DC: American Psychiatric Press, 1994.
6. Lyness JM, Caine ED, King DA *et al.* Psychiatric disorders in older primary care patients. *J Gen Intern Med* 1999; **14**: 249–54.

7. Lyness JM, King DA, Cox C et al. The importance of subsyndromal depression in older primary care patients: prevalence and associated functional disability. *J Am Geriat Soc* 1999; **47**: 647–52.

8. Gallo J, Rabins PV, Iliffe SI. The "research magnificent" in late life: psychiatric epidemiology and the primary health care of older adults. *Int J Psychiat Med* 1967; **27**: 185–204.

9. Woolley DC. Geriatric psychiatry in primary care: a focus on ambulatory settings. *Psychiat Clin N Am* 1997; **20**: 241–60.

10. Alexopoulos GS. Geriatric depression in primary care. *Int J Geriat Psychiat* 1996; **11**: 397–400.

11. Oxman TE. New paradigms for understanding the identification and treatment of depression in primary care. *Gen Hosp Psychiat* 1997; **19**: 79–81.

12. Schulberg HC, Mulsant B, Schulz R et al. Characteristics and course of major depression in older primary care patients. *Int J Psychiat Med* 1998; **28**: 421–36.

13. Borson S, Barnes, RA, Kukull WA et al. Symptomatic depression in elderly medical outpatients. I. Prevalence, demography, and health service utilization. *J Am Geriat Soc* 1986; **34**: 341–7.

14. Oxman TE, Barrett FE, Barrett J, Gerber P. Symptomatology of late-life minor depression among primary care patients. *Psychosomatics* 1990; **31**: 174–80.

15. Beekman ATF, Deeg DJH, Braam AW et al. Consequences of major and minor depression in later life: a study of disability, well-being and service utilization. *Psychol Med* 1997; **27**: 1397–409.

16. Copeland JRM, Davidson IA, Dewey ME et al. Alzheimer's disease, other dementias, depression and pseudo-dementia. Prevalence, incidence and three-year outcome in Liverpool. *Br J Psychiat* 1992; **161**: 230–9.

17. Horwath E, Johnson J, Klerman GL, Weissman MM. Depressive symptoms as relative and attributable risk factors for first-onset major depression. *Arch Gen Psychiat* 1992; **49**: 817–23.

18. Kukull WA, Koepsell TD, Inui TS et al. Depression and physical illness among elderly general medical clinic patients. *J Affect Disord* 1986; **10**: 153–62.

19. Callahan CM, Hui SL, Nienaber NA et al. Longitudinal study of depression and health services use among elderly primary care patients. *J Am Geriat Soc* 1994; **42**: 833–8.

20. Katz IR. On the inseparability of mental and physical health in aged persons. Lessons from depression and medical comorbidity. *Am J Geriat Psychiat* 1996; **4**: 1–16.

21. Lyness JM, Bruce ML, Koenig HG et al. Depression and medical illness in late life: report of a symposium. *J Am Geriat Soc* 1996; **44**: 198–203.

22. Williamson GM, Schulz R. Physical illness and symptoms of depression among elderly outpatients. *Psychol Aging* 1992; **7**: 343–51.

72

Neurochemistry

L. S. Schneider, updated by M. T. Abou-Saleh[1]

St George's Hospital Medical School, London, UK

As a preface to this chapter, it is important to consider that major depression is characterized and defined by descriptive, not biological, criteria, making it unlikely that a neurochemical finding could adequately characterize the disorder. The underlying validity of the diagnosis is assessed against other descriptive features of the illness such as symptoms, course, treatment outcome and biological changes. Yet people who manifest similar clinical phenomenology may not necessarily share similar pathophysiology. Major depression is heterogeneous in its expression, possessing various phenomenology, family history and course. Therefore, the underlying biology of each subtype would be expected to be distinct from others. This, however, is often not the case.

In the elderly, a neurochemical characteristic of depression would have to be sufficiently specific to distinguish depression from dementia or from secondary depression. In addition, neurochemical differences would be expected between late-onset and early-onset depression, or delusional and non-delusional depression, thus helping to validate these putative subtypes.

PRIMARY DEMENTIA VS. PRIMARY DEPRESSION IN THE ELDERLY

Both of these disorders share certain neurochemical characteristics and behavioural symptoms. For example, noradrenergic deficits are common to both disorders. Interestingly, greater neuronal loss in the nucleus locus coeruleus, the main noradrenergic outflow to the cortex, occurred in Alzheimer's disease (AD) patients who showed clinical manifestations of depression before death than in those who did not[1,2]. Similarly, primary dementia patients with major depression had over a 10-fold greater reduction in norepinephrine (noradrenaline) than non-depressed dementia patients[3], suggesting that, at least among elderly patients, noradrenergic functions may play a role in secondary depression.

Cerebrospinal fluid (CSF) studies demonstrate decreased concentrations of somatostatin in both major depression and AD patients, often with no differences in monoamine metabolites[4].

SECONDARY VS. PRIMARY DEPRESSION

Significant depressive symptomatology is common in older groups, who are more likely to be medically ill, and depressive symptoms in medically ill patients range from 10% to 50%[5]. However, the neurochemistry associated with depression in the elderly, such as the dexamethasone suppression test (DST), thyroid releasing hormone (TRH) test and platelet monoamine oxidase (MAO) activity, as discussed below, may change in physical disease as well as in depression, so that their adequate evaluation requires consideration of the effects of medical illness[6–8].

LATE-ONSET VS. EARLY-ONSET DEPRESSION

Early-onset depressives, i.e. patients with depression first occurring earlier in life, may be biologically distinguished from similarly-aged patients with late-onset depression. For example, late-onset elderly patients have a lower sedation threshold to amobarbital (both before and after treatment) than early-onset depressives[9]; they may have greater cortical atrophy and ventricular enlargement; and they may have relatively increased platelet MAO activity (see below).

DELUSIONAL VS. NON-DELUSIONAL DEPRESSION

Delusional depression may represent a distinct clinical subgroup and be more common among patients with late-onset depression[10]. Yet there is little evidence for biological differences between groups of depressed patients with and without delusions. For example, urinary MGPG (3-methoxy-4-hydroxy-phenylglycol), a metabolite of norepinephrine, has been reported to be reduced[11], increased[12] and not different[13] in delusionally depressed patients. Similarly, serum levels of dopamine-β-hydro-oxylase have been reported to be both lower[14] and not different[15] in delusional depression.

BIOLOGICAL CHANGES IN AGING AND DEPRESSION

Many of the neurobiological changes associated with aging are similar to those that occur with depression. For example, normal aging and depression are both associated with decreased brain concentrations of serotonin, dopamine, norepinephrine, their metabolites, increased brain MAO-B activity, increased hypothalamic–pituitary–adrenal (HPA) activity and increased sympathetic nervous system activity[16].

Principles and Practice of Geriatric Psychiatry, 2nd edn. Edited by J. R. M. Copeland, M. T. Abou-Saleh and D. G. Blazer
©2002 John Wiley & Sons, Ltd

HYPOTHALAMIC–PITUITARY–ADRENAL (HPA) AXIS

Depression across the age range is associated with hyperactivity and dysregulation of the HPA axis, characterized, in part, by elevated plasma and urinary cortisol, increased corticotropin-releasing hormone (CRH), blunted corticotropin (ACTH) response to CRH and resistance of cortisol to suppression by dexamethasone. Increased cortisol secretion is probably the most consistently observed physiological abnormality in patients with major depression (see Chapter 81 on dexamethasone suppression test).

Total urinary free cortisol may reliably distinguish depressed from non-depressed individuals in clinical studies of mixed-aged adults. The levels of cortisol, furthermore, appear to correlate with the severity of depression, the presence of psychotic features, and with cognitive impairment[17]. Anatomical imaging research shows correlations of cortisol with brain ventricular enlargement[18].

One way in which aging and depression may interact is as follows. It is possible that normal aging is associated with enhanced limbic–hypothalamic–pituitary–adrenal axis activity, possibly due to age-associated neuronal degeneration in the hippocampus. The neuronal degeneration, in turn, may result from increased levels of glucocorticoids associated with both depression and aging. Depressive illness in the elderly may exacerbate this condition, as may repetitive stressful life events.

PLATELET MONOAMINE OXIDASE (MAO) ACTIVITY

MAO catalyses the oxidative deamination of several monoamines and exists in two forms, identified by relative substrate specificity. In the brain, both MAO-A and MAO-B are present; in platelets, only MAO-B is present. In the brain, MAO-B may be more responsible for the degradation of dopamine and MAO-A for norepinephrine.

Platelet MAO activity increases with age, nearly doubles between ages 30 and 80, and is higher in females than males[19]. Platelet and brain MAO-B activity is increased in AD, over and above the increase associated with age[20,21]. Some medical conditions, including liver disease, anaemia, epilepsy and cancer, are also associated with increased MAO activity, whereas in diabetes this may be lower[7]. Although not specific for a particular psychiatric disorder, differences in platelet MAO activity seem to distinguish certain depression populations. Among subgroups of mixed-age, depressed subjects, MAO activity has been reported to be higher in primary depressed, non medically-ill outpatients than in controls, and also higher in secondary than in primary depression[22,23]. MAO activity may not distinguish endogenous from non-endogenous or delusional from non-delusional depression[22], but it may be lower in bipolar compared with unipolar depression[24].

Post mortem studies of MAO in the brain have shown that the quantitative distribution of MAO-A in brainstem monoamine nuclei is normal in major depression[25]. However the density of brain MAO-B in suicide victims showed a positive correlation with age, but was not different between suicides and age-matched controls[26].

Elderly female inpatients with primary, unipolar depression, predominately endogenous, whose illness onset was in mid-life, may have lower platelet MAO activity than either later-age-onset depressed females of controls[27], suggesting that despite similar clinical presentation, decreased MAO activity may be associated with early-onset depression in the elderly. On the other hand, in elderly depressed female outpatients, MAO activity was higher than controls, but age of onset was not assessed[28]. In a depressed population, lower platelet MAO activity predicted the occurrence of neurotic depression (ICD-9) 10 years later[29].

In a group of elderly, depressed outpatients, higher platelet MAO activity was correlated with anhedonia, anxiety, a positive family history of depression and response to MAO inhibitors[30]. Depressed patients with reversible cognitive impairment have higher MAO activity than depressed patients without cognitive impairment[31]. Also, among elderly outpatients, MAO activity was increased in a group with depression secondary to mental illness compared with a primary depression group[32]. Thus, changes in platelet MAO activity are complex among the elderly depressed population.

Platelet MAO activity may serve as a vulnerability marker for pyschopathology in general. Association studies suggested that in the population with age over 40 years, presence of the 165 bp allele of DXS7 at the MAO locus was significantly associated with unipolar depression[33]. Both high- and low-MAO activity are associated with increased risk of bipolar disorder, depression and alcoholism in family members.

SEROTONIN

Deficits in the serotonin neurotransmitter system have been implicated both in major depression and in suicide. Numerous studies have demonstrated an association between low platelet 5-HT uptake and depression and a recent study showed higher uptake efficiency in depressed patients with high net uptake rate but similar 5-HT content to normal controls[34]. Many studies suggest that the serotonin metabolite 5-hydroxyindole acetic acid (5-HIAA) is decreased in the CSF of depressed patients; presynaptic serotonin function is decreased as well[35]. Specific brain ^{3}H-imipramine binding sites are correlated with serotonin patterns of innervation and are located on presynaptic serotonergic nerve terminals[36]. The active component for this binding site has a role in modulating neuronal serotonin uptake. Among suicide victims, at least, there is evidence for a decrease in the number of imipramine receptors[35], and an increase in the number of postsynaptic serotonin$_2$ receptors[37]. This latter finding may represent upregulation due to decreased intrasynaptic serotonin.

The role of 5-HT has also been investigated in genetic, neuroimaging, neuroendocrine and post mortem studies. Serotonin transporter gene polymorphism was not associated with old-age depression[38]. However, in patients with Parkinson's disease, those with the short allele of the 5-HT transporter promoter region—associated with low 5-HT transporter density—had higher depression and anxiety scores than those without this polymorphism[39]. Secondary depression to Parkinson's disease, stroke and Huntington's disease in the elderly is associated with low cerebral blood flow and metabolic rate in orbital frontal cortex and basal ganglia, suggesting that, as in primary depression, there is disruption in cortical–basal ganglia–thalamic neuronal loops[40], abnormalities that are under 5-HT control[41]. Poststroke depression is associated with blunted prolactin response to buspirone indicating low 5-HT activity[42]. Serotonin transporter density, measured using paroxetine binding in midbrains of suicides with major depression, were comparable to values obtained in normal controls[43].

Although a considerable literature evaluating CSF markers in mixed-age depressed and suicidal patients exists, only one study has focused specifically on elderly depressed subjects. In this study, both CSF 5-HIAA and the dopamine metabolite homovanillic acid (HVA) were lower in elderly depressed patients who attempted suicide than in depressed non-suicidal patients and controls[44].

PLATELET ^{3}H-IMIPRAMINE BINDING

The ^{3}H-imipramine binding site is found in brain and on platelets, the two sites sharing many characteristics with each other. The binding site is closely related to the presynaptic serotonin-uptake site. Thus, during the last decade, platelet ^{3}H-imipramine binding density (β_{max}) has been examined extensively as a biological marker for mood disorder. Approximately two-thirds of the studies have reported β_{max} among certain depressive subtypes[46,47], including those with a family history of depression[47,48]. However, β_{max} values seem also to be decreased in obsessive–compulsive disorder, anorexia and enuresis. ^{3}H-imipramine binding defined by desmethylimipramine was lower in the putamen of non-violent depressed suicides and those who were antidepressants-treated than normal controls[49].

The effect of age on platelet binding density has not been systematically investigated. A few studies suggest an increase, decrease, or no change in density with age, but the age ranges have been limited. Animal studies suggest that brain binding sites increase with age[36]. Elderly unipolar depressed patients also show a 20–42% decrease in binding density when compared to age-appropriate controls, although, again, this is not always so[50].

Differences among specific depression subtypes in the elderly have not been widely studied; platelet receptor density seems to be somewhat lower in elderly depressed patients compared to a younger depressed cohort[51]. Platelet ^{3}H-imipramine β_{max} may discriminate between depression secondary to medical illness and primary major depression, with density decreased in primary depression patients compared to secondary depression patients and controls[32].

It is not known whether this marker represents a trait or a state characteristic. The evidence suggesting state dependence is that depressed patients treated with electroconvulsive therapy showed an increase in binding density[52]. The administration of various medications such as fluoxetine, paroxetine, citalopram and chlorimipramine affect imipramine binding.

Platelet ^{3}H-imipramine binding density does not seem to be affected, overall, in groups of AD patients[51,53,54] compared to controls, but AD patients with agitation and delusions may have a lower density than AD patients without these symptoms[53].

NORADRENERGIC FUNCTION

Studies in depression have failed to demonstrate consistent differences in brain of CSF norepinephrine (NE) or MHPG levels. Normal aging is associated with a decrease in brain NE and a loss of neurons from the noradrenergic nucleus locus coeruleus. In addition, there are decreases in two enzymes required for norepinephrine synthesis, tyrosine hydroxylase and dopa decarboxylase. A post mortem study of depressed patients reported lower NE transporter binding of ^{3}H-nisoextine in the midcaudal portion of the locus coeruleus (LC) than normal controls, which may be related to low NE availability[55]. Tyrosine hydroxylase (TH) immunoreactivity is reduced in LC in depressed non-suicidal patients indicating low NE availability[56], whilst its expression is elevated in LC of depressed patients indicating premortem overactivity or deficiency in NE[57]. Neurotrophin 3 which was shown to prevent the death of central NE neurons is low in CSF of elderly patients with major depression[58].

Platelet α_2-Adrenergic Binding

Presynaptic α_2-receptors, in general, seem to function as noradrenergic modulators by regulating NE through a feedback mechanism. Activation of the receptor decreases NE function, while antagonism increases it. Decreased α_2-receptor density in brain and platelets may indicate a subsensitive autoreceptor system with increased NE activity, whereas increased α_2-autoreceptor density may be a characteristic of the putative deficits in central NE function in depression. However, a post mortem study of α_2-receptor activity in prefrontal cortex and hippocampal cortex in depressed patients showed similar levels to values in normal controls[59].

α_2-Adrenergic receptors exist peripherally on platelets, and in most studies, appear increased in depressed patients[60]. Increased platelet α_2-receptors have also been found in elderly depressed compared to age-appropriate controls[61] (studies that report increased α_2-receptors tend to use α_2-agonists in the assay while studies showing no difference tend to use antagonists).

CONCLUSION AND METHODOLOGICAL LIMITATIONS

Limited work has been done in specifically assessing the neurochemistry of depression in the elderly. The biological characteristics discussed here generally discriminate depressed from non-depressed in older as well as in younger groups, but often occur in other disorders as well. Therefore, neurochemistry characterizing depression in the elderly has limited generalizability and validity.

Some of the neurochemical findings described may not be specific to affective disorder in the elderly, but indicate traits that are over represented in groups of depressed patients when compared to the general population. For example, decreased platelet imipramine binding density may characterize people with relative serotonin system deficits, who may be at increased risk for depression, or who have symptoms related to depression. Or, increased platelet α_2-receptor binding may identify individuals who possess noradrenergic or arousal defects associated with depression.

Whereas platelet, plasma and CSF are sources of assayable human tissue, the relationship of their biochemistry is not well understood. The similar embryological origin of megakaryocytes and neurons has been used to justify or explain platelet research findings. However, these cells and their platelets have differentiated considerably from neurons and are exposed to significantly different physiological influences. Thus, it could be considered remarkable that it is possible to use platelets at all in the manner discussed here.

The majority of these studies are based on cross-sectional assessments during an acute phase of illness, or at death. Longitudinal studies are needed to assess test–retest reliability, state vs. trait and other characteristics. An adequate understanding of the neurochemistry of depression in the elderly must address age effects and the effects of depression subtypes, and must adequately explain how the neurochemistry is related to the depression.

ACKNOWLEDGEMENT

Partial support was provided by the State of California Mental Health Research Program, and by NIMH Grant No. 19074.

REFERENCES

1. Zubenko GS, Moosy J. Major depression in primary dementia: clinical and neuropathologic correlates. *Arch Neurol* 1988; **45**: 1182–6.
2. Zweig RM, Ross CA, Hedreen JC *et al*. The neuropathology of aminergic nuclei in Alzheimer's disease. *Ann Neurol* 1988; **24**: 233–2.

3. Zubenko GS, Moossy J, Kopp U. Neurochemical correlates of major depression in primary dementia. *Arch Neurol* 1990; **47**: 209–14.

4. Molchan SE, Lawlor BA, Hill JL *et al*. CSF monoamine metabolites and somatostatin in Alzheimer's disease and major depression. *Biol Psychiat* 1991; **29**: 1110–18.

5. Rodin G, Voshar K. Depression in the medically ill: an overview. *Am J Psychiat* 1986; **143**: 696–705.

6. American Psychiatric Association Task Force on Laboratory Tests in Psychiatry. The dexamethasone suppression test: an overview of its current status in psychiatry. *Am J Psychiat* 1987; **114**: 1253–62.

7. Fowler CJ, Tipton KF, MacKay AVP, Youdim MB. Human platelet monoamine oxidase—useful enzyme in the study of psychiatric disorders? *Neuroscience* 1982; **7**: 1577–94.

8. Loosen PT. The TRH stimulation test in psychiatric disorders: a review. In Nemeroff C, Loosen PT, eds, *Handbook of Clinical Psychoneuroendocrinology*. New York: Guilford, 1987; 336–60.

9. Cawley RH, Post F, Whitehead A. Barbiturate tolerance and psychosocial functioning in elderly depressed patients. *Psychol Med* 1973; **3**: 39–52.

10. Meyers BS, Kalayam B, Mei-Tal V. Late onset delusional depression: a distinct clinical entity? *J Clin Psychiat* 1984; **45**: 347–9.

11. Sweeney D, Nelson C, Bowers M *et al*. Delusional vs. non-delusional depression—neurochemical differences. *Lancet* 1978; **ii**: 100–101.

12. Maes MH, De Rutyer M, Suy E. Prediction of subtype and severity of depression by means of dexamethasone suppression test, L-tryptophan: competing amino acid ratio, and MHPG flow. *Biol Psychiat* 1987; **22**: 177–88.

13. Edwards DJ, Spiker DG, Neil JF *et al*. MHPG excretion in depression. *Psychiatry Res* 1980; **2**: 295–305.

14. Meltzer HY, Hyong WC, Carroll BJ *et al*. Serum dopamine-β-hydrozylase activity in the affective psychoses and schizophrenia. *Arch Gen Psychiat* 1976; **33**: 585–91.

15. Lykouras E, Markioanos M, Malliaras D, Stefanis C. Neurochemical variables in delusional depression. *Am J Psychiat* 1988; **145**: 214–17.

16. Veith RC, Raskind MA. The neurobiology of aging: does it predispose to depression? *Neurobiol Aging* 1988; **9**: 101–17.

17. Kellner CH, Rubinow DR, Post RM. Cerebral ventricular size and cognitive impairment in depression. *J Affect Disord* 1986; **10**: 2215–19.

18. Kellner CH, Rubinow DR, Gold DW, Post RM. Relationship of cortisol hypersection to brain CT scan alterations in depressed patients. *Psychiat Res* 1983; **8**: 191–7.

19. Bridge TP, Soldo BJ, Phelps BH *et al*. Platelet monoamine oxidase activity: demographic characteristics contribute to enzyme activity variability. *J Gerontol* 1985; **40**: 23–8.

20. Adolffson R, Gottfries CG, Oreland L *et al*. Increased activity of brain and platelet monoamine oxidase in dementia of Alzheimer type. *Life Sci* 1980; **27**: 1029–34.

21. Alexopoulos GS, Lieberman KW, Young RC. Platelet MAO activity in primary degenerative dementia. *Am J Psychiat* 1984; **141**: 97–99.

22. Davidson JRT, McLeod MN, Turnbull CD *et al*. Platelet monoamine oxidase activity and the classification of depression. *Arch Gen Psychiat* 1980; **37**: 771–3.

23. White K, Shih J, Fong TL *et al*. Elevated platelet monoamine oxidase activity in patients with non-endogenous depression. *Am J Psychiat* 1980; **137**: 1258–9.

24. Belmaker RH, Bracha HS, Ebstein RP. Platelet monoamine oxidase in affective illness and alcoholism. *Schizophren Bull* 1980; **6**: 320–3.

25. Ordway GA, Farley JT, Dilley GE *et al*. Quantitative distribution of monoamine oxidase A in brainstem monoamine nuclei is normal in major depression. *Brain Res* 1999; **847** (1): 71–9.

26. Sastre M, Garcia-Sevilla, JA. Densities of 12-imidazoline receptors, α_2-adrenoceptors and monoamine oxidase B in brains of suicide victims. *Neurochem Int* 1997; **30** (1): 63–72.

27. Alexopoulos GS, Lieberman KW, Young RC. Platelet MAO activity and age at onset of depression in elderly depressed women. *Am J Psychiat* 1984; **141**: 1276–8.

28. Schneider LS, Severson JA, Pollock V *et al*. Platelet monoamine oxidase activity in elderly depressed outpatients. *Biol Psychiat* 1986; **21**: 1360–64.

29. Wahlund B, Saaf J, Wetterberg L. Clinical symptoms and platelet monoamine oxidase in subgroups and different states of affective disorders. *J Affect Disord* 1995; **35**: 75–87.

30. Georgotas A, McCue RE, Friedman E *et al*. Relationship of platelet MAO activity to characteristics of major depressive illness. *Psychiat Res* 1986; **19**: 247–56.

31. Alexopoulos GS, Lieberman KW, Yound RC, Shamoian CA. Monoamines and monoamine oxidase in primary degenerative dementia. In *Biology and Treatment of Dementia in the Elderly*. Washington, DC: American Psychiatric Press, 1984, 59–71.

32. Schneider LS, Severson JA, Sloane RB, Fredrickson E. Decreased platelet ^{3}H-imipramine binding in elderly outpatients with primary depression compared to secondary depression. *J Affect Disord* 1988; **15**: 195–200.

33. Qian Y, Lin S, Jiang S *et al*. Studies of the DXS7 polymorphism at the MAO loci in unipolar depression. *Am J Med Genet* 1999; **88**: 598–600.

34. Franke L, Schewe HJ, Muller B *et al*. Serotonergic platelet variables in unmedicated patients suffering from major depression and healthy subjects: relationship between 5-HT content and 5 HT-uptake. *Life Sci* 2000; **67**: 301–5.

35. Stanley M, Virgilio J, Geshon S. Tritiated imipramine binding sites are decreased in frontal cortex of suicides. *Science* 1982; **216**: 1337.

36. Severson JA. ^{3}H-Imipramine binding in aged mouse brain: regulation by ions and serotonin. *Neurobiol Aging* 1986; **7**: 83–7.

37. Stanley M, Mann JJ. Serotonin-2 binding sites are increased in the frontal cortex of suicide victims. *Lancet* 1983; **i**: 214–16.

38. Zill P, Badberg F, de Jonge S *et al*. Serotonin transporter (5-HTT) gene polymorphism in psychogeriatric patients. *Neurosci Lett* 2000; **284**: 113–15.

39. Menza MA, Palermo B, DiPaola R *et al*. Depression and anxiety in Parkinson's disease: possible effect of genetic variation in the serotonin transporter. *J Geriat Psychiat Neurol* 1999: **12**: 49–52.

40. Robinson RG, Chemerinski E, Jorge R. Pathophysiology of secondary depressions in the elderly. *J Geriat Psychiat Neurol* 1999: **12**: 128–36.

41. Nobler MS, Mann JJ, Sackeim HA. Serotonin, cerebral blood flow, and cerebral metabolic rate in geriatric major depression and normal aging. *Brain Res Brain Res Rev* 1999; **30**: 250–63.

42. Sevincok L, Erol A. The prolactin response to buspirone in poststroke depression: a preliminary report. *J Affect Disord* 2000; **59**: 169–73.

43. Bligh-Glover W, Killi TN, Shapiro-Kulnane L *et al*. The serotonin transporter in the midbrain of suicide victims with major depression. *Biol Psychiat* 2000; **47**: 1015–24.

44. Jones JS, Stanley B, Mann JJ *et al*. CSF 5-HIAA and HVA concentrations in elderly depressed patients who attempted suicide. *Am J Psychiat* 1990; **147**: 1225–7.

45. Langer SZ, Galzin AM, Poirier MF *et al*. Association of ^{3}H-imipramine ^{3}H-paroxetine binding with the 5-HT transporter in brain and platelets: relevance to studies in depression. *J Receptor Res* 1987; **7**: 499–521.

46. Baron M, Barkai A, Gruen R *et al*. Platelet ^{3}H-imipramine binding in affective disorders: trait vs. state characteristics. *Am J Psychiat* 1986; **143**: 711–17.

47. Lewis DA, McChesney C. Tritiated imipramine binding distinguishes among subtypes of depression. *Arch Gen Psychiat* 1985; **42**: 485–8.

48. Schneider LS, Fredrickson E, Severson J, Sloane RB. ^{3}H-imipramine binding in depressed elderly: relationship to family history and clinical response. *Psychiat Res* 1986; **19**: 257–66.

49. Lawrence KM, Kanagasundaram M, Lowther S *et al*. [^{3}H]-imipramine binding in brain samples from depressed suicides and controls: 5-HT uptake sites compared with sites defined by desmethylimipramine. *J Affect Disord* 1998; **47**: 105–12.

50. Georgotas A, Schweitzer J, McCue RE *et al*. Clinical and treatment effects on ^{3}H-clonidine and ^{3}H-imipramine binding in elderly depressed patients. *Life Sci* 1987; **40**: 2137–43.

51. Nemeroff CB, Knight DL, Krishnan KRK *et al*. Marked reduction in the number of platelet ^{3}H imipramine binding sites in geriatric depression. *Arch Gen Psychiat* 1988; **45**: 919–23.

52. Langer SZ, Sechter D, Loo H *et al*. Electroconvulsive shock therapy and maximum binding of platelet tritiated imipramine binding in depression. *Arch Gen Psychiat* 1986; **43**: 949–52.

53. Schneider LS, Severson J, Chui HC *et al*. ^{3}H-imipramine binding and MAO activity in Alzheimer's patients with agitation and delusions. *Psychiat Res* 1988; **25**: 311–22.

54. Suranyi-Cadotte BE, Gauthier S, Lafaille F *et al*. Platelet ^{3}H-imipramine binding distinguishes depression from Alzheimer dementia. *Life Sci* 1985; **37**: 2305–11.

55. Klimek V, Stockmeier C, Overholser J *et al*. Reduced levels of norepinephrine transporters in the locus coeruleus in major depression. *J Neurosci* 1997; **17**: 8451–8.

56. Baumann B, Danos P, Diekmann S *et al*. Tyrosine hydroxylase immunoreactivity in the locus coeruleus is reduced in depressed non-suicidal patients but normal in depressed suicide patients. *Eur Arch Psychiat Clin Neurosci* 1999; **249**: 212–19.

57. Zhu MY, Klimek V, Dilley GE *et al*. Elevated levels of tyrosine hydroxylase in the locus coeruleus in major depression. *Biol Psychiat* 1999; **46**: 1275–86.

58. Hock C, Heese K, Muller-Spahn F *et al*. Increased cerebrospinal fluid levels of neurotrophin 3 (NT-3) in elderly patients with major depression. *Mol Psychiat* 2000; **5**: 510–13.

59. Klimek V, Rajkowska G, Luker SN *et al*. Brain noradrenergic receptors in major depression and schizophrenia. *Neuropsychopharmacology* 1999; **21**: 69–81.

60. Garcia-Sevilla JA, Guimon J, Garcia-Vallejo P, Fuster MJ. Biochemical and functional evidence of supersensitive platelet α_2-adrenoceptors in major affective disorders. *Arch Gen Psychiat* 1986; **43**: 51–7.

61. Doyle MC, George AJ, Ravindran AV, Philpott R. Platelet α_2-adrenoreceptor in major affective disorders. *Am J Psychiat* 1985; **142**: 1489–90.

Neuro-imaging

Neuro-imaging Studies of Depression

Mohammed T. Abou-Saleh

St George's Hospital Medical School, London, UK

The use of neuro-imaging techniques in the study of depression has provided a major advance in the elucidation of its functional neuro-anatomy, metabolic correlates and biochemistry. Structural neuro-imaging techniques, such as computed axial tomography (CT) and magnetic resonance imaging (MRI) have demonstrated an association between structural brain abnormalities and depression in patients with unipolar and bipolar disorder[1]. Whilst these abnormalities are non-specific, there is evidence that volume reduction in the caudate[2] and frontal lobe[3] are specific abnormalities in depression, particularly in late-life depression. MRI studies have consistently shown an increase in the number and/or severity of signal hyperintensities in the white matter in both unipolar and bipolar disorder[4]. Deep white matter lesions have been shown in elderly patients with unipolar depression predominantly in the frontal lobes and basal ganglia, supporting the notion of frontostriatal dysfunction in depression. These lesions have been shown to be associated with poor long-term outcome[5]. A recent population-based study of over 1000 elderly people showed that those with severe periventricular white matter lesions were three to five times more likely to have depressive symptoms than those with only mild or no white matter lesions, whilst those with severe subcortical but not periventricular white matter lesions were more likely to have had a history of late-onset depression after the age of 60 years than those with only mild or no white matter lesions[6]. Severe white matter lesions are thought to represent vascular abnormalities, findings that support the notion that vascular pathology contributes to the aetiology of late-life depression.

Functional neuro-imaging techniques have also advanced our knowledge of the pathophysiology and chemical pathology of depression with the introduction of single-photon emission computed tomography (SPECT), positron emission tomography (PET) and magnetic resonance spectroscopy (MRS). Several studies have shown an association between depression, low cerebral blood flow and low metabolic activity. An extensive review of the literature showed evidence for low cerebral activity in the frontal lobes in unipolar and bipolar depressive patients, with an inverse correlation with increased severity of depressive symptoms and an association with low activity in basal ganglia and temporal and limbic regions[7]. Low neurostriatal cerebral blood flow was particularly associated with psychomotor slowing[8] and an association between hypofrontality and negative symptoms in depressive patients[9]. This abnormality is of special interest in the elderly because of the interface between depression and dementia in this age group.

We compared the cerebral perfusion in a group of elderly depressed patients with that in age matched healthy subjects and Alzheimer's disease (AD) patients, using SPECT methodology and hexamethyl propleneamine oxime (HMPAO) as the radio-ligand[10]. The regional cerebral perfusion values of depressed patients were intermediate between those of the healthy control subjects and the AD patients. This is consistent with the intermediate position of the depressed group on other measures, e.g. radioattenuation on CT scan. In addition to the global impairment in cerebral perfusion, there are topographical abnormalities but the cerebral region thus affected is seen to vary in different studies. Sackeim *et al.*[11] have argued that the traditional statistical paradigms, concentrating on identifying specific brain regions with higher or lower perfusion compared to control subjects, have failed to examine the important issue of identifying the abnormal patterning of regional activity, which would reflect the activity of functional neural networks. Using a novel scaled subprofile model based on factor analytic technique, they demonstrated topographical abnormalities in the temporo-parietal area, largely consisting of polymodal association cortex with strong reciprocal connection with the prefrontal polymodal association cortex. The study by Baxter *et al.*[12] on glucose metabolism using PET strongly suggests that the biological substrate common to depressive states in different patient groups is a reduction in glucose metabolism in the left prefrontal cortex.

The impairment in cerebral perfusion correlates positively with the endogenicity score but not necessarily with the severity of depressive illness[13]. This is in contrast with studies on cerebral glucose metabolism using PET, reporting a positive correlation between the severity of depressive symptoms and glucose metabolic rate. There are some reports on abnormality in the anteroposterior gradient in cerebral perfusion in depressive illness, but these are not consistent.

The temporal sequence of the perfusion abnormality and clinical depression is yet unclear. The impairment in cerebral perfusion improved with clinical recovery, suggesting that the continuing impairment can predict chronicity of the course or frequent relapse of depression. This notion can be examined in further longitudinal studies.

SPECT and PET techniques have also been utilized to investigate the chemical pathology of dopamine and serotonin systems in depression. SPECT studies of D2 receptors showed increased D2 receptor density in the striatum, reflecting reduced dopamine function[14], and an association between increased D2 receptor binding in the left striatum in the anterior cingulate gyrus and clinical recovery with selective serotonin reuptake inhibitors[15]. Studies of the dopamine transport receptors in depression showed increased receptor density in the basal ganglia[16]. Studies

Principles and Practice of Geriatric Psychiatry, 2nd edn. Edited by J. R. M. Copeland, M. T. Abou-Saleh and D. G. Blazer

of the serotonin system showed a number of interesting associations. A SPECT study of the brain serotonin transport receptor reported reduced density in depression[17], whilst a PET study of the serotonin type 2 receptor function showed a decrease in receptor density following treatment with desipramine, particularly in the frontal region[18]. Studies of the 5-HT_{1A} system showed a reduction in receptor density in the mesiotemporal cortex in bipolar patients, and in unipolar patients with bipolar relatives[19] and an association between widespread reduction of 5-HT_{1A} receptor binding and depression in medicated and non-medicated depressed patients[20]. Finally, studies of MRS depicting biochemical changes have detected an association between depression and reduced glutamine and glutamate, using proton-MRS[21], and increased phosphomonoesters and decreased ATP values in the frontal lobes of patients with major depression using $^{31}\text{P-MRS}$[22].

In summary, the findings of neuro-imaging studies in depression add credence and support to the biological basis of depression, refine its diagnostic subgroups and inform its treatment with more specific pharmacological treatments.

REFERENCES

1. Videbech P. MRI findings in patients with affective disorder: a meta-analysis. *Acta Psychiat Scand* 1997; **96**: 157–68.
2. Krishnan KRR, McDonald WM, Escalona PR *et al*. Magnetic resonance imaging of the caudate nuclei in depression. *Arch Gen Psychiat* 1992; **49**: 553–7.
3. Drevets WC, Price JL, Simpson JR Jr *et al*. Subgenual prefrontal cortex abnormalities in mood disorders. *Nature* 1997; **386**: 824–7.
4. O'Brien JT, Desmond P, Ames D *et al*. A magnetic resonance imaging study of white matter lesions in depression and Alzheimer's disease. *Br J Psychiat* 1996; **168**: 477–85.
5. O'Brien JT, Chiu E, Schweitzer I *et al*. Severe deep white matter lesions on MRI brain scan predict poor outcome in elderly patients with major depressive disorder. *Br Med J* 1998; **317**: 982–4.
6. De Groot JC, de Leeuw FE, Oudkerk M *et al*. Cerebral white matter lesions and depressive symptoms in elderly adults. *Arch Gen Psychiat* 2000; **57**: 1071–6.
7. Soares JC, Mann JJ. The functional neuroanatomy of mood disorders. *J Psychiat Res* 1997; **31**(4): 393–432.
8. Hickie I, Ward P, Scott E *et al*. Neo-striatal rCBF correlates of psychomotor slowing in patients with major depression. *Psychiat Res* 1999; **92**: 75–81.
9. Galynker II *et al*. Hypofrontality and negative symptoms in major depressive disorder. *J Nucl Med* 1998; **39**: 608–12.
10. Upadhyaya AK, Abou-Saleh MT, Wilson K *et al*. A study of depression in old age using single photon emission computerised tomography. *Br J Psychiat* 1990; **9**: 76–81.
11. Sackeim HA, Prohovnik I, Moeller JR *et al*. Regional cerebral blood flow in mood disorders. 1. Comparison of major depressives and normal controls at rest. *Arch Gen Psychiat* 1990; **47**: 60–70.
12. Baxter LR Jr., Schwartz JM, Phelps ME *et al*. Reduction of prefrontal cortex glucose metabolism common to three types of depression. *Arch Gen Psychiat* 1989; **46**: 243–50.
13. Abou-Saleh MT, Al Suhaili AR, Karin L *et al*. Single photon emission tomography with $^{99m}\text{Tc-HMPAO}$ in Arab patients with depression. *J Affect Disord* 1999; **55**: 115–23.
14. Shah PJ, Ogilvie AD, Goodwin GM *et al*. Clinical and psychometric correlates of dopamine-D2 binding in depression. *Psychol Med* 1997; **27**: 1247–56.
15. Larisch R, Klimke A, Vosberg H *et al*. *In vivo* evidence for the involvement of dopamine-D2 receptors in striatum and anterior cingulate gyrus in major depression. *Neuroimaging* 1997; **5**: 251–60.
16. Laasonen-Balk T, Kuikka J, Viinamaki H *et al*. Striatal dopamine transporter density in major depression. *Psychopharmacology (Berl)* 1999; **144**: 282–5.
17. Malison RT, Price LH, Berman R *et al*. Reduced brain serotonin transporter availability in major depression as measured by [123I]-2 β-carbomethoxy-3 β-(4-iodophenyl) tropane and single photon emission computed tomography. *Biol Psychiat* 1998; **44**: 1090–8.
18. Yatham LN, Liddle PF, Dennie J *et al*. Decrease in brain serotonin 2 receptor binding in patients with major depression following desipramine treatment: a positron emission tomography study with fluorine-18-labeled setoperone. *Arch Gen Psychiat* 1999; **56**: 705–11.
19. Drevets WC, Frank E, Price JC *et al*. PET imaging of serotonin 1A receptor binding in depression. *Biol Psychiat* 1999; **46**: 1375–87.
20. Sargent PA, Kjaer KH, Bench CJ *et al*. Brain serotonin 1A receptor binding measured by positron emission tomography with [11C]WAY-100635: effects of depression and antidepressant treatment. *Arch Gen Psychiat* 2000; **57**: 174–80.
21. Auer DP, Putz B, Kraft E *et al*. Reduced glutamate in the anterior cingulate cortex in depression: an *in vivo* proton magnetic resonance spectroscopy study. *Biol Psychiat* 2000; **15**: 305–13.
22. Volz HP, Rzanny R, Riehemann S *et al*. ^{31}P magnetic resonance spectroscopy in the frontal lobe of major depressed patients. *Eur Arch Psychiat Clin Neurosci* 1998; **248**: 289–95.

Is Imaging Justified in the Investigation of Older People?

D. McWilliam

Ribbleton Hospital, Preston, UK

Dementia is still diagnosable only by clinical examination, but a further battery of diagnostic tests may then be required to clarify the aetiology and identify potentially treatable cases. Any assessment of the cost-effectiveness of these further tests, including neuro-imaging, must compare the relative value of routine testing in all patients against selective testing in cases where there is a high index of suspicion or diagnostic doubt.

Routine testing will detect the small number of patients (about 1%) with a reversible cause for their dementia, but is burdensome, especially in the elderly, and may raise false expectations and lead to false-positive results. It would also identify early cases suitable for drug therapy. Selective testing will result in some treatable cases being missed, but causes less general risk and discomfort and may be more cost-effective, especially in those countries where neuro-imaging remains expensive and difficult, or even impossible, to access[1,2].

Providing cost-effective and accurate diagnosis of dementia therefore presents the clinician with a dilemma. Can neuro-imaging be included in a battery of ancillary investigations devised for routine use in all cases of dementia, or need such tests be carried out only as clinically indicated? The fact that definitive data on the sensitivity, specificity and cost-effectiveness of various neuro-imaging techniques are still needed[3] only adds to the problem.

The advent of treatments for dementia and the consequent need to identify early and potentially treatable cases has shifted the assessment of cost-effectiveness from investigation to treatment. The cost-benefit assessment of early treatment of dementia to a health economy has yet to be fully assessed but is likely to far exceed that of any neuro-imaging screening programme. A recent review[4] neatly encapsulates what is now as much a socioeconomic as a medical dilemma in a single statement: "How much is society willing to spend?".

Given that these socioeconomic drivers are unlikely to change, clinicians are now seeking to devise assessment protocols for dementia that best address the conflict. Unfortunately, we are still some distance from achieving a consensus view. Some authors[4] advocate routine neuro-imaging as part of a screening procedure in all patients in order to "include in" all treatable cases, perhaps avoiding litigation. Others, when attempting to define practice parameters, have regarded neuro-imaging as optional in the differential diagnosis of dementia[5]. Subsequent analysis showed that imaging studies did improve diagnostic accuracy but only with a significant increase in cost[6].

Considerations of cost and, in less well-developed countries, of access continue to determine whether neuro-imaging in dementia is used as a universal screen or only when clinically indicated. Various protocols indicating that neuro-imaging is not required in all patients, but should be a first-line test, especially in younger patients and those cases where there is diagnostic doubt on clinical grounds, have been suggested[7-10]. It is likely that, as costs of treatment increase relative to those of investigation, the use of neuro-imaging as a screening tool rather than a diagnostic aid in dementia will increase.

REFERENCES

1. van Crevel H, van Gool WA, Walstra GJM. Early diagnosis of dementia: which tests are indicated? What are their costs? *J Neurol* 1999; **246**: 73–8.
2. Chaves ML, Ilha D, Maia AL *et al*. Diagnosing dementia and normal ageing: clinical relevance of brain ratios and cognitive performance in a Brazilian sample. *Braz J Med Biol Res* 1999; **32**(9): 1133–43.
3. Small GW, Leiter F. Neuroimaging for diagnosis of dementia. *J Clin Psychiat* 1998: **59**(suppl 11): 4–7.
4. Ajax E, de Leon MJ, Golomb J *et al*. Imaging the brain in dementia: expensive and futile? *Am J Neuroradiol* 1997; **18**: 1847–50.
5. Quality standards subcommittee of the American Academy of Neurology Practice parameters for diagnosis: an evaluation of dementia (summary statement). *Neurology* 1994; **44**: 2203–6.
6. Chiu H, Zhang Q. Evaluation of dementia: a systematic study of the American Academy of Neurology's practice parameters. *Neurology* 1997; **49**(4): 925–35.
7. Hollister LE, Shah NN. Structural brain scanning in psychiatric patients: a further look. *J Clin Psychiat* 1996; **57**(6): 241–4.
8. Stahelin HB, Monsch AU, Spiegel R. Early diagnosis of dementia via a two-step screening and diagnostic procedure. *Int Psychogeriat* 1997; **9**(suppl 1): 123–30.
9. Cammer Paris BE. The utility of CT scanning in diagnosing dementia *Mt Sinai J Med* 1997; **64**(6): 372–5.
10. Galton CJ, Hodges JR. The spectrum of dementia and its treatment. *J R Coll Physicians Lond* 1999; **33**(3): 234–9.

Clinical Features of
Depression and Dysthymia

David G. Folks[1] **and Charles V. Ford**[2]

[1]*University of Nebraska College of Medicine, Omaha, NE and*
[2]*University of Alabama School of Medicine, Birmingham, AL, USA*

Depression *per se* is not characteristic of later life and should not be interpreted as "normal". Most normal adults make a satisfactory adjustment to the fact of growing older; after all, it is preferable to the alternative. Depression in old age may represent a continuation of a process that began in early life. For example, dysthymia as a chronic condition may extend into later life, or a continuation of cyclical changes of mood may be experienced, with periodic exacerbations of unipolar or bipolar depression. Additionally, some types of depression may originate in later life and the symptomatic presentation may or may not vary from the classical symptomatology. Depression and dysthymia may arise as a component of other psychiatric disturbances. Misdiagnosis or lack of referral for treatment of depression and dysthymia in older adults is due both to the context in which depression appears and the manner of presentation of symptoms[1]. Depression is a spectrum of disorders, rather than a unitary construct, and multiple biopsychosocial factors will influence how clinical features are manifested, as well as response to treatment. A depressive disorder may be diagnosed in accordance with current clinical criteria only if the depressive symptoms actually interfere with work, family or social functioning, or if the individual seeks professional treatment or has received medication for the disturbance[2].

The existing nomenclature may not accurately reflect depressive syndromes in late life. A number of well-established clinical syndromes are documented in the literature, for example depressive pseudodementia, somatization with underlying depression, and other forms of masked depression in individuals who deny depressive symptomatology. Subsyndromal depression may also occur in old age and can progress to a full syndrome of depression. Because of these potential differences in the presentation of depression in late life, epidemiologic data suggest that the elderly have a lower prevalence of major depression than do younger populations[1–4]. The literature has also consistently reported that a low proportion of clinically depressed elderly individuals seek or are referred for psychiatric care[6]. However, despite the inherent problems of describing depression and dysthymia in late life, and the presumed low rates of recognition or referral, depression is probably the most common psychiatric disorder in late life[7–10].

The clinical features of various forms of depression will be described using an outline form. The three clinical entities relevant to the current nomenclature and older adults are: *major depression*, unipolar or bipolar, single episode or recurrent, with or without melancholia, with or without psychotic features; *dysthymic disorders* or depressive neurosis; and *other atypical forms of depression*, i.e. somatization, cognitive impairment, including the reversible syndrome of dementia (pseudodementia) mood syndromes secondary to a general medical condition, and subsyndromal depression. The fact remains that in clinical practice considerable overlap exists for these syndromes, boundaries are often not distinct, and a spectrum of symptomatology is observed.

CLINICAL FEATURES OF THE DEPRESSIVE SPECTRUM

Symptoms of Grief and Pathological Bereavement

The hypothesis that demoralization and despair result from losses or incapacities due to aging seems to have no basis in empirical data. In fact, most surveys of older adults show older individuals to be more contented with their life situations than are those in earlier stages of the life cycle[9–11]. Perhaps when life events are anticipated and rehearsed, grief work can be completed before the loss with effective coping strategies. Grief, a psychologic response to the loss of a loved one, of possessions or of health itself, is associated with feelings of sadness, transient symptoms of gastrointestinal complaints, weight loss and difficulty in sleeping. Symptoms are often intense for several weeks and then typically begin to improve[12]. Many losses can lead to fear, demoralization or loneliness. In vulnerable individuals they may result in the onset, worsening or persistence of a mood disturbance. Pathological grief may include overactivity without a sense of loss, acquisition of symptoms belonging to the last illness of the deceased, frank psychosomatic illness, an alteration of relationships with family and friends with hostility towards specific individuals, and a persistent loss of patterns of social interactions[13–15].

Because older persons themselves, their families or even healthcare professionals can understand the difficulties experienced, depression occurring in the wake of such significant loss may be considered as "normal". This uninformed perspective works against making the diagnosis of clinical depression and interferes with the effective treatment of this painful and potentially life-threatening condition. Spousal bereavement is a common occurrence of late life, associated with prolonged personal suffering, declining mental and physical health and increased risk of mortality[16]. Among elderly widows and widowers, 20% meet the criteria for major depressive syndrome 2 months after their loss, and one-third of these individuals develop persistent depression for a year or longer[17]. Generally, individuals who are at greatest risk for persistent depression have worse health, more functional and social difficulties and more protracted grief than do bereaved individuals who are not depressed. Whenever major depression occurs, even if precipitated by a significant loss, it should be considered an illness and treated accordingly. As a rule of thumb, if a depressive syndrome occurs within the first 2 months after bereavement and lasts less than 2 months, it should be considered part of the normal grief process and not aggressively treated. However, even within the first 2 months, the depression should be considered a clinically important, treatable syndrome if it is severe or, associated with psychomotor retardation, is accompanied by feelings of worthlessness or suicidal ideation, or occurs in a person with a history of previous major depressive episode[5]. Persistence of severe symptoms beyond several months suggests a condition more severe than the normal grief process.

Symptoms Reflecting Adjustment

Disorders with Depressive Symptoms

The role of social or situational stressors contributing to depression in late life is not well established[18]. Situational stressors may include limited mobility, sensory deprivation, retirement, economic constraint, changing or unsatisfactory living conditions, social isolation, marital difficulty, loss of significant loved ones and/or rejection by children[19].

Of much greater frequency, however, is the development of depressive symptomatology secondary to general medical conditions. When the depressive symptoms accompanying physical illness dramatically exceed the level of symptoms expected, then the diagnosis of adjustment disorder is appropriate. General medical illness resulting in functional disabilities is believed to represent the more significant stressor, contributing to the loss of resources necessary for the maintenance of self-esteem[11,20]. Essentially, depression interferes with basic abilities to think, eat, sleep, love, interact with others, maintain a sense of purpose, experience gratification and maintain self-responsibility[21]. Consistent with the medical outcomes studies[22], depressive symptoms are associated with much social and physical dysfunction, days spent in bed and even physical pain as adverse as any general medical condition. Co-morbid medical illness increases the chronicity and refractoriness to treatment and it may slow recovery rates for patients with various conditions, including heart disease, stroke, hip fracture and dementia[5].

The resolution of stressful events probably depends on a variety of factors, including genetic predisposition, prevailing early life experiences, adequacy of previous adaptive and coping mechanisms, patterns and profiles of premorbid personality and the presence or absence of the support system. Not only may family or social dysfunction influence whether depressive symptoms are experienced by an older adult, but family and social support is apparently critical to the successful outcome in treating the depressed elderly. Blazer has outlined six critical areas as follows: (a) the presence of members of the family or social network who will be available; (b) the interaction of the older adult with family members and other individuals within their community; (c) the integrity of the overall family system and social system; (d) the family and social values regarding the psychiatric disorder; (e) the degree of family and social support with respect to tolerance of symptoms; and (f) other coincidental stressors or life events encountered by the family and social system[23].

Symptoms of Dysthymia

Dysthymic disorder is believed to be less frequent in older adulthood[3]. Co-morbid general medical conditions, cognitive disorders and frequent adverse life events, e.g. bereavement, make the diagnosis of dysthymic disorder quite difficult. Some associated features may include the presence of major chronic stressors, increased physical impairment and more symptoms of anxiety[24]. Generally, dysthymia is less associated with co-morbid Axis I or co-morbid Axis II disorders, and patients with dysthymia tend to be seen in primary care settings rather than by psychiatric specialists[25]. The usual psychologic mechanisms of dysthymia, i.e. self-reproach, guilt and the turning inward of hostile feelings towards loss, are not prominent in later life. However, psychodynamic explanations, i.e. loss of self-esteem and the inability to defend oneself against threats to security, are important in the pathogenesis of late-life dysthymia[26]. The role of narcissistic pathology in the etiology of late-life depression may also contribute significantly to episodes of recurrent depression or defensive grandiosity in response to minor disappointments, or due to self-consciousness or overdependence on approval from others for maintenance of self-esteem, and as a consequence of transitory periods of fragmentation and discohesiveness of the self[27]. Cultural or developmental factors may also contribute to dysthymia. For example, the development of habit patterns emphasizing activity, productivity and achievements can lead to depression and despair at retirement or with the cessation of parenting[28]. Also, as opportunities to interact with cohorts decline, an older individual may not reconcile generative disappointments, and may not proceed from Erikson's[29] developmental stage of generativity to that of integrity (vs. despair)[29].

Symptoms of Major Depression

Major depression is characterized by a persistently depressed mood, loss of interest in usual activities, guilt or other pessimistic thoughts, with accompanying vegetative symptoms reflecting preoccupation with somatic complaints, persistent sleep disturbance, decreased appetite with weight loss, decreased libido, anhedonia and inability to concentrate. Psychotic and delusional symptoms have been reportedly observed with greater frequency in major depressions occurring in later life[4]. Delusional themes are frequently either somatic or persecutory, and are less often characterized as delusions of guilt, sin, poverty, nihilism or jealousy[30]. Feelings of guilt, obsessive rumination, agitation and ideas of reference are frequently found in older adults with major depression. Perceptual disturbances, e.g. hallucinations, may be present but are less frequent than other psychotic symptoms. The prevalence of major depression in the oldest-old is lower than for persons in mid-life, but may be somewhat higher for those who are "young-old", usually estimated at 2–5%[31,32]. Patients with major depression are thought to be more likely to exhibit suicidal ideation. Suicidal ideation is strongly associated with completed suicide. One study has suggested that correlates of suicidal ideation include psychomotor retardation, a history of dysthymia, a previous psychiatric inpatient stay, being a "younger-elder" and having symptoms that reflect feeling "guilty, sinful or worthless"[33]. These correlates of suicidal ideation may be present among individuals who have dysthymia and other minor forms of depression as well.

Symptoms of Bipolar Affective Disorder

Bipolar disorder may be more common in the elderly population than currently recognized. Symptoms of the depressed bipolar elderly patient may include profound psychomotor retardation, even to the point of frank stupor. This psychomotor retardation mimics both dementia and the inanition associated with physical disease. Mood can be elevated or irritable but may be rather labile, showing a picture of depressive admixture[34,35]. These depressed patients may be unable to provide a meaningful history and/or cooperate with diagnostic procedures. Similarly, the elderly, manic patient may make inappropriate sexual comments and/or advances, or be agitated and/or assaultive, and as a result be regarded as cognitively impaired. Although bipolar patients have usually had a history of mood disturbances in the past, these episodes may have been "forgotten" or repressed by both the patients and primary relatives[36].

LATE-ONSET DEPRESSIVE ILLNESS

Depression in late life may be characterized as of early or late onset. Early-onset depression which recurs in later life may have symptoms similar to previous episodes. Differences in the clinical presentation may be observed in both early-onset and late-onset depressives[37]. Genetic predisposition, significant losses or multiple life stressors may interact with age-related biological vulnerabilities. Biological changes due to the physiologic effects of aging have been verified by the study by Schneider[38], showing that unmedicated, elderly depressed subjects demonstrated higher monoamine oxidase (MAO) activity than sex- and age-comparable controls.

Recent studies have proposed that neurobiologic and/or psychosocial factors may predispose an older individual to depression or dysthymia[39]. MRI-defined vascular depression has been identified as a late-onset, non-psychotic type of depression, seen more often in individuals with no family history of depression, together with symptoms of anhedonia and increased psychosocial impairment[40]. Other studies have verified the increasing incidence of depression among individuals with cerebrovascular risk factors, MRI findings associated with vascular disease and symptoms of apathy, together with diminished life quality[41]. Central nervous system degeneration, for example, from the biochemical changes in Alzheimer's disease or other complaints may predispose to an increased incidence of depression[42].

Age of onset has been used as a correlate for late-life depressive symptomatology. Depressive symptoms may be found to be more frequent among the old-old compared to the young-old, with approximately 20% compared to less than 10% in the community[43]. This higher frequency of depression among the old-old may be explained by a higher proportion of women, more general medical problems, more cognitive impairment and lower socioeconomic status. When these factors are controlled, no relationship exists between depressive symptoms and advancing age[44]. Nonetheless, depression is associated with disability among the old-old and a number of studies have illustrated the association between depression and frailty, functional disability and co-morbid general medical problems and/or cognitive impairment[45-47]. Essentially, having more than two previous episodes as compared to two or less is related to younger age, earlier age of onset, dysthymia, feelings of worthlessness, difficulty concentrating, slowed thoughts, suicidal ideation, symptoms of anxiety and decreased perception of social support. Patients with multiple recurrent episodes are also thought to be at higher risk for more severe illness[48]. Late-onset depression is more frequently associated with structural brain changes and cerebrovascular disease, while early-onset depression seems to be more influenced by family and genetic factors. Compared with early-onset depressives, patients with late-onset depression tend to show more loss of interest, less pathological guilt, more psychosis and more generalized anxiety. These correlates of depressive symptomatology based on age of onset suggest a certain heterogeneity in depression of old age.

Table 74.1 Somatization: principles of clinical management

1. The presentation is considered in the context of psychosocial factors, both current and past.
2. The diagnostic procedures and therapeutic interventions are based on objective findings.
3. A therapeutic alliance is fostered and maintained involving the primary care and/or psychiatric physician.
4. The social support system and relevant life quality domains* are carefully reviewed during each patient contact.
5. A regular appointment schedule is maintained for outpatients, irrespective of clinical course.
6. The patient dialogue and examination and the assessment of new symptoms or signs are engaged judiciously, and usually primarily address somatic rather than psychologic concerns.
7. The need for psychiatric referral is recognized early, especially for cases involving chronic symptoms, severe psychosocial consequences or morbid types of illness behavior.
8. Any associated, coexisting or underlying psychiatric disturbance is assiduously evaluated and steadfastly treated.
9. The significance of personality features, addictive potential and self-destructive risk is determined and addressed.
10. The patient's case is redefined in such a way that management, rather than cure, is the goal of treatment.

* Quality of life is an elusive concept but includes the psychosocial domains of occupation, leisure, family, marital, health, sexual and psychological functioning. From Folks et al.[55], with permission.

Atypical Forms of Depression

Depressive illness, particularly of late onset, may present without prominent mood disturbance[19]. Atypical forms of depression, or masked depression, are thus common among older individuals[19]. Masked depression is characterized by the denial of feelings of depression or the lack of complaints of sadness or dysphoria. The dysphoric affect is often prominently masked by somatic complaints, e.g. fatigue, pain, gastrointestinal upset, concentration difficulties or diminished energy[49]. These individuals who manifest prominent somatic symptoms of depression are prone to attribute symptoms of depression to their medical illnesses[10]. Two forms of somatization, hypochondriasis and conversion, may predominate in the clinical picture. The clinical approach to somatization is outlined in Table 74.1.

Hypochondriasis is a common form of masked depression in the elderly and may increase the risk for attempted suicide[50]. This "secondary" form of hypochondriasis must be differentiated from primary hypochondriasis, a persistent somatoform disorder that tends to have its onset in the third or fourth decade of life and persists. Hypochondriasis per se is not more prevalent in the elderly and its onset in later life should not be considered a part of normal aging, but rather reflective of psychologic distress, particularly depression[51-53]. Conversion symptoms or pain that occurs in an elderly person should also raise the question as to the presence of underlying depression, even when no prominent mood disturbance is found[54,55]. In the nursing home setting, a patient may not meet the clinical criteria for depression on patient interview but be observed to have depressive symptoms in the context of somatic complaints. Apathy, withdrawal and isolation may be clues that depression is present. On the other hand, a patient in a long-term care facility may become abruptly agitated with sleep disturbance and prominent somatic complaints, which should increase an index of suspicion for depression.

Table 74.2 Diagnostic features distinguishing depression from dementia

Depression	Dementia
Depressive symptoms	Euthymia
Subacute onset	Insidious onset
History of depression more	History of depression less
Aphasia, apraxia, agnosia absent	Aphasia, apraxia, agnosia present
Orientation intact	Orientation impaired
Concentration impaired	Recent memory impaired
Patient emphasis on memory complaint	Patient minimizes memory complaint
Patient gives up on testing	Patient makes effort on testing

Adapted from Wells[56].

Table 74.3 Medications reportedly associated with depression

Cardiovascular drugs	Hormones	Psychotropics
α-Methyldopa	Conjugal estrogens	Analgesics
Reserpine	ACTH (corticotropin)	Anti-parkinsonian
Propranolol	and glucocorticoids	Antihistamines
Guanethidine	Anabolic steroids	Benzodiazepines
Clonidine		Other sedative
Thiazide diuretics		hypnotics
Digitalis		Typical neuroleptics
	Anti-inflammatory/	
Anticancer agents	anti-infective agents	Others
Cycloserine	Non-steroidal anti-	Cocaine (withdrawal)
	inflammatory agents	Amphetamines
	Ethambutol	(withdrawal)
	Disulfiram	L-dopa
	Sulfonamides	Cimetidine
	Baclofen	Ranitidine
	Metoclopramide	

Adapted from Agency for Health Care Policy and Research[78].

Depression in late life may be masked not only by somatic complaints but also by cognitive difficulties, reflecting yet another atypical form of depression observed in older adults. Difficulty in concentrating or memory loss may result in the clinical picture of "depressive pseudodementia"[56]. This *dementia syndrome of depression* represents a reversible syndrome of dementia that may be clinically indistinguishable from irreversible dementias (Table 74.2)[57,58]. These individuals frequently make little effort to cooperate with mental status examination and the patient answers "Don't know" to many questions. However, notable losses of both recent and remote memory are observed, and these patients may show marked variability on the performance of tasks of similar difficulty. In some cases, depression may be diagnosed retrospectively after a favorable response to a trial of antidepressant medication[19]. Further complicating the issue, in about 20% of cases of true dementia a major depression may coexist[59]. In these cases, both mood and function may improve when treated with an antidepressant therapy, but the basic cognitive impairment remains.

Depression Secondary to a General Medical Condition

Depression may be intimately related to general medical disease or other "organic" influences. Of course, the relationship between somatic symptoms in the medically ill elderly and complaints of depression may be complex; older individuals are presumably more vulnerable to the stresses of poor health and disability that interfere with body image, self-esteem and autonomy. Co-morbidity is the rule, rather than the exception, and linked significantly to functional decline across multiple parameters with increasing age. Co-morbidity of depression with medical illness is associated with poor physical, mental and social functioning, all of which compound the patient's ability to enjoy the quality of life. Not only may medical problems act as precipitators of depression, but many direct effects of medical conditions induce a secondary form of depression (Table 74.3)[9,10]. Medications, including anxiolytics, antihypertensives and neuroleptics, may induce a syndrome of depression. Polypharmacy and drug interaction may further serve to culminate in a depressive illness. The association between depression and general medical–surgical problems may be summarized as follows: (a) physical disease is associated with narcissistic injury, loss of autonomy, pain and fear of impending death, frailty (to be discussed) and diminished quality of life; (b) physical illness may directly (e.g. a cerebrovascular accident) or indirectly (e.g. hypercalcemia) cause a depressive syndrome; or (c) medications used to treat medical diseases may themselves induce depression. These parameters are more significantly affected than in an individual with depression alone or general medical illness without depression[60]. Thus, among individuals with depression in the context of dementia, individuals who experience co-morbid depression and general

medical illness are less active, with fewer social contacts that explain increased disability risk[45]. Physical immobility and social isolation in turn increases disability over time, which further decreases mobility and social interactions, placing the person at risk for physical, psychological and social impairment[61,62]. For some individuals, the end result is a downward spiral in health, functioning and quality of life, a syndrome described by geriatricians as "frailty and failure to thrive". This manifestation is characterized by weight loss, weakness, fatigue, inactivity, decreased food intake and depression. Physical signs that may accompany these symptoms include sarcopenia, balance and gait abnormalities, deconditioning and decreased bone mass[63,64]. Failure to thrive specifies an end-stage of frailty that is characterized by unchecked weight loss, severe muscle wasting, apathetic depression and a host of physiologic abnormalities, including hypoalbuminemia, low creatinine, anemia, bicuspid ulcers and untimely death[65]. Indeed, depression in the elderly is closely related to the state of one's physical health.

Subsyndromal Depression

Subsyndromal depression is defined as depressive symptoms that do not qualify for a formal mood disorder using current clinical criteria. However, several studies have revealed that subthreshold depressive states can be associated with adverse clinical outcome. Additionally, subsyndromal depression may be a risk factor for subsequent major depression[66]. Subthreshold depressive disorder tends to be a heterogenous group of milder forms of depression with symptom patterns qualitatively distinct from more severe depressions such as major depression. According to the Berlin aging study, a subthreshold depression can be characterized in two ways among the elderly[67]; first, as a quantitatively minor variant of depression or a depression-like state, with fewer symptoms or with less continuity; second, as a condition qualitatively different from major depression, with fewer suicidal thoughts or feelings of guilt or worthlessness, while worries about health and weariness of living occur with a similar frequency.

CLINICAL FEATURES AND PROGNOSTIC FACTORS

The paucity of controlled studies in the diagnosis and phenomenology of depression and dysthymia in older adults restricts meaningful prognostication. Depression may be reflected in behavioral changes in the elderly, for example increased clinging, dependent behavior, phobias or avoidance of previously enjoyable activities, perhaps representing a variant of anhedonia. No conclusive evidence has shown that major depression is more chronic in later life; in fact, most psychogeriatricians are convinced that the outcome of adequately treated depression, uncomplicated by medical disease, is as good as the outcome from younger individuals. A caveat is that the risk of recurrence may be greater for older depressives[68,69]. Blazer[26] has noted the tendency for some older individuals to show only partial improvement not fully recovering from an episode of major depression. Thus, in some cases residual symptoms may persist even when response to treatment is definitive—this treatment resistance is more attributed to co-morbidity than to age *per se*.

Accurate and early diagnosis and adequate and aggressive treatment are important considerations in late-life depression and dysthymia. Patients should be screened, with history, questionnaires, observation, collateral information and the use of screening devices, such as the Geriatric Depression Scale[70] or the Center for Epidemiological Studies Depression Scale (CESD)[71], both of which are validated in older depressives and useful in the overall assessment process. These self-assessment instruments, together with the Hamilton Depression Rating Scale[72], an interviewer assessment agent, are useful for assignment of psychiatric diagnosis of depression. Other questions, designed to establish cognitive, nutritional and functional status, social function and general health perceptions, together with review of medications, medical work-up and laboratory assessment as indicated, are necessary in early intervention. Keller *et al.*[73] reported that depressed patients who did not receive treatment until long after the onset of depressive symptoms had the worst prognosis. These investigators suggested that early intervention is indeed the most effective means of reducing chronicity. Therapy must proceed across multiple domains simultaneously. This includes the mobilization of the social support system, the use of antidepressant medications, psychotherapy and efforts to improve physical or social functioning[74,75]. Among psychotherapeutic options, cognitive–behavioral therapy has been utilized most, with a few reports involving interpersonal psychotherapy. Other behavioral interventions range from prescribing regular group activities, physical exercise such as walking, and training exercises for increased independent functioning. Although few in number, studies of comprehensive interventions using all of the approaches outlined above have demonstrated efficacy comparable to that found in younger adults[76,77]. These existing studies are preliminary but promising, in view of the reduction in functional disability and symptomatic relief, together with improved quality of life and, ultimately, reduction in the healthcare cost associated with late-life depression.

CONCLUSION

The categorical approach to depression and dysthymia in late life continues to reflect the current nomenclature. Ultimately, the diagnosis and management of depression and dysthymia is allied with the traditional medical model. This approach enables the clinician to provide specific therapies for distinct diagnostic entities and provides the patient with a number of excellent biological and psychosocial interventions. However, classical symptoms may be overshadowed or replaced by a variety of other symptoms, in which the mood disturbance is not prominent. Thus, the key to the diagnosis and effective intervention of depression in old age is to maintain a high index of suspicion and attend to the functional disability and quality of life issues posed by late-life depression.

REFERENCES

1. Hendrie HC, Crosset JHW. An overview of depression in the elderly. *Psychiat Ann* 1990; **20**: 64–9.
2. *Diagnostic and Statistical Manual of Mental Disorders, 3rd edn, Revised.* Washington DC: American Psychiatric Association, 1987.
3. Meyers BS, Kalayam B, Mei-tal V. Late-onset delusional depression: a distinct clinical entity? *J Clin Psychiat* 1984; **45**: 347–9.
4. Blazer D, Hughes DC, George LK. The epidemiology of depression in an elderly community population. *Gerontologist* 1987; **27**: 281–7.
5. Zisook S, Downs NS. Diagnosis and treatment of depression in late life. *J Clin Psychiat* 1998; **59**(suppl 4): 80–91.
6. Shapiro S, Skinner EA, Kessler WA *et al.* Utilization of health and mental health services. *Arch Gen Psychiat* 1984; **41**: 10.
7. Blazer D, Williams CD. Epidemiology of dysphoria and depression in an elderly population. *Am J Psychiat* 1980; **137**: 439–44.
8. Mei-Tak V, Meyers BS. Major psychiatric illness in the elderly: empirical study on an inpatient psychogeriatric unit. Part I: diagnostic complexities. *Int J Psychiat Med* 1985; **15**: 91–109.
9. Folks DG, Ford CV. Psychiatric disorders in geriatric medical/surgical patients. Part I: report of 195 consecutive consultations. *South Med J* 1985; **78**: 239–41.
10. Ford CV, Folks DG. Psychiatric disorders in geriatric medical/surgical patients part II: review of clinical experience in consultation. *South Med J* 1985; **78**: 397–402.
11. Neugarten BL. Adaption and the life cycle. *J Geriatr Psychol* 1970; **4**: 41–87.
12. Clayton PJ. Clinical insights into normal grief. *Ri Med J* 1980; **63**: 107-9.
13. Brown JT, Stoudemire A. Normal and pathologic grief. *J Am Med Assoc* 1983; **250**: 378.
14. Bruce ML, Kim K, Leaf P *et al.* Depressive episodes and dysphoria resulting from conjugal bereavement in a prospective community sample. *Am J Psychiat* 990; **147**: 608–11.
15. Vargas LA, Loya F, Hodde-Vargas KC. Exploring the multidimensional aspects of grief reactions. *Am J Psychiat* 1989; **146**: 484–8.
16. Kaprio J, Koskenvuo M, Rita H. Mortality after bereavement; prospective study of 95 647 widowed persons. *Am J Publ Health* 1987; **77**: 282–7.
17. Zisook S, Shuchter SR. Major depression associated with widowhood. *Am J Geriatr Psychiat* 1993; **147**: 316–26.
18. George LK, Blazer D, Hughes DC *et al.* Social support and the outcome of major depression. *Br J Psychiat* 1989; **154**: 478–85.
19. Ruegg RG, Zisook S, Swerlow NR. Depression in the aged: an overview. *Psychiatr Clin N Am* 1988; **11**: 83–108.
20. Murphy E. Social origins of depression in old age. *Br J Psychiat* 1982; **141**: 135–42.
21. Diagnosis and treatment of depression in late life: NIH consensus development panel on depression in late life. *J Am Med Assoc* 1992; **268**(8): 1018–24.
22. Wells KB, Stewart A, Hays RD *et al.* The functioning and well-being of depressed patients: results from the Medical Outcomes Study. *J Am Med Assoc* 1989; **262**: 914–19.
23. Blazer DG. *Depression in Late Life.* St Louis, MO: CV Mosby, 1982.
24. Kirby M, Bruce L, Coakley D, Lawlor BA. Dysthymia among community-dwelling elderly. *Int J Geriat Psychiat* 1999; **14**: 440–5.
25. Bellino S, Bogetto F, Veschetto P *et al.* Recognition and treatment of dysthymia in elderly patients. *Drugs Aging* 2000; **16**: 107–21.
26. Blazer D. Depression in the elderly. *N Engl J Med* 1989; **320**: 164–5.
27. Lazarus LW, Weinberg J. Treatment in the ambulatory care setting. In Busse EW, Blazer DG, eds, *Handbook of Geriatric Psychiatry.* New York: Van Nostrand Reinhold, 1980: 427–53.
28. Wigdor BT. Drives and motivations with aging. In Birren JE, Sloane RB, eds, *The Handbook of Aging and Mental Health.* Englewood Cliffs, NJ: Prentice Hall, 1980.
29. Erikson EH. *Eight Ages of Man in Childhood and Society.* New York: WW Norton, 1963: 247–74.
30. Kalayam B, Shamoian CA. Geriatric psychiatry: an update. *J Clin Psychiat* 1990; **51**: 177–83.
31. Blazer D, Burchett B, Service C, George L. The association of age and depression among the elderly: an epidemiologic study. *J Gerontol Med Sci* 1991; **46**: M210–15.

32. Henderson A, Jorm A, MacKinnon A. The prevalence of depressive disorders and the distribution of depressive symptoms in later life: a survey using draft ICD-10 and DSM-III-R. *Psychol Med* 1993; **23**: 719–29.

33. Lynch TR, Mendelson T, Robins CJ et al. Perceived social support among depressed elderly, middle-aged, and young adult samples: cross-sectional and longitudinal analyses. *J Affect Disord* 1999; **55**: 159–70.

34. Himmelhoch JM, Mulla D, Neil JF. Incidence and significance of mixed affective states in a bipolar population. *Arch Gen Psychiat* 1976; **33**: 1062.

35. Shulman KI. Mania in old age. In Murphy E, ed., *Affective Disorders in the Elderly*. Edinburgh: Churchill Livingstone, 1986: 203–13.

36. Spar JE, Ford CV, Liston EH. Bipolar affective disorder in aged patients. *J Clin Psychiat* 1979; **40**: 504–7.

37. Alexopoulos GS, Young RC, Meyers BS et al. Late-onset depression. *Psychiatr Clin N Am* 1988; **II**: 115.

38. Schneider LS, Severson JA, Pollock V et al. Platelet monoamine oxidase activity in elderly depressed outpatients. *Biol Psychiat* 1986; **21**: 1360–63.

39. Veith RC, Raskind MA. The neurobiology of aging: does it predispose to depression? *Neurobiol Aging* 1988; **9**: 101–17.

40. Krishnan KR, Hays JC, Blazer DG. MRI-defined vascular depression. *Am J Psychiat* 1997; **15**: 497–501.

41. Lavretsky HM, Lesser IM, Wohl M et al. Clinical and neuroradiologic features associated with chronicity in late life depression. *Am J Geriat Psychiat* 1000; **7**: 309–16.

42. Zubenko GS, Henderson R, Stiffler JS et al. Association of the APOE ε4 allele with clinical subtypes of late-life depression. *Biol Psychiat* 1996; **40**: 1008–16.

43. White L, Blazer D, Fillenbaum G. Related health problems. In Cornoni-Huntley J, Blazer D, Lafferty M et al., eds, *Established Populations for Epidemiologic Studies of the Elderly* (NIH Publication No. 90-495). Bethesda, MD: National Institute on Aging, 1990: 70–85.

44. Blazer D, Burchett B, Service C, George L. The association of age and depression among the elderly: an epidemiologic study. *J Gerontol Med Sci* 1991; **46**: M210–15.

45. Pennix B, Leveille S, Ferrucci L et al. Exploring the effect of depression on physical disability: longitudinal evidence from the Established Populations for Epidemiologic Studies of the Elderly. *Am J Publ Health* 1999; **89**: 1346–52.

46. Broe G, Jorm A, Creasey H et al. Impact of chronic systemic and neurological disorders on disability, depression and life satisfaction. *Int J Psychiat* 1998; **13**: 667–73.

47. Parmelee P, Lawton M, Katz I. The structure of depression among elderly institution residents: affective and somatic correlates of physical frailty. *J Gerontol Med Sci* 1998; **53**: M155–62.

48. Steffens DC, Hays JC, George LK et al. Sociodemographic and clinical correlates of number of previous depressive episodes in the depressed elderly. *J Affect Disord* 1996; **52**: 99–106.

49. Salzman C, Shader RI. Depression in the elderly. I. Relationship between depression, psychologic defense mechanisms and physical illness. *J Am Geriatr Soc* 1978; **27**: 253–60.

50. Dealarcon R. Hypochondriasis and depression in the aged. *Gerontol Clin* 1964; **6**: 266–77.

51. Costs PT, McGae RR. Somatic complaints in males as a junction of age and neuroticism, a longitudinal study. *J Behav Med* 1980; **3**: 245–57.

52. Gianturco DG, Busse EW. Psychiatric problems encountered during a long-term study of normal aging volunteers. In Isaacs AG, Post F, eds, *Studies in Geriatric Psychiatry*. Chichester: Wiley, 1978: 1–17.

53. Goldstein SE, Birnbom F. Hypochondriasis and the elderly. *Am Geriatr Soc J* 1976; **24**: 150–54.

54. Levitan M, Bruni J. Repetitive pseudoseizures incorrectly managed as status epilepticus. *Can Med Assoc J* 1986; **134**: 1029–31.

55. Folks DG, Ford CV, Houck CA. Somatoform disorders, factitious disorders and malingering. In Stoudemire A, ed., *Clinical Psychiatry for Medical Students*. Philadelphia, PA: JB Lippincott, 1990: 237–68.

56. Wells CE. Pseudodementia. *Am J Psychiat* 1979; **136**: 895–900.

57. Feinberg T, Goodman B. Affective illness, dementia and pseudodementia. *J Clin Psychiat* 1984; **45**: 99–103.

58. Grunhaus L, Dilsaven S, Greden JF et al. Depressive pseudodementia: a suggested diagnostic profile. *Biol Psychiat* 1983; **18**: 215–25.

59. Reifler BV, Larson E, Henley R. Coexistence of cognitive impairment and depression in geriatric outpatients. *Am J Psychiat* 1982; **39**: 623–26.

60. Wells K, Sherbourne C. Functioning and utility for current health of patients with depression or chronic medical conditions in managed, primary care practices. *Arch Gen Psychiat* 1999; **56**: 897–904.

61. Von Korff M, Ormle J, Katon W, Liu E. Disability and depression among high utilizers of health care. A longitudinal study. *Arch Gen Psychiat* 1991; **49**: 91–100.

62. Hays J, Saunders W, Flint E et al. Depression and social support as risk factors for functional disability in late life. *Aging Ment Health* 1997; **3**: 209–20.

63. Fried L, Walston J. Frailty and failure to thrive. In Hazzard W, Blass J, Ettinger W et al., eds, *Principles of Geriatric Medicine and Gerontology*. New York: McGraw Hill, 1999; 1387–402.

64. Verdery R. Failure to thrive in older persons. *J Am Geriat Soc* 1996; **44**: 465–6.

65. Katz FR, Difilippo S. Neuropsychiatric aspects of failure to thrive in late life. *J Clin Geriat Med* 1997; **13**: 623–38.

66. Judd LJ, Rappaport MH, Paulus MP, Brown JL. Subsyndromal symptomatic depression: a new mood disorder? *J Clin Psychiat* 1994; **55**(suppl 4): 18–28.

67. Geiselmann B and Bauer M. Subthreshold depression in the elderly: qualitative or quantitative distinction? *Comp Psychiat* 2000; **41**(2): 32–8.

68. Baldwin RC, Jolley DJ. The prognosis of depression in old age. *Br J Psychiat* 1986; **149**: 475–583.

69. Reynolds C, Frank E, Dwe M et al. Treatment of 70+-year olds with recurrent major depression. Excellent short-term but brittle long-term response. *Am J Geriatr Psychiat* 1999; **7**: 64–9.

70. Yesavage J, Brink T, Rose T. Development and validation of a geriatric depression screening scale; a preliminary report. *J Psychiat Res* 1983; **17**: 37–49.

71. Radloff L. The CES-D scale; a self-report depression scale for research in the general population. *Appl Psycholol Meas* 1977; **1**: 385–401.

72. Hamilton M. A rating scale for depression. *J Neurol Neurosurg Psychiat* 1960; **23**: 56–62.

73. Keller MB, Klerman GL, Lavori PW et al. Long-term outcome of episodes of major depression. *J Am Med Assoc* 1984; **252**: 788–92.

74. Mossy J, Knott K, Higgins M, Talerico K. Effectiveness of a psychosocial intervention, interpersonal counseling, for dysthymic depression in medically ill elderly. *J Gerontol Biol Sci Med Sci* 1996; **51**: M172–8.

75. Lincoln N, Flannaghan T, Sutcliffe L, Rother L. Evaluation of cognitive behavioral treatment for depression after a stroke: a pilot study. *Clin Rehab* 1997; **11**: 114–22.

76. Cuijpers P. Psychological outreach programmes for the depressed elderly: a meta-analysis of effects and dropout. *Int J Geriatr Psychiat* 1998; **13**: 41–8.

77. Banerjee S, Shamash K, Macdonald A, Mann A. Randomized controlled trial of the effect of intervention by a psychogeriatric team on depression in frail elderly people at home. *Br Med J* 1997; **313**: 1058–61.

78. Agency for Health Care Policy and Research, Depression Guideline Panel. *Depression in Primary Care*. 1993; AHCPR No 93-0550.

Outcome of Depressive Disorders: Findings of a Longitudinal Study in the UK

Vimal Kumar Sharma

University of Liverpool, UK

A high prevalence of depressive disorders among the elderly has been reported by different community studies (*see* reviews[1,2]). More recent epidemiological studies[3-9] using standardized methods have also reported similar prevalence rates of depressive disorders in the range 8–15% in randomly selected community samples. It is not clear whether the high prevalence rate is due to chronicity of the disorder or to a high incidence rate of depression in this age group.

So far there have been few large-scale longitudinal studies of community-based elderly depressed subjects. Most of these studies have reported that 30–60% of the depressed elderly were continually ill[10-15]. Some studies have examined the prognostic factors associated with the poor outcome. Physical illness, handicap, female sex, poor social support, high depression score and anxiety and neuroticism, lack of satisfaction with life and feelings of loneliness are some of the factors reported to be associated with the poor outcome[12,14,16-21]. Kivela[22], in her 5 year follow-up study, reported organic outcome in 12% for major depression and 9% for dysthymic disorder. In contrast, Henderson *et al.*[16] found none of their 24 community cases of depression (ICD 10) to be organic cases after 3–4 years. Many of the studies have also reported that the majority of the depressed elderly never receive appropriate treatment[10,13,23-25].

Community studies[15,16,22,26,27] have reported increased mortality in depression. There have been a few relatively shorter (1–3.5 years) follow-up studies[10,29] which found no significant association between depression and mortality. In another study, when factors such as age, physical health and social conditions were taken into account, depression did not predict increased mortality[18].

Tannock and Katona[30] reviewed the literature and concluded that subsyndromal depression is common among the elderly and that very little is known about its nature and outcome.

Where the symptoms of an illness appear to lie on a continuum of severity with normal behaviour, as in depressive illness, variations in disease level might be found between studies because they use different cut-off points and/or record different types of symptoms, rather than because there are true differences in illness levels. Such spurious differences may also arise between different waves of interviewing in the same longitudinal study if the interpretation of symptoms is not standardized, and may also occur if the interviewers of subsequent waves are not blind to the findings of previous waves.

A further problem with such studies is that some psychiatrists assume depression to be a unitary disease but nevertheless do not agree on what conditions are to be excluded; e.g. some would include bereavement and adjustment disorder if the principal symptom is one of depression. Others would distinguish between major depressive disorders and dysthymia, or between endogenous and reactive, or neurotic and psychotic depression and might or might not recognize brief recurrent depression.

Cole and Bellovance[31], in their review of five community-based studies of depression in old age, highlighted such methodological limitations. They recommended that a large number of depressed elderly (based on explicit diagnostic criteria and reliable measures) should be followed up for a longer duration with specific outcome categories. Outcome assessments should be blind and reported at specific time points (e.g. every 6 months) during the follow-up interval. A continuously depressed elderly cohort should be examined closely to determine the sustaining factors of their depression.

This special article contains findings of the outcome data of the depressed elderly in the Liverpool longitudinal study.

The subsample for this study included 120 index AGECAT cases of depression and 47 of subcases of depression and 82 other subjects. The age distribution of each diagnostic group was similar. More women were present among the cases compared to subcases of depression and non-cases. Most subjects were in social class 3, 4 and 5. Around 40% of both cases and subcases of depression were living alone and this was higher than for non-cases. Stressful events, such as bereavement, illness in the family, house break-ins, family disputes in the preceding month, were more often recorded for subjects of the depressive neurosis group.

The overall dropout rate at 5 years was 28% for cases of depression, 30% for subcases of depression and 26% for other non-cases.

Over 5 years, 41 of 120 cases (34%) died, also 12 of 47 subcases of depression (26%) and 9 of 54 non-cases (17%). The risk of dying within 5 years was 2.1 times higher for the cases of depression compared to non-cases (95% CI, 1.1–3.9). Of the surviving and available cases of depression, 54% (43/79) at year 3, 43% (23/53) at year 4 and 54% (25/46) at year 5 had sufficient psychopathology to reach AGECAT case levels for some kind of mental illness. A further 18% (14/79) at year 3, 17% (9/53) at year 4 and 9% (4/46) at year 5 had psychopathology at the subcase level of depression.

LONGITUDINAL OUTCOME

The outcome of the cases of depression is given in Figure 1. Forty-six of the cases of depression had a complete 5 year evaluation. Eleven (24%) had sufficient symptoms to reach AGECAT case levels at all follow-up assessments. Another 11 (24%) reached AGECAT case levels at two of the three follow-up waves, whilst the other 14 (33%) reached case levels at only one. The remaining 10 (22%) never reached AGECAT case levels at any of the 3, 4 and 5 year follow-up waves. The AGECAT diagnosis at any follow-up wave was depression in 70% of the interviews. Those (30%) who were diagnosed as another type of case, other than depression, had a high depression score. Only one of the year 3 cases of depression was on antidepressant treatment and none of year 4 and 5 cases of depression were on antidepressants at the time of their interviews.

Outcome of the Subcases of Depression

As many as 16 (34%) of the 47 subcases of depression were AGECAT cases at year 3, most of them cases of depression. Their 5 year outcome is given in Figure 2.

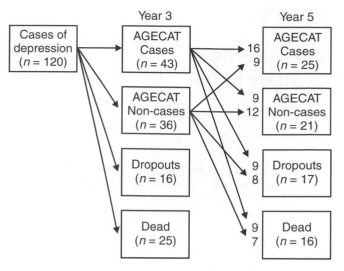

Figure 1 Outcome of the cases of depression (from ref. 34, with permission)

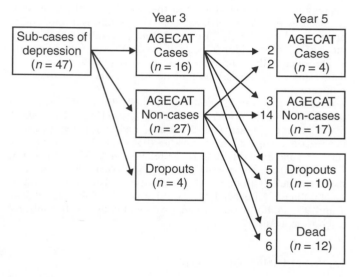

Figure 2 Outcome of the subcases of depression (from ref. 34, with permission).

Organicity and Outcome of the Cases of Depression

In all, 30 (25%) of the 120 cases of depression had co-morbid organic symptoms (AGECAT levels 1–2) at the index assessment. By year 5, nine (30%) had died and seven (23%) had dropped out. Of the remaining 14, 12 (40%) were AGECAT cases and two were non-cases. Seven (6%) of the 120 cases of depression (15% of the surviving cases) had become organic cases at the 5 year follow-up. Five of them had already had some organic symptoms (AGECAT levels 1 or 2) at the start of the study.

Predictors of Outcome

Univariate analyses were done to see which index variables (age, gender, marital status, social class, stressful events, living conditions, social support, physical illness, depression type (DP and DN), depression score and psychiatric co-morbidity) were predictive of a poor outcome for the depression cases that had survived. Anxiety caseness and a depression score of 30 were particularly predictive of a poor outcome in this sample. Those aged under 75 years did better than those 75 years and older.

A prospective follow-up of the cases of depressive disorders at shorter intervals is the strength of this study. Its findings highlight the importance of the mental health needs of this population. Further studies are needed to discover whether drug treatments or other psychosocial interventions can alleviate depression in elderly people living in the community.

REFERENCES

1. Blazer DG. Epidemiology. In Blazer DG, ed., *Depression in Late Life*. St. Louis, MO: C.V. Mosby, 1982; 103–17.
2. Eastwood MR, Corbin SL. The epidemiology of mental disorders in old age. In Arie THD, ed., *Recent Advances in Psychogeriatrics*. London: Churchill Livingstone, 1985; 17–32.
3. Copeland JRM, Dewey ME, Wood N *et al*. Range of mental illness among the elderly in the community: prevalence in Liverpool using the GMS–AGECAT package. *Br J Psychiat* 1987; **150**: 815–23.
4. Kay DWK, Henderson AS, Scott R *et al*. Dementia and depression among the elderly living in the Hobart community: the effect of the diagnostic criteria on the prevalence rates. *Psychol Med* 1985; **15**: 771–88.
5. Livingston G, Hawkins A, Graham N *et al*. The Gospel Oak Study: prevalence rates of dementia, depression and activity limitation among elderly residents in Inner London. *Psychol Med* 1990; **20**: 137–46.
6. Lindesay J, Briggs K, Murphy E. The Guys'/Age Concern Survey, prevalence rates of cognitive impairment depression and anxiety in an urban elderly community. *Br J Psychiat* 1989; **155**: 317–29.
7. Ben-Arie O, Swartz L, Dickman BJ. Depression in the elderly living in the community. Its presentation and features. *Br J Psychiat* 1987; **150**: 169–74.
8. Saunders PA, Copeland JR, Dewey ME *et al*. The prevalence of dementia, depression and neurosis in later life: the Liverpool MRC-ALPHA Study. *Int J Epidemiol* 1993; **22**(5): 838–47.
9. Kirby M, Bruce I, Radic A *et al*. Mental disorders among the community-dwelling elderly in Dublin. *Br J Psychiat* 1997; **171**: 369–72.
10. Ben-Arie O, Welman M, Teggin AF. The depressed elderly living in the community—a follow-up study. *Br J Psychiat* 1990; **157**: 425–7.
11. Kivela SL, Kongas-Saviaro P, Kesti E *et al*. Five-year prognosis for depression in old age. *Int Psychogeriat* 1994; **6**(1): 69–78.
12. Beekman ATF, Deeg DJH, Smit JH, Tilburg WV. Predicting the course of depression in the older population: results from a community based study in The Netherlands. *J Affect Disord* 1995; **34**: 41–9.
13. Copeland JRM, Davidson IA, Dewey ME *et al*. Alzheimer's disease, other dementias, depression and pseudodementia prevalence: incidence and three year outcome in Liverpool: GMS–HAS AGECAT. *Br J Psychiat* 1992; **161**: 230–9.
14. Kua EH. The depressed elderly Chinese living in the community: a five-year follow-up study. *Int J Geriat Psychiat* 1993; **8**: 427–30.
15. Prince MJ, Harwood RH, Thomas A, Mann AH. A prospective population-based cohort study of the effects of disablement and social milieu on the onset and maintenance of late-life depression. The Gospel Oak Project VII. *Psychol Med* 1998; **28**: 337–50.
16. Henderson AS, Korten AE, Jacomb PA *et al*. The course of depression in the elderly: a longitudinal community-based study in Australia. *Psychol Med* 1997; **27**(1): 119–29.
17. Livingston G, Manela M, Katona C. Cost of community care for older people. *Br J Psychiat* 1997; **171**: 56–9.
18. Pulska T, Pahkala K, Laippala P, Kivela SL. Six-year survival of depressed elderly Finns: a community study. *Int J Geriat Psychiat* 1997; **12**(9): 942–50.

19. Green BH, Copeland JR, Dewey ME *et al.* Risk factors for depression in elderly people: a prospective study. *Acta Psychiat Scand* 1992; **86**(3): 213–17.
20. Prince MJ, Harwood RH, Blizard RA *et al.* Impairment, disability and handicap as risk factors for depression in old age. The Gospel Oak Project. *Psychol Med* 1997; **27**(2): 311–21.
21. Copeland JR, Chen R, Dewey ME *et al.* Community-based case-control study of depression in older people. Cases and sub-cases from the MRC-ALPHA Study. *Br J Psychiat* 1999; **175**: 340–7.
22. Kivela SL. Long-term prognosis of major depression in old age: a comparison with prognosis of dysthymic disorder. *Int Psychogeriat* 1995; **7**: 69–82.
23. Beekman AT, Deeg DJ, Braam AW *et al.* Consequences of major and minor depression in later life: a study of disability, well-being and service utilization. *Psychol Med* 1997; **27**(6): 1397–409.
24. Livingston G, Watkin V, Milne B *et al.* The natural history of depression and the anxiety disorders in older people: the Islington community study. *J Affect Disord* 1997; **46**(3): 255–62.
25. Wilson KC, Copeland JR, Taylor S *et al.* Natural history of pharmacotherapy of older depressed community residents. The MRC-ALPHA Study. *Br J Psychiat* 1999; **175**: 439–44.
26. Enzell K. Mortality among persons with depressive symptoms and among responders and non-responders in a health check-up. *Acta Psychiat Scand* 1984; **69**: 89–102.
27. Davidson IA, Dewey ME, Copeland JRM. The relationship between mortality and mental disorder: evidence from the Liverpool longitudinal study. *Int J Geriat Psychiat* 1988; **3**: 95–8.
28. Markush RE, Schwab JJ, Farris P *et al.* Mortality and community mental health. *Arch Gen Psychiat* 1977; **34**: 1393–401.
29. Fredman L, Schoenbach VJ, Kaplan BH *et al.* The association between depressive symptoms and mortality among older participants in the epidemiologic catchment area—Piedmont Health Survey. *J Gerontol* 1989; **44**(4): 149–56.
30. Tannock C, Katona C. Minor depression in the aged. Concepts, prevalence and optimal management. *Drugs Aging* 1995; **6**(4): 278–92.
31. Cole MG, Bellavance F. The prognosis of depression in old age. *Am J Geriat Psychiat* 1997; **5**: 4–14.
32. Copeland JRM, Kelleher MJ, Kellett JM *et al.* A semi-structured clinical interview for the assessment of diagnosis and mental state in the elderly. The Geriatric Mental State Schedule, 1. Development and reliability. *Psychol Med* 1976; **6**: 439–49.
33. Copeland JRM, Dewey ME, Griffith-Jones HM. Computerised psychiatric diagnostic system and case nomenclature for elderly subjects: GMS and AGECAT. *Psychol Med* 1986; **16**: 89–99.
34. Sharma VK, Copeland JR, Dewey ME *et al.* Outcome of the depressed elderly living in the community in Liverpool: a 5-year follow-up. *Psychol Med* 1998; **28**(6): 1329–37.

Longitudinal Studies of Mood Disorders in the USA

Dan G. Blazer

Duke University Medical Center, Durham, NC, USA

Depressive disorders in late life tend to recur or persist and change the course of a person's life through time. For this reason, the assessment of depression through time necessitates an accurate understanding of the longitudinal course of depressive disorders. For this reason, when the Psychobiology of Depression Study Group began their extensive study of inpatient and outpatient persons in adulthood (but not including old age), they incorporated an extensive longitudinal study into their methodology. Results from this study revealed that 1 year following identification of an index episode of major depression, 50% of the cohort 59 years of age and younger had recovered, but the annual rate of recovery decreased to 28% by the second year and to 22% by the third year. These investigators determined that recovery from an index episode of major depression was most likely to occur within the year following identification of the episode. Among those individuals who do recover, 24% suffered a relapse within 3 months of the recovery; 16% of the individuals who identified suffering from an index episode remained ill throughout the first year. The cohort has now been followed for 15 years (original age of 18–59 with the current cohort now between 33–74); 85% of those who recovered from the index episode relapsed at least once over the 15 years and 58% of persons who recovered and remained well for 5 years relapsed over the next 10 years. Female gender, a longer index episode of depression, more prior episodes and never marrying all contributed to an increased likelihood of relapse.

There has been no equivalent study of the outcome of late-life depression within the USA that has currently been reported in the literature. However, an ongoing study by Duke University investigators has found that rates of chronicity, recovery and relapse are virtually identical to those reported by Keller and colleagues for younger age groups. The remainder of studies in North America have concentrated primarily upon outcome in controlled treatment trials. The Pittsburgh group found that over 3 years, subjects treated with optimal doses of antidepressant medications relapsed at a rate of between 30% and 40% over 3 years.

REFERENCES

1. Keller MB, Shapiro RW, Lavori PW, Wolf N. Recovery in major depressive disorders: analysis with the lifetable and aggression models. *Arch Gen Psychiat* 1982; **39**: 905–10.
2. Keller MB, Shapiro RW, Lavori PW, Wolf N. Relapse in major depressive disorder: analysis with the life-table. *Arch Gen Psychiat* 1982; **39**: 911–15.
3. George LK, Blazer DG, Hughes DC, Fowler N. Social support and the outcome of major depression. *Br J Psychiat* 1989; **154**: 478–85.
4. Mueller TI, Leon AC, Keller MB *et al.* Recurrence after recovery from major depressive disorder during 15 years of observational follow-up. *Am J Psychiat* 1999; **156**: 1000–6.
5. Reynolds CF III, Perel JM, Frank E *et al.* Three-year outcomes of maintenance nortriptyline treatment in late-life depression: a study of two fixed plasma levels. *Am J Psychiat* 1999; **156**: 1177–81.

Outcome of Depression in Finland

Sirkka-Liisa Kivelä

University of Turku, Finland

In the early 1980s, an epidemiological study of depression was carried out among the population aged 60 years or over ($n = 1529$) living in the municipality of Ähtäri in south-western Finland. DSM-III criteria were used to diagnose depression in interviews and examinations and 264 depressed persons (91 men and 173 women) were discovered; 42 met the criteria for major depression, 199 for dysthymic disorder, 21 for atypical depression and two for cyclothymic disorder.

The depressed persons were intensively treated in a primary care setting for about 2 years after the epidemiological study. The treatment consisted of individual psychological support by a general practitioner, antidepressive medication, counselling about nutrition and physical exercise and social support from the families, relatives, neighbours and home care personnel. Later, a less intensive treatment schedule, consisting of psychological support by a general practitioner and antidepressive medication, was arranged for those who had not recovered.

1 YEAR AND 5 YEAR CLINICAL OUTCOMES

Nearly half of both major depressive and dysthymic patients were non-depressed after 1 year (Table 1). The proportion of depressed subjects tended to be higher among the dysthymic patients, while the proportions of demented subjects and deaths tended to be higher among the major depressive patients. After 5 years, the proportion of recoveries was higher among the dysthymic patients, and the death rate was higher among the major depressive patients. Every fourth subject was depressed in both groups.

FACTORS RELATED TO RELAPSES OR LONG-TERM COURSE

Major depression had a definite tendency for a relapsing course during the 5 year follow-up, even without any special stressors in life or physical illnesses after recovery. The depressed patients who developed a physical disease and whose physical health deteriorated during the treatment had a high risk for non-recovery and a long-term course of depression. Many of these patients had suffered from poor self-appreciation and diurnal variation of symptoms at the onset of the treatment.

The results support the following proposals for clinical practice. Major depressive patients should be followed up after recovery in order to detect their possible relapse and to increase the probability of recovery. Intensive antidepressant and psychotherapeutic treatment and adequate treatment of physical diseases should be arranged for depressed patients who develop a physical disease or whose somatic condition deteriorates due to a previous physical disease. Cooperation between psychiatrists and general practitioners is needed in the above two cases.

MORTALITY

Major depressive patients had a high death rate, which was not explained by their poor physical health. These results suggest that there may be biological factors associated with major depression that increase the risk of death or the risk of the development of physical diseases leading to death. The mortality of dysthymic patients was

Table 1 One year and 5 year outcomes of major depressive and dysthymic older patients treated in primary health care

	1 Year outcome		5 Year outcome	
	n	(%)	*n*	(%)
Major depressive patients				
Non-depressed	19	(45)	5	(12)
Depressed	11	(26)	11	(26)
Demented	6	(14)	5	(12)
Dead	6	(14)	19	(45)
Refused to participate			2	(5)
Total	42	(100)	42	(100)
Dysthymic patients				
Non-depressed	79	(40)	71	(36)
Depressed	91	(45)	52	(26)
Demented	6	(3)	18	(9)
Dead	20	(10)	50	(25)
Refused to participate	3	(2)	8	(4)
Total	199	(100)	199	(100)

also higher than that of non-depressed persons, but their high mortality was explained by the high number of physical diseases.

Longstanding depression was a predictor for high mortality, independently of the physical diseases present at the onset of the treatment of depression. The physical diseases that occur during the treatment and predict a longstanding course may explain the high death rate seen here.

These results also underline the need for intensive and adequate treatment of depression and physical diseases in depressed older persons.

REFERENCES

1. American Psychiatric Association. *Diagnostic and Statistical Manual*, 3rd edn (DSM-III). Washington, DC: APA.
2. Kivelä S-L, Pahkala K, Laippala P. Prevalence of depression in an elderly population in Finland. *Acta Psychiat Scand* 1988; **78**: 401–13.
3. Kivelä S-L, Pahkala K, Laippala P. A one-year prognosis of dysthymic disorder and major depression in old age. *Int J Geriat Psychiat* 1991; **6**: 81–7.
4. Kivelä S-L, Köngäs-Saviaro P, Pahkala K *et al.* Five-year prognosis for dysthymic disorder in old age. *Int J Geriat Psychiat* 1993; **8**: 939–47.
5. Kivelä S-L. Long-term prognosis of major depression in old age: a comparison with prognosis of dysthymic disorder. *Int Psychogeriat* 1995; suppl 7: 69–82.
6. Kivelä S-L, Viramo P, Pahkala K. Factors predicting the long-term course of depression in old age. *Int Psychogeriat* 2000; **12**: 183–94.
7. Kivelä S-L, Viramo P, Pahkala K. Factors predicting the relapse of depression in old age. *Int J Ger Psychiat* 2000; **15**: 112–19.
8. Pulska T, Pahkala K, Laippala P, Kivelä S-L. Major depression as a predictor of premature deaths in elderly people in Finland: a community study. *Acta Psychiat Scand* 1998; **97**: 408–11.
9. Pulska T, Pahkala K, Laippala P, Kivelä S-L. Survival of elderly Finns suffering from dysthymic disorder: a community study. *Soc Psychiat Epidemiol* 1998; **33**(7): 319–25.
10. Pulska T, Pahkala K, Laippala P, Kivelä S-L. Follow-up study of longstanding depression as predictor of mortality in elderly people living in the community. *Br Med J* 1999; **318**: 432–3.

Physical Illness and Depression

Mavis E. Evans

Wirral and West Cheshire Community NHS Trust, Bebington, UK

EPIDEMIOLOGY

The prevalence of depression in the general population worldwide is usually found to be 3–8%[1–3]. The prevalence of major depression has been shown to be no higher in the elderly than the young, although these findings do not allow for the co-morbidity of physical illnesses or dementias[4]. Subthreshold or minor depressions have many different names and definitions, thus causing widely differing prevalence rates to be quoted. Categorical definitions of depression do not fit well with the range of symptoms and severity seen in normal clinical practice. However, it is generally accepted that the burden of depression among the elderly is high and an accepted measure of diagnosis is necessary to allow communication with patients, relatives and professional colleagues.

"Caseness" can be considered to be the severity of depression at which the majority of professionals would consider some form of intervention appropriate. Prevalence of this degree of depression is reported as 10–15% of the elderly in the community[5–6], 15–30% of those attending primary care facilities[7–8], 15–50% of those in hospital[8–10] and 30–40% of those in institutional care[8,11].

DIAGNOSIS

Depression cannot be diagnosed unless it is first considered a possibility, neither will it be appropriately treated unless it is considered pathological. Depression may be missed when too much emphasis is placed on the presenting complaints of, for example, lethargy, anorexia or pain[12]. Depression and feelings of worthlessness may cause failure to complain of symptoms of physical illness or to ask for help. It may cause non-compliance with medication and other treatments, self-neglect or non-attendance at clinics. Alternatively, the lowering of self-esteem and decreased ability to cope can lead to increased attendance at clinics.

The lack of a concise definition for depression in the elderly makes the establishment of validity a difficult task, which can only be examined by longitudinal follow-up of patients to see what happens to their symptoms[13]. Somatic symptoms, e.g. lack of energy, poor concentration and weight loss, may be due to the physical illness or ageing, not depression; even experienced clinicians may have difficulty attributing such symptoms to physical or psychiatric causes. Even feelings of life not being worth living and wishing to die are not always associated with depressed mood; poor subjective health, disability, pain, sensory impairment and living in an institution have been shown to be associated factors in the absence of depressive illness[14].

The elderly tend not to admit to feelings of depression and relatives may be unaware of the condition[15]. Somatization, "the tendency to experience and communicate somatic distress and somatic symptoms unaccounted for by relevant pathological findings, to attribute them to physical illness and to seek medical help for them"[16] is increasingly recognized. Somatization can still occur in those with genuine physical illness. The somatic symptoms of depression are similar to those of a chronic illness, such as cancer, and it must be remembered that depression and physical illness often coexist[17].

Hypochondriasis is a recognized symptom of depression in the elderly population[18]. However, in this age group, rigorous steps must be undertaken to exclude physical problems before ascribing symptoms to hypochondriasis or somatization[17,19]. That such patients are depressed is inferred from their good response to standard treatments for depression[20].

The 1991 NIH Consensus Statement on diagnosis and treatment of depression in late life concluded: "What makes depression in the elderly so insidious is that neither the victim nor the health provider may recognize its symptoms in the context of the multiple physical problems of many elderly people". DSM-4 allows somatic symptoms to be counted towards the diagnosis of depression if there is any possibility of psychological aetiology, a more inclusive and accurate means of diagnosis than previously.

MORBIDITY AND MORTALITY

Psychiatric morbidity in hospitals is higher than in the general population. Surveys of wards and clinics do not completely establish an association between psychiatric and physical morbidity because they may be biased for selective referral patterns: psychological symptoms can lead to help-seeking behaviour for physical illness in an individual who had previously been able to tolerate his/her physical problems. Similarly, they may influence a GP on whether or not to refer to hospital. Stress may be as important in triggering help-seeking behaviour as in triggering actual illness. In addition to the degree of distress, many other factors determine whether or not an individual will seek help, including religious and social values, socioeconomic background and personality.

Affective disorder in the elderly is strongly associated with physical ill-health[19]: "whether or not such an illness has a direct aetiological relationship to the affective disorder, its practical importance must be considered, for it is bound to influence the course and outcome of the psychiatric condition". Other studies have found that depression leads to increased mortality[21–23] over and above age effects, the prognosis worsening with severity of depression. Depression in the elderly may be due partly to a biological ageing process, which would directly increase mortality and morbidity[20,24]. Burvill and Hall[25] showed increased mortality in depressed elderly patients ($n = 103$, age 60+) followed for 5 years if they were aged 75+, had impaired mobility or showed poor recovery with residual symptoms or chronicity. There were two peaks of increased mortality, one early in the disease and one late. Cardiovascular or pulmonary disease and malignancies were the predominant causes of death. The results are similar to those of Murphy et al.'s 4 year follow-up[26], who also postulate that increased mortality seen in the depressed elderly (especially the men) was not due to differences in physical health alone. They suggest:

1. Inadequate treatment of the depression, leading to cardiovascular complications from the antidepressant but no benefit to the patient; the depression itself can also provoke cardiac death, especially in men.
2. "Subintentional suicide" in those who "turn their faces to the wall".
3. Residual depressive invalidism, causing poor nutrition and decreased mobility; with attendant complications of susceptibility to infection, fractures, bedsores, etc., all contribute to the increased mortality.

Mortality in hospital was found to be significantly higher in those depressed but over 30% of those discharged had died within, on average, 5 months, whether depressed or not[27]. The authors also noted that survivors with depression consumed more healthcare resources than did the non-depressed survivors. Among the depressed elderly, 40% have chronic poor physical health[28]; they use and need more medical services[29,30] than the non-depressed, but also use fewer social and recreational services[29]. An association has been found between poor mental health and subsequent physical disease, suggesting that positive mental health may significantly retard the decline in physical health with increasing age[31].

Physical illness affects the capacity for independent living, resulting in altered relationships with others, lowered self-esteem and vulnerability to depression. Serious illness may be seen by some as an unpleasant reminder of mortality, bringing apprehension and fear. Continuing physical illness is a poor prognostic factor for depression, although whether this is due to a biological relationship or to the psychological strain of being ill is uncertain.

Mortality in acute medical inpatients is significantly higher in those with associated depression, although the direction of causality is not established, e.g. Silverstone[32] followed consecutive admissions for myocardial infarction, subarachnoid haemorrhage, pulmonary embolus or upper gastrointestinal haemorrhage for 28 days post-admission; 34% were depressed and 47% of these had life-threatening complications or died, compared with 10% of those not depressed.

PHYSICAL ILLNESS AND DEPRESSION

Mood disturbance can result from structural brain disease, alterations in neurotransmitter concentration or activity caused by drugs or biochemical disturbance. These affective symptoms may present during a physical illness or be the initial symptom of an otherwise occult physical disorder. Depression may be:

1. The result of an illness, especially a painful or disabling one.
2. Iatrogenic, e.g. the result of steroid treatment.
3. A symptom of the physical illness, e.g. hypothyroidism.
4. An aetiological factor, e.g. alcohol abuse secondary to depression.

5. A depressed patient adopting the sick role as a coping mechanism.
6. A common aetiological factor, such as bereavement, may cause both depression and physical illness.
7. Coincidental.

The elderly are particularly susceptible to the side effects of drug treatment[33], especially as they are often subject to polypharmacy[34,35]. Patients with drug-induced depression often have a past or family history of depression and the drug may have precipitated the disease by affecting the levels of available neurotransmitters[34]. Depression can often be alleviated by cessation of the drug, although some patients will also require antidepressant treatment. The combination of a susceptible patient and a depressogenic drug may precipitate a depression sufficiently severe to lead to suicide[34].

Subjective rating of general health has been shown to be independently associated with depression in the elderly, including the very old[36–38]. This can lead to presentation at primary care or emergency facilities, unnecessary investigations and risk of iatrogenic disease, and lower quality of life. Recognition and treatment of the depression may lead to improvement in the patient's subjective perception of his/her health.

Physically ill depressed patients are more likely to be admitted to hospital than those who are not depressed[39]. Depressed patients have higher use of all categories of medical care, including admissions, laboratory tests and emergency department visits[30].

The presence of significant psychiatric disorder has been shown to adversely affect the course of medical admission[40,41], affective disorders in particular prolonging length of stay[42–44] (although the study by Ramsay[45] did not confirm this) and increasing the likelihood of admission to residential care[46]. Psychiatric intervention has been shown to increase recovery rate, reduce duration of stay, reduce the need for residential care after discharge and therefore reduce costs[47,48].

ADJUSTMENT DISORDER

Lipowski[49] has proposed that the subjective significance of an illness and its treatment, e.g. amputation, cancer, combined with the patient's personality and social circumstances, is the key to the psychological response. The variety of physical illnesses found with depression would support this view. Depression may be a reaction to physical problems; it occurs more frequently in those with increasing numbers of medical diagnoses and may be precipitated by developing new physical illnesses[21,50]. All illnesses except the very trivial involve an element of psychological adjustment. Serious medical illness is likely to be a potent psychological stressor, affecting body image, self-esteem, the sense of identity and the capacity to work and to maintain social, family and marital relationships[51]. However, the majority of people adapt their lives to the demands of their illness, maximizing their prospects of recovery and return to previous levels of activity.

In the elderly, physical illness is frequently chronic and may worsen with time. This, combined with the losses suffered by many elderly people, such as loss of status and income on retirement, loss of friends and family by death and the fear of loss of independence and dignity due to the illness itself, can lead to the adjustment disorder merging imperceptibly into a depressive illness. This can be considered secondary depression[52], the depression following or paralleling a life-threatening or incapacitating medical illness. However, the prevalence of this type of depression is unknown, as it is difficult to differentiate from depression related to other stressors and previous history. Patients with this type of depression tend to have fewer suicidal thoughts but have more feelings of helplessness, pessimism and anxiety[53].

SOMATIZED DEPRESSION

This is more common than medical illness presenting as depression, especially in the current generation of elderly, who tend to somatize their psychological symptoms, having been brought up in a society which did not encourage the expression of emotion. Somatic symptoms in the elderly may represent physical illness, depression or emotional responses to physical illness. The somatic symptoms will need investigation, but depression, if suspected, should be treated.

Pseudodementia is a specific type of masked depression. One of the most important differentiating factors is that the severity of cognitive impairment fluctuates in depressed patients, remaining constant or worsening in the evenings in dementia. Depressed patients tend not to try to succeed in tasks, giving up with "I don't know" or "I can't". Demented patients will try, delighting in success but possibly becoming very distressed by failure—the so-called catastrophic reaction. Biological symptoms of appetite and weight loss, sleep disturbance and headache are typical of depression and not dementia. However, depression and dementia can coexist and the differentiation of the two conditions is not always easy. If in doubt, a trial of antidepressant treatment will help elucidate the diagnosis. The pathognomic symptoms of masked or somatized depression include:

1. Diurnal variation (symptoms usually worse in the mornings).
2. Mild impairment of cognitive processes and concentration.
3. Dysthymic mood changes.
4. Fatigue, feeling tired, lack of energy.
5. Sleep disturbance (waking up early and being unable to get back to sleep).
6. An anxious sense of failure or of "impending disaster".

LIAISON

Consultation-liaison psychiatry is becoming well established as an important specialty within general hospitals on both sides of the Atlantic. In an ideal situation, psychiatrists would attend ward rounds in the general hospital, particularly on rehabilitation wards, where prevalence of depression is high and the effect on delayed discharge well documented[42-44]. However, restricted resources prevent this: psychiatric morbidity is too high for a psychiatrist to see all the patients affected—his main role should be educational[54], only taking an active part in the management of more difficult cases. In many areas there is increasing development of specialist liaison nurses who are able to advise on diagnosis and treatment, reducing delay before assessments. The liaison nurse is likely to be more permanent than junior doctors on rotation and can often help a patient who refuses to see a psychiatrist or whose physician refuses psychiatric referral[55]. Liaison nurses can educate general nurses in the recognition of psychiatric disorder and can in turn encourage junior medical staff to institute appropriate referral or treatment. Their development and use has been compared with that of community psychiatric nurses[56].

The most common reasons for requesting a psychiatric consultation in a general hospital are[57]:

1. Diagnostic uncertainty.
2. Recognition of a gross psychiatric disorder.
3. Excessive emotional reactions, e.g. fear, anger, depression.
4. A patient's deviant behaviour disturbing ward or medical procedures.
5. Delayed convalescence, i.e. disability incompatible with observed pathology, relapse on mention of discharge.
6. Crisis in the doctor–patient relationship (e.g. refusing consent!).

7. Patient's admission of serious psychosocial difficulties.
8. Selection and/or preparation of patients, e.g. pre-transplant, cosmetic surgery.

It can be seen from the above list that the depressed patient, sitting quiet and withdrawn on the ward or in a home, may not be referred for a psychiatric opinion. In practice, only about 2% of geriatric patients are referred to the liaison services[58-60]. Suggested reasons for the discrepancy between liaison rate and psychiatric morbidity are[58,61]:

1. High prevalence of transient self-limiting psychiatric disease.
2. Physician's failure to recognize psychiatric disease[62]. Many studies have highlighted the unrecognized psychiatric problems on medical wards[61] and the underdiagnosis of major depression in particular has been well documented[63].
3. Medical and nursing staff may actively avoid questioning for psychological problems, due to fear of precipitating emotional distress with which they have not been trained to deal.
4. The low priority of psychiatric disease compared to physical, especially in a busy medical ward with acutely ill patients.
5. Poor access to, or dissatisfaction with, psychiatric services.
6. Physician resistance to psychiatric consultation[47], due to stigma or underestimating the severity or the potential for treatment.

Use of screening scales is appropriate for assessing depression in the physically ill: it is common, can be a difficult diagnosis and has significant morbidity and mortality if untreated. Care must be taken to differentiate between short-lived adjustment disorders, occurring as a reaction to the admission itself, or the crisis which precipitated it. Diagnosis in acute admissions should therefore include enquiry into symptoms before admission. If none can be elicited, the patient should be reassessed at a later date, either during rehabilitation or after discharge.

Screening scales serve a dual function[64-66]—they identify patients in need of further assessment and also serve as an educational tool if given by general staff during routine admission procedures. They emphasize the associated symptoms and signs of depression in the elderly, who may not show depressed affect and will deny feeling sad. It is important, however, that education about the treatment of depression goes hand in hand with education to recognize it, or the liaison services will be swamped.

TREATMENT

The fact that one can intuitively "understand" why the physically-ill elderly are depressed does not mean that it should be accepted as normal and treatment not attempted. Continuing physical illness is recognized as both a precipitant of depression and a poor prognostic factor, yet despite this, ~80% of elderly general hospital patients are not depressed[42,67,68]. Successful coping mechanisms can prevent the emergence of clinical depression. Even in the terminal patient, depression or dysphoria can be relieved by euphoriants, such as oral or parenteral opiates, reducing the distress of patient and relatives[69] without significantly reducing the length of life remaining to the patient.

It is important that the diagnosis is not missed, as this condition usually responds well to treatment, at least initially, thus improving quality of life. Follow-up and early treatment of any relapses will further improve the prognosis. Increased self-esteem and ability to cope will reduce demand on families and possibly on services.

Even when the correct diagnosis is made, the depression may not be treated adequately, if at all: physically ill patients who are also depressed are more likely to be assigned to the "not to be resuscitated" group, compared with those elderly who are not depressed. The lack of effort and motivation caused by depression may be regarded as "not trying" or "giving up" by nurses and rehabilitation staff, who withdraw from this group of patients for more emotionally rewarding non-depressed elderly subjects on the same ward.

The elderly as a group have approximately twice as many adverse drug reactions as younger adults[70]. They are frequently already on polypharmacy, so drug interactions are a real possibility. It is therefore important that physicians are advised and supported by the psychiatric services in the use of safe, well-tolerated antidepressants and other treatments to reduce the impact of this disease on both the individual and society.

Electroconvulsive therapy (ECT) is an effective treatment of depression[71,72]. The response to treatment in older people is better than in the young[73,74]. With the increasing safety of anaesthesia, very few patients, even those with severe physical disease, are unable to tolerate a course of treatment. It is more rapid in effect than medication alone, but the improvement is rarely sustained unless antidepressants are also given to prevent relapse.

A review of psychological treatments in chronic illness[75] found very little empirical evidence of benefit when therapeutic interventions were applied indiscriminately. However, some evidence was found to show benefit in patients with somatization disorders rather than physical illness, and also that brief interventions following the onset of acute physical illness reduced longer-term psychological morbidity. A suggested general approach to the treatment of physically ill depressed patients is:

1. Investigate and give appropriate treatment to all physical problems, either curative treatment or to minimize persistent morbidity. Explain the illness, treatment and prognosis to the patient in as much detail as he/she wishes. Make sure the explanation is understood and repeat as often as necessary.
2. Give general social support, e.g. home help services, financial assistance if relevant, or residential or nursing home care.
3. Give psychological support—encouragement, continued interest in the patient, e.g. outpatient follow-up. Support groups are often beneficial for chronic conditions such as rheumatoid arthritis, Parkinson's disease, etc.
4. Consider antidepressant therapy if the symptoms are sufficiently severe that they would be considered to warrant medication if seen in a patient without physical problems. Monitor the response to treatment; this may take 7–8 weeks[76]. If no response is seen to a therapeutic dosage of antidepressant, consider a trial of an alternative antidepressant or adjunctive treatment, or specialist referral.

PROGNOSIS

Little is known of the prognosis of psychiatric disorder identified in the medical setting[77], except that concomitant physical illness is a poor prognostic factor. Psychiatric disturbance often persists[78-80], especially in patients with a previous history of psychiatric disorder. Those with affective disorder on admission have increased mortality and make greater demands on medical, social and psychiatric services[77,81].

In one series of consecutive acute medical admissions[80], fewer than 45% of those patients with concomitant depression had received antidepressants at all, 20% had been given benzodiazepines, and less than 25% had been treated for more than one week. The authors concluded that an effective treatment for depression in elderly patients needed to be found, with widespread education of geriatricians in the diagnosis and treatment of depression.

In psychiatric patients, relapse has been linked with supervening physical illness[82]. The presence or development of cerebral or any other irreversible physical disorder indicates poor future mental health in the great majority of patients, as well as the likelihood of early death[83].

The prognosis of the physical illness, for both morbidity and mortality, is also inextricably linked with that of the depression. Increased mortality from physical illness, especially cardiovascular disease, has been reported[84,85]. This excess of deaths is significantly associated with groups who have been only partially treated, e.g. have not responded to antidepressants[86], especially in older men[87].

Explanations for the apparent association of physical illness with poor treatment outcome might include[88]:

1. Age as a confounding factor—most of the trials of treatment in the physically ill are in the elderly.
2. Medically ill patients may be given inadequate doses of antidepressants because of problems with side effects or over-cautious physicians.
3. Different subtypes of depression exist, some medication-responsive, some not. Organic mood disorder (depression induced by physical illness or a specific organic factor) has been shown to have a worse prognosis at 4 year follow-up[89].

The prognosis of depression in the physically ill elderly is therefore dependent on accurate diagnosis, intensive treatment, follow-up and early treatment of any relapses[82,84,90]. Increased self-esteem and ability to cope will reduce demand on families and possibly on services. No studies have yet convincingly identified predictors of response in physically ill populations, although pre-existing depression prior to admission with physical problems appears to predict persistent depression, rather than if the depression develops in hospital[78,91].

SUICIDE

Suicide is the most dramatic of poor outcomes, and the elderly are over-represented in suicide statistics. Although the elderly are less likely to attempt suicide, they are more likely to complete it[92,93]. The presence of physical illness, especially if associated with chronic pain and disability, increases the risk; elderly men living alone are at the highest risk. The individual's adjustment to ill-health and his associated feelings of hopelessness and demoralization are obviously important[94]. Many elderly suicide victims are suffering from their first episode of major depression, which is typically only moderately severe but the diagnosis is missed[95], and the potential for recovery following intervention therefore lost.

Depression has been linked to decreased compliance and to voluntary refusal of life-saving essential medical treatments[96,97]. This may reflect either conscious or unconscious suicidal motivation.

SERVICE IMPLICATIONS

It is important to note that the aging population itself is growing older, with large numbers of very old individuals. It is this old-old group who have the highest physical and psychiatric morbidity and who make the greatest demands on services.

Undergraduate teaching programmes must be tightly integrated in order for students to develop a holistic approach to the elderly, together with an understanding of the psychosocial and economic factors that will affect presentation and treatment. Joint postgraduate meetings between the two specialties are becoming more common and should be encouraged, each maintaining their separate identities and training but working closely together in clinical practice.

Interdisciplinary research continues to grow in amount, but is mostly directed at psychiatric problems on medical wards. Little seems to be researched in the other direction, medical illnesses on psychiatric wards. All research is obviously relevant to both specialties and in practice helps to strengthen links between them.

CONCLUSION

Depression in the elderly physically ill can present a difficult problem of diagnosis. To avoid the increased morbidity and mortality of untreated depression, it is necessary to be aware of the possibility of depression causing somatic symptoms, the physical illness causing depressive symptoms, or both conditions coexisting, and then to treat the depression effectively. Close liaison between psychogeriatric and geriatric teams is thus very important if this vulnerable group is to receive the correct diagnosis and treatment.

REFERENCES

1. Myers JK, Weissman MM, Tischler GL. Six month prevalence of psychiatric disorders in three communities 1980–1982. *Arch Gen Psychiat* 1984; **41**: 959–67.
2. Mavreas VG, Beis A, Bouyias A. Psychiatric disorders in Athens: a community study. *Soc Psychiat* 1986; **21**: 172–81.
3. Bebbington PE, Hurry J, Tennant C. Epidemiology of mental disorders in Camberwell. *Psychol Med* 1981; **11**: 561–79.
4. Blazer D. EURODEP consortium and late life depression. *Br J Psychiat* 1999; **174**: 284–5.
5. Copeland JRM, Dewey ME, Wood N et al. Range of mental illness among the elderly in the community: prevalence in Liverpool using the GMS–AGECAT package. *Br J Psychiat* 1987; **150**: 815–23.
6. Blazer D, Williams CD. Epidemiology of dysphoria and depression in an elderly population. *Am J Psychiat* 1980; **137**: 439–44.
7. Callahan CM, Hendrie HC, Dittus RS et al. Depression in late life: the use of clinical characteristics to focus screening efforts . *J Gerontol* 1994; **9**: M9–14.
8. Katona CLE. The epidemiology of depression in old age: the importance of physical illness. *Clin Neuropharmacol* 1992; **15** (suppl): 281–2.
9. Fenton FR, Cole MG, Engelsman N, Mansouri I. Depression in older medical inpatients. *Int J Geriat Psychiat* 1994; **9**: 279–84.
10. Hammond MF, Evans ME, Lye M. Depression in medical wards. *Int J Geriat Psychiat* 1993; **8**: 957–8.
11. Harrison R, Savla N, Kafetz K. Dementia, depression and physical disability in a London Borough: a survey of elderly people in and out of residential care and implications for future developments. *Age Aging* 1990; **19**: 97–103.
12. Kidd CB. Misplacement of the elderly in hospital. A study of patients admitted to geriatric and mental hospitals. *Br Med J* 1962; **253**: 1491–5.
13. Koenig HG, Pappas P, Holsinger T, Bachar JR. Assessing diagnostic approaches to depression in medically ill older adults: how reliably can mental health professionals make judgements about the cause of symptoms? *J Am Geriat Soc* 1995; **43**: 472–8.
14. Jorm AF, Henderson AS, Scott R et al. Factors associated with the wish to die in elderly people. *Age Ageing* 1995; **24**: 389–92.
15. Hanley I, Baikie E. Understanding and treating depression in the elderly. In Hanley I, Hodge J, eds, *Psychological Approaches to the Care of the Elderly*. New York: Methuen, 1984.
16. Lipowski ZJ. Somatisation: the concept and its clinical application. *Am J Psychiat* 1988; **145**: 1358–68.
17. Sweer L, Rairin DC, Ladd RA et al. The medical evaluation of elderly patients with major depression. *J Gerontol* 1988; **3**: M53–8.
18. Kramer-Ginsberg E, Greenwald BS, Aisen PS, Brod-Miller C. Hypochondriasis and the elderly depressed. *J Am Geriat Soc* 1989; **37**: 507–10.
19. Roth M, Kay DWK. Affective disorders arising in the senium II: physical disability as an aetiological factor. *J Ment Sci* 1956; **102**: 141–50.
20. Jacoby RJ. Depression in the elderly. *Br J Hosp Med* 1981; 40–7.
21. Murphy E. The prognosis of depression in old age. *Br J Psychiat* 1983; **142**: 111–19
22. Baldwin RC, Jolley DJ. The prognosis of depression in old age. *Br J Psychiat* 1986; **149**: 574–83.
23. Robinson JR. The natural history of mental disorder in old age: a long term study. *Br J Psychiat* 1989; **154**: 783–9.
24. Post F. The management and nature of depressive illness in late life: a follow-through study. *Br J Psychiat* 1972; **121**: 393–404.
25. Burvill PW, Hall WD. Predictors of increased mortality in elderly depressed patients. *Int J Geriat Psychiat* 1994; **9**: 219–27.
26. Murphy E, Smith R, Lindesay J, Slattery J. Increased mortality rates in late-life depression. *Br J Psychiat* 1988; **152**: 347–53.
27. Koenig HG, Shelp F, Goli V et al. Survival and health care utilization in elderly medical inpatients with major depression. *J Am Geriat Soc* 1989; **37**: 599–606.
28. Murphy E. Social origins of depression in old age. *Br J Psychiat* 1982; **141**: 135–42.
29. Badger TA. Depression, physical health impairment and service use among older adults. *Publ Health Nurs* 1998; **15**: 136–45.
30. Unutzer J, Patrick DL, Simon G et al. Depressive symptoms and the cost of health services in HMO patients aged 65 years and older. *J Am Geriat Assoc* 1997; **277**: 1618–23.
31. Vaillant GE. Natural history of male psychologic health. *N Engl J Med* 1979; **301**: 1249–55.
32. Silverstone PH. Depression increases mortality and morbidity in acute life-threatening medical illness. *J Psychosom Res* 1990; **34**: 651–7.
33. Ouslander JG. Physical illness and depression in the elderly. *J Am Geriatr Soc* 1982; **30**: 593–9.
34. Whitlock FA. *Systematic Affective Disorders*. London: Academic Press, 1982.
35. Braithwaite R. The pharmakokinetics of psychotropic drugs in the elderly. In Wheatley D, ed., *Pharmacology of Old Age*. Oxford: Oxford University Press, 1982.
36. Evans ME, Copeland JRM, Dewey ME. Depression in the elderly in the community: effect of physical illness and selected social factors. *Int J Geriat Psychiat* 1991; **6**: 787–95.
37. Meller I, Fichter MM, Schroppel H. Risk factors and psychosocial consequences in depression of octo- and nonagenarians: results of an epidemiological study. *Eur Arch Psychiat Clin Neurosci* 1997; **247**: 278–87.
38. Mulsant BH, Ganguli M, Seaberg EC. The relationship between self-rated health and depressive symptoms in an epidemiological sample of community-dwelling older adults. *J Am Geriat Soc* 1997; **45**: 954–8.
39. Kay DWK, Beamish R, Roth M. Old age mental disorders in Newcastle upon Tyne. Part 1: a study of prevalence. *Br J Psychiat* 1964; **110**: 146–58.
40. Johnston M, Wakeling A, Graham N, Stokes F. Cognitive impairment, emotional disorder and length of stay of elderly patients in a district general hospital. *Br J Med Psychol* 1987; **60**: 133–9.
41. Coid J, Crome P. Bed blocking in Bromley. *Br Med J* 1986; **292**: 1253–6.
42. Bergmann K, Eastham EJ. Psychogeriatric ascertainment and assessment for treatment in an acute medical ward setting. *Age Ageing* 1974; **3**: 174–87.
43. Mossey JM, Mutran E, Knott K, Craik R. Determinants of recovery 12 months after hip fracture: the importance of psychosocial factors. *Am J Publ Health* 1989; **79**: 279–86.
44. Verbosky LA, Franco KN, Zrull JP. The relationship between depression and length of stay in the general hospital patient. *J Clin Psychiat* 1993; **54**: 177–81.
45. Ramsay R, Wright P, Katz A et al. The detection of psychiatric morbidity and its effects on outcome in acute elderly medical admissions. *Int J Geriat Psychiat* 1991; **6**: 861–6.
46. Lindesay J, Murphy E. Dementia, depression and subsequent institutionalisation—the effect of home support. *Int J Geriat Psychiat* 1989; **4**: 3–9.
47. Steinberg R, Torem M, Saravay SM. An analysis of physician resistance to psychiatric consultations. *Arch Gen Psychiat* 1980; **37**: 1007–12.
48. Levitan SJ, Kornfeld DS. Clinical and cost benefits of liaison psychiatry. *Am J Psychiat* 1981; **138**: 790–3.

49. Lipowski ZJ. Review of consultation psychiatry and psychosomatic medicine. I: general principles. *Psychosom Med* 1967; **29**: 153–71.

50. Kukull WA, Koepsall T, Inui T *et al.* Depression and physical illness among elderly general medical clinic patients. *J Affect Disord* 1986; **10**: 153–62.

51. Rodin GM, Voshart K. Depression in the medically ill: an overview. *Am J Psychiat* 1986; **143**: 696–705.

52. Feighner JP, Robins E, Guze SB *et al.* Diagnostic criteria for use in research. *Arch Gen Psychiat* 1972; **26**: 57–63.

53. Lloyd GG. Emotional aspects of physical illness. In Granville-Grossman K, ed., *Recent Advances in Clinical Psychiatry*, vol 5. London: Churchill Livingstone, 1985.

54. Anderson DN, Philpott RM. The changing pattern of referrals for psychogeriatric consultation in the general hospital: an eight year study. *Int J Geriat Psychiat* 1991; **6**: 801–7.

55. Collinson Y, Benbow SM. The role of an old age psychiatry consultation liaison nurse. *Int J Geriat Psychiat* 1998; **13**: 159–63.

56. Benbow SM. Liaison services for elderly people. In Benjamin S, House A, Jenkins P, eds, *Liaison Psychiatry: Defining Needs and Planning Services*. London: Gaskell, 1994.

57. Lipowski ZJ. Review of consultation liaison psychiatry and psychosomatic medicine. II: Clinical aspects. *Psychosom Med* 1967; **29**: 201–24.

58. Popkin MK, MacKenzie TB, Callies AL. Psychiatric consultation to geriatric medically ill patients in a university hospital. *Arch Gen Psychiat* 1984; **41**: 703–7.

59. Ruskin PE. Geropsychiatric consultation in a University hospital: a report on 67 referrals. *Am J Psychiat* 1985; **142**: 333–6.

60. Poynton AM. Psychiatric liaison referrals of elderly inpatients in a teaching hospital. *Br J Psychiat* 1988; **152**: 45–7.

61. Maguire GP, Julier DL, Hawton KE, Bancroft JHJ. Psychiatric morbidity and referral on two general medical wards. *Br Med J* 1974; **1**: 268–70.

62. Gurland B. The comparative frequency of depression in various adult age groups. *J Gerontol* 1976; **31**: 283–92.

63. Koenig HJ, Meador KG, Cohen HJ, Blazer DG. Self rated depression scales and screening for major depression in the older hospitalised patient with medical illness. *J Am Geriat Soc* 1988; **36**: 699–706.

64. Yesavage JA, Brink TL. Development and validation of a geriatric depression screening scale: a preliminary report. *J Psychiat Res* 1983; **17**: 37–49.

65. Adshead F, Cody DD, Pitt B. BASDEC: a novel screening instrument for depression in elderly medical inpatients. *Br Med J* 1992; **305**: 397.

66. Evans ME. Development and validation of a screening test for depression in the elderly physically ill. *Int Clin Psychopharmacol* 1993; **8**(4): 333–6.

67. Schneider L, Plopper M. Geropsychiatry and consultation liaison services. *Am J Psychiat* 1984; **141**: 721–2.

68. Schuckit MA, Miller PL, Hahlbohm D. Unrecognised psychiatric illness in elderly medical–surgical patients. *J Gerontol* 1975; **30**: 655–60.

69. Ban T. Chronic disease and depression in the geriatric population. *J Clin Psychiat* 1984; **45**: 18–23.

70. Bazire S. *Psychotropic drug directory*. Wiltshire: Mark Allen, 1995.

71. West ED. Electroconvulsive therapy in depression: a double blind controlled trial. *Br Med J* 1981; **282**: 355–7.

72. Brandon S, Cowley P, McDonald C *et al.* Electroconvulsive therapy: results in depressive illness from the Leicestershire trial. *Br Med J* 1984; **288**: 22–5.

73. Benbow SM. The role of electroconvulsive therapy in the treatment of depressive illness in old age. *Br J Psychiat* 1989; **155**: 147–52.

74. Wilkinson DG. ECT in the elderly. In Levy R, Howard R, Burns A, eds, *Treatment and Care in Old Age Psychiatry*. Petersfield: Wrightson Biomedical, 1993.

75. Guthrie E. Emotional disorder in chronic illness: psychotherapeutic interventions. *Br J Psychiat* 1996; **168**: 265–73.

76. Georgotas A, McCue R. The additional benefit of extending an antidepressant trial past seven weeks in the depressed elderly. *Int J Geriat Psychiat* 1989; **4**: 191–5.

77. Mayou R, Hawton K, Feldman E. What happens to medical patients with psychiatric disorder? *J Psychosom Res* 1988; **32**: 541–9.

78. Hawton K. The long-term outcome of psychiatric morbidity detected in general medical patients. *J Psychosom Res* 1981; **25**: 237–43.

79. Feldman E, Mayou R, Hawton K *et al.* Psychiatric disorder in medical inpatients. *Qu J Med* 1987; **241**: 405–12.

80. Koenig HG, Goli V, Shelp F *et al.* Major depression in hospitalised medically ill older men: documentation, management and outcome. *Int J Geriat Psychiat* 1992; **7**: 25–34.

81. Cooper B. Psychiatric disorders among elderly patients admitted to hospital medical wards. *J R Soc Med* 1987; **80**: 13–16.

82. Gordon WF. Elderly depressives, treatment and follow-up. *Can J Psychiat* 1981; **26**: 110–13.

83. Post F. *The Significance of Affective Symptoms in Old Age*, Chapter X: conclusions. Maudsley Monograph No. 10. London: Oxford University Press, 1962.

84. Baldwin RC, Jolley DJ. The prognosis of depression in old age. *Br J Psychiat* 1986; **149**: 574–83.

85. Rabins PV, Harvis K, Koven S. High fatality rates of late life depression associated with cardiovascular disease. *J Affect Disord* 1985; **9**: 165–7.

86. Avery D, Winokur G. Mortality in depressed patients treated with ECT and antidepressants. *Arch Gen Psychiat* 1976; **33**: 1029–37.

87. Rorsman B, Hagnell O, Lanke J. Mortality and hidden mental disorder in the Lundby study: age-standardised death rates among mentally ill "non-patients" in a total population observed during a 25 year period. *Neuropsychobiology* 1983; **10**: 83–9.

88. Gregory RJ, Jimmerson DC, Walto BE *et al.* Pharmacotherapy of depression in the medically ill: directions for future research. *Gen Hosp Psychiat* 1992; **14**: 36–42.

89. Yates WR, Wesner RB, Thompson R. Organic mood disorder: a valid psychiatry consultation diagnosis. *J Affect Disord* 1991; **22**: 37–42.

90. Burvill PW, Hall WD, Stampfer HG, Emmerson JP. The prognosis of depression in old age. *Br J Psychiat* 1991; **158**: 64–71.

91. Lloyd GG, Cawley RH. Distress or illness? A study of psychological symptoms after myocardial infarction. *Br J Psychiat* 1983; **142**: 120–5.

92. Gurland BJ, Cross P. Epidemiology of psychopathology in old age. *Psychiat Clin N Am* 1982; **5**: 11–25.

93. Gurland BJ, Meyers B. Geriatric psychiatry. In Talbott J, Hales R, Yudofsky S, eds, *A Textbook of Psychiatry*. Washington, DC: American Psychiatric Press, 1987.

94. Cattell H. Suicidal behaviour. In Copeland JRM, Abou-Saleh MT, Blazer DG, eds, *Principles and Practice of Geriatric Psychiatry*. 1st edn. Chichester: Wiley, 1994.

95. Alexopoulos GS, Chester JG. Outcomes of geriatric depression. *Clin Geriat Med* 1992; **8**: 363–76.

96. Stoudmire A, Thompson TL. Medication non-compliance: systematic approaches to evaluation and intervention. *Gen Hosp Psychiat* 1983; **5**: 223–39.

97. Rodin GM, Chmara J, Ennis J. Stopping life-sustaining medical treatment: psychiatric considerations in the termination of medical dialysis. *Can J Psychiat* 1981; **26**: 540–4.

Physical Illness and Depression: a Number of Conundrums

M. Robin Eastwood

Formerly at St Louis University Medical School, MO, USA

One of the clinical conundrums in modern medicine is that psychiatric patients complain frequently in somatic terms and yet *truly* suffer from an excess of physical illness[1]. In a review conducted as part of a European Science Foundation Study (EMRC), Hafner and Bickel[2] concluded that "Studies of mortality in mental patients have shown that...these patients still have an excess risk for natural causes of death which is not restricted to patients or to certain diagnostic groups...However, the evidence for *specific* associations between psychiatric diagnosis and natural causes of death is not yet conclusive". In a commentary, Rorsman[3] said that two out of three major *longitudinal* studies indicate, at least in men, that mental illness strongly affects the risk of dying from natural causes. Murphy *et al.*[4], from the Stirling County study, found death to be significantly associated with affective, not physical disorder, and depression, not anxiety. Rorsman *et al.*[5], from the Lundby study, found that psychiatric patients have a significantly increased natural death risk, and *untreated* psychiatric males in particular.

An issue of the *International Journal of Geriatric Psychiatry*[6] dealt with physical illness and depression in the elderly. Burvill, from Australia, pointed out that physical illness worsens the prognosis of depressive illness in the elderly. Lindesay, from the Guy's/Age Concern Survey in the UK, found that 70% of depressed subjects reported one or more serious physical problems. Sadavoy *et al.*, from Canada, found that about 75% of the elderly with chronic physical illness had cognitive impairment and 35% were depressed. There was a significant correlation between cognitive deficit and depression.

Eastwood and Corbin[7], in a review of the connection between depression and physical illness in the elderly, addressed another conundrum. While physical disease increases with age, depression may not do so. In community surveys of the elderly, fewer than 25% are disease-free and over 50% have at least one activity-limiting disorder[8]. While the findings are disputed, depressive illness apparently declines with age, while depressive symptoms increase. Snowdon[9] argued that depressive symptoms and syndromes are difficult to distinguish in the medically ill. He thought that, since conditions which significantly correlate with depression, such as dementia, physical disability, physical illness, bereavement and so on, increase with age, then so must depression. Recently, Mann[10] argued that, "if other depressive, diagnostic terms are included—'minor depression', 'subthreshold syndrome' or 'depressive symptoms'—then the total rate of depression is, in fact, higher than in the younger age groups". The truth probably lies in some complex multivariate relationship. Notwithstanding, there are some fascinating and relatively direct relationships, such as stroke causing depression[11] and grief causing increased coronary heart disease[12]. Fascinatingly, Glassman and Shapiro[13] consider that we have reached the point where we can state that depression is an independent risk factor for coronary heart disease. While taking this as an interesting postulate, it has to be remembered that atherosclerosis could be a cause of both depression and heart disease. At this stage we do not know whether intervention with antidepressants would reduce the risk of depression on heart disease.

Finally, as Hafner and Bickel suggest, prospective studies with disease registers will help sort out general and specific relationships and direct and indirect risk factors, and help confirm Rorsman's statement, that this all means that psychiatry is a branch of medicine.

REFERENCES

1. Eastwood MR. The relationship between physical and psychological morbidity. In Williams P, Wilkinson G, Rawnsley K, eds, *The Scope of Epidemiological Psychiatry—Essays in Honour of Michael Shepherd*. London: Routledge, 1989.
2. Hafner H, Bickel H. Physical morbidity and mortality in psychiatric patients. In Vhman R *et al.*, eds, *Interaction between Mental and Physical Illness: Needed Areas of Research*. Berlin: Springer-Verlag, 1989.
3. Rorsman B. Discussion in connection with Hafner and Bickel's paper. Physical mortality and morbidity in psychiatric patients. In Vhman R *et al.*, eds, *Interaction between Mental and Physical Illness: Needed Areas of Research*. Berlin: Springer-Verlag, 1989.
4. Murphy JM, Monson RR, Olivier DC *et al.* Affective disorders and mortality. A general population study. *Arch Gen Psychiat* 1987; **44**: 473–80.
5. Rorsman B, Hagnell O, Lanke J. Mortality and hidden mental disorder in the Lundby study. Age-standardized death rates among mentally ill "non-patients" in a total population observed during a 25-year period. *Neuropsychobiology* 1983; **10**: 83–9.
6. Special Issue. *Int J Geriat Psychiat* 1990; **5**(3).
7. Eastwood MR, Corbin SL. The relationship between physical illness and depression in old age. In Murphy E, ed., *Affective Disorders in the Elderly*. London: Churchill Livingstone, 1986.
8. Jarvik L, Perl M. Overview of physiologic dysfunctions related to psychiatric problems in the elderly. In Levenson AJ, Hall RCW, eds, *Neuropsychiatric Manifestations of Physical Disease in the Elderly*. New York: Raven, 1981.
9. Snowden J. Editorial: the prevalence of depression in old age. *Int J Geriat Psychiat* 1990; **5**: 141–4.
10. Mann A. Old age disorders in primary care. In Tansella M, Thornicroft G, eds, *Common Mental Disorders in Primary Care*. London: Routledge, 1999.
11. Robinson R, Starkstein S. Current research in affective disorders following stroke. *J Neuropsychiat* 1990; **2**(1): 1–14.
12. Parkes CM, Benjamin B, Fitzgerald RG. Broken heart: a statistical study of increased mortality among widowers. *Br Med J* 1969; **1**: 740.
13. Glassman AH, Shapiro PA. Depression and the course of coronary artery disease. *Am J Psychiat* 1998; **155**(1): 4–10.

Depression after Stroke

Peter Knapp and Allan House

University of Leeds, UK

It is now accepted that stroke patients have high rates of all types of depressive disorder. However, estimates of the prevalence of depression within the first month of stroke vary greatly[1,2], according to the type of measure used and the way the sample was derived. The consensus seems to be that 20–25% of patients after stroke will suffer a major depressive disorder within the first month[3]. Rates of depression later on after stroke are less certain, because of patient attrition in studies. Depression remits in some patients, while in others it persists: one study reported that 50% of those depressed within 3 weeks of stroke remained depressed 1 year later[4]. Depression not only affects quality of life: patients with depression after stroke may be at greater risk of mortality[5], cognitive impairment[6] and poorer functional or social recovery[7,8].

There are claims that post-stroke depression is a distinct sub-type[9]. There is little unequivocal evidence to support this claim, since psychological and biological symptoms reported by patients are found in depression seen in non-stroke patients[10]. What does appear to be distinctive is the increased prevalence of persistent crying (emotionality) among stroke patients. A small number of patients suffer *pathological laughing and crying*, a syndrome which is probably neurological in origin, in which emotional expression arises after minor provocation that often appears meaningless[11]. A more common syndrome, *emotionalism*, is also characterized by increased tearfulness, but is more complex. The emotional episodes are provoked by meaningful stimuli, but the crying is characterized by a lack of warning and control. There appears to be a psychological component to its origin[12]. *Emotionalism* is associated with an increased risk of depression[13], but patients with emotionalism may be at greater risk of psychological problems not explained by concurrent depression[14]. This syndrome is probably under-recognized.

Reaching a diagnosis of depression after stroke can be complicated by the presence of problems such as communicative or cognitive impairment[15]. Patients with expressive communication problems can often be assessed by the careful use of closed questions. The assessment of those with receptive communication problems or significant cognitive impairment is much more complex: a non-language-based assessment of depression shows promise but is insufficiently reliable in its present form for accurate diagnosis[16]. The diagnosis of depression might also be confused by facial palsy and a disturbance of speech prosody (rhythm in speech), both of which are relatively common after stroke and which give the patient the appearance of a person with depression[17]. The dexamethasone suppression test is not sufficiently sensitive to be used as a diagnostic tool[18].

The high rate of depression reported in some stroke research has led to the suggestion that the neurological damage is a key factor in its aetiology[19]. As a result, many studies have attempted to link depression after stroke with lesion location. A series of studies proposed, first, that patients with left hemisphere lesions were at greater risk of depression[20], and later, that those with left anterior lesions were at most risk[21,22]. Other researchers[23–25] have not replicated these findings, suggesting that patient sampling and the timing of assessment might explain the differences.

Even if lesion location is associated with greater risk of depression, the context of this relationship is important. First, it is clear that stroke patients with all sorts of lesions can suffer depression[9], so factors other than lesion location must also be at work. Second, stroke location is extremely varied[26], so those with any particular lesion (such as left anterior lesions) will be a minority of patients, making the attributable risk due to any one type of lesion small. Last, although the rate of depression in stroke patients is higher than in age-matched non-stroke controls, it is about the same rate as in patients with non-neurological disabling illness[17,27], suggesting that non-neurological factors are as important. Relevant non-neurological aetiological factors are likely to include the threat of disability and a sense of loss.

That psychosocial factors are likely to be relevant to both the onset and persistence of depression has been illustrated in several studies. For example, one study found that depression at 4 months after stroke onset was commoner among those with greater disability, those who were divorced and those with higher pre-stroke alcohol intake[24]. Depression is more likely in those patients who perceive their stroke as a greater threat, and in those who have fewer psychological resources to deal with that threat.

Patients with depression after stroke might be considered for pharmacological or psychological treatments. Two small trials showed beneficial effects of antidepressants, although both studies had high rates of patient dropout[28,29]. The evidence for treating emotionalism with antidepressants is rather stronger—both tricyclics and SSRIs have been shown to reduce the frequency of crying episodes[30–32]. There is no good trial evidence to draw upon in assessing whether psychological interventions are effective in treating depression after stroke[33].

Some services aim to intervene in an attempt to prevent the onset of depression after stroke. A recent small trial found that patients prescribed mianserin as a prophylactic had greater improvement in depression scores, but the drug did not reduce rates of major depression 6 months after stroke[34]. A variety of preventive psychosocial interventions have been evaluated in clinical trials. The interventions, including education, leisure therapy and specialist stroke nurse visits, have shown no effect in reducing the prevalence of depression. However, many of the trials are small and imperfectly designed, so the conclusion should be lack of evidence, rather than evidence of no effect[35].

Our own recently completed study suggests that a brief psychological treatment (problem-solving therapy) may be beneficial[36,37]. Patients who received therapy visits from a community psychiatric nurse had lower rates of depression 6 and 12 months after stroke than those in the treatment-as-usual group, and lower scores on a measure of psychological distress at 12 months. This finding is encouraging, since it shows that a brief, structured psychological intervention is beneficial to patients after stroke, albeit in a sample selected to participate in a clinical trial. There are disadvantages to psychological management: it may be difficult to implement in patients with significant speech and cognitive impairment[38], and some patients find psychological treatments unacceptable, both before and after the treatment has started.

In summary, depression after stroke is common, and its causes are probably multiple—biological, psychological and social—as is the case in other physical illnesses. The evidence for benefit from antidepressant drugs is surprisingly poor, considering their problematic side effects and how widely they are prescribed. The potential for psychological therapies has been underevaluated, which is a deficit that badly needs correcting. Pending further research, clinicians will need to rely on evidence from other areas of physical medicine to inform their treatments.

REFERENCES

1. Kotila M, Numminen H, Waltimo O, Kaste M. Depression after stroke: results of the FINSTROKE Study. *Stroke* 1998; **29**: 368–72.
2. Pohjasvaara T, Leppavuori A, Siira I *et al.* Frequency and clinical determinants of poststroke depression. *Stroke* 1998; **29**: 2311–17.
3. House A, Dennis M, Mogridge L. Mood disorders in the year after first stroke. *Br J Psychiat* 1991; **158**: 83–92.
4. Wade DT, Legh-Smith J, Hewer RA. Depressed mood after stroke. A community study of its frequency. *Br J Psychiat* 1987; **151**: 200–205.
5. Morris PL, Robinson RG, Samuels J. Depression, introversion and mortality following stroke. *Aust N Z J Psychiat* 1993; **27**: 443–9.
6. House A, Dennis M, Warlow C *et al.* Intellectual impairment after stroke and its relation to mood disorder. *Psychol Med* 1990; **20**: 805–14.
7. Starkstein SE, Parikh RM, Robinson RG. Post-stroke depression and recovery after stroke. *Lancet* 1987; **1**: 743.
8. Feibel JH, Springer CJ. Depression and failure to resume social activities after stroke. *Arch Phys Med Rehab* 1982; **63**: 276–8.
9. Robinson RG. Neuropsychiatric consequences of stroke. *Ann Rev Med* 1997; **48**: 217–29.
10. House A. Depression associated with stroke. *J Neuropsychiat Clin Neurosci* 1996; **8**: 453–7.
11. Andersen G. Treatment of uncontrolled crying after stroke. *Drugs Aging* 1995; **6**: 105–11.
12. Allman P, Hope T, Fairburn CG. Crying following stroke: a report on 30 cases. *Gen Hosp Psychiat* 1992; **14**: 315–21.
13. Calvert T, Knapp P, House A. Psychological associations with emotionalism after stroke. *J Neurol Neurosurg Psych* 1998; **65**: 928–9.
14. Eccles S, House A, Knapp P. Psychological adjustment and self reported coping in stroke survivors with and without emotionalism. *J Neurol Neurosurg Psychiat* 1999; **67**: 125–6.
15. Spencer KA, Tompkins CA, Schulz R. Assessment of depression in patients with brain pathology: the case of stroke. *Psychol Bull* 1997; **122**: 132–52.
16. Sutcliffe LM, Lincoln NB. The assessment of depression in aphasic stroke patients: the development of the Stroke Aphasic Depression Questionnaire. *Clin Rehab* 1998; **12**: 506–13.
17. House A. Mood disorders after stroke: a review of the evidence. *Int J Geriat Psychiat* 1987; **2**: 211–21.
18. Harvey SA, Black KJ. The dexamethasone suppression test for diagnosing depression in stroke patients. *Ann Clin Psychiat* 1996; **8**: 35–9.
19. Castillo CS, Robinson RG. Depression after stroke. *Curr Opin Psychiat* 1994; **7**: 87–90.
20. Robinson RG, Lipsey JR, Price TR. Diagnosis and clinical management of post-stroke depression. *Psychosomatics* 1985; **26**: 769–78.
21. Parikh RM, Lipsey JR, Robinson RG, Price TR. Two-year longitudinal study of post-stroke mood disorders: dynamic changes in correlates of depression at one and two years. *Stroke* 1987; **18**: 579–84.
22. Astrom M, Adolfsson R, Asplund K. Major depression in stroke patients. A 3-year longitudinal study. *Stroke* 1993; **24**: 976–82.
23. Andersen G, Vestergaard K, Ingemann-Nielsen M, Lauritzen L. Risk factors for post-stroke depression. *Acta Psychiat Scand* 1995; **92**: 193–8.
24. Burvill P, Johnson G, Jamrozik K *et al.* Risk factors for post-stroke depression. *Int J Geriat Psychiat* 1997; **12**: 219–26.
25. MacHale SM, O'Rourke S, Dennis MS, Wardlaw JM. Depression and its relation to lesion location after stroke. *J Neurol Neurosurg Psychiat* 1998; **64**: 371–4.
26. Bamford J, Sandercock P, Dennis M *et al.* Classification and natural history of clinically identified subtypes of cerebral infarction. *Lancet* 1991; **337**: 1521–6.
27. Kennedy G, Kelman H, Thomas C. The emergence of depressive symptoms in later life: the importance of declining health and increasing disability. *J Commun Health* 1990; **15**: 93–104.
28. Lipsey J, Robinson R, Pearlson G *et al.* Nortriptyline treatment of post-stroke depression: a double-blind study. *Lancet* 1984; **1**: 297–300.
29. Andersen G, Vestergaard K, Lauritzen L. Effective treatment of poststroke depression with the selective serotonin reuptake inhibitor citalopram. *Stroke* 1994; **25**: 1099–104.
30. Andersen G, Vestergaard K, Riis JO. Citalopram for post-stroke pathological crying. *Lancet* 1993; **342**: 837–9.
31. Brown K, Sloan R, Pentland B. Fluoxetine as a treatment for post-stroke emotionalism. *Acta Psychiat Scand* 1998; **98**: 455–8.
32. Robinson RG, Parikh RM, Lipsey JR *et al.* Pathological laughing and crying following stroke: validation of a measurement scale and a double-blind treatment study. *Am J Psychiat* 1993; **150**: 286–93.
33. Lincoln NB, Flannaghan T, Sutcliffe L, Rother L. Evaluation of cognitive behavioural treatment for depression after stroke: a pilot study. *Clin Rehab* 1997; **11**: 114–22.
34. Palomaki H, Kaste M, Berg A *et al.* Prevention of poststroke depression: 1 year randomised placebo controlled double blind trial of mianserin with 6 month follow up after therapy. *J Neurol Neurosurg Psychiat* 1999; **66**: 490–94.
35. Knapp P, Young J, House A, Forster A. A review of non-drug strategies to address psychosocial difficulties after stroke. *Age Ageing* 1999; November (in press).
36. House A, Knapp P, Dempster C, Vail A. A randomised controlled trial of psychological treatment after stroke. Conference of the British Stroke Research Group, Newcastle 1999.
37. Dempster C, Knapp P, House A. The collaboration of carers during psychological therapy. *Ment Health Nurs* 1998; **18**: 24–7.
38. Gainotti G. Emotional, psychological and psychosocial problems of aphasic patients: an introduction. *Aphasiology* 1997; **11**: 635–50.
39. Hibbard MR, Gordon WA. Post-stroke depression: an examination of the literature. *Arch Phys Med Rehab* 1997; **78**: 658–63.
40. Hosking SG, Marsh NV, Friedman PJ. Post-stroke depression: prevalence, course, and associated factors. *Neuropsychol Rev* 1996; **6**: 107–33.
41. House A. Mood disorders in the physically ill—problems of definition and measurement. *J Psychosom Res* 1988; **32**: 345–53.

Treatment of Depression in Older People with Physical Disability

Sube Banerjee[1] **and Florian A. Ruths**[2]

[1]*Institute of Psychiatry, London, and* [2]*Queen's Resource Centre, Croydon, UK*

THE CASE FOR TREATMENT

As discussed elsewhere, depression is the most common mental disorder in the over-65s, with a prevalence of 13–16%[1,2]. It is a serious disorder, associated with profound decrease in quality of life[3], suicide[4], non-suicidal excess mortality unexplained by physical disorder[5], and excess health and social service use not explained by disability[6,7]. Depression in the elderly also has a substantial financial impact, costing community health and social services in the UK in excess of £1 billion/year in depression-dependent service use[8].

Depression in the elderly therefore has a serious impact on the people suffering from it, their families, and health and social services. Despite this, it is a consistent finding that few older people with depression receive appropriate treatment from primary or secondary care services. Only 10–20% of cases of depression are prescribed antidepressants[7,9,10], with no evidence of their receiving non-drug treatment instead. The reasons for this lack of appropriate action is unclear, some implicating low GP recognition[11] and some a lack of action when depression is found[12]. Whatever the mechanism, there are clear discontinuities on the path from contact, through recognition to action[13].

Older people with physical illness or disablement are a high-risk group for the development of depression[14]. One particular high-risk group consists of those maintained at home, receiving social service home care; 26% of these have clinical depression[15] and, adjusting for age and gender, they have twice the prevalence of depression of the general elderly population, with a four-fold excess of the most severe forms[7]. One possible determinant of therapeutic inactivity may be a perception that depression is untreatable in frail older people, and an important element in clinical behaviour change is evidence of the effectiveness of intervention. Meta-analyses suggest that antidepressants have efficacy in the treatment of depression in those with a variety of physical illnesses[16], with the same sort of effect sizes as those observed in the physically well. However, the evidence for the effectiveness of treatment for depression in the disabled elderly is sparse, since they are often systematically excluded from drug trials[17]. We therefore completed a randomized controlled trial (RCT) to investigate whether depression in home-care clients was treatable by community old age psychiatric services[18].

THE EFFECTIVENESS OF OLD AGE PSYCHIATRIC COMMUNITY TEAM INTERVENTION

Sixty-nine cases of depression were identified by screening the home-care population and randomly allocating them to treatment as usual by their GP, or to treatment by the local old age psychiatric community team, with blind follow-up at 6 months. There was a powerful treatment effect, with 58% of the intervention group recovering, compared with only 25% of the control group (adjusted odds ratio 9.0 [95% CI, 2.1–41.5]). The intervention was pragmatic, involving the multidisciplinary team formulating an individualized management plan and this being implemented by a research worker working as a generic team member. Analyses were carried out on an intention-to-treat basis.

This study's results suggest that therapeutic nihilism, based on an assumed poor response to treatment in the disabled elderly, may not be justified. There are similarly encouraging data for the general population of older adults with depression from GP practice-based community psychiatric nurse intervention[19,20] and nurse-based outreach programmes[21]. However, all these interventions are complex and delivered by secondary care services, and are therefore not directly transferable into primary care settings. Given that there may be 500 000 disabled older adults with clinically significant depression in the UK alone at any one time, secondary care intervention for all is not feasible. It would also be unnecessary if depression in the disabled elderly were to be managed successfully by primary healthcare teams. These are questions which require further research.

Elements of Effective Intervention

The dysjunction in the system of care from disorder to recognition to action has been outlined above. What, therefore, does this mean for the formulation of effective interventions for older people with depression, and where might change be focused best to achieve maximum health gain? These questions can be addressed by considering the pathway from depressed state to resolution, using the data we have for disabled elderly home-care recipients.

Figure 1 presents a simple model. In it, the outcome of depression depends on two parameters, the natural history of the disorder and the effectiveness of intervention. The extent to which an intervention is deployed depends on there being both recognition and action. In Figure 1, the data from the home-care studies are applied to a standard population of 100. In the first stage, the current 15% rate of any active management for depression in this population[7] is applied to divide the group into a "treated" and a "not treated" group. The second stage is to apply the spontaneous recovery rate of 25% to the "not treated" group and the 60% recovery rate from our RCT with active management to the "treated" group[18]. When these filters are applied, only

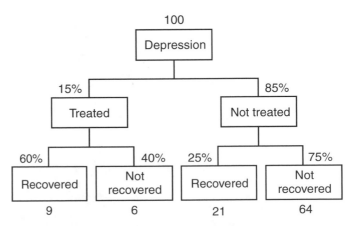

Figure 1

30 of the 100 recover (only nine in the "treated" group and 21 spontaneously recovering in the "not treated" group).

Where, then, should effort be focused to address this situation? The spontaneous recovery rate will be fairly resistant to change and the gain from trying to improve the efficacy of treatment would appear to be relatively limited. For example, an increase in the efficacy from 60% to 80% (an increase unlikely to be possible at present) would only increase the numbers recovering by 3 to 12 in the "treated" group. What is clear from Figure 1 is that the main determinant of the poor population outcome is the low rate of recognition/active management. This would suggest that resources should be focused on increasing the proportion that enter the "treated" group, since there is the greatest scope for improvement at this point and any benefit at this stage will cascade down the system. So, if the proportion "treated" were to be raised by 20% to 35%, the numbers recovering in the "treated" arm would rise to 21 (with 37% recovering overall). If only half of the population of people with depression were identified and treated, then this would rise further to 30 (with 43% recovering overall) and a 75% treatment rate would yield 45 recoveries (51% overall).

CONCLUSIONS

These data demonstrate that, on a population level, there is likely to be far greater health gain from attending to the processes of recognition of depression in the elderly, and of linking this recognition to action, than there is by simply focusing resources on attempting to develop interventions with greater efficacy. This is supported by the emerging evidence base, which endorses the feasibility, acceptability and effectiveness of screening for and treating depression in older adults in the community[18–21].

REFERENCES

1. Copeland JRM, Dewey ME, Wood N et al. Range of mental illness among the elderly in the community prevalence in Liverpool using the GMS–AGECAT package. Br J Psychiat 1987; 150: 815–23.
2. Livingston G, Hawkins A, Graham N et al. The Gospel Oak Study: prevalence rates of dementia, depression and activity limitation among elderly residents in inner London. Psychol Med 1990; 20: 137–46.
3. Gurland B. The impact of depression on quality of life of the elderly. Clin Geriat Med 1992; 8: 377–86.
4. Conwell Y, Rotenberg M, Caine ED. Completed suicide at age 50 and over. J Am Geriat Soc 1990; 38: 640–44.
5. Murphy E, Smith R, Lindesay J, Slattery J. Increased mortality rates in late life depression. Br J Psychiat 1988; 152: 347–53.
6. Blanchard MR, Wattereus A, Mann AH. The nature of depression among older people in Inner London, and their contact with primary care. Br J Psychiat 1994; 164: 396–402.
7. Banerjee S, Macdonald A. Mental disorder in an elderly home care population: associations with health and social service use. Br J Psychiat 1996; 168: 750–56.
8. Livingston G, Manela M, Katona C. Cost of community care for older people. Br J Psychiat 1997; 171: 56–69.
9. Copeland JRM, Gurland BJ, Dewey ME et al. Is there more dementia, depression and neurosis in New York? A comparative study of the elderly in New York and London using the computer diagnosis AGECAT. Br J Psychiat 1987; 151: 466–73.
10. Skoog I, Nilsson L, Landahl S, Steen B. Mental disorders and the use of psychotropic drugs in an 85-year-old urban population. Int Psychogeriat 1993; 5: 33–47.
11. Crawford MJ, Prince M, Menezes P, Mann AH. The recognition and treatment of depression in older people in primary care. Int J Geriat Psychiat 1998; 13: 172–6.
12. Macdonald AJD. Do general practitioners 'miss' depression in elderly patients? Br Med J 1986; 292: 13650–8.
13. Banerjee S. The needs of special groups: the elderly. Int Rev Psychiat 1998; 10: 130–33.
14. Prince M, Harwood R, Thomas A, Mann AH. A prospective population-based cohort study of the effects of disablement and social milieu on the onset and maintenance of late-life depression. Psychol Med 1998; 28: 337–50.
15. Banerjee S. Prevalence and recognition rates of psychiatric disorder in the elderly clients of a community care service. Int J Geriat Psychiat 1993; 8: 125–31.
16. Gill D, Hatcher S. Antidepressants for depression in people with physical illness (Cochrane Review). In The Cochrane Library, Issue 4. Oxford: Update Software, 2000.
17. Banerjee S, Dickinson E. Evidence-based old age psychiatry. Int J Psychiat Med 1997; 27: 2803–92.
18. Banerjee S, Shamash K, Macdonald A, Mann A. Randomised controlled trial of effect of intervention by psychogeriatric team on depression in frail elderly people at home. Br Med J 1996; 313: 1058–61.
19. Waterreus A, Blanchard M, Mann A. Community psychiatric nurses for the elderly: well tolerated, few side-effects and effective in the treatment of depression. J Clin Nurs 1994; 3: 299–306.
20. Blanchard MR, Waterraus A, Mann A. The effect of primary care nurse intervention upon older people screened as depressed. Int J Geriat Psychiat 1995; 10: 289–98.
21. Rabins PV, Black BS, Roca R et al. Effectiveness of a nurse-based outreach program for identifying and treating psychiatric illness in the elderly. J Am Med Assoc 2000; 283: 2802–9.

76

Acute Management of Late-life Depression

Veronica Gardner and David C. Steffens

Duke University Medical Center, Durham, NC, USA

The acute management of late-life depression may require hospitalization, both for accurate diagnosis and for effective treatment. Ambulatory management is frequently favored because of rising hospital costs in a managed care environment. However, the elderly present special challenges that may require that diagnosis and/or treatment be undertaken in a hospital setting. The hospital provides an environment for the monitoring of symptoms for accurate diagnosis and proper personnel for regular and accurate treatment administration. Several factors may interfere with both accurate diagnosis and effective treatment on an ambulatory basis[1], including underlying chronic medical illness, pain, neurodegenerative changes, dementia, adverse life events, inadequate family support, secret self-medication, substance abuse, bereavement, interpersonal conflicts and social isolation of the elderly patient.

Actually, the elderly patient who is cognitively intact may be reliably managed on an ambulatory basis and can be instructed about medication side effects. Similarly, the more impaired elderly patient who has adequate social support for observation and medication management may only need the community support of a visiting psychiatric nurse, assuming one is available. Varying levels of care are also implemented in the hospital environment. A patient may have the usual care of routine monitoring or may have more intense one-to-one monitoring if he/she is an imminent risk to him/herself or others.

As a general rule, the more the physical and psychiatric impairments and fewer psychosocial resources, the greater the need to hospitalize for accurate diagnosis and effective treatment. When deciding safe and effective management, the following factors favor hospitalization: poor or unstable physical health, high suicide risk, impaired judgment and reality testing, likelihood of poor compliance, impaired cognitive functioning, lack of social support, and severe anorexia and weight loss.

CO-MORBIDITY OF PHYSICAL ILLNESS: THE INTERFACE OF PRIMARY CARE AND PSYCHIATRY

Accurate diagnosis is a prerequisite for effective treatment. Elderly patients with depression present to their primary care physicians and psychiatrists in a complex manner, and signs and symptoms of physical illness and depression overlap. Even the normal effects of aging may cause diagnostic difficulties and restrict treatment options. Many primary care physicians diagnose and treat late-life depression without referral. However, those patients who fail two or three trials with antidepressants, usually selective serotonin-reuptake inhibitors (SSRIs) or newer agents, are commonly referred to a psychiatrist for further management. These patients represent a treatment challenge and may require complex medication regimens that are more successful with hospitalization. Primary care physicians also refer for the following reasons: suicidality, co-morbidity with substance abuse, dementia, anxiety disorder, presence of psychosis (delusions, hallucinations), catatonia, bipolar disorder, and inability to tolerate antidepressant treatment[2,3]. Such patients often need to be managed in the hospital.

Depression is often co-morbid with other physical diseases. Approximately 80% of older adults suffer from at least one chronic health problem[4]. The prevalence of co-morbid depression may be up to 30% in stroke patients, 18% in myocardial infarction patients, 51% in patients with hip fracture, and 50% in patients with chronic pain[1]. Existence of an undiagnosed and untreated depression with these illnesses leads to higher disability[5]. The diagnosis of depression with certain illnesses is complex, and the hospital environment provides the necessary monitoring and support staff when complicated medication changes are required.

For example, a patient with cardiovascular disease may present with decreased energy and apathy. Determining whether this is caused by a compromised cardiac status, a medication side effect, or is actually a symptom of depression may be difficult without hospitalization, close monitoring and various medication trials. Formerly, hospitalization was favored for the initiation of tricyclic antidepressant therapy in elderly patients with unstable cardiac disease. First-line treatment with SSRIs is now available and proved safe for use in cardiac disease[6].

Co-morbid neurological illness is also common in geriatric depression. Patients with depressive symptoms following a cerebrovascular accident also present a diagnostic challenge. There may be communication difficulties or other neurologic abnormalities. Depression may be diagnosed only by the report of the nursing staff and family, who observe apathy, irritability, tearfulness and weight loss[7]. Patients with Parkinson's disease may develop an affective illness or psychosis, which may be secondary to treatment with L-dopa. Hospitalization may be required for medication changes if outpatient support is inadequate.

Severe anorexia, weight loss and refusal to eat are indications for hospitalization for safe and effective treatment[8,1]. Poor oral intake commonly accompanies severe depression, but it may also result from a variety of medical conditions. For example, individuals with active rheumatoid arthritis may experience insomnia, fatigue and poor appetite equally from their physical illness or an associated depression[9].

SUICIDE RISK AND THE DECISION TO HOSPITALIZE

Suicidality is the most common reason for psychiatric hospitalization. According to Jacobson[29], three goals for inpatient treatment are: (a) the preservation of life and safety; (b) the elimination of suicidal intent and ideation and treatment of underlying disorders; and (c) the improvement of intrapsychic capabilities, personal factors and psychosocial circumstances to facilitate coping after discharge and decreasing risk of the return of suicidality. However, implementation of these treatment plans is predicted on the initial detection of suicidality.

Careful assessment of suicide risk in depressed older adults is thus vital. The elderly are less likely to have made a prior suicide attempt, but they consistently demonstrate a higher rate of completed suicides[10]. The ratio of attempted to completed suicides decreases with age from 200:1 in young adulthood to 4:1 in the elderly[11]. The higher rate is due primarily to the increased frequency of deaths among older, White males. In 1992, persons 65 and older accounted for 13% of the population but almost 20% of suicides. Even though the frequency of suicide has increased among older persons in the USA, the prevalence is not as high as that of other industrialized societies[10].

Recognition of variables such as gender and race may influence management decisions. Risk factors for suicide in late life include increased age, with the highest prevalence of suicide of persons older than 85[10]. Also, being male, White, single, separated or divorced, or widowed are risk factors for suicide. Other risk factors implicated in late-life suicide include: a positive psychiatric history (especially depression and alcohol abuse and dependence); physical illness and functional disability (especially diseases of the central nervous system, malignancies, cardiopulmonary conditions, and urogenital diseases in men); previous suicide attempts; psychological factors (i.e. hopelessness); social factors (stressful life events, e.g. bereavement); and biological susceptibility (dysregulation of the hypothalamic–pituitary–adrenal axis or the serotonin system).

Most older people who commit suicide have seen a primary care provider within 30 days of death[11]. This observation stresses the need for collaborative efforts with primary care physicians and the need to make careful assessment based on risk factors.

A number of assessment guidelines have been developed to aid in the evaluation of potentially suicidal patients. A four-item screen for identification of suicidal ideation among general medical patients was developed by Cooper-Patrick et al.[12].

1. Have you ever felt that life is not worth living?
2. Have you ever thought of hurting or harming yourself?
3. Have you considered specific methods for harming yourself?
4. Have you ever made a suicide attempt?

This four-fold layered approach to assessment is useful in obtaining the necessary data without disrupting the therapeutic relationship. If the answer to the first or second question is negative, then the inquiries can cease and the older person may be considered at low risk for suicide[10]. This approach has advantages over other assessment tools, which usually suggest one question to be asked to assess suicidal risk.

DELUSIONS AND LATE-LIFE DEPRESSION

Accurate diagnosis and effective treatment of depressed elderly patients with delusions can be hindered by their impairment of reality testing. Their sometimes well-organized and complex delusions may make them distrust medicine and the physician who prescribes it. This disorder is less frequent in the community and more prevalent in the hospital setting[13,14]. Accurate diagnosis is necessary, as some studies have suggested that the depression is more severe[14,15] and it has been associated with suicide[13]. Varying reports also demonstrate decreased cognitive functioning and social functioning among patients with delusional depression[16]. These patients are best treated in the hospital. They cannot be relied upon to take accurate doses of medications. Effective pharmacologic treatment for delusional depression requires combination treatment with high-dose antipsychotic medication and antidepressants[15]. ECT has been successful for the treatment of delusional depression[17–19] and can be performed on an outpatient basis only with adequate social support.

COGNITIVE DYSFUNCTION AND LATE-LIFE DEPRESSION

A full discussion of how depression is distinguished from dementia is given elsewhere in this book. To summarize, diagnosis is difficult because several symptoms of depression and dementia overlap, such as a flattened affect, psychomotor retardation and presence, at times, of delusions[20]. Delusions are reported to occur in up to 40%[13] of Alzheimer's disease patients, although they are described as transient and less organized than in delusional depression[13]. Major depression occurs in over 20% of patients with Alzheimer's disease and vascular dementia[4,21]. This significant co-morbidity may lead to profound disability[22].

The diagnosis of depression in dementia usually requires the input of family members or nursing personnel[23,24]. The patient with cognitive dysfunction and impaired reality testing cannot reliably report symptoms, take medication accurately, or reliably report side effects.

Dementia with depression and behavioral disturbance is frequently too complex to treat on an outpatient basis. These patients may even require involuntary commitment. Aggression may be verbal or physical. Aggression and agitation in dementia may be as high as 50% in the outpatient population[25,26]. The hospital environment is the only setting with constant monitoring to make an accurate diagnosis, contain behavior and monitor medication.

The reversible cognitive impairment that may accompany depression also increases disability[27]. With treatment, the cognitive impairment usually improves. However, these patients are at higher risk to develop an irreversible dementia in the future[28].

CONCLUSIONS

The patient with late-life depression frequently presents in a complex manner that may require hospitalization. Accurate diagnosis and treatment of these patients is essential to prevent disability, caregiver burden and nursing home placement. Confusion, suicidality and aggression represent psychiatric emergencies in the elderly and may require hospitalization for effective management.

REFERENCES

1. Montano CB. Primary care issues related to the treatment of depression in elderly. J Clin Psychiat 1999; 60(suppl. 20): 45–51.
2. Mulsant B, Ganguli M. Epidemiology and diagnosis of depression in late life. J Clin Psychiat 1999; 60(20): 9–14.
3. Unutzer J, Katon W et al. Treating depressed older adults in primary care: narrowing the gap between efficacy and effectiveness. Millbank Qu 1999; 77(2): 225–56.
4. Edelstein B, Kalish K et al. Assessment of depression and bereavement in older adults. In Lichtenberg P, ed., Handbook of Assessment in Clinical Gerontology. New York: Wiley, 1999; 11–58.
5. Das Gupta K. Treatment of depression in elderly patients: recent advances. Arch Fam Med 1998; 7(3): 274–80.
6. Roose S, Spatz E. Treatment of depression in patients with heart disease. J Clin Psychiat 1999; 60(20): 34–7.

7. Mather R. Old age psychiatry in a general hospital. In Jacoby R, Oppenheimer C, eds, *Psychiatry in the Elderly*. New York, NY: Oxford University Press, 1997; 536–73.

8. Joseph S. Practical diagnostic and management guidelines. In Joseph S, ed., *Symptom Focused Psychiatric Drug Therapy for Managed Care*. Binghamton, NY: Haworth Medical, 1997; 25–45.

9. Baldwin RC. Depressive illness. In Jacoby R, Oppenheimer C, *Psychiatry in the Elderly*. New York: Oxford University Press, 1997; 336–54.

10. Steffens DC, Blazer DG. Suicide in the elderly. In Jacobs DG, ed., *Guide to Suicide Assessment and Intervention*. San Francisco, CA: Jossey-Bass. 1999; 443–62.

11. Conwell Y. Management of suicidal behavior in the elderly. *Psychiat Clin N Am* 1997; **20**(3): 667–83.

12. Cooper-Patrick L, Crum RM *et al*. Identifying suicidal ideation in general medical patients. *J Am Med Assoc* 1994; **272**: 1757–62.

13. Meyers BS. Geriatric delusional depression. *Clin Geriat Med* 1992; **8**(2): 299–308.

14. O'Brein J, Ames D *et al*. Magnetic resonance imaging and endocrinological differences between delusional and non-delusional depression in the elderly. *Int J Geriat Psychiat* 1999; **12**: 211–18.

15. Chiu HF. Antidepressants in the elderly. *Int J Clin Pract* 1997; **51**(6): 369–74.

16. Blazer DG. Severe episode of depression in late life: the long road to recovery. *Am J Psychiat* 1996; **153**(12): 1620–3.

17. Spar JE, LaRue A. Mood disorders: treatment. In Spar JE, LaRue A, eds, *Concise Guide to Geriatric Psychiatry*. Washington, DC: American Psychiatric Press, 1990; 65–88.

18. Alexopoulos GS. Affective disorders. In Sadavey J, Lazarus LW, Jarvik LF, Grossberg GT, eds, *Comprehensive Review of Geriatric Psychiatry*, vol II. Washington, DC: American Psychiatric Press, 1996; 563–92.

19. Small GW. Treatment of geriatric depression. *Depress Anxiety* 1998; **8**(1): 32–42.

20. Reisberg B, Kluger A. Assessing the progression of dementia: diagnostic considerations. In Salzman C, ed., *Clinical Geriatric Psychopharmacology*. Baltimore, MD: Williams and Wilkins, 1998; 432–62.

21. Newman S. The prevalence of depression in Alzheimer's disease and vascular dementia in a population sample. *J Affect Disord* 1999; **52**: 169–76.

22. Simpson S, Allen H *et al*. Neurological correlates of depressive symptoms in Alzheimer's disease and vascular dementia. *J Affect Disord* 1999; **53**: 129–36.

23. Plopper M. Common psychiatric disorders. In Yoshikawa TT, ed., *Ambulatory Geriatric Care*. St. Louis, MO: Mosby Year Book, 1993; 346–62.

24. Harwood D, Barker WW *et al*. Association between premorbid history of depression and current depression in Alzheimer's disease. *J Geriat Psychiat Neurol* 1999; **12**: 72–5.

25. Kunick ME, Yudofsky SC *et al*. Pharmacologic approach to management of agitation associated with dementia. *J Clin Psychiat* 1994; **55**(2): 13–17.

26. Tueth M, Zuberi P. Life-threatening psychiatric emergencies in the elderly: overview. *J Geriat Psychiat Neurol* 1999; **12**: 60–66.

27. Katz IR, Miller D *et al*. Diagnosis of late-life depression. In Salzeman C, ed., *Clinical Geriatric Psychopharmacology*. Baltimore, MD: Williams and Wilkins, 1998; 153–83.

28. Alexopoulos GS, Meyers BS *et al*. The course of geriatric depression with reversible dementia: a controlled study. *Am J Psychiat* 1993; **150**(11): 1693–9.

77

Electroconvulsive Therapy (ECT)

David G. Wilkinson

Moorgreen Hospital, Southampton, UK

Those who decry it in the elderly are sentimental and ill-informed. ECT for suitable patients not only relieves intolerable anguish but saves lives (Brice Pitt[1]).

Despite continued opposition to its use, ECT remains a fundamental tool in the armamentarium of the psychiatrist treating the severely mentally ill. There have now been thousands of papers and articles published concerning its use and we have a wealth of accumulated wisdom, and yet the controversy continues[2].

In geriatric psychiatry there is no controversy: papers continue to confirm that in the elderly ECT is an effective treatment for severe affective disorders[3-6] and is the treatment of choice in severe delusional depression[7-10]. It is safe, despite the likelihood of multiple system disorders and medications[11]. It is well tolerated, if not always well liked[12], but does sometimes exacerbate confusion. There is no convincing evidence of brain damage or even of lasting memory impairment, particularly if brief pulse right unilateral ECT is used[13]. ECT should be considered in every patient who has either failed to respond to other treatments, or who is suffering intolerable distress, or who may die through inanition or dehydration as a result of his/her depression. It is probably for these reasons that ECT continues to be used six to seven times more frequently in the elderly than in their younger counterparts[14]. The fact that in the USA it has also been shown that early use of ECT reduces inpatient costs may have also been an influential factor in its greater use[15].

INDICATIONS

Studies on the efficacy of ECT, which have largely been conducted on younger patients[7], all emphasize that ECT appears to be more effective than placebo, single-drug therapy and tricyclic/neuroleptic combinations, and that patients with more florid symptoms of recent onset fare best[7,16-18]. Experience with the elderly would confirm these findings. Indicators of response are perhaps less clear in the elderly, with some authors finding psychomotor disturbance and psychosis a positive predictor of response[10] and others suggesting that patients without these features can also do well[19]. That the classic distinction between neurotic and psychotic depression appears less helpful in this group as a predictor of good response is nothing new. Post[20] in 1976 stressed the practical irrelevance of any subclassification of elderly depressives, as he found that ECT rendered severe psychotic depressives fit for discharge only slightly more often than neurotic depressives. The presenting picture of hysterical illness, hypochondriasis or other apparent neurotic illness may well be caused by an underlying functional psychosis, often depressive in the elderly. More recently, in a study of 163 elderly patients given ECT, it was found that 27% had predominantly neurotic depressive features and yet had a good response to treatment[3]. In fact, in the study by Fraser and Glass[21], psychic anxiety, along with the more expected features of short duration, severity of illness, guilt and agitation, was one of the symptoms correlated with a favourable response to ECT, whereas the typical endogenous features of late insomnia and diurnal variation in mood were not. Treatment resistance in the elderly will respond to ECT, although not as well as non-resistant patients[22]. However, they do respond better to ECT than SSRIs[18] and Flint[5] found that ECT was significantly superior to tricyclic/neuroleptic combinations, even when the former had been augmented with lithium. A pragmatic consensus would suggest that in the elderly a trial of ECT is indicated in any depressed patient who might otherwise be regarded as a treatment non-responder, and if the illness is severe and of short duration there is likely to be a good response, regardless of the presenting symptoms. If the illness has been present for some time, or even years, it still may respond if there is a clear history of a change for the worse in the patient who had previously maintained a stable personality and had coped normally with the vicissitudes of life. Prolonged or abnormal bereavement reactions with marked depressive features not responding to antidepressants or talking therapies may need to be treated with ECT before psychotherapy or counselling can be effective. ECT may need to be given within a few months of the loss if hopelessness and suicidal ideation suggest a risk to life, and should not be withheld due to the feeling that the patient must work through his/her grief naturally, as he/she may never get that chance.

Mania is another indication for a trial of ECT[23], particularly in the elderly, where neuroleptics may fail to control the symptoms and yet produce unsteadiness, postural hypotension or falls, and lithium may not be tolerated due to toxicity problems.

Paraphrenia will often respond to ECT[24], although this is more likely if there are obvious depressive symptoms or delusions.

ECT is certainly useful in the depressed patient with Parkinson's disease, as the motor symptoms will improve as well as the depression, and indeed, some authors advocate ECT as the treatment of choice for certain stages of Parkinson's disease, whether or not depression is a major problem[25,26]. I have given daily ECT with excellent results to a parkinsonian patient who had developed severe paranoid delusions. His refusal to accept his medication rendered him rigid and immobile with pressure sores, he needed intravenous fluids and nasogastric feeding until he had four treatments, whereupon his physical and emotional improvement was dramatic.

Principles and Practice of Geriatric Psychiatry, 2nd edn. Edited by J. R. M. Copeland, M. T. Abou-Saleh and D. G. Blazer

Fogel[16] suggests that ECT might be more readily used in the elderly if we were more objective about its virtues as compared with the severe side effects often associated with neuroleptics, which are quite readily used in the agitated elderly patient. Extrapyramidal effects were usually the limiting factor but are not so noticeable with atypical neuroleptics. However, he postulates that the demented patient who is very agitated and screaming might suffer less indignity and fewer side effects if treated with ECT, rather than tranquillizers, as the patient may have an underlying affective disturbance manifest only by the agitation and negativism that one often sees in this condition.

CONTRAINDICATIONS

There are no absolute contraindications, only relative risks, relative that is to the morbidity and mortality of untreated depression. The limiting factor is whether the patient is fit for the light anaesthetic that ECT requires. The majority of risk factors are therefore associated with the cardiovascular system. Many people are denied treatment due to irrational caution. For example, pacemakers are not barriers to treatment; the bodily tissues, being highly resistant, prevent the ECT stimulus from reaching the pacemaker in any case. The patient should remain insulated from the ground, however, to prevent the unlikely event of the current leaking to earth and being conducted down the pacemaker wire to the heart. Equally, myocardial infarction is not a contraindication to treatment if the depression is so severe as to threaten life; in less severe cases, an interval, governed by sentiment rather than science, of 4–6 weeks is usually left. The risks are greatest during the first 10 days post-infarct, and probably negligible after 3 months. I have treated a patient with treated hypothyroidism who had two prosthetic heart valves, was therefore on anticoagulants and had a pacemaker, with no special precautions or untoward effects. Patients with osteoporosis or with recent femoral neck fractures can be treated, provided an adequate muscle relaxant is given. Stroke is certainly not a contraindication, and ECT given as soon as 1 month after does not present a major risk to patients. There is now a growing body of literature attesting to the usefulness of ECT in treating post-stroke depression[27].

The case of deep venous thrombosis (DVT) is less clear. I have given ECT to a patient who had a DVT in his calf during his depressive illness, once he was adequately anticoagulated. In fact, the risk of pulmonary embolism seems, in my practice, greater in the dehydrated immobile depressive than in those receiving ECT. Arterial hypertension is often regarded as a contraindication, as blood pressure is well known to rise during ECT. This can sometimes be controlled and the pressor response avoided by using sublingual nifedipine or short-acting β-blockers shortly before treatment[28]. Chronic glaucoma is another condition in which ECT causes fewer problems than tricyclic antidepressants; in fact, intraocular pressures are said to reduce ECT[29]. Insulin-dependent diabetes is a condition, like Parkinson's disease, which alters during ECT. Insulin requirements may decrease quite substantially during the course of ECT, so more careful monitoring of blood glucose levels is needed. It is also necessary to avoid hyperglycaemia prior to treatment, which may significantly raise the fit threshold, and the timing of ECT administration may need consideration to prevent undue fluctuations in diabetic control. Transient asystole occasionally occurs, for some reason less frequently in the old-old, but it is not of any consequence and need not prevent further treatments[30,31].

Epileptic patients on anticonvulsants should not stop their medication during ECT, as that might increase the risk of status epilepticus. However, they may need higher than usual electrical dosages to produce an adequate response.

It is interesting that the seizure during ECT is invested with great powers of harm compared with epileptic seizures *per se*, which can of course occur in patients with any disease or at any time and seldom result in death. It seems understandable, then, that a seizure in the controlled conditions of the ECT room is probably even less likely to result in fatality. There is, of course, a mortality rate associated with ECT but, as noted by Fink[32], the treatment rate of 0.002% compares favourably with the rate for anaesthetic induction alone (0.003–0.04%).

ADMINISTRATION

The responses of senior psychiatrists to the process of ECT vary from those who simply prescribe six treatments and leave the administration to the newest recruit, who has often had no training at all, to those surgeons *manqués* who may overstate the risks and precautions in order to increase the perceived risk of their jobs. Clearly, the ideal path lies somewhere between, but nearer the latter than the former! ECT is the only psychiatric treatment in the elderly that involves significant medical intervention with general anaesthesia, and as such, the psychiatrist should have a clear understanding of what he/she is prescribing and regular involvement in its administration. As much attention should be paid to the prescription of ECT as to any other prescription.

A clear decision as to whether bilateral or unilateral electrode placement is wanted should be made; the ECT record sheet should be reviewed to ensure that an adequate convulsive response has occurred without excessive stimulus; treatments should not be in blocks of six, but, provided that the illness is one with a good prognosis, treatment should be continued until the expected degree of improvement is obtained, whether that is after three or 23 treatments.

There is no evidence that the habit of giving one or two extra ECTs after full recovery is effective in preventing relapse[33]. The decision to give unilateral or bilateral ECT in the elderly is made easier by the fact that high dose unilateral ECT does seem to produce less confusion, memory loss and headache and appears to be equally effective in many patients[34,52]. However, there is a great deal of discrepancy in the results of comparative studies, possibly due to differences in diagnosis, age and gender, together with variance in the technique of administration of unilateral ECT. The consensus seems to indicate that, for many patients, both treatments are equally effective; some patients require more right unilateral treatments than bilateral to achieve the same result and some patients who do not respond to right unilateral ECT will respond when switched to bilateral treatment. Male gender and older age are also associated with better response to bilateral treatment.

It is my practice to use bilateral treatment initially in very severe psychotic depressives but right unilateral treatment in most other cases, particularly if there is evidence of prior cognitive impairment, switching to bilateral treatment if there is no response after six to eight right unilateral treatments. Brief pulse ECT at a moderately supra-threshold stimulus (which is often only around 275–350 millicoulombs) appears to offer efficacy, with the advantage of much less memory loss and confusion than the modified sine wave stimulus, and should be used in all cases, with a record of dosage received by the patient to ensure adequate technique[53].

There is considerable debate about the necessity to use a dose-titration technique to establish seizure threshold prior to treatment, with some viewing this as unnecessary and even detrimental in those patients requiring several non-convulsive stimuli. Adequate seizure response can be measured using inter-ictal EEG monitoring. Some clinicians seem to have developed an over-weaning interest in stimulus intensity, seizure threshold and seizure duration. It is clear that seizure threshold will increase by about 40% during the course of ECT and the seizure duration will tend to decrease by about one-third. However, while it seems that outcome is not correlated with either seizure duration or threshold for bilateral ECT[35], it may be more important to keep the stimulus intensity above seizure threshold in unilateral treatment[36]. Seizure duration is more difficult to evaluate, as some patients regularly have brisk and brief responses with good results. The use of propofol to induce anaesthesia consistently reduces seizure duration, although apparently without affecting efficacy[37,38]. The use of caffeine prior to treatment to prolong seizure activity has been associated with improved efficacy in some patients[39]. It would seem that, as a rule of thumb, we should aim for a seizure length of around 25 s and any seizure less than 15 s or more than 120 s is likely to adversely affect response[40]. Cumulative seizure duration again seems less interesting now than it once was as a measure of the length of a course of treatment, and clinical response still seems the best measure.

There is no evidence that routine atropine premedication improves cardiac stability or lessens secretions. Theoretically it could cause confusion, but there is no convincing evidence of this either. Glycopyrrolate, which does not cross the blood–brain barrier, may be a better drug to use as a drying agent. Methohexitone for the induction of anaesthesia at a dosage of 30–50 mg is adequate to ensure sleep without hangover, and muscle relaxation with a suxamethonium dosage of 20–40 mg is enough to modify the convulsion without abolishing all evidence of motor activity. If the minimum amount of anaesthetic is combined with treatment early in the morning, the patient is not required to starve any longer than usual, he/she is less likely to be dehydrated, is less likely to break his/her fast, has less time to become anxious and agitated and will recovery quickly enough to enjoy a breakfast with the other patients on the ward. If this routine is combined with regular supervision of treatment by the prescribing psychiatrist, the patient will derive the maximum benefit from each treatment and the course will not be unnecessarily prolonged or ineffective. Outpatient ECT does not appear to be as effective in the elderly, except occasionally as maintenance, and consequently most patients will require admission to a specialist unit, where the effects of ECT combined with the therapeutic milieu will hasten improvement. Familiar staff administering the treatment and a well-designed ECT suite will help reduce anxiety.

MAINTENANCE AND CONTINUATION ECT

In 1990 the American Psychiatric Association task force on ECT defined continued administration of ECT over a 6 month period to prevent relapse after induction of remission as continuation ECT (C-ECT); treatment beyond 6 months was termed maintenance ECT (M-ECT). This was felt to be a viable form of management for selected patients.

Maintenance ECT has been used for many years: a survey of British psychogeriatricians in 1991[47] found that 20% were using it but there is little more than anecdote to support its use in the literature. Such studies as there are consist mainly of case-studies and small series of hospitalized patients, all of a "naturalistic" nature.

In a 1 year follow-up of nine elderly patients, continuation treatment, even if discontinued fairly quickly seemed to confer some lasting advantage in prevention of relapse[48], as did Petrides et al.'s study, looking at 33 courses of C-ECT[49]. The conclusion seemed to be that where patients have responded to acute ECT but previously failed on continuation pharmacotherapy there was compelling evidence for C-ECT and little therapeutic alternative.

The four patients in this study[49] who continued with M-ECT remained well and the five who had previously stopped did not. Naturally this result is open to other interpretations, but it does suggest that C-ECT should be considered for those with recurrent depression who respond well to ECT acutely but receive no prophylaxis from pharmacotherapy. The practicalities of using outpatient M-ECT have prevented my using it more. Bringing elderly patients to hospital for outpatient ECT early in the day, from a rural catchment area some distance from the hospital, can be problematic, they soon lose enthusiasm for the treatment and consequently often withdraw consent. This is an issue recently addressed by Kim[50]. However, Schwarz's findings, that rehospitalization rates were reduced by 67% after instituting M-ECT, suggest that we should try and overcome the practical difficulties[51].

CONSENT

Popular myths about ECT are always more readily believed than the reality and can be part of what the patient believes they are consenting to. Occasionally patients consent as part of their death wish. I use a video of myself administering ECT to a patient seen before and after treatment, to show anxious or interested relatives and patients; no-one having seen it has then declined the treatment. There is one study suggesting that understanding is not enhanced by this method. The issue of informed consent in depressed patients is complex. As I have suggested, many care little and are prepared to do anything their doctor suggests, and patients' recollection of what was explained to them, after the ECT and when the depression has lifted, is often vague. A careful explanation should be made and recorded, and if there are doubts on either side a chance to preview the ECT room or an explanatory video may be helpful. However, it is doubtful whether the explanation of ECT is any less detailed than that of most surgical procedures and most people are willing to consent without seeing a video of the operation in question. Passive acceptance of ECT is often the case in the severely depressed but this should not prevent a full explanation, including consulting relatives if appropriate.

Involuntary ECT should never be given except within the guidelines of the relevant Mental Health legislation if we are to ensure the availability of ECT as a treatment option in the future. Nevertheless, depression is such a serious and debilitating illness that the chance of a cure through use of ECT should never be denied to a patient whose prognosis is favourable, simply through difficulty in obtaining actual written consent.

SIDE EFFECTS

As already mentioned, confusion and memory loss are often regarded as an inevitable corollary of ECT in the elderly, but this is clearly not the case and there are well conducted studies showing no objective permanent effects on memory, and in fact this often improves as a result of improvement in the depression[21,41,42]. Nevertheless, there is no doubt that some patients who were given bilateral sine wave ECT experienced long-term, even permanent, memory loss, and bland reassurances that this or even brief pulse bilateral ECT will not cause any memory loss is foolish and counterproductive. Some patients given bilateral brief pulse ECT may have amnestic gaps, but can be assured that no lasting effect on memory function, i.e. new learning or intelligence, will occur. The situation with right unilateral brief pulse ECT is different, with any subjective memory impairment being transient and undetectable 6 months later[43,44]. Patients with existing dementia may well show signs of memory impairment, even with unilateral ECT. This may be acceptable in view of the relief from distress and agitation and improvement in behaviour and performance.

The cognitive side effects can be minimized by reducing concomitant medications, particularly benzodiazepines, anticholinergic antidepressants and lithium[45], although a recent study found no problems with the administration of ECT and lithium[46]. Benzodiazepines, given intravenously as the seizure ends, can be of use in controlling emergence delirium, which can last for 15–30 min after treatment and be very difficult to control otherwise[13]. Dementia *per se* does not preclude the use of ECT, provided that the coexisting depression is circumscribed. A history of depression before the dementia adds weight to the decision, particularly if there was a good response to ECT previously. Other side effects of treatment, such as headache and dizziness or muscle pain, usually only after the first anaesthetic, are minimal and soon forgotten as the depression lifts.

ECT is a valuable and as yet essential tool in the treatment of depression in old age, a disease which untreated carries a significant mortality. It is interesting that in my practice elderly patients who have attempted suicide are nearly all offered ECT. This is because those, albeit only very few in number, who have subsequently killed themselves during a depressive illness have all been patients who have either refused ECT or not been given it at the time of their index suicide attempt. However, whilst there are many compelling arguments for the use of ECT, it is not a universal panacea. ECT, like any potent treatment, should be prescribed with accuracy and its use monitored carefully by those prescribing it.

Depression in the elderly presents with protean manifestations. ECT should be part of an eclectic approach to treatment and as such will continue to relieve distress and save lives.

REFERENCES

1. Pitt B. *Psychogeriatrics*. Edinburgh: Churchill Livingstone, 1974.
2. Wilkinson DG, Daoud J. The stigma and enigma of ECT. *Int J Geriat Psychiat* 1998; **13**: 833–5.
3. Godber C, Rosenvinge H, Wilkinson DG *et al.* Depression in old-age: prognosis after ECT. *Int J Geriat Psychiat* 1987; **2**: 19–24.
4. Stroudemire A, Hill CD, Maarquardt M *et al.* Recovery and relapse in geriatric depression after treatment with antidepressants and ECT in a medical–physical population. *Gen Hosp Psychiat* 1998; **20**(3): 170–4.
5. Flint AJ, Rifat SL. The treatment of psychotic depression in later life: a comparison of pharmacotherapy and ECT. *Int J Geriat Psychiat* 1998; **13**(1): 23–8.
6. Williams JH, O'Brian JT, Cullum S. Time course of response to electroconvulsive therapy in elderly depressed subjects. *Int J Geriat Psychiat* 1997; **12**(5): 563–6.
7. Johnstone EC, Deakins JF, Lawler P *et al.* The Northwick Park electroconvulsive therapy trial. *Lancet* 1980; **ii**: 1317–20.
8. Baldwin RC. Delusional and non-delusional depression in late life. Evidence of distinct sub-types. *Br J Psychiat* 1988; **152**: 39–44.
9. Ottoson J. Use and misuse of electroconvulsive treatment. *Biol Psychiat* 1985; **20**: 933–46.
10. Hickie I, Mason C, Parker G, Brodaty H. Prediction of ECT response; validation of a refined sign-based (CORE) system for defining melancholia. *Br J Psychiat* 1996; **169**(1): 68–74.
11. Gaspar D, Samarasinghe LA. ECT in psychogeriatric practice—a study of risk factors, indications and outcomes. *Comp Psychiat* 1982; **23**: 170–5.
12. Hughes J, Barraclough B, Reeve W. Are patients shocked by ECT? *J R Soc Med* 1981; **74**: 283–5.
13. Abrams R. *Electronconvulsive Therapy*. New York: Oxford University Press, 1988.
14. Flint AJ. Electroconvulsive therapy in the elderly. *Curr Opin Psychiat* 1999; **12**: 481–5.
15. Olfson M, Marcus S, Sackeim HA *et al.* Use of ECT for the inpatient treatment of recurrent major depression. *Am J Psychiat* 1998; **155**: 22–9.
16. Fogel B. Electroconvulsive therapy in the elderly: a clinical research agenda. *Int J Geriat Psychiat* 1988; **3**: 181–90.
17. Kroessler D. Relative efficacy rates for therapies of delusional depression. *Convuls Ther* 1985; **1**: 173–82.
18. Folkerts HW, Michael N, Tolle R *et al.* Electroconvulsive therapy vs. paroxetine in treatment-resistant depression—a randomised study. *Acta Psychiat Scand* 1997; **96**: 334–42.
19. Sobin C, Prudic J, Devanand DP *et al.* Who responds to electroconvulsive therapy? A comparison of effective and ineffective forms of treatment. *Br J Psychiat* 1996; **169**(3): 322–8.
20. Post F. The management and nature of depressive illness in late life: a follow-through story. In Gallant D, ed., *Depression*. New York: Spectrum, 1976.
21. Fraser R, Glass I. Unilateral and bilateral ECT in elderly patients. A comparative study. *Acta Psychiat Scand* 1980; **62**: 13–31.
22. Prudic J, Haskett RF, Mulsant B *et al.* Resistance to antidepressant medications and short term clinical response to ECT. *Am J Psychiat* 1996; **153**(8): 985–92.
23. Black D, Winokur G, Nasrallah A. Treatment of mania: naturalistic study of electroconvulsive therapy versus lithium in 438 patients. *J Clin Psychiat* 1987; **48**: 132–9.
24. Turek I. Combined use of ECT and psychotropic drugs: antidepressive and antipsychotics. *Comp Psychiat* 1973; **14**: 495–502.
25. Lebensohn Z, Jenkins R. Improvement of Parkinsonism in depressed patients treated with ECT. *Am J Psychiat* 1975; **132**: 283–5.
26. Douyon R, Sorby M, Klutchko B *et al.* ECT and Parkinson's disease revisited: a naturalistic study. *Am J Psychiat* 1989; **146**: 1451–5.
27. Murray G, Shea V, Conn D. Electroconvulsive therapy for post stroke depression. *J Clin Psychiat* 1986; **47**: 258–60.
28. Wells D, Davies G, Rosewarne F. Attenuation of electroconvulsive therapy-induced hypertension with sublingual nifedipine. *Anaes Intens Care* 1989; **17**: 31–3.
29. Kalinowsky L, Hippius H, Klein H. *Biological Treatments in Psychiatry*. New York: Grune and Stratton, 1982.
30. Burd J, Kettl P. The incidence of asystole in electroconvulsive therapy in elderly patients. *Am J Geriat Psychiat* 1998; **6**(3): 203–11.
31. McCall WV. Asystole in electroconvulsive therapy: Report of four cases. *J Clin Psychiat* 1996; **57**(5): 199–203.
32. Fink M. *Convulsive Therapy: Theory and Practice*. New York: Raven, 1979.
33. Barton J, Mahta S, Snaith R. The prophylactic value of extra ECT in depressive illness. *Acta Psychiat Scand* 1973; **49**: 386–92.
34. Weiner R. The role of electroconvulsive therapy in the treatment of depression in the elderly. *J Am Geriat Soc* 1982; **30**: 701–12.
35. Shapira B, Lidsky D, Garfine M, Lever B. Electroconvulsive therapy and resistant depression: clinical implications of seizure threshold. *J Clin Psychiat* 1996; **57**(1): 32–8.
36. Krystal AD, Coffey CF, Weiner RD *et al.* Changes in seizure threshold over the course of electroconvulsive therapy affect therapeutic response and are detected by vital EEG ratings. *J Neuropsychiat Clin Neurosci* 1998; **10**(2): 178–86.
37. Kirkby KC, Beckett WG, Matters RM *et al.* Comparison of propofol and methohexitone in anaesthesia for ECT: effect on seizure duration and outcome. *Aust NZ J Psychiat* 1995; **29**(2): 229–303.
38. Malsch E, Gratz I, Mani S *et al.* Efficacy of electroconvulsive therapy after propofol and methohexital anesthesia. *Convuls Ther* 1994; **10**(3): 212–19.
39. Kelsey MC, Grossberg GT. Safety and efficiency of caffeine-augmented ECT in elderly depressives: a retrospective study. *J Geriat Psychiat Neurol* 1995; **8**(3): 168–72.
40. Haas S, Nash K, Lippmann SB. ECT-induced seizure durations. *J Kentucky Med Assoc* 1996; **94**(6): 233–6.
41. Squire L, Chace P. Memory functions six to nine months after electroconvulsive therapy. *Arch Gen Psychiat* 1975; **32**: 1557–64.
42. Freeman C, Weeks D, Kendall R. ECT: II: Patients who complain. *Br J Psychiat* 1980; **137**: 17–25.
43. Weiner R, Rogers H, Davidson J. Effects of stimulus parameters on cognitive side effects. *Ann NY Acad Sci* 1986; **462**: 315–25.
44. Abrams R, Taylor M. A prospective follow-up study of cognitive functions after ECT. *Convuls Ther* 1985; **1**: 4–9.

45. Summers W, Robins E, Reich T. The natural history of acute organic mental syndrome after bilateral electroconvulsive therapy. *Biol Psychiat* 1979; **14**: 905–12.

46. Jha AK, Stein GS, Fenwick P. Negative interaction between lithium and electroconvulsive therapy—a case-control study. *Br J Psychiat* 1996; **168**(2): 241–3.

47. Benbow SM. Old age psychiatrists' views on the use of ECT. *Int J Geriat Psychiat* 1991; **6**: 317–22.

48. Mirchandani I, Abrams R, Young R, Alexopoulos G. One-year follow-up of continuation convulsive therapy prescribed for depressed elderly patients. *Int J Geriat Psychiat* 1994; **9**: 31–6.

49. Petrides G, Dhossche D, Fink M, Francis A. Continuation ECT: relapse prevention in affective disorders. *Convuls Ther* 1994; **10**: 189–94.

50. Kim E, Zisselman M, Pelchat R. Factors affecting compliance with maintenance electroconvulsive therapy: a preliminary study. *Int J Geriat Psychiat* 1996; **11**: 473–6.

51. Schwarz T, Loewenstein J, Isenberg K. Maintenance ECT: indications and outcome. *Convuls Ther* 1995; **11**: 14–23.

52. Sackeim HA, Prudic J, Devanand DP *et al*. A prospective, randomized, double-blind comparison of bilateral and right unilateral electroconvulsive therapy at different stimulus intensities. *Arch Gen Psychiat* 2000; **57**(5): 425–34.

53. McCall WV, Reboussin DM, Weiner RD, Sackheim HA. Titrated moderately suprathreshold vs fixed high-dose right unilateral electroconvulsive therapy: acute antidepressant and cognitive effects. *Arch Gen Psychiat* 2000; **57**(5): 438–44.

78

Pharmacological Treatment of Depression

Mohammed T. Abou-Saleh

St George's Hospital Medical School, London, UK

A recent review[1] identified mood disorders as a major public health problem, with poor recognition, diagnosis and treatment despite the availability of reasonably safe, effective, economical treatments and the established effectiveness of continuing educational programmes for care providers. The magnitude of the following problems is greater in the elderly with mood disorders: poor recognition for most somatic and cognitive symptoms; increased physical morbidity and disability; and high mortality from suicide and other causes. This situation, however, is balanced by the availability of effective pharmacological treatments, which are successful in two-thirds of patients within few weeks of treatment, who remain well 1 year later. However, the temporal profiles of the course of late-life depression during treatment shows marked variation in rate, stability and direction of recovery with reliable pretreatment predictors of outcome[2]. The usefulness of pharmacological treatment for patients with subsyndromal depression has not, however, been investigated[3].

PRETREATMENT CONSIDERATIONS

There are a number of pretreatment considerations before starting specific pharmacological treatment of mood disorders in the elderly[4,5]. With advancing age, there are important and clinically significant changes in distribution, metabolism and elimination of these drugs[6]. The age-related increase in volume of distribution results in a longer half-life for all psychotropic drugs. Hepatic drug metabolism decreases with age, also resulting in a prolonged half-life, which may be two to three times longer than in younger patients, and the decrease in renal function with advancing age is particularly relevant with regard to lithium, which also results in two to three times higher plasma levels than those in younger patients on the same daily dose. Of particular importance, however, has been the study of the inhibitory effects of the selective serotonin reuptake inhibitors (SSRIs) on the cytochrome p450 enzymes; these pharmacodynamic actions have pharmacokinetic consequences for co-administered drugs, such as tricyclic antidepressants (TCAs), which are dependent on these enzymes for biotransformation.

To determine the best pharmacological treatment options for individual patients requires careful consideration of a number of clinical factors, which include the following: type of mood disorder; degree of urgency for treatment; previous response to treatment; concurrent medical problems; concurrent drug therapy; risk of overdose; reasonable half-life; dosing flexibility, and affordability[7].

TREATMENT OF DEPRESSION

Elderly patients with depression could be successfully treated with conventional TCAs, monoamine oxidase inhibitors (MAOIs), SSRIs and atypical antidepressants. A recent update of the evidence reported the results of 26 RCTs of pharmacological treatments and 21 of these were placebo-controlled. People were recruited mainly from outpatient clinics. Significant benefits were found for fluoxetine, trazodone and phenelzine. Of the 17 drug vs. drug comparisons (mainly involving heterocyclic drugs), none showed significant benefit above the others. In people with depression plus a physical illness vs. placebo, one systematic review of 18 RCTs found that antidepressants were more effective than placebo in people with depression and a physical illness. TCAs have the major limitations of anticholinergic effects, postural hypotension, excessive daytime sedation and cardiotoxicity in overdose. Their advantages, however, are their established efficacy and low cost. A number of recent reviews[4,6,7] identified the secondary amines desipramine and nortriptyline among the TCAs having more favourable side-effect profiles, with desipramine having the fewest anticholinergic effects and nortriptyline causing the least postural hypotension. The secondary amines also have the advantage of therapeutic drug monitoring, with an established therapeutic window for nortriptyline and a therapeutic plasma level of desipramine. Therapeutic drug monitoring enables the clinician to determine the minimal therapeutic dose and to monitor compliance. Nortriptyline has been well investigated for use in elderly patients, including patients older than 80 years[8] and patients who have had strokes[9].

Among the MAOIs, phenelzine has been shown to be effective in treating elderly patients with depression[10,11], particularly for patients who could not tolerate TCAs and those with resistant depression. Their main limitation is their interaction with tyramine-rich foods, causing hypertensive crisis. For this, they are superseded by moclobemide, a reversible and selective inhibitor of monoamine oxidase type A. Comparative trials in the elderly have established its efficacy compared with imipramine[12], nortriptyline[13] and placebo[14]. Moclobemide also showed enhancing effects on cognition in patients who had dementia and depressive symptoms[14].

The SSRIs, however, have provided a major advance in the successful and safe management of depression in late life. These include fluoxetine, fluvoxamine, sertraline, paroxetine and citalopram. The advantages of SSRIs over TCAs are the absence of anticholinergic effects, orthostatic hypotension and arrhythmia in the side-effect profiles, and their safety in overdose[7]. The consensus statement update from the US National Institutes of Health[3] on the diagnosis and treatment of depression in late life concluded that the SSRIs are roughly equivalent to TCAs in

Principles and Practice of Geriatric Psychiatry, 2nd edn. Edited by J. R. M. Copeland, M. T. Abou-Saleh and D. G. Blazer

efficacy in the elderly, with 60–80% of patients responding to treatment. The authors concluded that the efficacy data are not robust when an SSRI is compared with placebo; the only available report from a randomized placebo-controlled trial of fluoxetine in outpatients[15] found a lower drug–placebo difference than that found for many studies with TCAs. Moreover, comparison of fluoxetine with nortriptyline in inpatients with severe depression and heart disease showed that nortriptyline may be more effective in this population[16]. A meta-analysis of the comparative efficacy and safety of SSRIs and TCAs in elderly patients[17] showed no differences in safety and dropout rates.

The side-effects profile of SSRIs includes nausea, diarrhoea, insomnia, headaches, agitation, anxiety and sexual dysfunction. The SSRIs also seem to worsen parkinsonism. As with other antidepressants[18] there have been case reports of hyponatraemia, hypomania and seizures[7]. An important aspect of their use is their drug–drug interactions, and their inhibitory effects on hepatic cytochrome p450 isoenzymes, the route through which many drugs commonly prescribed for elderly people are metabolized[19]. Paroxetine, norfluoxetine and sertraline have clinically important inhibitory effects (in vivo) on cytochrome P2D6, resulting in increased plasma concentrations of co-administered TCAs, such as desipramine, and antipsychotics, such as haloperidol[20]. Sertraline, however, had a modest effect on plasma nortriptyline levels in depressed elderly patients[21]. Fluoxetine increases plasma levels of co-administered carbamazepine; alprazolam and fluvoxamine increase plasma concentration of co-administered TCAs and antipsychotics by inhibiting cytochrome P1A2[9]. An extensive list of drugs metabolized by various p450 isoenzyme types is provided in the reviews by Catterson et al.[5] and Rivard[7].

CONTINUATION AND PROPHYLACTIC TREATMENT

Early studies indicated a poor outcome of late-life depression[25], with high relapse, recurrence and chronicity. This view was based on naturalistic observation without monitoring of compliance, adequate dosage and duration of treatment, including prophylactic treatment, and was therefore challenged[26]. Controlled studies of maintenance antidepressant medication, however, showed better outcome for late-life depression[27]. The Pittsburgh group reported a 3 year follow-up study of maintenance treatment with nortriptyline or placebo with or without interpersonal psychotherapy (IPT)[28] and showed that 80% of patients assigned to nortriptyline, with or without IPT, remained in remission. The Pittsburgh group also identified the elderly patients who remained well after placebo-controlled discontinuation of antidepressant medication for a period of 1 year. Recovery of good subjective sleep quality by early continuation treatment was useful in identifying which remitted elderly depressed patients remained well with monthly IPT after discontinuation of antidepressant medication[29]. Moreover, effective maintenance treatment with nortriptyline was associated with enhancement in the rate of delta-wave production in the first non-rapid eye movement sleep and of rapid movement activity throughout the night[30].

A recent study of the effect of treatment on the 2 year course of late-life depression[31] showed a 74% survival rate without relapse. This good outcome was obtained by the use of full-dose anti-depressant medication, frequent follow-up and rigorous treatment of relapse.

The US National Institute of Mental Health consensus statement update[3] concluded that recent evidence supports the recommendation for at least 6 months of treatment beyond recovery for those with first onset in late life, and for at least 12 months for those with a recurrent illness[32]. Moreover, prophylactic treatment should be of the same type and of same dosage as that which was successful in the initial acute phase. The consensus statement also concluded that treatment response and long-term outcome for all the patients is generally similar to that observed in younger adults, but the temporal course may be somewhat slower in the elderly and risk of relapse somewhat greater[3]. The use of lithium in continuation and prophylactic treatment of depression in the elderly has also been recommended[27,33,34], with the use of lower doses/plasma levels[34]. Lithium may be a more favourable prophylactic treatment than antidepressants in recurrent depression with melancholia and in depression with psychotic features (delusional depression), which are particularly common among the elderly, with a tendency to respond less well to antidepressants[26,34]. The other advantage of lithium therapy is the evident decreased mortality, whether from suicide or other causes[35]. A recent 1 year prospective, placebo-controlled study of maintenance lithium in conjunction with cognitive–behavioural psychotherapy in elderly depressed patients[36] showed that, although cognitive–behavioural psychotherapy reduced depression severity during follow-up, lithium therapy was no better than placebo. This appears to be related to poor compliance, a finding that highlights the serious difficulties in undertaking prophylactic studies in elderly depressed patients.

TREATMENT OF BIPOLAR DISORDER

Elderly patients with late presentation or late-onset mania respond well to standard antimanic treatment with neuroleptics, lithium and anticonvulsants[37]. Neuroleptic treatment is best avoided in the elderly because of its known extrapyramidal side effects, except for floridly psychotic, agitated and behaviourally disturbed patients who need rapid control of symptoms. Lithium remains the treatment of choice, followed by valproic acid[37]. The evidence for the efficacy of lithium in late-life mania is based on retrospective and uncontrolled studies; there have been no controlled studies, and there have been no controlled studies of the efficacy of anticonvulsants in late-life mania. It has been suggested that valproate is a safer alternative treatment to lithium than carbamazepine, whether used as single or adjunct treatment, in elderly manic patients[37]. There are no guidelines regarding the optimal plasma concentration of valproate in relation to efficacy[37].

A recent evidence-based review of the treatment of mania, mixed state and rapid cycling in younger populations[38] concluded that lithium and divalproex sodium are effective in mania, whereas divalproex sodium and carbamazepine are more effective in mixed states. Divalproex sodium is the drug of choice for rapid cycling disorder. With bipolar depression, lithium is recommended as a first-line treatment and the addition of a second mood stabilizer or the TCA would be an appropriate next step[39].

The guidelines for the continuation and prophylactic treatment of bipolar illness in late life are similar to those advocated for younger patients, except for the notion of high recurrence rates necessitating prophylactic treatment, even after a first-onset manic episode. Lithium remains the medication of choice for prophylaxis[34]. An open naturalistic study of lower doses/plasma-lithium levels of lithium[34] showed efficacy in the elderly comparable to that in younger patients at plasma lithium levels as low as 0.4 mmol/l, with fewer side effects and renal and thyroid adverse effects.

TREATMENT-RESISTANT DEPRESSION

Treatment-resistant depression occurs in one-third of elderly depressed patients[40] and can only be ascertained after adequate recognition, compliance with treatment and effective treatment[41].

It has also been related to cognitive impairment, physical and psychiatric co-morbidity, late onset and presence of melancholic and psychotic features[41]. Moreover, elderly patients with anxious depression are less responsive to nortriptyline than are those without significant anxiety symptoms[42].

Although TCAs[16] and MAOIs[43] have shown efficacy, the SSRIs are specifically advocated[41]. Fluvoxamine has shown efficacy (70% good response) in desipramine non-responders[44,45], and patients who were intolerant of fluoxetine completed a trial of sertraline with a response rate of 76%[46]. Efficacy has also been shown for trazodone[47], bupropion[48] and venlafaxine[49]. Combination and augmentation strategies have been advocated[41]. Lithium augmentation in TCA non-responders is effective in 20–65% of cases[50–52]. It is, however, conducive to cognitive and neurological side effects in 50% of patients[50,51,53,54]. Lithium has been successfully added to SSRIs, notwithstanding the risk of neurotoxicity with an SSRI–lithium combination[41]. Advocated augmentation/combination strategies includes TCA/triodo-thyronine; SSRI/TCA; SSRI/anticonvulsants; and SSRI/oestrogen[41], and elderly patients requiring adjunctive medication to achieve remission may need continuation of adjunctive medication to remain well and to avoid early relapse[55].

For refractory bipolar disorders, a recent review[56] concluded that the safest combination of mood stabilizers is valproate plus lithium. This was also shown in a series of elderly patients with lithium-resistant rapid cycling mania[57].

CONCLUSION

Although there have been impressive advances in the pharmacological treatment of mood disorders in general, there has been a relative paucity of controlled studies in the elderly, particularly in maintenance and prophylaxis. Generalization from the results of studies of younger patients may be inappropriate in view of the significant changes associated with normal ageing and concomitant medical illness, which affect the pharmacokinetics and pharmacodynamics of psychotropic drugs.

Nevertheless, there has been a change of culture. The nihilism that had prevailed in the treatment of mood disorders in late life has been replaced by cautious optimism with regard to the results of controlled trials in naturalistic settings, as well as studies in high-risk groups, including patients with multiple medical conditions and subsyndromal states.

A large majority of elderly patients with depression could be treated successfully with antidepressants, particularly the SSRIs, because of their favourable side-effect profiles and their low toxicity in overdose. The SSRIs, however, challenge the clinician with their clinically significant drug–drug interactions. Patients who improve should receive continuation of prophylactic treatment with the same dose. For mania, lithium remains the optimal treatment, with anticonvulsants, particularly divaloproex, providing a second-line treatment. The efficacy and safety of atypical neuroleptics remain to be evaluated in both acute and long-term management of bipolar illness. There is also hope for those with resistant-mood disorders with the design of augmentation/combination strategies, which require further evaluation.

REFERENCES

1. Bland RC. Epidemiology of affective disorders: a review. *Can J Psychiat* 1997; **42**: 367–77.
2. Dew MA, Reynolds CF III, Houck PR *et al*. Temporal profiles of the course of depression during treatment. *Arch Gen Psychiat* 1997; **54**: 1016–24.
3. Lebowitz BD, Pearson JL, Schneider LS *et al*. Diagnosis and treatment of depression in late life: consensus statement update. *J Am Med Assoc* 1997; **278**: 1186–90.
4. Salzman C, DuRand C. Pharmacological treatment of depression. In Copeland JRM, Abou-Saleh MT, Blazer D, eds, *Principles and Practice of Geriatric Psychiatry* 1st edn. Chichester: Wiley, 1994: 575–80.
5. Catterson ML, Preskorn SH, Martin RM. Pharmacodynamic and pharmacokinetic considerations in geriatric psychopharmacology. *Geriat Psychiat* 1997; **20**: 205–19.
6. Hermann N, Bremner EK, Naranjo CA. Pharmacotherapy of late life mood disorders. *Clin Neurosci* 1997; **4**: 41–7.
7. Rivard MFT. Pharmacotherapy of affective disorders in old age. *Can J Psychiat* 1997; **42**(suppl 1): 10–18S.
8. Salzman C, Schneider L, Alexopoulos G. Pharmacological treatment of depression in late life. In Bloom F, Kupfer D, eds, *Psychopharmacology: the Fourth General of Progress*. New York: Raven, 1995; 1771–7.
9. Robinson RG, Morris PH, Fedoroff JP. Depression and cerebrovascular disease. *J Clin Psychiat* 1990; **51**: 26–33.
10. Georgotas A, McCue RE, Hapworth W *et al*. Comparative efficacy and safety of MAOI vs. TCAs in treating depression in the elderly. *Biol Psychiat* 1986; **21**: 1155–66.
11. Lazarus LW, Groves L, Gierl B *et al*. Efficacy of phenelzine in geriatric depression. *Biol Psychiat* 1986; **21**: 699–701.
12. Pancheri P, Delle CR, Donnini M *et al*. Effects of moclobemide on depressive symptoms and cognitive performance in a geriatric population: a controlled comparative study vs. imipramine. *Clin Neuropharmacol* 1994; **17**(suppl 1): 58S–73S.
13. Nair NP, Amin M, Holm P *et al*. Moclobemide and nortriptyline in elderly depressed patients: a randomised multicentre trial against placebo. *J Affect Disord* 1995; **33**: 1–9.
14. Roth M, Mountjoy CQ, Amrein R. The International Collaborative Study Group. Moclobemide placebo-controlled trial. *Br J Psychiat* 1996; **16**: 149–57.
15. Tollefson GD, Holman SL. Analysis of the Hamilton Depression Rating Scale factors from a double-blind, placebo-controlled trial of fluoxetine in geriatric major depression. *Int Clin Psychopharmacol* 1993; **8**: 253–9.
16. Roose SP, Glassman AH, Attia E, Woodring S. Comparative efficacy of selective serotonin reuptake inhibitors and tricyclics in the treatment of melancholia. *Am J Psychiat* 1994; **151**: 1735–9.
17. Mittmann N, Shear NH, Busto VE *et al*. Comparative evaluation of the efficacy and safety of tricyclic antidepressants and serotonin reuptake inhibitors in the elderly: a meta-analysis. *Clin Invest Med* 1994; **18**: B53.
18. Spigset O, Hedenmalm K. Hyponatremia in relation to treatment with antidepressants: a survey of reports in the World Health Organization database for spontaneous reporting of adverse drug reactions. *Pharmacotherapy* 1997; **17**: 348–52.
19. Nemeroff CB, DeVane CL, Pollock BG. Newer antidepressants and the cytochrome P450 system. *Am J Psychiat* 1996; **153**: 311–20.
20. Preskorn SH. Reducing the risk of drug–drug interactions: a goal of rational drug development. *J Clin Psychiat* 1996; **57**(suppl 1): 3–6S.
21. Solai LK, Mulsant BH, Pollock BG *et al*. Effect of sertraline on plasma nortriptyline levels in depressed elderly. *J Clin Psychiat* 1997; **58**: 440–43.
22. Volz HP, Moller HJ. Antidepressant drug therapy in the elderly: a critical review of controlled clinical trials conducted since 1980. *Pharmacopsychiatry* 1994; **27**: 93–100.
23. Mahapatra SN, Hackett D. A randomised double-blind, parallel-group comparison of venlafaxine and dothiepin in geriatric patients with major depression. *Int J Clin Pract* 1997; **51**: 209–13.
24. Fontaine R, Ontiveros A, Elie R *et al*. A double-blind comparison of nefazodone, imipramine and placebo in major depression. *J Clin Psychiat* 1994; **55**: 234–41.
25. Murphy E. The prognosis of depression and response to anti-depressive therapies. *Br J Psychiat* 1983; **142**: 111–19.
26. Abou-Saleh MT, Coppen A. Classification of depression and response to anti-depressive therapies. *Br J Psychiat* 1983; **143**: 601–3.
27. Stoudemire A. Recurrence and relapse in geriatric depression: a review of risk factors and prophylactic treatment strategies. *J Neuropsychiat* 1997; **9**: 209–21.

28. Reynolds CF. Treatment of depression in late life. *Am J Med* 1994; **97**(suppl 6A): 39–46S.

29. Reynolds CF III, Frank E, Houck PR *et al*. Which elderly patients with remitted depression remain well with continued interpersonal psychotherapy after discontinuation of antidepressant medication? *Am J Psychiat* 1997; **154**: 958–62.

30. Reynolds CF III, Buysse DJ, Brunner DP *et al*. Maintenance nortriptyline effects on electroencephalographic sleep in elderly patients with recurrent major depression: double-blind, placebo- and plasma level-controlled evaluation. *Soc Biol Psychiat* 1997; **42**: 560–67.

31. Flint AJ, Rifat SL. The effect of treatment on the two-year course of late-life depression. *Br J Psychiat* 1997; **170**: 268–72.

32. Reynolds CF, Frank E, Perel J *et al*. Maintenance therapies for late life recurrent major depression: research and review circa 1995. *Int Psychogeriat* 1995; **7**(suppl): 27–40.

33. Coppen A, Abou-Saleh MT. Lithium therapy: from clinical trials to practical management. *Acta Psychiat Scand* 1988; **78**: 759–62.

34. Abou-Saleh MT. Long-term management of affective disorder. In Copeland JRM, Abou-Saleh MT, Blazer DG, eds, *Principles and Practice of Geriatric Psychiatry* 1st edn. Chichester: Wiley, 1994; 587–96.

35. Coppen A. Depression as a lethal disease: prevention strategies. *J Clin Psychiat* 1994; **55**(suppl): 37–45.

36. Wilson KCM, Scott M, Abou-Saleh MT *et al*. Long-term effects of cognitive–behavioural therapy and lithium therapy on depression in the elderly. *Br J Psychiat* 1995; **167**: 653–8.

37. Young RC. Bipolar mood disorders in the elderly. *Geriat Psychiat* 1997; **20**: 121–36.

38. Kusumakar V, Yatham LN, Haslam DRS *et al*. Treatment of mania, mixed state, and rapid cycling. *Can J Psychiat* 1997; **42**(suppl 2): 79–86S.

39. Yatham LN, Kusumakar V, Parikh SV *et al*. Bipolar depression: treatment options. *Can J Psychiat* 1997; **42**(suppl 2): 87–91S.

40. Goff DC, Jenike MA. Treatment-resistant depression in the elderly. *J Am Geriat Soc* 1986; **34**: 63–70.

41. Kamholz BA, Mellow AM. Management of treatment resistance in the depressed geriatric patient. *Psychiat Clin N Am* 1997; **19**: 269–87.

42. Flint AJ, Rifat SL. Anxious depression in elderly patients. Response to antidepressant treatment. *Am J Geriat Psychiat* 1997; **5**: 107–15.

43. Georgotas A, Friedman E, McCarthy M *et al*. Resistant geriatric depressions and therapeutic response to monoamine oxidase inhibitors. *Biol Psychiat* 1983; **18**: 195–205.

44. Delgado PL, Price LH, Charney DS, Heninger GR. Efficacy of fluvoxamine in treatment-refractory depression. *J Affect Disord* 1988; **15**: 55–60.

45. White K, Wykoff W, Tynes LL *et al*. Fluvoxamine in the treatment of tricyclic resistant depression. *Psychiat J Univ Ottawa* 1990; **15**: 156–8.

46. Brown WA, Harrison W. Are patients who are intolerant to one SSRI intolerant to another? *Psychopharmacol Bull* 1992; **28**: 253–6.

47. Cole JO, Schatzberg AF, Sniffin C *et al*. Trazodone in treatment-resistant depression: an open study. *J Clin Psychopharmacol* 1981; **1**(suppl): 49–54.

48. Ferguson J, Cunningham L, Meredith C *et al*. Bupropion in tricyclic antidepressant non-responders with unipolar major depressive disorder. *Ann Clin Psychiat* 1994; **6**: 153–60.

49. Nierenberg AA, Feighner JP, Rudolph R *et al*. Venlafaxine for treatment-resistant unipolar depression. *J Clin Psychopharmacol* 1994; **14**: 419–23.

50. Finch EJL, Katona CIE. Lithium augmentation in the treatment of refractory depression in old age. *Int J Geriat Psychiat* 1989; **4**: 41–6.

51. Flint AJ. Recent developments in geriatric psychopharmacotherapy. *Can J Psychiat* 1994; **39**(suppl 1): S9–S18.

52. Zimmer B, Rosen J, Thornton JE *et al*. Adjunctive lithium carbonate in nortriptyline-resistant elderly depressed patients. *J Clin Psychopharmacol* 1991; **11**: 254–6.

53. Flint AJ, Rifat SL. A prospective study of lithium augmentation in antidepressant-resistant geriatric depression. *J Clin Psychopharmacol* 1994; **14**: 353–6.

54. Lafferman J, Solomon K, Ruskin P. Lithium augmentation for treatment-resistant depression in the elderly. *J Geriat Psychiat Neurol* 1998; **1**: 49–52.

55. Reynolds CF III, Frank E, Perel JM *et al*. High relapse rate after discontinuation of adjunctive medication for elderly patients with recurrent major depression. *Am J Psychiat* 1996; **153**: 1418–22.

56. Freeman MP, Stott AL. Mood stabiliser combinations: a review of safety and efficacy. *Am J Psychiat* 1998; **155**: 12–21.

57. Schneider AL, Wilcox CS. Divalproate augmentation in lithium-resistant rapid cycling mania in four geriatric patients. *J Affect Disord* 1998; **47**: 201–5.

Treatment-resistant Depression

Alastair J. Flint

Toronto General Hospital, Toronto, Ontario, Canada

Treatment resistance is a common clinical problem, reported in up to one-third of older depressed patients[1]. Many patients labelled as "treatment-resistant" in fact have not had an adequate course of treatment[2]. Therefore, the first step in achieving remission of depressive symptoms is to ensure that the patient has been given, and has complied with, an optimum dose of antidepressant for a sufficient length of time (at least 6 weeks). In treatment-resistant depression, it is also important to investigate the patient for unidentified physical conditions (such as hypothyroidism, vitamin B_{12} or folate deficiency, or hypercalcemia) that could be contributing to poor antidepressant response[2].

In patients who have failed to respond to an adequate trial of antidepressant medication, the following options can be considered: (a) augment the antidepressant with another drug that is not primarily an antidepressant, such as lithium, triiodothyronine, methylphenidate, pindolol, buspirone or valproate; (b) add a second antidepressant to the first (combination therapy), e.g. add

a tricyclic antidepressant (TCA) or bupropion to a selective serotonin-reuptake inhibitor (SSRI); (c) switch to a different antidepressant medication; or (d) switch to electroconvulsive therapy (ECT). The advantage of augmentation or combination therapy is that they do not require discontinuation of the original antidepressant and, therefore, patients who have partially responded to treatment are not put at risk of returning to their baseline severity of depression. Also, response may at times be faster with augmentation/combination than with a new trial of antidepressant medication. The disadvantage of these strategies, especially in older people, is that the combination of medications increases the risk of side effects and drug–drug interactions. Also, there have been no placebo-controlled trials of augmentation or combination therapy in elderly depressed patients and so their efficacy has not yet been established in this population[2,3].

There are virtually no research data on switching from one antidepressant medication to another in refractory geriatric depression. Flint and Rifat[4] found that seven of 15 elderly patients (47%) who had failed to respond to 6 weeks of nortriptyline followed by 2 weeks of lithium augmentation subsequently responded to a 6 week trial of phenelzine. This rate of response is comparable to that reported among younger patients refractory to TCAs[5]. Data obtained from mixed-aged patients with resistant depression suggest that switching to an antidepressant within the same class is less effective than switching to one from another class[5]. If a patient has failed to respond to an SSRI or nefazodone, then switching to an antidepressant with dual neurotransmitter action (e.g. venlafaxine, mirtazapine or nortriptyline) is a reasonable approach.

Although substitution of treatment usually involves switching from one antidepressant medication to another, switching from an antidepressant to ECT should also be considered. The efficacy of ECT in patients who have failed to respond to adequate antidepressant pharmacotherapy is lower than in patients without established medication resistance[6]. Nevertheless, no antidepressant, alone or in combination, has been shown to be more effective than ECT in treatment-resistant depression and ECT remains a valuable option in this situation.

REFERENCES

1. Schneider LS. Pharmacologic considerations in the treatment of late-life depression. *Am J Geriat Psychiat* 1996; **4**(suppl 1): S51–65.
2. Mulsant BH, Pollock BG. Treatment-resistant depression in late life. *J Geriat Psychiat Neurol* 1998; **11**: 186–93.
3. Flint AJ. Augmentation strategies in geriatric depression. *Int J Geriat Psychiat* 1995; **10**: 137–46.
4. Flint AJ, Rifat SL. The effect of sequential antidepressant treatment on geriatric depression. *J Affect Disord* 1996; **36**: 95–105.
5. Thase ME, Rush AJ, Kasper S, Nemeroff CB. Tricyclics and newer antidepressant medications: treatment options for treatment-resistant depressions. *Depression* 1994/1995, **2**: 152–68.
6. Prudic J, Haskett RF, Mulsant B *et al*. Resistance to antidepressant medications and short-term clinical response to ECT. *Am J Psychiat* 1996; **153**: 985–92.

79

Psychotherapy of Depression and Dysthymia

Thomas R. Lynch[1] **and Christine M. Vitt**[2]

[1]*Duke University Medical Center and* [2]*Duke University, Durham, NC, USA*

BACKGROUND

Depression in the elderly is a treatable disorder. Although antidepressant medication has traditionally been considered a first-line intervention, psychotherapy has been shown to be *at least* equally effective[1-3]. The NIH Consensus Development Conference on Diagnosis and Treatment of Depression in Late Life concluded that psychotherapy was an important treatment option for elderly depression, although not sufficient by itself[4-6]. This conclusion has been challenged in the literature, with reviews of psychotherapy research finding a powerful effect of psychotherapy alone on depression as compared to wait-list controls[1,3,7]. Additional research on the combination of medication and psychotherapy for elderly depression has shown promising results for both acute treatment and relapse prevention[8]. Less is known about the treatment of dysthymic disorder, although its similarities to major depressive disorder suggest that aggressive treatment is the most powerful treatment option.

This chapter reviews the theoretical elements and empirical evidence supporting the use of psychotherapy to treat elderly depression. First, we examine special issues associated with treating elderly depression using psychotherapy. Next, we review the theoretical foundations and evidence for the use of psychotherapy with older adults, including cognitive-behavioral, psychodynamic, interpersonal and group interventions. Finally, we examine recent theoretical developments and research that have addressed problems associated with relapse prevention, treatment-resistant depression, and co-morbid personality disorders.

SPECIAL ISSUES IN PSYCHOTHERAPY WITH OLDER PATIENTS

Psychotherapy is a particularly useful option for depressed patients who cannot or will not tolerate medication, or who are dealing with stressful conditions, interpersonal difficulties, limited levels of social support and/or recurrent episodes of depression[6,8,9]. Although it has been established that psychotherapy and medication are effective treatments for major depression, there is a sizeable literature highlighting the underdiagnosis and undertreatment of late-life depression[10-16]. Consequently, millions of older persons deserving of mental health care go untreated[17]. Friedhoff[14] indicated that only 10% of older adults in need of psychiatric services actually receive professional care and there

has been minimal utilization of mental health services in this age group[16,18,19].

Under Diagnosis

Older adults are more likely to see general practitioners than mental health professionals, essentially leaving the responsibility for diagnosis of late-life depression in primary care. Although physicians are more likely than mental health professionals to see depressed older adults, this does not mean that elderly patients will purposefully present with depressive symptoms. Studies have shown that up to 75% of older adults who complete suicide had seen their physician in the previous month, emphasizing the important role general practitioners play in diagnosing clinical depression[20]. In a non-depressed community sample of 462 older adults, 40% indicated they would keep depressive symptoms to themselves and not report them to anyone[21]. Of those who would seek help, over half (52%) indicated they would talk to their regular doctor. Allen *et al.*[22] surveyed attitudes toward treatments for depression in older and younger inpatients. The older group, particularly those identified as depressed, was less likely to approach anyone for help. In addition, the older adults had more negative attitudes about approaching their physician than the younger group.

Hesitation to seek help for mental health problems should not be considered unfounded. Link and colleagues[23] have identified a social stigma associated with undergoing treatment for psychiatric dysfunction. However, treatment outcome research suggests that gains in well-being likely outweigh any stigma associated with the disorder. Hence, coming to an understanding of the origins of these attitudes may assist in developing educational interventions addressing the needs of this age group.

This descriptive research highlights several issues of concern for the diagnosis of depression. First, general practitioners typically bear the responsibility for the diagnosis of depression in their older patients, despite the possibility that patients may not feel comfortable about discussing depressive symptoms with others. Making this more difficult have been reports that older patients may not recognize that they have symptoms, or may pass off symptoms as signs of other physical conditions[10]. Second, not all older patients regularly see general practitioners. For these older adults, informal resources (family, friends, religious sources) are left with the responsibility of identifying changes in moods and the need for professional intervention. Third, psychiatrists and psychologists have greater expertise for accurate diagnosis, yet typically only encounter a potential patient after referral from a general practitioner. In addition, mental health professionals specializing in work with geriatric populations are still in the minority and most training programs for both psychology and medicine do not emphasize geriatric mental heath issues. This only exacerbates the factors that make recognition less likely to occur[24,25]. In order for improvements in detection to occur, all three areas discussed above will need to be addressed. Physicians will need to enhance their ability to detect depressive symptoms and make quick treatment decisions during increasingly short office visits. Relatives and other informal sources of referral will require greater education regarding depressive symptoms and encouragement to report those symptoms. Finally, a greater number of mental health professionals will need to obtain specific training in geriatric issues and increase their visibility among potential referral sources.

Under Treatment

Ideally, if the dilemma of underdiagnosis of late-life depression could be resolved, under treatment would not be a problem. However, this does not appear to be the case. Research indicates that even cases that are diagnosed are not necessarily treated. Koenig et al.[13] reported that 34% of hospitalized medically ill elderly patients with a diagnosis of depression in their charts were not treated with antidepressant medication during their inpatient stay or during a 45 week follow-up period, neither were these patients referred to psychotherapy. Only 12.4% of the sample had documented psychotherapeutic intervention in their medical charts at discharge[13]. Thus, not only does recognition appear to be a difficulty, but under-treatment as well. The question is why?

Many practitioners assume that older adults have negative attitudes toward psychotherapy as a treatment for depression. However, research on attitudes toward treatment in elderly samples is not conclusive, with considerable descriptive research suggesting that older adults may prefer counseling over medica-tion treatment for depression. Sixty-eight percent of the previously mentioned non-depressed community-dwelling older adult sample agreed with a statement that professional counseling or therapy helps most depressed people feel better. Interestingly, 56% of the same sample reported that they believed antidepres-sant medications to be addictive, and only 4% disagreed[21]. Older adults have also been shown to report a greater number of positive attitudes toward mental health professionals, and to be less concerned with stigma attached to seeking treatment for depression relative to younger adults[26]. On the other hand, Allen et al.[22] found attitudinal barriers to treatment in a survey of both younger adult and older adult inpatient samples. However, in the older sample, the pattern of preference for counseling and psychotherapy over medication persisted, with 95% of the older group agreeing that "people with depression should be offered counseling", and 46% agreeing that "people with depression should be treated with antidepressant tablets"[22]. Hence, it appears that interventions addressing these issues must educate practi-tioners to evaluate their assumptions about elderly preferences for treatment, as well as educate older and younger adults about available treatment options.

PSYCHODYNAMIC THERAPY

This type of treatment is based on psychoanalytic theory that views current interpersonal and emotional experience as influenced by early childhood experience. This experience results in the development of a complex inner world shaped by both unconscious and conscious mental processes. There have been a variety of theoretical formulations developed over the years that have utilized a psychodynamic formulation to treat depression, including classic psychoanalytic theory[27], ego-psychology[28], self-psychology[29] and object-relations theory[30]. Revised conceptuali-zations have emphasized understanding how relationships are internalized and transformed into a sense of self[29–32]. Because early interactions with caregivers are so tied up with emotional gratification and deprivation, the interaction with mother is viewed as a template for all subsequent relationships. Psycho-pathology is theorized as related to arrests in the development of the self and depression is viewed as a symptom state resulting from unresolved intrapsychic conflict, which may be activated by life events such as loss.

There have been several indications in the geriatric depression literature that short-term psychodynamic therapy, particularly as conducted by Thompson, Gallagher-Thompson and collea-gues[33,34], is an effective means to treat depression in older samples. In studies with random assignment to wait-list control, short-term psychodynamic therapy or cognitive-behavioral ther-apy, there were no significant differences between the types of psychotherapy at the end of treatment or at 12 and 24 month follow-ups. Additional research on depressed caregivers demon-strated an interaction between mode of therapy and length of caregiving, such that those who had been providing care for less than 44 months appeared to improve more from dynamic therapy, whereas longer-term caregivers seemed to benefit most from CBT[35]. The authors suggested that the long-term caregivers needed the skills learned in CBT in order to care for family members with more pronounced deficits and requiring more complicated care. These interesting results call for additional controlled trials comparing different treatment modalities, con-tinued component analysis research, and continued research that examines which type of treatment works best with which type of patient.

LIFE REVIEW AND REMINISCENCE THERAPY

Life review and reminiscence therapies are psychoanalytically orientated approaches to psychotherapy for depression. Life review therapy includes a review of life experiences in order to revisit and resolve old conflicts and reintegrate life experiences[36,37]. Conflicts emerge in interviews about past life experiences, in both acknowledgment and omission. Reminiscence therapy differs from life review in that the focus is on enhancing self-esteem and social intimacy by recounting past experiences, rather than directly resolving past conflicts[2,38]. Lewis and Butler[37] suggest several techniques to encourage elderly clients to participate in the life review process. Written and taped autobiographies, pil-grimages to the place of childhood, reunions, scrapbooks and photographs are tools that can stimulate past memories. A crucial component of any life review therapy is careful, attentive listening on the part of the therapist[36,38].

Results on empirical research of life review and reminiscence therapies are promising, but inconsistent. Teri and McCurry[2] reviewed 12 empirical studies using reminiscence techniques. Results were mixed, likely due to the range of patient populations (institutionalized, homebound, community-dwell-ing), treatment duration (1–10 sessions), type of therapy (group, individual) and diagnosis (major depression, no diag-nosed psychopathology). Also, the distinction between life review and reminiscence therapy has not been clearly operation-ally defined, resulting in an ambiguous designation of the differences between the two therapies.

Research does suggest that the amount of structure in reminiscence therapy may influence outcome[39]. Fry[39] compared individual structured reminiscence therapy, non-structured reminiscence and non-reminiscence visits in a sample of moderately depressed elderly. Subjects in the non-reminiscence control group had significantly higher post-treatment depression scores than those in either reminiscence group; the subjects in the structured reminiscence groups had lower depression scores than those in the unstructured reminiscence groups. Reminiscence group therapy has also been tested in nursing home residents with dementia and has been found to reduce self-reported symptoms of depression to a greater degree than subjects in supportive therapy or control groups[40]. However, the therapy did not improve cognitive or behavioral outcomes, and the reduction in depression was short-lived[40]. Rattenbury and Stones[41] found that both reminiscence and current event discussion groups showed positive changes on measures of psychological well-being when compared to non-treatment controls. However, because subjects were not selected for high depression scores, this was not an empirical test of treatment for *clinical depression*. Yet the results do suggest that there is something beneficial about client-focused interaction, a fundamental component of any form of psychotherapy.

INTERPERSONAL PSYCHOTHERAPY

Interpersonal psychotherapy (IPT) is a manualized, time-limited outpatient treatment for depression, focusing on current interpersonal issues in four problem areas: interpersonal disputes, role transitions, interpersonal deficits and abnormal grief[42]. The therapist and client collaborate to identify which problem area to focus on in treatment; commonly, more than one problem area is chosen. Klerman *et al.*[42] pointed out that, regardless of the origin of depression (genetic, biochemical, developmental vulnerability, personality), the condition is expressed within an interpersonal context. The initial goal of therapy is to reduce symptoms of depression, but the overarching goal is to improve the patient's social functioning and interpersonal relationships[43]. With its emphasis on addressing interpersonally relevant problems, IPT appears particularly well suited to the life changes that many older people experience. Techniques utilized in treatment include: role playing, communication analysis, clarification of the patient's wants and needs, and links between affect and environmental events[44]. Frank and colleagues[45] have developed separate treatment manuals for IPT in late life (IPT-LL) and interpersonal maintenance therapy for older patients (IPT-LLM) (cited in ref 44). These manuals include adaptations specific for use in elderly patients, including, but not limited to, flexibility in length of sessions, long-standing role disputes, and the need to help the patient with practical problems.

Controlled trials in adult depressed populations have demonstrated the efficacy of IPT for the treatment of acute depression (reviewed in refs 43, 44). IPT has also been found as effective in the acute treatment of major depressive disorder in elderly patients as nortriptyline[46]. Of additional importance were findings that elderly patients in IPT treatment were less likely to drop out of treatment than those taking nortriptyline, because of the medication's side effects.

Research from the Reynolds group at the University of Pittsburgh has shown IPT in combination with nortriptyline to be an effective treatment for elderly depression in geriatric samples[47,48]. In an attempt to understand more regarding the treatment of elderly patients with recurrent depression, Reynolds *et al.*[47] selected patients only if they reported at least one prior episode of depression. The authors reported that 78.4%

(116/148) remitted during the acute phase of treatment (8–14 weeks). During the continuation phase, 15.5% (18/116) experienced relapse of major depression; thus, a total of 66.2% patients recovered fully[47,48]. Consequently, the authors concluded that older patients with recurrent major depression can successfully be treated with a combination of antidepressant medication and interpersonal psychotherapy, and that older patients respond as well, albeit more slowly, than middle-aged patients[49].

COGNITIVE-BEHAVIORAL THERAPY

The cognitive model of depression[50] is based on the notion that, as a consequence of early learning, depressed individuals develop stable cognitive schemas or core beliefs which predispose them to negative interpretations of life events (i.e. cognitive distortions). This distorted style of thinking is hypothesized to result in depressive behavior and experience.

Cognitive-behavioral interventions for depression typically involve three active components. First is a behavioral activation component, in which the patient is exhorted to increase activities that are reinforcing, and thus increase the amount of pleasurable experience in life. Second, automatic dysfunctional thoughts are identified, explored, challenged and replaced with more accurate cognition, based on a thorough assessment of the patient's contextual environment. Third, underlying cognitive schemas or structures, which are hypothesized to drive automatic cognitive distortions and limit access to experiences that may alter these schemas, are identified and altered to more accurately reflect the patient's actual environmental, social and personal experience. Recent component analysis research suggests that behavioral activation and automatic thought modification are equally effective, and both components together are no more effective in preventing relapse than when used alone[51,52].

More purely behavioral interventions are derived from classic learning theory, in which problem behaviors are viewed as the result of specific antecedent stimuli and consequential events that reinforce, punish or maintain behavioral responses[53]. This therapeutic approach views depression as a state in which there is a relative shift toward an increase in certain aversive affective reactions (respondent processes) and a concomitant reduction in the frequency of overt activities (operant extinction or punishment). In addition, histories of pervasive inescapable punishment, reinforcement of distressed behavior, classically conditioned dysphoric responses, and the evocative salience of certain stimuli depending on mood, may be examined as part of a functional analysis of depressed behavior[53,54]. For example, a previously active person suffering from a serious illness may experience a reduction in the frequency of self-esteem-generating activities and positive social contacts, as well as increased dependency on others for the provision of positive reinforcers, and may feel bored, helpless and pessimistic. Restoration of the predictability and availability of positive reinforcers, and reduction in negative reinforcers (i.e. avoidance behaviors), is seen as linked to the curative process, with goals of symptom reduction and increased skill at identifying and obtaining appropriate reinforcement. Techniques used might include monitoring behavior and affect patterns, assigning pleasant events, stimulus control, limiting worry and depressive ruminations with time limits, behavioral exposure, and skills training (relaxation, problem-solving, interpersonal skills).

A related therapy for elderly depression, which utilizes elements associated with both cognitive and behavioral interventions described above, examines problems associated with social problem solving. Social problem-solving therapy (PST) is based on a model in which ineffective coping under stress is hypothesized to lead to a breakdown of problem-solving abilities and subsequent depression[55,56]. Therapeutic approaches involve identifying and modifying maladaptive beliefs or attitudes associated with ineffective problem-solving while increasing motivation to generate alternative solutions, make decisions, implement solutions and assess solution utility.

Outcome studies have supported the use of cognitive and behavioral psychotherapy in treatment of depression in elderly samples (see reviews[1,7,33,57]). In a study comparing cognitive, behavioral and brief psychodynamic therapy to wait-list controls, Thompson et al.[33] found that all of the treatment modalities led to comparable and clinically significant reductions of depression. All three treatment regimens included individual treatment twice weekly for 4 weeks and weekly thereafter, totaling 16–20 sessions. Overall, 52% of the sample attained complete remission after treatment, and 18% showed significant improvement, with some enduring depressive symptoms. These rates are comparable to treatment outcomes in younger adult populations and response to pharmacotherapy[33,58]. Follow-up research indicated that at 12 months after treatment 58% of the sample was depression-free, and at 24 months 70% of the sample was not depressed. As in acute treatment, there were no differences between treatment modalities at follow-up[34], although in previous research with a smaller sample size depressed geriatric patients in cognitive and behavioral therapies maintained the gains longer than those treated in brief psychodynamic therapy[59]. Arean et al.[60] examined the efficacy of PST in a randomized controlled trial of 74 clinically depressed older adults (age 55 and over). Patients were assigned to one of three treatment conditions: problem-solving therapy (PST); reminiscence therapy (RT); or a waiting-list control. Following 12 weekly sessions, both therapies showed significant reductions in depressive symptoms at post-treatment and at a 3 month follow-up, relative to controls. However, PST showed a significantly greater number of patients, compared to RT, who were classified as improved or in remission following treatment.

Subsequent research on the same sample used in the Thompson[33] study examined the role of change expectancies relative to outcome[61]. Of those who were assigned to cognitive therapy, subjects who originally indicated that they expected a change from cognitive and behavioral processes attained greater improvement. In addition, some elderly patients, more familiar with the "doctor takes care of patient" mentality pervasive in medicine, may not be accustomed to the hard work involved on the part of the patients for the success of cognitive-behavioral therapy. Thompson et al.[62] recommend addressing such views directly, while helping the patient to gain insight into how his/her thoughts influence mood and how new skills can help in coping with stressful events and automatic thoughts.

GROUP INTERVENTIONS

Group therapy has been shown efficacious for depression in adult samples[63] and in geriatric samples[64]. Non-specific treatment factors that may influence positive outcomes include diffusing dependence on individual therapists, as well as providing a supportive social network. In addition, with the relative dearth of coverage for mental health care among many insurance providers, and the relative lack of parity for mental health care in Medicare, the lower cost of group therapy may be a more appealing option in older patient populations.

Beutler and colleagues[64] tested the relative and combined effectiveness of alprazolam and group cognitive therapy in a sample of 56 depressed older adults. Subjects were assigned to one of four groups: alprazolam and weekly management sessions; placebo and weekly management sessions; cognitive therapy plus alprazolam; and management and cognitive therapy plus placebo. The cognitive therapy groups were held in 12 weekly 90 min sessions. Patients in group therapy showed a significant and consistent decline in BDI scores, while those not in group therapy failed to produce significant changes. Also, a significantly higher proportion of those in group cognitive therapy were asymptomatic at the end of follow-up (29% vs. 12%). Although the results indicate that the cognitive therapy group was more effective in reducing depressive symptoms than alprazolam, this drug (a type of benzodiazepine) is not a recommended medication for depression. However, it appears that benzodiazepines remain a relatively commonly prescribed medication in medical practice. In a sample of depressed inpatients at a large university medical center during 1993–1996, 25% of patients diagnosed with depression by a geriatric psychiatrist were prescribed only benzodiazepines by their physicians[13]. Koenig et al.[13] also found that newer and older antidepressants were prescribed with the same frequency, suggesting that the prescribing practices of many physicians do not include the newer, safer antidepressants. Despite the fact that benzodiazepines are still used in clinical practice for depression, a revised research project using one of the newer antidepressants in Beutler's design would be informative for today's clinicians.

Steuer et al.[65] investigated cognitive-behavioral therapy (CBT) and psychodynamic group therapy in a sample of 33 depressed elders. The investigators assigned members to each condition on the basis of time entering the study and did not include a control group in their study design. Both treatment groups evidenced significant clinical improvement over 9 months of therapy. Of the 13 subjects who dropped out of treatment before the end of the 9-month period, 10 showed improvements in depression on the HAM-D, with mean improvement being 34%. There were no differences between treatments on the clinician-rated Hamilton Rating Scale (HAM-D), although the CBT group had lower scores on the self-report Beck Depression Inventory (BDI).

Lynch et al.[66] have reported unpublished pilot work using dialectical behavior therapy (DBT) skills training to treat elderly depression. Twenty-seven participants were randomly assigned to DBT skills training plus medication or medication alone plus clinical management. All participants were on antidepressant medication and all met criteria for MDD at baseline. DBT included weekly 2 h group skills training and weekly half-hour telephone check-in calls by a therapist for 28 weeks. Approximately 29% of the sample met strict criteria for a SCID-II diagnosis of personality disorder. Although there was a trend for DBT patients to show lower desires to please others from pre- to post-treatment relative to medication alone, there were no significant differences between treatments on outcome measures. Both DBT and medication alone showed significant reductions in HAM-D and BDI scores. Within-group analyses revealed that the medication alone group showed significant improvement over time on only one variable that the DBT condition did not, namely fear of sadness. The DBT condition showed: significant decreases in hopelessness and in total adaptive, avoidant, detached, and emotional coping; significantly lower sociotropy/dependency; lower desires to please others; and lower autonomy scores from pre- to post-treatment.

MAINTENANCE THERAPY AND RELAPSE PREVENTION

Despite the effective treatments available for depression in the elderly, it has been established that elderly patients who recover from an episode of major depression are at high risk for relapse. Reynolds et al.[8] used a combination of medication and psychotherapy for the acute treatment of depression in order to empirically test the most effective maintenance therapy for remitted elderly. In their study, the 107 patients who fully recovered in open acute treatment with nortriptyline and interpersonal therapy were randomly assigned to one of four maintenance therapies: nortriptyline and IPT; nortriptyline and medication clinic; placebo and IPT; or placebo and medication clinic. Combined psychotherapy (IPT plus medication) was superior (80% effect) to medication alone (57% effect), psychotherapy alone (43% effect) or placebo (10% effect) for the maintenance of treatment gains and prevention of relapse. Reynolds et al.[8] concluded that combined psychotherapy and medication treatment appears to be the optimal long-term strategy in preserving depression remission and recommended that all older patients with recurrent depression be referred for psychotherapy. Research is currently under way testing the hypothesis that combination treatment is the most cost-effective way to treat recurrent depression in the elderly.

TREATMENT-RESISTANT POPULATIONS

While Reynolds and colleagues have established that combination therapy is the preferred means for maintenance of remission, there is an alarming number of elderly depressed patients who do not respond to medication, psychotherapy or the combination. Although acute remission rates of 50–70% are impressive, there remains another 30–50% of patients who do not respond. It has been found that elderly patients with co-morbid personality disorder, irrespective of level of depression, are less likely to benefit from short-term therapy than patients without co-morbidity[67] (see review[68]); hence, part of the population not responding to treatment may have personality disorders. However, with the exception of case studies, no outcome study has specifically focused on treating late-life personality disorders, and those studies reporting outcomes for personality-disordered elderly have suffered from varied methodological problems[68]. Nevertheless, poorer outcome and increased likelihood of relapse among personality-disordered elders, as well as continued observations that depression in the elderly is often a recurring phenomenon, require that revisions to existing treatments be made and implemented.

DYSTHYMIA

Despite the growing interest in studying treatment of depression in the elderly, we did not find any research specifically investigating the treatment of dysthymia in elderly patients. Although the research on treatment of recurrent old-age depression[8] may reflect issues associated with treating dysthymic individuals, research protocols up to now have focused primarily on a diagnosis of major depression. However, minor depression or less severe forms of depression remain important areas of investigation. Partial responses to treatment are associated with higher rates of relapse[69] and minor depression is more prevalent than MDD and subsequently has a greater number of disability days associated with it[70]. In addition, researchers have found that patients with endogenous depression (an older term with a symptom profile similar to dysthymia) responded less favorably to psychotherapy than non-endogenous depression patients, and that improvement occurred more quickly for the non-endogenous subtype[57]. Thus, more research is needed to examine the public health challenges posed by old-age chronic recurring depressive experience, partial responses to treatment, and minor depression.

CONCLUSIONS

There is a growing body of research demonstrating that psychotherapy offers significant promise for the treatment of elderly depression, preventing depressive relapse, and at times may be the preferred treatment modality in terms of both efficacy and patient choice. Referral to psychotherapy remains a problem, and current research on underdiagnosis and undertreatment of depression in older adults focuses more on describing the problem than on understanding it. However, with more insight into the reasons why elderly depression is inadequately diagnosed and treated, health providers can begin to develop operative means to ensure that this disabling yet treatable disorder is not ignored. General practitioners and mental health professionals do have the means to treat depression in the elderly with medication and/or psychotherapy; the work now lies in getting out into the "real world" and putting these techniques into practice.

REFERENCES

1. Scogin F, McElreath L. Efficacy of psychosocial treatments for geriatric depression: a quantitative review. J Consult Clin Psychol 1994; **62**: 69–74.
2. Teri L, McCurry SM. Psychosocial therapies. In Coffey CE, Cummings JL et al., eds, American Psychiatric Press Textbook of Geriatric Neuropsychiatry. Washington, DC: American Psychiatric Press, 1994: 662–82.
3. Zeiss AM, Breckenridge JS. Treatment of late life depression: a response to the NIH Consensus Statement. Behav Ther 1997; **28**: 3–21.
4. Schneider LS, Reynolds CF, Lebowitz BD, Friedhoff AJ. Diagnosis and Treatment of Depression in Late Life. Washington DC: American Psychiatric Press, 1994.
5. Schneider LS. Meta-analysis from a clinician's perspective. In Schneider LS, Reynolds CF, Lebowitz BD, Friedhoff AJ, eds, Diagnosis and Treatment of Depression in Late Life. Washington DC: American Psychiatric Press, 1994: 361–73.
6. Lebowitz BD, Pearson JL, Schneider LS et al. Diagnosis and treatment of depression in late life: consensus statement update. J Am Med Assoc 1997; **278**: 1186–90.
7. Koder D, Brodaty H, Anstey KJ. Cognitive therapy for depression in the elderly. Int J Geriat Psychiat 1996; **11**: 97–107.
8. Reynolds CF III, Frank E, Perel JM et al. Nortriptyline and interpersonal psychotherapy as maintenance therapies for recurrent major depression: a randomized controlled trial in patients older than 59 years. J Am Med Assoc 1999; **281**: 39–45.
9. Koenig HG. Late-life depression: how to treat patients with co-morbid chronic illness. Geriatrics 1999; **54**: 56–61.
10. Hirschfeld R, Keller M, Panico S et al. The National Depressive and Manic Depressive Association consensus statement on the under-treatment of depression. J Am Med Assoc 1997; **277**: 333–40.
11. Bortz J, O'Brien K. Psychotherapy with older adults: theoretical issues, empirical findings and clinical applications. In Nussbaum P, ed., Handbook of Neuropsychology and Aging: Critical Issues in Neuropsychology. New York: Plenum, 1997: 431–51.
12. Cooper-Patrick L, Powe NR, Jenckes MW et al. Identification of patient attitudes and preferences regarding treatment of depression. J Geriat Intern Med 1997; **12**: 431–8.
13. Koenig HG, George LK, Meador KG. Use of antidepressants by non-psychiatrists in the treatment of medically ill hospitalized depressed elderly patients. Am J Psychiat 1997; **154**: 1369–75.
14. Friedhoff A. Consensus Development Conference statement: diagnosis and treatment of depression in late life. In Schneider LS, Reynolds CF, Lebowitz BD, Friedhoff AJ, eds, Diagnosis and Treatment of Depression in Late Life. Washington DC: American Psychiatric Press, 1994: 491–511.

15. Schonfeld L, Garcia J, Streuber P. Factors contributing to mental health treatment of the elderly. *J Appl Gerontol* 1985; **4**: 30–9.

16. Weissman M, Myers J, Thompson W. Depression and its treatment in a US urban community, 1975–1976. *Arch Gen Psychiat* 1981; **38**: 417–21.

17. Rosen AL, Pancake JA, Rickards L. Mental health policy and older Americans: historical and current perspectives. In Gatz M, ed., *Emerging Issues in Mental Health and Aging*. Washington DC: American Psychological Association, 1995: 1–18.

18. Abrahams R, Patterson R. Psychological distress among the community elderly: prevalence, characteristics and implications for service. *Int J Aging Hum Dev* 1978; **9**: 1–18.

19. Rogers WH, Wells KB, Meredith LS *et al*. Outcomes for adult depressed outpatients under pre-paid and fee-for-service financing. *Arch Gen Psychiat* 1993; **50**: 517–25.

20. Conwell Y. Suicide in elderly patients. In Schneider LS, Reynolds CF, Lebowitz BD, Friedhoff AJ, eds, *Diagnosis and Treatment of Depression in Late Life*. Washington DC: American Psychiatric Press, 1994: 397–418.

21. Vitt CM, Idler EL, Leventhal H, Leventhal EA. Attitudes toward treatment and help-seeking preferences in an elderly sample. Poster presented at the Annual Meeting of the Gerontological Society of America, San Francisco, CA, November 1999.

22. Allen R, Walker Z, Shergill P, Katona C. Attitudes to depression in hospital inpatients: a comparison between older and younger subjects. *Aging Ment Health* 1998; **2**: 36–9.

23. Link BG, Struening EL, Rahav M *et al*. On stigma and its consequences: evidence from a longitudinal study of men with dual diagnoses of mental illness and substance abuse. *J Health Soc Behav* 1997; **38**: 177–90.

24. Gatz M, Finkel SI. Education and training of mental health service providers. In Gatz M, ed., *Emerging Issues in Mental Health and Aging*. Washington, DC: American Psychological Association, 1995.

25. Knight B. *Older Adults in Psychotherapy: Case Histories*. Newbury Park, CA: Sage, 1992.

26. Rokke PD, Scogin F. Depression treatment preferences in younger and older adults. *J Clin Geropsychol* 1995; **1**: 243–57.

27. Freud S. Mourning and melancholia. In *Collected Papers*. London: Hogarth, 1917.

28. Bibring E. Mechanisms of depression. In Greenacre P, ed., *Affective Disorders*. New York: International Universities Press, 1953.

29. Kohut H, Wolf E. The disorders of the self and their treatment: an outline. *Int J Psychoanal* 1978; **59**: 413–24.

30. Kernberg O. *Object Relations Theory and Clinical Psychoanalysis*. New York: Jason Aronson, 1976.

31. Klein M. Some theoretical conclusions regarding the emotional life of the infant. In Klein M, ed., *Envy, Gratitude and Other Works, 1946–1963*. New York: Delacorte Press, 1972.

32. Mahler M. On child psychosis and schizophrenia: autistic and symbiotic infantile psychoses. *Psychoanal Study Child* 1952; **7**: 206–305.

33. Thompson LW, Gallagher D, Breckinridge JS. Comparative effectiveness of psychotherapies for depressed elders. *J Consult Clin Psychol* 1987; **55**: 385–90.

34. Gallagher-Thompson D, Hanley-Peterson P, Thompson LW. Maintenance of gains vs. relapse following brief psychotherapy for depression. *J Consult Clin Psychol* 1990; **58**: 371–4.

35. Gallagher-Thompson D, Steffen AM. Comparative effects of cognitive-behavioral and brief psychodynamic psychotherapies for depressed family caregivers. *J Consult Clin Psychol* 1994; **62**: 543–9.

36. Butler RN. The Life Review: an interpretation of reminiscence in the aged. *Psychiatry* 1963; **26**: 65–76.

37. Lewis ML, Butler RN. Life-review therapy: putting memories to work in individual and group therapy. *Geriatrics* 1974; **29**: 165–73.

38. Soltys FG, Coats L. The SolCos Model: facilitating reminiscence therapy. *J Gerontol Nurs* 1994; **20**: 11–16.

39. Fry PS. Structured and unstructured reminiscence training and depression among the elderly. *Clin Gerontol* 1983; **1**: 15–37.

40. Goldwasser AN, Auerbach SM, Harkins SW. Cognitive, affective and behavioral effects of reminiscence group therapy on demented elderly. *Int J Aging Hum Dev* 1987; **25**: 209–22.

41. Rattenbury C, Stones MJ. A controlled evaluation of reminiscence and current topics discussion groups in a nursing home context. *Gerontologist* 1989; **29**: 768–71.

42. Klerman GL, Weissman MM, Rounsaville BJ, Chevron E. *Interpersonal Psychotherapy of Depression*. New York: Basic Books, 1984.

43. Frank E, Spanier C. Interpersonal psychotherapy for depression: overview, clinical efficacy and future directions. *Clin Psychol Sci Pract* 1995; **2**: 349–69.

44. Hinrichsen GA. Interpersonal psychotherapy for depressed older adults. *J Geriat Psychiat* 1997; **30**: 239–57.

45. Frank E, Frank N, Cornes C. Interpersonal psychotherapy in the treatment of late-life depression. In Klerman GL, Weissman MM, eds, *New Applications of Interpersonal Psychotherapy*. Washington DC: American Psychiatric Press, 1993: 167–98.

46. Sloane RB, Stapes FR, Schneider LS. Interpersonal therapy versus nortriptyline for depression in the elderly. In Burrows GD, Normal TR, Dennerstein L, eds, *Clinical and Pharmacological Studies in Psychiatric Disorders*. London: John Libby, 1985: 344–6.

47. Reynolds CF III, Frank E, Perel JM *et al*. Combined pharmacotherapy and psychotherapy in the acute and continuation treatment of elderly patients with recurrent major depression: a preliminary report. *Am J Psychiat* 1992; **149**: 1687–92.

48. Reynolds CF III, Frank E, Perel JM *et al*. Treatment of consecutive episodes of major depression in the elderly. *Am J Psychiat* 1994; **151**: 1740–3.

49. Reynolds CF III. Treatment of major depression in later life: a life cycle perspective. *Psychiat Qu* 1997; **68**: 221–46.

50. Beck AT. *Depression: Clinical, Experimental and Theoretical Aspects*. New York: Harper and Row, 1967.

51. Jacobson NS, Dobson KS, Truax PA *et al*. A component analysis of cognitive-behavioral treatment for depression. *J Consult Clin Psychol* 1996; **64**: 295–305.

52. Gortner ET, Gollan JK, Dobson KS, Jacobson NS. Cognitive-behavioral treatment for depression: relapse prevention. *J Consult Clin Psychol* 1998; **66**: 377–84.

53. Dougher MJ, Hackbert L. A behavioral-analytic account of depression and a case report using acceptance-based procedures. *Behav Anal* 1994; **17**: 321–34.

54. Kohlenberg RJ, Tsai M. *Functional Analytic Psychotherapy: Creating Intense and Curative Therapeutic Relationships*. New York: Plenum, 1991.

55. Nezu AM. A problem-solving formulation of depression: a literature review and proposal of a pluralistic model. *Clin Psychol Rev* 1987; **7**: 121–44.

56. Nezu AM, Perri MG. Social problem-solving therapy for unipolar depression: an initial dismantling investigation. *J Consult Clin Psychol* 1989; **57**: 408–13.

57. Thompson LW, Gallagher D. Efficacy of psychotherapy in the treatment of late-life depression. *Adv Behav Res Ther* 1984; **6**: 127–39.

58. O'Rourke N, Hadjistavropoulos T. The relative efficacy of psychotherapy in the treatment of geriatric depression. *Aging Ment Health* 1997; **1**: 305–10.

59. Gallagher D, Thompson LW. Treatment of major depressive disorder in older adult outpatients with brief psychotherapies. *Psychother Theor Res Pract* 1982; **19**: 482–90.

60. Arean PA, Perri MG, Nezu AM *et al*. Comparative effectiveness of social problem-solving therapy and reminiscence therapy as treatments for depression in older adults. *J Consult Clin Psychol* 1993; **61**: 1003–10.

61. Gaston L, Marmar CR, Gallagher D, Thompson LW. Impact of confirming patient expectations of change processes in behavioral, cognitive and brief dynamic psychotherapy. *Psychotherapy* 1989; **26**: 296–302.

62. Thompson LW, Davies R, Gallagher D *et al*. Cognitive therapy with older adults. *Clin Gerontol* 1986; **5**: 245–79.

63. DeRubeis RJ, Crits-Christoph P. Empirically supported individual and group psychological treatments for adult mental disorders. *J Consult Clin Psychol* 1998; **66**: 37–52.

64. Beutler LE, Scogin F, Kirkish P *et al*. Group cognitive therapy and alprazolam in the treatment of depression in older adults. *J Consult Clin Psychol* 1987; **55**: 550–6.

65. Steuer JL, Minta J, Hammen CL *et al.* Cognitive-behavioral, psychodynamic group psychotherapy in the treatment of geriatric depression. *J Consult Clin Psychol* 1984; **52**: 80–9.

66. Lynch TR, Morse JQ, Mendelson T *et al.* Dialectical behavior therapy for treatment of elderly depression: a randomized controlled trial. In Robins CJ (Chair), *Dialectical Behavior Therapy for Multi-problem Patients: Findings from Controlled Studies.* Symposium conducted at the Association for the Advancement of Behavior Therapy 33rd Annual Convention, Toronto, 1999.

67. Frank E, Kupfer DJ, Jacob M, Jarnett D. Personality features and response to acute treatment in recurrent depression. *J Pers Disord* 1987; **1**: 14–26.

68. Morse JQ, Lynch TR. Personality disorders in late life. *Curr Psychiat Rep* 2000; **2**: 24–31.

69. Thase ME, Simons AD, McGeary J *et al.* Relapse after cognitive behavior therapy for depression: potential implications for longer courses of treatment. *Am J Psychiat* 1992; **149**: 1046–52.

70. Broadhead WE, Blazer DG, George LK, Tse CK. Depression, disability days, and days lost from work in a perspective epidemiologic survey. *J Am Med Assoc* 1990; **264**: 2524–8.

80

Long-term Management of Affective Disorders

Mohammed T. Abou-Saleh

St George's Hospital Medical School, London, UK

Depressive illness is a public health problem. One in five individuals will suffer from one form of depression or another, four-fifths of those will suffer further episodes of illness and a fifth will die by suicide or cardiovascular disorders. Affective disorders are the most commonly diagnosed psychiatric conditions in the elderly in both general and hospital practice. Their incidence and prevalence increases with age, particularly in their more severe forms, with endogenous and psychotic features. It would be true to say that non-bipolar depressive illnesses with endogenous and psychotic features are essentially illnesses of old age. Depressive illnesses are often recurrent and are associated with high continuing morbidity and mortality. Their acute and long-term management is often successful and rewarding, with the availability of highly specific and effective physical and psychological treatments.

The focus of this chapter is on the strategies of long-term management of affective disorders, starting with a review of studies of their natural history and the usefulness of antidepressants and lithium as continuation and prophylactic therapies. Particular emphasis is laid on lithium therapy, its efficacy and safety, optimal dosage and dosage regimen and important aspects of its routine in psychiatric practice.

In essence, the usefulness of any treatment with established effectiveness also applies to the elderly with depressive illness, and the evidence marshalled to support the use of these treatments often derives from studies done on younger patients. In this chapter, reference will be made to whether the study was done on younger or older patients.

NATURAL HISTORY

Studies of the natural history of depressive illness in old age have been relatively few compared with studies in younger patients. The literature on both hospital and community-based studies have been critically reviewed[1].

Post[2] studied patients over 60 years of age who were followed up for a period of 3 years after discharge from hospital: a quarter of the patients had lasting recovery, whilst the other three-quarters were equally subdivided into a group who had recurrences and a group who continued to be ill over the entire study period. Factors that predicted poor outcome were age over 70 and a duration of illness of more than 2 years prior to admission. Blessed and Wilson[3] reported a 2 year follow-up study of a hospital cohort: one in five of their patients with affective psychosis had either not been discharged or had been re-admitted within the follow-up period. In a similar study, however, Christie[4], found that only 6% of the patients were still in hospital within the

2 years of follow-up. The study by Murphy[5] involving patients over the age of 65, treated in a variety of settings and followed up 1 year later, found that 43% had recovered by 1 year and 57% either had an early relapse of illness or had not recovered. Predictors of poor outcome were increased severity of illness, the presence of physical illness, longer duration of illness and the occurrence of life events during the follow-up year. Ninety per cent of patients with delusional depression had poor outcome. The study by Baldwin and Jolley[6], using a similar methodology to that by Murphy[5], reported a more favourable outcome: 50% of patients were fully recovered, 15% had a relapse following recovery and 18% were continuously ill. Poor prognosis was predicted by being male with physical illness, but was not associated with delusions. Longer follow-up studies over 20 years, involving elderly patients with depressive illness, showed that three-quarters of patients had recurrences[7,8]. Remarkably, the study by Ciompi[8] found that only 11% were totally free from psychiatric symptoms and one-third of patients had chronic depressive illness.

The year 3 follow-up of 1070 persons aged 65 and over living in the community in Liverpool[9] showed that 72% of patients with depressive psychosis and 62% of patients with depressive neurosis were either dead or had some kind of psychiatric illness 3 years later.

In conclusion, these studies, despite differences in methodology and duration of follow-up, clearly indicate the high continuing morbidity of depression in old age: the majority of patients with depression occurring or recurring in old age will suffer further episodes of illness, with one-fifth to one-third of patients experiencing chronic illness, particularly those who present with more severe illness and those with physical conditions leading to high mortality by suicide and cardiovascular conditions (see Chapters 83, 87 on suicide and prognosis, this volume).

ACUTE MANAGEMENT

Acute management of depression in old age is often successful and rewarding, with the introduction of highly effective and specific treatment. In his review of the efficacy of antidepressants in elderly patients, Peet[10] concluded that efficacy is established for drugs such as imipramine, amitriptyline, nortriptyline, phenelzine and mianserin with placebo control. Of the new antidepressants, trazodone and bupropion also show convincing efficacy in comparison with placebo. About two-thirds of patients respond well to these antidepressants. The effectiveness of psychological treatment in the acute management of depression in the elderly has not been satisfactorily established (see Chapter 79). However, reference is made to studies done on younger patients. A recent study from the National Institute of Mental Health (NIMH)[11] established the efficacy of brief interpersonal psychotherapy in comparison with standard treatment with imipramine plus clinical management, particularly with patients who are more severely depressed and functionally impaired. Cognitive–behavioural therapy (CBT) was found to be less effective than these two treatments when compared with placebo plus clinical management. This study was the first comparative study of the effectiveness of interpersonal psychotherapy and CBT. Its results, however, are disappointing to those who advocate the supremacy of CBT for the treatment of depression in general and hospital practice. However, there is evidence for its long-term effectiveness in preventing relapses or recurrences of illness[12]. The evidence for the efficacy of antidepressants (26 RCTs) and psychological treatment (RCTs) in older adults with depression has been critically reviewed[13]. Compared to placebo, efficacy has been established for fluoxetine, trazodone and phenelzine but no evidence for the superiority of any antidepressant over any other. In depressive patients with physical illness (18 RCTs), antidepressants were more effective than placebo. For psychological treatments in 40 controlled trials, treatments (cognitive therapy or CBT) were shown to be more effective in mild to moderate depression. However, these treatments were no more effective than non-specific attention.

The evidence for the efficacy of electroconvulsive therapy (ECT) in the severe forms of depression is overwhelming, although this derives mainly from studies done on younger patients. Of note was that the only predictor of good response to real vs. simulated (sham) ECT is the presence of delusions. There is, however, a high rate of relapse following recovery by ECT, indicating the need for continuation treatment following recovery. Post[2], in his 3 year follow-up study of depressed elderly patients, noted that 75% of patients relapsed when dosages of antidepressant were lowered after 3 months, and that it had been possible to discontinue treatment permanently in only 18% of patients; 38% of patients required tricyclic antidepressants (TCAs) intermittently or continuously and others had to be given lithium or had a further course of ECT. The study by Murphy[5] had no patients on prophylactic lithium.

Continuation Therapy Following ECT

The efficacy of ECT in the management of depression in old age is often compromised by the high relapse rate following recovery. Abou-Saleh and Coppen[14] critically reviewed the evidence for the efficacy of continuation therapy with antidepressants and lithium following recovery with ECT. It was shown that in four prospective placebo-controlled studies over a period of 6 months to 1 year, these drugs substantially reduced the relapse–recurrence rates during follow-up. The conclusion was that lithium would be particularly effective in those with delusional depression, bipolar depression and in the elderly.

LONG-TERM MANAGEMENT

Long-term management occurs in two phases: a continuation therapy phase to prevent early relapse of illness and a maintenance–prophylactic phase to prevent recurrence (Figure 80.1). Studies of the value of continuation therapy after recovery have established the efficacy of antidepressants and lithium in preventing relapse of illness. Continuation therapy with drugs appears to reduce the relapse rate by half compared to placebo within 4–6 months from recovery from the acute illness[13].

The American Psychiatric Association Guidelines[15] recommend antidepressant continuation therapy for 16–20 weeks following remission, using the dose used in the acute phase. There is also evidence to support the use of specific psychotherapy during the continuation phase. The patient's clinical condition, as well as the specific treatment being provided, determine the frequency of visits. The decision to discontinue treatment should be based on the factors considered in the decision to initiate maintenance treatment, including the probability of recurrence, frequency and severity of past episodes, the persistence of dysthymic symptoms after recovery, the presence of co-morbid disorders and patient preference, in addition to consideration of the benefits and adverse effects of maintenance treatment.

In a number of controlled investigations of variable stringency, TCAs and lithium were shown to reduce the long-term morbidity and mortality in patients with unipolar illness, including the elderly. The results of these studies have, however, been disappointing, with only 48% success rate (absence of a relapse–recurrence) in the NIMH study with imipramine maintenance therapy over 2 years. The Medical Research Council study showed a success rate for amitriptyline of 32% over a period of 3 years' maintenance therapy[16].

Prophylactic Treatment

Early studies indicated a poor outcome of late-life depression[5], with high relapse, recurrence and chronicity. This view was based on naturalistic observation without monitoring the compliance, adequate dosage and duration of treatment, including prophylactic treatment, and was therefore challenged[17]. Controlled studies of maintenance antidepressant medication, however, showed better outcome for late-life depression[18]. The Pittsburgh group reported a 3 year follow-up study of maintenance treatment with nortriptyline or placebo, with or without interpersonal psychotherapy (IPT)[19] and showed that 80% of patients assigned to nortriptyline, with or without IPT, remained in remission. The Pittsburgh group also identified the elderly patients who remained well after placebo-controlled discontinuation of antidepressant medication for a period of 1 year. Recovery of good subjective sleep quality by early continuation treatment was useful in identifying which remitted elderly depressed patients remained well with monthly IPT after discontinuation of antidepressant medication[20]. Moreover, effective maintenance treatment with nortriptyline was associated with enhancement in the rate of delta-wave production in the first non-rapid eye movement (REM) sleep and of REM activity throughout the night[21].

A recent study of the effects of treatment on the 2 year course of late-life depression[22] showed a 74% survival rate without relapse. This good outcome was obtained by the use of full-dose antidepressant medication, frequent follow-up and rigorous treatment of relapses. In a prospective 1 year uncontrolled study in elderly depressed and dysthymic patients, reboxetine was shown to be effective and well tolerated[23].

The US National Institute of Mental Health consensus statement update[24] concluded that recent evidence supports the recommendation for at least 6 months of treatment beyond recovery for those with first onset in late life, and for at least 12 months for those with a recurrent illness[25]. Moreover, prophylactic treatment should be of the same type and of same dosage as that which was successful in the initial acute phase. The consensus statement also concluded that treatment response and long-term outcome for all patients is generally similar to that observed in younger adults, but the temporal course may somewhat be slower in the elderly and risk of relapse somewhat greater[24]. The use of lithium in continuation and prophylactic treatment of depression in the elderly has also been recommended[18,26], with the use of lower doses/plasma levels. Lithium may be a more favourable prophylactic treatment than antidepressants in recurrent

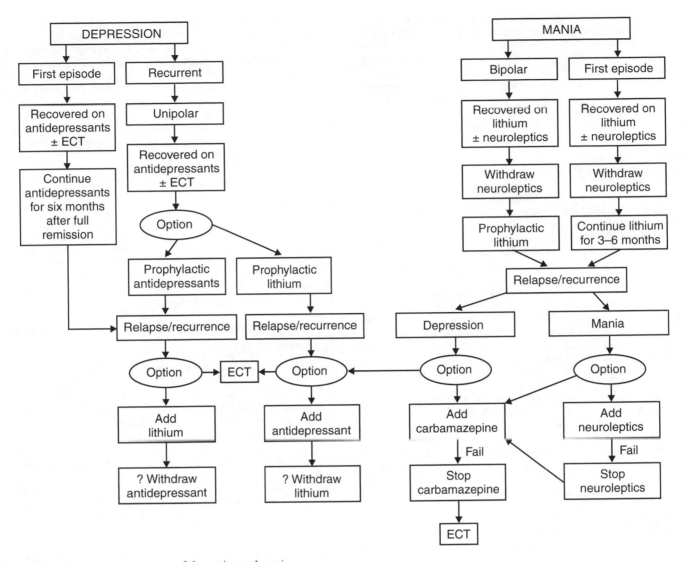

Figure 80.1   Long-term management of depression and mania

depression with melancholia and in depression with psychotic features (delusional depression), which are particularly common among the elderly, with a tendency to respond less well to antidepressants[17]. The other advantage of lithium therapy is the evident decreased mortality, whether from suicide or other causes[27]. A recent 1 year prospective, placebo-controlled study of maintenance lithium in conjunction with CBT in elderly depressed patients[28] showed that, although CBT reduced depression severity during follow-up, lithium therapy was no better than placebo. This appears to be related to poor compliance, a finding that highlights the serious difficulties in undertaking prophylactic studies in elderly depressed patients.

Lithium Therapy

The use of lithium in the management of affective disorders has proved to be one of the most rewarding therapeutic strategies in medical practice. In the management of bipolar disorders, it has provided one of the most specific psychotropic drugs in

psychiatry. Lithium is the treatment of choice for mania and has comparable efficacy to neuroleptics, except in disturbed and agitated manic patients, who respond more dramatically to neuroleptic medication. The advantage of lithium, however, is that patients do not complain of the "strait-jacket" effect they experience with neuroleptics. Moreover, intermittent exposure to neuroleptics has been shown to be associated with a high incidence of tardive dyskinesia, particularly in the elderly, who are often less tolerant of neuroleptics and more commonly develop parkinsonian side effects. Lithium is also strongly recommended for the treatment of bipolar depression, rather than tricyclics, which may provoke hypomanic episodes and increase the risk for the development of rapid-cycling illness. There is evidence that lithium alone is effective in depression that has failed to respond to tricyclic medication, and in combination with other antidepressants in the management of resistant depression (see below).

Affective disorders are recurrent illnesses and the discovery of the prophylactic effects of lithium opened a new era in their management. In a number of controlled investigations of varying stringency, done mostly on younger patients, lithium was shown to substantially reduce the long-term morbidity of both unipolar and bipolar disorder[14,29]. Prospective controlled studies showed that lithium was superior to placebo and tricyclics in the prophylaxis of bipolar illness. The majority of studies evaluating its prophylactic efficacy in unipolar illness found it superior to placebo, as effective as imipramine or amitriptyline, and more effective than mianserin and maprotiline. This may be related to the greater heterogeneity of unipolar illness.

Treatment of Bipolar Disorder

Elderly patients with late presentation or late-onset mania respond well to standard antimanic treatment with neuroleptics, lithium and anticonvulsants[30,31]. Neuroleptic treatment is best avoided in the elderly because of its known extrapyramidal side effects, except for floridly psychotic, agitated and behaviourally disturbed patients, who need rapid control of symptoms. Lithium remains the treatment of choice, followed by valproic acid[30]. The evidence for the efficacy of lithium in late-life mania is based on retrospective and uncontrolled studies, and there have been no controlled studies of the efficacy of anticonvulsants in late-life mania. It has been suggested that valproate is a safer alternative treatment to lithium than carbamazepine, whether used as single or adjunct treatment in elderly manic patients[30,31]. There are no guidelines regarding the optimal plasma concentration of valproate in relation to efficacy[30].

A recent evidence-based review of the treatment of mania, mixed state and rapid-cycling illness in younger populations[32] concluded that lithium and divalproex sodium are effective in mania, whereas divalproex sodium and carbamazepine are more effective in mixed states. Divalproex sodium is the drug of choice for rapid-cycling disorder. With bipolar depression, lithium is recommended as a first-line treatment and the addition of a second mood stabilizer or a TCA would be an appropriate next step[33].

The guidelines for the continuation and prophylactic treatment of bipolar illness in late life are similar to those advocated for younger patients, except for the notion of high recurrence rates necessitating prophylactic treatment even after a first onset manic episode. Three sets of guidelines for the treatment of patients with bipolar disorder were reviewed[35]: the American Psychiatric Association Practice Guideline[15], the Expert Consensus Guideline Series (1996) and the Clinical Practice Guidelines for Bipolar Disorder from the Department of Veterans Affairs[36]. Lithium remains the medication of choice for prophylaxis. A comparative audit of the prevalence of lithium therapy and the quality of monitoring in over-65s in Cambridge and Southampton showed a wide variation and indicated that a dedicated monitoring service leads to a better quality of treatment supervision[37].

Who Responds to Prophylactic Lithium?

Response to lithium varies between complete, with no further episodes of illness, to partial, with the frequency and severity of episodes reduced, to failure to respond, when morbidity continues unabated. Overall, 50–70% of patients with bipolar and severe unipolar illness show favourable responses to lithium, with a small minority who are total non-responders. The latter are often patients with rapid-cycling bipolar illness (those who suffer four episodes of illness per annum or more). The main reasons for failure of prophylaxis are poor compliance and side effects such as weight gain, increased thirst, difficulties with memory, poor concentration and loss of enthusiasm.

A recent study examined the clinical and psychological characteristics of elderly patients receiving prophylactic lithium in relation to long-term outcome of treatment (Abou-Saleh, unpublished). Elderly patients with bipolar illness had better outcome than those with unipolar illness. In their personality characteristics, those who had an excellent response showed higher scores on extraversion and energy output than those who responded less well. The most powerful predictor of long-term response, however, was their response during the first 6 months of therapy, confirming the results obtained in younger patients[34].

Treatment Compliance

Compliance with treatment is a major problem in the elderly. A study by Johnson[38] showed that the dropout rate from a group of depressed patients treated in general practice increased from 16% at the end of the first week to 68% at the end of 1 month. This was related to doubts about the benefits and less related to the occurrence of side effects. Of particular importance are the cognitive and sensory impairments of the elderly, low motivation, and poor communication by doctors of the benefits and risks to patients and their relatives. In the background lurks a nihilistic attitude and doubts about the effectiveness of treatment in both patients and doctors.

Prophylactic Lithium in the Elderly

Himmelhoch[39], in an open study of the efficacy of lithium in elderly patients, reported a favourable response rate in two-thirds of these patients. The majority of poor responders, however, had neurological conditions, which probably impaired the efficacy of lithium. The present author reported the results of a series of open and controlled studies of the efficacy of lithium in conventional and lower doses in the prophylactic management of affective disorders in old age[40]. In the Lithium Clinic at the Medical Research Council Neuropsychiatry Laboratory in Epsom, UK, 44 male and 104 female patients with affective disorders were followed up for a period of 1–14.5 years (mean 4.9 years). They all received a slow-release lithium preparation at bedtime. Plasma lithium concentrations were maintained at 0.8–1.2 mmol/l 12 h after dosing. Prophylactic lithium was started in 47 of these patients after 60 years of age. There was no significant difference in the Affective Morbidity Index (a composite index of severity and duration of affective episodes) between the younger and these elderly patients, as shown in Table 80.1. Side effects in the older group were similar to these in younger patients. In a further study[34], 22 elderly patients over 60 years of age who started lithium in late life received 25–50% reduction in lithium dosage in a double-blind situation. The elderly group of patients fared as well on lower doses of lithium as younger patients and had a significant reduction in subjective side effects, such as tremor and thirst (Table 80.2). However, results for the whole group, with a majority of younger patients, showed that a reduction of 50% in daily dosage was safe: patients who had the reduced dose of lithium and plasma lithium levels of 0.45–0.59 mmol/l showed reduced morbidity during the year of follow-up, compared with the year preceding the trial, and showed fewer subjective side effects and adverse effects on thyroid and renal function.

Side Effects

Subjective Side Effects

The occurrence of subjective side effects during lithium therapy is well documented[41]. Side effects in the early stage (within 6 weeks

Table 80.1 General details of patients and relationship between age and morbidity during lithium therapy (results expressed as mean ± SEM)

Age when lithium started (years)	n	Episodes prior to lithium	Years on lithium	AMI[b]
> 60	47	4.9 ± 0.6	3.8[a] ± 0.4	0.18 ± 0.03
40–60	79	4.2 ± 0.3	5.5 ± 0.4	0.17 ± 0.02
< 40	22	4.4 ± 0.6	5.3 ± 0.7	0.14 ± 0.03

[a]Significantly lower than (40–60 years) group $p < 0.01$ and (less than 40 years) group $p < 0.05$.
[b]Affective Morbidity Index.

Table 80.2 Morbidity and plasma lithium level in 22 elderly patients before and during trial period (results expressed as mean ± SEM)

Plasma lithium level (mmol/l)	n	AMI	
		Before trial	During trial
> 0.8	8	0.16 ± 0.08	0.17 ± 0.06
0.60–0.79	6	0.40 ± 0.17	0.36 ± 0.12
0.45–0.59	8	0.22 ± 0.15	0.36 ± 0.20

of starting lithium) include nausea, loose stools, fatigue, muscle weakness, polydipsia, polyuria and hand tremor.

During maintenance, weight gain, mild memory impairment and hand tremor are common complaints and polydipsia and polyuria may persist. The rate of occurrence of these side effects and their severity is related to plasma lithium concentrations. The elderly are particularly vulnerable to side effects. Smith and Helms[42] examined the incidence and severity of side effects in elderly patients receiving lithium in comparison with younger patients. Whilst there was no difference in the total incidence of side effects, there was a trend for more serious side effects to occur more frequently in the elderly: 33% of the elderly experienced "confusion" vs. 12% of the younger group. Worthy of note is that the patients were maintained on relatively high plasma concentrations for this age group, 0.86–1.26 mmol/l. Patients with neurological conditions (parkinsonism and facial dyskinesia) develop neurotoxicity at relatively low plasma levels of less than 0.65 mmol/l[39]. In a recent investigation, Coppen and Abou-Saleh[26] reported that prevalence rates of subjective side effects in elderly patients receiving low-dose lithium (plasma lithium levels of 0.52–0.6 mmol/l) were similar to those of younger patients maintained on similar plasma levels.

Thyroid Effects

Elderly patients on prophylactic lithium are more likely to develop hypothyroidism than younger ones and women are more susceptible than men. This may be related to the increased disposition of women to develop autoimmune thyroid disease in middle and old age. Indeed, pre-existing thyroid disease is the major vulnerability factor for the development of hypothyroidism during lithium therapy. Coppen and Abou-Saleh[26] studied thyroid function in 125 patients receiving low-dose plasma levels of lithium. Women had significantly higher levels of thyroid stimulating hormone (TSH) than men, and all four patients with abnormally high TSH levels were unipolar women. Of the 11 patients who received replacement thyroxine, 10 were unipolar patients. Thyroid function has been related to increased affective

morbidity during receipt of prophylactic lithium and has been implicated in the development of rapid-cycling bipolar disorder.

Renal Effects

Overall, 5–10% of patients on prophylactic lithium develop tubular kidney damage complicated with glomerular pathology. There is no evidence that these changes are conducive to renal insufficiency, which rarely occurs in patients who have suffered lithium intoxication or had pre-existing renal disease. Lithium dose requirements show a decrease with age, which could be accounted for by the age-dependent fall in glomerular filtration rate and lithium clearance. With age, there is a decrease in muscle mass, which limits the value of measuring serum creatinine levels as an indicator of renal function. Age-related decrease in the volume of distribution of lithium also contributes to higher plasma levels in the elderly. The daily dosage of lithium required to achieve a given plasma level may be half the dose required for a younger patient. A number of studies have evaluated renal function in relation to the dosage regimen, comparing a once per day dosage regimen to a twice-daily regimen. Contrary to the conventional wisdom, of avoiding higher peak plasma levels associated with a single daily dosage regimen, this regimen was found to be safer for renal function than a divided daily dosage regimen: functional and structural abnormalities were more pronounced in the group of patients who received lithium in divided doses than those who received it in the single daily dosage regimen, suggesting that it may be more important to have regular periods with lower levels than it is to have lower peaks.

Optimum Plasma Levels

In an open trial of lithium in elderly patients with mania (age 65–77 years), two-thirds of patients responded at levels of 0.52–0.8 mmol/l (mean 0.58 mmol/l). Two weeks after obtaining that range, two patients developed neurotoxicity and two patients only responded when the levels were raised to 0.9 mmol/l[44]. Several retrospective and prospective controlled trials have evaluated the efficacy and safety of variable lithium dosage levels in bipolar and unipolar disorder[45]. Some of these studies have included elderly patients. Overall, the minimal effective lithium level of the majority of patients is 0.4–0.8 mmol/l. Bipolar patients may require higher dosages/levels than unipolar patients[46]. It is evident that lower dosages/levels are associated with less severe subjective side effects and adverse effects on thyroid and renal function. A prospective open study examined the ongoing morbidity of 128 patients with unipolar, bipolar and schizoaffective disorders maintained at low doses of lithium (mean level 0.56 mmol/l) over a period of 1 year[26]. Affective morbidity was measured for three age brackets: < 60 years; 66–70; and > 70 years. Elderly patients aged 70+ had remarkably less morbidity than the two younger groups, but similar side effects (Table 80.3).

Shulman et al.[48] followed up 43 elderly patients (mean age 74 years) maintained on 12-hourly lithium levels of 0.5 mmol/l for an average period of 2 years. The majority of patients responded well to lithium, which was well tolerated, and compliance was excellent. The most common side effects were hand tremor in one-third of the patients and polyuria or polydipsia in one-quarter.

Lithium Interactions

Special consideration should be given to lithium interactions with drugs commonly prescribed for the elderly. Lithium may interact

Table 8.3 Affective morbidity and side effects in patients on lithium, divided according to age (results shown as mean $\pm$ SEM)

Age (years)	n	AMI	BDI[a]	Side effects
< 59.9	61	0.16 $\pm$ 0.02	6.3 $\pm$ 0.9	8.8 $\pm$ 1.0
60.0–69.9	51	0.14 $\pm$ 0.02	5.8 $\pm$ 0.7	8.7 $\pm$ 1.3
> 70.0	16	0.06 $\pm$ 0.01[a]	6.9 $\pm$ 1.7	7.6 $\pm$ 1.4

[a]Beck Depression Inventory.

with β-blockers, resulting in the slowing of heart rate, and similar interactions have been noted when lithium is combined with digoxin, with reports of increased risk of sudden cardiovascular death on this combination in predisposed patients. The elderly, however, are commonly prescribed thiazide diuretics for hypertension, which reduce lithium clearance and increase plasma lithium levels by reducing plasma volume, causing an increase in lithium and sodium reabsorption. This interaction is not observed with potassium-sparing diuretics and loop diuretics, such as frusemide. Amiloride, however, has been used for treating lithium-induced polyuria and diabetes insipidus. Finally, the widely used non-steroidal anti-inflammatory drugs have been reported to reduce lithium clearance and increase plasma levels, except for aspirin and sulindac. Ibuprofen was shown to cause significant decrease in renal lithium clearance and was linked to cases of lithium intoxication. Indomethacin, however, has been used to treat lithium-induced polyuria.

CONCLUSION

Good management calls for a comprehensive reassessment of the patient's condition to review diagnosis and to identify the reasons for treatment failure by a diligent assessment of the adequacy of previous treatments.

With regard to therapeutic strategies, these involve two concepts: alternative and adjunct therapy (Figure 80.1). The adjunct approach takes primacy over the alternative treatment approach. Adjunct treatments include lithium[49,50], folate and T4/T3, and also cognitive or interpersonal psychotherapy. Alternative basic treatment involves changing the conventional antidepressant to a new one, such as a selective serotonin reuptake inhibitor (SSRI) or the use of ECT. In mania, adjunct or alternative treatments are essentially anticonvulsants, principally valproate added to lithium or neuroleptics.

GUIDELINES FOR LONG-TERM THERAPY IN THE ELDERLY

The long-term management of recurrent affective disorders in the elderly starts with a careful assessment of the patient's psychiatric, physical and social condition. This involves full psychiatric examination and physical investigation for careful diagnosis, including the pattern of symptoms, previous episodes and their nature and treatment. Patients who have recovered from an acute episode of illness should be maintained for a minimum of 6 months at the same dosage, and those with a delusional first episode in late life, or who had recurrent (minimum of two episodes in 5 years) illnesses, should be considered for prophylaxis with antidepressants or lithium. The choice of antidepressant will depend on the physical condition of the patient. Conventional antidepressants should only be considered for the physically well. Otherwise, the new generation of antidepressants, including the SSRIs, should be considered. Lofepramine, fluoxetine, fluvoxamine, paroxetine and sertraline are safer antidepressants,

with no cardiotoxic effects. Fluoxetine and sertraline have been successfully evaluated as maintenance and prophylactic treatments. It is prudent to start with low doses and build up the dose gradually, with careful monitoring of side effects. Lithium is particularly effective in bipolar illness and in delusional unipolar illness, either given alone or as an adjunct in those who are already receiving antidepressants with incomplete response. Carbamazepine and valproate is a useful adjunct in bipolar patients who have failed to respond to lithium. ECT is a highly effective treatment for relapses–recurrences, whilst continuing on maintenance or prophylactic medication. The elderly require regular follow-up, to monitor their physical, psychiatric and social conditions and to deal with any emergent problems and complications, with careful attention to their social network.

REFERENCES

1. Katona CLE. The epidemiology and natural history of depression in old age. In Ghose K, ed., *Antidepressants for Elderly People*. London: Chapman and Hall, 1989; 27–40.
2. Post F. The management and nature of depressive illnesses in late life: a follow-through study. *Br J Psychiat* 1972; **121**: 393.
3. Blessed G, Wilson ID. The contemporary natural history of depression in old age. *Br J Psychiat* 1982; **141**: 59.
4. Christie AB. Changing patterns in mental illness in the elderly. *Br J Psychiat* 1982; **140**: 154.
5. Murphy E. The prognosis of depression in old age. *Br J Psychiat* 1983; **142**: 111–19.
6. Baldwin RC, Jolley DJ. Prognosis of depression in old age. *Br J Psychiat* 1986; **151**: 129.
7. Gianturco DT, Busse EW. Psychiatric problems encountered during a long-term study of normal ageing volunteers. In Isaacs AD, Post F, eds, *Studies in Geriatric Psychiatry*. New York: John Wiley, 1978; 1–16.
8. Ciompi L. Follow-up studies on the evolution of former neurotic and depressive states in old age. *J Geriat Psychiat* 1969; **3**: 90.
9. Copeland JRM, Davidson IA, Dewey ME *et al*. Alzheimer's disease, other dementias, depression and pseudodementia, prevalence, incidence and three year outcome in Liverpool: GMS–HAS AGECAT. *Br J Psychiat* 1992; **161**: 230–39.
10. Peet M. Which antidepressant? In Ghose K, ed., *Antidepressants for Elderly People*. London: Chapman and Hall, 1989; 137–62.
11. Mood disorders: pharmacologic prevention of recurrences (NIMH/NIH Consensus Development Conference Statement). *Am J Psychiat* 1985; **142**(20): 469–76.
12. Blackburn IM, Eunson KM, Bishop S. A two-year naturalistic follow-up of depressed patients treated 21 with cognitive therapy, pharmacotherapy and a combination of both. *J Affect Disord* 1986; **10** 67–75.
13. Geddes J, Butler R, Warner J *et al*. Depressive Disorders. *Clinical Evidence*. *Br Med J* 2000; **4**: 520–35.
14. Abou-Saleh MT, Coppen A. Who responds to prophylactic lithium? *J Affect Disord* 1986; **10**: 115–25.
15. American Psychiatric Association Guidelines. *Am J Psychiat* 2000; **157**: 1–45.
16. Glen AI, Johnson AL, Sheperd M *et al*. Continuation therapy with lithium and amitriptyline in unipolar depressive illness: a randomized, double-blind, controlled trial. *Psychol Med* 1984; **14**: 37–50.
17. Abou-Saleh MT, Coppen A. Classification of depression and response to anti-depressive therapies. *Br J Psychiatr* 1983; **143**: 601–3.
18. Stoudemire A. Recurrence and relapse in geriatric depression: a review of risk factors and prophylactic treatment strategies. *J Neuropsychiat* 1997; **9**: 209–21.
19. Reynolds CF. Treatment of depression in late life. *Am J Med* 1994; **97**(suppl 6A): 39–46S.
20. Reynolds CF III, Frank E, Houck PR *et al*. Which elderly patients with remitted depression remained well with continued interpersonal psychotherapy after discontinuation of antidepressant medication? *Am J Psychiat* 1997; **154**: 958–62.

21. Reynolds CF III, Buysse DJ, Brunner DP *et al*. Maintenance nortriptyline effects on electroencephalographic sleep in elderly patients with recurrent major depression: double-blind, placebo- and plasma level-controlled evaluation. *Soc Biol Psychiat* 1997; **42**: 560–67.

22. Flint AJ, Rifat SL. The effect of treatment on the two-year course of late-life depression. *Br J Psychiat* 1997; **170**: 268–72.

23. Aguglia E. Reboxetine in the maintenance therapy of depressive disorder in the elderly: a long-term open study. *Int J Geriat Psychiat* 2000; **15**: 784–93.

24. Lebowitz BD, Pearson JL, Schneider LS *et al*. Diagnosis and treatment of depression in late life: consensus statement update. *J Am Med Assoc* 1997; **278**: 1186–90.

25. Reynolds CF, Frank E, Perel J *et al*. Maintenance therapies for late life recurrent major depression: research and review circa 1995. *Int Psychogeriat* 1995; **7**(suppl): 27–40.

26. Coppen A, Abou-Saleh MT. Lithium therapy: from clinical trials to practical management. *Acta Psychiat Scand* 1988; **78**: 759–62.

27. Coppen A. Depression as a lethal disease: prevention strategies. *J Clin Psychiat* 1994; **55**(suppl): 37–45.

28. Wilson KCM, Scott M, Abou-Saleh M *et al*. Long-term effects of cognitive–behavioural therapy and lithium therapy on depression in the elderly. *Br J Psychiatr* 1995; **167**: 653–8.

29. Elkin I, Shea T, Watkins JT. National Institute of Mental Health Treatment of Depression Collaborative Research Programme: general effectiveness of treatments. *Arch Gen Psychiat* 1989; **46**: 971–82.

30. Young RC. Bipolar mood disorders in the elderly. *Geriat Psychiat* 1997; **20**: 121–36.

31. Shulman KI, Hermann N. The nature and management of mania in old age. *Psychiat Clin N Am* 1999; **22**: 549–65.

32. Kusumakar V, Yatham LN, Haslam DRS *et al*. Treatment of mania, mixed state, and rapid cycling. *Can J Psychiat* 1997; **42**(suppl 2): 79–86S.

33. Yatham LN, Kusumakar V, Parikh SV *et al*. Bipolar depression: treatment options. *Can J Psychiat* 1997; **42**(suppl 2): 87–91S.

34. Abou-Saleh MT, Coppen AJ. Predictors of long-term outcome of mood disorders on prophylactic lithium. *Lithium* 1990; **1**: 27–35.

35. Snowdon J. The relevance of guidelines for treatment mania in old age. *Int J Geriat Psychiat* 2000; **15**: 779–83.

36. Bauer MS, Callahan AM, Jampala C *et al*. Clinical practice guidelines for bipolar disorder from the Department of Veterans Affairs. *J Clin Psychiat* 1999; **60**: 9–21.

37. Fielding S, Kerr S, Godber C. Lithium in the over-65s—a dedicated monitoring service leads to a better quality of treatment supervision. *Int J Geriat Psychiat* 1999; **14**: 985–7.

38. Johnson DAW. Treatment of depression in general practice. *Br Med J* 1973; **2**: 18–20.

39. Himmelhoch JM, Neil JF, May SJ *et al*. Age, dementia, dyskinesias and lithium response. *Am J Psychiat* 1980; **137**: 941–5.

40. Abou-Saleh MT, Coppen A. The prognosis of depression in old age: the case for lithium therapy. *Br J Psychiat* 1983; **143**: 527–8.

41. Abou-Saleh MT, Coppen A. Subjective side-effects of amitriptyline and lithium in affective disorders. *Br J Psychiatry* 1983; **142**: 391–7.

42. Smith RE, Helms PM. Adverse effects of lithium therapy in the acutely ill elderly patient. *J Clin Psychiat* 1982; **43**: 94–9.

43. Coppen A, Abou-Saleh MT. Lithium therapy: from clinical trials to practical management. *Acta Psychiat Scand* 1982; **78**: 754–62.

44. Schaffer CB, Garvey MJ. Use of lithium in acutely manic elderly patients. *Clin Gerontol* 1984; **3**: 58–60.

45. Abou-Saleh MT. The dosage regime. In Johnson FN, ed., *Depression and Mania: Lodem Lithium Therapy*. Washington, DC: IRL Press, 1987; 99–105.

46. Gelenberg AJ, Kane JM, Keller MB. Comparison of standard and low serum levels of lithium for maintenance treatment of bipolar disorders. *N Engl J Med* 1989; **321**: 1489–93.

47. Coppen A, Peet M, Bailey J. Double-blind and open prospective studies of lithium prophylaxis in affective disorders. *Psychiat Neurol Neuroclin* 1973; **76**: 501–10.

48. Shulman KI, MacKenzie S, Hardy B. The clinical use of lithium carbonate in old age: a review. *Prog Neuropsychopharmacol Biol Psychiat* 1987; **11**: 159–64.

49. van Marwijk HWJ, Bekker FM, Nolen WA *et al*. Lithium augmentation in geriatric depression. *J Affect Disord* 1990; **20**: 217–23.

50. Katona CL. Lithium augmentation in refractory depression. *Psychiat Dev* 1977; **6**: 153–71.

81

Laboratory Diagnosis:
Dexamethasone Suppression Test

Mohammed T. Abou-Saleh

St George's Hospital Medical School, London, UK

There is little doubt that the application of the dexamethasone suppression test (DST) for the management of depressive illness has provided one of the most dramatic developments in biological psychiatry. Extensive investigations of this test began in the late 1960s and culminated in its introduction as a highly specific diagnostic test for endogenous depression[1]. There have been hundreds of studies on its use in diagnosis, in management and as a paradigm for investigating the pathophysiology of depressive illness.

Carroll[2] proposed that the DST was a highly specific diagnostic test for endogenous depression, with a specificity of 96% and a sensitivity of 50%. This claim has not been substantiated by other investigators, who reported high rates of non-suppression in a variety of psychiatric conditions, including non-endogenous depression[3], dementia[4], schizophrenia and alcoholism[5]. Abnormal DST results have also been obtained in mania[6] and eating disorders[7]. These findings have been repeatedly confirmed by other investigators and the clinical utility of the DST in the diagnosis and management of depression has been critically reviewed[1].

METHODOLOGICAL CONSIDERATIONS

Most studies have used the overnight DST, with 1 mg dexamethasone administered before midnight for cortisol estimation at 4 p.m. the following day. A cortisol of 50 ng/ml and above is taken as the criterion for non-suppression. A number of methodological aspects have been investigated, including sampling time, dexamethasone dose, the cortisol criterion for non-suppression, the assay technique and the bio-availability of dexamethasone. The criterion for non-suppression has been empirically determined by trading off the test's sensitivity and specificity, aiming for a specificity of over 90% and a sensitivity of 50%. Carroll's criterion of 50 ng/ml for non-suppression has been universally adopted, in spite of the great variation in sensitivity and specificity achieved in various centres.

Perhaps the most important contributing variable to the DST results is the dose of dexamethasone administered: the 1 mg DST has higher sensitivity and lower specificity than 2 mg DST. A corollary of the dose of dexamethasone is the corresponding plasma concentration achieved and its relationship to the results of the dexamethasone test: levels of dexamethasone in non-suppressors are lower than in suppressors[8]. The extent to which differences in bio-availability of oral dexamethasone account for differences in sensitivity and specificity of the DST for depression is variable. The application of dexamethasone "windows" could reduce this source of test variance[8]. Dexamethasone metabolism is influenced by liver function in males and by body mass in females[9]. The combination of DST with corticotropin releasing factor has been shown to be more closely associated with hypothalamic–pituitary–adrenal (HPA) activity than DST in depressed and normal subjects[10].

The influence of non-specific factors on the results of the DST has been reviewed[1]; factors studied included the degree of stress, ageing, the presence of physical illness, marked weight loss, and the effects of administration and withdrawal of psychotropic drugs.

An association between increasing age and non-suppression has been shown in depressive and demented patients and in normal controls[11]. However, a longitudinal study in elderly normal subjects followed up for a period of 2.5 years showed no effect of age and suggested that genetic factors may influence the set point of the HPA axis[9]. Physical illness is associated with non-suppression, particularly diabetes mellitus and hypothalamic disorders.

The list of drugs that interfere with the DST has been increasing, and includes hormonal preparations, liver enzyme-inducing drugs such as barbiturates, anticonvulsants and alcohol. Test results are not affected by normal doses of benzodiazepines, antidepressants and neuroleptics. High doses of benzodiazepines have been associated with normal suppression. The effects of withdrawing psychotropic medication have also been studied, with higher rates of non-suppression being observed in patients who discontinued antidepressants, neuroleptics and benzodiazepines. These non-specific factors have important effects on test results and must be ascertained when the DST is carried out in the clinical situation. They have undoubtedly contributed to the considerable variation in the rate of non-suppression in normal controls and psychiatric patients.

DIAGNOSTIC VALUE

The claim that the DST is a highly specific diagnostic test for endogenous depression (melancholia) has not been substantiated. Rates of non-suppression in endogenous depression varied (18–81%), a variation that may be partly related to the criteria used to define endogenous depression. An early review found that in 12 out of 20 studies, significant increases in non-suppression rates were found in endogenous compared with non-endogenous depressives, with the Newcastle Scale providing

Principles and Practice of Geriatric Psychiatry, 2nd edn. Edited by J. R. M. Copeland, M. T. Abou-Saleh and D. G. Blazer

better discrimination than studies using the Research Diagnostic Criteria and DSM-III criteria[12].

The Research Diagnostic Criteria for distinction between endogenous and non-endogenous depression have been validated by the DST[13]. Mitchell[14] studied the DST in relation to the Core system (objective signs of psychomotor disturbance), Newcastle scale and DSM-III-R melancholia: all three definitions were associated with DST results. The Core index, but not the Newcastle scale, was associated with cortisol levels and dexamethasone levels after partialling out the effects of age and baseline cortisol levels. A meta-analysis of studies of the DST in relation to psychotic/non-psychotic depression (14 studies) and melancholic/non-melancholic depression (19 studies) reported a strong association of DST non-suppression and psychotic depression (64.1%) vs. non-psychotic depression (41%)[15]. The DST has good discriminating power between patients with severe psychiatric disorders, including major affective disorders, acute psychoses and dementia and patients with chronic conditions, such as dysthymic disorders (neurotic depression), chronic schizophrenia, anxiety, panic disorders and acute grief. The specificity of the test is higher in normal controls (93%) and lowest in manic patients (51%). It has satisfactory sensitivity and specificity for diagnosing secondary depression in patients with stroke. DST non-suppression after 3 months from acute stroke predicts the occurrence of depression 3 years later[16]. A review of nine studies reported a median sensitivity of 47% and specificity of 87%, suggesting the DST's utility for the evaluation of post-stroke depression[17]. However, an interesting feature is the higher rate of non-suppression in demented patients with depressive symptoms than in those without.

PROGNOSTIC VALUE

The prognostic value of the DST has been evaluated by examining the clinical outcome following antidepressive treatments in suppressors and non-suppressors, by examining changes in suppression status in relation to clinical change, and by evaluating differences in long-term outcome between non-suppressors who later converted to normal suppression and those who remained non-suppressors. Initial studies of the predictive value of the test indicated a more favourable response to antidepressant treatment in non-suppressors than in suppressors. Coppen et al.[18], however, failed to find a difference in therapeutic outcome between suppressors and non-suppressors, classified on the basis of the traditional cut-off point (50 ng/ml) for cortisol level, but found that non-suppressors had more favourable responses to both antidepressants and electroconvulsive therapy (ECT) when the criterion for non-suppression was taken as a plasma control concentration of 100 ng/ml and above. Non-suppression confers a small advantage (1%) over suppression in predicting a more favourable response to antidepressant therapy. DST status predicted improvement on nortriptyline, but not moclobemide or placebo[19].

Changes in DST status have also been examined in relation to long-term outcome: persistent non-suppression has been associated with a greater risk of relapse within several months of treatment. Depressive patients who continued to be non-suppressors had a relapse or a fatal outcome in 77% of cases, while only 19% of those who had a conversion to normal suppression had such outcome[20]. In depressive disorders, Coryell and Schlesser[21] recently reported DST non-suppression to be more powerful than clinical factors in predicting completed suicides: survival analyses over 15 years showed that the estimated risk for eventual suicide was 27% in those with DST non-suppression compared to 3% in those with normal DST. In elderly depressive patients, post-dexamethasone cortisol levels

were associated with clinical improvement and high cortisolism (150 mg/ml), and predicted improvement in delusional depression[22]. In six out of nine studies, patients with DST non-suppression following ECT had a higher rate of relapse than suppressors[23]. The value of the DST in predicting outcome following discharge has also been investigated in patients with schizophrenia and mania: non-suppressors had a more favourable clinical outcome after 6 months, and those manic patients who became suppressors before discharge had better outcomes after discharge than those who continued to be non-suppressors. In patients with senile dementia of the Alzheimer type who had depressive symptoms and who were non-suppressors, a trial of citalopram, a highly specific 5-hydroxytryptamine (5-HT)-uptake inhibitor was associated with improvement in these depressive symptoms and normalization of the DST[24].

COMMENT AND CONCLUSIONS

The introduction of the DST for the investigation of the psychobiology of depression has been a landmark development in biological psychiatry: it has had unprecedented evaluation and has been shown to be one of the most reproducible findings in the search for biological markers for depression. The balance of evidence indicates that the overnight 1 mg DST, with one plasma cortisol estimation in the afternoon of the next day and a cut-off point of 50 ng/ml has satisfactory sensitivity for depressive illness and high specificity when its results are compared with those obtained in normal controls and patients with minor psychiatric conditions and chronic schizophrenia. The specificity of the test for depression is unsatisfactory in comparison with other psychoses, including mania, schizophrenia and dementia. The sensitivity of the test is highest for severe depression with endogenous/psychotic features, mixed affective states and depression in old age. The test has little value in predicting response to antidepressants and ECT but provides a useful monitor of clinical progress and is a good predictor of long-term outcome: continued non-suppression or reversion from suppression to non-suppression during treatment or follow-up is an ominous sign that indicates a greater risk of relapse in the months following treatment. The influence of non-specific factors on the DST is considerable. Factors such as age, stress, weight loss, alcohol misuse, administration of anticonvulsants, withdrawal of psychotropic medication, presence of diabetes mellitus and the bio-availability of dexamethasone are important contributing factors to the test results. These factors, however, do not account for the variation in test results that appear to be essentially related to the biological process underlying depression. The 2 mg test has greater specificity, but lower sensitivity, than the 1 mg test and its diagnostic and prognostic value requires further investigation. The DST is only an aid to diagnosis and prognosis, aspects that should be essentially based on careful clinical assessment. The abnormal result provides a "physical sign" indicating biological depression. The DST test, like any other laboratory investigation, may increase the diagnostic confidence of the clinical diagnosis, but could never replace careful clinical assessment. The test is particularly useful in the assessment of biological depression associated with neurotic disorders, personality disorders, grief reaction and physical illness. Moreover, the presence of this "physical sign" indicates the necessity for vigorous physical treatment, or at least the use of a combined physical–psychological approach to such conditions as agoraphobia, obsessional illness and grief reaction, and the test may be particularly useful in monitoring the course of the illness and predicting its long-term outcome. Patients who continue to be non-suppressors are likely to relapse following recovery, and to require more intensive follow-up and continuation or maintenance of prophylactic medication. The test may also be useful in determining when to discontinue medication: continuing non-suppression may reflect continuing vulnerability or activity of the illness, in spite of apparent recovery, and medication should only be discontinued if the test results change to normal suppression. When using the test in clinical practice, it is important to assess the presence of confounding non-specific factors and to interpret the presence of this "sign" accordingly in guiding diagnosis and prognosis. The value of the test for the clinician, like the value of a new drug, can only be empirically determined by its trial in routine clinical practice.

THE DST IN PSYCHOGERIATRIC PRACTICE

The diagnostic and prognostic value of the DST is enhanced in the psychogeriatric setting. This is related to the higher prevalence of depressive illness, endogenous type, and delusional depressions in the elderly and hence the higher prevalence of DST non-suppression (higher sensitivity) in this population. This increased sensitivity, however, is slightly impaired by the influence of age *per se* on the performance of the test, lowering its specificity; i.e. 10–20% of normal elderly patients show non-suppression. Its specificity is even lower when performed in patients with dementia, who show similar rates of non-suppression to depressive patients, which renders the DST less useful in the differential diagnosis of depressive pseudodementia. Moreover, the contribution of physical factors, including the presence of physical illness and the influence of interfering medication, further impairs its specificity for the diagnosis of endogenous depressive illness. There is, however, evidence that DST non-suppression in dementia is related to the presence of concomitant depressive symptoms[4,25], suggesting the usefulness of treatment with anti-depressant medication. The evidence for this is, however, inconsistent: other studies have found no association between non-suppression and concomitant depressive symptoms and treatment with antidepressant medication has not consistently improved these symptoms or normalized the abnormal DST[26]. Whether the DST has diagnostic and prognostic value in milder forms of depression, which are common in the elderly, remains to be investigated.

REFERENCES

1. Abou-Saleh MT. How useful is a dexamethasone suppression test? *Curr Opin Psychiat* 1988; **1**: 60–645.602.
2. Carroll BJ. The dexamethasone test for melancholia. *Br J Psychiat* 1982; **140**: 292–304.
3. Coppen A, Abou-Saleh MT, Milln P *et al*. Dexamethasone suppression test in depression and other psychiatric illness. *Br J Psychiat* 1983; **142**: 498–504.
4. Abou-Saleh MT, Spalding EM, Kellett JM, Coppen A. Dexamethasone suppression test in dementia. *Int J Geriat Psychiat* 1987; **2**: 59–65.
5. Abou-Saleh MT, Merry J, Coppen A. Dexamethasone suppression test in alcoholism. *Acta Psychiat Scand* 1984; **2**: 112–16.
6. Graham PM, Booth J, Boranga G *et al*. The dexamethasone suppression test in mania. *J Affect Disord* 1982; **4**: 201–11.
7. Abou-Saleh MT, Olesky D, Crisp AH, Lacey JH. Dexamethasone suppression and energy balance in eating disorders. *Acta Psychiat Scand* 1986; **73**: 242–51.
8. Cassidy F, Ritchie JC, Verghese K, Carroll BJ. Dexamethasone metabolism in dexamethasone suppression test suppressors and nonsuppressors. *Biol Psychiat* 2000; **47**(7): 677–80.
9. Huizenga NA, Koper JW, de Lange P *et al*. Interperson variability but intraperson stability of baseline plasma cortisol concentrations and its relation to feedback sensitivity of the hypothalamo–pituitary–adrenal axis to a low dose of dexamethasone in elderly individuals. *J Clin Endocrinol Metab* 1998; **83**(1): 47–54.
10. Deuschle M, Schweiger U, Gotthardt U *et al*. The combined dexamethasone/corticotropin-releasing hormone stimulation test is more closely associated with features of diurnal activity of the hypothalamo–pituitary–adrenocorticol system than the dexamethasone suppression test. *Biol Psychiat* 1998; **43**(10): 762–6.
11. O'Brien JT, Ames D, Schweitzer I *et al*. Clinical and magnetic resonance imaging correlates of hypothalamic–pituitary–adrenal axis function in depression and Alzheimer's disease. *Br J Psychiat* 1996; **168**(6): 679–87.
12. Braddock L. Dexamethasone suppression test: fact or artefact? *Br J Psych* 1986; **148**: 363–71.
13. Rush AJ, Giles DE, Schlesser MA *et al*. The dexamethasone suppression test in patients with mood disorders. *J Clin Psychiat* 1996; **57**(10): 470–84.
14. Mitchell P, Hadzi-Pavlovic D, Parker G *et al*. Depressive psychomotor disturbance, cortisol, and dexamethasone. *Biol Psychiat* 1996; **40**(10): 941–50.
15. Nelson JC, Davis JM. DST studies in psychotic depression: a meta-analysis. *Am J Psychiat* 1997; **154**(11): 1497–503.
16. Astrom M, Olsson T, Asplund K. Different linkage of depression to hypercortisolism early versus late after stroke. A 3-year longitudinal study. *Stroke* 1993; **24**(1): 52–7.
17. Harvey SA, Black KJ. The dexamethasone suppression test for diagnosing depression in stroke patients. *Ann Clin Psychiat* 1996; **8**(1): 35–9.
18. Coppen A, Milln P, Harwood J, Wood K. Does the dexamethasone suppression test predict antidepressant treatment success? *Br J Psychiat* 1985; **42**: 193–204.
19. Kin NM, Nair NP, Amin M *et al*. The dexamethasone suppression test and treatment outcome in elderly depressed patients participating in a placebo-controlled multicenter trial involving moclobemide and nortriptyline. *Biol Psychiat* 1997; **42**(10): 925–31.
20. Arana CW, Baldessarini RJ, Ornsteen M. The dexamethasone suppression test for diagnosis and prognosis in psychiatry. *Arch Gen Psychiat* 1985; **42**: 193–204.
21. Coryell W, Schlesser M. The dexamethasone suppression test and suicide prediction. *Am J Psychiat* 2001; **158**(5): 748–53.
22. Meyers BS, Alpert S, Gabriele M *et al*. State Specificity of DST abnormalities in geriatric depression. *Biol Psychiat* 1993; **34**(1–2): 108–14.
23. Bourgon LN, Kellner CH. Relapse of depression after ECT: a review. *J ECT* 2000; **16**(1): 19–31.
24. Balldin JF, Gottfries CG, Karlsson I *et al*. Relationship between DST and the serotonergic system. Results from treatment with two 5-HT re-uptake blockers in dementia disorders. *Int J Geriat Psych* 1988; **3**: 7–26.
25. Katona CLE, Aldridge CR. The dexamethasone suppression test and depressive signs in dementia. *J Affect Disord* 1985; **8**: 83–9.
26. Slotkin TA, Hays JC, Nemeroff CB, Carroll BJ. Dexamethasone suppression test identifies a subset of elderly depressed patients with reduced platelet serotonin transport and resistance to imipramine inhibition of transport. *Depress Anxiety* 1997; **6**: 19–25.

82

Bereavement

Robert J. Kastenbaum

Arizona State University, Tempe, AZ, USA

Advanced age and bereavement are circumstances, not psychiatric syndromes. An octogenarian may have a variety of concerns, such as remembering which medication to take when, fear of falling on icy pavement, and worry about remaining financially independent on a fixed income. A recently bereaved octogenarian is likely to have additional concerns: "Who can I share my day with?"; "Who will do the driving/cooking?"; "Where do I go from here?". These are all essentially human rather than geriatric problems. Therefore, the psychiatry of bereavement in old age does not assume pathology or the necessity for professional intervention. Hastily prescribing psychotropic medication for a "geriatric patient" can all too easily become part of the problem, rather than the solution. Instead, we ask ourselves such questions as, "Who is this person?"; "What was the nature of this unique relationship that has been ended by death?"; "What does this loss mean to the bereaved person—and what coping skills and resources can be called upon to make it through?".

A perspective on bereavement in old age can be developed by following the sequence of events and challenges. Fortunately, a growing number of clinical observations and research findings are available to guide this overview.

THE PRE-BEREAVEMENT SITUATION

Four questions are particularly useful in approaching an understanding of the situation that existed prior to a bereavement in old age.

1. What Was the Nature and Status of the Relationship at This Time?

This question should be answered both structurally and substantively, e.g. "He was her older brother; she relied on him for advice and support more than on any other person, including her husband"; or "She was his second wife; he had expected her to look after him—actually, to wait on him hand and foot!—and suddenly he had to be the caring person . . .". It is useful to explore both the affective and pragmatic dimensions of the relationship. Was the survivor or the deceased heavily dependent on the other person? Had the relationship been in serious trouble? If so, was this shown by silent coexistence or stormy disputes? Did the deceased provide most of the couple's link to society? Had the survivor organized his/her life around taking care of the deceased?

Particular sensitivity may be required in understanding an elderly person's response to the death of an adult child or a grandchild. Recent studies suggest a highly individualized deep interiorization of grief after the first shock of the loss[1,2]. There may be little apparent behavioral change but much continued inner processing of the loss and an intensified life review. Researchers are reaching consensus on the multidimensionality of the older person's response to bereavement and caution against simplistic characterizations, such as "depression".

2. How Was the Prospect of Death Integrated into the Life Scenario?

The possibility of *anticipatory grief* should be explored, rather than assumed. Fatal accidents (especially falls and motor vehicle accidents) are far more common among people 65 and older than in any other age group (in fact, data from the US Center on Health Statistics indicate that there are more fatal accidents at 65+ than in all other age groups combined). This means that many an elderly spouse or sibling has no opportunity to prepare for the death of a person who did not seem to be in imminent danger of death. Others may have coped so long with chronic health problems that it seemed as though they might continue to go on forever. Furthermore, obvious risks may have been strongly defended against by compartmentalization or other common mechanisms. The bereavement may also take the form of the completely unexpected death of a younger family member or friend.

Despite many exceptions, however, there is a greater probability that the death will have been expected. Not only do an increasing proportion of deaths occur in old age, but modern health care has lengthened the interval between development of a life-threatening condition and the day of death. The four leading causes of death for elderly people in the USA (heart disease, malignant neoplasms, cerebrovascular disease and respiratory conditions) all involve a long period of living with progressive life-threatening conditions and, therefore, opportunity for both prolonged stress and adaptation to the prospect of death. Anticipatory grief is similar in many respects to the grief that is experienced after a death[3]. There are affective, cognitive and somatic components, e.g. sadness, obsession, exhaustion, etc. Clinical experience suggests that a period of anticipatory grief often helps the survivor to cope with the loss, by avoiding the element of surprise and providing the opportunity for preliminary adjustment. Traumatic grief reactions are more common when bereavement is sudden and unexpected[4].

However, awareness of an impending loss is not an invulnerable shield against the first impact. "I thought I had cried all the tears there were to cry. I had myself under control", one woman reported. "Not a bit of it! I went all to pieces, feeling Sammy's hand so cold". We are beginning to learn that anticipatory grief

Principles and Practice of Geriatric Psychiatry, 2nd edn. Edited by J. R. M. Copeland, M. T. Abou-Saleh and D. G. Blazer
©2002 John Wiley & Sons, Ltd

has both its advantages and its risks. Did this survivor start to detach him/herself emotionally while the spouse was still alive, depriving them both of the support they needed? Or did both partners use this time to affirm their love and consult with each other in making plans and decisions?

Physicians and other caregivers have the opportunity to make valuable contributions to the survivor's ability to cope with grief by sensitive response to the situation as it exists prior to the death. Offering accurate information, suggesting other options and improving the lines of communication within the family are among the ways in which one can help to shape the anticipatory grief period into a source of strength rather than intensified anxiety. The age differential between most caregivers and the elderly bereaved people they are trying to help sometimes interferes with communication, e.g. when elders are patronized and their ability to cope with bad news is underestimated. There is also an underappreciated connection between quality of terminal care and grief recovery. A hospice physician reports that, "The pain relief we achieve for an old man in his last weeks of life helps his wife to be more of her normal self when he really needs her— and a widow with fewer regrets and nightmares later"[5].

3. What Was the Survivor's Own Health Status Previous to the Bereavement?

This is a particularly useful question to ask with respect to the older bereaved person. The spouse was the most frequent principal family caregiver in the 40 hospices studied by Mor *et al.*[6]. About two-thirds of the spouses taking responsibility for care were people above the age of 55 and it was not unusual for the caregiver to be over 75. The elderly caregiver seldom developed new physical problems over the course of the spouse's final illness, but there was a tendency to ignore his/her existing conditions. During the first months of bereavement, the survivor's health was sometimes impaired by exacerbation of previous illnesses and impairments. It would be helpful, then, to encourage the spouse and other elderly family members and friends to look after their own health during the pre-bereavement period, and to see that health status is carefully assessed afterward. Symptoms that might appear to be part of an anxious depression syndrome could be related to physical health problems that have not received the attention they deserved.

4. Who Else Was There and What Else Was Happening?

Explored diligently, this line of inquiry may reveal significant sources of concern or potential strength that bear on adjustment to the loss. "Well, Frank's brother had come to live with us again. And he was drinking again. I could have killed him"; "The people from the church were over all the time. They really cared. We were so far from the rest of the family, but they were just like family to us . . ."; "I couldn't get anything from the doctor—what was really going on with George, what else I could do. I felt like telling him, 'I'm old—not stupid!', but you don't do that, do you?". Some of the problems that beset the survivors after the death may be the continuation or outcome of difficulties that occurred earlier. Strained interpersonal relationships and unanswered questions create more of a burden for some survivors than the death itself.

AT THE TIME OF DEATH

Learning what happened around the time of death can help us understand the bereaved elder's state of mind. Consider, for

example, the difference between death at home and in a hospital setting. A terminally ill woman was being looked after at home by her elderly mother, with support from a local hospice service. The mother had accepted her daughter's wish to be allowed to die at home without intubation and other futile procedures. But when the daughter appeared to be actively dying, the mother panicked and called not the hospice but a visiting nursing service. Now, as a survivor, the old woman is haunted by memories of her suctioned, intubated and drugged daughter accusing her with her eyes[7]. In a more frequent scenario, an elderly person will call for assistance from paramedics when his/her spouse appears to have died. But when the paramedic team arrives, the caller may have second thoughts about seeing the spouse's body subjected to resuscitation procedures. Some bereaved elderly persons remain troubled not by the fact of the death itself, but by unanswered questions about whether or not they did the right thing at the right time.

Knowing only that the death took place in a hospital does not tell us whether supportive nurses encouraged a woman to be with her husband right through to the end and to have time with him afterward—or whether she was made to feel unwelcome and hustled away. Perhaps, again, she had not been notified until some time after the death. The particularities of the final scene can either provide an acceptable conclusion to the story of a marriage or friendship, or torment the survivor with resentment, self-doubt and other disturbing thoughts.

The psychiatrist often has the opportunity to increase the sensitivity of physicians, nurses, and other caregivers in their communication patterns around the time of death. Survivors may hold on to a word or a gesture, either as a cherished or an infuriating/depressing memory. Often one can be helpful simply by validating the survivor-to-be's feelings and giving him/her the opportunity to clarify his/her own thoughts by active listening. The generational difference between the bereaved person and the psychiatrist can be a source of misunderstanding. A widow, for example, may first respond according to the models of grief that were prevalent in her youth. It may take patience and encouragement to help her discover, express and cope with her own feelings. It is also helpful to be aware of ethnic differences in expectations for behavior around the time of death. Caregivers whose own tradition involves subdued behavior and restraint of emotions may not be prepared for families in which intense expressions of grief are expected, even required.

EARLY PHASES OF BEREAVEMENT

The idea that there are fixed "stages" of either dying or grief has attracted more believers than it deserves. One can select and force observations to fit stage theories, but to what purpose? Individual responses to grief deviate markedly from the models: this is even more common in old age, where uniqueness has been deeply engraved and polished to a high gloss.

It does make sense, though, to differentiate between responses to earlier and later periods subsequent to bereavement. Indicators of a potentially intense, disabling and protracted reaction often appear within a short time. Parke and Weiss[8] found that those who had the most difficult time coping with the spouse's death tended to smoke and drink more heavily, use tranquilizers and express depressive mood (e.g. "Life is a strain for me . . . I wonder whether anything is worthwhile any more"). These and other investigators have found that the way the survivor responds to the loss within the first few months provides a fairly reliable forecast of what kind of adjustment will be made over a longer period of time. The obvious lesson here is that early-appearing indicators, such as loss of appetite, withdrawal from friends and activities, sleep disturbances and escape into alcohol and drugs (including the hoarding of prescription or over-the-counter elixirs) should be taken seriously. Time alone will not necessarily prove the healer.

Dependency needs frequently come to the fore when the survivor is having great difficulty in coping. Counselors and therapists face the challenge of helping survivors to rekindle their sense of competency and autonomy. This is likely to be a step-by-step progression, in which the therapist may have to play the roles of protector and mentor for some time. The advanced age of the bereaved person does not necessarily stand in the way of therapeutic success. It has been observed in clinical practice and confirmed by research (e.g. Duran *et al.*[9]) that both the individual's personality and his/her social support often make the crucial difference in recovery from bereavement.

It is not unusual to see an elderly person appear relatively unresponsive to a death. In some situations this is the observer's failure to notice subtle but significant changes. But the lack of a strong overt response is sometimes associated with bereavement overload[10]. So much active and re-activated grief from previous bereavements has commanded the person's attention that there is not enough emotional energy available to respond fully to the most recent death. Survivors of the Holocaust and other disasters have often been afflicted in this way.

LATER PHASES OF BEREAVEMENT

Many senior adults have proved highly resilient after experiencing bereavement. Studies do not invariably find that widows sit around weeping and feeling helpless. The gender dimension is important here. Women outnumber men in the upper age echelons and often show themselves more skillful in providing social and emotional support. By contrast, the bereaved older man runs more risk of becoming isolated. In some environments, such as the retirement community with its high density of older women, the widower may be looked after and valued. Nevertheless, there is a major problem of hidden grief among older men, a problem that often persists for years after the loss. Quiet, keeping to himself, expressing little obvious emotion, the older bereaved man is more likely to be suffering intensely than his female peer, with her greater facility in self-expression and more sensitive support network[11]. This not yet well appreciated fact suggests that psychiatrists and other caregivers should explore the possibility of bereavement—even a fairly remote bereavement—as the underlying factor in a variety of behavioral and somatic problems experienced by older men. Unfortunately, some of the most traumatic bereavements leave the elderly survivor with the most limited social support. This is especially the case with suicide[12]. The high rate of suicide among elderly white men each year often leaves their spouses and siblings alone with their grief.

A FEW SPECIAL CONSIDERATIONS

1. Bereavement is a status marker: in spousal death, for example, the survivor is no longer a husband or a wife. From that day forward, society tends to treat him/her in a different way. We can be helpful in supporting survivors' movement to meaningful new roles and the restoration of self-confidence.
2. The "little deaths" that often accompany the later years of life can both anticipate and intensify grief reactions. The old man may have been mourning the loss of his mobility even before his wife died; the old woman who has been relieved of her starring role as a church soloist may have felt abandoned and rejected long before her husband's death.
3. Both elders and young children are sometimes regarded as incapable of grief, although for different reasons. This unfounded assumption results in the additional suffering involved in *disenfranchized grief*[13]. Instead of being a core part of the family communication network and helping to support others in their grief, the elder may be shunted aside, thereby becoming increasingly vulnerable to depression.
3. The death of animal companions can lead to authentic grief reactions[14]. The grief syndrome may be very similar to what is experienced upon the death of a human companion, although the intensity is less likely to endure as long. Rage joins with grief when an elderly person is placed in a nursing home (loss of independence, loss of choice) and then learns that his/her animal companion has been taken to the pound and destroyed.

In a sense, there are no "little griefs", and there may be no "getting over" the greatest losses we experience in our lives. But most elderly adults have learned to live with disappointments, limitations and suffering. When bereavement comes, as a rule they do not need drugs, hospitalization and the whole rigmarole of the health care system. To be offered companionship and to see in that companion's eyes that one is still valued and needed is often all that is needed for the survivor to get on with life.

REFERENCES

1. de Vries B, Davis CG, Wortman B, Lehman DR. Long-term psychological and somatic consequences of later life parental bereavement. *Omega* 1997; **35**: 97–118.
2. Fry PS. Grandparents' reactions to the death of a grandchild: an exploratory factor analytic study. *Omega* 1997; **35**: 119–40.
3. Gilliland G, Fleming S. A comparison of spousal anticipatory grief and conventional grief. *Death Studies* 1998; **22**: 541–70.
4. Prigerson HG, Shear MK, Bierhals AJ *et al.* Case histories of traumatic grief. *Omega* 1997; **35**: 9–24.
5. Silverman H. Phoenix: Hospice of the Valley. Private communication, 1990.
6. Mor V, Greer DS, Kastenbaum R, eds. *The Hospice Experiment*. Baltimore, MD: Johns Hopkins University Press, 1988.
7. Kastenbaum R. *The Psychology of Death*, 3rd edn. New York: Springer, 2000.
8. Parkes CM, Weiss RS. *Recovery from Bereavement*. New York: Basic Books, 1983.
9. Duran A, Turner CW, Lund DA. Social support, perceived stress, and depression following the death of a spouse in late life. In Lund DA, ed., *Older Bereaved Spouses*. New York: Hemisphere, 1989; 69–78.
10. Kastenbaum R. Death and bereavement in later life. In Kutscher AH, ed., *Death and Bereavement*. Springfield, CT: Charles C. Thomas, 1969; 28–54.
11. Stroebe MS, Stroebe W. Who participates in bereavement research? A review and an empirical study. *Omega* 1989–1990; **20**: 1–30.
12. Farberow NL, Gallagher-Thompson D, Gilewski M, Thompson L. The role of social supports in the bereavement process of surviving spouses of suicide and natural deaths. In Leenaars AA, Maris RW, McIntosh JL, Richman J, eds, *Suicide and the Older Adult*. New York: Guilford, 1992; 107–24.
13. Weisman AD. Animal companions and human grief. *Omega* 1990–1991; **22**: 22–43.

83

Suicidal Behaviour

Howard Cattell

Wrexham Maelor Hospital, Wrexham, UK

This chapter concerns itself with completed and attempted suicide in the elderly. It is a major public health problem and the clinician has a crucial influence in determining outcome in suicidal patients. We shall discuss the epidemiological, social, physical and psychiatric factors involved and conclude with a consideration of preventive measures.

EPIDEMIOLOGY

Although there are significant international variations in the official completed suicide rates reported by countries throughout the world, the overall rates continue to remain among the highest in the elderly, as rates increase with age. Males aged 75 and over have the highest rates of suicide in nearly all industrialized countries, with rates for men throughout the elderly lifespan exceeding those for women. However, suicide rates in the elderly, for both sexes, have declined in recent years in many countries, with rates declining by over 30%, for example, in the UK for both sexes between 1982 and 1996[1]. Explanations for such trends are largely speculative.

The prevalence of suicidal thoughts in the elderly has been investigated in some recent studies. Skoog *et al.* examined a population of non-demented 85-year-olds with the finding that among the mentally well, none had seriously considered suicide, but that the presence of mental disorder, especially major depression, was strongly correlated with suicidal feelings[2]. The study by Forsell *et al.*[3] of almost 1000 over-75-year-olds similarly found that those with frequent suicidal thoughts had a strong association with major depression. The conclusion from studies such as these is similar, notably that a careful assessment of the mental state, focused especially on the possibility of depression, is essential before any rational basis for suicidal thoughts be considered.

Little attention has been focused on non-fatal suicidal acts in the elderly, due probably to the phenomenon in recent decades being one of younger people. No countries keep national statistics, but data from centres with well-defined catchment areas allow examination of numbers, rates and trends. Cases of elderly self-harm account for about 5% of the total number of self-harm admissions to general hospitals in the UK and North America.

SOCIAL FACTORS

Studies of individual elderly suicides have drawn attention to a number of social variables. With regard to marital status, widowed, single or divorced individuals seem to be more at risk, with marriage appearing to offer a protective factor. The great majority of elderly suicides occur in a community setting, usually in the person's home. The method of suicide varies over time, with age, gender and other sociocultural factors. It is generally found that men adopt more violent methods than women, e.g. deaths due to hanging and firearms are commoner in men. In the USA, firearms are used by over 60% of all completed suicides, with elderly White men employing this method most frequently.

The role of social isolation as a risk factor has traditionally been considered an important variable[4], although several subsequent studies[5,6] have found no difference between living alone and number of social contacts compared to younger suicides. Bereavement appears as a significant risk factor, with studies of attempted and completed suicide citing its relevance. The first year of widowhood seems to be a vulnerable period, with elderly widowed men being at greater relative risk.

The antecedents in terms of precipitating life events appear to differ in the elderly population compared with younger and middle-aged groups. The latter are associated more closely with interpersonal and relationship problems, financial, legal and occupational difficulties, and less with physical illness, fear of dependency and loss of function, as is often the situation in the elderly. Although complaints of "loneliness" are frequent, a recent Scandinavian study revealed that a similar proportion of younger victims (around 38%) also complained of this difficulty[7].

PSYCHIATRIC ILLNESS

The major finding in the clinical studies of suicide and attempted suicide in the elderly is the presence of psychiatric disorder in the period prior to the event. Among the elderly, however, depressive illness is the most important predictor of suicide and this needs to be emphasized. Most comprehensive studies of completed suicide employing the psychological autopsy method report the prevalence of major depression and other mood disorders to be 60–90%. For example, Conwell *et al.*[8], examining the relationship between age and Axis 1 diagnoses in a sample of 141 completed suicides aged 21–92 years, found 71% and 64% of the 75–92- and 55–77-year-old cohorts, respectively, to exhibit mood disorders, compared with 30% of the 21–34-year-old group. Major depression was diagnosed in almost 60% of the most elderly suicides, with other mood disorders accounting for 10–20% of the sample in this study. The elderly constituted the most homogeneous group, in which non-affective psychoses were rare, addictive disorders less common and late-onset depression the rule.

Principles and Practice of Geriatric Psychiatry, 2nd edn. Edited by J. R. M. Copeland, M. T. Abou-Saleh and D. G. Blazer
©2002 John Wiley & Sons, Ltd

The symptom profile of elderly suicides prior to the event has been described in earlier studies. Barraclough[4], in examining 30 elderly suicides, reported complaints of insomnia (90%), weight loss (75%), guilt feelings (50%) and hypochondriasis (50%) in the month prior to death. The existence of suicidal ideation often lacks spontaneous expression and it is important that such ideas are explored. Suicidal intent may be less evident, particularly where physical ill-health complaints are prominent. For example, in a recent study from Finland[7] of over 200 elderly suicides, suicidal intent was communicated to attending healthcare professionals in only 18%. The lesson to be learnt is that the presence of somatic symptoms should not detract from a close examination of the mental state with particular regard to a depressive illness and coexistent suicidal thoughts.

Primary substance misuse disorders account for a smaller proportion of suicides than in younger age groups, with prevalence estimates of 5–40%. Similarly, non-affective psychoses are uncommonly reported compared to younger suicides. The association between suicide and dementing illnesses has received limited attention. Although advanced dementia is likely to be a protective factor, the significance of an early dementia as a risk factor for suicide is largely speculative. Individual case studies, however, indicate that in some people the fear of progressive dependency and "institutionalization" is an important dynamic, irrespective of the presence of evident cognitive deficits. There are similarly few reports on the association between personality and suicide in the elderly. Earlier studies described a personality profile of inflexibility, "failure to adjust" and poor adaptation to change. More recently, Duberstein[9] reported a lower openness to experience (OTE) score in elderly compared to younger suicides. This profile may be summarized as a cognitive propensity to perceive problems in dichotomous, black-and-white terms, a rigidly defined self-concept and a diminished behavioural repertoire, thus decreasing the capacity to adapt to loss and change.

BIOLOGICAL FACTORS

Suicide as a distinct neurobiological entity has been investigated in the search to identify potential biological markers, although this research has been almost exclusively undertaken on a younger population. This may be partly attributable to the inherent and often contradictory data on the effect of ageing on central nervous system neurotransmitter systems. Jones et al.[10], however, in a study of the suicidal elderly, found significant lower concentrations of cerebrospinal fluid 5-hydroxyindoleacetic acid and homovanillic acid, compared to non-suicidal and normal controls, which is in keeping with other studies in younger suicides.

PHYSICAL ILLNESS

The importance of physical illness as a major antecedent to suicide and attempted suicide in the elderly has long been emphasized. Not only does the older suicide have a higher prevalence of illness compared to his younger counterpart, but the incidence of physical illness greatly exceeds that found in the non-suicidal elderly. Several early studies reported medical illness directly contributing to suicide in around 60–70% of cases, with evidence of higher rates of physical illness among elderly males compared to females. In a recent Scandinavian study[5], the importance of physical ill-health as a life event in the 3 months before death was demonstrated, with elderly men displaying an excess of serious somatic illness compared to elderly females (55% vs. 31%), suggesting gender differences in coping with such age-normative stressors.

Several central nervous system and systemic disorders have been linked with increased risk of suicide. These include epilepsy, multiple sclerosis, Huntington's chorea, head injury, peptic ulcer and rheumatoid arthritis. The association of suicide with cancer is inconsistent with some studies supporting such an association, while others refute the risk, especially among hospitalized patients. In a study from Canada[11] involving 543 elderly suicides, with information obtained from coroners' inquests, those with medical illnesses were significantly less likely to be referred to psychiatric services than those without a medical illness, and those with a terminal illness, comprising almost 9% of the total, were least likely of all to receive a psychiatric assessment. A number of studies have drawn attention to the importance of subjective complaints of pain prior to suicide in the elderly[12,13], with nearly 20% of the samples indicating it to be a major concern prior to death. The point to be reiterated is that the presence of physical illness or presentation with somatic or hypochondriacal concerns may mask the underlying depression, and this type of presentation may be of importance in elderly men, who may be less likely to verbalize their depressed mood or admit to suicidal thoughts.

These findings for completed suicide have their parallel in attempted suicide in the elderly. In a study of 100 elderly suicide attempts, 53% were considered to be suffering from significant physical illness at index assessment following the attempt[14]. The cohort demonstrated an increased mortality from natural causes compared to an age- and gender-matched population and, after an average of 3.5 years, 42% of the original subjects had died.

PREVENTION

Any strategy designed to prevent suicidal behaviour needs to take account of the following factors. Which individuals are likely to be at risk, how are they to be identified, and by whom? To what extent may training and education influence detection and management of vulnerable elderly individuals? How may services be improved to effect a reduction in rates of suicidal behaviour?

Risk Assessment

The act of suicide is a complex phenomenon, involving multiple psychological, physical and social factors operating at a crucial moment in the life of a vulnerable individual, and any risk assessment procedure needs to reflect these varied antecedents. A typical high-risk individual, for example, may be described as an elderly male, living alone following recent bereavement, who may have painful, chronic health problems, who is currently depressed and who has made previous suicide attempts. The problem with applying risk factors lies in the generation of high false-positive predictions associated with the relatively low base rate of completed suicide, and as yet no instruments exist with sufficient sensitivity or specificity to be clinically useful as a risk assessment scale in the elderly. It is the clinical interview that remains the cornerstone of such assessment and needs to clarify key variables. These considerations should not, however, detract the assessor from the real increased susceptibility of the elderly to eventual suicide. This can be seen particularly in elderly attempters, where suicidal intent, as measured by the Beck intent scale, is at its highest for any age group[15]. Attempts in the elderly are also a much stronger predictor of subsequent completed suicide, compared with attempts in younger people, with a ratio of attempts to completion estimated to be around 4:1 compared with between 8:1 and 200:1 for younger attempters. All attempts should be taken seriously.

Recognition

Despite the unique multifactorial precipitants that contribute to individual cases of suicide, opportunities for recognition exist. Suicidal intent, for example, is frequently directly expressed, albeit in different contexts, and should be taken seriously. In the recent study from Finland[2], for example, although nearly half of the victims, men as often as women, had brought up their suicidal ideation or intent to their next of kin, the same intent had only been communicated to healthcare professionals in 18%, despite the great majority (70%) being in contact with health services in the month before their death. The study, however, also reported that in only 24% of the cases had the healthcare professionals even asked about suicidal intentions. It is a misconception to suppose that discussion of suicidal ideas generates attempts. Most individuals feel grateful for a discussion of their suicidal feelings, about which they may feel unduly guilty.

The role of primary care services in suicide prevention is of considerable interest. Most studies report substantial levels of contact: 40–70% of elderly suicides seeing their general practitioner (GP) in the month preceding their death and between 20–50% attending in the preceding week. This raises the important issue of effective intervention at a time when the individual is particularly vulnerable. The importance of training and education programmes for GPs in the recognition and treatment of depression as a means of reducing the suicide rate arises from the Gotland Study[16], in which in the year following training, suicide rates on the island fell significantly compared with other parts of Sweden, and the fall was accounted for largely by the proportion of suicides with major depression. Although not specific to the elderly, such research requires replication.

Research evidence also suggests that a minority of elderly suicides have been in contact with secondary psychiatric services prior to death. Several studies report that around 20% of their series of completed elderly suicides had contact within 6 months and around 10–15% in the preceding 1 month[17,18]. It is important to realize that around 30–60% have no contact with health professionals prior to death, despite the high prevalence of psychiatric disorder.

The issue of treatment adequacy is of significance, given the importance of depressive illness in completed and attempted suicide, with several studies revealing inadequate or inappropriate treatment with psychotropic medication. Conwell[19], for example, described the recognition and treatment of psychiatric symptoms in primary care settings for 51 elderly suicides and found only two who had received adequate treatment, with men and those with coexistent physical illness presenting the greatest challenge. Information from several Coroner's Inquest studies reveal low levels of antidepressant treatment of around 10–25%[11,12,17], although a more optimistic finding has been reported from Sweden, where 50% of a cohort of 75 elderly suicides had a documented history of treatment for affective disorder in the 6 months prior to death[20].

Preventive Strategies

Strategies for the prevention of elderly suicide have been recently reviewed from an international perspective[21]. It would be fair to say that there are limited data on the effectiveness of specific assertive outreach programmes targeting the elderly, although some encouraging initiatives have been described. DeLeo et al.[22] described a Tele-Help/Tele-Check service for a population of 12 000 over-65-year-olds in Padua, Italy. The service provides active contacts to clients by trained staff giving information, support and prompt intervention in medical and psychological emergencies. After 4 years of this service, only one suicide was reported, which was significantly lower than expected.

In the USA, the Gatekeepers Program of Spokane, Washington, addresses the need to contact non-self-referrals by training business personnel in the recognition and referral to health professionals of elderly distressed individuals. Such personnel include apartment managers, pharmacists, meter readers, etc. In the UK, the implementation of screening policies for the elderly, the development of community-based old age psychiatry services maintaining close links with primary care facilities, improved education and liaison links with general hospital services, and local and national audit programmes, are likely to be useful.

CONCLUSION

Although there has been a recent decline in elderly suicide rates in several Western countries, the rates remain among the highest for any age group in most societies throughout the world. Despite this, the phenomenon receives little public attention. A common assumption is that suicide in these individuals is an understandable, normal reaction to hopeless, irreversible situations and is consequently unavoidable. There is increasing debate over the individual's "right to die" and self-determination and euthanasia advocates have adopted a more prominent position.

Whatever an individual's personal views are towards the morality of suicidal behaviour, it is incumbent on the physician to pay close attention to the mental and physical state. Available evidence suggests that the great majority of individuals who attempt or commit suicide suffer from both potentially treatable psychiatric conditions (mainly depression) and associated physical and social difficulties for which much can be done. To condemn the elderly by adopting a negative approach is to succumb to the dangers of "ageism".

REFERENCES

1. Kelly S, Bunting J. Trends in suicide in England and Wales 1982–1996. *Population Trends* 1998; **92**: 29–41.
2. Skoog I, Aevarsson O, Beskow J *et al.* Suicidal feelings in a population sample of non-demented 85 year olds. *Am J Psychiat* 1996; **153**: 1015–20.
3. Forsell Y, Jorm A, Winblad B. Suicidal thoughts and associated factors in an elderly population. *Acta Psychiat Scand* 1997; **95**: 108–11.
4. Barraclough B. Suicide in the elderly. In Kay DWK, Walks A, eds, *Recent Developments in Psychogeriatrics*. Headley: Royal Medico-Psychological Association, 1971; 87–97.
5. Heikkinen ME, Lonnqvist JK. Recent life events in elderly suicide: a nationwide study in Finland. *Int Psychogeriat* 1995; **7**: 287–300.
6. Carney SS, Rich CL, Burke PA *et al.* Suicide over 60: the San Diego Study. *J Am Geriat Soc* 1994; **42**: 174–80.
7. Pitkala K, Isometsa ET, Henriksson MM, Lonnqvist JK. Elderly suicide in Finland. *Int Psychogeriat* 200; **12**: 209–20.
8. Conwell Y, Duberstein PR, Cox C *et al.* Relationship of age and axis 1 diagnoses in victims of completed suicide: a psychological autopsy study. *Am J Psychiat* 1996; **153**: 1001–8.
9. Duberstein PR. Openness to experience and completed suicide across the second half of life. *Int Psychogeriat* 1995; **7**: 183–98.
10. Jones JS, Stanley B, Mann JJ *et al.* CSF 5-HIAA and HVA concentrations in elderly depressed patients who attempted suicide. *Am J Psychiat* 1990; **147**: 1225–7.
11. Duckworth G, McBride H. Suicide in old age: a tragedy of neglect. *Can J Psychiat* 1996; **41**: 217–22.
12. Cattell H. Elderly suicide in London: an analysis of coroners inquests. *Int J Geriat Psychiat* 1988; **3**: 251–61.
13. Purcell D, Thrush CRN, Blanchette PL. Suicide among the elderly in Honolulu County: a multiethnic comparative study (1987–1992). *Int Psychogeriat* 1999; **11**: 57–66.

14. Hepple J, Quinton C. One hundred cases of attempted suicide in the elderly. *Br J Psychiat* 1997; **171**: 42–6.

15. Merrill J, Owens J. Age and attempted suicide. *Acta Psychiat Scand* 1990; **82**: 385–8.

16. Rutz W, von Knorring L, Walinder J. Frequency of suicide on Gotland after systematic postgraduate education of general practitioners. *Acta Psychiat Scand* 1989; **30**: 151–5.

17. Cattell H, Jolley DJ. One hundred cases of suicide in elderly people. *Br J Psychiat* 1995; **169**: 451–7.

18. Osuna E, Perez-Carceles M, Conejero J *et al*. Epidemiology of suicide in elderly people in Madrid, Spain (1990–1994). *Forens Sci Int* 1997; **87**: 73–80.

19. Cornwell Y. Management of suicidal behaviour in the elderly. *Psychiat Clin N Am* 1997; **20**: 667–83.

20. Waern M, Beslow J, Rumeson B *et al*. High rate of antidepressant treatment in elderly people who commit suicide. *Br Med J* 1996; **313**: 1118.

21. Pearson JL, Conwell Y, Lindesay J *et al*. Elderly suicide: a multinational view. *Ageing Ment Health* 1997; **1**: 107–11.

22. DeLeo D, Carollo G, Buono MD. Lower suicide rates associated with a Tele-Help/Tele-Check service for the elderly at home. *Am J Psychiat* 1995; **15**: 632–4.

84

Genetics and Aetiology

Thomas R. Thompson and William McDonald

Emory University School of Medicine, Atlanta, GA, USA

The literature surrounding the genetics of psychiatric illness and bipolar disorder is expanding, but is limited and often contradictory. Great advances have been made regarding DNA analysis and mapping the human genome. Despite these advances, it is difficult to adequately analyze the available data because the genes studied are complex and exhibit significant heterogeneity in genotype and subsequent phenotype.

There is clear evidence from family studies that bipolar disorder is inherited[1–5]. However, the genetic foundation of this disorder is not well understood. Leonhard's[6] early hypothesis, that bipolar and unipolar illnesses are distinct clinical entities and do not share a common genetic vulnerability, has been supported by empirical data. However, Roglev's[7] recent study supported the polygenic threshold model of transmission, giving credence to the hypothesis that unipolar and bipolar disorder may be one illness. Angst[8] first demonstrated the greater prevalence of both unipolar and bipolar illness in the probands of bipolar patients, compared to unipolar probands who only showed an excess number of unipolar relatives. These data have been replicated in a number of studies[9]. Following up on earlier research demonstrating a linkage between an X chromosome marker (color blindness) and manic depressive illness[10], additional chromosomal studies have linked markers on the X chromosome to bipolar disease and pedigrees from Belgium and Israel[11]. Yet, clearly this mode of genetic transmission could not be solely responsible for bipolar illness. Families with both fathers and sons with the illness are not explained by this mode of transmission, since the father only gives the son the Y chromosome. Other researchers have demonstrated linkage between bipolar disorder and the H-ras-1 locus of chromosome 11 in a pedigree of North American Amish[12,13]. However, separate investigations fail to confirm this linkage in Icelandic, Irish and North American[14] pedigrees. Baron and Egeland later published an update and re-evaluation of their data, essentially reversing their original findings supporting linkage between chromosomes X and 11 with bipolar disorder[15,16]. More recent studies suggest links between bipolar disorder and expanded trinucleotide repeats, potassium channel gene hKCa3, Darier's disease and velo-cardio-facial syndrome[17,18–21]. However, other research can be found that questions some of these links[22–23]. Other chromosomes, including 18, 21, 22, 5, 12 and X, have been implicated in bipolar disorder[17]. The consensus has evolved that the constellation of symptoms making up the phenotypic expression of bipolar disorder are probably due to genetic heterogeneity, and that subtypes within the bipolar spectrum may exist.

The discrepancy in the literature can be best understood using the model of bipolar illness as a genetically heterogeneous disorder. Probably, these are complex genes with variable penetrance that do not exhibit true Mendelian genetics[17]. Because of these factors, it is difficult to obtain significant "power" to demonstrate gene linkage, explaining some of the conflicting results found in the literature[24].

In the elderly, bipolar disorder can be divided into those patients with an early onset of their manic symptoms and those patients for whom symptoms first appear in late life, thereby underscoring possible genetic etiology vs. environmental factors contributing to the expression of manic symptoms. Mania in geriatric patients may be due to bipolar disorder, with early onset and later recurrence or chronic course, or to the first episode of mania occurring in late life. In Shulman and Post's[25] review of bipolar patients admitted to the hospital after age 60, the mean age of onset of the manic symptoms is 60 years. Similarly, in a group of manic hospitalized patients over 65 years old, Stone[26] found that 26% had no prior history of affective disorders. Other larger epidemiologic studies with patient populations of all ages have demonstrated that the onset of bipolar disorder peaks at an early age and declines throughout an individual's lifetime[27–30].

Older adults presenting with the same phenotype (i.e. manic symptoms) may therefore have a very different past clinical course of their illness and may possibly fit into different subtypes of bipolar disorder (e.g. early and late onset).

Stone's[26] review of elderly patients with mania demonstrates that patients with a family history of affective disorder have an earlier average age of onset of their manic symptoms (53 years, compared to 60 years for patients with no family history of affective disorder). Further studies have also supported the notion that patients with early-onset mania (usually defined as less than 30 years old) have an increased number of relatives with affective disorder and possibly an increased genetic loading for bipolar disorder[31–33]. However, other authors have not found a relationship between age of onset of manic symptoms and family history[28,34].

There is also evidence that females are more likely to develop early-onset mania[28,35]. This evidence would provide support for the notion that genetic loading and the X chromosome may play a significant role in early-onset mania. As Winokur[28] points out, other studies indicate that women are more common than men in both the early- and late-onset groups[36–38]. However, recent epidemiological studies in the USA show approximately equal risk of bipolar disorder in males and females[39]. Additionally, Spicer notes an increase in first episodes of mania among men but not women over 60[40].

Clinical studies would also suggest that late-onset mania is more often precipitated by organic factors than mania, which has its onset early in life[41]. Krauthammer and Klerman[42] were the first to review causes of secondary mania (mania directly related to organic illness, rather than an idiopathic cause). These researchers describe manic symptoms that were secondary to drugs, infection, neoplasia, epilepsy and metabolic disturbances. The patients in their study had a later onset of symptoms (average age of onset 41 years) and fewer family members with affective illness than is commonly reported in the literature describing bipolar subjects.

Stasiek and Zetin[43] have updated Krauthammer and Klerman's original study with additional organic causes of manic symptoms. These authors again emphasize the importance of looking for an organic cause of mania when there is a negative family history for affective disorder or a later onset to the bipolar disorder. Neurological disease, particularly cerebrovascular disease, is also associated with secondary late-life mania[44-46]. Neuroimaging of manic geriatric patients has shown differences in the basal ganglia morphology and the putamen volume when compared to control subjects[47,48].

McDonald et al. demonstrate a correlation between bipolar disorder and subcortical hyperintensities, as evidenced on magnetic resonance images in patients with the onset of manic symptoms after the age of 50 years[49,50]. Only two of the 10 patients in this study had a family history of affective disorders[49]. The significance of subcortical hyperintensities has been debated, although they are thought to result from a focal loss of brain parenchyma, due to ischemia from any cause including hypertension, vasculopathy, atherosclerosis or thromboembolism[51].

Finally, Yassa et al.[52] find a low incidence of organic factors precipitating mania in an elderly population. However, seven of their 10 geriatric bipolar patients demonstrated a stressful event in the 6 month period prior to their manic episode. None of these patients had a family history of affective disorders.

AFFECTIVE DISORDERS

In summary, there is evidence from family studies and chromosomal linkage studies that manic depressive illness is transmitted genetically and may have more than one mode of genetic transmission. There is also evidence from clinical studies that there may be a different etiology for bipolar disorder, which has an onset early in life, compared to those which begin in older adults. Late-onset mania is more often associated with organic precipitants and, as in other types of mania, may be closely associated with stressful events. Patients with an earlier onset to their symptoms more often have a family history of affective disorder. Clinically, patients who present with manic symptoms after the age of 50 years should be given careful consideration for an organic cause to their symptoms, particularly if there is no evidence of affective disorders in other family members.

REFERENCES

1. Mendlewicz J, Rainer JD. Adoption study supporting genetic transmission in manic-depressive illness. Nature 1974; 268: 327–9.
2. Bertelson AA. Danish twin study of manic-depressive disorders. In Schou M, Stromgren E, eds, Origin, Prevention and Treatment of Affective Disorder. London: Academic Press, 1979; 227–39.
3. Gershon ES, Hamovit J, Guroff JJ et al. A family study of schizoaffective, bipolar I, bipolar II, unipolar, and normal control probands. Arch Gen Psychiat 1982; 39: 1157–67.
4. Wender PH, Kety SS, Rosenthal D et al. Psychiatric disorders in the biological and adoptive families with affective disorders. Arch Gen Psychiat 1986; 43: 923–9.
5. Tsuang MT, Faraone SV. The Genetics of Mood Disorders. Baltimore, MD: Johns Hopkins University Press, 1990.
6. Leonhard K, Korff I, Shulz H. Unipolar proband temperaments in the families of monopolar and bipolar psychoses. Psychiat Neurol 1962; 143: 416–34.
7. Roglev M. Application of polygenic threshold models in the etiology of affective disorders. Folia Med 1997; 39(2): 64–70.
8. Angst J. Atiologie und Nosologie endogener depressiver Psychosen. Berlin: Springer-Verlag, 1966.
9. Clayton PJ. The epidemiology of bipolar affective disorder. Comp Psychiat 1981; 22: 31–43.
10. Reich T, Clayton PJ, Winokur G. Family history studies: V. The genetics of mania. Am J Psychiat 1969; 125: 1358–69.
11. Baron M, Risch N, Hamburger N et al. Genetic linkage between X-chromosome markers and bipolar affective illness. Nature 1987; 326: 289–92.
12. Gerhard DS, Egeland JA, Pauls DL et al. Is a gene for affective disorder located on the short arm of chromosome 11? Am J Hum Genet 1984; 36(suppl): abstr 1.
13. Egeland JA, Gerhard DS, Pauls DL et al. Bipolar affective disorders linked to DNA markers on chromosome 11. Nature 1987; 325: 783–6.
14. Detera-Wadleigh SD, Berrettini WH, Goldin LR et al. Close linkage of c-Harvey-ras-1 and the insulin gene to affective disorder is ruled out in three North American pedigrees. Nature 1987; 325: 806–9.
15. Baron M, Freimer NF, Risch N et al. Diminished support for linkage relationship between manic-depressive illness and X-chromosome markers in three Israeli pedigrees. Nature Genet 1993; 3: 49–55.
16. Kelsoe JR, Grinns EI, Egeland JA et al. Re-evaluation of the linkage relationship between chromosome 11p loci and the gene for bipolar affective disorder in the Old Order Amish. Nature 1989; 342: 238–43.
17. Papolos D, Veit S, Shprintzen R. Chromosomal abnormalities and bipolar affective disorder: velo-cardio-facial syndrome. Medscape Ment Health 1997; 2(8).
18. Dawson E. Linkage studies of bipolar disorder in the region of the Darier's disease gene on chromosome 12q23-24.1. Am J Med Geriat 1995; 60(2): 94–102.
19. Speight G. Exclusion of CAG/CTG trinucleotide repeat loci which map in chromosome 4 in bipolar disorder and schizophrenia. Am J Med Genet 1997; 74(2): 204–6.
20. Mendlewicz J, Lindbald K, Souery D et al. Expanded trinucleotide CAG repeats in families with affective disorder. BioPsychiat 1997; 42: 115–22.
21. Chandy KG. Isolation of a novel potassium channel gene hsKCa3 containing a polymorphic CAG repeat: a candidate for schizophrenia and bipolar disorder? Mol Psychiat 1998; 3(1): 32–7.
22. Craddock N. Expanded CAG/CTG repeats in bipolar disorder: no correlation with phenotypic measures of illness severity. Biol Psychiat 1997; 42(10): 876–81.
23. Guy C. No association between a polymorphic CAG repeat in the human potassium channel gene hKCa3 and bipolar disorder. Am J Med Genet 1999; 88(1): 57–60.
24. Gershon E. Bipolar illness and schizophrenia as oligogenic diseases: implications for the future. Biol Psychiat 2000; 47(3): 240–51.
25. Shulman K, Post F. Bipolar affective disorder in old age. Br J Psychiat 1980; 136: 26–32.
26. Stone K. Mania in the elderly. Br J Psychiat 1989; 155: 220–4.
27. Petterson U. Manic-depressive illness: a clinical, social and genetic study. Acta Psychiat Scand 1977; 269(suppl): 73–80.
28. Winokur G. The Iowa 500: heterogeneity and course in manic-depressive illness (bipolar). Comp Psychiat 1975; 16: 125–31.
29. Carlson GA, Kotin J, Davenport YB et al. Follow-up of 53 bipolar manic-depressive patients. Br J Psychiat 1974; 124: 134–9.
30. Angst J, Baastrup P, Grof P et al. The course of monopolar depression and bipolar psychosis. Psychiat Neurol Neurochir (Amst) 1973; 76: 489.
31. Mendlewicz J, Fieve RR, Rainer JD et al. Manic-depressive illness: a comparative study of patients with and without a family history. Br J Psychiat 1972; 120: 523–30.
32. James NM. Early- and late-onset bipolar affective disorder: a genetic study. Arch Gen Psychiat 1977; 34: 715–17.
33. Taylor M, Abrams R. Manic states: a genetic study of early and late onset affective disorders. Arch Gen Psychiat 1973; 28: 656–8.
34. Gershon ES, Mark A, Cohen N et al. Transmitted factors in the morbid risk of affective disorders: a controlled study. J Psychiat Res 1975; 2: 283.
35. Perris C. A study of bipolar (manic-depressive) and unipolar recurrent depressive psychoses. Acta Psychiat Scand 1966; 194: 21.
36. Lundquist G. Prognosis and course in manic-depressive psychoses. Acta Psychiat Neurol 1945; 45(suppl): 88–92.

37. Winokur G. Genetic findings and methodological considerations in manic depressive disease. *Br J Psychiat* 1970; **117**: 267–74.

38. Stenstedt A. A study in manic-depressive psychosis: clinical, social and genetic investigations. *Acta Psychiat Neurol Scand* 1952; **79**(suppl): 78–85.

39. American Psychiatric Association: DSM-IV, 4th edn. Washington, DC: American Psychiatric Association, 1994.

40. Spicer CC, Hare EH, Slater E. Neurotic and psychotic forms of depressive illness: evidence from age incidence in a national sample. *Br J Psychiat* 1973; **123**: 535.

41. Broadhead J, Jacoby R. Mania in old age: a first prospective study. *Int J Geriat Psychiat* 1990; **5**: 215.

42. Krauthammer C, Klerman GL. Secondary mania: manic syndromes associated with antecedent physical illness or drugs. *Arch Gen Psychiat* 1978; **35**: 1333–9.

43. Stasiek C, Zetin M. Organic manic disorders. *Psychosomatics* 1985; **26**: 394–402.

44. Shulman KI. Neurologic co-morbidity and mania in old age. *Clin Neurosci* 1997; **4**: 37–40.

45. Cummings JL, Mendez MF. Secondary mania with focal cerebrovascular lesions. *Am J Psychiat* 1984; **141**: 1084–7.

46. Berthier ML, Kulisevsky J, Gironell A *et al*. Poststroke bipolar affective disorder: clinical subtypes, concurrent movement disorders, and anatomical correlates. *J Neuropsychiat Clin Neurosci* 1996; **8**: 160–7.

47. Bocksberger JPH, Young RC, Elkin A *et al*. Basal ganglia morphology in geriatric mania (abstr). Presented at the Annual Meeting of the Society of Biological Psychiatry, New York City, 1996.

48. Young RC, Bocksberger JP, Alexopoulos G *et al*. Putamen volume and age at onset in geriatric mania (abstr). Presented at the New Research Program of the Annual Meeting of the American Psychiatric Association, 1996.

49. McDonald W, Krishnan R, Doraiswamy M *et al*. Subcortical hyperintensities in elderly subjects with mania. *Biol Psychiat* 1990; **27**: 162A.

50. McDonald WM, Tupler LA, Marsteller FA *et al*. Hyperintense lesions on magnetic resonance images in bipolar disorder. *Biol Psychiat* 1999; **45**(8): 965–71.

51. Drayer BP. Imaging of the aging brain. Part 11: pathologic conditions. *Radiology* 1988; **166**: 797–803.

52. Yassa R, Nair V, Nastase C *et al*. Prevalence of bipolar disorder in a psychogeriatric population. *J Affect Disord* 1988; **14**: 197–201.

85

Epidemiology and Risk Factors

S. Lehmann and P. Rabins

Johns Hopkins Medical Institutions, Baltimore, MD, USA

In recent years there has been renewed research and clinical interest in the syndrome of mania in the elderly. Much of the current work in this area has been focused on the following issues: can mania first present in late life?; do the causes, features, clinical course, and responsiveness to treatment differ in older manic patients compared to younger persons with mania?; how do elderly manic patients with an early age of onset of illness differ from those with onset of illness in late life?

EPIDEMIOLOGY

The manic phase of bipolar affective disorder, or mania, is an uncommon disorder in the elderly. In the five-site Epidemiologic Catchment Center study of more than 20 000 non-institutionalized individuals, 1 month prevalence rates for mania were 0.4–0.8% for 18–44-year-olds and 0.2% in the 45–64-year-old group. Notably, no cases of mania were identified among people over age 64[1].

Nevertheless, elderly patients with mania are seen in significant numbers in a variety of clinical settings. In Roth's[2] retrospective review of 464 psychogeriatric patients over age 60 in a long-term hospital, 14 cases were manic. This represented 6% of the total number of cases of affective disorder. Two studies of first admissions to British psychiatric hospitals, using Department of Health statistics, found that the number of first admissions with mania either remained steady with age[3] or increased with advancing age[4]. In the USA, other studies in short-stay hospitals have reported that mania accounted for approximately 5% of elderly psychiatric admissions[5,6]. Similarly, one recent study identified 39 patients over age 60 with bipolar, manic or mixed state disorder out of 791 inpatient admissions (approximately 5%) over a 4 year period[7]. Most studies of elderly manic patients have found more females than males[5–8] but one recent report found a slight male preponderance[9].

For the majority of elderly bipolar patients, the first episode of affective disorder is usually a depression. Indeed, it is quite common for a first manic episode to occur 10 years or more after an initial depressive episode and to be preceded by multiple depressive episodes over many years[5,10,11]. Generally, elderly patients have been found to have suffered more episodes of depression before a first manic episode and to have had a long gap between an initial depression and a first manic episode than young manic patients[11].

It must be noted that, at the present time, there is no agreed-upon standard regarding which age should serve as the dividing line between early and late onset of bipolar illness. Furthermore, age of onset itself is often difficult to determine with exactitude.

Different criteria have been used among various investigators to identify age of onset, including first onset of symptoms, first hospitalization and first time at which the patient met full criteria for the disorder[7]. Several recent studies have observed bi-modality in age of onset of mania among elderly patients. In these studies, one subgroup of patients was found to have developed bipolar disorder in early life with a mean age in their 30s, and another subgroup developed a first manic episode after age 60[7,11]. Late-onset bipolar patients tend to have had a longer gap between first depression and first mania than early-onset bipolar patients[11], and in one study were more likely to be married or living with a significant other[7].

RISK FACTORS

A number of studies have reported that elderly bipolar patients who had an early age of onset were more likely to have had first degree relatives with affective disorder than late-onset elderly bipolar patients[11,12]. This trend holds across studies that have used ages between 20 and 60 years to divide early and late cases and suggests that genetics plays a greater role in the disease of early-onset bipolar disorder. At the same time many investigators have reported associations between late-onset mania and cerebrovascular and neurologic disease. A cohort study comparing 50 elderly patients with mania to 50 age- and sex-matched patients with unipolar depression found that 36% of the manic patients had neurological disorders compared with only 8% of the depressed patients[13]. Interestingly, among these neurologically impaired manic patients, 33% had a positive family history of affective disorder in first-degree relatives. In another recent study comparing elderly patients with early- and late-onset bipolar disorder, researchers found that patients with late-onset illness were more likely to demonstrate cerebrovascular risk factors or clinical evidence of cerebrovascular disorders[7]. In a prospective study of mania in 35 patients over age 60, the elderly manic patients had more cortical atrophy on CT scans than age-matched controls[11]. However, no significant difference in cortical atrophy was found between elderly patients with early- and late-onset mania. In addition, subcortical hyperintensities have been reported on magnetic resonance imaging (MRI) in elderly patients with mania[14]. These hyperintensities are believed to be due to focal loss of brain parenchyma but they do not seem to be specific to elderly patients with mania, since subcortical hyperintensities have also been found in late-onset depression as well as late-onset paranoid disorders[15].

Krauthammer and Klerman[16] proposed criteria for secondary mania, which included cases of no prior family history, no prior psychiatric history, and a definable medical or neurological etiology. While it is true that organic factors may precipitate mania in some elderly patients, these cases appear to be in the minority. Manic episodes can be caused by such widely prescribed medications as levodopa, procyclidine, pergolide, selegiline and bromocriptine[17]. A variety of steroids have been reported to produce manic syndromes, as have thyroid supplements, and there have been case reports of mania associated with H2-antagonists, antiarrhythmics, estrogen and antitubercular agents[18]. In addition, mania can occur in association with systemic infections, such as influenza, Q fever and St Louis type A encephalitis. Cases of mania secondary to space-occupying lesions, such as meningiomas, subarachnoid hemorrhages and metastases (usually in the non-dominant hemisphere), have also been reported[6]. In these cases, mania usually resolves with removal of the offending pharmacologic agent or treatment of the underlying disorder.

More commonly, mania has been reported in elderly patients with cerebrovascular and neurological disorders. One prospective study found that 20% of patients with mania over the age of 60 had a first manic episode closely temporally related to a cerebral organic disorder[11]. Another prospective study of 20 manic patients with onset over age 50 found that 65% developed bipolar disorder after a silent cerebral infarction[19]. In particular, injury to the right hemisphere appears to be strongly associated with the development of mania. There have been reports of secondary mania in patients with ischemic injury to right-sided basal ganglia, orbitofrontal cortex, and right basotemporal cortex[20]. It has been hypothesized that these brain areas may be significant because of their connections to the limbic system and the modulation of emotion. Overall, however, mania following stroke is much less common than depression after a stroke. In one large study of 700 stroke victims only three developed manic syndromes[21]. There have been two case reports of mania secondary to infarctions in the thalamic and perithalamic areas[22]. Starkstein et al.[23] studied 11 patients who developed mania after stroke and found that eight had lesions involving limbic areas and nine had right hemispheric involvement. These patients also had significantly larger bifrontal and third ventricular brain ratios than matched control patients, indicating pre-existing anterior subcortical atrophy. Moreover, almost half of the patients had a family history of affective disorder in a first-degree relative. Taken together, the current literature on mania in patients with neurologic and cerebrovascular disorders underscores that genetic loading is also a factor contributing to the development of mania in these patients as well. Furthermore, while up to a quarter of elderly manic patients in various studies have been found to have some evidence of concurrent cerebral disease, it is still unclear to what extent these impairments play an etiological role in the development of mania. If cases in which subjects with a known previous history of affective disorder are excluded, few cases of clear secondary mania are found[6,11,12]. An exception to this is Shulman et al.[13], who felt that 36% of elderly patients they studied who were hospitalized with mania had true secondary mania associated temporally with clearly documented neurological disorders.

Mania can occur in the setting of dementia. In a chart review of 134 patients with Alzheimer's disease, 2% were found to have had mania[24], although others have reported higher rates[25]. Broadhead and Jacoby[11] found that 32% of elderly manic patients studied scored in the demented range on cognitive testing, even though they had no history of progressive cognitive decline. Furthermore, more extensive cortical atrophy on head CT correlated with poorer test scores, but there was no significant difference between early- and late-onset manic patients with respect to CT findings or cognitive changes. It is unknown at this time whether these patients have progressed to develop true dementia. In one retrospective study of 92 elderly patients with mania, only three went on to develop documented dementia over a 10 year follow-up period[12]. To date, there does not appear to be an increased risk for elderly manic patients to develop dementia compared to the rest of the population.

As in younger patients, stressful life events have been felt by some investigators to precipitate mania in elderly patients. One study that reported on 10 elderly manic patients found that 70% had major changes in lifestyle in the 6 months preceding onset of mania. Stresses included marital discord and disruption of living arrangements[5].

REFERENCES

1. Regier DA, Boyd JH, Burke JD Jr. *et al.* One-month prevalence of mental disorders in the United States. *Arch Gen Psychiat* 1988; **45**: 977–86.
2. Roth M. The natural history of mental disorder in old age. *J Ment Sci* 1955; **101**: 281–301.
3. Eagles JM, Whalley LJ. Ageing and affective disorders: the age at first onset of affective disorders in Scotland. *Br J Psychiat* 1985; **147**: 180–7.
4. Spicer CC, Hare EH, Slater E. Neurotic and psychotic forms of depressive illness: evidence from age-incidence in a national sample. *Br J Psychiat* 1973; **123**: 535–41.
5. Yassa R, Nair V, Nastase C *et al.* Prevalence of bipolar disorder in a psychogeriatric population. *J Affect Disord* 1988; **B14B**: 197–201.
6. Glasser M, Rabins P. Mania in the elderly. *Age Ageing* 1983; **13**: 210–13.
7. Wylie ME, Mulsant BH, Pollock BG *et al.* Age at onset in geriatric bipolar disorder. *Am J Geriat Psychiat* 1999; **7**: 77–83.
8. Shulman K, Post F. Bipolar affective disorder in old age. *Br J Psychiat* 1980; **136**: 26–32.
9. Tohen M, Shulman KI, Satlin A. First-episode mania in late life. *Am J Psychiat* 1989; **151**: 130–2.
10. Snowdon J. A retrospective case-note study of bipolar disorder in old age. *Br J Psychiat* 1991; **158**: 485–90.
11. Broadhead J, Jacoby R. Mania in older age: a first prospective study. *Int J Geriat Psychiat* 1990; **5**: 215–22.
12. Stone K. Mania in the elderly. *Br J Psychiat* 1989; **1155**: 220–4.
13. Shulman KI, Tohen M, Satlin A *et al.* Mania compared with unipolar depression in old age. *Am J Psychiat* 1992; **149**: 341–5.
14. McDonald WM, Krishnan KRR, Doraiswamy PM, Blazer DG. Occurrence of subcortical hyperintensities in elderly subjects with mania. *Psychiat Res Neuroimag* 1991; **40**: 211–20.
15. Schulman K. Recent developments in the epidemiology, co-morbidity and outcome of mania in older age. *Rev Clin Gerontol* 1996; **6**: 249–54.
16. Krauthammer C, Klerman GL. Secondary mania. *Arch Gen Psychiat* 1978; **35**: 1333–9.
17. Factor SA, Molho BS, Podskalny GD *et al.* Parkinson's disease: drug-induced psychiatric states. *Behav Neurol Movement Disorders* 1995; **65**: 115–38.
18. Ganzini L, Millar SB, Walsh JR. Drug-induced mania in the elderly. *Drugs Aging* 1993; **3**: 428–35.
19. Fujikawa T, Yaamawaki S, Touhouda Y. Silent cerebral infarctions in patients with late-onset mania. *Stroke* 1995; **26**: 946–9.
20. Starkstein SE, Mayberg HS, Berthier ML *et al.* Mania after brain injury: neuroradiological and metabolic findings. *Ann Neurol* 1990; **27**: 652–9.
21. Robinson RG, Staff LB, Price TR. A two-year longitudinal study of mood disorders following stroke: prevalence and duration at six months follow-up. *Br J Psychiat* 1984; **144**: 256–62.
22. Cummings JL, Mendez MF. Secondary mania with focal cerebrovascular lesions. *Am J Psychiat* 1984; **141**: 1084–7.
23. Starkstein SE, Pearlson GD, Boston JB, Robinson RG. Mania after brain injury: a controlled study of causative factors. *Arch Neurol* 1987; **44**: 1069–73.
24. Lyketsos C, Corazzini K, Steele C. Mania in Alzheimer's disease. *J Neuropsychiat* 1995; **150**: 350–2.
25. Burns A, Jacoby R, Levy R. Psychiatry phenomena in Alzheimer's disease, III: disorders of mood. *Br J Psychiat* 1992; **157**: 81–6.

86

Mania: Clinical Features and Management

S. Lehmann and P. Rabins

Johns Hopkins Medical Institutions, Baltimore, MD, USA

Descriptions of manic syndromes in elderly patients published during the 1960s and 1970s tended to emphasize differences in clinical features compared to younger manic patients. Post felt that elderly manic patients had more depressive features and more mood-incongruent persecutory delusions, but were less likely to have flight of ideas[1]. Slater and Roth noted that euphoric states in older manic patients tended to be less "infectious" and had more expressed "hostility and resentment"[2].

More recent retrospective and prospective studies, on the other hand, suggest that symptoms are actually quite similar across the age span. For example, two studies have reported that hyperactivity, insomnia and thought disorder (e.g. flight of ideas) occur in 60% of elderly manic patients. Other common manic symptoms include grandiose delusions, irritability, hypersexuality and paranoid delusions[3,4]. Similarly, a more recent study of 14 patients over age 65 hospitalized with a first manic episode found that 43% had psychotic features, including grandiose and persecutory delusions[5]. In a prospective study comparing hospitalized manic patients over age 60 to those under age 40, no differences were found between young and old patients in the time course or outcome of the manic episode. However, the authors had the clinical impression that younger patients tended to experience a more severe illness than older patients. The authors also noted that more elderly patients relapsed into a depressive episode after discharge from the hospital[6].

There has been little research to date comparing elderly manic patients with early- and late-onset bipolar disorder in terms of clinical presentation, response to treatment or clinical course. One intriguing study of patients over age 60 hospitalized with bipolar, manic, mixed or depressed states found that elderly patients with late-onset bipolar disorder were more likely to have psychotic features compared to patients with early-onset bipolar disorder. However, early- and late-onset bipolar patients did not differ in terms of pharmacological treatment, hospital stay length, or likelihood to be admitted for a manic, mixed-state or depressed episode[7].

Although several authors have noted that cognitive dysfunction is common in elderly patients with mania, the relationship between mania and dementia in older patients remains complex. Broadhead and Jacoby[6] found that 32% of elderly manic patients scored within the demented range on a cognitive assessment, even though none of the patients had a history of progressive intellectual decline. Moreover, there was no significant difference between manic patients with early- and late-onset bipolar disorder in terms of cognitive impairment. In a 5–7 year follow-up study of 25 elderly patients previously hospitalized for acute mania, 32% had developed a clinically significant cognitive disorder[8]. In contrast, an earlier 10 year follow-up study of 92 elderly patients

with mania found that only 3% had developed dementia[9]. Clearly this is an area that warrants further study.

TREATMENT AND MANAGEMENT

A recent study of mental health service use by elderly patients with bipolar disorder and unipolar major depression found that the bipolar patients used more case-management services, were three times more likely to use partial hospitalization and three times more likely to have had at least one psychiatric hospitalization over the 6 months prior to the assessment[10]. This study highlights the importance of effective treatment and mental health monitoring for elderly patients with bipolar disorder.

As with younger patients, lithium carbonate is the mainstay of pharmacological treatment in the older manic patient. There are clear changes in the pharmacokinetics of lithium with age, due to age-related decline in creatinine clearance. In people with no renal disease there is a 30–50% decline in glomerular filtration rate (GFR) between the third and eighth decades. Since lithium is almost exclusively excreted through the kidneys, this leads to decreased clearance of lithium with age. As a result, the biological half-life in the serum increases from 18 h in adolescents to 36 h in people over age 60 and may be even longer in elderly patients with renal disease[11].

In addition, there is considerable agreement that both the toxic and therapeutic effects of lithium occur at lower plasma levels in the elderly compared to younger patients. Plasma levels of lithium that would be considered therapeutic for a young manic patient cause delirium in some elderly patients. The reasons behind this are unclear but it has been hypothesized that this phenomenon reflects an increase in brain sensitivity to lithium. Fine hand tremor secondary to lithium also seems to occur more frequently in people over age 60 than in younger patients. In summary, therefore, it is prudent to begin elderly manic patients on lower doses of lithium than one would for younger patients, and to aim for lower plasma levels of 0.5–0.6 mmol/l, even in the acute phase of treatment. For long-term maintenance and prophylaxis, even lower plasma levels of lithium of 0.4–0.5 mmol/l are often effective for this older age group.

Studies of patients taking lithium over many years indicate that lithium rarely causes changes in glomerular filtration rate or renal failure[12]. Furthermore, lithium does not appear to decline in efficacy over the lifespan[13]. However, for a variety of reasons, some patients become unable to tolerate lithium as they age. In these cases lithium treatment must be replaced or supplemented by other mood-stabilizing medications. As with younger patients, anticonvulsants such as carbamazepine,

Principles and Practice of Geriatric Psychiatry, 2nd edn. Edited by J. R. M. Copeland, M. T. Abou-Saleh and D. G. Blazer

valproate and clonazepam are being used more frequently as an alternative or adjunct to lithium treatment[14]. Although systematic data regarding the efficacy and toxicity of carbamazepine treatment in elderly manic patients are lacking, there are a few reports indicating that it can be safe and effective in older patients[15]. The major risk of carbamazepine is the rare occurrence of aplastic anemia or agranulocytosis[11]. However, many older patients have difficulty tolerating this medication, due to its propensity to cause sedation and ataxia.

In recent years valproate has been widely prescribed for the acute treatment of mania in both young and elderly patients with bipolar disorder. A case series study of seven older patients with long-standing bipolar disorder who had failed to respond to conventional medications reported at least minimal improvement in six out of seven patients after valproate was added adjunctively to the medication regimen[16]. Two retrospective studies of valproate treatment of patients over age 60 hospitalized with mania found valproate effective in improving symptoms of mania at serum levels of 31–106 μg/ml[17,18]. In another retrospective study assessing the efficacy of lithium compared to valproate in patients over age 55 hospitalized for mania, 38% of elderly patients receiving valproate were improved at discharge compared to 67% of patients receiving lithium. However, the authors note that fewer patients on valproate therapy were within the therapeutic range and valproate serum levels of 65–90 μg/ml correlated with a better therapeutic response than did lower serum levels[19].

Gabapentin is a new anticonvulsant with gaba-ergic and glutaminergic properties that has been shown to have antimanic effects and may be effective as an adjunctive agent in the treatment of mania[20]. It has not yet been studied systematically in elderly patients. Similarly, in a mixed-age population of patients with acute mania, olanzapine, a novel neuroleptic, was found to be more effective than placebo[21]. Novel neuroleptics such as risperidone and olanzapine have the potential to be particularly useful adjuncts in the treatment of mania in the elderly because of their lower rates of extrapyramidal side effects and tardive dyskinesia, compared with traditional neuroleptics[22]. As a result, they may be better tolerated by elderly manic patients than traditional neuroleptics, such as haldol, for adjunctive treatment of psychosis and agitation. More research is needed on both the short- and long-term effects of these newer mood-stabilizing and antipsychotic medications in older persons.

Finally, the clinical management of older patients with mania must always include attention to psychosocial support issues and psychotherapy. As with younger patients, individual counseling, emotional support and illness education are critical to a successful outcome. Additionally, involvement of family members and significant others in the acute treatment and long-term management of the illness helps to ensure compliance with treatment recommendations and early detection of signs of relapse.

REFERENCES

1. Post F. *The Clinical Psychiatry of Late Life*. Oxford: Pergamon, 1965.
2. Slater E, Roth M. In Mayer-Gross W, Slater E, Roth M (eds), *Clinical Psychiatry*, 3rd rev. edn. London: Baillière Tindall & Cassell, 1977, pp 571–2, 600.
3. Yassa R, Nair V, Nastase C et al. Prevalence of bipolar disorder in a psychogeriatric population. *J Affect Disord* 1988; **B14B**: 197–201.
4. Glasser M, Rabins P. Mania in the elderly. *Age Ageing* 1983; **13**, 210–13.
5. Tohen M, Shulman KI, Satlin A. First-episode mania in late life. *Am J Psychiat* 1994; **151**: 130–2.
6. Broadhead J, Jacoby R. Mania in older age: a first prospective study. *Int J Geriatr Psychiat* 1990; **5**: 215–22.
7. Wylie ME, Mulsant BH, Pollock BG et al. Age at onset in geriatric bipolar disorder. *Am J Geriat Psychiat* 1999; **7**: 77–83.
8. Dhingra U, Rabins PV. Mania in the elderly: a five to seven year follow-up. *J Am Geriat Soc* 1991; **39**: 581.
9. Stone K. Mania in the elderly. *Br J Psychiat* 1989; **155**: 220–4.
10. Bartelss SJ, Forester B, Miles KM, Joyce T. Mental health service use by elderly patients with bipolar disorder and unipolar major depression. *Am J Geriat Psychiat* 2000; **8**: 160–6.
11. Jenike MA. Side effects of lithium. In *Geriatric Psychiatry and Psychopharmacology*. New York: Yearbook Medical, 1989; 85–6.
12. Schou M. Forty years of lithium treatment. *Arch Gen Psychiat* 1997; **54**: 9–13.
13. Murray N, Hopwood S, Balfour DJK et al. The influence of age on lithium efficacy and side effects in outpatients. *Psychol Med* 1983; **13**: 53–60.
14. Keck PE, McElroy SL, Nemeroff CB. Anticonvulsants in the treatment of bipolar disorder. *J Neuropsychiat Clin Neurosci* 1992; **4**: 395–405.
15. Shulman KI, Herrmann N. The nature and management of mania in old age. *Psychiat Clin N Am* 1999; **22**: 649–65.
16. McFarland BH, Miller MM, Straumfjord AA. Valproate use in the older manic patient. *J Clin Psychiat* 1990; **51**: 479–81.
17. Mordecai DJ, Sheikh JI, Glick ID. Brief report: divalproex for the treatment of geriatric bipolar disorder. *Int J Geriat Psychiat* 1999; **14**: 494–6.
18. Noaghiul S, Narayan M, Nelson JC. Divalproex treatment of mania in elderly patients. *Am J Geriat Psychiat* 1998; **6**: 257–62.
19. Chen ST, Altshuler LL, Melnyk KA et al. *J Clin Psychiat* 1999; **60**: 181–6.
20. Ghaemi SN, Katzow JJ, Desai SP, Goodwin FK. Gabapentin treatment of mood disorders: a preliminary study. *J Clin Psychiat* 1998; **59**: 426–9.
21. Tohen M, Jacobs TG, Grundy SL et al. Efficacy of olanzapine in acute bipolar mania: a double-blind, placebo-controlled study. *Arch Gen Psychiat* 2000; **57**: 841–9.
22. Van Gerpen MW, Johnson JE, Winstead DK. Mania in the geriatric patient population: a review of the literature. *Am J Geriat Psychiat* 1999; **7**: 188–202.
23. Krauthammer C, Klerman GL. Secondary mania. *Arch Gen Psychiat* 1978; **35**: 1333–9.

87

Prognosis

Mustafa M. Husain

University of Texas, Dallas, TX, USA

In a follow-up study of approximately 400 bipolar patients, Grof *et al.*[1] found that virtually every patient experienced recurrence of the illness. The course of the recurring episode was predicted by the course of the previous episode. The first recurrence usually occurs 40–48 months after the initial episode, but later in the course of the illness, there may be more frequent relapses and the interval between episodes may shorten up to 50%.

Winokur[2], using IOWA-500 data from a long-term follow-up study, suggested that bipolar illness may burn itself out with time; thus, aging may be a mitigating factor. Cutler and Post[3], however, in a review of a small number of untreated patients with severe and prolonged bipolar disorder, found a tendency for more rapid recurrences late in the history of the illness with decreasing periods of normality. In other words, if bipolar illness emerges in later years, then the episodes of mania or mania mixed with depression may tend to cluster with each other.

The course of the illness also depends on the age of onset. Mania, in general, is an illness of early onset. The mean age of onset is 30 years with a range from teens through 50 years. However, there are several patients who experience their first episode of manic illness in the later years of life[4–7]. Unfortunately, the prognosis of mania in the elderly has not been studied as systematically as in the younger population.

Post[8,9] suggested that the first onset of affective illness in late life carried a less favorable prognosis than early-onset patients. He further stated that elderly manic patients tend to remain disturbed somewhat longer. Although most episodes may subside in a few weeks, some may last up to 6 months. In the elderly, recurrent episodes of mania tend to occur more frequently, most commonly every 1 to 2 years, as compared to longer intervals between episodes in younger patients. Post also noted that late-onset patients displayed a significantly less frequent family history of affective disorder compared to early-onset patients.

In another retrospective study of 67 elderly bipolar patients, Shulman and Post[10] found that the first manic episode occurred at about 60 years of age, often after a latency period of 10 years from the first affective symptoms. There was an average of three depressive episodes before the occurrence of the first manic episode in these patients.

More recently, Kit Stone[11], in a retrospective study of 92 patients admitted with mania over the age of 65, reported that 26% had no prior history of mood disorder, 30% had previously only experienced depression, half of them had at least three episodes of depression before the onset of mania and the mean latency period for the first depressive symptoms to the onset of first manic episode was 16 years. He also noted that patients with a family history of affective disorders had a significantly earlier age of onset.

In a prospective, comparative study of 35 elderly manic patients over the age of 60 and 35 young patients below the age of 40, Broadhead and Jacoby[12] reported that elderly manic patients suffered more depression before the first manic episode and had a longer interval between the first depression and the first manic episode than the young bipolar patients. They also reported clinical differences between the young and the old manic patients; although the young experienced more severe illness than the old, the elderly patients appeared to have a more fragile recovery and were more likely to relapse into a depressive episode during resolution of their manic illness. Within the elderly group, 50% of the early-onset subgroup had a family history of affective disorder in first-degree relatives as compared to only 14% in the late-onset subgroup.

In a study describing the relationship between age, signs and symptoms of mania in 40 inpatients, Young and Falk[13] reported that increasing age is associated with attenuated manic response characterized by less intense level of over-activity and sexual drive, while thought processes are generally less disrupted. They also noted greater residual psychopathology in elderly patients as compared to younger patients over a period of time. These findings are similar to previous follow-up studies by McDonald[14], Wertham[15] and Lundquist[16], who found that duration or chronicity of manic illness increases with age.

Ameblas[17] reported a special relationship between life events and the onset of the first manic episode. This finding suggests that later in life, less stressful events may precipitate mania, and therefore late-onset manic episodes may be related to increased cerebral vulnerability in the elderly.

There has been a recent interest in the concept of secondary mania. Krauthammer and Klerman[18] described secondary manias in heterogeneous groups of illnesses, including metabolic disturbance, drugs, infections, neoplasms and epilepsy. There is also increasing evidence that elderly patients with coarse brain changes secondary to stroke, head trauma and other neurological conditions appear to be more vulnerable to mania. Elderly subjects are more prone to develop these conditions and the prognosis of these secondary manias depends in part on the prognosis of the conditions causing such manic episodes.

Spicer[19], in an attempt to explain the increased incidence of mania with old age (a finding not replicated in most studies), suggested that manic episodes might occur on the basis of dementia. Shulman and Post[20], Stone[11] and Broadhead and Jacoby[12], however, did not find an association between mania and dementia in elderly patients. In a retrospective clinical study of mania and old age, Shulman and Post[12] did find a temporal association between onset of mania and history of cerebral disease in 16 out of 67 (24%) of their patients. Glasser and Rabins[21]

Principles and Practice of Geriatric Psychiatry, 2nd edn. Edited by J. R. M. Copeland, M. T. Abou-Saleh and D. G. Blazer
©2002 John Wiley & Sons, Ltd

suggested from their study that elderly men with coarse brain changes as a result of stroke, head trauma and other neurological conditions, appear to be most vulnerable to developing mania. Kit Stone[11] reported that 24% of his elderly patients developed mania following some sort of cerebral insult. In their comparative study of young and old manic patients, Broadhead and Jacoby[12] found that 20% of their elderly patients had first manic episodes that were closely related temporally to cerebral organic disease, in contrast to none in the younger manic group. In other words, manic episodes in late life may derive not only from a predisposition to bipolar disorder but also from cerebral pathological changes, and therefore the prognosis of the brain disease may determine the prognosis of mania in these patients.

Shukla *et al.*[22] studied 20 patients with mania after head injury. They suggest a significant relationship between post-traumatic seizures and development of mania. Elderly individuals are more prone to falls and subsequently at a higher risk for developing mania after head injuries. In a recent magnetic resonance imaging (MRI) study of elderly manic patients, McDonald and Blazer[23] found an increased incidence of sub-cortical hyperintensities in the right middle third of the brain parenchyma.

Young and Falk[13] noted a less vigorous response to lithium in older than in younger manic patients. This difference, based on age, was even more impressive since their sample maximum age was 66 with a mean of 36 years. Their data suggest that increased age may be associated with attenuation of aspects of manic psychopathology and response to pharmacotherapy. Himmeloch *et al.*[24], in a study of 81 bipolar patients over the age of 55, demonstrated that neurological status rather than age is the critical factor determining the natural course of the illness. Neurological status not only determined the evolution of chronic mania; it also predicted poor treatment response and lithium-induced neurotoxicity.

Despite the possible difference in the clinical presentation and response to treatments of mania in young and old age, evidence indicates a good therapeutic response to lithium for both an acute manic episode and prophylaxis in elderly patients, but close monitoring is required, with particular attention to interactions with other illness and medications. Contrary to the general belief, the prognosis of mania in old age is good and comparable to that of the young manic patient.

REFERENCES

1. Grof P, Angst J, Haines T. The clinical course of depression: practical issues. In Angst J, ed., *Classification and Prediction of Outcome in Depression*. New York: F. K. Shatlaur Village, 1973.
2. Winokur G. The Iowa 500: heterogeneity and course in the manic–depressive illness (bipolar). *Comp Psychiat* 1975; **16**: 125–31.
3. Cutler NR, Post RM. Life course of illness in untreated manic–depressive patients. *Comp Psychiat* 1982; **23**: 101–15.
4. Perris C. The course of depressive psychosis. *Acta Psychiat Scand* 1968; **44**: 238–48.
5. Winokur G, Clayton P, Reich T. *Manic Depressive Illness*. St Louis: CV Mosby, 1969.
6. Taylor M, Abrams R. Manic states: a generic study of early and late onset affective disorders. *Arch Gen Psychiat* 1973; **28**: 656–8.
7. Loranger AW, Levine PM. Age at onset of bipolar affective disorder. *Arch Gen Psychiat* 1978; **35**: 1345–8.
8. Post F. *The Significance of Affective Symptoms in Old Age*. London: Oxford University Press, 1962.
9. Post F. *The Clinical Psychiatry of Late Life*. Oxford: Pergamon, 1965.
10. Shulman K, Post F. Bipolar affective disorder in old age. *Br J Psychiat* 1980; **136**: 26–32.
11. Kit Stone. Mania in the elderly. *Br J Psychiat* 1989; **155**: 220–24.
12. Broadhead J, Jacoby R. Mania in old age: a first prospective study. *Int J Geriatr Psychiat* 1990; **51**: 215–22.
13. Young RC, Falk NR. Age, manic psychopathology and treatment response. *Int J Geriat Psychiat* 1988.
14. MacDonald JB. Prognosis in manic–depressive insanity. *J Nerv Ment Dis* 1918; **47**: 20–30.
15. Wertham FI. A group of benign chronic psychoses: prolonged manic excitements. *Am J Psychiat* 1928; **9**: 17–78.
16. Lundquist G. Prognosis and course in manic depressive psychosis. *Acta Psychiat Scand* 1945; **35**(suppl 1): 1–96.
17. Ameblas A. Life events and mania. *Br J Psychiat* 1987; **150**: 235–40.
18. Krauthammer C, Klerman C. Secondary mania: manic syndromes associated with antecedent physical illness or drugs. *Arch Gen Psychiat* 1978; **35**: 1333–9.
19. Spicer CC, Hare EH, Slater E. Neurotic and psychotic forms of depressive illness: evidence from age incidence in a national sample. *Br J Psychiat* 1973; **123**: 535–41.
20. Shulman K, Post F. Bipolar affective disorder in old age. *Br J Psychiat* 1980; **136**: 26–32.
21. Glasser M, Rabins P. Mania in the elderly. *Age Ageing* 1984; **13**: 210–13.
22. Shukla S, Cook BL, Mukherjee S *et al*. Mania following head injury. *Am J Psychiat* 1987; **144**: 93–6.
23. McDonald and Blazer 1990.
24. Himmelhoch JM, Neil JF, May SJ *et al*. Age, dementia, dyskinesia and lithium response. *Am J Psychiat* **137**: 941–5.

88

The Management of Acute Mania

John L. Beyer and K. Ranga R. Krishnan

Duke University Medical Center, Durham, NC, USA

Primary acute mania in the elderly (>65 years) is rare, its prevalence being much less than 1%[1]. Kramer *et al.*[2] reported that no patients with mania were identified out of 923 elderly persons interviewed in the Epidemiologic Catchment Area study. However, other researchers[3] have reported that 5%–10% of elderly patients presenting with mood disorders have mania or hypomania. Further, approximately 4%–5% of geriatric patients hospitalized for acute conditions in a state psychiatric facility were noted to have bipolar disorders[4]. Most elderly bipolar patients appear to be individuals who had an early onset of bipolar disorder and now have reached an older age. However, a first episode of mania in late life is not unknown and appears to be more commonly associated with underlying neurological/medical illnesses[5] and the absence of family history of affective disorders[6].

Clinicians who treat the elderly are aware that late-life mania presents unique treatment challenges. Older patients with mania who require hospitalization tend to have a slower course of improvement than younger patients[7]. This often results in longer hospitalizations and the appearance of increased treatment resistance. Further, rates of cognitive and functional impairment were found to be much higher in elderly bipolar patients over a 5 year period than seen in the general population[8].

Complicating treatment guidelines is the observation that, as opposed to bipolar disorder in younger populations, the treatment of bipolar disorders in the elderly remains an understudied area[9]. The treatment of late-life bipolar disorder is primarily extrapolated from data obtained in studies of younger patients or mixed patient populations, uncontrolled studies of elderly patients and case reports.

TREATMENT GOALS

Management of acute mania initially begins with the treatment of the acute symptoms and assessment of cause. This can be done either in the hospital or in an outpatient setting. However, since the manic patient frequently presents with excessive energy, irritability, grandiosity, impulsiveness or even psychosis, the physician must first determine the appropriate level of care required for treatment. Usually, hospitalization is required when patients present with severe symptoms or psychosis which affects functioning and requires behavior management. This may be especially true for the patient with cognitive impairment. Hospitalization can often be useful in facilitating the evaluation of first episodes and increasing both acute and long-term medical compliance. Elderly patients in nursing care facilities may be able to be treated without hospitalization if the support system is sufficient. A hypomanic patient can usually be treated as an outpatient as long as he/she demonstrates adequate compliance and the primary caregiver does not feel overwhelmed.

Before a primary manic episode is diagnosed, a potential medical or substance-induced etiology must be ruled out. Therefore, comprehensive evaluation, physical work-up and diagnosis are necessary prior to treatment of mania in the older person. After stabilizaton, the focus of treatment is then directed to the maintenance phase, relapse prevention and other necessary social interventions.

PRIMARY MEDICATIONS FOR ACUTE MANIA

Lithium

Efficacy

As in younger patients, lithium is indicated in elderly manic patients for both treatment of acute manic episodes and prophylactic maintenance. Although it has been suggested that lithium may not be as effective in older patients, most studies have demonstrated that lithium is equally effective in elderly patients. However, lithium does require special precautions for use in the general adult population and especially the geriatric population. In fact, underlying dementia, cardiovascular disease or kidney disease in the elderly can increase the potential for neurotoxicity, cardiotoxicity and nephrotoxicity[10,11]. Lithium is not considered an ideal choice for patients with these problems, despite their positive response to the drug.

Treatment Considerations

Prior to starting patients on lithium, the patient's medical history should be reviewed with special attention to systems that may be affected by lithium. Laboratory tests should include a complete blood count (CBC), serum chemistry panel [with plasma sodium, potassium, blood urea nitrogen (BUN) and creatinine levels] thyroid function tests [iodothyronine (T3), thyroxine (T4), and thyrotropin-stimulating hormone (TSH) levels] and an electrocardiogram (ECG). If the elderly patient is suspected of having renal dysfunction, a 24-hour urine collection measuring creatinine clearance is the best way of assessing glomerular filtration rate (GFR). However, if this is not feasible, a less precise estimate of GFR and renal clearance can be calculated by measurements of BUN and creatinine. Unfortunately, in patients with low muscle mass, the values may be overestimated. An electroencephalogram (EEG), computed tomography (CT) head scan or magnetic resonance image (MRI) of the brain are unnecessary unless specific neurological deficits are found in these patients on physical examination.

Principles and Practice of Geriatric Psychiatry, 2nd edn. Edited by J. R. M. Copeland, M. T. Abou-Saleh and D. G. Blazer
©2002 John Wiley & Sons, Ltd

Dose

Older patients may be started on low doses of 150–300 mg/day, usually divided into two doses. The dose should be gradually increased according to the patient's response and ability to tolerate side effects. Lithium pharmacokinetics are affected by the aging process. As one ages, there is a decrease in total body water, renal blood flow and glomerular surface area. Therefore, the excretion of lithium decreases with age. This tendency is parallel to the reduction in creatinine clearance with age. Several studies have shown that elderly patients require one-third to one-half the lithium dose suitable for young adults[12]. A longer elimination half-life (<36 h) seen in the elderly suggests that a steady state may be reached within 7–10 days of initiation of therapy. Initially, lithium levels should be monitored at least once a week, with the blood level estimated at least 12 h after the last dose (the most convenient time would be early morning prior to the first dosage).

The target for lithium concentration level should always be based on individual therapeutic response. However, studies have indicated that lithium levels of 0.8–1.2 mEq/l are generally recommended. Those studies have predominately been done on mixed-age populations. Some researchers have suggested that the elderly may respond to relatively lower serum lithium levels (0.3–0.5 mEq/l)[13].

Side Effects

General Side Effects.   Common side effects with lithium therapy are a benign fine tremor, metallic taste, polyuria, polydipsia, gastric irritability, nausea, weight gain and mild sedation. The presence of tremor is an especially common and bothersome side effect in all adults taking lithium, but it tends to increase with age[14]. The tremor occurs at relatively low serum concentrations, and may worsen as the concentration increases[9]. Various researchers have found the incidence of tremor in the elderly to be between 17.5–58%[15–17].

Lowering the dosage may reduce most of these side effects. Taking the lithium with food or using the enteric coated form can reduce the problem of gastric irritation. If lithium tremor is persistent, propranolol may be helpful, although its use should be closely monitored because of the potential for other side effects to which elderly patients may be susceptible. Low-dose thiazide diuretics may improve polyuria and polydipsia, but should be used with caution (see below).

Signs of lithium toxicity include the significant exacerbation of the above symptoms, as well as vomiting, diarrhea, ataxia, slurred speech, severe lethargy, weakness, blurred vision, severe drowsiness or, at times, agitation. Lithium toxicity is often seen in the acute treatment of a manic episode in an older adult as the lithium dose is being regulated. Therefore, frequent monitoring of blood levels and side effects is essential. If symptoms are present, lithium should be stopped immediately. Dialysis may be used to remove excessively high levels of lithium from the blood. Recovery from lithium toxicity may be prolonged in the elderly due to slow renal clearance, the presence of an underlying dementia, or possibly subclinical brain changes[18].

Neurotoxicity.   Excessive amounts of lithium may result in neurotoxic effects, characterized by confusion, disorientation, memory loss, ataxia and akathisia. However, several reports have shown that neurotoxic effects may develop at relatively low serum concentrations of lithium in the elderly. Himmelhoch et al.[10] found that the presence of an underlying neurological disorder that produces parkinsonian symptoms, dementia or episodic confusion is highly predictive of lithium-induced neurotoxicity, even with low serum lithium concentrations.

Cardiovascular Toxicity.   Lithium may cause both non-specific and specific ECG changes associated with repolarization. Some of the specific ECG changes are T-wave flattening or inversion (which may be caused by potassium depletion) and the appearance of U waves. Adverse effects of cardiotoxicity can present as conduction defects, irregular and slowed sinus rhythm, first degree atrioventricular (AV) block, or premature ventricular complexes (PVCS). Ventricular tachycardia is a sign of severe cardiotoxicity. Older patients are at a higher risk for these cardiovascular effects, even with milder degrees of lithium toxicity. Regular comparison of the ECG with baseline measures is important once the patient starts treatment with lithium.

Nephrogenic Diabetes Insipidus.   Lithium may also cause symptoms of nephrogenic diabetes insipidus in up to 20–40% of patients on maintenance lithium therapy[19]. This condition is caused by the inability of the patient to concentrate his/her urine. The result is the excretion of large quantities (>3 l/day) of urine, which can cause dehydration if comparable fluid intake is not maintained. This syndrome is usually reversible and is not dose-related[20]; however, there appears to be a risk of persistent concentrating defects even after the lithium is stopped[21,22]. Diabetes insipidus can be treated effectively with amiloride or hydrochlorothiazide (HCTZ), but each of these also has the possibility of causing electrolyte imbalance, particularly in geriatric patients.

Thyroid Abnormalities.   Lithium therapy can interfere with thyroid functioning, such as synthesis, degradation and release of T3 and T4. Decrease in thyroid hormone can stimulate TSH by negative feedback. Even though compensation may occur initially, some patients develop signs of hypothyroidism[23] with goiter. If detected early, hypothyroidism is reversible, either by stopping the lithium or by the use of thyroid supplements. Lithium should be discontinued if the patient develops goiter, as this can be reversed if detected sufficiently early.

Drug Interactions

Lithium is eliminated from the body through the kidneys. Therefore any medication which may alter kidney function (especially glomerular filtration or electrolyte balance) will change lithium concentration. Medications frequently prescribed to elderly patients that may have significant drug interactions with lithium include anti-hypertensive medications [thiazide diuretics, loop diuretics, angiotensin-converting enzyme (ACE) inhibitors, and calcium antagonists], non-steroidal anti-inflammatory drugs (NSAIDs), carbamazepine, theophylline, caffeine and aciclovir. Selective serotonin-reuptake inhibitors (SSRIs) have been noted to increase the risk of lithium toxicity when used in conjunction with tricyclic antidepressants (Salama, Noveske, Vesely). Aspirin (acetylsalicylic acid) has not been shown to affect lithium concentrations.

Carbamazepine (CBZ)

Efficacy

Carbamazepine, a tricyclic anticonvulsant drug, has proven efficacy in treating adults with acute mania[24–28]. However, all of these studies were done in mixed age adult populations. Systematic studies of carbamazepine in the elderly are lacking. Although lithium remains the preferred treatment for patients with the classic presentation of bipolar disorder, the response rate drops to 50% when the full bipolar spectrum is considered[29]. Greil et al.[30,31] have found that carbamazepine may be useful in patients with non-classical features (mixed or rapid cycling bipolar disorder) or subgroups with depressive or schizophrenia-like features. A few investigators have identified increased benefit with carbamazepine when they treated patients who had EEG abnormalities associated with symptoms of rage and violent behavior[32].

Treatment Considerations

Prior to starting patients on carbamazepine, the patient's medical history should be reviewed, with special attention to previous episodes of blood dyscrasias or liver disease. Laboratory tests should include a complete blood count (CBC), serum chemistry panel, and liver function tests [lactate dehydrogenase (LDH), ALT, AST, bilirubin and alkaline phosphatase levels].

Dose and Administration

Treatment in older patients should be initiated with low doses, starting with 200–400 mg/day by mouth. The dose should be increased gradually and slowly. Carbamazepine therapeutic levels are in the range 4–12 ng/ml; however, these parameters are based on the anticonvulsant effect. There is no standard blood level recommendation for the treatment of bipolar disorder. The ideal therapeutic blood level is subjectively determined and depends on the patient's clinical response and the appearance of side effects. During the initial 6–8 weeks of treatment, blood levels may decrease despite maintaining a regular dose, due to carbamazepine's ability to induce its own metabolism. Checking blood levels and adjusting appropriately is important for maintenance of the treatment effect. Geriatric patients may be able to maintain adequate therapeutic levels on lower doses (400–600 mg) due to slower metabolism.

Side Effects

Bone marrow depression (aplastic anemia, decreased cell counts, agranulocytosis) and hepatotoxicity can occur with carbamazepine. Risk of bone marrow depression is estimated at 1/125 000. Weekly monitoring of blood counts, liver profile and carbamazepine levels is indicated during the early weeks of treatment. Idiosyncratic reactions are rare; however, patients should be asked to report immediately reactions such as fever, sore throat or severe fatigue of sudden onset.

The most common adverse effects of carbamazepine are dizziness, drowsiness, vertigo, ataxia, diplopia, nystagmus and blurred vision[9]. These effects are usually dosage-related and may be minimized by reducing the dose. Skin rash, urticaria, Stevens–Johnson syndrome, Lyell's syndrome, photosensitivity and dermatitis have also been reported, so that carbamazepine should be discontinued if these symptoms appear.

Other side effects include cardiovascular complications, such as congestive heart failure, hypertension, hypotension, arrhythmias, AV block and thrombophlebitis[33] as may occur with other tricyclic agents. The risk is greatest if patients already have underlying cardiovascular disease.

Drug Interactions

Carbamazepine interacts with a variety of other medications. Serum carbamazepine concentrations are markedly increased when carbamazepine is given with SSRIs, erythromycin, isoniazid, calcium channel blockers and danazol. Blood levels will also increase to a lesser degree with cimetidine, valproate, phenobarbital, phenytoin and theophylline. Carbamazepine decreases neuroleptic blood levels, which may lead to a lower efficacy of the neuroleptic in combined therapy.

Valproate (Valproic Acid)

Efficacy

Valproate is an anticonvulsant also shown to be effective in the treatment of bipolar disorder in the general adult population. It has also been documented to be effective for the elderly bipolar patient[34–44]. Valproate primarily works through the GABA system, and has recently been used to treat patients with acute mania who are resistant to traditional drugs such as lithium and carbamazepine[36,45]. It remains the drug of choice in patients who have failed to respond to lithium or carbamazepine or who are unable to tolerate these medications because of their side effects. Valproic acid may be used effectively in combination with lithium if there is only a partial response to either drug. Like carbamazepine, valproate causes minimal cognitive side effects, which is of particular advantage in the elderly patient.

Treatment Considerations

Valproate appears to be very well tolerated by elderly patients. Prior to starting patients on valproate, liver function tests and a CBC should be performed. Albumin levels should be performed on the frail elderly. Valproate may be used in combination with lithium, although experience suggests that a trial of monotherapy is usually indicated initially[9].

Dose and Administration

Valproic acid is available in three forms: valproic acid, sodium valproate and divalproate sodium. Gastric irritation is not uncommon with valproic acid or sodium valproate treatment. In such patients, the use of divalproate sodium may reduce gastrointestinal (GI) irritability. This medication is available in three strengths, 125 mg, 250 mg and 500 mg. Treatment should begin with low divided doses (125 mg twice a day) and be gradually increased to 500–1000 mg/day, depending on tolerance, side effects and blood levels. Most studies evaluating the effectiveness of valproate in bipolar disorder have used the target drug concentrations found effective in the treatment of epilepsy (50–100 mg/ml)[46]. Higher blood levels may sometimes be required to achieve optimal clinical response.

Valproate is rapidly absorbed from the gastrointestinal system and has a half-life of 6–16 h in younger patients, although this could be longer in geriatric patients. In serum it is predominantly protein-bound after absorption. The decrease in serum albumin levels associated with aging may result in lower dosages being required for elderly patients to achieve adequate blood levels. It is metabolized in the liver prior to elimination.

Side Effects

Gastrointestinal side effects of valproate include nausea, vomiting and indigestion. Occasionally abdominal cramps, constipation and diarrhea are reported. Anorexia has also been observed, although weight gain appears more common. These effects are usually transient, diminishing with continued treatment. Persistent GI symptoms may respond to a reduction in the dose or changing to the enteric-coated form.

Common central nervous system (CNS) effects are sedation and ataxia, which are generally dose-related. Nystagmus, headache, diplopia and asterixis are less common side effects. Dizziness and lack of coordination can occur and are also dose-related.

Minor elevations of liver transaminases (SGOT, SGPT and LDH) can occur as side effects of treatment. Hepatotoxicity with hepatic failure has been reported in children but less frequently in adults. Baseline and periodic monitoring of hepatic function is indicated during the initial phase of treatment.

Idiosyncratic reactions may cause alopecia, which can be treated effectively with vitamin supplements containing zinc and selenium. Other side effects, such as thrombocytopenia, leukocytosis, edema, weakness and skin rash, have been reported but are generally rare.

Drug Interactions

Because valproate is extensively metabolized in the liver, it may interact with other medications. Valproate may inhibit the metabolism of phenobarbital, ethosuximide, phenytoin and some tricyclic antidepressants, resulting in higher blood levels of these drugs. Frequent monitoring of blood levels and appropriate adjustment of dosage may be needed to maintain therapeutic blood levels during the initial stages of treatment. Combinations of valproate and clonazepam may produce lapse of memory, which could present a significant problem in elderly patients. The use of anticoagulants such as aspirin and warfarin should be closely monitored, as the potency of these drugs may be enhanced.

Newer Anticonvulsants

Gabapentin

Gabapentin is a novel anticonvulsant agent structurally related to γ-aminobutyric acid (GABA), currently approved as an adjunctive therapy in patients with partial seizures. Its mechanism of action is not yet fully understood. Gabapentin has been increasingly used for the treatment of bipolar disorder, behavioral disturbances in Alzheimer's disease, and social phobia. Multiple case reports and small open-label studies in the general adult population have demonstrated gabapentin to be effective as monotherapy or as an adjunct therapy for the treatment of acute mania, or as a prophylactic therapy for bipolar illness[47–52]. Experience in the non-demented elderly bipolar patient is limited.

Gabapentin is not metabolized and is not protein-bound. It is excreted in the kidneys essentially unchanged. It has few pharmacokinetic interactions with other medications. Some researchers have reported a small increase in Depakote levels when used together[53]. Gabapentin is not associated with any hematologic or hepatic problems and does not require monitoring of serum concentration. In addition, gabapentin has a relatively benign side-effect profile. The most commonly reported adverse effects are sedation, dizziness, ataxia and fatigue[54]. These are usually minor and transient. These properties have made gabapentin a very attractive medication choice for use in bipolar patients who are receiving multiple medications, experience blood or liver problems, or in whom blood level monitoring is a problem[55]. Some researchers[51], however, have suggested that gabapentin may only exert a "moderate" antimanic effect, and that its onset of effect may be delayed when compared with other mood stabilizers. Thus, gabapentin may be less effective in the acute treatment of mania, and is recommended as adjunctive therapy in severe mania.

The effective dose of gabapentin in the treatment of bipolar disorder is not yet known. Most trials in young adults have used a dosage range of 300–2400 mg/day, although the use of larger doses has also been documented. Ferrier[55] has suggested that gabapentin may be particularly efficacious in rapid-cycling bipolar disorder (dose range 1500–2400 mg/day). Elderly patients would presumably require less, due to age-related decreases in creatinine clearance. The usual starting dose is 300–600 mg/day in divided doses.

Lamotrigine

As the use of anticonvulsant medications for treatment of bipolar disorder has proved successful, other anticonvulsants have also been increasingly used. Lamotrigine is an anticonvulsant approved as an adjunctive treatment for refractory epilepsy. The exact mechanism of action is not yet known, although evidence suggests that it reduces the release of excitatory amino acids (by blocking voltage-dependent sodium channels) and may act as a calcium channel antagonist[56,57]. Early studies and case reports in young adults have suggested that lamotrigine may be useful as a monotherapy or as an adjunctive therapy for bipolar disorder[58–61,95,96,98] and is particularly effective in rapid-cycling bipolar disorder and bipolar depression[62–66]. Lamotrigine has not been studied in elderly bipolar patients.

Lamotrigine is metabolized in the liver, with a half-life of 25–30 h. Protein binding is 55%. Lamotrigine does not appear to induce the P450 system and it has little interactions with other psychotropic medications. However, carbamazepine may decrease lamotrigine levels while valproate may increase them.

The most common side effects are headache, nausea, diplopia, dizziness and ataxia. A skin rash may occur in 5% of patients, more commonly with older age, rapid escalation of dose and the concomitant use of valproate. In most cases the rash is mild and transient; however, a few patients have developed Stevens–Johnson syndrome. Therefore, the medication is usually titrated very slowly (beginning at 12.5 mg/day) and is discontinued if a rash develops. Lamotrigine has also been reported to cause confusion or psychosis or to induce mania. There are no current standard dosage recommendations and routine measurement of serum concentrations is not required.

ADJUNCTIVE MEDICATIONS FOR ACUTE MANIA

Clonazepam

Efficacy

Clonazepam is a nitrobenzodiazepine derivative indicated in the treatment of absence seizures, infantile spasms, myoclonus and atonic seizures. It has proven efficacy in reducing seizure frequency and has also been used effectively in restless leg syndrome, panic disorder and Tourette's disorder. Clonazepam has also been used with success in treating acute mania[67,68]. It has also been used to augment mood stabilizers during the acute treatment of manic episodes, allowing a decrease in the use of neuroleptics in non-psychotic mania[69–71]. Clonazepam has not been well studied for use in geriatric patients with bipolar disorder.

Dose and Metabolism

The antimanic effect is attained in younger adults with a dose range of 2–16 mg/day in divided doses[67]. The half-life in younger adults is 20–80 h. Older patients require much lower doses for clinical efficacy because of delayed metabolism and therefore a much longer half-life. A clinical response is usually seen in the dose range 2–6 mg in divided doses in such patients.

Side Effects

The most common side effects are ataxia, disinhibition, drowsiness and sedation. A paradoxical effect (excitation, agitation, irritability) has been observed, and is more likely to occur in patients with underlying neurological illness. Clonazepam can potentiate other sedating drugs, such as antihistamines and alcohol.

Benzodiazepine use is always recommended as short-term therapy only. Patients maintained on clonazepam may develop tolerance and dependence after 6 months of consistent use. The use of benzodiazepines in the elderly is of special concern, due to the potential to cause decrease in cognition, alertness or balance. Clonazepam should always be gradually tapered to avoid withdrawal symptoms.

Lorazepam

Efficacy

Lorazepam is a short-acting benzodiazepine that has proved effective in the treatment of acute mania[72,73,97,99]. Lorazepam is frequently used as an adjunctive medication for the control of symptoms of acute mania until the mood-stabilizer becomes effective. Like clonazepam, the use of lorazepam has decreased the use of neuroleptics for agitation during the acute manic episode[74,75]. This medication is not indicated for maintenance treatment. The use of lorazepam in the elderly bipolar patient is not well studied.

Dose and Metabolism

Lorazepam is available in both oral and intramuscular forms, and absorbed rapidly with either route of administration. It is the most common benzodiazepine used in geriatric populations due to its short half-life (10–20 h), large therapeutic index, no metabolites, gluconoride conjugation and rapid onset of action. The dose range is generally 1–4 mg/day in divided doses for a geriatric population, titrated by individual response side effects.

Side Effects

Like all benzodiazepines, increased and persistent sedation may increase the risk of falling, especially in the elderly. Paradoxical behaviors and disinhibition can occur in a small percentage of patients, most commonly those with underlying neurological illness. Lorazepam also potentiates other sedating drugs; therefore, close monitoring is required when using lorazepam in the elderly.

ANTIPSYCHOTIC MEDICATIONS

Acute manic episodes of moderate to severe degree, or manic episodes associated with symptoms such as hallucinations, delusions, paranoia or severe irritability or agitation, can be treated initially with antipsychotic medications. Most typical antipsychotic medications effect clinical improvement by blocking dopamine pathways in the brain and provide sedation through antihistamine effects. Atypical antipsychotic medications are thought to effect clinical change through a combination of dopamine-blocking effects and serotoninergic activity. Clozapine, risperidone and olanzapine have been reported to be effective in the treatment of acute mania, both as single agents and in adjunctive treatment[76–81]. These studies, however, have not involved elderly patients.

High-potency typical antipsychotics tend to cause significant extrapyramidal symptoms, such as rigidity, bradykinesia, tremor, dystonia, akathisia and a Parkinson-like syndrome, but a low incidence of hypotension, cardiovascular toxicity and sedation. Low-potency typical antipsychotics cause significant sedation, postural hypotension and peripheral anticholinergic effects. The newer atypical antipsychotics have less severe side effects, but still may cause sedation, orthostasis or extrapyramidal side effects. Given the high risk of such side effects in geriatric patients, low-potency neuroleptics should generally be avoided. The atypical antipsychotics are increasingly being used, due to their preferred side-effect profile. The use of antipsychotic medications in conjunction with other medications appears to have limited adverse interactions; however, a few studies have reported the development of neurotoxicity from the combined use of typical antipsychotic medications and lithium[82–84].

Geriatric patients typically require lower doses than middle-aged patients. Lower doses also minimize important side effects, particularly the risk of tardive dyskinesia in the long-term use of neuroleptics. Once acute symptoms improve, the antipsychotic dosage can be lowered or even discontinued while stabilizing patients on antimanic medications.

ELECTROCONVULSIVE THERAPY (ECT)

Electroconvulsive therapy (ECT) has been shown to be a highly effective treatment for acute mania[85–87]. Several studies of both geriatric and general adult manic patients have shown an improvement in approximately 80% with ECT[88,89]. This is especially significant, since ECT is frequently used for patients who have been resistant to other treatments or who have significant medical co-morbidities.

Contraindications

Even though there are no absolute contraindications for ECT, the risk of morbidity and mortality is increased in certain conditions. These include space-occupying intracerebral lesions or other conditions that may increase intracranial pressure, unstable vascular aneurysms or malformations, intracerebral hemorrhage, recent acute myocardial infarction or severe uncontrolled hypertension[90]. However, if ECT is required, risks can usually be minimized by pharmacologic treatment during ECT.

Risks and Adverse Effects

Usually, elderly patients tolerate ECT very well. The mortality rate for elderly patients is 0.01%, roughly the same as for the anesthesia induction itself[88,91,92]. Two-thirds of the deaths are from cardiac complications, such as ischemia, arrhythmias and transient severe increases in blood pressure. Most incidents occur immediately after the treatment or in the recovery period.

Side effects commonly observed during ECT include confusion and short-term memory loss. The latter is generally temporary, but occasionally some patients complain of prolonged loss, although no organic or irreversible changes in the brain have been found[93]. The risk of confusion and memory loss tends to be associated with high stimulus intensity, bilateral electrode placement, increased number and/or frequency of treatments, older age and pre-existing cognitive deficiencies. Adjustment of the stimulus waveform, decreasing the stimulus intensity, using unilateral electrode placement or increasing the interval between treatment may decrease the cognitive side effects.

Other somatic side effects include headaches, nausea, and muscle soreness. Prophylactic treatment with analgesics or using an increased dose of the muscle relaxants during ECT may minimize these symptoms. ECT patients are also at a higher risk for falls.

Treatment Considerations

Prior to initiating ECT treatment, a focused medical history and physical examination is necessary to assess and minimize any potential risk factor. Laboratory tests should include a hematocrit or hemoglobin, serum electrolytes and an electrocardiogram (ECG)[90]. Most practitioners also obtain either an EEG, CT of the head, or brain MRI prior to ECT. If a patient has a history of musculoskeletal disease or osteoporosis, spinal X-rays may be obtained to evaluate the presence of underlying compression fractures, so that anesthetic/muscle relaxant medication may be properly adjusted. Dental evaluation is of particular importance in aged patients and attention should be given to patients who have loose teeth or none or only partial dentures.

An informed consent should be obtained prior to initiating ECT. In geriatric patients whose judgement and insight are compromised by their illness, the family should be involved in treatment decision making and consent. In the case of patients not competent to give consent, the legal guardian must be identified and approve consent.

The use of psychiatric medications during ECT should be minimized. Lithium should be discontinued prior to ECT, since it may increase the risk of status epilepticus and prolonged muscular blockade with succinylcholine. The anticonvulsants (valproate, carbamazepine) should also be discontinued, since they inhibit the ECT seizure. It should also be remembered that all benzodiazepines increase seizure threshold. They can be tapered prior to ECT or a benzodiazepine antagonist can be used just prior to the procedure.

Early reports suggested that mania was more resistant to ECT or required more frequent treatments than depression. Recent research has found this not to be true. The patient's clinical improvement is the best guide in deciding the optimal number of treatments. An average of 6–12 treatments is usually required for optimal response. Recommendations for treatment parameters may be found in several other texts[90,91,94].

REFERENCES

1. Young RC, Klerman GL. Mania in late-life: focus on age at onset. *Am J Psychiat* 1992; **149**: 867–76.
2. Kramer M, German PS, Anthony JC *et al*. Patterns of mental disorders among the elderly residents of eastern Baltimore. *J Am Geriat Soc* 1985; **33**(4): 236–45.
3. Yassa R, Nair V, Nastase C *et al*. Prevalence of bipolar disorder in a psychogeriatric population. *J Affect Disord* 1988; **14**: 197–201.
4. Stevick CP. Some demographic and diagnostic characteristics of a geriatric population in a state geriatric facility. *J Am Geriat Soc* 1980; **28**(9): 426–9.
5. Snowdon J. A retrospective case-note study of bipolar disorder in old age. *Br J Psychiat* 1991; **158**: 485–90.
6. Rice J, Reich T, Andreasen NC *et al*. The familial transmission of bipolar illness. *Arch Gen Psychiat* 1987; **44**(5): 441–7.
7. Young RC, Falk JR. Age, manic psychopathology and treatment response. *Int J Geriat Psychiat* 1989; **4**: 73–8.
8. Dhingra U, Rabins P. Mania in the elderly: a 5–7 year follow-up. *J Am Geriat Soc* 1991; **39**: 581–3.
9. Eastham JH, Jeste DV, Young RC. Assessment and treatment of bipolar disorder in the elderly. *Drugs Aging* 1998; **12**(3): 205–24.
10. Himmelhoch JM, Neil JF, May SJ *et al*. Age, dementia, dyskinesias, and lithium response. *Am J Psychiat* 1980; **137**(8): 941–5.
11. Jefferson JW. Lithium and affective disorders in the elderly. *Comp Psychiat* 1983; **24**: 166–78.
12. Hardy BG, Shulman K, MacKenzie SE *et al*. Pharmacokinetics of lithium in elderly. *J Clin Psychopharmacol* 1987; **7**: 153–8.
13. Vestergaard P, Shou M. The effect of age on lithium dosage requirements. *Pharmaco-Psychiatry* 1984; **17**: 199–201.
14. Murray N, Hopwood S, Balfour DJK *et al*. The influence of age on lithium efficacy and side-effects in outpatients. *Psychol Med* 1983; **13**: 53–60.
15. Chacko RC, Marsh BJ, Marmion J *et al*. Lithium side effects in elderly bipolar outpatients. *Hillside J Clin Psychiat* 1987; **9**(1): 79–88.
16. Smith RE, Helms PM. Adverse effects of lithium therapy in the acutely ill elderly patient. *J Clin Psychiat* 1982; **43**(3): 94–9.
17. Holroyd S, Rabins PV. A retrospective chart review of lithium side effects in a geriatric outpatient population. *Am J Geriat Psychiat* 1994; **2**(4): 346–51.
18. Nambudiri DE, Meyers BS, Young RC. Delayed recovery from lithium neurotoxicity. *J Geriat Psychiat Neurol* 1991; **4**(1): 40–3.
19. Swaminathan R. Hyperosmolar coma due to lithium-induced diabetes insipidus. *Lancet* 1995; **346**: 413–17.
20. Angrist BM, Gershon RG, Leir RV *et al*. Lithium-induced diabetes insipidus like syndrome. *Comp Psychiat* 1970; **11**: 141–6.
21. Bucht G, Wahlin A. Renal concentrating capacity in long-term lithium treatment and later withdrawal of lithium. *Acta Med Scand* 1980; **207**: 309–14.
22. Stone KA. Lithium-induced nephrogenic diabetes insipidus. *J Am Board Fam Pract* 1999; **12**(1): 43–7.
23. Jefferson JW. Lithium carbonate induced hypothyroidism—its many faces. *J Am Med Assoc* 1979; **242**: 271–2.
24. Lerer B, Moore N, Meyendorff E *et al*. Carbamazepine vs. lithium in mania. A double-blind study. *J Clin Psychiat* 1987; **48**: 89–93.
25. Grossi E, Sachetti E, Vita A *et al*. CBZ vs. chlorpromazine in mania: a double-blind trial. In Enrich EM, Okuma T, Mullera F, eds, *Anticonvulsants in Affective Disorders*. Amsterdam: Excerpta Medica, 1984; 177–87.
26. Brown D, Silverstone T, Cookson J. Carbamazepine vs. haldol in acute mania. *Soc Biol Psychiat* 1986; **28**: 229.
27. Ballenger JC. Use of anticonvulsants in manic depressive illness. *J Clin Psychiat* 1988; **49**(suppl): 21–4.
28. Post RM, Unde TW, Roy Berne PP *et al*. Correlates of antimanic responses to carbamazepine. *Psychiat Res* 1987; **21**: 71–83.
29. Calabrese JR, Fatemi SH, Kujawa M, Woyshville MJ. Predictors of response to mood stabilizers. *J Clin Psychopharmacol* 1996; **16**(2 Suppl 1): 24–31S.
30. Greil W, Ludwig-Mayerhofer W, Erazo N *et al*. Lithium vs. carbamazepine in the maintenance treatment of schizoaffective disorder: a randomised study. *Eur Arch Psychiat Clin Neurosci* 1997; **247**(1): 42–50.
31. Greil W, Kleindienst N, Erazo N, Muller-Oerlinghausen B. Differential response to lithium and carbamazepine in the prophylaxis of bipolar disorder. *J Clin Psychopharmacol* 1998; **18**(6): 455–60.
32. Hakola HPA, Lauluman BAO. Carbamazepine in treatment of violent schizophrenics. *Lancet* 1982; **i**: 1358.
33. Ladefoged SD, Mogelvang JC. Total atrioventricular block with syncopes complicating carbamazepine therapy. *Acta Med Scand* 1982; **212**(3): 185–6.
34. Yassa R, Cvejic J. Valproate in the treatment of posttraumatic bipolar disorder in a psychogeriatric patient. *J Geriat Psychiat Neurol* 1994; **7**: 55–7.
35. Rinsinger RC, Risby ED, Risch SC. Safety and efficacy of divalproex sodium in elderly bipolar patients. *J Clin Psychiat* 1994; **55**(5): 215.
36. McFarland BH, Miller MR, Straumfjord AA. Valproate use in the older manic patient. *J Clin Psychiat* 1990; **51**(11): 479–81.

37. Sharma V, Persad E. Augmentation of valproate with lithium in a case of rapid cycling affective disorder. *Can J Psychiat* 1992; **37**(8): 584–5.

38. Pope HG, McElroy SL, Satlin A. Head injury, bipolar disorder, and response to valproate. *Comp Psychiat* 1988; **29**: 34–8.

39. Kando JC, Tohen M, Castillo J *et al.* The use of valproate in an elderly population with affective symptoms. *J Clin Psychiat* 1996; **57**(6): 238–40.

40. Gnam W, Flint AJ. New onset rapid cycling bipolar disorder in an 87 year old woman. *Can J Psychiat* 1993; **38**: 324–6.

41. Schneider AL, Wilcox CS. Divalproate augmentation in lithium-resistant rapid cycling mania in four geriatric patients. *J Affect Disord* 1998; **47**: 201–5.

42. Mordecai DJ, Sheikh JI, Glick ID. Divalproex for the treatment of geriatric bipolar disorder. *Int J Geriat Psychiat* 1999; **14**: 494–6.

43. Puryear L, Kunik M, Workman JR. Tolerability of divalproex sodium in elderly psychiatric patients with mixed diagnoses. *J Geriat Psychiat Neurol* 1995; **8**: 234–7.

44. Noaghuil S, Narayan M, Nelson J. Divalproex treatment of mania in elderly patients. *Am J Geriat Psychiat* 1998; **6**: 257–62.

45. McElroy SL, Keek PE, Pope HG. Sodium valproate: its use in primary psychiatric disorders. *J Clin Psychopharmacol* 1987; **7**: 16–24.

46. Bowden CL, Janicak PG, Orsulak P *et al.* Relation of serum valproate concentration to response in mania. *Am J Psychiat* 1996; **153**(6): 765–70.

47. McElroy SL, Soutullo CA, Keck PE, Kmetz GF. A pilot trial of adjunctive gabapentin in the treatment of bipolar disorder. *Ann Clin Psychiat* 1997; **9**: 99–103.

48. Schaffer CB, Schaffer LC. Gabapentin in the treatment of bipolar disorder (letter). *Am J Psychiat* 1997; **154**: 291–2.

49. Stanton SP, Keck PE, McElroy SL. Treatment of acute mania with gabapentin (letter). *Am J Psychiat* 1997; **154**: 287.

50. Young LT, Robb JC, Patelis-Siotis I *et al.* Acute treatment of bipolar depression with gabapentin. *Biol Psychiat* 1997; **42**: 851–3.

51. Erfurth A, Kammerer C, Grunze H *et al.* An open label study of gabapentin in the treatment of acute mania. *J Psychiat Res* 1998; **32**: 261–4.

52. Hatzimanolis J, Lykouras L, Oulis P, Christodoulou GN. Gabapentin as monotherapy in the treatment of acute mania. *Eur Neuropsychopharmacol* 1999; **9**(3): 257–8.

53. Riva R, Albani F, Contin M, Baruzzi A. Pharmacokinetic interactions between antiepileptic drugs. Clinical considerations. *Clin Pharmacokinet* 1996; **31**: 470–93.

54. Dichter MA, Brodie MJ. New antiepileptic drugs. *N Engl J Med* 1996; **334**: 1583–90.

55. Ferrier IN. Lamotrigine and gabapentin: alternatives in the treatment of bipolar disorder. *Neuropsychobiology* 1998; **38**:192–7.

56. Leach MJ, Marsden CM, Miller AA. Pharmacological studies on lamotrigine, a novel potential antiepileptic drug. II. Neurochemical studies on the mechanism of action. *Epilepsia* 1986; **27**: 490–7.

57. Xie X, Hagan RM. Cellular and molecular actions of lamotrigine: Possible mechanisms of efficacy in bipolar disorder. *Neuropsychobiology* 1998; **38**(3): 119–30.

58. Sporn J, Sachs G. The anticonvulsant lamotrigine in treatment-resistant manic-depressive illness. *J Clin Psychopharmacol* 1997; **17**: 185–9.

59. Kusumakar V, Yatham LN. An open study of lamotrigine in refractory bipolar depression. *Psychiat Res* 1997; **72**: 145–8.

60. Kusumakar V, Yatham LN. Lamotrigine treatment of rapid cycling bipolar disorder (letter). *Am J Psychiat* 1997; **154**: 1171–2.

61. Fogelson DL, Sternbach H. Lamotrigine treatment of refractory bipolar disorder (letter). *J Clin Psychiat* 1997; **58**: 271–3.

62. Calabrese JR, Fatemi SH, Woyshville MJ. Antidepressant effects of lamotrigine in rapid cycling bipolar disorder (letter). *Am J Psychiat* 1996; **153**: 1236.

63. Labbate LA, Rubey RN. Lamotrigine for treatment-refractory bipolar disorder (letter). *Am J Psychiat* 1997; **154**: 1317.

64. Walden J, Hesslinger B, van Calker D, Berger M. Addition of lamotrigine to valproate may enhance efficacy in the treatment of bipolar affective disorder. *Pharmacopsychiatry* 1996; **29**: 193–5.

65. Bowden CL, Calabrese JR, McElroy SL *et al.* The efficacy of lamotrigine in rapid cycling and non-rapid cycling patients with bipolar disorder. *Biol Psychiat* 1999; **45**(8): 953–8.

66. Fatemi SH, Rappaport DJ, Calabrese JR, Thuras P. Lamotrigine in rapid-cycling bipolar disorder. *J Clin Psychiat* 1997; **58**(12): 522–7.

67. Chourinard G, Young SN, Annable L. Antimanic effect of clonazepam. *Biol Psychiat* 1983; **18**: 451–66.

68. Bottai T, Hue B, Hillaire-Buys D *et al.* Clonazepam in acute mania: time-blind evaluation of clinical response and concentrations in plasma. *J Affect Disord* 1995; **36**(1–2): 21–7.

69. Sachs GS. Use of clonazepam for bipolar affective disorder. *J Clin Psychiat* 1990; **51**(suppl): 31–34, 50–53.

70. Edwards R, Stephenson U, Flewett T. Clonazepam in acute mania: a double blind trial. *Aust N Z J Psychiat* 1991; **25**(2): 238–42.

71. Chouinard G, Annable L, Turnier L *et al.* A double-blind randomized clinical trial of rapid tranquilization with i.m. clonazepam and i.m. haloperidol in agitated psychotic patients with manic symptoms. *Can J Psychiat* 1993; **38**(suppl 4): S114–21.

72. Modell JG, Lenox RH, Weiner S. Inpatient clinical trial of lorazepam for the management of manic agitation. *J Clin Psychopharmacol* 1985; **5**: 109–13.

73. Modell JG. Further experience and observations with lorazepam in management of behavioral agitation. *J Clin Psychopharmacol* 1986; **6**: 385–6.

74. Lenox RH, Newhouse PA, Geelman WL, Whitaker TM. Adjunctive treatment of manic agitation with lorazepam versus haloperidol: a double blind study. *J Clin Psychiat* 1992; **53**(2): 47–52.

75. Lenox RH, Newhouse PA, Creelman WL, Whitaker TM. Adjunctive treatment of manic agitation with lorazepam vs. haloperidol: a double-blind study. *J Clin Psychiat* 1992; **53**(2): 47–52.

76. Frankenburg FR. Clozapine and bipolar disorder. *J Clin Psychopharmacol* 1993; **13**(4): 289–90.

77. Calabrese JR, Kimmel SE, Woyshville MJ *et al.* Clozapine for treatment-refractory mania. *Am J Psychiat* 1996; **153**: 759–64.

78. Zarate CA Jr, Tohen M, Baldessarini RJ. Clozapine in severe mood disorders. *J Clin Psychiatry* 1995; **56**: 411–17.

79. Zarate CA Jr, Tohen M, Banov MD. Is clozapine a mood stabilizer? *J Clin Psychiat* 1995; **56**: 108–12.

80. Frye MA, Ketter TA, Altshuler LL *et al.* Clozapine in bipolar disorder: treatment implications for other atypical antipsychotics. *J Affect Disord* 1998; **48**: 91–104.

81. Tohen M, Sanger TM, McElroy SL *et al.* Olanzapine vs. placebo in the treatment of acute mania. *Am J Psychiat* 1999; **156**(5): 702–9.

82. Mirchandani I, Young RC. Management of mania in the elderly: an update. *Ann Clin Psychiat* 1993; **5**(1): 67–77.

83. Cohen WF, Cohen NH. Lithium carbonate, haloperidol, and irreversible brain damage. *J Am Med Assoc* 1974; **230**(9): 1283–7.

84. Miller F, Menninger J, Whitcup SM. Lithium-neuroleptic neurotoxicity in patients given lithium and a neuroleptic. *Hosp Commun Psychiat* 1987; **38**(11): 1219–21.

85. McCabe MS. ECT in treatment of mania, a controlled study. *Am J Psychiat* 1976; **133**: 688–91.

86. McCabe MS, Norris B. ECT vs. chlorpromazine in mania. *Biol Psychiat* 1977; **12**: 245–54.

87. Small JG, Small IF, Milstein V *et al.* Manic symptoms: an indication for bilateral ECT. *Biol Psychiat* 1985; **20**: 125–34.

88. Greenberg L, Fink M. The use of electroconvulsive therapy in geriatric patients. *Clin Geriat Med* 1992; **8**(2): 349–54.

89. Muckherjee S, Sackeim HA, Schnur DB. Electroconvulsive therapy of acute manic episodes: a review of 50 years' experience. *Am J Psychiat* 1994; **151**: 169–76.

90. APA Task Force Report on ECT. *The Practice of Electroconvulsive Therapy. Recommendations for Treatment and Privileging.* Washington, DC: American Psychiatric Press, 1990.

91. Abrams R. *Electroconvulsive Therapy*, 2nd edn. New York: Oxford University Press.

92. Burke WJ, Rubin EH, Zorumski CF *et al.* The safety of ECT in geriatric psychiatry. *J Am Geriat Soc* 1987; **35**(6): 516–21.

93. Weiner RD. The role of electroconvulsive therapy in the treatment of depression in the elderly. *J Am Geriat Soc* 1982; **30**: 710–12.

94. Beyer JL, Weiner RD, Glenn MD. *Electroconvulsive Therapy: A Programmed Text*, 2nd edn. Washington, DC: American Psychiatric Press, 1998.

95. Calabrese JR, Bowden CL, McElroy SL *et al.* Spectrum of activity of lamotrigine in treatment-refractory bipolar disorder. *Am J Psychiat* 1999; **156**(7): 1019–23.

96. Calabrese JR, Bowden CL, Sachs GS. A double-blind placebo-controlled study of lamotrigine monotherapy in outpatients with bipolar I depression. Lamictal 602 study group. *J Clin Psychiat* 1999; **60**(2): 79–88.

97. Bradwejn J, Shriqui C, Koszycki D *et al*. Double-blind comparison of the effects of clonazepam and lorazepam in acute mania. *J Clin Psychopharmacol* 1990; **10**(6): 403–8.

98. Suppes T, Brown ES, McElroy SL *et al*. Lamotrigine for the treatment of bipolar disorder: a clinical case series. *J Affect Disord* 1999; **53**(1): 95–8.

99. Cohen S, Khan A, Johnson S. Pharmacological management of manic psychosis in unlocked setting. *J Clin Psychopharmacol* 1987; **7**: 261–4.

Part G

Schizophrenic Disorders and Mood-incongruent Paranoid States

Late-life Psychotic Disorders:
Nosology and Classification

Lisa T. Eyler Zorrilla and Dilip V. Jeste

University of California, San Diego, and VA San Diego Healthcare System, CA, USA

The notion that mental disorders could occur in particular periods of life, such as old age, appeared only in the second half of the nineteenth century[1]. During this short history, there has been little agreement, and much confusion, regarding the nosology and classification of late-life mental disorders, particularly in the area of psychotic disorders.

One group of individuals with late-life non-affective psychotic disorders consists of those with onset of a psychotic illness (e.g. schizophrenia, delusional disorder) early in life, who have now aged. Debates about the classification of these patients have followed the same lines as those regarding younger adults (e.g. degree of overlap between psychosis and affective disorders, issues of duration and course) but most would agree that these patients should retain their original diagnosis into old age unless symptoms change dramatically enough to warrant a different diagnosis. A second group of patients consists of those individuals with new onset of non-affective psychosis late in life. In a majority of such cases, psychosis is secondary to a general medical condition such as dementia. There has been little controversy about the classification of these "organic" psychoses in the elderly, and this group of individuals will not be discussed further in the present chapter. In contrast, the classification systems for late-onset non-affective, non-organic psychoses are replete with overlapping terms, multiple definitions of the same nomenclature and different methods of conceptualizing similar disorders. Only recently, with the publication of an international consensus statement[2], has at least the geriatric psychiatry community come to some agreement on a set of terms to describe late-onset psychotic disorders.

EARLY HISTORY

Kraepelin was one of the first clinical researchers to recognize that non-affective psychoses could arise in middle age or later in life. Although the term "dementia praecox", with its inherent emphasis on an early age of onset, would seem to exclude late-onset cases, Kraepelin himself reported that one-third of his patients had symptom onset after age 30[3]. Kraepelin also studied a group of patients he described as suffering from "paraphrenia". This term had been used earlier by Guislain as a synonym for the syndrome of "folly"[4] and was used by Kraepelin to characterize a group of patients with minimal volitional and affective disturbance, prominent paranoia and a relatively preserved personality. While some of the subgroups of paraphrenia he described had a relatively later age of onset,

Kraepelin did not consider paraphrenia to be exclusively a late-onset disorder. Furthermore, follow-up studies of these patients showed that they did not differ greatly from those classified as dementia praecox[5,6]. Thus, many of Kraepelin's followers ultimately came to believe that dementia praecox and paraphrenia were the same disorder and that this disorder could arise early or late in life.

Other clinician investigators working during this time, however, felt that psychotic disorders arising for the first time in late life should be classified separately. The history of these classifications has been thoroughly reviewed[7]. Gaupp[8] distinguished between dementia praecox and a disorder diagnosed for the first time in post-menopausal women that was characterized by depressive agitation, resulting in "mental weakness". Stransky[9] used the term "dementia tardiva" to describe late-onset dementia praecox. Some authors emphasized the prevalence of paranoid symptoms among those with onset of psychosis late in life by using terms such as "paranoia chronica"[10] or "involutional paranoia"[11]. Following this tradition, Albrecht's[12] classification of late-onset psychotic patients distinguished between patients with paranoid symptoms and little personality disturbance ("presenile paraphrenia") and those with "depressive madness resulting in imbecility". The latter category seemed somewhat similar to a late-onset form of dementia praecox. Others who described syndromes of late-onset dementia praecox used the terms "involutional paraphrenia"[13], "stiffening involutional psychosis"[14] and "paraphrenia"[15]. Unfortunately, the use of "paraphrenia" to indicate an age of onset distinction led to a great deal of later confusion. Some psychiatrists employed the term to indicate a separate phenomenology independent of age of onset (much like Kraepelin's original use; e.g. Leonhard[16]), while others used that diagnosis to encompass most late-onset psychoses.

1940–1970

Using his father's term for dementia praecox, "schizophrenia", Manfred Bleuler[17] described individuals with "late-onset schizophrenia" as those with onset after age 40 exhibiting symptoms similar to those with an earlier onset of the disorder and no evidence of brain disease. Very few of these patients had onset after the age of 60. This classification was adopted by most subsequent German authors[7].

In the UK during this period, however, the classification of late-onset psychotic disorders took a somewhat different path. Studying a group of patients with onset after age 60, Roth and

Morrissey[18] described a syndrome of paranoid delusions and hallucinations in the context of preserved intellect, personality and affect. Because of the phenomenological similarity to Kraepelin's "paraphrenia" and due to its late onset, Roth and colleagues termed this disorder "late paraphrenia"[19,20], a name that was designed to encompass all late-onset, non-affective, non-organic psychoses in which paranoid symptoms were prominent. Thus, the term was both broader than late-onset schizophrenia, in that it encompassed late-onset delusional disorder, and more restrictive, in that it did not include non-paranoid forms of late-onset psychosis. Post[21] developed a different descriptive system. He divided late-onset (after age 50) psychoses into paranoid hallucinosis, schizophreniform syndrome, and schizophrenic syndrome. Based on a 3 year follow-up, however, he concluded that these three diseases were actually a continuum of the same disorder with slightly different symptom profiles.

European debates and developments were slow to influence the classification system used in the USA. The first *Diagnostic and Statistical Manual of the Mental Disorders* (DSM-I)[22] used the term "involutional psychotic reaction", which encompassed both paranoid ideation and depression in older patients. This amalgam of affective and psychotic symptoms in the elderly was split in the second edition (DSM-II)[23] in favor of "involutional paranoid state (involutional paraphrenia)" and "involutional melancholia". The former disorder, like Roth's late paraphrenia, was characterized by "delusion formation with onset in the involutional period . . . The absence of conspicuous thought disorders typical of schizophrenia distinguishes it from that group"[23]. Schizophrenia could be diagnosed in individuals with any age of onset.

1970–PRESENT

As European psychiatrists began to study patients with late paraphrenia more systematically, new classification systems in the USA were restricting the diagnosis of late-onset psychosis. One of the five Feighner Research Criteria[24] for schizophrenia was age of onset before age 40. In the third edition of the DSM (DSM-III)[25], a diagnosis of schizophrenia could not be made if the onset of symptoms was after age 45. Late-onset psychosis that involved persistent persecutory delusions with prominent hallucinations could be given a diagnosis of "paranoid disorder". This classification system was in stark contrast to both earlier RDC criteria[26] and to the 9th version of the *International Classification of Diseases* (ICD-9)[27], neither of which imposed age-of-onset restrictions for schizophrenia. The ICD-9 also allowed for a diagnosis of paraphrenia at any age. The revised version of DSM-III (DSM-III-R)[28] rectified the omission of late-onset schizophrenia by providing a separate diagnostic category for those diagnosed with schizophrenia after age 45. In the most recent version of the DSM (DSM-IV)[29] and the ICD (ICD-10)[30], no special categories exist for late-onset psychoses, although schizophrenia may be diagnosed at any age.

TOWARD A CONSENSUS

It is clear from this historical review that there has been little consensus regarding the classification of late-onset non-affective non-organic psychoses. Two opposing lines of thought have pulled the terminology in different directions. On the one hand, some authors have preferred to emphasize the similarity of late-onset psychoses to the corresponding early-onset disorders. This has resulted either in the use of terms such as "late-onset schizophrenia" and "late-onset delusional disorder" or has prompted a move toward ignoring age of onset altogether in

classification (e.g. DSM-IV, ICD-10). On the other hand, some members of the psychiatry community (mainly those in the UK) have preferred to emphasize differences between the phenomenology of late- and early-onset psychosis and thus have tended to use distinct terminology, such as "paraphrenia" or "late paraphrenia".

Thus, questions remain about which terminology would optimally serve the clinical and research communities. There are at least two overlapping issues to consider. First, how similar or different is the late-onset, non-affective, non-organic psychosis from early-onset disorders? If late-onset patients are no different from early-onset patients in terms of demography, phenomenology, etiological factors, prognosis and treatment, then it would be redundant to classify them in a separate category. If, however, such features differ between early-onset and late-onset individuals, then it would seem important to preserve a distinct diagnostic category in order to encourage further research and allow for optimal prognostic evaluation and treatment. The magnitude or extent of the differences between early- and late-onset individuals should also influence the terminology chosen for the diagnostic categorization. If a majority of critical clinical features are shared with an early-onset disorder, then it would make sense to adopt a term such as "late-onset schizophrenia". If the extent of differences is sufficiently large, a separate term would be warranted. A second issue to consider in determining the best classification scheme is what age of onset should be called "late". Most of the American studies of late-onset non-affective, non-organic psychosis have included patients with onset after 45 and generally before age 65. In addition, among the patients in Bleuler's late-onset schizophrenia studies, only 4% had an onset after age 60[7]. In contrast, most studies of late paraphrenia have been conducted with patients whose onset was after age 65. Differences in age-of-onset between late-onset schizophrenia and late paraphrenia studies may help to explain some of the diagnostic confusions that have persisted.

Only recently has the weight of evidence become sufficiently great in the field of late-life psychoses to allow for adequate consideration of these issues. In July 1998, the International Late-Onset Schizophrenia Group met to present reviews of published data on late-onset non-affective, non-organic psychosis and to develop a consensus statement regarding diagnostic categories[2]. The statement recognizes two illness classifications: late-onset (onset after the age of 40 years) schizophrenia and a very-late-onset (onset after 60) schizophrenia-like psychosis. Thus, the group determined that it was important to recognize a diagnostic distinction based on age of onset, due to differences between late- and early-onset patients, but that the disorders were not sufficiently different to warrant a separate nomenclature. In addition, the group felt that a further distinction was warranted within late-onset patients between those with onset in middle age and those with very late onset, based on major differences between these groups.

The similarities and differences among early-onset schizophrenia, late-onset schizophrenia and very-late-onset schizophrenia-like psychosis are summarized in Table 89.1. There are many areas of similarity between both late-onset groups and early-onset schizophrenia, such as symptoms[31–33], family history[32], brain imaging findings[34–36], and the nature of cognitive deficits[35]. The decision to retain the word "schizophrenia" in the nomenclature of both disorders was driven by these strong similarities. On the other hand, the consensus statement's distinction between those with middle-age-onset and old-age-onset psychoses was motivated by epidemiological, etiological and symptom differences between these two groups. Very-late-onset schizophrenia-like psychosis is different from both early- and late-onset schizophrenia, in that these cases tend to be associated with sensory impairment and social isolation[20], are less likely to exhibit formal thought disorder and

Table 89.1 Comparison of typical-onset (age 15–40) schizophrenia, middle-age-onset (age 41–65) schizophrenia, and very late-onset (age >65) schizophrenia-like psychosis

	15–40	41–65	>65
Female:male ratio	0.6:1	2:1	up to 8:1
Poor premorbid functioning	+ +	+	−
Family history of schizophrenia	+ +	+ +	−
Sensory deficits	−	−	+
Negative symptoms	+ + +	+ +	−
Thought disorder	+ + +	+ + +	−
Strokes, tumors	−	−	+
Neuroleptic dose	+ + +	+ +	+

+, presence; −, absence; number of symbols indicates degree of presence or absence.

affective blunting but more likely to have visual hallucinations[26,34,37] and have less familial aggregation of schizophrenia[40]. It should be emphasized that the members of the International Late-onset Schizophrenia Group were not unanimous in their support of the particular age cut-offs given in the consensus statement and also felt that the proposed nomenclature was not an end but a beginning of future research into this important topic.

Late-onset schizoaffective disorder and late-onset delusional disorder are not specifically addressed in the consensus statement. Based on recent research[38], late-onset schizoaffective disorder appears to share a majority of critical clinical and demographic features with late-onset schizophrenia. Thus, late-onset schizoaffective disorder appears to be a subgroup of late-onset schizophrenia in which mood symptoms are also present. Late-onset delusional disorder, by contrast, can be distinguished from late-onset schizophrenia by a unique preoccupation with non-bizarre delusions in the context of preserved affective and personality functioning in other domains[29]. In addition, treatment of these individuals may be more challenging than in schizophrenia due to a difficulty in establishing rapport with therapists[39]. Cognitive function, however, is somewhat more preserved in older patients with delusional disorder than in those with schizophrenia[39]. Unfortunately, there is a lack of research comparing early- and late-onset delusional disorder.

Further research is needed to clarify the classification of late-onset psychotic disorders. Specifically, longitudinal follow-up studies are necessary to determine whether the course of illness is different in the three groups of patients and how the course of late-onset disorders compares to that of early-onset syndromes. Such an enterprise is greatly aided by the consensus classification recently proposed. In summary, despite a tumultuous history, the future for research and clinical work in late-onset psychotic disorders appears to be on firmer footing for the new millennium.

ACKNOWLEDGEMENTS

This work was supported, in part, by the National Institute of Mental Health Grants MH43695, MH49671, MH45131 and MH19934 and by the Department of Veterans Affairs.

REFERENCES

1. Berrios GE. Late-onset mental disorders: a conceptual history. In *Late-Onset Mental Disorders: The Potsdam Conference*. Bell & Bain, 1999; 1–23.
2. Howard R, Rabins PV, Seeman MV, Jeste DV and the International Late-onset Schizophrenia Group. Late-onset schizophrenia and very-late-onset schizophrenia-like psychosis: an international consensus. *Am J Psychiat* 2000; **157**: 172–8.
3. Kraepelin E. *Dementia Praecox and Paraphrenia*. Chicago: Chicago Medical Book, 1919.
4. Campbell RJ. *Psychiatry Dictionary*, 7th edn. New York: Oxford University Press, 1996.
5. Mayer W. On paraphrenic psychoses (in German). *Zeitschr Gesamt Neurol Psychiat* 1921; **71**: 187–206.
6. Mayer-Gross W. Die Schizophrenie (IV. Die Klinik: V. Erkennung und Differential Diagnose). In Bumke O, ed., *Handbuch der Geiskrankheiten*, special 5th edn. Berlin: Springer, 1932.
7. Reicher-Rossler A. Late onset schizophrenia: the German concept and literature. In Howard R, Rabins PV, Castle DJ, eds, *Late Onset Schizophrenia*. Basel: Wrightson Biomedical, 1999; 3–16.
8. Gaupp R. Depression des hoheren Lebensalters. *Münch Med Wochenschr* 1905; **52**; 1531–7.
9. Stransky E. Dementia tardiva. *Mschr Psychiat* 1906; **18**: 1–38.
10. Berger H. Klinische Beitrage zur Paranoiafrage. *Mschr Psychiat* 1913; **34**: 181–229.
11. Kleist K. Die Involutionsparanoia. *Allg Z Psychiat* 1913; **70**: 1–134.
12. Albrecht H. Die funktionellen Psychosen des Ruckbildungsalters. *Z Neurol Psychiat* 1914; **22**: 306–44.
13. Serko A. Die Involutionsparaphrenie. *Mschr Psychiat* 1919; **45**: 245–86.
14. Medow. Eine Gruppe depressiver Psychosen des Ruckbildungsalters mit ungunstiger Prognose. *Arch Psychiat* 1922; **64**: 480–506.
15. Kolle K. *Die primare Verrucktheit: psychopathologische, klinische und genealogische Untersuchungen*. Leipzig: Thieme, 1931.
16. Leonhard K. *Aufteilung der endogenen Psychosen*. Berlin: Akademie, 1957.
17. Bleuler M. Late schizophrenic clinical pictures. *Fortschr Neurol Psychiat* 1943; **15**: 259–90.
18. Roth M, Morrissey JD. Problems in the diagnosis and classification of mental disorder in old age: with a study of case material. *J Ment Sci* 1952; **98**: 66–80.
19. Roth M. The natural history of mental disorder in old age. *J Ment Sci* 1955; **101**: 281–301.
20. Kay DWK, Roth M. Environmental and hereditary factors in the schizophrenias of old age ("late paraphrenia") and their bearing on the general problem of causation in schizophrenia. *J Ment Sci* 1961; **107**: 649–86.
21. Post F. *Persistent Persecutory States of the Elderly*. London: Pergamon, 1966.
22. American Psychiatric Association. *Diagnostic and Statistical Manual of Mental Disorders*, 1st edn. Washington, DC: American Psychiatric Press, 1952.
23. American Psychiatric Association. *Diagnostic and Statistical Manual of Mental Disorders*, 2nd edn. Washington, DC: American Psychiatric Press, 1968.
24. Feighner JP, Robins E, Guze SB *et al*. Diagnostic criteria for use in psychiatric research. *Arch Gen Psychiat* 1972; **26**: 57–63.
25. American Psychiatric Association. *Diagnostic and Statistical Manual of Mental Disorders*, 3rd edn. Washington, DC: American Psychiatric Press, 1980.
26. Spitzer RL, Endicott J, Robins E. *Research Diagnostic Criteria for a Selected Group of Functional Disorders*. New York: New York State Psychiatric Institute, 1978.
27. World Health Organization. *ICD-9. The International Statistical Classification of Diseases and Related Health Problems*. Geneva: WHO, 1978.
28. American Psychiatric Association. *Diagnostic and Statistical Manual of Mental Disorders*, 3rd edn, revised. Washington, DC: American Psychiatric Press, 1987.
29. American Psychiatric Association. *Diagnostic and Statistical Manual of Mental Disorders*, 4th edn. Washington, DC: American Psychiatric Association, 1994.
30. World Health Organization. *ICD-10. The International Statistical Classification of Diseases and Related Health Problems*. Geneva: WHO, 1991.
31. Howard R, Castle D, Wessely S, Murray RM. A comparative study of 470 cases of early and late-onset schizophrenia. *Br J Psychiat* 1993; **163**: 352–7.
32. Jeste DV, Symonds LL, Harris MJ *et al*. Non-dementia non-praecox dementia praecox? Late-onset schizophrenia. *Am J Geriat Psychiat* 1997; **5**: 302–17.

33. Pearlson GD, Kreger L, Rabins RV *et al*. A chart review study of late-onset and early-onset schizophrenia. *Am J Psychiat* 1989; **146**: 1568–74.

34. Howard RJ, Almeida O, Levy R *et al*. Quantitative magnetic resonance imaging volumetry distinguishes delusional disorder from late-onset schizophrenia. *Br J Psychiat* 1994; **165**: 474–80.

35. Jeste DV, McAdams LA, Palmer BW *et al*. Relationship of neuropsychological and MRI measures with age of onset of schizophrenia. *Acta Psychiat Scand* 1998; **98**: 156–64.

36. Pearlson GD, Tune LE, Wong DF *et al*. Quantitative D$_2$ dopamine receptor PET and structural MRI changes in late onset schizophrenia. *Schizophr Bull* 1993; **19**: 783–95.

37. Rabins P, Pauker S, Thomas J. Can schizophrenia begin after age 44? *Comp Psychiat* 1984; **25**: 290–3.

38. Evans JD, Heaton RK, Paulsen JS *et al*. Schizoaffective disorder: a form of schizophrenia or affective disorder. *J Clin Psychiat* 1999; **60**: 874–82.

39. Evans JD, Paulsen JS, Harris MJ *et al*. A clinical and neuropsychological comparison of delusional disorder and schizophrenia. *J Neuropsychiat Clin Neurosci* 1996; **8**: 281–6.

40. Howard R, Graham C, Sham P *et al*. A controlled family study of late-onset non-affective psychosis (late paraphrenia). *Br J Psychiat* 1997; **170**: 511–14.

90

Clinical Assessment and Differential Diagnosis

D. N. Anderson

Mossley Hill Hospital, Liverpool, UK

The schizophrenias of late life, previously called late paraphrenia[1] and paranoid states in old age, present fascinating, complex, biopsychosocial problems that span the whole of psychiatry and medicine. The characteristic features of late-onset schizophrenia have been summarized by several authors[2-10], although never better than in the seminal paper by Kay and Roth[2].

These conditions usually present with paranoid ideation, most commonly persecutory in nature, with or without other schizophrenia-like symptoms. The central abnormality implied by the term "paranoid" is a morbid distortion of beliefs, but not all distorted beliefs are delusions and not all elderly people expressing them are mentally ill. Many aspects of old age increase vulnerability, exposing elderly people to abuse and victimization, and a sensitive appreciation of this situation is needed when assessing the paranoid elderly patient.

Furthermore, not all patients with delusions have schizophrenia[11] and the first aim of assessment will be to clarify the nature of paranoid symptoms and consider a differential diagnosis. In most cases a diagnosis will be clear from the detailed historical account of symptoms and their course, abnormalities of mental state and simple physical investigations. Assessment must, then, evaluate the individual's level of functioning, independence, vulnerability, social and family support and physical health, which will all be of relevance to aetiology and management. The assessment will aim to consider patients and their symptoms within the wider context of their social environment, physical and psychological limitations. It is, therefore, necessary to have knowledge of premorbid personality, life style, life experience and cultural background, remembering that young and older generations have important cultural differences.

Ideally, the assessment will take place in the patient's home, when environment may be maximally appreciated. Home assessment provides a more complete picture of the patient's circumstances and helps put the problem into a living context. Commonly, paranoid ideas in old age relate to the patient's immediate, local environment and people within it. Herbert and Jacobson[3] used the term "partition delusions" to describe the belief that things were happening just the other side of the wall, floor or ceiling. Post[12] found that paranoid symptoms often temporarily disappeared when the patient was removed from the hostile environment and this can give a misleading impression of their nature.

The floridly deluded and hallucinated patient is easily recognized, but in old age paranoid ideation may be almost plausible when complaints of being abused, victimized, stolen from or manipulated are not beyond the bounds of possibility. Trying to establish the validity of such claims requires observation and information from a variety of sources.

Table 90.1 Differential diagnosis

Delirium
Dementia
Organic delusional/hallucinatory disorder, secondary to physical illness or drugs
Late-onset schizophrenia
Delusional disorder
Depression
Mania
Schizoaffective disorder
Paranoid personality disorder
Factual (basis in fact)
Sensory impairment

We need, first, to consider the differential diagnosis of paranoid symptoms (Table 90.1) and how clinical assessment helps to differentiate diagnostic categories before discussing the process of assessment in more detail.

DIFFERENTIAL DIAGNOSIS

Christensen and Blazer[13] found the prevalence of paranoid ideas in a community sample to be 4%. Leuchter and Spar[14] retrospectively reviewed 880 psychogeriatric admissions and the 8% who suffered a first episode psychotic illness met DSM-III criteria for major affective disorder (36%), organic mental disorder (43%) and primary paranoid disorder (21%). The more common conditions will be reviewed briefly from the point of clinical differentiation, although for detailed consideration reference should be made to the relevant chapters.

Delirium (Acute Confusion)

The history is short, usually days or a few weeks, and the onset rapid. Paranoid ideas and hallucinations occur in 40–50%[15]. These are typically poorly organized, fluctuating and variable in content, while hallucinations most commonly occur in the visual modality. Other features of delirium will normally be present.

Dementia (Chronic Confusion)

Ballinger et al.[16] found delusions and hallucinations in 38% and 34% of 100 dementia admissions. The study by Burns et al.[17] of

178 Alzheimer patients revealed persecutory ideation (20%), delusions (16%) and hallucinations (17%) to be common. Fifty per cent of patients with multi-infarct dementia may have delusions at some time[18] and the clinical course of diffuse Lewy body disease is particularly characterized by paranoid ideation and hallucinations[19].

The manifestations of progressive, global, cognitive impairment will usually be present, although dementia may present with paranoid symptoms that can be indistinguishable from function illness[20]. Paranoid ideas are frequently related to cognitive deficits, especially memory, leading to accusations of theft[17] or problems arising from perceptual difficulties and misidentification[8]. Like delirium, these fluctuate and may be ferociously denied, or forgotten, at interview, although the theme and content remain fairly consistent.

Depression

If depression is of delusional proportions, biological and characteristic depressive symptoms are usually marked. Delusions and hallucinations, occurring in all sensory modalities, are normally mood-congruent but incongruent symptoms occur and may be difficult to distinguish from those of primary paranoid disorders.

Kay et al.[21] suggested six historical variables that help distinguish affective and paranoid psychoses: life events and family history of affective illness favoured an affective diagnosis, while low social class, few surviving children and social deafness favoured paranoid disorder. Premorbid personality proved the best discriminator, with paranoid patients being solitary, shy, touchy, suspicious and emotionally aloof, and patients with affective disorders reporting subjective ratings of high premorbid anxiety.

Mania

Traditional teaching suggested that mania in old age was both rare and atypical in presentation. Broadhead and Jacoby's[22] prospective study found that young and older-onset patients were clinically very similar. The onset of mania in old age is more common than once thought[23] and the majority of patients will have a history of affective disorder, some 50% having had three or more depressive episodes, with a latency of 15–17 years from first depression to mania[22–25].

Organic Delusional/Hallucinatory Disorder

Paranoid hallucinatory disorders have been associated with a variety of organic conditions[8,11,26–29] and pharmacological agents[5,8,11,30]. The symptoms may be typical of functional disorders[26,31] and the diagnosis depends on establishing a clear aetiological link and temporal relationships between a physical disorder or drug and mental disturbance. As Kay[32] put it, "Had the organic diagnosis not been reached independently of the psychiatric symptomatology, most of the cases would have been regarded as, indubitably, schizophrenic".

The more common causes encountered in clinical practice include hypothyroidism, intra- and extracerebral tumours, epilepsy and cerebrovascular disease, and pharmacological agents such as psychostimulants, anti-parkinsonian and dopaminergic drugs and steroids. Alcohol intoxication and withdrawal from alcohol, benzodiazepines and barbiturates may all cause paranoid states, and withdrawal syndromes should be particularly considered when psychosis develops shortly after a hospital admission.

Paranoid Personality Disorder

This is necessarily a life-long problem which must be demonstrable from early adulthood. It is characterized by a sensitive and defensive attitude that causes people to feel they are victims of life and interpret events in a self-referential way[14]. The effects of ageing and the vicissitudes of later life may accentuate these traits and, if dementia or functional illness supervene, will colour the symptomatology.

Late-onset Schizophrenia

Kay and Roth's[2] description of the characteristic features of this condition has never been surpassed. Schizoid and paranoid premorbid personality, reduced likelihood of marriage and fertility, living alone with few surviving relatives, and deafness contributing to social isolation, and a limited but significant hereditary predisposition for schizophrenia with female preponderance, all characterize this disorder. The whole range of psychopathology typical of schizophrenia may be evident, although personality is more often preserved and negative features less prevalent[2,3,20,33,34]. Roth and Kay[35] provide a thoughtful discussion of the apparent similarities and differences of the associated features of late- and early-onset schizophrenia.

Delusional Disorders

These are conditions characterized by a persistent, circumscribed delusional theme and if hallucinations occur they are not prominent. They are defined by their delusional content, which may be erotic, jealous, hypochondriacal, persecutory or grandiose. These conditions have not been the subject of systematic study in old age, when they are thought to be relatively rare[8]. Onset is usually in middle age but as patients normally function well outside their particular delusion and symptoms frequently persist they may present in old age. Unlike late-onset schizophrenia, delusional disorder seems not to be associated with premorbid paranoid personality or deafness[36], although querulent paranoia has been related to deviant personality structure[65]. Familially they appear unrelated to affective or schizophrenic illnesses[37,38]. Howard et al.[39] found dilatation of lateral and third ventricle volumes by magnetic resonance imaging (MRI) to be more a feature of delusional disorder than schizophrenia in old age, as defined by ICD-10 criteria.

A small retrospective study comparing paraphrenia (schizophrenia of late onset) with paranoia (delusional disorder of late onset) found cerebral infarction on CT brain scan to be a feature of paranoia rather than paraphrenia. Furthermore, social isolation and being unmarried was not a feature of paranoiacs, with cerebral infarction suggesting separate groups defined by organic or social associations. Response to antipsychotic drugs was worse for paranoia[40].

ASSESSMENT

Interview

Interviewing paranoid elderly people may be complicated by deafness, speech problems or visual handicap, so time and patience are essential. An informant history is mandatory and often several sources may be required.

It is crucial to establish the interview situation, explain its purpose, allay anxieties and put patients at their ease. The patients should decide whether they prefer to be seen in private or with a confidant(e) as another's presence may equally inhibit or encourage the disclosure of sensitive material. For similar reasons an informant may wish to speak privately though discussions should never appear clandestine.

Deafness and communication problems should be openly acknowledged, hearing aids worn and working, and extraneous noise eliminated, otherwise false impressions of cognitive state may be formed[41]. If a patient is seen in a hospital setting, insist on a separate, quiet interview room, otherwise conversation will be inhibited and information lost. Posture and attitude convey sincerity, concern and how seriously problems are considered. The patient needs to form a trusting relationship, and a respectful, honest but never patronizing approach is normally accepted. A sympathetic hand can reassure and encourage an anxious or suspicious patient.

The importance of establishing a positive therapeutic relationship at this early stage cannot be overstated, as it can have far-reaching effects, not only for the openness of discussion but also for future compliance and prognosis[12].

History

The nature of psychotic symptoms, their form, content and course must be detailed. Late-onset schizophrenia may develop insidiously over months or a year or more[2,3], delusional depression over a few months, delirium over days and dementia over 1–2 years. The intensity of paranoid ideas and their effect on behaviour assist diagnosis and the evaluation of risk. Associated symptoms, particularly affective and cognitive, should then be elicited.

Current and past medical problems and their temporal relationship to the onset of paranoid symptoms must be clearly established, including visual or auditory failure. Aetiologically significant hearing loss in late-onset schizophrenia is typically of long duration, severe and due to bilateral middle ear disease, often originating in early life[42–45]. Details of prescribed and non-prescribed drugs, dosages and recent alterations are essential.

Previous episodes of mental disorder should be confirmed from medical records, when past diagnoses and response to treatment may quickly clarify a diagnostic dilemma. Careful enquiry might uncover past episodes of untreated, self-limiting illness[3,31] and changes in behaviour may date the onset of current problems.

Premorbid personality and behaviour are important because departures from these in old age usually signify the onset of a morbid process. Forty to fifty per cent of late-onset schizophrenics have schizoid or paranoid premorbid traits[2,3] and the diagnosis of personality disorder depends on establishing a life-long attitude, Brenes Jette and Winnett[46] emphasized the interaction of narcissistic personality traits and the psychosocial consequences of ageing in their psychodynamic formulation of late-onset paranoid disorder.

The genetic loading of schizophrenia in old age is less marked than with younger patients but a positive family history is often found[2,7,20,47]. Odd behaviour or suicide among family members may be discovered when formal psychiatric treatment is absent.

Current social circumstances and recent change are of relevance to aetiology and management. The schizophrenias of late life are particularly associated with social isolation, but rarely with precipitating life events[2,3]. Paranoid patients frequently have poor socioeconomic status and multiple difficulties[13] and social support has prognostic implications[12]. Enquiring about alcohol and drug abuse must not be avoided for fear of offending a respectable elderly person. The elderly are not without vice and may be less inclined to confess it.

Mental State Examination

The detailed psychopathology of these conditions is described elsewhere and only points relevant to the process of mental state examination will be mentioned here.

It is important to ensure that the patient understands the terminology used to elicit abnormal experiences and that a common language is being used. Eliciting paranoid and psychotic symptoms can be difficult, but with tact and careful choice of words most patients will participate in an exchange of ideas about their experiences. This must be an unthreatening process for the patient and it is unwise to challenge or trivialize complaints at an early stage. A neutral position is advisable until a firm relationship is established, when complaints may be gradually reframed so that they can be viewed by the patient as problems that can be relieved, rather than immovable realities that are not amenable to therapeutic intervention. Suggesting that "it's all imagination" will be considered insulting and the patient's confidence will be lost.

Insight is rarely retained and patients may not volunteer experiences if they interpret questions as purely an enquiry into the state of their health. Patients have limited ability to accept the presence of illness or recognize psychiatric experiences as pathological[48]. Needless to say, the mental state examination must be thorough.

Physical Examination

A complete physical examination should be performed routinely, with particular emphasis on neurological status and sensory function. The association between sensory impairment and late-onset schizophrenia[44,49] makes attention to this area important and remediable conditions may be found. Visual impairment, particularly due to cataracts, is often found in association with delusions and deafness[43,50] and visual hallucinations may be as much to do with ocular pathology as psychiatric diagnosis[51]. A particular form of acute, elaborate visual hallucinosis, the Charles–Bonnet syndrome, is usually related to eye disease or cerebral organic disorder[52]. Simple clinical interview and self-reporting seriously underestimate sensory impairment and more detailed ophthalmic and audiometric examination may be necessary[53–55]. A simple battery of laboratory investigations is required for all patients, including haematology, biochemistry, thyroid function, urinalysis and chest radiography.

Advanced neuroradiological techniques promise much for the future but have limited clinical application at the present time. Some authors recommend the routine use of computed tomography (CT) and MRI. These procedures frequently reveal structural cerebral abnormalities, including increased ventricular size and periventricular and deep white matter hyperintensities[56,57], although their clinical significance is uncertain[58,59] and they appear to bear little relationship to clinical state or outcome[60,61]. These findings have no diagnostic value and the role of neuroimaging in clinical practice, at present, is to exclude specific intracranial pathology, particularly space-occupying lesions suggested by clinical examination. Similarly, non-specific electrophysiological abnormalities are common[5] and the EEG will only be of value in a minority of cases.

Psychometric testing may provide a useful baseline measure that can be serially repeated when the possibility of dementia arises[62]. Psychometric testing certainly reveals cognitive deficits in late-onset schizophrenic patients, particularly affecting frontal lobe and memory function[56]. These rarely signify dementia[60] and are more like the deficits found with early-onset schizophrenia than Alzheimer's disease[56]. They do not correlate with severity of psychosis or other clinical parameters[60,62].

CONCLUSION

Most patients with late-onset schizophrenia or primary delusional disorders will be adequately and preferably managed from home[12,63]. The need to admit to hospital seems to be declining[64] and may be determined as much by social and physical factors or treatment compliance as degree of psychopathology. For the patient requiring more than outpatient treatment, a day hospital can provide the necessary facilities for more intensive assessment of mental state, physical health and functional level.

The multifactorial contributions from ageing, physical disability, sensory impairment and social factors demand a multi-professional approach and all relevant disciplines must be available and involved[8]. The evaluation of these conditions requires clinical skill, rigorous attention to detail and an holistic approach. The accuracy of diagnosis and success of management will depend on the quality of initial assessment and if diagnostic doubts exist, treatment should be postponed until the situation becomes clear. Occasionally a diagnostic trial of treatment will be justified.

The paranoid disorders of old age are stimulating, complex, challenging clinical problems that encompass the breadth of psychiatry, medicine and social sciences and their assessment and management will continue to appeal to the enquiring clinical mind.

REFERENCES

1. Roth M. The natural history of mental disorder in old age. *J Ment Sci* 1955; **101**: 281–301.
2. Kay DWK, Roth M. Environmental and hereditary factors in the schizophrenias of old age (late paraphrenia) and their bearing on the general problems of causation in schizophrenia. *J Ment Sci* 1961; **107**: 649–86.
3. Herbert ME, Jacobson S. Late paraphrenia. *Br J Psychiat* 1967; **113**: 461–9.
4. Tanna VL. Paranoid states: a selected review. *Comp Psychiat* 1974; **15**: 452–70.
5. Bridge TP, Wyatt RJ. Paraphrenia: paranoid states of late life. I European research. *J Am Geriat Soc* 1980; **5**: 193–200.
6. Grahame PS. Late paraphrenia. *Br J Hosp Med* 1985; **27**: 522–8.
7. Volavka J. Late-onset schizophrenia. *Comp Psychiat* 1983; **26**: 148–56.
8. Stoudemire A, Riether AM. Evaluation and treatment of paranoid syndromes in the elderly: a review. *Gen Hosp Psychiat* 1987; **9**: 267–74.
9. Pearlson G, Rabins P. The late onset psychoses: possible risk factors. *Psychiat Clin N Am* 1988; **11**: 15–32.
10. Harris MJ, Jeste DV. Late-onset schizophrenia: an overview. *Schizophren Bull* 1988; **14**: 39–55.
11. Manschreck TC, Petri M. The paranoid syndrome. *Lancet* 1978; **ii**: 251–3.
12. Post F. *Persistent Persecutory States of the Elderly*. Oxford: Pergamon, 1966.
13. Christenson R, Blazer D. Epidemiology of persecutory ideation in an elderly population in the community. *Am J Psychiat* 1984; **141**: 1088–91.
14. Leuchter AF, Spar JE. The late onset psychoses: clinical and diagnostic features. *J Nerv Ment Dis* 1985; **173**: 488–94.
15. Lipowski ZJ. Delirium in the elderly patient. *N Engl J Med* 1989; **320**: 578–82.
16. Ballinger BR, Reid AH, Heather BB. *Br J Psychiat* 1982; **140**: 257–62.
17. Burns A, Jacoby R, Levy R. Psychiatric phenomena in Alzheimer's disease. I. Disorders of thought content. II. Disorders of perception. *Br J Psychiat* 1990; **157**: 72–81.
18. Cummings JL, Miller B, Hill MA, Neshkes R. Neuropsychiatric aspects of multi-infarct dementia and dementia of the Alzheimer type. *Arch Neurol* 1987; **44**: 389–93.
19. McKeith IG, Perry RH, Fairbairn AF et al. Operational criteria for senile dementia of Lewy Body type [SDLT]. *Psychol Med* 1992; **22**: 911–22.
20. Holden NL. Late paraphrenia or the paraphrenias? A descriptive study with a 10 year follow-up. *Br J Psychiat* 1987; **150**: 635–9.
21. Kay DWK, Cooper AF, Garside RF, Roth M. The differentiation of paranoid from affective psychoses by patients' premorbid characteristics. *Br J Psychiat* 1976; **129**: 207–15.
22. Broadhead J, Jacoby R. Mania in old age: a first prospective study. *Int J Geriat Psychiat* 1990; **5**: 215–22.
23. Eagles JM, Whalley LJ. Ageing and affective disorders: the age at first onset of affective disorders in Scotland, 1969–1978. *Br J Psychiat* 1985; **147**: 180–7.
24. Shulman K, Post F. Bipolar affective disorder in old age. *Br J Psychiat* 1980; **136**: 26–32.
25. Stone K. Mania in the elderly. *Br J Psychiat* 1989; **155**: 220–4.
26. Davison K, Bagley CR. Schizophrenia-like psychoses associated with organic disorders of the central nervous system: a review of the literature. In Herrington RN, ed., *Current Problems in Neuropsychiatry*. British Journal of Psychiatry Special Publication No. 4. Ashford: Headley Brothers, 1969; 113–84.
27. Miller BL, Benson DF, Cummings JL, Neshkes R. Late life paraphrenia: an organic delusional syndrome. *J Clin Psychiat* 1986; **47**: 204–7.
28. Dupon RM, Munro Cullum C, Jeste DV. Post-stroke depression and psychosis. *Psychiat Clin N Am* 1988; **11**: 133–49.
29. Galasko D, Kwo-On-Yuen PF, Thal L. Intracranial mass lesions associated with late onset psychosis and depression. *Psychiat Clin N Am* 1988; **11**: 151–66.
30. Wood KA, Harris MJ, Morreale A, Rizos AL. Drug induced psychosis and depression in the elderly. *Psychiat Clin N Am* 1988; **11**: 167–93.
31. Kay DWK. Schizophrenia and schizophrenia-like states in the elderly. *Br J Hosp Med* 1972; **7**: 369–76.
32. Kay DWK. Late paraphrenia and its bearing on the aetiology of schizophrenia. *Acta Psychiat Scand* 1963; **39**: 156–69.
33. Howard R, Castle D, Wessely S, Murray R. A comparative study of 470 cases of early-onset and late-onset schizophrenia. *Br J Psychiat* 1993; **163**: 352–7.
34. Castle DJ, Wessely S, Howard R, Murray R. Schizophrenia with onset at the extremes of adult life. *Int J Geriat Psychiat* 1997; **12**: 712–17.
35. Roth M, Day DWK. Late paraphrenia: a variant of schizophrenia manifest in late life or an organic clinical syndrome? A review of recent evidence. *Int J Geriat Psychiat* 1998; **13**: 775–84.
36. Watt JAG. Hearing and premorbid personality in paranoid states. *Am J Psychiat* 1985; **142**: 1453–5.
37. Winokur G. Delusional disorder (paranoia). *Comp Psychiat* 1977; **18**: 511–21.
38. Watt JAG. The relationship of paranoid states to schizophrenia. *Am J Psychiat* 1985; **142**: 1456–8.
39. Howard RJ, Almeida O, Levy R et al. Quantitative magnetic resonance imaging volumetry distinguishes delusional disorder from late-onset schizophrenia. *Br J Psychiat* 1994; **165**: 474–80.
40. Flint AJ, Rifat SL, Eastwood MR. Late-onset paranoia: distinct from paraphrenia? *Int J Geriat Psychiat* 1991; **6**: 103–9.
41. Ohta RJ, Carlin MR, Harmon BM. Auditory activity and performance on the Mental State Questionnaire in the elderly. *J Am Geriat Soc* 1981; **29**: 376–8.
42. Cooper AF, Curry AR, Kay DWK et al. Hearing loss in paranoid and affective psychoses of the elderly. *Lancet* 1974; **ii**: 851–61.
43. Cooper AF, Curry AR. The pathology of deafness in the paranoid and affective psychoses of later life. *J Psychosomat Res* 1976; **20**: 97–105.
44. Cooper AF. Deafness and psychiatric illness. *Br J Psychiat* 1976; **129**: 216–26.
45. Cooper AF, Garside RF, Kay DWK. A comparison of deaf and non-deaf patients with paranoid and affective psychoses. *Br J Psychiat* 1976; **129**: 532–8.
46. Brenes Jette CC, Winnett RL. Late-onset paranoid disorder. *Am J Orthopsychiat* 1987; **57**: 485–94.
47. Howard RJR, Graham C, Sham P et al. A case controlled family study of late-onset non-affective psychosis [late paraphrenia]. *Br J Psychiat* 1997; **170**: 511–14.

48. Almeida OP, Levy R, Howard RJ, David AS. Insight and paranoid disorders in late life (late paraphrenia). *Int J Geriat Psychiat* 1996; **11**: 653–8.

49. Corbin SL, Eastwood MR. Sensory deficits and mental disorders of old age: causal or coincidental associations? *Psychol Med* 1986; **16**: 251–6.

50. Cooper AF, Porter R. Visual acuity and ocular pathology in the paranoid and affective psychoses of later life. *J Psychosom Res* 1976; **20**: 107–14.

51. Berrios GE, Brook P. Visual hallucination and sensory delusions in the elderly. *Br J Psychiat* 1984; **144**: 662–4.

52. Damas-Mora J, Skelton-Robinson M, Jenner FA. The Charles Bonnet syndrome in perspective. *Psychol Med* 1982; **12**: 251–61.

53. Gilholme-Herbst K, Humphrey C. Hearing impairment and mental state in the elderly living at home. *Br Med J* 1980; **281**: 903–5.

54. Corbin S, Reed M, Nobbs H *et al.* Hearing assessment in homes for the aged: a comparison of audiometric and self reporting methods. *J Am Geriat Soc* 1984; **32**: 396–400.

55. Eastwood R, Corbin-Rifat S. Hearing impairment, mental disorders and the elderly. *Stress Med* 1987; **3**: 171–3.

56. Miller BL, Lesser IM, Boone KB *et al.* Brain lesions and cognitive function in late-life psychosis. *Br J Psychiat* 1991; **158**: 76–82.

57. Howard R, Cox T, Almeida O *et al.* White matter abnormalities in the brains of patients with late paraphrenia and the normal community living elderly. *Biol Psychiat* 1995; **38**: 86–91.

58. Naguib M, Levy R. Late paraphrenia: neuropsychological impairment and structural brain abnormalities on computed tomography. *Int J Geriat Psychiat* 1987; **2**: 83–90.

59. Rabins P, Pearlson G, Jayaram G *et al.* Increased ventricle to brain ratio in late-onset schizophrenia. *Am J Psychiat* 1987; **144**: 1216–18.

60. Hymas N, Naguib M, Levy R. Late paraphrenia—a follow-up study. *Int J Geriat Psychiat* 1989; **4**: 23–9.

61. Burns A, Carrick J, Ames D *et al.* The cerebral cortical appearance in late paraphrenia. *Int J Geriat Psychiat* 1989; **4**: 31–4.

62. Munro-Cullum C, Heaton RK, Nemiroff B. Neuropsychology of late life psychoses. *Psychiat Clin N Am* 1988; **11**: 47–59.

63. Berger KS, Zarit SH. Late life paranoid states: assessment and treatment. *Am J Orthopsychiat* 1978; **48**: 528–37.

64. Christie AB, Wood ERM. Further change in the pattern of mental illness in the elderly. *Br J Psychiat* 1990; **157**: 228–31.

65. Astrup C. Querulent paranoia: a follow-up. *Neuropsychobiology* 1984; **11**: 149–54.

91

Aetiology, Genetics and Risk Factors

David J. Castle[1] and Robin M. Murray[2]

[1]*Mental Health Research Institute and University of Melbourne, Melbourne, Australia and* [2]*Institute of Psychiatry, London, UK*

There is considerable controversy about the classification of the late-onset non-affective psychoses, and their relationship to "typical" early-onset schizophrenia. Kraepelin delineated "paraphrenia", a late-onset delusional state with prominent hallucinations, as distinct from dementia praecox. Mayer performed a follow-up study of a number of patients diagnosed by Kraepelin as having paraphrenia, and found that a high proportion had a longitudinal course of illness similar to that of dementia praecox patients. This study challenged the distinction between paraphrenia and dementia praecox and, once the Bleulerian label "schizophrenia" had been widely adopted, "paraphrenia" became a neglected term.

The term was resurrected by Roth[1] as "late paraphrenia", although he used it to describe a rather different group of patients, namely those manifesting a paranoid delusional state with prominent hallucinations for the first time in very late life. Confusingly, ICD-9 retained Roth's category, relabelled it "paraphrenia", and subsumed it under "paranoid states"; this has been dropped altogether from ICD-10. Furthermore, definitions of "late onset" range from over the age of 40 (after Feighner *et al.*[2]) to over 60 (after Roth[1]). The 3rd edition of the American Psychiatric Association's *Diagnostic and Statistical Manual* (DSM-III) set an age cut-off of 45 years for schizophrenia, so that later-onset paranoid states were labelled "atypical psychosis" or "paranoid (delusional) disorder". The revised editions of the manual (DSM-III-R and DSM-IV) removed this age stipulation, and it is now widely believed that schizophrenia can manifest for the first time at any age.

These changing conceptions make comparison across studies difficult. In this chapter, we refer to studies where a 40 year or later cut-off is used. We employ the term "late paraphrenia" for those patients with an illness akin to Roth's description, with first manifestation usually after the age of 60. Delusional (paranoid) disorder is not specifically addressed here.

GENETICS

It is generally accepted that schizophrenia tends to run in families. Gottesman and Shields[3], pooling data from a number of family studies, calculated the average morbid risk for schizophrenia (broadly defined) in first-degree relatives of schizophrenia probands to be around 10%, compared with about 1% in the general population. Rates are generally lower when operational criteria such as those of DSM-III are applied, but the higher relative risk in first-degree relatives compared with the general population remains. Twin studies consistently report higher concordance rates for schizophrenia in monozygotic (MZ) compared with

dizygotic (DZ) twin pairs, suggesting that, in part at least, this familial aggregation is due to genetic factors. This conclusion is supported by adoption studies, which show that biological risk for schizophrenia is carried with the proband, irrespective of family environment (i.e. "adopted-away" offspring).

Few studies have specifically assessed familial aggregation in late-onset schizophrenia (see Table 91.1) and these all have methodological shortcomings. Authors have often failed to give a clear definition of illness in either probands or relatives; standardized diagnostic instruments have not been employed; and assessments have not been blind to proband diagnosis. Furthermore, proband numbers are mostly small, and it is often unclear exactly how many family members were assessed, and whether adjustments were made for those who were not. Also, because of the late onset of illness, many family members (siblings, parents) would have died and thus have been unavailable for interview; it is also difficult to know whether relatives had passed through the period of risk for illness-onset. Controls have rarely been employed, reliance being placed on results from independent studies of earlier-onset patients, which have again used different methodologies and diagnostic criteria.

Thus, the conclusions that can be drawn are limited. Overall, studies of "late paraphrenia" patients show rates of schizophrenia in siblings that are intermediate between those for siblings of early-onset probands and the general population. The discrepancy in rates quoted for parents is probably due to problems in assessing the parental generation. Those studies with an earlier age cut-off report higher risks for schizophrenia in relatives approaching those in the relatives of early-onset probands. However, these studies have used broad, non-specific definitions of schizophrenia, and have thus probably overestimated rates. The very high rate in the study of Huber and colleagues (see Table 91.1) is probably due to the misdiagnosis of patients with affective disorders, as they report no relatives with affective illness. The more recent study of Howard *et al.*[4], who employed a controlled family interview methodology, is more sound. These researchers assessed lifetime risk of schizophrenia and other psychiatric disorders in 269 relatives of 47 late paraphrenia patients, and compared the rates with those in 272 relatives of 42 elderly general population controls. The results, shown in Table 91.1, reveal no difference in the risk between the two groups of relatives with respect to schizophrenia, but do show the relatives of the schizophrenia probands to have a significantly elevated risk of depression (16.3% vs. 4.4% in controls).

Kendler *et al.*[5] in a review of family and twin studies, found no strong consistent relationship between age at onset of schizophrenia and risk for the illness in relatives. However, they did not specifically investigate late-onset schizophrenia patients, and the

Table 91.1 Family studies in late-onset schizophrenia

Reference No.	No.	Age	Definition of illness	Risk of schizophrenia	Risk of affective disorder
53[a]	65	>40	Schneiderian first rank	Siblings: 9.8% Parents: 4.4% (9 of 24 late-onset)	Not stated
25	57	>60	"Late paraphrenia"	Siblings: 2.5% Parents: 0 Children: 7.3% Nephews/nieces: 3.1%	Not stated
14	93	>60	"Late paraphrenia"	5 relatives (2 late-onset)	16 relatives
43	45	>65	Systematized delusions with or without hallucinations	Siblings: 2.3% Fathers: 2.2% Mothers: 4.4%	Not stated
44[a]	110	>40	Schneiderian first rank	19.4%	0%
54[a]	62 cases: 58 early-onset controls	>50	Late- vs. early-onset schizophrenia (definition of illness not stated)	10.8% vs. 17.7% in early-onset patients	2.0% vs. 6.6% in early-onset patients
48	35 cases; 35 affective disorder controls	>44	"Persistent delusions" with no affective features	5 relatives vs. 3 relatives of controls	0 relatives vs. 12 relatives of controls
4	47 cases; 42 controls	>60	"Late paraphrenia" (cases) vs. non-psychiatric controls	Narrow age range (15–50 years): 1.3% in cases and controls; wide age range (15–90 years): 2.3% cases, 2.2% controls	21 relatives of cases vs. 6 relatives of controls ($p = 0.003$)

[a]Quoted by Volavka[55] (1985).
From ref. 56, with permission.

data reviewed here suggest that there may indeed be a gradient of familial risk, dependent upon age of onset of the proband. Such a notion is compatible with the idea that late-onset patients have a smaller genetic loading than those with early onset and thus require more "environmental events" to manifest the illness. This conception presumes a multifactorial "vulnerability/stress" or "continuum of liability" model of schizophrenia that is useful in as far as it produces testable hypotheses. For example, Holden[6], in a study of 47 cases of paranoid psychosis with onset after the age of 60, found that deafness, which is considered a risk factor for late-onset schizophrenia (see below), was inversely related to family history of psychiatric illness.

An equally parsimonious explanation for the intermediate family risk in late-onset probands is that it is due to the greater proportion of such patients who have a less genetic subtype of illness. For example, paranoid ideation is common in late-onset schizophrenia patients, and Tsuang and Winokur[7] and Tsuang et al.[8] have reported that patients with the paranoid subtype of schizophrenia have later onset and fewer affected relatives than do the more disorganized "hebephrenia" patients. Furthermore, at least some patients labelled "late-onset schizophrenics" have an organic illness (see below), and such patients would be expected to have a low family risk for schizophrenia. Also, the family loading for affective disorder found in some studies (see above) suggests that at least some patients with late-onset schizophrenia have aetiological links with affective disorder.

FEMALE GENDER

All studies of late-onset schizophrenia that have included both sexes have attested to an excess of women. Table 91.2 shows data from a representative sample of such studies, which confirm that this female excess is robust to more- or less-restrictive definitions of illness. This excess cannot be explained on the basis of the relative longevity of women.

What is also evident from the data in Table 91.2, is that the older the sample, the greater the female excess. Few studies have assessed gender differences in non-affective psychoses in an epidemiologically-based sample of patients, ascertained across all ages at onset. The Camberwell Register First Episode Study[9]

afforded an opportunity to do this. The sample consisted of 91% of all patients ($n = 477$) with a non-affective psychotic disorder, from a defined catchment area, who made their first contact with the psychiatric services over the period 1965–1984. Patients were rediagnosed according to a range of operational definitions for psychotic disorders, using the OPCRIT diagnostic system. Age-at-onset incidence curves were established for both sexes, using the base population figures as the denominator. Not only was the mean age at onset later for females, but the distributions of onset age for the two sexes were not isomorphic; males showed a dramatic early peak and a lesser mid-life peak, whilst females showed three peaks of onset, one in very late life. When subjected to an admixture analysis, the distributions for males showed two age distributions, with modal ages at onset of 21 and 39 years, whilst for females there were three distributions, with modal onsets at 22, 37 and 62 years[10].

A possible explanation for the female excess in late-onset schizophrenia is that female schizophrenia patients are somehow "protected" from the manifestations of disease at earlier ages. For example, Seeman[11] has suggested that the antidopaminergic action of oestrogen has such a protective function, with the illness manifesting perimenopausally when oestrogen levels fall. This theory gains support from animal and clinical studies that show that oestrogen has antidopaminergic properties. However, as described above, the incidence curves for schizophrenia in women do not mirror the menopausal fall in oestrogen levels, and the disease can manifest for the first time at very advanced ages.

A further consideration in attempting to explain the female excess amongst late-onset schizophrenia patients is the fact that the brains of males and females age differently. Of particular interest is the differential rate of loss of dopamine D2 receptors, with loss being more precipitous in men than in women. Thus, young males have a relative excess of D2 receptors compared with females, but in older females this gender difference is reversed[12]. This differential loss of D2 receptors between the sexes could conceivably play a part in the vulnerability of females to the manifestation of schizophrenia in late life and might also account, in part at least, for the particular female vulnerability to the development of tardive dyskinesia on exposure to neuroleptic medication in late life.

Table 91.2 Selected series of late-onset schizophrenia patients reporting gender ratio

Reference No.	No. of cases	Ascertainment method	Diagnosis	Age (years)	Ratio female:male
25	57	Hospital admissions	Late paraphrenia[a]	>60	5.3:1
43	47	Hospital admissions	Systematized delusion $\pm$ hallucinations; not demented	>65	22.5:1
44	644	Hospital admissions	Late-onset schizophrenia; not organic	>40	1.8:1
45	6064	First admissions	ICD-8 schizophrenia	>40	1.6:1
46	320	Hospital admissions	Late paraphrenia[a]	>65	6:1
47	25	Consecutive referrals	Late paraphrenia[a]	>60	3.2:1
48	35	Hospital admissions	Persistent delusional state; absence of mood or cognitive disorder	Onset >40	10.7:1
49	106	First admissions	ICD-8 schizophrenia, paranoid state, reactive psychosis, other psychoses	>60	2.2:1
6	37	Case register	Late paraphrenia[a] (13 cases considered "organic" at follow-up)	>60	7:1–3:1[b]
50	477	Case register	ICD-9 schizophrenia and related disorders, paraphrenia, atypical psychoses	>60	4.4:1
51	47	Referrals from a number of psychiatric settings	Late paraphrenia[a]	>65	9:1

[a]Akin to Roth's[1] criteria.
[b]Dependent on whether "organic" cases included.
From ref. 52, with permission.

PREMORBID CHARACTERISTICS

It has been consistently reported that a higher proportion of patients with late-onset paranoid psychoses have abnormal premorbid personality traits, most commonly described as "suspicious", "hostile" and "reclusive". Some workers have considered that the occurrence of paranoid psychosis in individuals with such personality traits is an "understandable transition", while Retterstol[13] has suggested that psychotic breakdown is a reaction to stress in a "hypersensitive" personality. Post[14] proposed that the paranoid/schizoid personality traits reflect a long-standing latent schizophrenic disorder that manifests itself only when additional factors come into effect. Such factors might include social deprivation, sensory deprivation (deafness and possibly visual loss, as discussed below), frank cerebral pathology, or even ordinary ageing processes in the brain. Moreover, such personality traits could be expected to result in social isolation and reclusiveness, which in turn would exacerbate the paranoid imaginings characteristic of the illness.

In contrast to their early-onset counterparts, late-onset schizophrenia patients are generally neither educationally nor occupationally compromised. This again suggests that they may have a form of disease that is relatively distinct from the severe early-onset "dementia praecox" type.

SOCIAL ISOLATION

Ageing often results in increasing social isolation. It appears, however, that patients with late-onset schizophrenia have a greater likelihood of being socially isolated than age-matched normals or affective disorder patients. Low rates of marriage, few offspring and paranoid premorbid personality traits could all be expected to contribute to such isolation. Paranoid ideation in the disease itself is often directed at neighbours, resulting in further reclusiveness. Thus, social isolation in late-life psychosis might well be a consequence rather than a cause of the illness.

SENSORY DEFICITS

A number of general population studies have found an association between paranoid ideation and sensory impairment in the elderly. This perhaps understandable association has also been investigated as potentially causal in late-onset paranoid illnesses. For example, Post[14] reported that 25% of 72 elderly paranoid psychotic patients had hearing loss, compared with 11% of an affective disorder group; the mode of audiometric assessment was not stated. Cooper et al.[15] found that 25 (46%) of a group of 65 elderly paranoid patients were "socially deaf", compared with 12 (21%) of 67 patients with affective illness. Audiometry and otological examination of an enlarged sample (27 paranoid and 18 affective deaf subjects) revealed that the paranoid group were more likely to have long-standing conductive hearing loss, as opposed to later-onset sensorineural loss in the affective group. Visual impairment, mostly due to cataracts, was found in 30 (56%) of 54 of the paranoid group, and 21 (37%) of 57 of the affective group.

From such data, Kay et al.[16] and Cooper[17] concluded that in the elderly, long-standing conductive deafness is an independent risk factor for paranoid, as opposed to affective, psychosis. This probably does not apply in earlier-onset schizophrenia patients, neither are persons with profound (prelingual) deafness predisposed to schizophrenia. The association with visual impairment is less robust, possibly because determination of functional visual impairment is difficult.

More recently, however, Prager and Jeste[18] failed to confirm an excess of constitutional ("uncorrected") visual and hearing impairment in late-onset schizophrenia patients; they did, however, find that such patients were more likely than controls to have sensory deficits that were not adequately "corrected", e.g. by spectacles or hearing aids. Thus, these data are complex and interpretation of causality problematic. Furthermore, there is no consistent association between particular modalities of sensory loss and any specific psychotic symptom. For example, it is not the case that hearing impairment is necessarily associated with auditory hallucinosis. Likewise, the association between visual impairment and visual hallucinations, so dramatically represented in the Charles–Bonnet syndrome[19], does not appear to be found in late-life schizophrenia.

The social and psychological consequences of sensory impairments (social withdrawal and ostracization; misinterpretation of social cues) may result in suspiciousness and hostility, leading to paranoid ideation. Abnormal percepts associated with reduced sensory input might result in hallucinations, as in the Charles–Bonnet syndrome, although secondary delusional elaboration is considered unusual in such settings[19]. Moreover, Watt[20], in a study of 35 patients, found no association between hearing loss and paranoid psychosis manifesting in middle life. It might be that psychosis occurs only in individuals who are already prone to paranoid ideation, e.g. by virtue of mild cerebral damage. This is consonant with findings in an elderly general population sample[21], of an association between persecutory ideation, sensory impairment and cognitive dysfunction.

"ORGANIC" FACTORS

Acute paranoid ideation may result from cerebral or extracerebral organic factors, and the elderly are especially susceptible to such effects. More persistent delusional persecutory states are seen in association with a wide variety of structural brain changes and systemic toxic and metabolic disturbances. In particular, such states can occur in dementia. For example, Wragg and Jest[22], in a review of studies reporting the prevalence of psychotic phenomena in patients with Alzheimer's disease, found a rate of delusions of anything from 10% to 73% (aggregating to 30–38%, with a median of 33.5%). For hallucinations, the range was 21–49% (mean 28%). The importance of organic factors in the aetiogenesis of psychotic phenomena in the elderly is underlined by general population studies, which have consistently found the strongest predictor of paranoid ideation in the elderly to be cognitive impairment[23,24].

Kay[25] stated that a diagnosis of late-onset schizophrenia can be made only in the absence of "gross and persistent disorientation in time and place or severe failure of memory". Roth[1] claimed that his follow-up data validated the separation of such disorders from the dementias, while Kay and Roth[26] found only minimal evidence of organic cerebral damage in their late paraphrenic patients. Subsequently, Kay[25] reported survival rates for late paraphrenia patients of 0.97:1 (observed expected), compared with 0.3:1 for patients with dementia.

However, it is becoming increasingly clear that a significant number of elderly patients with "functional" paranoid states *do* have evidence of organic cerebral deterioration, not part of ordinary ageing. For example, Post[14] reported that some 15% of his patients were demented at follow-up, while Holden[6] found that 13 (35%) of 37 late paraphrenia patients had demented within 3 years of diagnosis; the only distinguishing feature on admission was a slight impairment on psychometric assessment in the "organic" group.

Neuroimaging investigations have revealed structural brain changes in a proportion of elderly patients with persistent psychosis and no obvious neurological or neuropsychological deficit. Miller and colleagues[27] reported three such patients who had CT scan evidence of cerebral infarction and one with normal pressure hydrocephalus. In a prospective CT and MRI study of 27 patients with late-life psychosis, Miller et al.[28] found silent vascular lesions in five (19%); subcortical frontal connections were most commonly involved. Similarly, Jernigan et al.[29] reported 13 patients with late-onset psychosis (10 schizophrenia, three delusional disorder) to have significantly more white-matter pathology on MRI than age-matched normal controls; and Breitner et al.[30] found significant leucoencephalopathy, especially affecting the temporoparietal and occipital regions, in eight late-onset schizophrenia patients; such lesions were minimal or absent in controls.

These findings may provide useful information about the pathogenesis of late-onset schizophrenia. However, the exact relationship of the reported lesions to the manifestation of the disease is unclear. There is little consistency in the site of the lesions, and white-matter changes have also been reported in elderly patients with severe depression[31]. Moreover, it appears that when late-onset schizophrenia patients are clinically screened fastidiously, so as to exclude any patients with potential "organic" aetiologies, they show no excess of white matter abnormalities compared to controls[32].

NON-SPECIFIC STRUCTURAL BRAIN ABNORMALITIES

Numerous neuroimaging studies have revealed an increase in ventricular:brain ratio (VBR) in younger schizophrenia patients compared with normal controls. These findings, and those suggesting temporal lobe dysplasia, appear to have a developmental origin. There are few such studies in late-onset patients. Rabins et al.[33] studied 29 schizophrenia patients with disease onset after the age of 44, and found mean VBR to be greater than for matched normal controls. Naguib and Levy[34] reported similar findings in 43 late paraphrenia patients; there was no correlation between illness duration and ventricular size, and ventricular size did not predict disease outcome at a mean of 3.7 years[35]. In an MRI study, Jeste and Harris[36] confirmed an increase in ventricular size in 20 late-onset schizophrenia patients compared with normals. Again, there was no relationship between illness duration and ventricular size, suggesting that the abnormality preceded disease onset and was not progressive. In an attempt to correlate brain imaging findings with clinical symptomatology, Howard and colleagues[37] reported that ventricular/sulcal enlargement was most dramatically evident in those late paraphrenia patients who did not manifest Schneiderian first-rank symptoms.

The relationship between neuroimaging findings in early- vs. late-onset schizophrenia patients remains a moot point. Pearlson et al.[38] compared 11 late-onset with 11 early-onset schizophrenia patients, and found no significant differences between the groups in terms of volume of a number of brain structures. Summarizing these and other such data, Pearlson[39] concluded that "early- and late-onset cases of schizophrenia share common structural ... brain abnormalities". But the significance of these findings is unclear. It seems very unlikely that they have a similar developmental origin to the equivalent abnormalities in early-onset schizophrenia. Indeed, a comparative study of very early (<25 years) and very late-onset (>60 years) schizophrenia patients found that the latter group did not seem prone to those risk factors (e.g. obstetric complications) that have been implicated in the aetiology of the neurodevelopmental form of schizophrenia[40]. Presumably, the ventricular enlargement is of little consequence in its own right, being merely an echo of some undetected cerebral lesion. Burns et al.[41] have suggested that there occurs, in late paraphrenia, an "uncoupling" of the normal association between ventricular and cortical size, but the exact mechanism whereby this results in psychotic symptoms is unclear. There is a place for further studies in this area. Specifically, further attempts should be made to find clinical correlates of enlarged ventricles, and to assess predictive value in longer-term follow-up studies. The use of more advanced neuroimaging techniques to search for more specific abnormalities will also be important.

CONCLUSIONS

Many authors consider late-onset schizophrenia to be "a form of schizophrenia, albeit attenuated and modified". One suggestion is that inherent genetic vulnerability, itself insufficient to cause psychosis, acts in concert with environmental factors (social isolation, sensory impairments, non-specific brain atrophy) to precipitate delusional breakdown. Paranoid/schizoid premorbid personality traits might be an expression of such intermediate genetic loading.

Alternatively, the late-onset schizophrenia-like states could be considered as comprising one or more subtypes, relatively distinct from early-onset schizophrenia. For example, Post[14] delineated "paranoid psychosis", "schizophreniform psychosis" and "late schizophrenia"; however, this schema has neither prognostic nor aetiological utility. A more useful approach might be subdivision based on biological parameters that have a bearing on pathogenesis, e.g. the finding of a subgroup of patients with subcortical white-matter changes has important heuristic implications.

Our own view is conditioned by our belief that early-onset schizophrenia is a neurodevelopmental disorder whose origins lie in faulty brain development in foetal or neonatal life[42]. It seems a long bow to draw to suggest that patients with the first manifestation of psychosis in late or very late life have a neurodevelopmental illness. In this context, we consider that those patients currently labelled "late-onset schizophrenia" form a heterogeneous group, some of whom have an illness relating to paranoid personality, some to sensory deprivation, some to late-onset organic change and some to affective illness. A degree of interaction will be expected between these factors. Careful clinical, neuroimaging and, ultimately, pathological examination of such patients will be required to further elucidate these issues.

REFERENCES

1. Roth M. The natural history of mental disorder in old age. *J Ment Sci* 1955; **101**: 281–301.
2. Feighner JP, Robins E, Guze SB *et al*. Diagnostic criteria for use in psychiatric research. *Arch Gen Psychiat* 1972; **26**: 57–63.
3. Gottesman II, Shields J. *Schizophrenia, the Epigenetic Puzzle*. Cambridge: Cambridge University Press, 1982.
4. Howard R, Graham C, Sham P *et al*. A controlled family study of late-onset non-affective psychosis (late paraphrenia). *Br J Psychiat* 1997; **170**: 511–14.
5. Kendler KS, Gruenberg AM, Tsuang MT. Psychiatric illness in first-degree relatives of schizophrenics and surgical control patients. A family study using DSM-III criteria. *Arch Gen Psychiat* 1985; **42**: 770–9.
6. Holden NL. Late paraphrenia or the paraphrenias? A descriptive study with 10-year follow-up. *Br J Psychiat* 1987; **150**: 635–9.
7. Tsuang MT, Winokur G. Criteria for subtyping schizophrenia. *Arch Gen Psychiat* 1974; **31**: 43–7.
8. Tsuang MT, Fowler RC, Cadoret RJ, Monnelly E. Schizophrenia amongst first-degree relatives of paranoid and non-paranoid schizophrenics. *Comp Psychiat* 1974; **15**: 295–302.
9. Castle DJ, Wessely S, VanOs J, Murray RM. *Psychosis in the Inner City: The Camberwell First Episode Study*. Hove: Psychology Press, 1998.
10. Castle DJ, Sham P, Murray RM. Differences in ages of onset in males and females with schizophrenia. *Schizophren Res* 1998; **33**: 179–83.
11. Seeman MV. Gender differences in schizophrenia. *Can J Psychiat* 1982; **27**: 107–111.
12. Wong DF, Wagner HN, Dannals RE *et al*. Effects of age on dopamine and serotonin receptors measured by positron tomography in the living human brain. *Science* 1984; **226**: 1393–6.
13. Retterstol N. Paranoid psychoses. *Br J Psychiat* 1968; **114**: 553–62.
14. Post F. *Persistent Persecutory States of the Elderly*. Oxford: Pergamon, 1966.
15. Cooper AF, Garside RF, Kay DWK. A comparison of deaf and non-deaf patients with paranoid and affective psychoses. *Br J Psychiat* 1976; **192**: 532–8.
16. Kay DWK, Cooper AF, Garside RE, Roth M. The differentiation of paranoid from affective psychoses by patients' premorbid characteristics. *Br J Psychiat* 1976; **129**: 207–15.
17. Cooper AF. Deafness and psychiatric illness. *Br J Psychiat* 1976; **129**: 216–26.
18. Prager S, Jeste DV. Sensory impairment in late life schizophrenia. *Schizophren Bull* 1993; **19**: 755–71.
19. Damas-Mora J, Skelton-Robinson M, Jenner FA. The Charles Bonnet syndrome in perspective. *Psychol Med* 1982; **12**: 153–61.
20. Watt JAG. Hearing and premorbid personality in paranoid states. *J Psychiat* 1985; **142**: 1453–5.
21. Christensen R, Blazer D. Epidemiology of persecutory ideation in an elderly population in the community. *Am J Psychiat* 1984; **141**: 1088–91.
22. Wragg RE, Jeste DV. Overview of depression and psychosis in Alzheimer's disease. *Am J Psychiat* 1989; **146**: 577–87.
23. Forsell Y, Henderson AS. Epidemiology of paranoid symptoms in an elderly population. *Br J Psychiat* 1998; **172**: 429–32.
24. Henderson AS, Korten AE, Levings C *et al*. Psychotic symptoms in the elderly: a prospective study in a population sample. *Int J Geriat Psychiat* 1998; **13**: 484–92.
25. Kayk DWK. Late paraphrenia and its bearing on the aetiology of schizophrenia. *Acta Psychiat Scand* 1963; **39**: 159–69.
26. Kay DWK, Roth M. Environmental and hereditary factors in the schizophrenias of old age ("late paraphrenia") and their bearing on the general problem of causation in schizophrenia. *J Ment Sci* 1961; **107**: 649–86.
27. Miller BL, Benson F, Cummings JL, Neshkes R. Late-life paraphrenia: an organic delusional syndrome. *J Clin Psychiat* 1986; **47**: 204–7.
28. Miller BL, Lesser IM, Boone K *et al*. Brain white-matter lesions and psychosis. *Br J Psychiat* 1989; **155**: 73–8.
29. Jernigan TL, Jeste DV, Harris JM, Salmon D. MRI abnormalities in late-onset schizophrenia. Presented at American Psychiatric Association Annual Meeting, New York, 1990.
30. Breitner JCS, Husain MM, Krishnan KRR *et al*. Leucoencephalopathy in late-onset schizophrenia. Presented at American Psychiatric Association Annual Meeting, New York, 1990.
31. Coffey CE, Figiel GS, Djang WT, Weiner RD. Subcortical hyperintensity of magnetic resonance imaging: a comparison of normal and depressed elderly subjects. *Am J Psychiat* 1990; **147**: 187–9.
32. Howard RJ, Cox T, Almeida O *et al*. White matter signal hyperintensities in the brains of patients with late paraphrenia and the normal, community-living elderly. *Biol Psychiat* 1995; **38**: 86–91.
33. Rabins P, Pearlson G, Jayaram G *et al*. Ventricle-to-brain ratio in late-onset schizophrenia. *Am J Psychiat* 1987; **144**: 1216–18.
34. Naguib M, Levy R. Late paraphrenia: neuropsychological impairment and structural brain abnormalities on computed tomography. *Int J Geriat Psychiat* 1987; **2**: 83–90.
35. Hymas N, Naguib M, Levy R. Late paraphrenia—a follow-up study. *Int J Geriat Psychiat* 1989; **4**: 23–9.
36. Jeste DV, Harris MH. Late-onset schizophrenia: subtype of schizophrenia. Presented at American Psychiatric Association Annual Meeting, New York, 1990.
37. Howard RJ, Forstl H, Almeida O *et al*. First-rank symptoms of Schneider in late paraphrenia: cortical structural correlates. *Br J Psychiat* 1992; **160**: 108–9.
38. Pearlson GD, Tune LE, Wong DF *et al*. Quantitative D2 receptor PET and structural MRI change in late-onset schizophrenia. *Schizophr Bull* 1993; **19**: 783–95.
39. Pearlson G. Brain imaging studies in late onset schizophrenia. In Howard R, Rabins PV, Castle DJ, eds, *Late-onset Schizophrenia*. Petersfield: Wrightson Biomedical, 1999; 191–204.
40. Castle DJ, Wessely S, Howard R, Murray RM. Schizophrenia with onset at the extremes of adult life. *Int J Geriat Psychiat* 1997; **12**: 712–17.
41. Burns A, Carrick J, Ames D *et al*. The cerebral cortical appearance in late paraphrenia. *Int J Geriat Psychiat* 1988; **4**: 31–4.
42. Murray RM, O'Callaghan E, Castle DJ, Lewis SW. A neurodevelopmental approach to the classification of schizophrenia. *Schizophren Bull* 1992; **18**: 319–32.
43. Herbert ME, Jacobsen S. Late paraphrenia. *Br J Psychiat* 1967; **113**: 461–9.
44. Huber G, Gross G, Schuttler R. Spatzschizophrenie. *Arch Psychiat Nervkrankheit* 1975; **221**: 53–66.
45. Bland RC. Demographic aspects of functional psychoses in Canada. *Acta Psychiat Scand* 1977; **55**: 369–80.
46. Blessed G, Wilson ID. The contemporary natural history of mental disorders in old age. *Br J Psychiat* 1982; **141**: 59–67.
47. Grahame PS. Schizophrenia in old age (late paraphrenia). *Br J Psychiat* 1984; **145**: 493–5.

48. Rabins P, Pauker S, Thomas J. Can schizophrenia occur after age 44? *Comp Psychiat* 1984; **25**: 290–3.
49. Jorgensen P, Munk-Jorgensen P. Paranoid psychoses in the elderly. *Acta Psychiat Scand* 1985; **72**: 358–63.
50. Castle DJ, Murray RM. The epidemiology of late onset schizophrenia. *Schizophren Bull* 1993; **19**: 691–700.
51. Almeida OP, Howard RJ, Levey R, David AS. Cognitive and clinical diversity in psychotic states arising in late life (late paraphrenia). *Psychol Med* 1995; **25**: 699–714.
52. Castle DJ. Gender and age at onset in schizophrenia. In Howard R, Robins P, Castle D, eds, *Late-onset Schizophrenia*. Petersfield: Wrightson Biomedical, 1999; 147–64.

53. Bleuler M. Late schizophrenic clinical pictures (in German). *Forschr Neurol Psychiat* 1943; **15**: 259–90.
54. Rokhlina ML. A comparative clinico-genetic study of attack-like schizophrenia with late and early manifestations with regard to age (in Russian). *Zhurnal Nevropatalogii i Psiikhiatrii Imeni SS Korsakova* 1975; **75**: 417–24.
55. Volavka J. Late-onset schizophrenia: a review. *Comp Psychiat* 1985; **26**: 148–56.
56. Castle DJ, Murray RM. Schizophrenia: aetiology and genetics. In Copeland JRM, Abou-Saleh MT, Blazer DG, eds, *Principles and Practice of Geriatric Psychiatry* 1st edn. Chichester: Wiley, 1994; 653–9.

Brain Imaging in Schizophrenia-like and Paranoid Disorders in Late Life

Robert Howard

Institute of Psychiatry and Maudsley Hospital, London, UK

Two general conclusions can be drawn from the results of brain-imaging investigations of patients with an onset in late life of a schizophrenia-like psychosis. First, the established neuroimaging abnormalities reported in early adult life-onset schizophrenia are also seen in later life-onset patients. Second, imaging has not implicated focal or generalized neurodegenerative abnormalities that can be implicated in psychosis aetiology, as has been the case for late-onset affective disorders.

STRUCTURAL IMAGING

Computed tomography (CT) studies of onset after 45 years[1] and 60 years[2] patients have shown lateral and third ventricle volume enlargement that does not approach the ventriculomegaly seen in Alzheimer's disease. Structural magnetic resonance imaging (MRI) has confirmed these findings, as well as indicating possible reductions in left temporal lobe and superior temporal gyrus volumes[3-5]. MRI studies of patients with so-called "late-life psychosis" have included patients with organic as well as schizophrenia-like psychoses and, not surprisingly, have reported an excess of focal structural abnormalities within deep grey and white matter structures[6]. Similar studies of patients with more rigorously defined late-onset schizophrenia, with exclusion of individuals who are cognitively impaired or have clinical evidence of focal cerebrovascular disease, have found no significant increase in such focal brain lesions compared to age-matched comparison subjects[7,8].

FUNCTIONAL IMAGING

Resting bloodflow abnormalities have been reported with single-photon emission computed tomography (SPECT) in "late-life psychosis", which may include patients with organic psychoses[9]. To date no bloodflow studies using cognitive activation paradigms have been reported in late-onset patients. A single neuroreceptor positron emission tomography study has reported increased binding values for dopamine D2 receptors[3], although age-matched control subjects were not examined for comparison. In a small group of drug-naive onset 60+ patients, we were unable to demonstrate any absolute increase in striatal D2 receptor number compared with elderly controls using SPECT[10]. Hence, the issue as to whether or not neuroreceptor levels are abnormal in late-onset cases mirrors the dispute in the early-onset schizophrenia literature.

Although brain imaging studies to date have supported the concept that early- and late-onset cases of schizophrenia share common structural and neuroreceptor brain abnormalities, more sophisticated future studies may show differences. These may help to settle which of two current hypotheses concerning the aetiopathology of late-onset schizophrenia and very late-onset schizophrenia-like psychosis are most likely to be correct. If schizophrenia arising at any point in life is essentially a unitary condition, then we cannot expect neuroimaging studies of even remarkable sophistication to reveal differences between early- and late-onset cases[11]. If (and the author favours this second hypothesis) the later-onset cases represent a subtle organic phenocopy of schizophrenia, then application of novel imaging methodologies, such as diffusion tensor imaging, which allow high resolution definition of white matter structures *in vivo* should be informative in the next few years.

REFERENCES

1. Rabins PV, Pearlson G, Jayaram G *et al*. Increased ventricle-to-brain ratio in late-onset schizophrenia. *Am J Psychiat* 1987; **144**: 1216–18.
2. Naguib M, Levy R. Late paraphrenia: neuropsychological impairment and structural brain abnormalities on computed tomography. *Int J Geriat Psychiat* 1987; **2**: 83–90.
3. Pearlson GD, Tune LE, Wong DF *et al*. Quantitative D2 receptor PET and structural MRI change in late-onset schizophrenia. *Schizophr Bull* 1993; **19**: 783–95.
4. Howard RJ, Almeida OP, Levy R *et al*. Quantitative magnetic resonance imaging volumetry distinguishes delusional disorder from late-onset schizophrenia. *Br J Psychiat* 1994; **165**: 474–80.
5. Howard RJ, Mellers J, Petty R *et al*. Magnetic resonance imaging volumetric measurements of the superior temporal gyrus,

hippocampus, parahippocampal gyrus, frontal and temporal lobes in late paraphrenia. *Psychol Med* 1995; **25**: 495–503.

6. Miller BL, Lesser IM, Boone KB *et al*. Brain lesions and cognitive function in late-life psychosis. *Br J Psychiat* 1991; **158**: 76–82.

7. Howard RJ, Cox T, Almeida O *et al*. White matter signal hyperintensities in the brains of patients with late paraphrenia and the normal community-living elderly. *Biol Psychiat* 1995; **38**: 86–91.

8. Symonds LL, Olichney JM, Jernigan TL *et al*. Lack of clinically significant gross structural abnormalities in MRIs of older patients with schizophrenia and related psychoses. *J Neuropsychiat Clin Neurosci* 1997; **9**: 251–8.

9. Lesser IM, Miller BL, Swartz JR *et al*. Brain imaging in late-life schizophrenia and related psychoses. *Schizophr Bull* 1993; **19**: 773–82.

10. Howard RJ, Cluckie A, Levy R. Striatal D2 receptor binding in late paraphrenia. *Lancet* 1993; **342**: 562.

11. Pearlson GD. Brain imaging in late onset schizophrenia. In Howard R, Rabins PV, Castle DJ, eds, *Late-onset Schizophrenia*. Petersfield: Wrightson Biomedical, 1999; 191–204.

92

Schizophrenic Disorder and Mood-incongruent Paranoid States: Epidemiology, Prevalence, Incidence and Course

Robert Howard

Institute of Psychiatry and Maudsley Hospital, London, UK

Although paranoid symptoms are commonly encountered in a range of psychiatric disorders that present to old age psychiatrists, remarkably few epidemiological studies of mood-incongruent paranoid states have been reported compared with cognitive and affective disorders[1]. Because these conditions are comparatively rare, it is difficult to determine their prevalence and incidence accurately. The epidemiological information that we do have on such states that have their onset in later life has come from two sources: studies based upon patients in contact with psychiatric services, and surveys of the elderly general population. Because of the nature of paranoid states, sufferers are unlikely to cooperate with community surveys and are often hidden from contact with psychiatric services. Thus, all the studies reviewed below are likely to represent underestimates of the true prevalence and incidence of these disorders.

PARANOID IDEATION AMONG COMMUNITY-LIVING ELDERLY

In 1173 subjects aged over 64 years in the Epidemiological Catchment Area survey, with a response rate of 85%, generalized persecutory ideation, as assessed on the paranoid scale of the Mini-Mult, was present in 4%[2]. There was a significant excess of unmarried individuals among those with persecutory ideation, but no association with gender or living alone. Other associated features were visual and hearing deficits, cognitive impairment, impaired physical health and disabilities in daily living, together with reduced social and economic resources. Among a community sample of 1420 individuals aged over 75 years, paranoid ideation (defined as recording of paranoid symptoms by both a physician and informant's interview) was found in 6.3%[3]. The prevalence of paranoid ideation in people with cognitive impairment was 12.1%, while it was only 2.6% in those who were cognitively intact. Once the effect of cognitive impairment has been controlled for, the variables significantly associated with paranoid ideation were being divorced, being female, having depressive symptoms, receiving psychotropic drugs, having no friends or visitors, using community care and being an immigrant. In a survey of 935 interviews with individuals aged 70 or over in Canberra and a neighbouring town[4], 65 had at least one psychotic symptom; 22 reported current auditory hallucinations only, 23 delusions only and three hallucinations and delusions: 25 of these individuals had cognitive impairment or dementia. The point prevalence of psychotic symptoms was 5.7% and the significantly associated risk factors, apart from cognitive impairment, were living alone, male gender, limited education, social isolation, poor health and depressive symptoms.

HALLUCINATIONS IN COMMUNITY-LIVING ELDERLY

Data from the Epidemiological Catchment Area study were used to estimate the self-reported age-specific prevalence of hallucinations in a sample of 15 258 individuals of all ages. Patients with dementia were not excluded, and although the prevalence of both auditory and visual hallucinations was highest in young subjects, an increase in auditory and visual hallucinations was found in the elderly, with a rate of visual hallucinations of 40/1000/year in males aged 80 + [5].

PSYCHOSIS DIAGNOSED IN COMMUNITY-LIVING ELDERLY

The prevalence of schizophrenia and delusional disorder in those aged 65 + in the community has varied widely from study to study, but on the whole low rates have been found. The Epidemiological Catchment Area survey found a prevalence of schizophrenia of 0.2%[6] and the 6 month prevalence rate of schizophrenia was 0.4–0.6% in a Danish survey[7]. In a sample of 612 elderly Chinese Singaporeans examined using GMS–AGECAT criteria, 0.5% had schizophrenia or paraphrenia diagnoses[8]. From a random sample of 5222 individuals aged 65 +, Copeland and colleagues[9] made estimates of the prevalence and incidence of DSM-III-R-defined delusional disorder and schizophrenia. The sample were chosen from the lists of general practitioners' patients and were interviewed by nurses trained in the use of the GMS–AGECAT computerized diagnostic system. The prevalence of DSM-III-R schizophrenia was estimated at 0.12% (95% CI, 0.04–0.25%) and delusional disorder at 0.04% (95% CI, 0.00–0.14%). The minimum incidence of schizophrenia for new cases was 3.0, for new and relapsed cases 45.0, and for delusional disorder 15.6/100 000/year. Two of the five cases of schizophrenia identified in the sample were found to have been first diagnosed before the age of 65.

Principles and Practice of Geriatric Psychiatry, 2nd edn. Edited by J. R. M. Copeland, M. T. Abou-Saleh and D. G. Blazer
©2002 John Wiley & Sons, Ltd

STUDIES BASED ON PSYCHIATRIC CONTACTS

From the 1966 official figures from England and Wales for individuals aged over 65 years, Kay[10] calculated annual incidence rates of schizophrenia of 10–15/100 000 for males and 20–25/100 000 for females. The annual incidence of DSM-III-R-defined schizophrenia in the over-65s on the Camberwell Case Register was estimated at 12.6 per 100 000[11]. van Os and colleagues[12] examined the annual incidence rate of late-onset (age 59+) non-affective, non-organic psychosis in 8010 elderly admissions to psychiatric hospitals in The Netherlands and 1777 elderly admissions in the UK. The incidence of psychosis showed a significant increase with age in both countries, the cases rising from around 10/100 000 person-years in the age group 60–65 years to just over 25/100 000 person-years in the 90+ age group. After adjustments for the possible confounding effects of time trend and gender, the linear trend in the association between increasing age and first admission rates corresponded to an 11% increase in incidence with each 5 year increase in age.

COURSE AND COGNITIVE PROGNOSIS

Long-term follow-up of those patients we used to call "late paraphrenics", but should now describe as suffering from "very late-onset schizophrenia-like psychosis"[13], has shown that in the absence of cognitive impairment at the outset, the mortality rate does not differ from expectation and the causes of death in these patients are similar to the general population[14]. When those patients with accompanying organic brain syndromes and associated cognitive impairment are included in follow-up studies, rates of progression to dementia and mortality are, not surprisingly, high[15].

REFERENCES

1. Castle DJ. Epidemiology of late-onset schizophrenia. In Howard R, Rabins PV, Castle DJ, eds, *Late-onset Schizophrenia*. Petersfield: Wrightson Biomedical, 1999: 139–46.
2. Christenson R, Blazer D. Epidemiology of persecutory ideation in an elderly population in the community. *Am J Psychiat* 1984; **141**: 59–67.
3. Forsell Y, Henderson AS. Epidemiology of paranoid symptoms in an elderly population. *Br J Psychiat* 1998; **172**: 429–33.
4. Henderson AS, Korten AE, Levings C *et al*. Psychotic symptoms in the elderly: a prospective study in a population sample. *Int J Geriat Psychiat* 1998; **13**: 484–92.
5. Tien AY. Distribution of hallucinations in the population. *Soc Psychiat Psychiat Epidemiol* 1991; **26**: 287–92.
6. Keith SJ, Regier DA, Rae DS. Schizophrenic disorders. In Robins LN, Regier DA, eds, *Psychiatric Disorders in America*. New York: Free Press.
7. Neilsen JA, Neilsen J. Prevalence investigation of mental illness in the aged in 1961, 1972 and 1977 in a geographically delimited Danish population group. *Acta Psychiat Scand* 1989; **79**: 95–104.
8. Kua EH. A community study of mental disorders in elderly Singaporean Chinese using the GMS–AGECAT package. *Aust N Z J Psychiat* 1992; **26**: 502–6.
9. Copeland JR, Dewey ME, Scott A *et al*. Schizophrenia and delusional disorder in older age: Community prevalence, incidence, comorbidity and outcome. *Schizoph Bull* 1998; **24**: 153–61.
10. Kay DWK. Schizophrenia and schizophrenia-like states in the elderly. *Br J Hosp Med* 1972: 369–75.
11. Castle DJ, Murray RM. The epidemiology of late-onset schizophrenia. *Schizophr Bull* 1993; **19**: 691–703.
12. van Os J, Howard R, Takei N, Murray R. Increasing age is a risk factor for psychosis in the elderly. *Soc Psychiat Psychiat Epidemiol* 1995; **30**: 161–4.
13. Howard R, Rabins PV, Seeman MV, Jeste DV. Late-onset schizophrenia and very late-onset schizophrenia-like psychosis. An International Consensus. *Am J Psychiat* 1999 (in press).
14. Kay DWK. Outcome and cause of death in mental disorders of old age: a long-term follow-up of functional and organic psychoses. *Acta Psychiat Scand* 1962; **38**: 249–76.
15. Holden NL. Late paraphrenia or the paraphrenias? *Br J Psychiat* 1987; **150**: 635–9.

93

The Fate of Schizophrenia with Advancing Age: Research Findings and Implications for Clinical Care

Robert Howard

Institute of Psychiatry and Maudsley Hospital, London, UK

Although approximately 20% of the long-stay population of psychiatric hospitals in the UK are aged over 65 years[1], and the large-scale closure of mental hospitals that began in the 1950s is nearing completion, old schizophrenic patients and the factors that might influence the success of their move into the community have only recently become the subject of serious study[2]. Ready availability of nursing-home places and a lack of public concern about the potential dangerousness of elderly people with schizophrenia in the community have fostered such disinterest, although the numbers of people involved are enormous: some 200 000 elderly people with schizophrenia have been discharged to nursing homes in the USA[3].

LONG-TERM OUTCOME IN SCHIZOPHRENIA

Enduring positive symptoms of psychosis, cognitive deficits, negative symptoms and adaptive problems may all contribute to long-term disability in schizophrenia. Although some long-term follow-up studies suggest that cognitive and social decline plateau after the age of 40 years and that some symptoms actually improve with increasing age[4-6], many patients experience multiple exacerbations of illness or spend many years in hospital[7]. Although we are traditionally taught that males have a generally worse prognosis in schizophrenia, the situation is complicated. At 2–13 years after initial diagnosis, females do seem to do better[8,9], but their advantage may be lost after 20 years[4,6]. From follow-up studies spanning three decades, Seeman[10] has suggested that males are typically more severely ill in the first 10 years of illness but then improve, while females, after a relatively need-free first decade, show increasing disability over time.

COGNITIVE IMPAIRMENT

The mean Mini-Mental State Examination (MMSE) score in a group of 38 chronic elderly schizophrenic inpatients in one study was 9.6[11]—well within the moderately demented range. Such cognitive deficit does not appear to be specifically linked to a history of brain-damaging treatments, such as leucotomy, insulin coma therapy or lifetime total neuroleptic dosing[7] and cannot be attributed to the appearance of Alzheimer-type neuropathological change, which is rare in the brains of such patients coming to neuropathology[12]. Indeed, in a neuropathological study of 66 patients with schizophrenia, 68% of whom had a history of marked cognitive impairment in life, only 8% had brain changes

that satisfied diagnostic criteria for AD[13]. Although cognitive impairment in such patients cannot therefore be attributable to AD, those patients with most severe impairment had significantly more plaques and tangles in their brains than did the unimpaired subjects examined. Severe cognitive impairment is the most important single predictor of poor outcome in chronic schizophrenia[14]. There is debate in the literature regarding whether or not schizophrenic cognitive impairment progresses within chronic illness. Although cross-sectional studies have tended to suggest that cognitive function does not decline over time in schizophrenia[15,16], there is no doubt that cognitive impairment does appear at some point in the illness. Either it is present as a static feature at or soon after illness onset, or it progresses insidiously or in limited subgroups of patients, so that the studies have missed it. This latter point is supported by the results of a large 30-month cognitive follow-up study of 326 chronic schizophrenic patients aged over 65 years[17]. In this study, 30% of patients who had baseline scores in the less impaired range of the Clinical Dementia Rating scale showed a worsening of this score at follow-up to moderate or more severely impaired levels. Only 7% of the sample with lower scores at baseline showed any improvement in functioning. Factors predicting cognitive decline included lower levels of education, older age and more severe positive symptoms. Although the cognitive and functional decline over 30 months demonstrated by this study was convincing and dramatic, it is important to remember that the patients involved were chronically institutionalized, with very adverse illness courses. Middle-aged poor-prognosis schizophrenic patients may also have neuroimaging evidence of progressive ventricular enlargement[18]—further support for the thesis that a subgroup of middle-aged or elderly schizophrenic patients with poorly controlled symptoms are at particular risk of declining cognitive function. Although cognitive deficits have received the most research attention, because they are relatively straightforward to measure reliably and appear to be so predictive of outcome, they represent only a single dimension of disability in chronic schizophrenia. In a study of 102 middle-aged or elderly outpatients with schizophrenia, assessed with the Direct Assessment of Functional Status (a standardized measure of behaviours during performance of simulated daily tasks), patients were significantly more limited than controls on all subscales, except for grooming and eating[19]. Schizophrenic patients were more disabled than outpatients with major depression, but less impaired than those with Alzheimer's disease. Lower levels of formal education, greater severity of extrapyramidal symptoms and cognitive deficits were all associated with lower functional assessment scores.

Principles and Practice of Geriatric Psychiatry, 2nd edn. Edited by J. R. M. Copeland, M. T. Abou-Saleh and D. G. Blazer
©2002 John Wiley & Sons, Ltd

THE EFFECTS OF INSTITUTIONALIZATION

Since poor long-term outcome in schizophrenia is associated with long institutionalization and cognitive impairments, could the deficits be a consequence of a non-stimulating psychiatric hospital environment or overtreatment with medication? One simple way to examine the possible causal relationship between these factors has involved comparing the cognitive and adaptive functioning deficits in groups of elderly schizophrenic patients cared for in different types of institutions in widely differing parts of the world. In a cross-national study of cognitive impairment in poor-outcome geriatric patients with schizophrenia[20] in London and New York, remarkable similarities in cognitive dysfunction between the US and UK patients were found, despite differences in the structure of institutional care provided. Mean MMSE scores in New York were 10.5 and in London 10.6. When the patients in the two centres were investigated with an adaptive functioning scale, however, differences emerged which were probably related to institutional differences. American patients were more impaired in social initiation, but less impaired in social competence and personal hygiene, than their English counterparts.

WHERE ARE PATIENTS BEST LOOKED AFTER?

It is probably unsafe to make generalized assertions about the ways in which the needs of elderly schizophrenic patients are best met because they are a heterogeneous group in terms of enduring psychotic symptoms, cognitive and adaptive deficits and family or other social support. In a cross-sectional study of 97 chronically hospitalized schizophrenic patients, 37 chronic schizophrenic residents in nursing homes and 31 acutely admitted geriatric patients with schizophrenia, patients in each of these groups had very different patterns of symptoms and impairments[21]. Whilst differences in positive and negative schizophrenic symptoms were small, nursing-home residents had the most severe adaptive deficits. Prospective studies of chronic schizophrenic patients successfully discharged to nursing homes, compared with those who are retained in long-term psychiatric care, have shown that it is not cognitive or adaptive deficits that prevent discharge but continuing belligerence and hostility[22]. Just as it appears unwise to generalize about the care needs of patients, it is rash to assume that all nursing homes or long-stay psychiatric facilities are the same. When 159 long-term schizophrenic inpatients within Veterans Administration hospitals were allocated to either a community nursing home, a Veterans Administration nursing home or another long-stay psychiatric ward, or allowed to remain on their original ward, at 12 months the patients with the best outcomes were those who had been transferred to another long-stay ward. The worst outcomes were seen in those who had been discharged to community nursing homes[23,24]. Rather than the location of care, particular features of the quality of care were the factors most strongly associated with good outcome. Staffing characteristics, e.g. the staff:patient ratio and the rate of staff turnover, together with the mean functional ability of fellow residents, were significantly linked to outcome. A similar study from the UK came to superficially conflicting conclusions. Elderly long-stay schizophrenic patients transferred to nursing homes showed slower functional decline over the next 2–3 years than those who remained on the wards[25]. The important difference from the situation in the Veterans Administration study was that in the UK study staff–patient contact was greater in community facilities than on the long-stay wards and this contributed to better outcome. Studies such as those reviewed above examine only the grosser disabilities and deficits of elderly schizophrenic patients and the few published investigations of quality of life give a rather depressing insight into exactly what the lives of these people are like. In a 10 year follow-up of 40 older patients with schizophrenia, overall subjective quality-of-life ratings did not improve from the low levels seen at the beginning of the study[26]. Ratings on a small number of items (contacts, inner experiences and knowledge/education) had improved slightly, but the reasons for these improvements were just as likely to be that patients had downgraded their expectations as that they were interacting more successfully with their environment or that housekeeping services received had improved.

MORTALITY IN CHRONIC SCHIZOPHRENIA

Excess mortality among patients with schizophrenia is a consistent and accepted research finding that cannot be fully explained by the observation that 10% of patients will kill themselves[27]. In a prospective study of 88 schizophrenic patients with a mean age of 62.6 years at study commencement, 39 had died after 10 years' follow-up—none through suicide[28]. The relative risk of death among the patients was 1.33 (95% CI, 1.01–1.65). Six variables, some of which have important clinical implications, affected independent prediction of reduced survival and these were: increasing age; male gender; the edentulous state; time since most recent neuroleptic withdrawal; maximum number of antipsychotics given concurrently; and the absence of anti-cholinergic treatment.

IMPLICATIONS FOR CLINICAL CARE

Since elderly patients with chronic schizophrenia have high levels of disability and dependence upon caring services, their apparent invisibility to mental health policy makers must largely be attributable to ageist assumptions that they should not expect much more than basic nursing home provision, and to a lack of general public concern about the safety of placing elderly (and therefore "low-risk") psychotic patients in the community. They also represent a group of patients who are poorly served by specialist psychiatric services. Sometimes rather grandly termed "graduates" because they are alumni of mental health services set up for younger patients, it is often not clear whether they have become the responsibility of local old age psychiatrists or whether they should continue to be looked after by the general adult psychiatry teams with whom they have been in contact. In a call to arms to all mental health professionals who may be involved in the care of these patients, Rodriguez-Ferrer and Vassilas have set out four objectives of importance in the establishment of a seamless and ideal service. First, general practitioners should be central in the coordination of service provision and should be involved in the assessment of physical needs, as well as psychiatric ones. Second, the organization and delivery of specialist mental health services should take into account the fact that, in the future, the majority of these patients will live in residential and nursing homes. Third, purchasers of mental health services need to be aware of the effects of the quality of the physical and staffing environment of residential and nursing homes on patient functioning. Finally, services should maintain clarity at all times as to exactly which agencies (psychiatric, social, voluntary) have responsibility for each individual's care. Now that we have an agenda for the management of this hitherto-neglected group, together with novel antipsychotic agents that are less likely to induce movement disorders and may even improve cognitive function[29], this really does represent a clinical population for whom recent research has positive implications. The most recent indications are that deinstitutionalization has been, on the whole, a modest success. At the end of a 5 year follow-up of 670 elderly chronic patients (80% of whom had schizophrenia), 89.6% were still living in the community and only one-third had required any kind of hospital readmission[30].

REFERENCES

1. Clifford P, Charman A, Webb Y, Best S. Planning for community care. Long-stay populations of hospitals scheduled for rundown or closure. *Br J Psychiat* 1991; **158**: 190–6.
2. Rodriguez-Ferrera S, Vassilas CA. Older people with schizophrenia: providing services for a neglected group. It's the quality of their environment that matters, not where it is. *Br Med J* 1998; **317**: 293–4.
3. Goldman HH, Feder J, Scanlon W. Chronic mental patients in nursing homes: re-examining data from the National Nursing Home Survey. *Hosp Commun Psychiat* 1986; **37**: 269–72.
4. Bleuler M. The long-term course of the schizophrenic psychoses. *Psychol Med* 1974; **4**: 244–54.
5. Huber G, Gross G, Schuttler R. A long-term follow-up study of schizophrenia. Psychiatric course of illness and prognosis. *Acta Psychiat Scand* 1975; **52**: 49–57.
6. Harding CM, Brooks GW, Ashikaga T et al. The Vermont longitudinal study of persons with severe mental illness. I. Methodology, study sample and overall status 32 years later. *Am J Psychiat* 1987; **144**: 718–26.
7. Davidson M, Harvey PD, Powchik P et al. Severity of symptoms in chronically institutionalised geriatric schizophrenic patients. *Am J Psychiat* 1995; **152**: 197–207.
8. Mason P, Harrison G, Glazebrook C et al. The characteristics of outcome in schizophrenia at 13 years. *Br J Psychiat* 1995; **167**: 596–603.
9. Harrison G, Croudace P, Mason C et al. Predicting the long-term outcome of schizophrenia. *Psychol Med* 1996; **26**: 697–705.
10. Seeman MV. Narratives of 20–30 year outcomes in schizophrenia. *Psychiatry* 1998; **61**: 249–61.
11. Davidson M, Harvey PD, Welsh K et al. Cognitive impairment in old-age schizophrenia: a comparative study of schizophrenia and Alzheimer's disease. *Am J Psychiat* 1996; **153**: 1274–9.
12. Powchik P, Davidson M, Haroutunian V et al. Postmortem studies in schizophrenia. *Schizophr Bull* 1998; **24**: 325–41.
13. Dwork AJ, Susser ES, Keilp J et al. Senile degeneration and cognitive impairment in chronic schizophrenia. *Am J Psychiat* 1998; **155**: 1536–43.
14. Perlick D, Mattis S, Stastny P, Teresi J. Neuropsychological discriminators of long-term inpatient or outpatient status in chronic schizophrenia. *J Neuropsychiat Clin Neurosci* 1992; **4**: 428–34.
15. Goldberg T, Hyde TM, Kleinman JE, Weinberger DR. Course of schizophrenia: neuropsychological evidence for static encephalopathy. *Schizophr Bull* 1993; **19**: 787–804.
16. Russell AJ, Munro JC, Jones PB et al. Schizophrenia and the myth of intellectual decline. *Am J Psychiat* 1997; **154**: 635–9.
17. Harvey PD, Silverman JM, Mohs RC et al. Cognitive decline in late-life schizophrenia: a longitudinal study of geriatric chronically hospitalised patients. *Biol Psychiat* 1999; **45**: 32–40.
18. Davis KL, Buchsbaum MS, Shihabuddin L et al. Ventricular enlargement in poor-outcome schizophrenia. *Biol Psychiat* 1998; **43**: 783–93.
19. Harvey PD, Leff J, Trieman N et al. Cognitive impairment in geriatric chronic schizophrenic patients: a cross-national study in New York and London. *Int J Geriat Psychiat* 1997; **12**: 1001–7.
20. Patterson TL, Klapow JC, Eastham JH et al. Correlates of functional status in older patients with schizophrenia. *Psychiat Res* 1998; **80**: 41–52.
21. Harvey PD, Howanitz E, Parrella M et al. Symptoms, cognitive functioning and adaptive skills in geriatric patients with lifelong schizophrenia: a comparison across treatment sites. *Am J Psychiat* 1998; **155**: 1080–6.
22. Trieman N, Leff J. Difficult to place patients in a psychiatric closure programme. The TAPS project 24. *Psychol Med* 1996; **26**: 765–74.
23. Linn MW, Gurel L, Williford WO et al. Nursing home care as an alternative to psychiatric hospitalisation. *Arch Gen Psychiat* 1985; **42**: 544–51.
24. Timko C, Nguyen AQ, Williford WO, Moos RH. Quality of care and outcomes of chronic mentally ill patients in hospitals and nursing homes. *Hosp Commun Psychiat* 1993; **44**: 241–6.
25. Trieman N, Wills W, Leff J. TAPS project 28. Does reprovision benefit elderly long-stay mental patients? *Schizophr Res* 1996; **21**: 199–208.
26. Skantze K. Subjective quality of life and standard of living: a 10 year follow-up of outpatients with schizophrenia. *Acta Psychiat Scand* 1998; **98**: 390–9.
27. Brown S. Excess mortality in schizophrenia: a meta-analysis. *Br J Psychiat* 1997; **171**: 502–8.
28. Waddington JL, Youssef HA, Kinsella A. Mortality in schizophrenia. Antipsychotic polypharmacy and absence of adjunctive anti-cholinergics over the course of a 10 year prospective study. *Br J Psychiat* 1998; **173**: 325–9.
29. Trieman N, Leff J, Glover G. Outcome of long-stay psychiatric patients resettled in the community: prospective cohort study. *Br Med J* 1999; **319**: 13–16.
30. Howard R. Cognitive impairment in late life schizophrenia: a suitable case for treatment? *Int J Geriat Psychiat* 1998; **13**: 400–4.

94

Rehabilitation and Long-term Management

Robert Pugh

St Luke's–Woodside Hospital, London, UK

THE LONG-TERM OUTCOME OF SCHIZOPHRENIA

Schizophrenia has been conventionally considered to be a disorder with a poor long-term prognosis. The concept of schizophrenia as a disorder with a poor prognosis was reflected by DSM-III[1], where features included a failure to return to premorbid functioning, recurrent acute exacerbation with increasing residual impairment between episodes, continued symptoms, unemployment, social isolation and an inability for self-care. DSM-IV[2] included a revised view of schizophrenia, stating that most studies of the outcome of schizophrenia suggest that the course may be variable, with some individuals displaying exacerbation and remission, whereas others remain chronically ill.

The pessimistic views on outcome had mainly been formed from the early longitudinal studies reported by Kraepelin[3] and Eugen Bleuler[4]. In the course of his work, Kraepelin became pessimistic about the outcome of dementia praecox, reporting that fewer than 5% of patients sustained a lasting recovery. When Eugen Bleuler originally described the concept of schizophrenia, an essential component of the diagnosis was that patients were not able to regain their premorbid abilities. These early studies have had a major effect on our concept of schizophrenia. Indeed, many psychiatrists[5,6] considered that if a patient makes a good recovery, then the validity of the diagnosis of schizophrenia may be in question. These views still persist and have had a major effect on service planning for people suffering from schizophrenia and their medical management. Five, large, long-term studies of schizophrenia patients have produced very different results from those of Kraepelin and Bleuler and have effectively challenged this view.

Harding et al.[7,8] carried out a 32 year follow-up study of a rehabilitation programme of comprehensive rehabilitation and community placement for those "backward" patients who had not improved sufficiently following the introduction of chlorpromazine. A total of 269 patients who were considered to be amongst the most severely disabled and chronically mentally ill in the hospital were referred to the programme. After an average of 32 years, 178 were still alive and were interviewed again; 71 patients had died and in these cases the family were interviewed; 13 other patients were still alive but refused participation; and the remaining seven could not be located. A battery of interview instruments described as the Vermont Community Questionnaire was used to evaluate outcome. Evidence of good inter-rater reliability and face and construct validity for the questionnaires are presented in their paper. The patients were rediagnosed using DSM-III classification retrospectively: 188 of the original subjects were considered to have met the DSM-III criteria for schizophrenia. The results showed that the long-term outcome was mixed, with many patients demonstrating various degrees of productivity, social involvements and competent functioning; 68% of the patients displayed neither positive nor negative symptoms of schizophrenia at follow-up and 45% of the sample displayed no psychiatric symptoms at all; 82% of patients had not been in hospital in the last year; 61% met with friends every week or two; 68% had one or more moderately/very close friends; 40% had been employed in the past year; 81% were rated as being able to meet basic needs; and 73% were felt to lead a moderate to very full life. The study also includes an assessment of income; 77% of the sample were assessed on the Community Care Schedule as having an adequate income. The schedule's definition of "adequate" was that "the amount of money received will cover the subject's basic needs comfortably". Four other studies report similar findings.

Manfred Bleuler[9] described a follow-up study of 208 patients who met his own and Eugen Bleuler's diagnostic criteria for schizophrenia, and reported a significant improvement in 53% at a 23 year follow-up.

Huber et al.[10] described the largest study, following up 502 patients over an average of 22.4 years, using the diagnostic criteria of E. and M. Bleuler[4,9,11] and Schneider[12]; 53% showed significant or total improvement.

Ciompi and Muller[13] followed up 289 patients admitted before the age of 65 who were over 65 by 1963. The mean length of follow-up was 36.9 years. The diagnostic criteria of E. and M. Bleuler were used; again, over 50% (57%) of patients showed significant improvement.

Tsuang et al.[14] followed 186 patients admitted to Iowa State Hospital between 1934 and 1944 for a period of 35 years. In this study, 46% showed significant improvement.

The results of these studies challenge the prevailing concept of outcome in schizophrenia and support the concept of heterogeneity of outcome. Together, these studies found that between one-half and two-thirds of more than 1300 patients studied for a period in excess of 20 years achieved recovery or significant improvement. This is not to deny the fact that many patients do not show an improvement over the years and require continuing medical and social support, but it clearly suggests that it is erroneous to view deterioration as an inevitable outcome.

The differences between these studies and those of Kraepelin and Bleuler have been attributed to sampling biases. The criticism has been that both Kraepelin and Bleuler chose samples of patients who were admitted to hospital for long-term care. In addition to this, Kraepelin's studies probably included patients with tertiary syphilis and other organic disorders for which tests were unavailable at the time. Certainly, Eugen Bleuler's son, Manfred Bleuler, attributed his father's pessimism about the outcome of schizophrenia to this bias.

Principles and Practice of Geriatric Psychiatry, 2nd edn. Edited by J. R. M. Copeland, M. T. Abou-Saleh and D. G. Blazer
©2002 John Wiley & Sons, Ltd

ENVIRONMENTAL, SOCIAL AND CULTURAL FACTORS AND OUTCOME OF SCHIZOPHRENIA

There is evidence that environmental factors play a major part in the outcome of schizophrenia, although this is clearly not as marked as was first claimed in the early descriptions of institutionalization by Barton[15] and Goffman[16]. They considered that the disabilities of long-stay patients were primarily due to the psychiatric institutions in which they lived. In a major study of these institutions, Wing[17] studied the outcome of patients who were managed in three hospitals with very different policies of care. He concluded that institutionalization had contributed significantly to the patients' disabilities.

The influence of environment and culture was also illustrated by the WHO international pilot study of schizophrenia[18], in which 1202 patients diagnosed as having schizophrenia in 10 different countries were followed up over a 2 year period. The heterogeneity of outcome was again underlined, but patients suffering from schizophrenia in the developing countries had a better outcome than those in the developed countries. The report concluded that the diagnosis of schizophrenia alone did not provide sufficient grounds for a firm statement about the patient's likely pattern or course, probability of relapses and admissions, or the degree of social impairment in the future.

Similar findings emerge from a 5 year follow-up study of patients living in the peasant society of Sri Lanka, described by Waxler[19]. She concluded that in Western society, expectation and a belief about mental illness and the process by which treatment is provided alienate patients suffering from schizophrenia from their normal roles, and thus prolong illness. In contrast, the beliefs and practices in non-industrial societies encourage a quick return to normality.

THE ROLE OF REHABILITATION

Although the recent outcome studies have shown that the prognosis of schizophrenia is not as poor as had previously been considered, it is also clear that outcome is mixed, with some patients showing no improvement and remaining severely disabled. Continuing care services for people suffering from schizophrenia should aim to reduce these disabilities wherever possible and to meet the needs of those who remain severely disabled into old age.

The care of patients with schizophrenia has moved from long-term hospital to care in the community. This international change occurred with very little contemporary evidence to support it. However, the controlled studies that exist[20,21] demonstrate that patients treated in the community did not experience increases in homelessness, mortality or suicide and did not need excessive readmissions to hospital. Importantly, patients taking part in these studies preferred treatment outside hospital.

Intercultural studies would support the concept that environmental factors can have an effect on outcome. However, although one would expect that the socioenvironmental factors involved in community care would improve the prognosis, this has been very difficult to demonstrate in practice. Wing's Three Hospital Study is one of the few papers that supports this view. There is little evidence that psychiatric symptomatology or psychosocial function improve when patients are treated in the community.

In the UK the view that all patients with schizophrenia can have long-term care in the community has been revised, and there is provision for 24 hour nursing care[22]. Treiman[23] demonstrated that this care can be successful in reducing severely disrupted behaviours. However, this group of patients are different from the long-stay hospital population. They are younger, suffer from more psychotic symptoms and often have multiple problems, such as cognitive deficits, substance misuse and violence. Their self-care skills are often intact.

CHANGES IN REHABILITATION

One problem in interpreting these studies is that the term "rehabilitation" may mean very different things to different people, and indeed, in recent years the term "rehabilitation" has sometimes even become synonymous with discharge from hospital. This use of the word is misleading. Bennett[24] considered that the goal of rehabilitation was to enable the individual "to make the best use of his residual abilities in order to function at an optimum level in as normal a social context as possible". He introduced the concept of rehabilitation as a continuous and recursive process, applicable in many service settings, which could be independent of the discharge process. He considered the interaction between the individual and the environment to be particularly important. Rehabilitation should entail both working with patients to enhance their confidence and coping skills and the provision of such "prosthetic environments" and social, emotional and material support as may be necessary to maintain their optimal level.

The concept of helping a patient to cope with his/her disability is central to rehabilitation and forms the basis of cognitive-behavioural therapy for schizophrenia[25]. Patients may deny that they are unwell and this may make engaging them in treatment difficult. It is important to approach their problems from their point of view and work with them to reduce the problems they perceive as important. Education about their illness and medication may be helpful. It is also helpful to discuss exacerbating factors, such as stress and substance misuse. Discussion of early signs of relapse, such as unusual behaviour or prodromal symptoms, may enable patients to prevent a serious relapse. The involvement of family and friends is often helpful. If assessment of risk reveals a substantial risk to the patient or others, then patients should be engaged in the process of reducing the risk.

The Royal College of Psychiatrists report on Rehabilitation emphasized the importance of primary, secondary and tertiary disability[26]. The primary disabilities are emotional, cognitive, motivational and behavioural dysfunction. Secondary handicaps include loss of self-esteem and confidence, social withdrawal and loss of social roles and networks. Unemployment, homelessness, poverty and stigmatization are the tertiary handicaps. Often patients' main concerns are about the secondary and tertiary problems and it is important to address these to achieve an effective treatment plan.

Deegan[27] has described how Mental Health Service users emphasize the importance for them of feeling "in the driver's seat"—empowerment. She uses the word "recovery" rather than "rehabilitation", highlighting the fact that patients recover and professionals rehabilitate. She describes the importance of people becoming experts in their own self-care.

THE PRACTICE OF REHABILITATION

Rehabilitation is based on assessment, development of treatment plans and monitoring. In the UK this forms the basis of the care programme approach. The assessments are based on patients' abilities and difficulties in a wide range of areas. These should include the following.

- *Psychiatric illness:* positive and negative symptoms; insight; compliance with medication; self-medication ability.

- *Physical illness:* specific problems, e.g. diabetes, heart disease; eyesight, hearing and dental problems; preventative medicine, e.g. blood pressure monitoring, breast examination.
- *Education:* literacy and numeracy.
- *Daily living skills:* personal hygiene; laundry skills; budgeting; shopping; cooking; use of public facilities; road safety.
- *Family and social contact:* contact with family; expressed emotion; social networks.
- *Day activities:* work; day hospital; day centre.
- *Financial:* welfare rights, Court of Protection.
- *Accommodation:* patients' wishes; needs based on abilities and difficulties.
- *Risk assessment:* assessment of risk to self and others, including children.

It is often difficult to collect all of the above information and it is important to set a date for an initial review, when the information that has been collected by that time is gathered together. The purpose of the initial review is to appraise the patients' strengths and difficulties and to decide what further information needs to be obtained. Preliminary treatment plans and goals should also be set at this stage. A review of medication, including the use of clozapine for treatment-resistant psychosis[28] and the possible use of cognitive-behavioural therapy[25] and family interventions[29] should be explored.

It is important to have a clear system for reviews, and each patient population or treatment environment requires different systems to be developed, but the essential areas that need to be covered remain the same. Within a district or service it is often helpful to standardize the order of the areas (or headings) in which the assessments are made, so that assessments made in one setting can be easily understood by other teams working in other settings. This leads to improved liaison throughout the service and in particular helps communication between the community and the hospital.

An important part of an initial review is to decide on the order in which problems may be tackled. Sometimes the most important problems are worked on first but on other occasions it may be an idea to start with an easy problem to enable the patient to develop some self-confidence. It is important to set and record practical attainable goals.

Sometimes the review forms or care plan forms that are developed automatically tag the assessment of all strengths and difficulties with treatment plans and goals. This practice can lead to difficulties, as many patients have a large number of problems and in practice only three or four treatment plans can be followed at one time.

The other two vital components of a review are to identify individual staff who have responsibility for components of care and to set a date for a further review when new information on abilities and difficulties can be discussed and the treatment plans and goals evaluated. It is helpful to have patients involved in their treatment programme and many review forms have a space for the patient's signature on them, which assists patient involvement.

RATING SCALES IN REHABILITATION

Although there is no alternative to thorough individual assessments, standardized rating scales can be useful. They are used for the planning of services, the coarse screening of populations to draw up short lists of long-stay patients who may benefit from more intensive assessment of resettlement potential, and for obtaining a quantified assessment of a patient's progress. There are many scales available for assessments in rehabilitation, but few of these have been subjected to investigations of their reliability and validity. The REHAB: Rehabilitation Evaluation[30] is an exception to this and is probably the most widely used scale in the UK at present. It is a scale that has been specifically designed for use with long-stay patients and was developed during the course of a 7 year research study. On the basis of behaviour, over 1 week raters complete 23 items in total; seven three-point response scales indicate the frequency of occurrence of difficult or embarrassing behaviours and produce a deviant behaviour score (DV); aspects of social and everyday behaviour are rated in 16 items, each using a visual analogue response format, with written descriptions at each end on which the rater makes a mark that is scored 0–9 using a template. These scores are aggregated to yield the general behaviour score (GB), which can be used to categorize patients as "discharge potential", "moderate handicap" or "severe handicap". There are also five scale scores—social activity, speech disturbance, speech skills, self-care and community skills. The Handbook for the scale is particularly useful, in that it enables one to compare the patient's scores with scores in other populations, so that one can estimate the proportion of people with similar scores in the hospital or the community. Sensitivity to change has also been demonstrated. Provided that raters are properly trained, good reliability levels can be achieved and, once training has been undertaken, the scale itself is brief and easy to complete and score.

CONCLUSION

In conclusion, long-term outcome studies have demonstrated that schizophrenia has a much more heterogeneous outcome than had previously been understood, with many patients making substantial improvements over the years. The effects of environment on outcome are complex and require further long-term evaluation. The aim of rehabilitation is to enable patients to cope with their illness and make the most of their lives, by reducing symptoms and increasing abilities whenever possible and by providing supportive services to match individual need. It is important to see problems from the patients' point of view. In practice this is achieved through a series of reviews which are a focus for assessment, goal planning and evaluation.

REFERENCES

1. American Psychiatric Association. *Diagnostic and Statistical Manual of Mental Disorders*, 3rd edn (DSM-III). Washington, DC: APA.
2. American Psychiatric Association. *Diagnostic and Statistical Manual of Mental Disorders*, 4th edn (DSM-IV). Washington, DC: APA.
3. Kraepelin E. *Clinical Psychiatry; A Textbook for Students and Physicians* (6th edn of *Lehrbruch der Psychiatrie*), transl Defendorf AR. New York: Macmillan, 1902.
4. Bleuler E. *Dementia Praecox or the group of Schizophrenias*, transl Zimkin J. New York: Macmillan International Universities Press, 1950.
5. Kleinst K. Schizophrenic symptoms and chronic pathology. *J Ment Sci* 1960; **186**: 246–53.
6. Leonhard K. The cycloid psychosis. *J Ment Sci* 1961; **187**: 633–48.
7. Harding CM, Zubin J, Strauss JS. Chronicity in schizophrenia: fact, partial fact, or fiction? *Hosp Commun Psychiat* 1987; **38**: 477–86.
8. Harding CM, Brooks GW, Ashikasga T *et al*. The Vermont Longitudinal Study of Persons with Severe Mental Illness. 1. Methodology: study sample and overall status 32 years later. 2. Long-term outcome of subjects who retrospectively met DSM-III criteria for schizophrenia. *Am J Psychiat* 1992; **144**(6): 718–35.
9. Bleuler M. *The Schizophrenic Disorders: Long-term Patient and Family Studies*, transl Clemens SM. New Haven, CT: Yale University Press, 1978.
10. Huber G, Gross G, Schuttler R. A long-term follow-up study of schizophrenia; psychiatric course of illness and prognosis. *Acta Psychiat Scand* 1975; **52**: 49–57.

11. Bleuler M. The long-term course of the schizophrenic psychosis. *Psychol Med* 1974; **4**: 244–254.

12. Schneider K. *Clinical Psychopathology*. New York: Grune & Stratton, 1959.

13. Ciompi L, Muller C. *Lebensweg und Alter der Schizophrenen; eine Katamnestische Langzeitstudies bis ins Senium*. Berlin: Springer-Verlag, 1976.

14. Tsuang MT, Woolson RF, Fleming JA. Long-term outcome of major psychoses. I: Schizophrenia and affective disorders compared with psychiatrically symptom-free surgical conditions. *Arch Gen Psychiat* 1979; **36**: 1295–301.

15. Barton R. *Institutional Neurosis*. Bristol: Wright, 1959.

16. Goffman E. *Asylums*. Harmondsworth: Penguin, 1961.

17. Wing JK. Pilot experiment in the rehabilitation of long-hospitalised male schizophrenic patients. *Br J Prev Soc* 1960; **14**: 173–80.

18. Sartorius N, Jablensky A, Shapiro R. Two year follow-up of patients included in the WHO International Pilot Study of Schizophrenia. *Psychol Med* 1977; **7**: 629.

19. Waxler NE. Is outcome for schizophrenia better in non-industrial societies? *J Nerv Ment Dis* 1979; **167**(3): 144–58.

20. Treiman N, Leff J, Glover G. Outcome of long stay patients resettled in the community: a prospective cohort study. *Br Med J* 1999; **319**: 13–16.

21. Test MA, Stein LI. The clinical rationale for community treatment; a review of the literature. In Stein LI, Test MA, eds, *Alternatives to Mental Hospital Treatment*. New York: Plenum, 1978.

22. Department of Health. *24-Hour Nursed Care for People with Severe and Enduring Mental Illness*. Leeds: NHS Executive, 1996.

23. Trieman N, Leff J. The TAPS project. 36. The most difficult to place long-stay psychiatric in-patients. Outcome one year after relocation. *Br J Psychiat* 1996; **169**(3): 289–92.

24. Bennett DH. The historical development of rehabilitation services. In Watts FN, Bennett DH, eds, *The Theory and Practice of Rehabilitation*. Chichester: Wiley, 1983.

25. Kuipers E, Garrety P, Fowler D. London–East Anglia randomized controlled trial of cognitive-behaviour therapy for psychosis; effects of treatment phase. *Br J Psychiat* 1997; **171**: 319–27.

26. Royal College of Psychiatrists. *Rehabilitation in the 1980s*. London: Royal College of Psychiatrists, 1981.

27. Deegan P. Recovery and empowerment for people with psychiatric disabilities. *Soc Work Health Care* 1997; **25**: 11–24.

28. Wahlbeck K, Cheine M, Essale MA. Clozapine vs. typical neuroleptic medication for schizophrenia. Oxford: Cochrane Library; Oxford Update Software, 1999.

29. Mari J, Streiner D. Family intervention for people with schizophrenia. Oxford: Cochrane Review; Oxford Update Software, 1996.

30. Baker R, Hall JN. *REHAB; Rehabilitation Evaluation*. Aberdeen: Vine, 1983.

31. Department of Health. *Building Bridges: a Guide to Arrangements for Inter-agency Working for the Care and Protection of Severely Mentally Ill People*. London: Department of Health, 1995.

95

Treatment of Late-onset Psychotic Disorders

Elsa M. Zayas and George T. Grossberg

St Louis University, St Louis, MO, USA

As the world population ages, a greater proportion of the population will be over the age of 65. Psychopathology can present in various ways in the elderly. Psychoses, as defined in DSM-IV, consist of "delusions or prominent hallucinations occurring in the absence of insight into their pathological nature"[1]. Hallucinations can be visual, auditory, tactile and/or olfactory in nature. Delusions or falsely-held beliefs are at times very difficult to distinguish from reality. They may require corroboration from caregivers to authenticate their psychotic nature.

Psychotic disorders can present in the elderly as either chronic or acute conditions. The disorders can include early- and late-onset schizophrenia, schizoaffective disorders, delusional disorder, mood disorders with psychotic symptoms, delirium and dementias with psychosis. Furthermore, the etiology of psychosis can be the result of medical conditions, such as Parkinson's disease or neoplasms, as well as drugs or other substances (Table 95.1).

Table 95.1 Psychotic disorders manifested in the elderly

Schizophrenia
    Late-onset
    Aging patients with early onset
Schizoaffective disorder
Psychosis NOS
Delusional disorder
Dementia with psychotic symptoms
    Alzheimer's dementia
    Vascular dementia
    Lewy body dementia
    Mixed dementias
Delirium
Psychoses due to a general medical condition
Psychoses due to a substance
Mood disorders with psychotic symptoms

EPIDEMIOLOGY

The geriatric data from the Epidemiologic Catchment Area study showed, at three sites, a 6 month prevalence for schizophrenia and schizophreniform disorders of 0.2–0.9%; cognitive impairment, including organic psychosis, was 16.8–23%[2]. Reported prevalences of psychotic disorders in a nursing home population was 10% and in a community-based sample in Sweden 4.7%[3,4]. Patients with Alzheimer's disease may also exhibit psychotic symptoms, with reported prevalences as high as 63%[5].

Patients with late-onset schizophrenia (LOS) present with their psychotic symptoms after the age of 45. LOS tend to be predominantly women, and have better premorbid functioning compared to younger schizophrenics[6]. Women with late-onset compared to early-onset schizophrenia tend to have more severe positive symptoms and fewer negative symptoms when compared to men with late onset of the disorder[7]. Women also tend to have less social withdrawal, better premorbid functioning and a gradual decline in functioning[8,9]. Patients with late-onset schizophrenia tend to have less affect flattening and formal thought disorder[6]. Aging patients who suffer from schizophrenia may have less intensity of their symptoms[10].

Delusional disorders are defined as non-bizarre falsely-held beliefs with minimal hallucinations[1]. Delusional disorders often have their onset in mid- or late life[11] and tend to affect men earlier than women[12]. Low socioeconomic status, immigration, hearing loss and bedfast status are some of the risk factors for developing a delusional disorder[13–16]. Psychotic symptoms seen in dementias can consist of hallucinations or delusions.

NEUROCHEMICAL HYPOTHESIS

The dopamine hypothesis of schizophrenia associates an increase in the activity of dopamine in various cortical areas that are concerned with positive, negative and cognitive symptoms of schizophrenia, as well as side effects seen with the use of neuroleptics. An increase in the level of dopamine activity in the mesolimbic pathways of the brain would be associated with the psychotic symptoms seen, i.e. hallucinations and delusions. Blockade in activity at the mesocortical pathway would be associated with cognitive symptoms and may account for worsening of the negative symptoms seen with conventional antipsychotics. Blockade of dopamine at the tubuloinfundibular tract is associated with increases in prolactin levels, a troublesome side effect which, in younger patients, may lead to non-compliance and discontinuation of treatment.

DIFFERENTIAL DIAGNOSIS

Prior to initiating treatment, it is essential to conduct a biopsychosocial evaluation of the patient. Delirium is often the cause of an acute onset of psychotic symptoms in the elderly and must be foremost in one's differential assessment. Delirium, defined as an acute mental status change with waxing and waning of the levels of consciousness, often presents with hallucinations, predominantly visual, as well as delusions.

Medical conditions in the elderly that can cause delirium include: infection (frequently urinary tract infections); metabolic disorders (thyroid disease, diabetes); electrolyte imbalances; pain;

Principles and Practice of Geriatric Psychiatry, 2nd edn. Edited by J. R. M. Copeland, M. T. Abou-Saleh and D. G. Blazer

Table 95.2 Differential diagnosis of psychotic disorders in the elderly

Medical conditions
  Infections
    Urinary tract infections
    Pneumonia
    Viral
  Electrolyte imbalance
  Endocrine disorders
  Cardiovascular events
    Myocardial infarctions
    Arrhythmias
  Neurological
    Transient ischemic attacks
    Seizures
    Strokes
    Neoplasms
  Other events
    Urinary retention
    Impaction

acute events, such as myocardial infarctions, strokes, transient ischemic attacks; and exacerbation of chronic conditions, such as chronic obstructive pulmonary disease. Furthermore, medications are frequently part of, if not the underlying etiological cause of, delirium. Medications may contribute as a result of their side-effects profile, toxicity or mechanism of action. Inquiries should be made about the use of other substances, including alcohol or illegal drugs. Corticosteroids, digoxin, anticholinergic drugs and dopaminergic agents are just some of the medications that may be implicated.

The elderly are very sensitive to the side effects of medications, especially to the anticholinergic side effects of drugs. Many medications have anticholinergic side effects, including many antipsychotics, both typical and atypical. The untoward peripheral anticholinergic effects of dry mouth, constipation, urinary retention and dry eyes are troublesome to the elderly and may further aggravate pre-existing physical conditions. Untoward central effects of these medications include the worsening of confusion and cognitive functioning.

TREATMENT OF PSYCHOSIS

One should keep in mind when treating the elderly the old axiom of "do no harm". The risk:benefit ratio of all treatments prescribed to elderly patients must always be assessed. When choosing an antipsychotic, one should take into account treatment history and susceptibility to potential side effects, as well as family history and familial response to medications. An important principle to apply when initiating treatment is to "start low and go slow". Treatment should be initiated with doses of half to one-third adult starting dose, remembering that most elderly patients with psychotic symptoms require much lower doses than younger patients.

Age-related bodily changes affect the pharmacokinetics of neuroleptics in the elderly. Absorption of medications may be altered by changes in gastric acidity and emptying and changes in blood flow. Age changes the body's composition, causing an increase in body fat with an associated decrease in lean body mass and total body water. In addition, there are decreases in liver mass and blood flow and changes in renal blood flow and function. All these changes affect the absorption, metabolism, distribution and clearance of neuroleptics.

The phenothiazines are lipophilic substances, well absorbed, with an extensive first-pass metabolism in the liver. In the elderly, as a result of the increase in total body fat, there is an increase in the volume of distribution of drugs. This leads to an increased half-life for those substances that are lipophilic. Thus, the elderly should be given lower doses of lipophilic drugs.

Neuroleptics are the treatment of choice for psychosis. They have recently been divided into typical (conventional) and atypical antipsychotics, based on their capacity to treat the positive and negative symptoms of schizophrenia as well as their potential to cause neurological side effects. All antipsychotics have the same level of efficacy. It may be relevant to recall that 100 mg chlorpromazine is equivalent to 1 mg haloperidol and 0.5 mg risperidone.

Typical or "conventional" antipsychotics can be divided into groups, based on their potency—high, intermediate and low potency. High-potency antipsychotics include haloperidol, fluphenazine and loxapine. High-potency neuroleptics have greater affinity for the dopamine receptors and less affinity for the muscarinic and α-receptors. High-potency neuroleptics are more likely to be associated with a higher incidence of extrapyramidal symptoms, akathisia, acute dyskinesia and parkinsonism, thus limiting their use in the elderly. Intermediate potency neuroleptics include perphenazine, loxapine and molidone. The atypical neuroleptics are clozapine, risperidone, olanzapine, quetiapine and ziprasidone. Low-potency antipsychotics, such as thioridazine and chlorpromazine, have a higher affinity for muscarinic, histaminic and α-adrenergic receptors and furthermore are more likely to produce increased sedation, orthostatic hypotension and anticholinergic side effects. They should be prescribed with caution in the elderly.

Limitations of Typical Neuroleptics in Geriatrics

Typical antipsychotics block various receptors that have the potential to cause side effects which can limit their use in the elderly. Dopaminergic blockade is associated with acute and long-term neurological side effects. Acute neurological side effects are extrapyramidal side effects (EPS), which include parkinsonism (resting tremors, rigidity, bradykinesia and gait disturbances), akathisia and dystonias and long-term effects of tardive dyskinesia, as well as the potential for neuroleptic malignant syndrome (NMS). Histaminergic blockade is associated with sedation and weight gain. Their quinidine-like cardiac effects are associated with the potential for arrhythmias. α-Adrenergic blockade leads to orthostatic hypotension. In addition, the muscarinic blockade leads to anticholinergic side effects.

Neuroleptic induced parkinsonism (NIP) is a potential concern with the use of neuroleptics in the elderly. The reported prevalence of NIP in patients aged over 60 on neuroleptics is 50%[17]. One study that looked at the use of low-dose neuroleptics and the incidence of NIP in the elderly found that 32% of patients developed NIP on an average daily dose of 43 mg chlorpromazine[17]. In addition, the risk factors contributing to the incidence of NIP were older age, instrumental tremor at baseline, EPS, the type of neuroleptic administered and the severity of dementia[17,18]. Parkinsonism can increase the risk of dependency, falls and fractures[19]. These often troublesome side effects can be treated either by reducing the neuroleptic dose, switching to an atypical agent, or using anticholinergics such as benztropine or trihexyphenidyl. Care needs to be taken when using antiparkinsonian medications in the elderly, who are very sensitive to the anticholinergic side effects.

Akathisia is another neuroleptic side effect that can be difficult to address. Akathisia is characterized by increased restlessness and psychomotor activity, with an inability to sit still. Akathisia is

Table 95.3 Medications/substances associated with delirium

Corticosteroids
Digoxin
Pain medications
Opioids
Muscle relaxants
H2 blockers
Anticholinergics
Benzodiazepine withdrawal
Alcohol withdrawal
Alcohol intoxication

often mistaken for worsening of the psychotic symptoms, leading one to erroneously increase the neuroleptic dose, when actually lowering the dose may address this troublesome side effect. In addition, akathisia can be treated with benzodiazepines and/or β-blockers.

Tardive dyskinesia (TD) is a potentially irreversible abnormal involuntary choreiform movement disorder. In the elderly, the 3 year cumulative incidence of severe TDs was found to be 2.5% after 1 year, 12.1% after 2 years and 22.9% after 3 years[20]. Another study reported the cumulative rates for TD to be 25% after 1 year, 35% after 2 years and 53% after 3 years[21]. Factors that were predictive of TD included higher daily dose at study entry, greater cumulative amounts of prescribed neuroleptics, greater severity of worsening negative symptoms, and the presence of early EPS[21,22]. Caution should be used when administering conventional neuroleptics in the elderly and they should only be prescribed when necessary and at the minimal effective dose[20].

Neuroleptic malignant syndrome (NMS) is a serious side effect with the potential to be lethal. NMS presents with symptoms of muscle rigidity, fever, autonomic instability, fluctuating levels of consciousness and elevations in CPK and white blood cell counts. NMS can be seen with the use of all neuroleptics, including the atypical[23].

The potential cardiovascular effects of these drugs include orthostatic hypotension and QRS prolongation, leading to an increased risk for torsade de pointe. Orthostasis is of especial concern in the elderly who, due to physiological changes, are already at increased risk. In addition, in those patients who are already suffering from orthostasis or who are being prescribed medications known to have pressure-lowering effects, low-potency neuroleptics should be avoided. Orthostatic hypotension places the elderly at increased risk of falls, leading to increased morbidity and mortality.

The anticholinergic effects of these drugs can have both troubling and undesired peripheral and central effects. Peripheral side effects include dry mouth and eyes, blurred vision, constipation, and urinary retention, which is of especial concern in males who have prostatic hypertrophy. Central effects include worsening of cognition, confusion and/or delirium[3,24]. One should be aware

Table 95.4 Recommended doses in the elderly

Drug	Initial dose	Maximum dose
Clozapine	6.25 mg/day	50–100 ng/day
Risperidone	0.25–0.50 mg/day	2 mg/day
Olanzapine	2.5 mg/day	5–10 mg/day
Quetiapine	25 mg/day	100–150 mg/day
Ziprasidone	20 mg/day	80–160 mg/day

that the atypical antipsychotics clozapine and olanzapine also have anticholinergic side effects.

An additional side effect of concern with the use of antipsychotics is photosensitivity in those patients who are on chlorpromazine. Patients may experience irreversible degenerative pigmentation retinopathy, caused by doses of thioridazine greater than 800 mg/day. Weight gain is of especial concern in those patients with an obesity problem or who are known to gain weight easily on medications. Weight gain can be seen with the use of both conventional and atypical antipsychotics.

Atypical Antipsychotics

Atypical antipsychotics are so defined because they are effective at treating both the positive and the negative symptoms of schizophrenia, while having a lower incidence of extrapyramidal symptoms and tardive dyskinesia. FDA-approved atypical antipsychotics are clozapine, risperidone, olanzapine, quetiapine and ziprasidone.

Clozapine

Clozapine was the first atypical antipsychotic approved for use in the USA. Compared to typical neuroleptics, it has a higher affinity for the dopamine D2 receptor, being more selective for the mesolimbic and mesocortical pathways. Clozapine continues to have a favorable neurological side-effect profile but is reported to have the following untoward effects: drowsiness, sedation, hypersalivation, tachycardia, dizziness, constipation, nausea and vomiting, the most concerning being agranulocytosis and seizures. It is recommended that clozapine treatment should be initiated only after a patient has failed two trials with conventional antipsychotics. In a double placebo-controlled study of six patients, clozapine was found to have similar efficacy as in younger patients. Although it was felt to be fairly safe in the elderly, the most frequent side effects were sedation, confusion and agranulocytosis[25].

Concern exists that the elderly may be at greater risk for agranulocytosis. In an Australian elderly study, the occurrence of agranulocytosis was found to be 4% compared to 0.25% in younger patients[25]. Increased sedation, hypersalivation, bradycardia, postural hypotension and delirium are frequent side effects reported in the elderly with the use of clozapine[26–28]. Another potential side effect is weight gain. One author found that 75% of the patients prescribed clozapine had gained an average of 7.5 kg[29]. The potential for agranulocytosis requires constant monitoring of blood, which may be difficult and costly in the elderly. Clozapine was tolerated as well as chlorpromazine in one study. In one open label report in 300 older adults, the discontinuation rate for clozapine was 43% and agranulocytosis occurred in two non-fatal cases[30].

Clozapine should be considered once a patient has failed two trials of conventional neuroleptics. When prescribing clozapine, it is prudent to initiate treatment with a dose of 6.25 mg/day, followed by weekly titration of 6.25 mg/day until a therapeutic effect is achieved and/or side effects develop[13,31]. Daily doses may range from 6.25 to 400 mg[31]. Clozapine should be initiated slowly and titrated slowly. Chengappa[26] has reported that the rapid titration of this drug can lead to drug intolerance and poor response.

Risperidone

Risperidone, a serotonin–dopamine antagonist, is an atypical antipsychotic that is a benzisoxasole derivative[32]. Risperidone has been found to be effective for the treatment of both positive and negative symptoms of schizophrenia, with minimal EPS. Risperidone has been studied extensively in the elderly[33,34]. It is a potent antagonist of the 5-HT receptor and less so of D2, with α-receptor blocking. In addition, it has minimal histaminergic blockade and practically no affinity for cholinergic receptors[35].

Side effects seen with this drug include orthostatic hypotension, sedation, fatigue and palpitations. Risperidone has dose-dependent incidence of EPS and TD. The incidence of sedation is in the range 6–15%[36–38]. There are no cardiac or laboratory abnormalities associated with this drug. Hypotension can be seen and should be carefully monitored in patients with pre-existing hypotension or who are on medications that have this effect. The 1 year incidence of TD seen in a large sample of elderly patients treated with risperidone was 2.6%[39].

Risperidone is the atypical antipsychotic most widely studied in the elderly. Most studies have favored the use of lower doses, finding them to be efficacious. In a study of patients who were diagnosed with dementia with behavioral disturbances, risperidone was found to be effective at doses of 1 mg/day; more adverse events were seen at doses of 2 mg/day[34]. These authors recommended the use of a serotonin–dopamine agonist when treating elderly patients with psychotic symptoms[34]. In a population of American veterans the average dose of risperidone was 3.6 mg/day compared to an average olanzapine dose of 10.2 mg/day[40] that EPS were reduced from baseline.

Risperidone has been found to be effective in treating both the negative and positive symptoms in patients with the diagnosis of schizophrenia and schizoaffective disorders. In a prospective open-label, 12 week study of 103 elderly patients who were diagnosed with schizophrenia or schizoaffective disorders the mean dose was 2.4 mg/day. An overall improvement of 45% was seen for both PANNS and CG[37]. The most frequently reported adverse events were dizziness, insomnia, agitation, somnolence, constipation and EPS. The authors concluded that risperidone was safe in this population but that doses should not be lower than 3 mg/day. Various authors have found risperidone to be a safe and efficacious treatment in this population[33,37,38]. In the medically ill elderly with psychotic symptoms, risperidone is also an effective and safe treatment. It does demonstrate dose-dependent EPS[37,41]. Risperidone treatment should be initiated at low doses (0.25 mg/day) and slowly titrated to a target dose of 1.5 mg/day for patients with dementia with psychotic symptoms. In elderly patients with psychosis, the optimal dose should be 2 mg/day. Risperidone in the elderly is an effective safe first-line treatment of psychosis.

Olanzapine

Olanzapine is a thienobenzodiazepine analog with an *in vitro* receptor affinity profile similar to clozapine. It is considered to be an atypical antipsychotic, as it is more effective than haloperidol in the treatment of both positive and negative symptoms of schizophrenia with minimal EPS[42]. Olanzapine affects the dopamine D1 and D4 receptors and the serotonin 2a and 2c receptors; it is well absorbed, with a mean half-life of 30 h, and is metabolized by the cyp 1a2, cyp2 D6 and flavin mono-oxygenase system. The CYP2D6 is a minimally involved system, thus there should be minimal concern for drug interactions with potent inhibitors of this system. Olanzapine has no active metabolite[42].

The most frequent untoward events seen with olanzapine are hypotension, constipation, weight gain, somnolence, agitation and dizziness[42]. It does have anticholinergic side effects, and can cause significant weight gain, which may be an advantage for those elderly patients who have suffered significant weight loss. The optimally recommended dose range is 2.5–15 mg/day.

An ad hoc study reviewing the olanzapine data in those over the age of 65 with psychotic disorders found no significant difference between the elderly and younger patients. Dose comparisons were similar for patients younger and older than 65[43,44]. A study using olanzapine in patients with dementia of the Alzheimer's type showed no difference in efficacy from the placebo group at doses in the range 1–8 mg/day. This same study found no difference in liver function test, EPS, leukopenia or orthostasis when compared to placebo[45]. Although olanzapine appears to have anticholinergic side effects, these were not significantly different from those seen in comparison to a placebo group[43]. Olanzapine was found to be well tolerated and safe in the elderly. Doses used are similar to those for younger patients; initial doses should be 2.5–5.0 mg/day. Olanzapine has the added advantage of once daily dosing.

Quetiapine

Another novel antipsychotic recently FDA-approved for use in the USA is quetiapine. Quetiapine is a dibenzothiazepine derivative. It exhibits higher affinity for 5-HT$_2$ receptors than for dopamine D2 receptors and is reported to have greater affinity for the mesolimbic than the nigrostriatal sites, thus accounting for its effect on positive symptoms with minimal EPS[46,47]. Quetiapine is reported to treat both the positive and negative symptoms of schizophrenia[46,47]. The incidence of EPS has been found to be minimally no different than placebo.

In a study of elderly patients with psychotic disorders, the average dose of quetiapine was 100 mg/day. In that same study the most frequent side effects found were somnolence (32%), dizziness (14%), postural hypotension (13%) and agitation (11%). However, from a cardiovascular perspective, the patients did exhibit a slight increase in their heart rate but there were no changes in the QRS complex. No hematological changes were noted, except for a non-significant slight increase in t4 not associated with substantial changes in the mean thyroid-stimulating hormone levels. Quetiapine was rarely associated with weight gain. These authors recommended starting at a dose of 25 mg/day and titrating to a target dose of 100 mg/day in divided doses. Most patients will be treated with doses in the range 100–300 mg/day, with an occasional patient requiring higher doses[46,48].

Ziprasidone

A new atypical antipsychotic currently awaiting FDA approval in the USA is ziprasidone. Ziprasidone is reported to have affinity for the dopamine D2 and D3 receptors and the agonist of 5-HT$_2$. It has negligible affinity for the other receptors of concern in the elderly, including α-2 and β-muscarinic; it moderately inhibits the reuptake of serotonin and norepinephrine but weakly effects the reuptake of dopamine[49,50]. This drug is potentially effective for both positive and negative symptoms and depression, with a low likelihood of causing EPS[49].

The following studies have looked at the use of ziprasidone in younger patients, the oldest being 64. Patients with acute exacerbation of schizophrenia and schizoaffective disorder had a better response than placebo on both 80 mg/day and 160 mg/day[50]. Often patients with these disorders are suffering from depression; in this same study 160 mg of ziprasidone was found to be effective to treat depression[50]. Other studies have reported that a dose of 120 mg/day was more effective than 40 mg/day. The side effects reported included dyspepsia, transient somnolence, constipation, nausea and abdominal pain[49]. Ziprasidone was associated with a lower incidence of EPS and postural hypotension, with no weight gain or laboratory abnormalities[49].

REFERENCES

1. American Psychiatric Association: *Diagnostic and Statistical Manual of Mental Disorders*, 4th edn. Washington, DC: American Psychiatric Association, 1994.

2. Myers JK, Weissman MM, Tischler G. Six month prevalence of psychiatric disorders in three communities. *Arch Gen Psychiat* 1984; **41**: 959–70.

3. Junginger J, Phelan E, Cherry K *et al.* Prevalence of psychopathology in elderly persons in nursing homes and in the community. *Hosp Commun Psychiat* 1993; **44**: 381–3.

4. Skoog I, Nilsson L, Landahl S *et al.* Mental disorders and the use of psychotropic drugs in an 85-year-old urban population. *Int Psychogeriat* 1993; **5**: 33–48.

5. Kotrla KJ, Chacko RC, Harper RG, Jhingran S, Doody R. SPECT findings on psychosis in Alzheimer's disease. *Am J Psychiat*. 1995; **152**(10): 147–5.

6. Burke D, Sushmita S. Early intervention in schizophrenia in the elderly. *Aust NZ J Psychiat* 1998; **32**: 809–14.

7. Lindamer LA, Lohr JB, Harris MJ *et al.* Gender related clinical differences in older patients with schizophrenia. *J Clin Psychiat* 1999; **60**: 61–7.

8. Lacro JP, Jeste DV. Geriatric psychosis. *Psychiat Qu* 1997; **68**: 247–60.

9. Harris MJ. Psychosis in late life spotting new-onset disorders in your elderly patients. *Postgrad Med* 1997; **102**: 139–42.

10. Ciompi L. Catamnestic long-term study on the course of life and aging of schizophrenics. *Schizophren Bull* 1980; **6**: 606–18.

11. Kim KY, Goldstein MZ. Treating older adults with psychotic symptoms. *Psychiat Serv* 1997; **48**: 1123–6.

12. Streim JE, Oslin D, Katz IR, Parmelee PA. Lessons from geriatric psychiatry in the long-term care setting. *Psychiat Q* 1997; **68**(3): 281–307.

13. Zayas E, Grossberg GT. The treatment of psychosis in late life. *J Clin Psychiat* 1998; **59**(5): 5–10.

14. Jeste DV, Harris MJ, Krull A *et al.* Clinical and neuropsychological characteristics of patients with late-onset schizophrenia. *Am J Psychiat* 1995; **152**: 722–30.

15. Ohi G, Kai I, Ichikawa S *et al.* Psychotic manifestation in the bed-fast elderly. *Hum Ergol* 1989; **18**: 237–40.

16. Eastwood MR, Corbin SL, Reed M *et al.* Acquired hearing loss and psychiatric illness: an estimate of prevalence and comorbidity in a geriatric setting. *Br J Psychiat* 1985; **147**: 552–6.

17. Caliguiri MP, Lacro JP, Jeste DV. Incidence and predictors of drug-induced parkinsonism in older psychiatric patients treated with very low doses of neuroleptics. *J Clin Psychopharmacol* 1999; **19**: 322–8.

18. Caliguiri MP, Rockwell E, Jeste DV. Extrapyramidal side effects in patients with Alzheimer's disease treated with low-dose neuroleptic medication. *Am J Geriat Psychiat* 1998; **6**: 75–82.

19. Tison F, Lecaroz J, Letenneur L *et al.* Parkinsonism and exposure to neuroleptic drugs in elderly people living in institutions. *Clin Neuropharmacol* 1999; **22**: 5–10.

20. Caliguiri MP, Lacro JP, Rockwell E *et al.* Incidence and risk factors for severe tardive dyskinesia in older patients. *Br J Psychiat* 1997; **171**: 148–53.

21. Woerner MG, Alvir JA, Saltz BL *et al.* Prospective study of tardive dyskinesia in the elderly: rates and risk factors. *Am J Psychiat* 1998; **155**: 1521–8.

22. Caliguiri MP, Lohr JB. Instrumental motor predictors of neuroleptic-induced parkinsonism in newly medicated schizophrenia patients. *J Neuropsychiat Clin Neurosci* 1997; **9**: 562–7.

23. Johnson V, Bruxner G. Neuroleptic malignant syndrome associated with olanzapine. *Aust NZ J Psychiat* 1998; **32**: 884–6.

24. Brown FW. Late-life psychosis: making the diagnosis and controlling symptoms. *Geriatrics*. 1998; **53**(12): 26–8, 37–8, 41–2.

25. Herst L, Powell G. Is clozapine safe in the elderly? *Aust NZ J Psychiat* 1997; **31**: 411–17.

26. Chengappa KNR, Baker RW, Kreinbrook SB *et al.* Clozapine use in female geriatric patients with psychoses. *J Geriat Psychiat Neurol* 1995; **8**: 12–15.

27. Salzman C, Vaccaro B, Lieff J *et al.* Clozapine in older patients with psychosis and behavioural disruption. *Am J Geriat Psychiat* 1995; **3**: 26–33.

28. Pitner JK, Mintzer JE, Pennypacker LC *et al.* Efficacy and adverse effects of clozapine in four elderly psychotic patients. *J Clin Psychiat* 1995; **56**: 180–5.

29. Briffa D, Meehan T. Weight changes during clozapine treatment. *Aust NZ J Psychiat* 1998; **32**: 718–21.

30. Sajatovic M, Ramirez LF, Garver D *et al.* Clozapine therapy for older veterans. *Psych Serv* 1998; **49**: 340–4.

31. Sajatovic M, Ramirez L. Clozapine therapy in patients with neurologic illness. *Int J Psychiat Med*. 1995; **25**(4): 331–44.

32. Janssen PA, Niemegeers CJ, Awouters F, Schellekens KH, Megens AA, Meert TF. Pharmacology of risperidone (R 64 766), a new antipsychotic with serotonin-S2 and dopamine-D2 antagonistic properties. *J Pharmacol Exp Ther*. 1988; **244**(2): 685–93.

33. Sajatovic M, Ramirez LF, Vernon L *et al.* Outcome of risperidone in the treatment of elderly patients with chronic psychosis. *Int J Psychiat Med* 1996; **57**(3): 39–45.

34. Katz IR, Jeste DV, Mintzer JE *et al.* Comparison of risperidone and placebo for psychosis and behavioral disturbances associated with dementia: a randomized, double-blind trial. *J Clin Psychiat* 1999; **60**: 107–15.

35. Grossberg GT, Manepalli J. The older patient with psychotic symptoms. *Psychiat Serv*. 1995; **46**(1): 55–9.

36. Madhusoodanan S, Brenner R, Araujo L, Abaza A. Efficacy of risperidone treatment for psychoses associated with schizophrenia, schizoaffective disorder, bipolar disorder, or senile dementia in 11 geriatric patients: a case series. *J Clin Psychiat*. 1995; **56**(11): 514–8.

37. Madhusoodanan S, Brecher M, Brenner R, Kasckow J, Kunik M, Negron AE, Pomara N. Risperidone in the treatment of elderly patients with psychotic disorders. *Am J Geriatr Psychiat*. 1999; **7**(2): 132–8.

38. Madhusoodanan S. Risperidone and Cognitive Functioning in Elderly Schizophrenic Patients (Dr. Madhusoodanan comments). *Am J Geriatr Psychiat*. 2000; **8**(2): 178–9.

39. Fischer P, Tauscher J, Kufferle B. Risperidone and tardive dyskinesia in organic psychosis. *Pharmacopsychiatry*. 1998; **31**(2): 70–1.

40. Voris JC, Glazer WM. Use of risperidone and olanzapine in outpatient clinics at six veterans affairs hospitals. *Psychiat Serv* 1999; **50**(2): 163–8.

41. Zarate CA, Baldessarini RJ, Siegel AJ *et al.* Risperidone in the elderly: a pharmacologic study. *J Clin Psychiat* 1997; **58**: 311–17.

42. Stephenson CM, Pilowsky LS. Psychopharmacology of olanzapine. A review. *Br J Psychiatry Suppl*. 1999; (38): 52–8.

43. Street JS, Tollefson GD, Tohen M *et al.* Olanzapine for psychotic conditions in the elderly. *Psychiat Ann* 2000; **30**(3): 191–6.

44. Tollefson GD, Beasly CM, Tran PV *et al.* Olanzapine vs. haloperidol in the treatment of schizophrenia and schizoaffective and schizophreniform disorders: results of an international collaborative trial. *Am J Psychiat* 1997; **154**: 457–65.

45. Beasley CM Jr, Sanger T, Satterlee W, Tollefson G, Tran P, Hamilton S. Olanzapine versus placebo: results of a double-blind, fixed-dose olanzapine trial. *Psychopharmacology (Berl)*. 1996; **124**(1–2): 159–67.

46. McManus DQ, Arvantis LA, Kowalcyk BB. Quetiapine, a novel antipsychotic: experience in elderly patients with psychotic disorders. *J Clin Psychiat* 1999; **60**: 292–8.

47. Tariot PN, Salzman C, Yeung PP, Pultz J, Rak IW. Long-Term use of quetiapine in elderly patients with psychotic disorders. *Clin Ther*. 2000; **22**(9): 1068–84.

48. Tariot PN, Salzman C, Yeung PP *et al.* Clinical improvement and tolerability is maintained long term in elderly patients with psychotic disorders treated with seroquel (quetiapine). *Eur Neuropsychopharmacol* 1999; **9**(5): S268.

49. Keck P, Buffenstein A, Ferguson J *et al.* Ziprasidone 40 and 120 mg/day in the acute exacerbation of schizophrenia and schizoaffective disorder: a 4 week placebo-controlled trial. *Psychopharmacology* 1998; **140**: 173–84.

50. Daniel DG, Zimbroff DL, Potkin SG *et al.* Ziprasidone 80 mg/day and 160 mg/day in the acute exacerbation of schizophrenia and schizoaffective disorder: a 6-week placebo-controlled trial. *Neuropsychopharmacology* 1999; **20**(5): 491–505.

51. Gregory C, McKenna P. Pharmacological management of schizophrenia in older patients. *Drugs Aging* 1994; **5**: 254–62.

52. McKeith I, Fairbain A, Perry R *et al.* Neuroleptic sensitivity in patients with senile dementia of the Lewy body type. *Br Med J* 1992; **305**: 673–8.

53. Schneider LS. Pharmacologic management of psychosis in dementia. *J Clin Psychiat* 1999; **60**(8): 54–60.

96

Risk Factors for Dyskinesia in the Elderly

Thomas R. E. Barnes

Imperial College School of Medicine, London, UK

TARDIVE DYSKINESIA

Clinical Features

In the mid-1950s, within a few years of the introduction of antipsychotic drugs, clinicians drew attention to "neurotoxic reactions" to this treatment. In addition to parkinsonian features, involuntary orofacial movements were noted[1,2]. Sigwald et al.[3] are usually credited with the first detailed description of "facio-bucco-linguomasticatory dyskinesia" associated with these drugs. In the early 1960s, Faurbye et al.[4] coined the term "tardive dyskinesia" for this condition.

Abnormal involuntary orofacial movements remain the most familiar and prevalent features of tardive dyskinesia. The movements are irregular, stereotyped and choreic in nature, and tend to involve the tongue, lips, jaw and face, including the peri-orbital areas. The movements observed include protrusion or twisting of the tongue, lip smacking, cheek puffing, pursing and sucking actions of the lips, and chewing and lateral jaw motions. The particular combinations of movement seen vary considerably between patients but tend to be relatively consistent for each individual.

In addition to these orofacial phenomena, most descriptions of tardive dyskinesia include a variety of trunk and limb movements. These are typically choreiform or choreoathetoid in type, although athetosis of extremities, and axial and limb dystonia, are often listed as part of the syndrome, as are abnormalities of gait and trunk posture, such as lordosis, rocking and swaying, shoulder shrugging and rotary movements of the pelvis. Grunting and respiratory arrhythmias are also seen.

The notion that orofacial and limb and trunk dyskinesia represent distinct pathophysiological entities with different risk factors and clinical correlates[5] seems to hold true in older patients[6]. For example, Paulsen et al.[7] studied middle-aged and elderly outpatients starting antipsychotic drug treatment and obtained systematic follow-up data over 2 years. They found that the cumulative incidences and the significant predictors identified differed for the two subsyndromes.

Prevalence, Incidence and Natural History

While tardive dyskinesia is a common problem in those individuals receiving antipsychotic drug treatment long-term, the majority will not exhibit the condition. The reported prevalence figures vary widely, from 0.5% to 56%[8,9], reflecting variables such as the age of the sample studied (see below) and the sensitivity of the rating instrument used. Overall, the literature suggests that

only 20% or so of drug treated patients will develop the problem, and of these, the dyskinesia is likely to be serious in less than 10%. Gardos et al.[10] concluded that the severe tardive dyskinesia is very uncommon, occurring in approximately 1/100–1/1000 patients with the condition. Nevertheless, in elderly psychiatric inpatients, prevalence figures of around 50% or greater are not uncommonly reported[6].

The prospective study of Kane et al.[11,12] suggested that new cases of tardive dyskinesia can occur at a rate of 3–4% a year in the first few years after starting antipsychotic medication. However, there is only limited information available to guide the clinician as to who might be most at risk. Tardive dyskinesia was originally considered irreversible, although follow-up studies[13,14] have revealed that it is not a progressive disorder, but rather tends to fluctuate in severity over time. Spontaneous remissions are relatively common, particularly in younger patients. Such a view of the natural history of tardive dyskinesia in patients on chronic drug treatment was reinforced by the results of two 10 year follow-up studies by Yagi and Itoh[15] and Casey and Gardos[16].

To some degree, these findings might be seen as relatively reassuring, allaying earlier fears that tardive dyskinesia was a major iatrogenic condition that would constrain the use of long-term antipsychotic drug therapy. However, while the condition itself is rarely disabling, it can be socially stigmatizing. Further, severe tardive dyskinesia can be a troublesome problem, particularly in the elderly. Orofacial dyskinesia can interfere with eating and swallowing, render speech unintelligible, and cause breathing difficulties, sometimes leading to dysphagia or choking[17–19]. Trunk and limb dyskinesia may be associated with disturbances of gait that can lead to falls and injury[20].

RISK FACTORS

Advancing Age

In numerous studies, advancing age has been clearly shown to be a major vulnerability factor for tardive dyskinesia. It is associated not only with an increased occurrence of tardive dyskinesia but also with greater severity and a reduced likelihood of spontaneous remission[9,21]. Studies involving geriatric patients have consistently found a higher incidence of tardive dyskinesia with conventional antipsychotics, even at low doses[22,23]. Examining pooled epidemiological data has revealed a strong linear correlation between age and both the prevalence and severity of tardive dyskinesia[24]. However, duration of exposure to antipsychotic drugs is a confounding variable, as older patients are likely to have received drug treatment for longer; i.e. age-group and length of time on drug treatment would be expected to be linked. Nevertheless, clinical studies have consistently shown an effect of age independent of that attributed to length of drug treatment[9,13]. Further, it would seem that the older patients are when they first receive antipsychotic medication, the more likely they are to develop the condition early in treatment[25]. This was dramatically demonstrated in a prospective study of tardive dyskinesia in patients 55 years or older who were just beginning antipsychotic drug treatment[26]. These investigators initially presented preliminary data on 160 patients[27] and subsequently reported on the complete study group of 261 patients[26]. Patients were assessed at 3 month intervals. After approximately 1, 2 and 3 years of cumulative exposure to antipsychotic medication, the incidence figures for tardive dyskinesia in the larger sample were 25%, 34% and 53%, respectively. These investigators concluded that the rate of tardive dyskinesia for patients over 50 years of age starting antipsychotic drug treatment was three to five times that reported in younger adults.

Much of the variation in incidence and prevalence figures reported in the published literature is likely to be due to age differences in the sample studied[9]. The results of a 3 year follow-up study of tardive dyskinesia by Barnes et al.[13] suggested that patients receiving antipsychotic drugs may be most likely to develop the condition in their sixth decade. Jeste et al.[28] calculated that in the sample of chronically ill, schizophrenic inpatients they studied, the probability of having tardive dyskinesia was greater than 0.4 in those patients over 65 years old. In their review of the literature, Smith and Baldessarini[24] pointed out that the rise in prevalence with age may partly reflect the relative persistence of tardive dyskinesia in older patients. They concluded that tardive dyskinesia in those less than 60 years of age was over three times more likely to remit spontaneously. However, as the relevant studies included patients either withdrawn from antipsychotic medication or on extended "drug holidays", this conclusion partly reflects the reversibility of the condition after drugs are discontinued. Younger patients appear to possess a greater recovery potential when medication is withdrawn, but whether they show a higher spontaneous remission rate than older patients when maintained on chronic antipsychotic drug therapy remains unconfirmed. Work with an animal model of tardive dyskinesia suggests that spontaneously remitting dyskinesia emerging early in drug treatment can become irreversible with prolonged drug therapy[29].

Antipsychotic Medication

While it seems plausible that the relationship between exposure to antipsychotic treatment and vulnerability to tardive dyskinesia varies with age, such a relationship has not been systematically tested. In the minority of studies where a relationship between specific drug variables and tardive dyskinesia has been found, it has tended to be within the first few years of treatment[9,11], particularly in studies of elderly populations[30–32]. For example, Jeste et al.[21] studied 266 patients over 45 years of age receiving conventional antipsychotic medication. At baseline, the median duration of total lifetime antipsychotic exposure was only 21 days. Over the first 3 years, the cumulative incidence of tardive dyskinesia was 26%, 52% and 60%, respectively. The main risk factors for the appearance of tardive dyskinesia included baseline duration of antipsychotic treatment of over 90 days, and the cumulative amount of antipsychotic medication prescribed, particularly "high-potency" drugs. This group of investigators[33] also examined risk factors specifically for severe tardive dyskinesia. In a prospective study of 378 older neuropsychiatric patients over 3 years, the incidence of severe tardive dyskinesia was 2.5%

in the first year, 12% in the second and 23% in the third. As in the earlier study, higher daily doses of antipsychotic medication at baseline and greater cumulative amount of prescribed antipsychotic emerged as risk factors. In the study by Woerner et al.[26] mentioned above, higher mean daily dose of antipsychotic and cumulative dosage were also found to be associated with a greater risk of developing tardive dyskinesia.

The mechanisms whereby advancing age exerts an influence on susceptibility to tardive dyskinesia remain speculative. It is possible that neuropathological and/or neurochemical changes occurring with age may be associated with an increasing prevalence of tardive dyskinesia. Neuronal damage or degeneration, receptor changes and the reduced efficiency of adaptive homeostatic processes may well underlie the vulnerability of certain drug-induced neurological side effects in older patients. The development of supersensitive post-synaptic dopamine receptors in the basal ganglia remains the accepted explanation of the pathophysiology of tardive dyskinesia. However, such supersensitivity would seem to be an inevitable consequence of prolonged antipsychotic drug treatment, and is therefore insufficient to explain why only a proportion of patients on long-term medication develop dyskinesia[34]. An interaction between drug-induced receptor changes in the striatum, and age-related degenerative effects in the nigrostriatal system may be necessary for the appearance of tardive dyskinesia.

Pharmacokinetic mechanisms could also be relevant. Age-related changes in the absorption, metabolism and excretion of drugs may lead to higher plasma drug levels and delayed clearance. Plasma levels of antipsychotic drugs have been found to be raised in the elderly, compared with younger patients[35,36].

Atypical Antipsychotics

The newer, atypical antipsychotics are characterized by a lower liability for extrapyramidal side effects and, for some of these agents, evidence is emerging for a lower risk of tardive dyskinesia[37]. However, thus far, there have only been a few studies addressing the safety and tolerability of these drugs, at appropriate dosage, in the elderly. For reasons addressed briefly above, the findings of clinical trials in young adults may not be reliably extrapolated to the elderly, for whom dosage requirements tend to be lower[38,39]. Preliminary clinical data suggest that newer agents such as risperidone and olanzapine may be relatively well tolerated in older people[40] and there have been similar claims for low-dose clozapine[41], but well-designed, controlled studies in the elderly are required[42,43].

In respect of tardive dyskinesia risk in the elderly, risperidone has been the atypical antipsychotic most commonly studied. Over a period of 9 months, Jeste et al.[44] found a significantly lower incidence of tardive dyskinesia in older patients treated with risperidone as opposed to haloperidol. The patients were middle-aged or elderly (mean age 66 years) and had not received previous treatment with antipsychotics. "Clinically comparable" groups receiving treatment with either risperidone or haloperidol were compared. The median dose for both drugs was 1 mg/day. The haloperidol-treated patients proved to be significantly more likely to develop tardive dyskinesia. A further study by the same group of investigators[45] addressed the risk of persistent tardive dyskinesia with risperidone in elderly patients with dementia. In an open study, a sample of 330 patients (mean age 82.5 years) received risperidone in flexible dosage (mean modal dose 0.96 mg/day) over a year. Amongst the 255 patients with no evidence of tardive dyskinesia at baseline, the 1 year cumulative incidence of the condition was 2.6%, and patients who had exhibited dyskinesia at baseline experienced significant improvement. The investigators concluded that such an incidence was much lower than would be expected with conventional antipsychotic treatment in such patients. A similar conclusion was reached by Davidson et al.[46], who conducted an open study of risperidone in a sample of 180 elderly, chronically-ill, psychotic patients (median age 72 years) over 1 year; 97 of those in the sample received risperidone for the full 12 months. At the endpoint, the mean dose of risperidone was 3.7 mg/day. Only six cases of persistent tardive dyskinesia emerged during the study period, representing an incidence of 4.3%.

Preliminary evidence also raises expectations of a relatively lower risk of tardive dyskinesia in the elderly with olanzapine[18,47] and possibly quetiapine[18].

Gender

A relatively consistent finding has been that women show a greater prevalence of severe dyskinesia, although there is evidence to suggest that this is limited to the geriatric age range, that is, over 60 years of age[9,48,49] and the more severe cases[50,51]. The ability to detect a significant effect for gender is probably related to the size of the study sample and the base rate of tardive dyskinesia in the population being studied. Nevertheless, Smith and Dunn[52] identified 13 studies reporting statistically significant differences supporting female vulnerability, with the average unweighted female:male prevalence ratio in the patient samples being 1.69.

For example, Ramsay and Millard[53], in a sample of 426 elderly subjects, predominantly geriatric or psychogeriatric inpatients, found dyskinetic movements in 12.5% of women but only 7.6% of men. In a sample of patients over 65 years with senile dementia of the Alzheimer type, O'Keane and Dinan[54] found that significantly more females (89%) had evidence of orofacial dyskinesia compared with the males (60%). However, the prospective study of tardive dyskinesia in the elderly, conducted by Woerner et al.[26], failed to find a significant relationship between sex and incidence of the condition. Indeed, the incidence was slightly higher for males, although they were significantly younger than the females.

Richardson et al.[55] reported that females showed an increase in prevalence of tardive dyskinesia in all age groups up to and beyond 75 years, while males only demonstrated an increase up to 75 years, with a decline subsequently. The differences in prevalence between the sexes was minimal up to 64 years using mild severity to define a case, but female prevalence was substantially higher when a criterion of moderate to high severity was applied. These findings support the view that the magnitude of sex differences in tardive dyskinesia is dependent on the severity of the criteria used to define the disorder, as well as the age of the sample[50,51].

As a vulnerability factor, gender is far weaker than age, with which there seems to be an interaction. There is no clear explanation for the female preponderance, although it has been suggested that neuroendocrine factors may be relevant. Oestrogen and prolactin may influence striatal dopamine function[56], and the reduced ovarian function in post-menopausal women, with low oestradiol levels, may increase vulnerability to tardive dyskinesia[57,58]. However, rather than a direct reflection of gender, it has been variously speculated that female sex is a proxy variable for longer duration of hospitalization, higher drug dose and longer duration of treatment.

Organicity

Reviews of the risk factors for tardive dyskinesia[59–61] suggest that in patients with schizophrenia, evidence of "organicity" is a marker of vulnerability to tardive dyskinesia. Putative, indirect indices of organicity, such as soft neurological signs and cognitive impairment, computed tomography (CT) evidence of structural brain pathology and the presence of negative symptoms, have all been found more commonly in patients with tardive dyskinesia than those without. Thus, ageing may be a predisposing factor for tardive dyskinesia only insofar as it increases the likelihood of organic brain dysfunction.

Hunter et al.[62] and Crane and Paulson[63] surveyed mixed psychiatric inpatient populations and found tardive dyskinesia to be more prevalent in patients with organic mental syndromes than in those with schizophrenia. Yassa et al.[64] conducted a similar study, assessing over 300 psychiatric patients treated with antipsychotic drugs. They also found that patients with organic mental syndromes, including those diagnosed as epilepsy with psychosis and mental retardation with psychosis or alcoholism, showed a significantly higher prevalence of tardive dyskinesia compared to those with schizophrenia. A number of organic mental syndromes and neuromedical conditions, such as multi-infarct dementia, strokes and cerebral tumour, are more common in older individuals, and this may partly explain why the prevalence of tardive dyskinesia is greater in elderly samples[65,66]. However, any such hypothesis should take account of the influence of the range of other psychiatric diagnosis in such samples. For example, Yassa et al.[64] found that patients with a primary bipolar affective disorder had the same prevalence of tardive dyskinesia as those with organic mental syndromes. In their prospective study in the elderly, Woerner et al.[26] reported that the risk of tardive dyskinesia in individuals with multi-infarct dementia was similar to that for people with mood disorder, while patients with Alzheimer's disease and other organic mental syndromes showed a lower rate.

Psychiatric Diagnosis

Affective Disorder

Recent work has highlighted affective disturbance as a possible relevant variable. Both a positive family history of affective disorder and the presence of depressive features in patients with schizophrenia have been mooted as markers of an increased likelihood of developing both parkinsonian side effects and tardive dyskinesia, but the evidence is tentative at present. However, there is accumulating evidence that patients with primary affective disorder may be at particular risk of tardive dyskinesia if administered antipsychotic drugs long-term. A report by Davis et al.[67] noted the relatively high prevalence of tardive dyskinesia among such patients and this has been confirmed by later studies[68–70].

The preliminary data from the prospective study of tardive dyskinesia by Kane et al.[19] provides additional support for a diagnosis of affective disorder as a vulnerability factor. A life-table analysis based on the length of drug administration, and comparing the cumulative incidence of tardive dyskinesia in patients with affective or schizoaffective disorder with that of inpatients with a diagnosis of schizophrenia, revealed that the former have a significantly greater incidence after 6 years of exposure to antipsychotic drugs. The incidence figures were 26% for the affective and schizoaffective patients compared with 18% for those with schizophrenia. Further evidence was provided by Mukherjee et al.[71], who found persistent tardive dyskinesia in 35% of a sample of bipolar patients who had received maintenance antipsychotic drugs, while no patients without such a drug history had persistent dyskinesia.

Schizophrenia

The schizophrenic illness itself may be a risk factor[59,61]. Long before the advent of antipsychotic drugs, a variety of motor disorders were described in psychiatric patients, particularly those with catatonic schizophrenia[72-74] and other types of schizophrenia[75-77]. These movements would seem to be principally disturbances of voluntary motor activity and may be classified as stereotypes and mannerisms, preservative movements, tics, grimaces and general clumsiness, awkwardness and lack of coordination. However, Kraepelin[78], and then later Farran-Ridge[75], observed spasmodic movements, mainly involving the orofacial muscles, which they considered choreiform in nature.

Nevertheless, Marsden et al.[79] concluded that true chorea and athetosis were scarce in chronic psychiatric patients before drug treatment, and that much of the motor disorder seen was attributable to organic neurological disorder, such as encephalitis and syphilis. Further, the terminology used is confused, reflecting various conceptual notions of the aetiology of the motor phenomena observed[80,81]. Kleist[73] and Farran-Ridge[75] commented that the similarity between the manifestations of dementia praecox and epidemic encephalitis was such that difficulties in differential diagnosis could arise. However, there is no doubt that some of the movements described would be scored on current rating scales for tardive dyskinesia if seen now in patients receiving antipsychotic drugs.

There would seem to be three possible interpretations of these observations[59]. First, the type of motor disturbance historically described is not specifically associated with schizophrenia, but rather the product of organic brain disease. The two conditions also occur together when the brain disease is also responsible for symptomatic schizophrenia, as, for example, when schizophrenia appears in patients with encephalitis, Wilson's disease or Huntington's disease, among other conditions[82]. Second, the association of motor disturbance and schizophrenia may be more specific, in that an underlying neuropathological process is capable of producing both psychological and motor impairments. Third, as Kraepelin and Bleuler tended to suggest, the movements may be secondary to the schizophrenic disturbance of will, thought and emotion. However, the distinctions between the three explanations cannot be too sharply drawn, and more than one may be relevant.

In a relevant contemporary study, Owens et al.[83] compared chronic schizophrenia inpatients with and without a history of antipsychotic drug treatment, and found a similar prevalence of abnormal involuntary movements in the two groups. This finding confirmed the occurrence of spontaneous movement disorder in schizophrenia. However, the contribution of drug therapy was acknowledged, in that when the age difference between the two patient samples was taken into account in further analysis of the data, there was a significant linear relationship between the prevalence of abnormal involuntary movements and exposure to antipsychotic drugs[84]. Grouping movements into clinically recognizable syndromes revealed a particular susceptibility to orofacial dyskinesia in the drug-treated patients. Nevertheless, the schizophrenic illness, at least in some forms, may be seen as a psychomotor disorder with an inherent, increased risk of dyskinesia. Antipsychotic drug treatment may interact with the disease process and age-related cerebral deterioration to hasten or provoke the appearance of such movement disorder[59,85].

Dementia

Accepting that organicity is a risk factor for tardive dyskinesia, it might be expected that the neurodegenerative changes of Alzheimer's disease would be associated with a relatively high risk of spontaneous dyskinesia and also a greater risk of tardive dyskinesia when antipsychotic drugs are administered. Molsa et al.[86] assessed abnormal involuntary movements in 177 patients with Alzheimer's disease, with a mean age of 75 years. In the 143 patients who had never received antipsychotic drugs, the prevalence of dyskinesia was 17%, while for the 34 patients treated with antipsychotic drugs the figure was 53%. As part of a larger study, Ramsay and Milard[53] looked at 40 patients on long-stay psychogeriatric wards. Of the 13 (32.5%) patients with dyskinesia, 12 had a history of treatment with antipsychotic drugs. These findings suggest a vulnerability to tardive dyskinesia in dementia patients receiving antipsychotic drugs.

O'Keane and Dinan[54] assessed 78 patients with an age range of 65–91 years, all of whom fulfilled DSM-III criteria for senile dementia of the Alzheimer type. The scales used included the Mini-Mental State (MMS)[87] and Abnormal Involuntary Movements Scale (AIMS)[88]. They reported that 62 patients (69%) had evidence of orofacial dyskinesia, a figure the authors noted to be over 10 times that reported in healthy elderly adults, and also considerably higher than the prevalence found in populations of patients with chronic schizophrenia. Orofacial dyskinesia was by far the most common abnormal movement rated. The mean doses of antipsychotic drug for those with and without abnormal movements were modest, and although the former group was receiving a higher mean dosage, the differences between the two groups was not statistically significant.

Molsa et al.[86] found that the severity of orofacial dyskinesia in their sample of patients with Alzheimer's disease increased with the degree of cognitive deficit. Bakchine et al.[89] studied a group of 91 patients with dementia of the Alzheimer type and examined the relationships between primitive reflexes, extrapyramidal symptoms and severity of cognitive impairment. They failed to find any significant relationship between "buccolinguofacial dyskinesias" and a low score on intellectual functioning, but their methodology was criticized by O'Keane and Dinan[54], who pointed out that they only rated abnormal movement as either present or absent, rather than qualifying the movements using a standardized scale. In their own study O'Keane and Dinan found that there were no significant differences in terms of age or length of illness between those patients with and without abnormal movements, and both groups showed evidence of severe intellectual impairment. However, those patients with abnormal movements had a significantly greater degree of cognitive impairment, as judged on mean MMS scores. On the basis of this finding, O'Keane and Dinan suggested that orofacial dyskinesia might prove to be a useful indicator of the severity of intellectual decline in patients with Alzheimer's disease.

Acute Extrapyramidal Side Effects: Parkinsonism and Akathisia

Susceptibility to acute drug-induced extrapyramidal side effects as a predictor of tardive dyskinesia was first suggested by Crane in 1972[90]. He considered that tardive dyskinesia was more likely to emerge in patients who had developed parkinsonism as an acute side effect of antipsychotic drug treatment than in those who had not.

Based on clinical observation, Chouinard et al.[91] suggested that patients with tremor or akathisia, which they described as "hyperkinetic" symptoms of parkinsonism, were more likely to manifest tardive dyskinesia than patients with "hypokinetic" symptoms, such as bradykinesia and rigidity. De Veaugh-Geiss et al.[92] elaborated on this idea, suggesting that in some cases akathisia represented a stage in a progression from parkinsonism to the development of orofacial and trunk and limb dyskinesia. Consistent with this notion, Barnes and Braude[93] reported two cases where the appearance of akathisia at the beginning of drug therapy, which then persisted despite the reduction of drug dosage to maintenance levels, seemed to herald the early onset of tardive dyskinesia.

Thus, a variety of study findings and case reports suggest that patients presenting with symptoms of parkinsonism and acute akathisia are more likely to manifest tardive dyskinesia. More convincing evidence is available from a prospective study of risk factors for tardive dyskinesia carried out by Kane et al.[11]. Analysis of the data from the first 5 years of their follow-up study suggested that a history of early, clinically significant parkinsonism indicated susceptibility to the subsequent development of tardive dyskinesia, particularly for those patients developing tardive dyskinesia within the first 2 years of exposure to antipsychotic drugs. The patients in this study were relatively young, the mean age of the 800 patients originally recruited being 27 years. Further supportive evidence was provided by the prospective studies of elderly patients conducted by these investigators[26,27]. Individuals exhibiting signs of acute extrapyramidal side effects, i.e. parkinsonism and akathisia, early in treatment with antipsychotic drugs showed a greater vulnerability to tardive dyskinesia.

If susceptibility to akathisia is associated with susceptibility to tardive dyskinesia, it might be expected that the two conditions would commonly coexist in patients chronically treated with antipsychotics. Several studies have found this to be the case[13,94]. For example, Barnes and Braude[95] reported that 39% of schizophrenic outpatients with chronic akathisia also had orofacial dyskinesia. Further, out of 52 cases of chronic akathisia, Burke et al.[96] found that all but one had either orofacial dyskinesia (63%), tardive dystonia (8%) or both (27%). Dufresne and Wagner[97] also reported an association between the two conditions. In 33 chronic schizophrenic patients, these investigators found that the mean AIMS score (see earlier) was significantly higher in those patients with akathisia compared with those without the condition.

SPONTANEOUS DYSKINESIA

A condition described as spontaneous or idiopathic orofacial dyskinesia has been noted in psychiatric inpatients, predominantly elderly, who have never received antipsychotic drugs[8,98–100]. The prevalence figures in the literature vary from 0% to around 37%, but it is not always clear whether the hyperkinetic movements disorders reported represent senile chorea, spontaneous orofacial dyskinesia or senile dyskinesia[101,102]. These spontaneous orofacial movements show an increase in incidence with age. In a sample of 661 patients, Klawans and Barr[103] found a prevalence of 0.8% between the ages of 50 and 59, 6% between 60 and 69 years, and nearly 8% in patients between 70 to 79 years.

Crane[104] has stated that "chronicity of disease and/or institutionalization with attendant emotional and physical deprivation" may be responsible for these abnormal movements, being a common factor in both drug-treated and non-drug-treated psychiatric inpatients. Nevertheless, Altrocchi[105] reported two outpatients presenting with spontaneous orofacial dyskinesia, and this condition has also been observed as a relatively rare phenomenon in non-psychiatric, drug-free residents in old-age homes[48,49]. It has been estimated that this condition is present in some 2% of the geriatric home population[106,107], although Varga et al.[108] surveyed a population of elderly people never exposed to antipsychotic drugs and discovered that 10% had clear evidence of oral dyskinesia. In a similar sample, Bourgeois et al.[109,110] found that 18% exhibited "buccolinguofacial dyskinesia". These cases of spontaneous orofacial dyskinesia are generally considered to be indistinguishable from orofacial tardive dyskinesia, although

subtle differences in the distribution of movements have been detected between elderly psychiatric patients who were receiving antipsychotic drugs and normal elderly individuals who were drug-naïve[111].

Blowers et al.[112] surveyed 500 elderly residents in local authority homes using the AIMS. Out of the 378 individuals who had never received antipsychotic drugs, 50 (15%) were diagnosed as having "tardive dyskinesia" as they scored 3 or more on the AIMS global assessment scale. However, the AIMS may have limitations as a diagnostic scale[113,114].

These data generally suggest that elderly individuals are at a greater risk of spontaneous dyskinesias and abnormal involuntary movements related to various neurological and medical conditions independent of antipsychotic drugs. Nevertheless, surveys of normal elderly subjects suggest that spontaneous dyskinesias are relatively uncommon in the absence of brain disease or dysfunction.

SUMMARY

Elderly individuals would seem to be particularly vulnerable to the development of tardive dyskinesia when administered antipsychotic drugs, with females and those patients with dementia, other neurodegenerative conditions and organic brain syndromes being perhaps especially at risk. A diagnosis of affective disorder and the development of acute extrapyramidal side effects, such as parkinsonism and akathisia, when starting antipsychotic medication should also serve as warnings of a higher risk for tardive dyskinesia observed in elderly populations. Preliminary data suggest that use of the newer atypical antipsychotics, rather than conventional antipsychotics, in the elderly may substantially reduce the proportion developing tardive dyskinesia. A proportion of the orofacial dyskinesia observed in elderly populations, between 5% and 15% according to the majority of studies, will be spontaneous dyskinesia of the elderly. This is a condition virtually indistinguishable from tardive dyskinesia.

REFERENCES

1. Ey H, Faure H, Rappard P. Les réactions de tolérance vis à vis de la chlorpromazine. L'Encéphale 1956; 45: 790–6.
2. Schonecker M. Ein eigentumliches Syndrome im oralen Bereich bei Megaphenappilkation. Nervenarzt 1957; 28: 35–42.
3. Sigwald J, Bouthier D, Raymondeaud U et al. Quatre cas de dyskinsie facio-bucco-linguomasticatrice à évolution prolongée secondaire a traitement par les neuroleptiques. Rev Neurol 1959; 100: 751–5.
4. Faurbye A, Rasch PJ, Petersen PB et al. Neurological symptoms in pharmacotherapy of psychoses. Acta Psychiat Scand 1964; 40: 10–27.
5. Barnes TRE. Movement disorder associated with antipsychotic drugs: the tardive syndromes. Int Rev Psychiat 1990; 2: 355–66.
6. Byne W, White L, Parella M et al. Tardive dyskinesia in a chronically institutionalized population of elderly schizophrenic patients: prevalence and association with cognitive impairment. Int J Geriat Psychiat 1998; 13: 473–9.
7. Paulsen JS, Caligiuri MP, Palmer B et al. Risk factors for orofacial and limbtruncal tardive dyskinesia in older patients: a prospective longitudinal study. Psychopharmacology 1996; 123: 307–14.
8. Tepper SJ, Haas JF. Prevalence of tardive dyskinesia. J Clin Psychiat 1979; 40: 508–16.
9. Kane JM, Smith JM. Tardive dyskinesia: prevalence and risk factors, 1959–1979. Arch Gen Psychiat 1982; 39: 473–81.
10. Gardos G, Cole JO, Salmon M et al. Clinical forms of severe tardive dyskinesia. Am J Psychiat 1987; 144: 895–902.
11. Kane JM, Woerner M, Lieberman J. Tardive dyskinesia: prevalence, incidence and risk factors. In Casey DE, Chase TN, Christensen AV, Gerlach J, eds, Dyskinesia Research and Treatment. Berlin: Springer-Verlag, 1985: 72–8.

12. Kane JM, Woerner M, Lieberman J. Epidemiological aspects of tardive dyskinesia. *L'Encéphale* 1988; **XIV**: 191–4.

13. Barnes TRE, Kidger T, Gore SM. Tardive dyskinesia: a 3-year follow up study. *Psychol Med* 1983; **13**: 71–81.

14. Richardson MA, Casey DE. Tardive dyskinesia status: stability or change. *Psychopharmacol Bull* 1988; **24**: 471–5.

15. Yagi G, Itoh H. Follow-up study of 11 patients with potentially reversible tardive dyskinesia. *Am J Psychiat* 1987; **144**: 1496–8.

16. Casey DE, Gardos G. Tardive dyskinesia: outcome at 10 years. *Schizophren Res* 1990; **3**: 11.

17. Yassa R, Lal S. Respiratory irregularity and tardive dyskinesia. *Acta Psychiat Scand* 1986; **73**: 506–10.

18. Gregory RP, Smith PT, Rudge P. Tardive dyskinesia presenting as severe dysphagia. *J Neurol Neurosurg Psychiat* 1992; **55**: 1203–4.

19. Feve A, Angelard B, Lacau-St-Guily J. Laryngeal tardive dyskinesia. *J Neurol* 1995; **242**: 455–9.

20. Jeste DV. Tardive dyskinesia in older patients. *J Clin Psychiat* 2000; **61**(4): 27–32.

21. Jeste DV, Caligiuri MP, Paulsen JS *et al.* Risk of tardive dyskinesia in older patients. A prospective longitudinal study of 266 outpatients. *Arch Gen Psychiat* 1995; **52**: 756–65.

22. Jeste DV, Lacro JP, Palmer B *et al.* Incidence of tardive dyskinesia in early stages of low-dose treatment with typical neuroleptics in older patients. *Am J Psychiat* 1999; **156**: 309–11.

23. Glazer WM. Review of the incidence studies of tardive dyskinesia associated with typical antipsychotics. *J Clin Psychiat* 2000; **61**(4): 15–20.

24. Smith JM, Baldessarini RJ. Changes in prevalence, severity and recovery in tardive dyskinesia with age. *Arch Gen Psychiat* 1980; **37**: 1368–73.

25. Jus A, Pineau R, Lachance R *et al.* Epidemiology of tardive dyskinesia. Part I. *Nerv Syst* 1976; **37**: 210–14.

26. Woerner MG, Alvir JMJ, Saltz BL *et al.* Prospective study of tardive dyskinesia in the elderly: rate and risk factors. *Am J Psychiat* 1998; **155**: 1521–8.

27. Saltz BL, Woerner MM, Kane JM *et al.* Prospective study of tardive dyskinesia incidence in the elderly. *J Am Med Assoc* 1991; **266**: 2402–6.

28. Jeste DV, Jeste SD, Wyatt RJ. Reversible tardive dyskinesia: implications for therapeutic strategy and prevention of tardive dyskinesia. In Bannet J, Belmaker RH, eds, *New Directions in Tardive Dyskinesia Research*, Vol 21. Basel: Karger, 1983: 34–48.

29. Domino EF, Kovacic B. Monkey models of tardive dyskinesia. In Bannet J, Belmaker RH, eds, *New Directions in Tardive Dyskinesia Research*, Vol 21, Basel: Karger, 1983: 21–33.

30. Crane GE, Smeets RA. Tardive dyskinesia and drug therapy in geriatric patients. *Arch Gen Psychiat* 1974; **30**: 341–3.

31. Toenissen LM, Casey DE, McFarland BH. Tardive dyskinesia in the aged. *Arch Gen Psychiat* 1985; **42**: 278–84.

32. Labbate LA, Lande RG, Jones F, Oleshansky MA. Tardive dyskinesia in older out-patients: a follow-up study. *Acta Psychiat Scand* 1997; **96**: 195–8.

33. Caligiuri MP, Lacro JP, Rockwell E *et al.* Incidence and risk factors for severe tardive dyskinesia in older patients. *Br J Psychiat* 1997; **171**: 148–53.

34. Jeste DV, Wyatt RJ. Changing epidemiology of tardive dyskinesia: an overview. *Am J Psychiat* 1981; **138**: 297–309.

35. Jeste DV, Rosenblatt JE, Wagner RL *et al.* High serum neuroleptic levels in tardive dyskinesia (letter). *N Engl J Med* 1979; **301**: 1184.

36. Yesavage JA, Holman CA, Becker J *et al.* Correlation of age and acute thiothixene levels. *Psychopharmacology* 1981; **74**: 117–20.

37. Barnes TRE, McPhillips MA. Critical analysis and comparison of the side-effect and safety profiles of the new antipsychotics. *Br J Psychiat* 1999; **174**(38): 34–43.

38. Maixner SM, Mellow AM, Tandon R. The efficacy, safety and tolerability of antipsychotics in the elderly. *J Clin Psychiat* 1999; **60**(8): 29–41.

39. Jeste DV, Rockwell E, Harris MJ *et al.* Conventional vs. newer antipsychotics in elderly patients. *Am J Geriat Psychiat* 1999; **7**: 70–6.

40. Madhusoodanan S, Suresh P, Brenner R, Pilai R. Experience with the atypical antipsychotics—risperidone and olanzapine in the elderly. *Ann Clin Psychiat* 1999; **11**: 113–18.

41. Barak Y, Wittenberg N, Naor S *et al.* Clozapine in elderly psychiatric patients: tolerability, safety, and efficacy. *Comp Psychiat* 1999; **40**: 320–5.

42. Chan YC, Pariser SF, Neufeld G. Atypical antipsychotics in older adults. *Pharmacotherapy* 1999; **19**: 811–22.

43. Tariot PN. The older patient: the ongoing challenge of efficacy and tolerability. *J Clin Psychiat* 1999; **60**(23): 29–33.

44. Jeste DV, Lacro JP, Bailey A *et al.* Lower incidence of tardive dyskinesia with risperidone compared with haloperidol in older patients. *J Am Geriat Soc* 1999; **156**: 309–11.

45. Jeste DV, Okamoto A, Napolitano J *et al.* Low incidence of persistent tardive dyskinesia in elderly patients with dementia treated with risperidone. *Am J Psychiat* 2000; **157**: 1150–5.

46. Davidson M, Harvey PD, Vervarcke J *et al.* A long-term, multicentre, open-label study of risperidone in elderly patients with psychosis. *Int J Geriat Psychiat* 2000; **15**: 506–14.

47. Street JS, Clark WS, Gannon KS *et al.* Olanzapine treatment of psychotic and behavioural symptoms in patients with Alzheimer disease in nursing care facilities. *Arch Gen Psychiat* 2000; **57**: 968–76.

48. Siede H, Muller HR. Choreiform movements as side effects of phenothiazine medication in geriatric patients. *J Geriat Soc* 1967; **15**: 517–22.

49. Kennedy PF, Hershon HI, McGuire RJ. Extrapyramidal disorders after prolonged phenothiazine therapy. *Br J Psychiat* 1971; **118**: 509–18.

50. Smith JM, Kucharski LT, Oswald WT *et al.* A systematic investigation of tardive dyskinesia in inpatients. *Am J Psychiat* 1979; **136**: 918–22.

51. Smith JM, Kucharski LT, Eblen C *et al.* An assessment of tardive dyskinesia in schizophrenic outpatients. *Psychopharmacology* 1979; **64**: 99–104.

52. Smith JM, Dunn DD. Sex differences in the prevalence of severe tardive dyskinesia. *Am J Psychiat* 1979; **136**: 1080–2.

53. Ramsay FM, Millard PH. Tardive dyskinesia in the elderly. *Age Ageing* 1986; **15**: 1145–50.

54. O'Keane V, Dinan TG. Orofacial dyskinesia and senile dementia of the Alzheimer type. *Int J Geriat Psychiat* 1991; **6**: 41–5.

55. Richardson MA, Pass R, Craig TJ *et al.* Factors influencing the prevalence and severity of tardive dyskinesia. *Psychopharmacol Bull* 1984; **20**: 33–8.

56. Hruska RE, Silbergeld EK. Estrogen treatment enhances dopamine receptor sensitivity in the rat striatum. *Eur J Pharmacol* 1980; **61**: 397–400.

57. Glazer WM, Naftolin F, Moore DC. The relationship of circulating estradiol to tardive dyskinesia in men and postmenopausal women. *Psychoneuroendocrinology* 1983; **8**: 429–34.

58. Dávila R, Andia I, Miller JC *et al.* Evidence of low dopaminergic activity in elderly women with spontaneous orofacial dyskinesia. *Acta Psychiat Scand* 1991; **83**: 1–3.

59. Barnes TRE, Liddle PF. Tardive dyskinesia: implications for schizophrenia? In Schiff AA, Roth M, Freeman HL, eds, *Schizophrenia: New Pharmacological and Clinical Development*. London: Royal Society of Medicine Services, 1985: 81–7.

60. Barnes TRE. Tardive dyskinesia: risk factors, pathophysiology and treatment. In Granville-Grossman K, ed., *Recent Advances in Clinical Psychiatry*, Vol 6. London: Churchill Livingstone, 1988: 185–207.

61. Waddington JL. Schizophrenia, affective psychoses, and other disorders treated with neurobiological determinants, and the conflict of paradigms. *Int Rev Neurobiol* 1989; **31**: 297–353.

62. Hunter R, Earl CJ, Thornicroft S. An apparently irreversible syndrome of abnormal movements following phenothiazine medication. *Proc R Soc Med* 1964; **54**: 758–62.

63. Crane GE, Paulson G. Involuntary movements in a sample of chronic mental patients and their relation to the treatment with neuroleptics. *Int J Neurol* 1967; **3**: 286–91.

64. Yassa R, Nair V, Schwartz G. Tardive dyskinesia and the primary psychiatric diagnosis. *Psychosomatics* 1984; **25**: 135–8.

65. Edwards H. The significance of brain damage in oral dyskinesia. *Br J Psychiat* 1970; **116**: 271–5.

66. Villeneuve A, Turcotte J, Bouchard M *et al.* Release phenomena and iterative activities in psychiatric geriatric patients. *Can Med Assoc J* 1974; **110**: 147–53.

67. Davis K, Berger P, Hollister L. Tardive dyskinesia and depressive illness. *Psychopharmacol Commun* 1976; **2**: 125.

68. Rosenbaum AH, Niven RG, Hanson HP et al. Tardive dyskinesia: relationship with primary effective disorder. Des Nerv System 1977; 38: 4223–6.

69. Rush M, Diamond F, Alpert M. Depression as a risk factor in tardive dyskinesia. Biol Psychiat 1982; 17: 387–92.

70. Casey DE, Keepers GA. Neuroleptic side effects: acute extrapyramidal syndromes and tardive dyskinesia. In Casey DE, Christensen AV, eds, Psychopharmacology: Current Trends. Berlin: Springer-Verlag, 1988: 74–93.

71. Mukherjee S, Rosen AM, Caracci G et al. Persistent tardive dyskinesia in bipolar patients. Arch Gen Psychiat 1986; 43: 342–6.

72. Kahlbaum KL. Die Katatonie oder das Spannungsirresein. Berlin: Hirschwald, 1874.

73. Kleist K. Studies of Psychomotor Symptoms in Mental Patients. Leipzig: Klinkhardt, 1908.

74. Bleur E. Dementia Praecox or the Group of Schizophrenias, 1911 edn. Translated by Zinkin Y. New York: International Universities Press, 1950.

75. Farran-Ridge C. Some symptoms referable to the basal ganglia occurring in dementia praecox and epidemic encephalitis. J Ment Sci 1926; 72: 513–23.

76. Jones M, Hunter R. Abnormal movements in patients with chronic psychiatric illness. In Crane GE, Gardner R, eds, Psychotropic Drugs and Dysfunction of the Basal Ganglia. Washington, DC: US Public Health Service Publication No 1938, 1969: 53–65.

77. Pfhol B, Winokur G. The evolution of symptoms in institutionalised hebephrenic/catatonic schizophrenics. Br J Psychiat 1982; 141: 567–72.

78. Kraepelin EP. Dementia Praecox and Paraphrenia. Translated by Barclay RM; Robertson GM, ed. Edinburgh: E and S Livingstone, 1919.

79. Marsden CD, Tarsy D, Baldessarini RJ. Spontaneous and drug-induced movement disorders in psychotic patients. In Benson DF, Blumer D, eds, Psychiatric Aspects of Neurological Disease. New York: Grune and Stratton, 1975.

80. Marsden CD. Is tardive dyskinesia a unique disorder? In Casey DE, Chase TN, Christensen AV, Gerlach J, eds, Dyskinesia—Research and Treatment. Berlin: Springer-Verlag, 1985: 64–71.

81. Rogers D. The motor disorders of severe psychiatric illness: a conflict of paradigms. Br J Psychiat 1985; 147: 221–32.

82. Davison K, Bagley C. Schizophrenia-like psychoses associated with organic disorders of the CNS: a review of the literature. In Herrington T, ed., Current Problems in Neuropsychiatry. British Journal of Psychiatry Special Publications No. 4. Ashford, Kent: Headley Brothers, 1969.

83. Owens DGC, Johnstone EC, Frith CD. Spontaneous involuntary disorders of movement. Arch Gen Psychiat 1982; 39: 452–61.

84. Owens DGC. Involuntary disorders of movement in chronic schizophrenia—the role of the illness and its treatment. In Casey DE, Chase TN, Christensen AV, Gerlach J, eds, Dyskinesia—Research and Treatment. Berlin: Springer-Verlag, 1985: 79–87.

85. Collinson SL, Pantelis C, Barnes TRE. Abnormal involuntary movements in schizophrenia and their association with cognitive impairment. In Pantelis C, Nelson HE, Barnes TRE, eds, Schizophrenia: A Neuropsychological Perspective. Chichester: Wiley, 1996: 237–58.

86. Mosla PK, Martilla RJ, Rinne UK. Extrapyramidal signs in Alzheimer's disease. Neurology 1984; 34: 1114–16.

87. Folstein MF, Folstein SE, McHugh P. Mini-Mental State: a practical method for grading the cognitive state of patients for the clinician. J Psychiat Res 1975; 12: 189–98.

88. Guy W. ECDEU Assessment Manual for Psychopharmacology. Department of Health, Education and Welfare Publication No. 76-338. Washington, DC: US Government Printing Office, 1976: 534–7.

89. Bakchine S, Lacomblez L, Palisson E et al. Relationship between primitive reflexes, extrapyramidal signs, reflective apraxia and severity of cognitive impairment in dementia of the Alzheimer type. Acta Neurol Scand 1989; 79: 38–46.

90. Crane GE. Pseudoparkinsonism and tardive dyskinesia. Arch Neurol 1972; 27: 426–30.

91. Chouinard G, Annable L, Ross-Chouinard A et al. Factors related to tardive dyskinesia. Am J Psychiat 1979; 136: 79–83.

92. De Veaugh-Geiss J, Smith JM, Borison RL et al. Prediction and prevention of tardive dyskinesia. In De Veaugh-Geiss J, ed., Tardive Dyskinesia and Related Involuntary Movement Disorders. Bristol: Wright, 1982: 161–6.

93. Barnes TRE, Braude WM. Persistent akathisia associated with early tardive dyskinesia. Postgrad Med J 1984; 60: 51–3.

94. Barnes TRE, Halstead SM, Little P. Akathisia variants: prevalence and iron status in an inpatient population with chronic schizophrenia (abst). Schizophren Res 1990; 3: 79.

95. Barnes TRE, Braude WM. Akathisia variants and tardive dyskinesia. Arch Gen Psychiat 1985; 42: 874–8.

96. Burke RE, Kang UJ, Jankovic J et al. Tardive akathisia: an analysis of clinical features and response to open therapeutic trials. Movem Disord 1989; 4: 157–75.

97. Dufresne RL, Wagner RL. Antipsychotic-withdrawal akathisia vs. antipsychotic-induced akathisia: further evidence for the existence of tardive akathisia. J Clin Psychiat 1988; 49: 435–8.

98. Kane JM, Weinhold P, Kinon B et al. Prevalence of abnormal involuntary movements ("spontaneous dyskinesia") in the normal elderly. Psychopharmacology 1982; 77: 105–8.

99. Casey DE, Hansen TE. Spontaneous dyskinesias. In Jeste DV, Wyatt RJ, eds, Neuropsychiatric Movement Disorders. Washington, DC: American Psychiatric Press, 1984: 68–95.

100. D'Allessandro R, Benass G, Christine E et al. The prevalence of lingual–facial–buccal dyskinesias in the elderly. Neurology 1986; 36: 1350–1.

101. Delwaide PJ, Desseilles M. Spontaneous buccolinguofacial dyskinesia in the elderly. Acta Neurol Scand 1977; 56: 256–62.

102. Lieberman J, Kane JM, Woerner M, Weinhold P. Prevalence of tardive dyskinesia in elderly samples. Psychopharmacol Bull 1984; 20: 22–6.

103. Klawans HL, Barr A. Prevalence of spontaneous lingual–facial–buccal dyskinesia in the elderly. Neurology 1982; 32: 558–9.

104. Crane GE. Persistent dyskinesia. Br J Psychiat 1973; 122: 395–405.

105. Altrocchi PH. Spontaneous oral-facial dyskinesia. Arch Neurol 1972; 26: 506–12.

106. Greenblatt DL, Dominick RN, Stotsky BA et al. Phenothiazine-induced dyskinesia in nursing home patients. J Am Geriat Soc 1968; 16: 27–34.

107. Marsden CD, Parkes JD. Abnormal movement disorders. Br J Hosp Med 1973; 10: 428–50.

108. Varga E, Sugerman AA, Varga V et al. Prevalence of spontaneous oral dyskinesia in the elderly. Am J Psychiat 1982; 139: 329–31.

109. Bourgeois M, Boueilh P, Tignol J. Dyskinesies spontanéous sénile idiopathiques et dyskinesies tardive des neuroleptiques. L'Encéphale 1980; VI: 37–9.

110. Bourgeois M, Boueilh P, Tignol J et al. Spontaneous dyskinesia vs. neuroleptic-induced dyskinesia in 270 elderly subjects. J Nerv Ment Dis 1980; 168: 177–8.

111. Barnes TRE, Rossor M, Trauer T. A comparison of purposeless movements in psychiatric patients treated with antipsychotic drugs, and normal individuals. J Neurol Neurosurg Psychiat 1983:

112. Blowers AJ, Borison RL, Blowers CM et al. Abnormal involuntary movements in the elderly. Br J Psychiat 1982; 139: 363–4.

113. Gardos G, Cole JO, La Brie R. The assessment of tardive dyskinesia. Arch Gen Psychiat 1977; 34: 1206–12.

114. Mackay AVP. Assessment of antipsychotic drugs. Br J Clin Pharmacol 1981; 11: 225–36.

Part H

Neuroses

97

Nosology and Classification of Neurotic Disorders

D. Bienenfeld

Wright State University School of Medicine, Dayton, OH, USA

The grouping of a variety of psychopathologic entities under the heading of "neurotic disorders" represents the current attempt to solve a nosological tangle dating back further than the time of Sigmund Freud. The contemporary categorization is controversial and less than satisfying to many. A brief look at its historical roots offers some explanation of the sense behind the current ICD-10 and DSM-IV structures.

HISTORY OF THE CLASSIFICATION OF THE NEUROSES

It was Hippolyte-Marie Bernheim who introduced the term "psychoneurosis" for hysteria and allied conditions. Freud, who studied with Bernheim, differentiated the "actual neuroses" (including neurasthenia, anxiety neurosis and hypochondria) from the psychoneuroses. The latter category included not only the "transference neuroses", such as hysteria and obsessive neurosis, but also the psychoses (paraphrenia, schizophrenia, paranoia and manic depression), perversions and neurotic character. Both types of neurosis were related to sexual disturbance; the actual neuroses were direct somatic consequences of a noxious physical influence resulting from misdirected sexual energy; the psychoneuroses were caused by unconscious conflict between instinctual and counter-instinctual forces[1]. Although Freud's thinking on the precise nature of the mental etiology of the psychoneuroses changed over the years from about 1894 to 1906, he remained consistent in his stance that the psychoneuroses were defined by their etiology rather than by their phenomenology[2]. Eventually, the psychoses were classified independently, consistent with the views of Kraepelin.

In 1952, the American Psychiatric Association published the first *Diagnostic and Statistical Manual of Mental Disorders* (DSM-I). It identified the subtypes of psychoneurotic disorders as anxiety, dissociative, conversion, phobic, obsessive-compulsive, and depressive reactions[3]. By the mid-1960s, the major diagnostic schemata, ICD-8 and DSM-II, codified the selection of the descriptive framework for identifying the neuroses. Anxiety was seen as the chief characteristic, whether felt and expressed directly or diverted unconsciously into other symptoms. The neuroses were also grouped by severity; they were more specifically symptomatic than the personality disorders, but entailed no gross distortion or impairment of reality testing, as in the psychoses. Categories included in the 300-code section were anxiety, hysterical, phobic, obsessive-compulsive, depressive, neurasthenic, depersonalization and hypochondriacal neuroses.

Transient situational disturbances constituted their own category (code 307)[4].

The descriptive focus was emphasized in ICD-9 with the substitution of the term "neurotic disorders" for "neuroses", although the categorization was not significantly modified[5]. In 1980, the American Psychiatric Association published the DSM-III[6], which took a substantial leap towards atheoretical descriptive diagnosis by adopting empirically validated criteria based on research diagnostic criteria. One of the most controversial changes was the elimination of the entire class of neuroses. The neurotic disorders were included in the affective, anxiety, somatoform, dissociative and psychosexual disorders[7]. The grouping by severity was abandoned in favor of clusters based on similarity of features. The diagnostic entities retained numerical codes compatible with ICD-9 and ICD-9-CM.

The other revolutionary change introduced with DSM-III was the use of a multiaxial system for diagnosis. Under this scheme, personality disorders, which often predispose individuals to the development of specific neurotic (and other) syndromes, were relegated to a separate and parallel Axis II. The 1987 revision, DSM-III-R, changed some names and criteria but retained the same hierarchy of the neurotic disorders and the same multiaxial formula[8]. DSM-IV, published in 1994, was a more substantive revision overall than DSM-III-R, with only a few changes relevant to the neurotic disorders. The diagnosis of Acute Stress Disorder was added for compatibility with ICD-10. Dissociative Identity Disorder was added to Axis I to replace Multiple Personality Disorder, which was removed from Axis II. Simple Phobia was renamed Specific Phobia for compatibility with ICD-10[9].

Neurotic Disorders in ICD-10 and DSM-IV

The creators of ICD-10 were faced with a formidable challenge, as this version, unlike its nine predecessors, was to be designed as the last of the series to be scheduled for regular revisions[10]. It therefore had to contain a format that would allow for flexibility in minor revisions while establishing a more permanent structure than versions 1–9. While following the lead of the phenomenological school in separating out a major category for mood disorders that includes both psychotic and neurotic levels of severity, it retains the major classification of neurotic disorders, including somatoform disorders and stress-related disorders[11]. This grouping solves the objection that the term "neurosis" groups together entities which could be better classified, e.g. by placing neurotic severities of depression together with other mood

Table 97.1 Relative positions of neurotic disorders in the diagnostic schemata

ICD-10	DSM-IV
F0 Organic mental disorders	Disorders usually first evident in infancy, childhood or adolescence
F1 Mental and behavioral disorders due to psychoactive substance uses	Delirium; dementia and amnestic and other cognitive disorders
F2 Schizophrenia, schizotypal states and delusional disorders	Mental disorders due to a general medical condition not elsewhere classified
F3 Mood disorders	Substance-related disorders
F4 NEUROTIC, STRESS-RELATED AND SOMATOFORM DISORDERS	Schizophrenia and other psychotic disorders
F5 Behavioral syndromes and mental disorders associated with physiological dysfunction and hormonal changes	Mood disorders
	ANXIETY DISORDERS
F6 Abnormalities of adult personality and behavior	SOMATOFORM DISORDERS
F7 Mental retardation	DISSOCIATIVE DISORDERS
F8 Developmental disorders	Factitious disorders
F9 Behavioral and emotional disorders with onset usually occurring in childhood or adolescence	Sexual and gender identity disorders
	Eating disorders
	Sleep disorders
	Impulse-control disorders not elsewhere classified

disorders, rather than with anxiety disorders. It does, however, retain the historical commonality that traces to Freud's original stress on the etiologic similarity of the psychoneuroses, acknowledging the current state of scientific knowledge that is, at best, ambiguous concerning the etiology of these disorders[12,13].

Table 97.1 compares the relative positions of the neurotic disorders in ICD-10 and Axis I of DSM-IV. The alphanumeric organization of the International Classification requires the constraint of all mental disorders to 10 major categories. DSM-IV, under no such limitation, separates out anxiety, somatoform and dissociative disorders but keeps them within the same gradient of severity between mood disorders and sexual disorders. Adjustment disorders are removed to a position implying less severity, as well as an implied direction that higher-ranking diagnoses are to be made or eliminated first. Personality disorders, of course, are assigned to Axis II.

Under the category of the neurotic disorders, the international and American systems differ in their organization, as outlined in Table 97.2. DSM-IV groups the phobic disorders, obsessive-compulsive disorder, post-traumatic stress disorder and generalized anxiety disorder together as anxiety disorders. ICD-10 separates phobic disorders, anxiety disorders, and obsessive-compulsive disorders. Post-traumatic stress disorders are classified with adjustment disorders. Both schemes separate dissociative and somatoform disorders. ICD-10 groups conversion disorder with dissociative states, consistent with the historical, etiologically-based classification of the hysterias. DSM-IV combines it with the somatoform disorders, based on their phenomenological similarities. ICD-10 retains the diagnosis of neurasthenia; while DSM-III-R refers the clinician to dysthymia, categorized unequivocally as a mood disorder, DSM-IV eliminates the term entirely[8,9,11].

DIAGNOSTIC FEATURES OF NEUROTIC DISORDERS

While each of the major categories of neurotic disorders is described in the chapters that follow, the clinical features of the seven ICD-10 groupings are presented here for overview and comparison[11].

Phobic disorders are a set of disorders in which anxiety is invoked only, or predominantly, by well-defined situations that are not in themselves dangerous. By definition, the object of the fear is external to the individual, so that fears of bodily processes are more appropriately relegated to the category of somatoform

disorders. The feared objects are characteristically avoided, and anticipatory anxiety is common.

Other anxiety disorders are those in which anxiety is the major symptom but which are not restricted to specific situations. They include panic disorder, generalized anxiety disorder, and mixed anxiety and depressive disorder. The latter is reserved for cases where symptoms of both are present, neither is predominant, and the depression is not severe enough to be classified under mild depressive disorder.

Obsessive-compulsive disorder is characterized by recurrent obsessional thoughts or compulsive acts, or both. These thoughts and acts are subjectively distressing. Subjective anxiety is usually present and depressive features are common.

Reactions to severe stress and adjustment disorders represent a unique category, in that the component disorders are identified on the grounds of both symptomatology and causation. In these disorders, anxiety follows an exceptionally stressful life event or a significant life change. While psychosocial stressors may precipitate a wide variety of psychiatric syndromes, they are elsewhere neither necessary nor sufficient to explain the occurrence and form of the disorder. The stress and adjustment disorders, however, are seen as arising as a direct consequence of the trauma or life change.

Dissociative disorder is a group of entities that share a partial or complete loss of the normal integration between memory of the past, awareness of identity and immediate sensations, and control of bodily movements. It is presumed that, in these disorders, the ability to exert conscious and selective control over memory, sensation or bodily function is impaired.

Somatoform disorders are those in which physical symptoms are repeatedly presented with requests for investigation or treatment, in spite of the absence of physical findings to substantiate the perception. Compared with patients who suffer from psychogenic movement or sensory disorders, those with somatoform disorders will demand attention and usually resent physicians who fail to believe in the physical nature of their illnesses. Even when the onset of symptoms is temporally related to a stressful life event, or when external manifestations of depression or anxiety are obvious to others, these patients will frequently resist speculation about psychological causation.

Other neurotic disorders feature two clinical entities, neurasthenia and depersonalization–derealization syndrome. The former, recalling the pre-Freudian nomenclature, is a controversial category in contemporary psychiatry. Its main feature is fatigue, which may occur upon either mental or physical exercise. The diagnosis is to be made only after depressive and anxiety

Table 97.2 Classification of neurotic disorders

ICD-10	DSM-IV
F40 *Phobic disorder*	*Anxiety disorders*
40.0 Agoraphobia	300.21 Panic disorder with
.00 Without panic disorder	agoraphobia
.01 With panic disorder	300.01 Panic disorder
40.1 Social phobias	without agoraphobia
40.2 Specific (isolated) phobias	300.22 Agoraphobia without
F41 *Other anxiety disorders*	history of panic disorder
41.0 Panic disorder	300.29 Specific phobia
41.1 Generalized anxiety disorder	300.23 Social phobia
41.2 Mixed anxiety and	300.3 Obsessive-compulsive
depressive disorder	disorder
F42 *Obsessive-compulsive disorder*	309.89 Post-traumatic stress
42.0 Predominantly obsessional	disorder
thoughts	308.3 Acute stress disorder
42.1 Predominantly compulsive	300.02 Generalized anxiety
acts	disorder
F43 *Reaction to severe stress and*	*Somatoform disorders*
adjustment disorders	300.81 Somatization disorder
43.0 Acute stress reaction	300.11 Conversion disorder
43.1 Post-traumatic stress	307 Pain disorder
disorder	300.7 Hypochondriasis
43.2 Adjustment disorder	300.7 Body dysmorphic disorder
.20 Brief depressive	*Dissociative disorders*
reaction	300.12 Dissociative amnesia
.21 Prolonged depressive	300.13 Dissociative fugue
reaction	300.14 Dissociative identity
.22 With predominant	disorder
disturbance of other	300.6 Depersonalization
emotions	disorder
.23 With predominant	*Adjustment disorder*
disturbance of conduct	309.0 With depressed mood
.24 With mixed	309.24 With anxiety
disturbance of	309.40 With mixed disturbances
emotions and conduct	of emotions and conduct
F44 *Dissociative and conversion*	309.28 With mixed anxiety and
disorder	depressed mood
44.0 Psychogenic amnesia	309.3 With disturbance of
44.1 Psychogenic fugue	conduct
44.2 Psychogenic stupor	
44.3 Trance and possession states	
44.4 Psychogenic movement	
disorders	
44.5 Psychogenic convulsions	
44.6 Psychogenic anaesthesia and	
sensory loss	
F45 *Somatoform disorders*	
45.0 Multiple somatization	
disorder	
45.1 Undifferentiated	
somatoform disorder	
45.2 Hypochondriacal syndrome	
45.3 Psychogenic autonomic	
dysfunction	
45.4 Psychogenic pain	
F48 *Other neurotic disorders*	
48.0 Neurasthenia	
48.1 Depersonalization–	
derealization syndrome	

disorders have been ruled out. Depersonalization–derealization syndrome is a rare disorder in which the patient feels that his/her own mental activity, body or surroundings are changed in quality so as to be unreal or remote. This phenomenon is more commonly observed as a feature of depression, phobias, obsessive-compulsive disorder and some psychoses.

Special Considerations in Geriatric Patients

Anxiety, both as a symptom and as a disorder, is common among the elderly, but not remarkably more or less so than at other ages. The nature of worry and its clinical manifestations, however, change with increasing age. The intricate relationships among psychosocial stress, physical illness, depression and anxiety in late life make the recognition, diagnosis and classification of neurotic disorders in the elderly quite complex[14–16].

The clinician can usually compare the fears and concerns of a younger patient against those of his/her own peers and arrive at a credible assessment of whether or not the anxieties are pathological. The aged, however have different fears; they worry about physical illness, crime, institutionalization, financial disaster, senility and physical dependency. It is often hard for the younger physician to determine whether the subjective interpretation of events, or the anticipation of future events, is in the realm of clinical anxiety or constitutes adaptive concern. Anxiety results from feelings of vulnerability, and the elderly are truly vulnerable in many ways. It is no easy task to diagnose agoraphobia in an 80-year-old person whose fear of crime in her neighborhood may exceed its statistical likelihood. The clinician walks a fine line between pathologizing a healthy response and failing to recognize neurotic dysfunction[14].

Physical illnesses with psychiatric manifestations increase in prevalence with age, as does the need to take medications with emotional or behavioral side effects. Emphysema, for example, may produce features indistinguishable from those of panic disorder. Hyperthyroidism is commonly accompanied by symptoms resembling those of generalized anxiety disorder. Further, the guiding symptom profiles for the underlying disorders may be absent or muted in the aging person. "Silent myocardial infarction" and afebrile pneumonia are fairly common. Finally, the elderly consume significantly more medication than do younger people and exhibit psychiatric side effects at lower doses and serum levels. Bronchodilators may produce the symptoms of many anxiety states; recommended doses of over-the-counter medications for sleep or colds may induce presentations resembling dissociative states[16].

As could be expected, the diagnosis of somatoform disorders and hypochondriasis is particularly complicated in the elderly. Somatic complaints are common. To some extent, the somatic presentation of emotional disorders is a sociocultural cohort phenomenon. The generation of people over 70 in the 2000s, for example, grew up in the 1940s and earlier. At that time, words such as "depression" and "anxiety" were not commonplace parts of everyday conversation. Emotional introspection was not culturally normative. Thus, the older person who complains today of having "butterflies in my stomach" may be aware of the physical concomitants of anxiety, but not of the emotional state underlying it. The clinician must "translate" somatically-phrased complaints to help determine the affective condition.

Furthermore, the increase in prevalence of almost all physical illnesses with age confounds the determination of pathological perception and behavior, necessary for making diagnoses of somatoform disorders. Both DSM-IV and ICD-10 leave room for a subjective judgment of whether the presence of physical symptoms is sufficient to explain the intensity of the patient's response. There are no objective grounds for deciding when a complaint of abdominal pain constitutes a somatoform disorder in a person with concurrent emphysema, arthritis and congestive heart failure[14,17].

While the delineation of the diagnosis and treatment of post-traumatic stress disorder (PTSD) followed the societal impact of returning Vietnam War veterans, the syndrome is not uncommon in older individuals. The trauma may have been a different war (World War II or Korea), a natural disaster, or a personal event such as physical assault. Symptoms may occur early and continue for decades. In many cases, symptoms may not even be manifest until many years after the traumatic event. Often, the symptoms of delayed PTSD are precipitated by a psychologically reminiscent contemporary event; a concentration camp survivor may not experience stress-related symptoms overtly until becoming widowed and being institutionalized half a century later[14,15].

SUMMARY

The current classification of neurotic disorders is the most recent step in the evolution of the nosological understanding of a diverse group of syndromes. The ICD-10 grouping represents a compromise between the phenomenological grouping of neurotic conditions on a scale of severity between healthy and psychotic function, and the etiological clustering of disorders presumed to arise from internal conflicts and vulnerabilities to external stressors. The ambiguities inherent in this system reflect the incomplete state of knowledge about the etiologies of the constituent conditions. The North American schema of DSM-IV sets aside questions of etiology, except in the case of adjustment disorders, and relies on ostensibly atheoretical phenomenological criteria.

Although the diagnostic criteria are technically independent of the age of the patient in both systems, aging affects the presentation of many of these disorders and makes clinical diagnosis challenging. The multiple biological and social stressors of late life blur the distinction between "normal" and "pathological" responses to these threats. Physical illnesses, which increase in frequency with aging, may produce clinical symptoms easily mistaken for neurotic anxiety. The prevalence of somatic pathology forces subjective judgments about the presence of somatoform and conversion disorders. Chronic and delayed stress reactions are clinically distinct from the acute forms seen in younger individuals.

The lack of clarity in the classification of these disorders, however, is probably less a manifestation of the shortcomings of the nosological systems than a reflection of the complicated function of the human mind. The neurotic disorders, as well as current science can determine, are a product not of brain disease but of human response to a complicated and stressful world. Simplicity in their nosology would belie the challenges they pose to patients and clinicians.

REFERENCES

1. Gray M. *Neuroses: A Comprehensive and Critical Review*. New York: Van Nostrand Reinhold, 1978: 1–32.
2. Brenner C. *An Elementary Textbook of Psychoanalysis*. Garden City: Doubleday, 1973: 171–92.
3. American Psychiatric Association. *Diagnostic and Statistical Manual of Mental Disorders* (DSM-I). Washington, DC: American Psychiatric Association, 1952.
4. American Psychiatric Association. *Diagnostic and Statistical Manual of Mental Disorders*, 2nd edn (DSM-II). Washington, DC: American Psychiatric Association, 1968.
5. World Health Organization. *Manual of the International Statistical Classification of Diseases, Injuries, and Causes of Death*, 9th revision. Geneva: WHO, 1977.
6. American Psychiatric Association. *Diagnostic and Statistical Manual of Mental Disorders*, 3rd edn (DSM-III). Washington, DC: American Psychiatric Association, 1980.
7. Spitzer RL. Introduction. In *Diagnostic and Statistical Manual of Mental Disorders*, 3rd edn (DSM-III). Washington, DC: American Psychiatric Association, 1980: 1–12.
8. American Psychiatric Association. *Diagnostic and Statistical Manual of Mental Disorders*, 3rd edn, revised (DSM-III-R). Washington, DC: American Psychiatric Association, 1987.
9. American Psychiatric Association. *Diagnostic and Statistical Manual of Mental Disorders*, 4th edn (DSM-IV). Washington, DC: American Psychiatric Association, 1994.
10. Sartorius N. International perspectives of psychiatric classification. *Br J Psychiat* 1988; **152**(1): 9–14.
11. World Health Organization. Tenth Revision of the International Classification of Diseases, Chapter V (F): Mental and Behavioural Disorders (Draft, revision 4). Geneva: WHO, 1987.
12. Freeman CP. In Kendell RE, Zeally AK eds, *Neurotic Disorders in Companion to Psychiatric Studies*, 4th edn. Edinburgh: Churchill Livingstone, 1988: 374–406.
13. Cooper JE. The structure and presentation of contemporary psychiatric classifications with special reference to ICD-9 and -10. *Br J Psychiat* 1988; **152**(1): 21–8.
14. Ruskin PE. In Bienenfeld D, ed., *Anxiety and Somatoform Disorders in Verwoerdt's Clinical Geropsychiatry*, 3rd edn. Baltimore, MD: Williams and Wilkins, 1990: 137–50.
15. Flint AJ. Management of anxiety in late life. *J Geriat Psychiat Neurol* 1998; **11**(4): 194–200.
16. Small GW. Recognizing and treating anxiety in the elderly. *J Clin Psychiat* 1997; **58**(suppl 3): 41–7.
17. Fogel BS, Sadavoy J. In Sadavoy J, Lazarus LW, Jarvik LF, Grossberg GT, *Somatoform and Personality Disorders in Comprehensive Review of Geriatric Psychiatry*, 2nd edn. Washington, DC: American Association for Geriatric Psychiatry, 1996: 637–58.

98

Epidemiology of Neurotic Disorders

Dan G. Blazer

Duke University Medical Center, Durham, NC, USA

Neurotic disorders are grouped as a special category (the 300 group) in ICD-9[1]. They are mental disorders without any demonstrable organic basis, in which the patient may have considerable insight, and has unimpaired reality testing, i.e. he/she usually does not confuse a morbid subjective experience and fantasies with external reality. Included within the neurotic disorders are anxiety states (both generalized anxiety and panic disorder), hysteria (including conversion reactions), phobic states, obsessive-compulsive disorder, neurotic depression, neurasthenia and depersonalization syndrome.

The Diagnostic and Statistical Manual of Mental Disorders[2] of the American Psychiatric Association, in contrast, does not recognize the neurotic disorders as a distinct entity. Rather, all mood disorders (including the more severe depressive disorders, such as bipolar disorder) are classified in the same category with dysthymia or neurotic depression. Anxiety disorders in DSM-IV include generalized anxiety, panic disorder, phobic disorders and obsessive-compulsive disorders. There is no category within DSM-IV for neurasthenia.

As the epidemiology of the mood disorders will be covered elsewhere, in this chapter current knowledge regarding the epidemiology of the neurotic disorders will be reviewed with especial attention to anxiety. All extant studies that provide useful estimates by age are prevalence studies. Few investigators have concentrated specifically on risk factors by age. In addition, a Medline search of prevalence and incidence studies of generalized anxiety, panic, phobic and obsessive-compulsive disorders in late life since 1996 uncovered only one study. Therefore, the focus of this chapter will be predominantly upon estimates of prevalence of the neurotic disorders by age. Much of the review will feature the Epidemiologic Catchment Area (ECA) studies in the USA.

HISTORICAL REVIEW

At least two early studies provide estimates of the prevalence of neurotic disorders by age. Leighton *et al.*[3], classifying "psychoneurotic" disorders according to DSM-I in the Sterling County study, found that women experienced a peak in psychoneurotic disorders in the 40–49 decade, while the largest percentage of male psychoneurotics were found in the 60–69 decade. For both groups, there was a significant decrease in prevalence in subjects over the age of 70. Pasamanic *et al.*[4] reported an overall prevalence of psychoneurotic disorders of 5.3%. The rates were lowest for subjects under the age of 15 but remained constant through most of adult life. For the 65+ age group, the prevalence estimate was 7%. These investigators of the epidemiology of psychoneurotic disorders found little evidence of an increased prevalence by age but neither did they find evidence for a decrease. In these studies, however, the number of subjects aged 65+ was generally too small to make accurate estimates.

Kay *et al.*[5], in their survey of older persons in Newcastle upon Tyne, which included both institutional cases and those individuals living in the community, found a prevalence of 10.2% for moderate to severe forms of neuroses in older persons. They did not compare the prevalence of neuroses by age. Bergmann[6] found that 11% of a community sample of 300 persons reported developing a neurosis after the age of 60. He also noted the association between neurotic disorders and physical health problems. Each of the above studies aggregated all psychoneurotic disorders and did not exclude depression.

Regarding specific neurotic disorders, few investigators have reported prevalence estimates by age (except for the Epidemiologic Catchment Area studies). The exception is generalized anxiety, one of the more common disorders regardless of age. Murphy[7] and colleagues estimated the prevalence of both anxiety disorders and conversion disorders in individuals less than 45 years of age vs. those 45 years of age and older in the Sterling County study described above. For these estimates, however, they applied diagnostic criteria similar to those used in the third edition of the *Diagnostic and Statistical Manual*[2] rather than the more inclusive category of psychoneurosis. The prevalence of generalized anxiety was 2.9% overall. In males the prevalence was 2.1% under the age of 45 but less than 1% in individuals 45 years of age and older. The prevalence of generalized anxiety in females 45 years of age and older was 2% compared to 6% for those under the age of 45.

Warheit *et al.*[8], in a study of community-dwelling adults in northern Florida, used a self-rating anxiety scale and found that 14.6% of the sample had significant symptoms of anxiety. Blacks, females, the elderly, those in the lower socioeconomic levels and those separated, widowed and divorced actually had the highest scores (in contrast to the ECA study). In a previous study using the Schedule of Affective Disorders and Schizophrenia–Lifetime Version (SADS-L), the overall prevalence of generalized anxiety was 2.5% and was slightly more common in middle-aged and younger women than in older adults.

Copeland *et al.*[9] in a survey of 1070 elderly persons (65+) living in Liverpool, using the Geriatric Mental State (GMS), found the overall levels of neurotic disorders in the elderly to be 2.4%. Anxiety disorder was the most prevalent of the neurotic disorders, with phobic disorder being the second most prevalent (see below). Hypochondriasis and obsessive-compulsive disorders were found in approximately 0.5% and 0.2%, respectively. During a 3 year follow-up[10], the incidence was 0.44%/year. Women were more

Principles and Practice of Geriatric Psychiatry, 2nd edn. Edited by J. R. M. Copeland, M. T. Abou-Saleh and D. G. Blazer
©2002 John Wiley & Sons, Ltd

Table 98.1 One year prevalence rates (%) of generalized anxiety (different exclusionary criteria) by age. ECA study[12]

Age	Generalized anxiety/no exclusions	Generalized anxiety/no panic or major depression	Generalized anxiety/no DSM diagnosis
<30	4.83	3.51	2.35
30–44	3.58	2.12	1.46
45–64	3.74	2.81	1.75
65+	2.22	1.92	1.05

Table 98.2 Cumulative prevalence by age of onset of cases of generalized anxiety (no panic or major depression). ECA study[12]

By age	Cumulative prevalence (%)
19	20.6
24	40.1
29	56.5
44	79.5
64	97.0

Table 98.3 Use of inpatient and outpatient general health services by age and diagnosis of generalized anxiety. ECA study[12]

	Outpatient use		Inpatient use	
Age	Generalized anxiety (%)	No generalized anxiety (%)	Generalized anxiety (%)	No generalized anxiety (%)
45–64	37.0	52.8	10.3	5.7
65+	53.5	60.8	38.4	12.0

likely to become cases than men. Many cases did remit during the 3 years between interviews, but most original cases continued to experience some symptoms at follow-up.

FINDINGS FROM THE EPIDEMIOLOGICAL CATCHMENT AREA SURVEY

The most detailed estimates of specific neurotic disorders are derived from the ECA surveys in the USA. The National Institute of Mental Health Multi-Site Epidemiologic Catchment Area (ECA) Program was a collaborative study that combined community and institutional surveys of five communities in the USA—New Haven, CT; Baltimore, MD; Durham, NC; St Louis, MO; and Los Angeles, CA. The large overall sample (over 18 000 subjects), coupled with oversamples of older persons in three of the five sites, provided the most comprehensive estimates of the

prevalence of specific anxiety disorders among community-dwelling elders from any extant study. The instrument used to establish cases was the Diagnostic Interview Schedule (DIS).

The prevalence of generalized anxiety disorder at three of the ECA sites by age is presented in Table 98.1. The patterns presented hold for both males and females and for Whites, Blacks and Hispanics (although the patterns for male Hispanics are less obvious than for the other age, sex and race groups). In all groups, the prevalence for generalized anxiety is relatively high, but is lower in the 65+ age group than for other ages. Prevalence is presented when the symptoms of generalized anxiety are present, regardless of the symptoms of other disorders, when generalized anxiety is present without evidence of panic or major depression, and when generalized anxiety is diagnosed with no other DIS/DSM-III disorders. The patterns by age are the same regardless. In a study from Liverpool, Copeland et al.[9] found the prevalence of cases of anxiety among females 65+ years of age to be 1.52%, yet nearly 16% of males and females were classified as subcases. Generalized anxiety is more frequent among persons with dementing disorders than without.

In a further analysis of the ECA data, the age of onset of generalized anxiety is presented in Table 98.2 for Durham, NC. Virtually all cases of generalized anxiety have their onset before the age of 65 in this community sample. Age of onset is evenly distributed across the life cycle except for individuals aged 65+.

In Table 98.3, the use of inpatient and outpatient general health service, with and without generalized anxiety disorder, are compared by age (persons 65+ years of age and persons 45–64). Older persons are more likely to report use of inpatient physical health services if they report a current episode of generalized anxiety. In contrast, older persons who suffer generalized anxiety are no more likely to use outpatient services. The trend in older persons is similar to trends in younger persons for both inpatient and outpatient use.

In Table 98.4, data are presented on other selected neurotic disorders by age and sex from the ECA study. In most cases, for both sexes, the prevalence of neurotic disorders decreases with age. Age differences in the rates of phobic disorder are not as pronounced as those seen for other disorders. Older persons have the lowest rates of panic disorder of any age group, whereas persons in the 30–44 age group have the highest rates. This trend occurs for Whites and Blacks but not for Hispanics. Not only do older persons appear to experience a lower prevalence of panic disorder in late life currently, they also appear to have a lower lifetime prevalence of panic disorder. This lower lifetime prevalence could be explained by the fact that persons with panic disorders are less likely to reach old age. In addition, the cohort phenomenon, which is described frequently throughout this book (i.e. persons in late life currently have been uniquely protected against a number of psychiatric disorders) may be operative for panic disorders as well. One must also consider, however, the possibility that older persons in these community surveys fail to recall episodes of panic in the distant past because they have not experienced them recently or they may find such episodes embarrassing to report.

Table 98.4 One year prevalence rates (%) of selected neurotic disorders by age and gender

	18–29		30–44		45–64		65+	
Disorder	Male	Female	Male	Female	Male	Female	Male	Female
Phobic disorder[13]	6.5	13.4	6.1	16.1	6.7	11.6	4.9	8.8
Panic disorder[13]	0.6	1.1	6.7	1.9	0.7	1.1	0.04	0.4
Obsessive-compulsive disorder[14]	1.8	2.6	1.9	2.2	0.8	1.2	0.8	0.9
Hypochondriasis[9]							0.5	0.5

REFERENCES

1. World Health Organization. *Mental Disorders: Glossary and Guide to their Classification in Accordance with the Ninth Revision of the International Classification of Diseases.* Geneva: WHO, 1978.
2. *Diagnostic and Statistical Manual of Mental Disorders*, 3rd edn revised. Washington, DC: American Psychiatric Association, 1987.
3. Leighton DC, Harding DS, Macklin DB *et al. The Character of Danger.* New York: Basic Books, 1963.
4. Pasamanic R, Roberts DW, Limkau PW, Krueger DB. A survey of mental disease in an urban population: prevalence by race and income. In Pasamanic B, ed., *Epidemiology of Mental Disorder.* Washington, DC: American Association for the Advancement of Science, 1959; 183–202.
5. Kay DW, Beamish P, Roth M. Old-age mental disorders in Newcastle upon Tyne. 1. A study of prevalence. *Br J Psychiat* 1964; **110**: 146–68.
6. Bergmann K. The neuroses of old age. In Kay DW, Walk A, eds, *Recent Developments in Psychogeriatrics.* Ashford: Headley Bros, 1971; 39–50.
7. Murphy JM, Sobol AM, Neff RK *et al.* Stability of prevalence—depression and anxiety disorders. *Arch Gen Psychiat* 1984; **41**: 990–7.
8. Warheit GJ, Bull RA, Schwab JJ, Buhl JM. The epidemiologic assessment of mental health problems in the south-eastern United States. In Weissman MM, Meyers JK, Ross CE, eds, *Community Surveys of Psychiatric Disorders.* New Brunswick: Rutgers University Press, 1980; 191–208.
9. Copeland JRM, Dewey ME, Wood H *et al.* Range of mental illness among elderly in the community: prevalence in Liverpool using GMS–AGECAT package. *Br J Psychiat* 1987; **150**: 815–23.
10. Larkin BA, Copeland JRM, Dewey ML *et al.* The natural history of neurotic disorders in an elderly urban population: findings from Liverpool longitudinal study of continuing health in the community. *Br J Psychiat* 1992; **160**: 681–6.
11. Robins LN, Regier DA (eds). *Psychiatric Disorders in America: The Epidemiologic Study.* New York: Free Press, 1990.
12. Blazer DG, Hughes D, George LK *et al.* Generalized anxiety disorder. In Robins LN, Regier DA, eds, *Psychiatric Disorders in America. The Epidemiologic Study.* New York: Free Press, 1990; 180–203.
13. Eaton WW, Dryman A, Weissman MM. Panic and phobia. In Robins LN, Regier DA, eds, *Psychiatric Disorders in America. The Epidemiologic Study.* New York: Free Press, 1990; 155–79.
14. Karno M, Golding JM. Obsessive-compulsive disorder. In Robins LN, Regier DA, eds, *Psychiatric Disorders in America: The Epidemiologic Study.* New York: Free Press, 1990; 204–19.
15. Forsell Y, Winblad B. Psychiatric disturbances and the use of psychotropic drugs in a population of nonagenarians. *Int J Geriat Psychiat* 1997; **12**: 533–6.
16. Blazer DG. Generalized anxiety disorder and panic disorder in the elderly: a review. *Harvard Rev Psychiat* 1997; **5**: 18–27.

99

Stress, Coping and Social Support

Lawrence R. Landerman and Dana Hughes

Duke University Medical Center, Durham, NC, USA

While a multitude of studies have examined the effects of social and environmental stressors, coping behaviors and social support on psychological distress, relatively little is known about their effects on neurotic disorders in the elderly. The effects of stress, support and coping on depression have been studied extensively in the general population and among those aged 65. A smaller number of studies examines their effects on the anxiety disorders in the general population. Very little work has been done with neurotic disorders as the outcome of interest among older persons. Recent reviewers conclude that the anxiety and panic disorders among the elderly have received little attention and that a systematic examination of the risk factors associated with late-life anxiety disorders has barely begun[1–3]. This is the case despite the fact that they are the most prevalent psychiatric conditions among the elderly, as they are among younger persons. Methodological problems involved with defining and operationalizing the anxiety disorders, disentangling anxiety from depression, and the transience of some symptom states account, in part, for the lack of attention they have received in epidemiologic studies[3,4].

Since the overwhelming majority of relevant studies deal with depression rather than the neurotic disorders, we will use these to examine the rationale and evidence for epidemiologic models linking stress, coping and support to psychiatric symptoms and disorder. Next, we will review a smaller but growing number of studies that have begun to examine whether stress, support and coping affect the anxiety disorders in a manner similar to their effects on depression. Since all but three of these anxiety studies are based on general population surveys rather than samples of the elderly *per se*, we will address the degree to which these studies are consistent with a conclusion that similar effects of stress, coping and support on neurosis are present among the elderly. Finally, we will point out key unresolved issues and the practical implications of the studies reviewed.

STRESS, COPING, SOCIAL SUPPORT AND DEPRESSION

Stress

Stressors refer to life experiences that may be perceived as threatening and/or challenging. They include discrete "stressful life events", such as changes in finances, health or marital status. They also include more enduring or chronic problems with regard to income, health or other areas of life. Reviewers are in accord that there is consistent evidence that stress is associated with an increased risk of psychiatric symptoms and disorder[5–7]. Findings for stress and depression are based on samples of older adults as well as the general population and include prospective studies where stress precedes the onset of symptoms[8–10].

Stressful life events are most likely to have negative health consequences if they are perceived as unexpected and undesirable[5]. Negatively-evaluated changes in health, family and living situations, work and finances have been shown to be strongly and positively related to depressive symptoms and major depressive episodes in the general population and in samples of older individuals[5,11,12]. Chronic stressors include poverty, deteriorated neighborhood conditions and ill health, which have been shown to predict both the onset of depression and the course of recovery[13–17]. While cross-sectional studies show an association between cognitive impairment and depression[4–17], prospective studies report mixed and inconclusive results regarding whether dementia or cognitive impairment are risk factors for the onset or duration of depression[17].

While older persons experience fewer potentially stressful life events[18], they experience a "changing landscape of stressors"[19], and are more likely to experience particular events that are strongly related to psychiatric morbidity[20]. These include poor health and disability, widowhood, and the death of other friends and family members[21,22]. While retirement *per se* is not associated with an increased risk of psychiatric disorder[23], a recent study[24] reports that driving cessation is strongly associated with an increased risk of depressive symptoms. Findings are mixed regarding whether stress associated with caring for a disabled person is a risk factor for depression. Initial studies of those (presumably more distressed) caregivers who sought services found high levels of depressive symptoms. A smaller number of community studies of caregiving and depression report inconsistent results[17].

Coping

Coping refers to steps the individual takes to avoid, solve or minimize the impact of life problems[25]. It serves two functions: problem solving and the regulation of emotions. Different coping strategies can have different consequences for psychological well-being generally, and for the impact of stress on well-being in particular. Rodin[26] contends that solving a problem without help from others may promote well-being by enhancing feelings of self-worth and personal control. Requesting help, on the other hand, may negatively affect well-being by generating interpersonal conflict if those asked are unwilling or unable to provide assistance[9]. This is especially true for financial help. One's social network is typically made up of persons in similar economic circumstances, whose financial resources may already be limited. There is evidence that most older people value independence and prefer to resolve problems by themselves, rather than depend upon others[27]. Systematic evidence for the impact of specific coping strategies on psychiatric morbidity is presently lacking. The number and variety of possible coping responses, together with the fact that assessments of appropriate coping behavior may vary across situations and social groups, has made research in this area difficult[20].

Social Support

Social support refers to a number of different aspects of social relations and includes: (a) social network: the size, stability, and structure of an individual's network of friends, relatives, and acquaintances; (b) social interaction: the presence and quantity of interaction with network members as well as organizational participation; (c) instrumental support: services and assistance provided by family and friends; and (d) perceived support: subjective satisfaction with one's social relationships and availability of support.

Two alternative models have guided most empirical studies of the relationship between social support and depression. With the "stress-buffering" model, a statistical interaction is hypothesized. The protective effect of support is expected to be at its maximum under conditions of stress and weaker when stress is absent[28,29]. Given the presence of a potentially stressful event or experience, social support is thought to influence the degree to which the situation is appraised as threatening, and an individual's capacity to cope. The impact of stress on depression will therefore be strongest among those lacking adequate support. In the absence of stress, the availability of support is of less importance, and the relationship between support and depression is expected to be weaker. With the "main effect" model of stress, support and depression, high levels of social support are hypothesized to promote mental health at all levels of stress. From this perspective, the effects of stress and support are not interactive—the effect of each does not depend upon the level of the other[30,31].

Reviewers report that the protective effect of support on depression varies across its different dimensions in the general population and among older persons[8,9,20,21]. Perceived support is most strongly and consistently protective for depression. There is also longitudinal evidence that the primary causal influence is from perceived support to depression, rather than the reverse. Findings for the protective effect of network size have been mostly negative. Amount of social interaction is associated with depression in several studies, but not with the onset of depression in longitudinal research. Received support can increase, as well as reduce, the risk of depression[9,12]. Krause et al.[9] reason that the receipt of assistance may reflect a failed attempt to solve a problem on one's own, and may be accompanied by hostility and resentment from those providing assistance. Reviewers are also in agreement that most (but not all) studies report a stress-by-support interaction consistent with the stress-buffering models[11,20]. Positive findings for stress buffering are most often present for perceived support, and recent findings suggest that anticipated support—the belief that others stand ready and able to help if called upon—is especially critical, as it promotes effective coping and confidence that a problem can be solved[9,13].

According to Kahn and Antonucci's convoy metaphor for social support[32], the size and composition of one's social network changes over the life course as individuals enter and leave a variety of social roles (e.g. spouse, parent, employee). Social networks change composition later in life in response to changes in one's health and employment, and to impairment and death among one's age peers[20]. For example, retirement can provide time to expand the scope of one's social participation, and even poor health, which limits some relationships, may enhance others as one's support network is mobilized to provide assistance[33]. Findings are mixed regarding whether there is a net decrease in network size and frequency of contact in old age, allowing different reviewers to draw different conclusions. However, there is general agreement that aging is not a time of social isolation, and that most older people have a significant number of relationships[20,33]. Studies of changes in social network and interaction after age 65 report considerable change, characterized by widely varying patterns of gains and losses rather than a trend toward isolation[33]. While it is unclear how these specific changes affect the psychological health of older adults, the notion that old age is a time of psychologically debilitating isolation is clearly not supported.

STRESS, COPING, SOCIAL SUPPORT AND THE NEUROTIC DISORDERS

The proposition that stress, support and coping may affect neurosis is consistent with existing theories that suggest that symptoms of anxiety and panic disorders represent a dysfunctional response to potentially stressful environmental events[10]. While anxiety is adaptive in the face of potentially threatening or unpleasant events, the anxiety disorders are characterized by unjustifiably intense and morbid anxiety and panic[2]. Endler's multidimensional interaction model of anxiety includes situational factors (stressors) and individual characteristics which interact to produce anxiety symptoms and disorder[34]. Relevant individual characteristics include "trait anxiety"—a predisposition to react to stressors generally, or to particular stressors, with dysfunctionally high and persistent levels of anxiety. Individual traits also include differentially effective coping styles and behaviors. One's appraisal and use of available resources, such as social support, is incorporated as part of coping.

There is also reason to expect differences in how stress and support might relate to anxiety as opposed to depression. The anxiety disorders, which include agoraphobia (with and without panic attack), social and simple phobia, panic disorder, generalized anxiety disorder and obsessive–compulsive disorder (OCD), are considerably more complex and diverse than the subtypes of depression. This has led reviewers to call for research that considers these subcategories separately in examining the effects of stress, support, coping and other risk factors[34,35]. The "multidimensional" aspect of Endler's model refers to the proposition that trait anxiety may be stressor-specific. Environmental danger might trigger anxiety only among those predisposed on this trait, while a symptomatic response to a job interview might be limited to those differently predisposed. The implication—that the effect of a stressor on anxiety would be greatly attenuated unless it is estimated separately for those with the corresponding trait anxiety—adds considerable complexity to the stress-support model. A related hypothesis—that stressors dealing with loss (of health, finances or social support) might result in sadness and depression, while stressors involving danger (severe future threat but not necessarily loss) might trigger anxiety—further complicates the picture[36].

Reviewers agree that most studies report a positive association between various stressors and one or another measure of anxiety[34,35,37]. Investigators report both transient and long-term symptoms of anxiety and depression following exposure to extreme experiences (e.g. combat missions and natural and man-made disasters)[34]. Chronic stressors and stressful life events are also related to anxiety[37,38] and negatively-evaluated stressful events have a stronger impact than the number of events *per se*[4]. Stressors included negative life events, physical decline, poor health, chronic financial stress, occupational stress and loss of a family member. Longitudinal findings show that various stressors precede the onset of anxiety[4,36,39,40] and influence treatment outcome over time[38]. There is also evidence that minor stressors ("daily hassles") may play a particularly important role in the onset of generalized anxiety disorder[41,42]. Three studies examined the stress–anxiety relationship in elderly populations and report various stressors, including stressful life events, health problems and loss of a loved one to be significant risk factors for phobic disorders, generalized anxiety disorder and the anxiety disorders generally[3,4,43].

Coping style and social support are related to one or another measure of anxiety in prior studies. Panic disorder has been found to be associated with less effective coping strategies in response to stress[44–46]. Those with panic disorder are more likely to use strategies involving escape, avoidance, wishful thinking and help-seeking, rather than focused problem-solving without help. Studies based on age-heterogeneous and elderly samples of the elderly report that external locus of control is positively related to anxiety[3,47]. Compared to others, those with generalized anxiety disorder are reported to perceive the same stressors as more stressful and threatening[35]. Several measures of social support have been found to be associated with anxiety symptoms and/or disorder. These include small network size, marital problems, not having a confidante, and loneliness[3,38,39,48]. In one study, death of a network member was found to affect depression but not anxiety[39]. Another study, which focused on stress-buffering, reports that a stress-by-support interaction effect is present for anxiety but weaker than the corresponding effect for depression[49].

CONCLUSION

While the above studies provide evidence that stress, coping and support affect the anxiety disorders as well as depression, they are limited in number and scope and do not permit any firm conclusions about the specific workings of the stress-vulnerability model derived from depression studies, or the more complex multidimensional model proposed by Endler[34]. This is especially true with respect to the elderly population, where we were able to locate only three relevant studies. The extensive literature on depression suggests that the effects of stress, support and coping on psychiatric disorder do not vary with age. However, researchers have only begun to address this issue with respect to neurosis. We located two studies comparing the effects of stress on anxiety in different age groups. One reported that the effects of different stressors were mostly the same in older and younger populations, while a second reported age differences in the impact of stressful life events[3,4].

Perhaps the most critical gap in the literature reviewed here is the absence of systematic knowledge about differences in the effects of stress, coping and support (and risk factors generally) across the specific subcategories of neurosis. Important in its own right, this information is especially critical if consistent and inconsistent findings across studies using different anxiety measures are to contribute to a cumulative understanding. Only one study has examined the effects of the same measures of stress, coping and support on the specific subtypes of anxiety, and reports that partner loss and poor health more strongly related to panic disorder and OCD, while network size and the exchange of emotional support affect only the phobias[3]. Their cross-sectional

data and the specificity of the sample (older adults in Holland) make this study an initial step in what needs to be an ongoing process.

Findings are also sparse and inconsistent with respect to other proposed links between neurosis and the risk factors considered. The hypothesis that anxiety and depression may result from different stressors (threat vs. danger) received support in an initial test[36]. Two subsequent studies report that most stressors affected both anxiety and depression, and that differences which did exist were not consistent with the threat vs. danger hypothesis[38,39]. Endler's proposition[34], that particular stressors may trigger anxiety only among those with a congruent susceptibility, has yet to be examined in representative community samples. While there is evidence that social support is protective for the neurotic disorders, we do not know which dimensions of support are critical, whether support exerts a generalized protective effect or whether stress-buffering is operative. Finally, as discussed in Monroe and Wade[35], substantial co-morbidity between anxiety and depression make it imperative that we examine the role of depression in the relationships of stress, coping and support to anxiety.

While epidemiologic examination of the effects of stress, coping and support on the neurotic disorders is still in an initial stage, the research reviewed here is not without practical import. As Sheikh[2] has observed, potential side effects, drug interactions and non-compliance among the elderly make effective non-pharmaceutical therapies particularly attractive[2]. In this regard, clinicians and researchers have reported that the success of exposure-based treatments for agoraphobia depends in part on the patient's marital relationship, and that including the spouse in therapy can be critical to successful treatment[50–52]. Findings reviewed here—that marital satisfaction is protective for anxiety symptoms in addition to agoraphobia—suggest that attention to the marital relationship may improve psychological and behavioral treatments for other anxiety disorders as well. Findings that other forms of social support are also protective suggest that focusing on relationships in addition to the marital one may also be useful. Additional studies of onset and recovery, which systematically related marital and other social relationships to onset and recovery for specific disorders among the elderly, would be especially useful in this area.

The studies reviewed also have implications at the social structural level. There is strong and consistent evidence that inequalities in education, occupation and income are major determinants of the public's mental health, and that the least privileged members of society are at increased risk for health, financial and work-related stressors, which contribute to both anxiety and depression[37,53]. The well-to-do, on the other hand, are less exposed and have more social and material reserves with which to overcome negative and unpredictable events. Treating mental disorder at the social as well as the individual level involves programs and policies designed to reduce inequality and/or reduce its impact on mental health. Among the elderly, improved coverage for mental health treatment under Medicare and Medicaid would enable the elderly, and particularly those with limited incomes, to obtain necessary and timely treatment[20]. Recognizing health problems as a major risk factor for depression among the elderly, Jorm advocates "improved geriatric care" to reduce depression[17]. While findings for the impact of health on neurosis are not nearly as extensive as for depression, poor health is a consistent risk factor for one or another measure of anxiety. In this regard, evidence is accumulating that expanded Medicare coverage for prescription drugs, preventive care and other services typically covered by supplemental private insurance would substantially reduce health problems and disability among older persons, especially those with limited financial resources[54].

Evidence that low income persons enter old age in considerably worse health than others[55] indicates that improving the mental health of the elderly will also require attention to social inequality and its link to physical and mental health throughout the life course.

REFERENCES

1. Blazer DG. Generalized anxiety disorder and panic disorder in the elderly: a review. *Harvard Rev Psychiat* 1997; **5**: 18–27.
2. Sheikh JI. Anxiety and panic disorders. In Busse EW, Blazer DG, eds, *Geriatric Psychiatry*, 2nd edn. Washington, DC: American Psychiatric Press, 1996: 279–89.
3. Beekman AT, Bremmer MA, Deeg DJ et al. Anxiety disorders in later life: a report from the Longitudinal Aging Study Amsterdam. *Int J Geriat Psychiat* 1998; **13**: 717–26.
4. Blazer DG, Hughes DC, George LK. Stressful life events and the onset of generalized anxiety syndrome. *Am J Psychiat* 1987; **144**: 1178–83.
5. Pearlin LI. The sociological study of stress. *J Health Soc Behav* 1989; **30**: 241–56.
6. George LK. Stress, social support, and depression over the life course. In Markides KS, Cooper CL, eds, *Aging, Stress and Health*. New York: Wiley, 1989: 241–67.
7. Eaton WW, Dohrenwend DP. Individual events. In Dohrenwend BP, ed., *Adversity, Stress, and Psychopathology*. New York: Oxford University Press, 1998: 77–9.
8. Krause N. Anticipated support, received support, and economic stress among older adults. *J Gerontol Psychol Sci* 1997; **52B**(6): 284–93.
9. Blazer DG, Hughes DC, George LK. The epidemiology of depression in an elderly community population. *Gerontologist* 1987; **27**: 281–7.
10. George LK. Social factors and the onset and outcome of depression. In Schaie KW, House JS, Blazer DG, eds, *Aging, Health Behaviors, and Health Outcomes*. Hillsdale, NJ: Erlbaum, 1992: 137–59.
11. Ranga RK, George LK, Peiper CF et al. Depression and social support in elderly patients with cardiac disease. *Am Heart J* 1998; **136**: 491–5.
12. Hayes JC, Landerman LR, George LK et al. Social correlates of the dimensions of depression in the elderly. *J Gerontol Psychol Sci* 1998; **53B**: 31–9.
13. Krause N. Chronic financial strain, social support, and depressive symptoms among older adults. *Psychol Aging* 1987; **2**: 185–92.
14. La Gory M, Fitzpatrick K. The effects of environmental context on elderly depression. *J Aging Health* 1992; **4**: 459–79.
15. Berkman LF, Berkman CS, Kasl S et al. Depressive symptoms in relation to physical health and functioning in the elderly. *Am J Epidemiol* 1986; **124**: 372–88.
16. Blazer DG, Burchette B, Service C et al. The association of age and depression among the elderly: an epidemiologic exploration. *J Gerontol* 1991; **46**: 210–15.
17. Jorm AF. The epidemiology of depressive states in the elderly. Implications for recognition, intervention, and prevention. *Psychiat Psychiat Epidemiol* 1995; **30**: 53–9.
18. Hughes DC, George LK, Blazer DG. Age differences in life event qualities: multivariate controlled analyses. *J Commun Psychol* 1988; **16**: 171–4.
19. Pearlin LI, Skaff MM. Stress and the life course: a paradigmatic alliance. *Gerontologist* 1996; **36**: 239–47.
20. George LK. Social and economic factors related to psychiatric disorders in late life. In Busse EW, Blazer DG, eds, *Geriatric Psychiatry*, 2nd edn. Washington, DC: American Psychiatric Press, 1996: 139–54.
21. Krause N. Stress and sex differences in depressive symptoms among older adults. *J Gerontol* 1986; **41**: 727–31.
22. Green BH, Copeland JRM, Dewey ME et al. Risk factors for depression in elderly people: a prospective study. *Acta Psychiat Scand* 1992; **86**: 213–17.
23. Atchley RC. *The Sociology of Retirement*. Cambridge, MA: Schenkmen, 1976.
24. Marotolli RA, Mendes de Leon CF, Glass TA et al. Driving cessation and increased depressive symptoms: prospective evidence from the New Haven EPESE. Established Populations for Epidemiologic Studies of the Elderly. *J Am Geriatr Soc* 1997; **45**(2): 202–6.
25. Pearlin L, Schooler C. The structure of coping. *J Health Soc Behav* 1978; **19**: 2–21.
26. Rodin J. Control by any name: Definitions, concepts, and processes. In Rodin J, Schooler C, Schaie KW, eds, *Self-directedness: Causes and Effects Throughout the Life Course*. Hillsdale, NJ: Erlbaum, 1990: 1–17.
27. Lee GR. Kinship and support of the elderly: the case of the United States. *Aging Soc* 1985; **5**: 19–38.
28. Cohen S, Wills TA. Social support, stress, and the buffering hypothesis. *Psychol Bull* 1985; **98**: 310–57.
29. Turner RJ. Social support as a contingency in psychological well being. *J Health Soc Behav* 1981; **22**: 357–67.
30. House JS. *Work Stress and Social Support*. Reading, MA: Addison-Wesley, 1981.
31. Thoits PA. Theoretical distinctions between causal and interaction effects of social support. *J Health Soc Behav* 1981; **22**: 357–67.
32. Kahn RL, Antonucci TC. Convoys over the life course: attachments, roles and social support. In Baltes PB, Brim O, eds, *Life Span Development and Behavior*. New York: Academic Press, 1980: 253–86.
33. van Tilburg TG. Losing and gaining in old age: changes in personal network size and social support in a four-year longitudinal study. *J Gerontol Soc Sci* 1998; **53B**: S313–23.
34. Endler NS, Edwards JM. Stress and vulnerability. In Last CG, Hersen M, eds, *Handbook of Anxiety Disorders*. New York: Pergamon, 1988: 278–92.
35. Monroe SM, Wade SL. Life events. In Last CG, Hersen M, eds, *Handbook of Anxiety Disorders*. New York: Pergamon, 1988: 293–305.
36. Finlay-Jones R, Brown GW. Types of stressful life events and the onset of anxiety and depressive disorders. *Psychol Med* 1981; **11**: 803–15.
37. Muntaner C, Eaton WW, Diala C, Kessler RC. Social class, assets, organizational control and prevalence of common groups of psychiatric disorders. *Soc Sci Med* 1998; **47**: 2043–53.
38. Wade SL, Monroe SM, Michelson LK. Chronic life stress and treatment outcome in agoraphobia with panic attacks. *Am J Psychiat* 1993; **150**: 1491–5.
39. Kendler KS, Karkowski LM, Prescott CA. Stressful life events and major depression risk period, long-term contextual threat, and diagnostic specificity. *J Nerv Ment Dis* 1998; **186**: 661–9.
40. Faravelli C, Pallanti S. Recent life events and panic disorder. *Am J Psychiat* 1989; **146**: 622–6.
41. Kanner AD, Coyne JC, Schaefer C, Lazarus RS. Comparison of two modes of stress measurement: daily hassles and uplifts vs. major life events. *J Behav Med* 1981; **4**: 1–39.
42. Brantley PJ, Mehan DJ Jr, Ames SC, Jones GN. Minor stressors and generalized anxiety disorder among low-income patients attending primary care clinics. *J Nerv Men Dis* 1999; **187**: 435–40.
43. Lindsey J. Phobic disorders in the elderly. *Br J Psychiat* 1991; **159**: 531–41.
44. Cox BJ, Endler NS, Swinson RP, Norton GR. Situations and specific coping strategies associated with clinical and non-clinical panic attacks. *Behav Res Ther* 1992; **30**: 67–9.
45. Vitaliano PP, Katon W, Russo J et al. Coping as an index of illness behavior in panic disorder. *J Nerv Ment Dis* 1987; **175**: 78–84.
46. Borden JW, Clum GA, Broyles SE, Watkins PL. Coping strategies and panic. *J Anxiety Disord* 1988; **2**: 339–52.
47. Borkovec TD, Shadick RN, Hopkins M. The nature of normal and pathological worry. In Rapee RM, Barlow DH, eds, *Chronic Anxiety: Generalized Anxiety Disorder and Mixed Anxiety–Depression*. New York: Guilford, 1991: 29–51.
48. Dalgard OS, Bjrk S, Tambs K. Social support, negative life events and mental health. *Br J Psychiat* 1985; **166**: 29–34.
49. Mathiesen KS, Tambs K, Dalgard OS. The influence of social class, strain and social support on symptoms of anxiety and depression in the mothers of toddlers. *Soc Psychiat Psychiat Epidemiol* 1999; **34**: 61–72.

50. Last CG, Hersen M. Overview. In Last CG, Hersen M, eds, *Handbook of Anxiety Disorders*. New York: Pergamon, 1988: 3–10.

51. Hafner RJ. Marital and family therapy. In Last CG, Hersen M, eds, *Handbook of Anxiety Disorders*. New York: Pergamon, 1988; 386–401.

52. Craske MG, Burton T, Barlow DH. Relationships among measures of communication, marital satisfaction and exposure during couples treatment of agoraphobia. *Behav Res Ther* 1989; **27**: 131–40.

53. Rogler LLH. Increasing socioeconomic inequality and the mental health of the poor. *J Nerv Ment Dis* 1996; **184**: 719–22.

54. Landerman LR, Fillenbaum GG, Pieper CF *et al.* Private health insurance and disability among older Americans. *J Gerontol Soc Sci* 1998; **53B**: S258–66.

55. House JS, Lepkowski JM, Kinney Mero RP *et al.* The social stratification of aging and health. *J Health Soc Behav* 1994; **35**: 213–34.

100

Clinical Features of Anxiety Disorders

Erin L. Cassidy[1,2], Pamela J. Swales[2] and Javaid I. Sheikh[1,2]

[1]*Stanford University School of Medicine, Stanford, CA, USA, and*
[2]*Veterans Affairs, Palo Alto Health Care System, CA, USA*

The subjective sense of trepidation or dread about some future event that can motivate one person to stay at work late to complete an important project, can send another to the hospital with the belief that he/she is going into cardiac arrest. As a normal human emotion, anxiety has adaptive value in helping one prepare for, and possibly avoid, deleterious events. This emotion, however, can manifest pathologically if it becomes excessive, inappropriate or maladaptive. Such morbid or clinically significant anxiety can range from excessive worry about mundane concerns to experiencing intense episodes of fear (panic attacks) for no apparent reason. Clinically significant anxiety is usually manifested by a variety of cognitive, behavioral and physiological symptoms. Table 100.1 lists some examples of these multidimensional features. When assessing such symptoms, the clinician will query the patient with regards to the duration, intensity and course to determine whether the cluster of symptoms meet criteria for any of the specific anxiety disorders.

Over the last two decades, researchers have made great strides in furthering the understanding of the phenomenology, co-morbidity and clinical course of anxiety disorders in the general population[1–4]. However, research with the geriatric population is lagging, forcing clinicians to use knowledge gained from studies that more commonly study a younger age group. In addition to utilizing these empirical studies, those treating the anxious elderly must rely mostly on their own observations and anecdotal information, in addition to the "youth-biased" literature base[5]. Some have expressed concern that the diagnosis of anxiety states may be particularly difficult in the elderly because of the frequent co-morbidity of depression or medical illness[6–7]. In addition, concerns are being raised regarding the *Diagnostic and Statistical Manual of Mental Disorders*, 4th edn (DSM-IV) of the American Psychiatric Association[8]. The DSM criteria for the anxiety disorders may not always allow for the correct identification of the anxiety-disordered elderly because many older adults display a tendency to deny cognitive symptomatology and instead somatize their distress[9]. Despite these limitations, analyses of the Epidemiologic Catchment Area (ECA) data (using the DSM-III-R criteria) indicate that anxiety disorders can be diagnosed successfully. Finally, the risk of developing an anxiety disorder does not fade in late life. For example, in a large sample of the 65+ age group, individuals experienced a rather high 6 month prevalence of 19.7% for all anxiety disorders[10].

This chapter presents the clinical features of various anxiety disorders based on the criteria set out in the DSM-IV. A list of the DSM-IV anxiety disorders appears in Table 100.2. Differential presentations and unique features of the anxiety disorders in the elderly will be discussed where appropriate.

PANIC DISORDER WITH/WITHOUT AGORAPHOBIA (PD/PDA)

Panic attacks are acute and discrete episodes of intense anxiety that result as a reaction to some perceived threat (emotional, environmental, etc.). The term "panic attack" is used when an individual experiences an intense and acute reaction to an internal or external cue, lasting between a few minutes and a half an hour. The physiological symptoms can include trembling, accelerated heart rate, sweating, shortness of breath, chest pain, dizziness, nausea and the sense that one is somehow detached from one's surroundings[11]. For example, an individual might have been trapped in a crowd of people entering an underground subway system, and will describe feeling "sick to their stomach" when entering one. Another individual might even report high levels of acute anxiety at the mere sight of the stairs leading to the subway. A clinically significant degree of panic symptoms are documented after a review of the patient's history, revealing recurrent and unpredictable panic attacks that precede at least 1 month spent with anticipated worry over possible recurrence.

Diagnostically, one needs also to consider whether there is the presence of agoraphobia in relation to the panic attacks. Agoraphobia involves the persistent fear of being in a situation that results in a panic attack. Individuals suffering from agoraphobia will commonly stay inside their house all day long to ensure the avoidance of the feared situation. Some of the common examples of frightening situations include being caught in traffic on a bridge or freeway. When comparing young and older adults with panic disorder (PD), one of the factors that can affect the clinical presentation appears to be the age of onset. Phenomenologically, it appears that late-onset PD (LOPD, onset of PD at or after age 55) patients report fewer panic symptoms, less avoidance, and score lower on somatization measures than do early-onset PD (EOPD, onset of PD prior to age 55) patients.

AGORAPHOBIA WITHOUT HISTORY OF PANIC DISORDER (AWOPD)

The literature is scant regarding this relatively rare disorder. Its distinguishing feature from Panic Disorder with Agoraphobia is a fear of being in public places or situations from which escape might be difficult, even though there is the *absence* of a history of panic attacks. There is a possibility that, although these patients may not experience full-blown panic attacks, they might suffer from milder ones with only one or two symptoms (limited symptom attacks). It is thus possible that some of these patients

Table 100.1 Multidimensional symptoms of anxiety

Cognitive	Behavioral	Physiological
Nervousness	Hyperkinesis	Muscle tension
Apprehension	Repetitive motor acts	Chest tightness
Worry	Avoidance (e.g. certain places)	Palpitations
Fearfulness	Pressured speech	Hyperventilation
Irritability	Increased startle response	Paresthesias
Distractibility	Lightheadedness	Lightheadedness
	Sweating	Sweating
	Urinary frequency	Urinary frequency

Table 100.2 DSM-IV anxiety disorders

- Panic disorder without agoraphobia (PD)
- Panic disorder with agoraphobia (PDA)
- Agoraphobia without history of panic disorder (AWOPD)
- Social phobia (social anxiety disorder, SAD)
- Specific phobia (formerly simple phobia)
- Obsessive-compulsive disorder (OCD)
- Acute stress disorder (ASD)
- Post-traumatic stress disorder (PTSD)
- Generalized anxiety disorder (GAD)
- Anxiety disorder not otherwise specified (ADNOS)
- Anxiety disorder due to a general medical condition
- Substance-induced anxiety disorder

are presenting with a variant of panic disorder. Multicenter studies suggest that AWOPD, GAD and Social Phobia are commonly co-morbid. Moreover, in general, AWOPD presents with worse global functioning than PD or PDA[12]. This syndrome has not been studied in the elderly.

SOCIAL PHOBIA (SOCIAL ANXIETY DISORDER)

Social Anxiety Disorder (SAD) is defined by a persistent fear in one or more social situations marked by fears of performance, excessive scrutiny or of acting in a way that will be embarrassing or bring shame. Frequently, the fear is that of trembling, blushing or sweating profusely in social situations. Other common concerns are of saying something stupid or "babbling or talking funny". Common examples include fears of public speaking, avoidance of dating, parties or other social gatherings. Social phobics typically experience marked anticipatory anxiety if they attempt to enter the phobic situation. SAD is associated with onset in early life—typically manifesting in adolescence. The two distinct subtypes, generalized and non-generalized, trigger different types of symptoms, course of illness, pathophysiology and response to treatment[13]. Although systematic studies of this disorder in the elderly are lacking, epidemiological data[11] indicate that it is chronic and persistent in old age. Common manifestations in old age include the inability to eat food in the presence of strangers and, especially in men, being unable to urinate in public lavatories. It is unlikely that an older adult will seek professional help with these complaints as primary. Although systematic studies of social phobia in older patients are lacking, our clinical experience suggests that eating or writing in public can be exceedingly difficult in older social phobics, exacerbated by the use of dentures or the presence of tremors. It is not uncommon to encounter social phobics who present with symptoms of panic disorder. Evidence suggests that this disorder is quite commonly co-morbid with panic disorder[14].

SPECIFIC PHOBIA (FORMERLY SIMPLE PHOBIA)

The distinguishing feature of this disorder is a marked and persistent fear of a specific object or situation (other than a fear of experiencing a panic attack or a fear of social situations). Typically, the patient experiences immediate and intense distress on encountering the phobic stimulus, and recognizes that the fear is excessive and/or unreasonable. Further, the avoidance or anxious anticipation of encountering the phobic stimulus must interfere with the person's daily routine, occupational functioning or social life, or the individual is markedly distressed about having the phobia. The level of anxiety or fear usually varies as a function of both the degree of proximity to the phobic stimuli and the degree to which escape is limited. Examples of common phobias include fear of animals (dogs, snakes, insects, etc.), closed spaces (claustrophobia), flying or heights. There is

frequent co-occurrence of Specific Phobia with PD and PDA. In the elderly, especially in urban settings, fear of crime seems to be particularly prevalent in the elderly population (although they are the least likely to be victimized). UK researcher Lindesay[15] looked at elderly phobics and matched them for age and sex to case controls without history of phobic disorders, and found that in the elderly phobic disorders are associated with considerably higher psychiatric and medical morbidity. It also appears that, despite higher rates of contact among the phobic elderly with general practitioners compared to controls, only 1 in 60 of the phobic elderly in this study was receiving psychiatric help. In general, systematic studies of specific phobias are lacking in the older population.

OBSESSIVE-COMPULSIVE DISORDER

Obsessive-compulsive disorder (OCD) involves persistent patterns of thoughts, obsessions and behaviors, compulsions that are performed in an effort to decrease the anxiety experienced as a result of the thoughts. Obsessions are thoughts or ideas that come to a person's mind, frequently during the process of completing a specific task, or that occur during a particular type of situation. For example, sufferers may find themselves washing their hands repeatedly, for hours at a time, as a result of shaking a stranger's hand. The unwanted thought is that they may have exposed themselves to a serious disease. The act of washing in this example is what is referred to as a compulsion. OCD is a disorder that is chronic and often disabling for the individual[16]. Depression and other symptoms of anxiety often accompany the symptoms of OCD.

POST-TRAUMATIC STRESS DISORDER (PTSD)

The distinctive feature of post-traumatic stress disorder (PTSD) is that the individual has experienced, either witnessed or was a victim of, a traumatic event to which they reacted with feelings of fear and helplessness. Examples of such events include those that involve actual or threatened death or serious injury, or other threat to one's integrity, or witnessing an event that involves death or serious injury of another, or hearing about death or serious injury to a family member or close associate. In addition, the individual's accompanying response must have involved extreme fear, helplessness or horror. Other essential features include a number of symptoms that cluster into three categories: (a) persistent *re-experiencing* of the traumatic event; (b) persistent *avoidance of stimuli* associated with the traumatic event and a numbing of general responsiveness; and (c) persistent symptoms of *increased arousal*. Symptoms of re-experiencing include distressing dreams of the event, and intense physical and/or psychological distress at exposure to internal or external cues that symbolize or resemble an aspect of the event. Symptoms of avoidance and numbing include efforts to avoid activities, people, places, and conversations associated with, or that would arouse recollections of, the trauma. Symptoms of hyperarousal include difficulty in falling or staying asleep, hypervigilance and exaggerated startle response. PTSD usually presents with co-morbid conditions such as depression, panic disorder and substance use disorders. Symptoms must be present for at least 1 month and cause clinically significant distress or impairment in social, occupational or other important area of functioning. Reports of PTSD in elderly Holocaust survivors[17] and among elders who were prisoners of war during World War II[18] indicate that PTSD can be a chronic disorder, continuing into old age. There is some evidence that the intensity of the physiological response to the original trauma may be the most significant predictor of a relatively poor outcome and a chronic course[19]. It also appears that ongoing life stressors may slow the recovery process.

ACUTE STRESS DISORDER (ASD)

Characteristic features of this disorder include the development of anxiety, dissociative and other symptoms that occur between 2 days and 1 month after exposure to an extreme traumatic stressor (such as natural or man-made disasters, rape, combat, assault). The symptoms are identical to those described in PTSD, therefore one should consider PTSD as the diagnostic descriptor after a month has passed.

GENERALIZED ANXIETY DISORDER

The distinctive symptoms of this disorder include intense worry about more than one area of one's life. This concern is accompanied by symptoms including: feeling easily tired, experiencing other physical symptoms, such as muscle tension, having trouble sleeping through the night, difficulty concentrating on a task, and feeling irritable or on edge. These symptoms need to be described as having occurred for at least 6 months and must be accompanied by the sense that one cannot control the feelings of anxiety. Many elderly patients with this syndrome may also present with features of depression, thus making it difficult to distinguish between the two diagnoses.

ANXIETY DISORDER DUE TO A GENERAL MEDICAL CONDITION/SUBSTANCE-INDUCED ANXIETY

The elderly as a group are probably most prone to developing this syndrome due to their high prevalence of medical illness and the relatively common occurrence of polypharmacy. Generalized anxiety and/or panic symptoms are the usual presentations among these patients. Among the more common medical disorders producing symptoms of anxiety are endocrine conditions (e.g. hyper- and hypothyroidism, hypoglycemia), cardiovascular conditions (e.g. congestive heart failure, pulmonary embolism, angina, arrhythmias), pulmonary conditions (e.g. chronic obstructive pulmonary disease, pneumonia) and neurological conditions (e.g. neoplasms, Parkinson's disease). Among the more common substances/medications producing symptoms of anxiety in the elderly are alcohol (intoxication or withdrawal), stimulants (caffeine, sympathomimetics in over-the-counter medications), steroids, thyroid preparations, anticholinergic medications and antidepressants. A thorough history, with an attempt to clarify temporal relationship of symptomatology with the onset of medical illness or the beginning of medication, goes a long way toward resolving the issue.

ANXIETY DISORDER NOT OTHERWISE SPECIFIED

This category includes disorders with prominent anxiety symptoms or phobic avoidance behaviors that do not meet criteria for any specific Anxiety or Adjustment Disorder with anxiety features.

MIXED ANXIETY DEPRESSIVE DISORDER (CATEGORY TARGETED FOR FURTHER STUDY IN DSM-IV)

This category of symptoms is included in the DSM-IV Criteria for Further Study. The essential feature of this proposed disorder is dysphoric mood that has been present for at least 1 month. This mood state must be associated with a minimum of four additional symptoms, such as irritability, worry, sleep disturbance, anticipating the worst, concentration or memory difficulties, and hopelessness. Clinicians working with the elderly have long observed the significant overlap in symptoms of anxiety and depression. In fact, it is quite common to see individuals with a combination of anxiety and depression, although one or both disorders might only be present at subsyndromal levels. Since the distinction between symptoms of anxiety and depression may be particularly difficult to make in older populations[20], this category has the potential for significant clinical utility. Further, making a distinction between a primary anxiety disorder and depression is not only of theoretical interest but also of considerable pragmatic value, since medications used for these disorders may have very different side-effect profiles.

ANXIETY/AGITATION IN DEMENTIA

Dementia patients, whether living at home or in a long-term care institution, commonly display behaviors described as agitation. Agitation is operationalized as verbal or motor activity that is either appropriate behavior but repeated frequently, or inappropriate behavior that suggests lack of judgment. As many as 85% of dementia patients go on to develop disruptive, agitated behavior. Early identification of triggers, including environmental stimuli, medication side effects and the inability to communicate internal needs, can lead to effective treatment and relief for already overburdened caregivers. One of the unique aspects in treating such patients is the need to also assess the health and function of the caregiver, which is frequently compromised due to the immense stress involved in performing the tasks to keep such patients safe and their needs attended to.

CONCLUSION

In summary, it appears that anxiety disorders are characterized by a chronic course, usually lasting into old age. Most of the research in the area of the phenomenology of anxiety disorders has been carried out in younger populations, and generalization to an older population is only extended by implication and a limited number of clinical studies and not on a broad-base of empirical data. Clinicians should keep in mind certain factors that can make assessment of anxiety in the elderly problematic. These include a higher rate of medical co-morbidity, which can confound the clinical picture in this population. In addition, a mixed symptom picture of anxiety and depression can make accurate assessment and specific treatment difficult at times. Finally, a tendency to deny psychopathology and a preference for somatic expression of distress may make it difficult at times to accurately assess the extent of anxiety. Studies designed to investigate any differential manifestations of anxiety disorders in the elderly are clearly needed.

REFERENCES

1. Sheikh JI. Anxiety disorders. In Coffey CE, Cummings JL, eds, *Textbook of Geriatric Neuropsychology*. Washington, DC: American Psychiatric Press, 2000: 274.
2. Sheehan DV. Current concepts in psychiatry: panic attacks and phobias. *N Engl J Med* 1982; **307**(3): 156–8.
3. Roth M. Anxiety and anxiety disorders—a general overview. In Roth M, Noyes JR, Burrow GD, eds, *Biological Clinical and Cultural Perspectives*. Amsterdam: Elsevier Science/North Holland, 1988: 1–44.
4. Marks IM. *Fears, Phobias, and Rituals: Panic, Anxiety, and their Disorders*. New York: Oxford University Press, 1987.
5. Sheikh JI, Salzman C. Anxiety in the elderly: course and treatment. *Psychiat Clin N Am* 1995; **18**(4): 871–83.
6. Shamoian CA. What is anxiety in the elderly? In Salzman C, Lebowitz B, eds, *Anxiety in the Elderly—Treatment and Research*. New York: Springer, 1991: 3–15.
7. Van Balkom AJ, Beekman AT, deBeurs E, Deeg DJ, van Dyck R, van Tilburg W. Comorbidity of the anxiety disorders in a community-based older population in The Netherlands. *Acta Psychiat Scand* 2000; **101**(1): 37–45.
8. American Psychiatric Association, Task Force and Work Groups on DSM-IV. *Diagnostic and Statistical Manual of Mental Disorders*, 4th edn. Washington, DC: American Psychiatric Association, 1994.
9. Gurian BS, Miner JH. Clinical presentation of anxiety in the elderly. In Saltzman C, Lebowitz B, eds, *Anxiety in the Elderly—Treatment and Research*. New York: Springer, 1991: 31–44.
10. Blazer D, George L, Hughes D. The epidemiology of anxiety disorders: an age comparison. In Salzman C, Liebowitz B, eds, *Anxiety in the Elderly—Treatment and Research*. New York: Springer, 1991: 17–30.
11. Ballenger JC, Davidson JRT, Lecrubier Y et al. Consensus statement on panic disorder from the International Consensus Group on Depression and Anxiety. *J Clin Psychiat* 1998; **59**(suppl 8): 47–54.
12. Goisman RM, Warshaw MG, Steketee GS et al. DSM-IV and the disappearance of agoraphobia without a history of panic: *Am J Psychiat* 1995; **152**(10): 1438–43.
13. Liebowitz MR. Update on the diagnosis and treatment of social anxiety disorder. *J Clin Psychiat* 1999; **60**(18): 22–6.
14. Goisman RM, Goldenberg I, Vasile RG, Keller MB. Comorbidity of anxiety disorders in a multicenter anxiety study. *Comp Psychiat* 1995; **36**: 303–11.
15. Lindesay J. Phobic disorders in the elderly. *Br J Psychiatry* 1991; **159**: 531–41.
16. Hantouche EG, Lancrenon S. Modern typology of symptoms and obsessive-compulsive syndromes: results of a large French study of 615 patients. *Encephale* 1996; **1**: 9–21.
17. Kuch K, Cox BJ. Symptoms of PTSD in 124 survivors of the Holocaust. *Am J Psychiat* 1992; **149**: 337–40.
18. Speed N, Engdahl B, Schwartz J, Eberly R. Posttraumatic stress disorder as a consequence of the POW experience. *J Nerv Ment Disord* 1989; **177**: 147–53.
19. Van der Kolk BA. The drug treatment of post-traumatic stress disorder. *J Affect Disord* 1987; **13**: 203–13.
20. Copeland JR, Davidson LA, Dewey ME. The prevalence and outcome of anxious depression in elderly people aged 65 and over living in the community. In Racagnia G, Smeraldi E, eds, *Anxious Depression—Assessment and Treatment*. New York: Raven, 1987: 43.

101

Prognosis of Anxiety Disorders

Pamela J. Swales[2], Erin L. Cassidy[1,2] and Javaid I. Sheikh[1,2]

[1]*Stanford University School of Medicine, Stanford, CA, and*
[2]*Veterans Affairs, Palo Alto Health Care System, CA, USA*

Anxiety disorders most commonly begin in early adulthood, seem to have a relatively protracted course and usually continue in later age[1]. As expected, relatively scant information exists at present about the prognosis of anxiety in the elderly. Therefore, this chapter will discuss research findings regarding the prognosis of anxiety disorders in the general population and, of necessity, make inferences about outcome in the elderly.

PANIC DISORDER (WITH AND WITHOUT AGORAPHOBIA)

Panic disorder is a common, usually chronic, illness with fluctuating symptomatology, which may be punctuated by periods of partial remission. Age of onset is typically in the mid-20s, but it may also develop in late life[2,3]. Panic disorder is commonly associated with considerable psychiatric co-morbidity including depression, obsessive–compulsive disorder, post-traumatic stress disorder and social anxiety disorder[4,5]. Nearly 50% of those with untreated panic disorder develop co-morbid depression and 43% of these have attempted suicide[6,7]. It is now quite well established that, if untreated, panic disorder may also lead to alcohol abuse[8], increased risk for suicide[7] and, in males, higher than average cardiovascular mortality[9]. Many untreated patients also develop multiple avoidance behaviors (agoraphobia), which are likely to produce serious impairments in social and occupational functioning[10].

Panic disorder rarely resolves without medical intervention[11]. Although both pharmacological and cognitive–behavioral interventions seem to be effective in the short term[11], the long-term effect of these treatments on the natural history of panic disorder is less established. Mounting clinical data favor the SSRIs as first-line treatment for patients with panic disorder. Patients should, in general, be treated for a minimum of 1 year. Those who have experienced previous relapses or who have co-morbid conditions should be considered for long-term therapy[12]. Patients who have more than two episodes should be maintained indefinitely.

OBSESSIVE–COMPULSIVE DISORDER

Obsessive–compulsive disorder (OCD) is a chronic and often disabling anxiety disorder that is characterized by recurring obsessions and uncontrolled compulsions. It often occurs co-morbidly with a number of depressive and anxiety disorders. Persons with obsessive–compulsive disorder often experience significant personal and social morbidity. Additionally, they may have difficulty finishing school, finding and maintaining a job and developing relationships[13].

Obsessive–compulsive disorder has a chronic course, and although symptoms may fluctuate over time, the disorder rarely resolves spontaneously without treatment[14,15]. Until relatively recently, many patients were refractory to conventional pharmacotherapy and obsessive–compulsive disorder was traditionally thought to have poor prognosis. However, of late, advances in both pharmacological and behavioral approaches and their combined use have become effective and important approaches in the management of this disorder. Specific psychopharmacological agents, clomipramine (a tricyclic antidepressant) and the selective serotonin reuptake inhibitors (SSRIs), have proved effective in controlled studies[16,17,18]. Thus, with appropriate diagnosis and treatments, most patients, including the elderly with OCD, will experience benefits and an improved quality of life.

SOCIAL PHOBIA (SOCIAL ANXIETY DISORDER)

Social anxiety disorder, an often-overlooked diagnosis, is characterized by a marked fear of social performance, excessive fear of scrutiny, and fear of acting in a way that will be embarrassing to oneself. Thus, exposure to social or public situations may provoke an anxiety response and be endured under extreme distress. The mean age of onset is 15.5 years and onset after age 25 years is uncommon[19]. Epidemiological data suggest that this disorder is chronic and persisting into old age, with most cases remaining untreated[20].

Social anxiety disorder is responsive to both pharmacological and psychological interventions and the two modalities appear to have complementary strengths. For example, cognitive–behavioral therapy[21] and social skills training have proven value. Pharmacological treatment includes the SSRIs, the monoamine oxidase inhibitors and the benzodiazepines, with the SSRIs as first-line treatment[22,23,24]. Information about long-term prognosis with these treatment strategies is lacking. A limitation of all medications is the substantial rate of relapse observed even after prolonged treatment. However, there appears to be a lower incidence of relapse following discontinuation of CBT[25]. Systematic studies of this disorder in the elderly are non-existent, although our clinical experience suggests that public speaking may seem less frightening, and a phobia such as fear of eating in public may be more bothersome, to the elderly than to younger people.

SIMPLE PHOBIA (SPECIFIC PHOBIA)

Generally, specific fears and phobias may be classified into the following groups: (a) situational phobias (lightning, enclosed spaces, darkness, flying, heights); (b) animal phobias (spiders, snakes); (c) blood-injury (injections, dentists, blood, injuries). An analysis of Epidemiological Catchment Area data suggests that the onset of social phobia is associated with female gender, low education and never having been married[26,27]. It is difficult to characterize the longitudinal course of simple phobias, principally due to the multiplicity of specific causal stimuli. In addition, individuals with one specific phobia may develop additional phobias or other psychopathology at some point in the course of their affliction.

Exposure and related desensitization techniques are the psychosocial treatments of choice for all variants of specific phobias and promise significant improvement[28]. These strategies also promise effective biobehavioral interventions for older individuals.

POST-TRAUMATIC STRESS DISORDER (PTSD)

This condition is commonly characterized by an acute-on-chronic course of multiple symptoms (e.g. emotional numbing, hyperarousal, hypervigilance, nightmares, avoidance behaviors) after a traumatic event. Most studies suggest that women are not at greater risk for traumatic exposure, but are more likely to develop PTSD when exposed to trauma, especially if experienced prior to age 15 years[29,30]. Intensity of the physiological response to the original trauma seems to be the most significant predictor of a relatively poor long-term outcome[31] (see also comments regarding acute stress disorder). Dissociative phenomena, sensation-seeking/high-risk behavior, emotional constriction, and drug and alcohol abuse also seem to indicate poor prognosis; in addition, on-going life stressors may slow the recovery process[31]. PTSD is frequently accompanied by obsessive–compulsive disorder, phobias, dissociative disorder, generalized anxiety disorder, panic disorder, depression and substance use disorders[13]. In addition, a number of somatic symptoms such as headaches, chronic pain, irritable bowel syndrome and fatigue, are commonly co-morbid.

There is accumulating evidence that pharmacotherapy is effective for the treatment of PTSD. For example, the selective serotonin reuptake inhibitors have demonstrated significant broad-spectrum effects in all the PTSD symptom clusters. They may be considered as first-line (preferred) pharmacological agents[32]. Other medications that may also be considered, are nefazodone, the tricyclic antidepressants and the monoamine oxidase inhibitors. Psychotherapy can be considered as either an alternative or an additive treatment to medications. Numerous psychotherapeutic techniques can help alleviate symptoms. These include cognitive–behavioral therapy, prolonged exposure, supportive–psychodynamic therapy and stress inoculation training[33].

Symptoms of the disorder are similar across age groups—re-experiencing the trauma, avoidance and hyperarousal—and there is no current evidence that aging affects the development of presentation of PTSD in older individuals. Elderly individuals do not appear any more predisposed to develop PTSD than do younger persons[34]. It is not uncommon for individuals who have experienced trauma (e.g. combat) to experience an exacerbation of PTSD, or for post-traumatic disorder to be reactivated, during later life[35,36]. As with other anxiety disorders, pharmacological and biobehavioral interventions found effective with younger populations can be incorporated into treatment for older adults.

GENERALIZED ANXIETY DISORDER (GAD)

GAD typically has an early onset with an acute-on-chronic course and is associated with increased utilization of medical and mental health services and increased consumption of psychotropic medications[37]. The presence of a co-morbid diagnosis is associated with a worsened prognosis and reduced remission rates compared with those patients with GAD alone[38,39]. Women with GAD are more likely to develop co-morbid conditions (e.g. depression) and the presence of such co-morbidity may reduce the likelihood of remission[40].

Treatments for GAD include both pharmacological and psychological interventions. Efficacy has been reported with buspirone, the benzodiazepines, the SSRIs and venlafaxine[41,42,43]. Cognitive–behavioral therapy (CBT) can be quite effective for this disorder in the short term[44]. Additionally, the benefits of CBT appear to be maintained at long-term follow-up and thus may provide a long-term and cost-effective intervention for GAD[45].

ANXIETY DISORDER DUE TO A MEDICAL CONDITION

This syndrome may be more common in the elderly due to more frequent medical illness. Prognosis depends on the nature and course of the underlying medical condition and its management.

ACUTE STRESS DISORDER

Acute stress disorder describes post-traumatic stress reactions that develop in the first month following a traumatic event. A review of the empirical literature on psychological reactions to trauma suggests that dissociative, intrusive, avoidance and arousal symptoms have often been identified across different kinds of traumatic events[46]. Of those individuals who experience trauma, a minority develops acute stress disorder. However, the literature suggests that a substantial majority of those who meet criteria for this disorder subsequently meet the criteria for ASD[47]. Symptoms with strong predictive power for the later development of PTSD include dissociation, re-experiencing, avoidance, acute numbing, and motor restlessness[48,49]. Therefore, in terms of prognosis, it is important to identify this pattern of reactions and to provide appropriate interventions to minimize their degree and duration.

SUBSTANCE-INDUCED ANXIETY DISORDER

A clinical picture of prominent anxiety, panic attacks, obsessions or compulsions characterizes this disorder. There must be evidence that medication use or substance intoxication or withdrawal are etiologically related to the symptoms. Symptoms must be clearly in excess of those customarily associated with the substance and these must cause clinically significant distress or impairment that warrants independent clinical attention. Once the substance is discontinued, the anxiety symptoms will usually remit within days to several weeks[13]. Symptom resolution is dependent upon the half-life of the substance, the presence of a withdrawal syndrome and other factors such as general health, medical co-morbidities and any psychiatric co-morbidities. For these reasons and the factor of aging, prognosis in the elderly may be more protracted.

CONCLUSION

In summary, it appears that anxiety disorders are characterized by a chronic course, with symptomatology becoming worse during periods of physical and emotional stress. Both pharmacological and psychotherapeutic approaches seem to be effective in the acute or short term. Definitive literature about the longer-term effects of treatments on the natural course of these disorders is still in progress. Not surprisingly, we know little about the natural course and prognosis of anxiety disorders in old age. Future studies designed to answer these questions are sorely needed.

REFERENCES

1. Sheikh JI, Salzman C. Anxiety in the elderly: course and treatment. *Psychiat Clin N Am* 1995; **18**(4): 871–83.
2. Weissman MM, Bland RC, Camino GJ *et al*. The cross-national epidemiology of panic disorder. *Arch Gen Psychiat* 1997; **54**: 305–9.
3. Sheikh JI, King R, Taylor CB. Comparative phenomenology of early vs. late-onset panic attacks: a pilot survey. *Am J Psychiat*, 1991; **148**: 1231–3.
4. Lydiard RB. Panic disorder and social phobia: possible implications of comorbid depression for drug therapy. *Anxiety* 1996; **2**: 61–70.
5. Lecrubier Y. Impact of comorbidity on the treatment of panic disorder. *J Clin Psychiat* 1998; **59**(suppl 8): 11–14.
6. Ballenger JC, Davidson JRT, Lecrubier Y *et al*. Consensus statement on panic disorder from the International Consensus Group on Depression and Anxiety. *J Clin Psychiat* 1998; **59**(suppl 8): 47–54.
7. Weissman MM, Klerman GL, Markovitz JS *et al*. Suicidal ideation and suicide attempts in panic disorder and attacks. *N Engl J Med* 1989; **321**: 1209–14.
8. Kushner MG, Sher KJ, Beitman BD. The relation between alcohol problems and the anxiety disorders. *Am J Psychiat* 1990; **147**: 685–95.
9. Coryell W. Mortality of anxiety disorders. In Noyes R Jr, Roth M, Burrows GD, eds, *Classification, Etiological Factors and Associated Disturbances*. Amsterdam: Elsevier Science/North Holland, 1988: 311–20.
10. Rubin HC, Rapaport MH, Levine B *et al*. Quality of well being in panic disorder: the assessment of psychiatric and general disability. *J Affect Disord* 2000; **57**: 217–21.
11. Sheehan DV. Current concepts in the treatment of panic disorder. *J Clin Psychiat* 1999; **60**(suppl 18): 16 21.
12. Davidson JRT. Long-term treatment of panic disorder. *J Clin Psychiat* 1998; **59**(suppl 8): 17–21.
13. American Psychiatric Association. *Diagnostic and Statistical Manual of Mental Disorders*, 4th edn. Washington, DC: American Psychiatric Association, 1994.
14. Rasmussen SA, Eisen JL. Treatment strategies for chronic and refractory obsessive-compulsive disorder. *J Clin Psychiat* 1997; **58**(suppl 13): 9–13.
15. Hantouche EG, Lancrenon S. Modern typology of symptoms and obsessive-compulsive syndromes: results of a large French study of 615 patients. *Encephale* 1996; **1**: 9–21.
16. Dolberg OT, Iancu I, Sasson Y *et al*. The pathogenesis and treatment of obsessive-compulsive disorder. *Clin Neuropharmacol* 1996; **19**: 129–47.
17. Ellingrod VL. Pharmacotherapy of primary obsessive-compulsive disorder: review of the literature. *Pharmacotherapy* 1998; **18**: 936–60.
18. Leonard HL. New developments in the treatment of obsessive-compulsive disorder. *J Clin Psychiat* 1997; **58**(suppl 14): 39–45.
19. Schneirer FR, Johnson J, Hornig CD *et al*. Social phobia: comorbidity and morbidity in an epidemiologic sample. *Arch Gen Psychiat* 1992; **49**: 282–8.
20. Blazer D, George L, Hughes D. The epidemiology of anxiety disorders: An age comparison. In Salzman C, Liebowitz B, eds, *Anxiety Disorders in the Elderly*. Hillsdale, NJ: Erlbaum, 1991.
21. Mersch PP, Emmelkamp PM, Bogels SM *et al*. Social phobia: Individual response patterns and cognitive interventions. *Behav Res Ther* 1989; **27**(4): 421–34.
22. Noyes R, Moroz G, Davidson J *et al*. Moclobemide in social phobia: a controlled dose–response trial. *J Clin Psychopharmacol* 1997; **17**: 247–54.
23. Katzelnick DJ, Kobak KA, Greist JH *et al*. Sertraline for social phobia: a double-blind placebo-controlled crossover study. *Am J Psychiat* 1995; **152**: 1368–71.
24. Stein MB, Liebowitz MR, Lydiard RB *et al*. Paroxetine treatment of generalized social phobia (social anxiety disorder): a randomized controlled trial. *J Am Med Assoc* 1998; **280**: 708–13.
25. Scholing A, Emmelkamp PMG. Treatment of generalized social phobia: results at long-term follow-up. *Behav Res Ther* 1996; **34**: 447–52.
26. Fredrikson M, Annas P, Fisher H. Gender and age differences in the prevalence of specific fears and phobias. *Behav Res Ther* 1996; **34**: 33–9.
27. Wells JC, Tien AY, Garrison R *et al*. Risk factors for the incidence of social phobia as determined by the Diagnostic Interview Schedule in a population-based study. *Acta Psychiat Scand* 1994; **90**: 84–90.
28. Zarate R, Agras WS. Psychosocial treatment of phobia and panic disorders. *Psychiatry* 1994; **57**: 133–41.
29. Breslau N, Davis G, Andreski P. Traumatic events and traumatic stress disorder in an urban population of young adults. *Arch Gen Psychiat* 1990; **48**: 218–22.
30. Breslau N, Davis GC, Andreski P *et al*. Sex differences in posttraumatic stress disorder. *Arch Gen Psychiat* 1997b; **54**: 1044–8.
31. van der Kolk BA. Posttraumatic stress disorder. In Hyman SE, Jenike MA, eds, *Manual of Clinical Problems in Psychiatry*. Boston, MA: Little, Brown, 1990.
32. Davidson JRT, Connor KM. Management of posttraumatic stress disorder: diagnostic and therapeutic issues. *J Clin Psychiat* 1999; **60**(suppl 18): 33–8.
33. Foa EB, Olasov Rothbaum B, Riggs DS *et al*. Treatment of posttraumatic stress disorder in rape victims: comparison between cognitive behavioral procedures and counseling. *J Consult Psychol* 1991; **59**: 715–23.
34. Weintraub D, Ruskin PE. Posttraumatic stress disorder in the elderly: a review. *Harvard Rev Psychiat* 1999; **7**: 144–52.
35. Macleod AD. The reactivation of posttraumatic stress disorder in later life. *J Psychosoc Nurs Ment Health Serv* 1995; **33**: 20–5.
36. Potts MK. Long-term effects of trauma; posttraumatic stress among civilian internees of the Japanese during WWII. *J Clin Psychol* 1994; **50**: 681–98.
37. Schweizer E. Generalized anxiety disorder: longitudinal course and pharmacologic treatment. *Psychiat Clin N Am* 1995; **18**(4): 843–57.
38. Woodman CL, Noyes R Jr, Black DW *et al*. A 5-year follow-up study of generalized anxiety disorder and panic disorder. *J Nerv Ment Dis* 1999; **187**(1): 3–9.
39. Yonkers KA, Warshaw MG, Massion AO. Phenomenology and course of generalized anxiety disorder. *Br J Psychiat* 1996; **168**: 308–13.
40. Kendler KS, Neale MC, Kessler RC *et al*. Major depression and generalized anxiety disorder: same genes, (partly) different environments? *Arch Gen Psychiat* 1992; **49**: 716–22.
41. Rickles K, Weisman K, Norstad N *et al*. Buspirone and diazepam in anxiety: a controlled study. *J Clin Psychiat* 1982; **43**: 81–6.
42. Rocca P, Fonzo V, Scotta M *et al*. Paroxetine efficacy in the treatment of generalized anxiety disorder. *Acta Psychiat Scand* 1997; **95**: 444–50.
43. Aguiar LM, Haskins T, Rudolph RL *et al*. Double-blind, placebo-controlled study of once-daily venlafaxine extended release in outpatients with GAD (NR-643). Paper presented at the 151st annual meeting of the American Psychiatric Association, Toronto, Canada, 1998.
44. Borkovec TD, Mathews AM, Chambers A *et al*. The effects of relaxation training with cognitive or non-directive therapy and the role of relaxation-induced anxiety in the treatment of generalized anxiety. *J Consult Clin Psychol* 1987; **55**(6): 883–8.
45. Harvey AG, Rapee RM. Cognitive-behavior therapy for generalized anxiety disorder. *Psychiat Clin N Am* 1995; **18**: 859–70.
46. Koopman C, Classen C, Cardena E *et al*. When disaster strikes, acute stress disorder may follow. *J Trauma Stress* 1995; **8**: 29–46.
47. Brewin CR, Andrews B, Rose S *et al*. Acute stress disorder and posttraumatic stress disorder in victims of violent crime. *Am J Psychiat* 1999; **156**: 360–6.
48. Classen C, Koopman C, Hales *et al*. Acute stress disorder as a predictor of posttraumatic stress disorder. *Am J Psychiat* 1998; **155**: 620–4.
49. Harvey AG, Bryant RA. The relationship between acute stress disorder and posttraumatic stress disorder: a prospective evaluation of motor vehicle accident survivors. *J Consult Clin Psychol* 1998; **66**: 507–12.

102

Acute Management of Anxiety and Phobias

Javaid I. Sheikh[1,2], **Erin L. Cassidy**[1,2] and **Pamela J. Swales**[2]

[1]*Stanford University School of Medicine, Stanford, CA, and*
[2]*Veterans Affairs, Palo Alto Health Care System, CA, USA*

Anxiety disorders are among the most common psychiatric conditions occurring in the elderly[1]. Although most of these disorders are of rather chronic nature, acute exacerbations, under a variety of conditions, can produce states of extreme anxiety and agitation that can require immediate attention. For example, patients in treatment for an anxiety disorder may seek an emergency appointment with their doctor/therapist due to a magnification of symptoms. Similarly, in a general hospital a psychiatrist may be called to consult on the management of acute anxiety of an elderly patient on a medical or surgical floor; or a resident may be called upon to evaluate and manage an acutely anxious elderly patient in the emergency room. It is also not unusual for patients with a primary anxiety disorder to present for emergency room services, thinking that they have acute medical problems[2], e.g. patients having a panic attack might fear an impending heart attack and seek medical treatment. Since older anxious patients are more likely to have concomitant medical problems than their younger counterparts, they may require a careful medical evaluation to rule out any organic causes of anxiety[3].

The goal of acute management is relief of marked distress; thus, the treatment approach described here will focus on decreasing patients' symptomatology to manageable proportions as expeditiously as possible. Therefore, treatment approaches for long-term management of anxiety and phobias will be omitted. Further, most situations requiring acute management will necessitate combined pharmacological and psychological interventions. Due to a lack of systematic studies of anxiety management in the elderly, much of our discussion will be based on evidence from studies in younger populations and our own clinical experience.

GENERAL PRINCIPLES OF ACUTE MANAGEMENT

Although acute management of various anxiety disorders may vary somewhat according to the diagnosis, certain guidelines can be useful in a majority of situations. To begin, it is important to remember that during states of extreme anxiety, patients can manifest grossly impaired judgment and might appear to be suffering from a psychotic condition, but a few minutes of questioning will usually clarify the issue. A supportive interaction with the patient is essential to successful treatment. A calm, reassuring manner can be very comforting in itself to alleviate the terror of extreme anxiety. Having a keen awareness of the unique psychosocial issues of the elderly, including retirement, possible deaths of close friends and loved ones and a gradual deterioration of physical functioning, is usually very helpful in developing the

Table 102.1 For patients: understanding your anxiety

- The intense physical symptoms you experience when you are highly anxious are those that are natural to the human body; they are not harmful to you as such. All people have an instinctive "fight-or-flight" response to danger. It is the apparent lack of real danger to you that makes your feelings of fear or anxiety seem so uncomfortable and overwhelming.
- A number of factors may have led to your anxiety experience(s). Your doctor or another clinician may have discussed some of these with you. You may have been given medication to help control your anxiety. It is important for you to take your medication exactly as directed. Anxiety may also be controlled by other methods. Some of these are breathing and muscle relaxation skills, visualization (imagination) techniques, and exposure to anxiety-producing situations with the aid of a therapist. No matter what type of treatment you receive, keep your therapist or doctor aware of any problems, questions or concerns you may notice.
- You and your doctor/therapist will be working together to help you in understanding and controlling your anxiety. In your efforts to cope (deal) with anxiety reactions, it is important to keep in mind that you are not alone. Many people suffer from intense and seemingly overwhelming periods of anxiety. Remember also, "there is light at the end of the tunnel". Anxiety symptoms can be controlled. This may take time, practice, courage and a "stick-to-it attitude", but it is definitely do-able.

initial rapport that will allow the patient to comply with subsequent treatment.

Patient education about their condition and various forms of treatment can be especially beneficial to geriatric patients. Patients with an anxiety disorder benefit from a discussion of thoughts, feelings and behaviors with their therapist or doctor, which can enhance rapport and facilitate patient understanding, decrease global anxiety and foster patient compliance. Information that may be provided to patients during acute management of anxiety reactions is included in Table 102.1.

The specific interventions may be pharmacological and/or psychological. Before describing specific treatments for various anxiety syndromes, it will be helpful to review general principles of pharmacological and psychological therapies with older adults.

PHARMACOLOGICAL MANAGEMENT

Common age-related changes in absorption, distribution, protein binding, metabolism and excretion of drugs and their implications have been covered in detail elsewhere in this book, and thus we will only address the relevance of these changes to anxiolytics, including benzodiazepines, β-blockers and buspirone. For benzodiazepines, the net effect of these changes is usually a relatively higher level of active medication or its metabolites compared to younger people. In addition, an increase in the proportion of body fat with aging may mean that a strongly lipophilic benzodiazepine, such as diazepam, will lead to a much higher accumulation in tissues, compared to less lipophilic drugs such as lorazepam and oxazepam, which are preferable in the elderly[4]. Of the β-blockers, propranolol is the most frequently used. One should note, however, that its adverse side effects are most common in patients over the age of 60, including its potential to cause depression and worsen cardiac failure and bronchial asthma, and its potentially troublesome interactions with various other drugs, such as calcium channel blockers, cimetidine and chlorpromazine[5]. Aging does not seem to significantly alter the pharmacokinetics of buspirone[6]. Appropriate usage of these agents in specific situations will be discussed in later sections.

PSYCHOLOGICAL MANAGEMENT

From a cognitive-behavioral perspective, anxiety can be understood to have three core components: psychological (e.g. cognitions and affects), physiological (e.g. increased heart rate, dizziness) and behavioral (e.g. ruminations, compulsions and avoidance behaviors). When unfounded, severe anxiety initiates and maintains maladaptive functioning and psychological disturbance. How an individual perceives, understands and functions with anxiety can be shaped by such factors as coping mechanisms, personality, social and environmental influences and past trauma. Cognitive-behavioral principles are very effective with a variety of psychiatric symptoms[7-8]. For example, breathing and muscle relaxation training, guided imagery, systematic desensitization, relabeling of anxiety reactions, insight into irrational beliefs and systematic homework assignments are effective interventions that may be utilized during acute presentations of anxiety. During acute management, elders may need a greater amount of reassurance and doctor/therapist contact time than their younger counterparts. Maintenance of such techniques through follow-up sessions will increase the internal support strategies of the patient and decrease the risk for future crises.

Diagnostic Categories Most Commonly Requiring Management

Panic Disorder

There are several management strategies that have shown some degree of success in panic disorder[9]. The therapeutic efficacy of antidepressants in panic disorder and agoraphobia is quite well established. Particularly effective are the tricyclic antidepressant imipramine, the monoamine oxidase inhibitor (MAOI) phenelzine, and the selective serotonin reuptake inhibitor (SSRI) sertraline[10-12]. Due to their rapid onset of therapeutic action, however, benzodiazepines should be considered the mainstay of acute management, as antidepressants usually take approximately 2–3 weeks for their therapeutic effects to take place. Although alprazolam is the most commonly used benzodiazepine in panic disorder[13], clonazepam[14] and lorazepam[13] have reportedly been effective.

Cognitive and behavioral therapies are inextricably intertwined in the acute treatment of panic disorder, with or without agoraphobia. Panic disorder may be managed acutely with breathing and muscle relaxation techniques, examination of cognitive beliefs and a series of progressive behavioral exercises. With therapist-assisted graded exposure beginning even during the acute management phase of treatment, frequent exposure sessions may facilitate the lessening of the anxiety symptoms.

Social Phobia (Fear of Public Speaking, Eating in Public, etc.)

β-Blockers have been shown to be superior to a placebo for treatment of a fear of public speaking or performance anxiety in the general population[15,16]. The espoused mechanism of such therapeutic response is the suppression of peripheral responses of anxiety (e.g. palpitations). We know of no studies or clinical reports that address the effectiveness of β-blockers in the socially phobic elderly; thus, it is hard to say whether this treatment will be equally effective in the elderly. It is also not clear whether a benzodiazepine in low dose (e.g. 0.5 mg lorazepam) will be helpful in encountering the phobic situations.

Office-based social skills training as well as exposure *in vivo* (individual or group treatment) can be very effective[17]. For acute management purposes, teaching a single, generally acceptable "coping strategy" is most useful to patients and can be implemented quite easily in a variety of situations. A skilled clinician may also consider the use of paradoxical intention, visualization and systematic desensitization in acute management interventions.

Specific Phobia (Crime, Medical and Dental Procedures, etc.)

A minority of individuals seek psychiatric treatment for simple phobias, and clinically significant improvement is usually obtained in 75–85% of specific phobias treated[18]. Common fears of older adults include being a crime victim and fears about medical and dental procedures. Although crime rates decrease with age, medical and dental procedures increase, therefore successful management strategies are warranted. We find that low-dose benzodiazepines before the medical or dental procedure in very fearful patients may be helpful in alleviating anxiety and producing better compliance with treatment.

Acute management of most simple phobias can be treated effectively, and with therapy gains maintained, with one (2–3 h) office-based, therapist-assisted exposure session[18]. Effective treatment requires focusing on one phobia-related avoidance behavior per session. Breathing and muscle relaxation techniques can also be quite effective in suppressing anxiety responses in older adults.

Generalized Anxiety

In certain instances, the symptomatology of patients with a generalized anxiety disorder can become extremely severe and may require immediate intervention with benzodiazepines. We recommend replacing benzodiazepines with buspirone and/or cognitive-behavioral interventions, including the range of relaxation exercises, until the acute symptomatology is under control.

CONCLUSION

Principles for the acute management of anxiety in the elderly remain more or less consistent over the range of anxiety disorders, although the contexts in which one is asked to evaluate and manage such cases may vary greatly. The importance of a good history, empathy to the patient's psychosocial situation, and awareness of a possibility of an underlying medical condition cannot be overemphasized. Finally, one needs to be cognizant of the great individual variation in this group and should be ready and willing to tailor the usage of medications and/or cognitive-behavioral techniques to each patient's special needs.

REFERENCES

1. Blazer D, George L, Hughes D. The epidemiology of anxiety disorders: an age comparison. In Salzman C, Liebowitz B, eds, *Anxiety in the Elderly: Treatment and Research*. New York: Springer, 1991: 17–30.
2. Boyd JH. Use of mental health services for the treatment of panic disorder. *Am J Psychiat* 1986; **143**(12): 1569–74.
3. Sheikh JI. Anxiety disorders. In Coffey CE, Cummings JL, eds, *Textbook of Geriatric Neuropsychology*. Washington, DC: American Psychiatric Press, 2000: 274.
4. Moran MG, Thompson TL II, Nies AS. Sleep disorders in the elderly. *Am J Psychiat* 1988; **145**(11): 1369–78.
5. *AHFS Drug Information*. Bethesda, MD: American Society of Hospital Pharmacists, 1990: 858–65.
6. Gammans RE, Westrick ML, Shea JP *et al*. Pharmacokinetics of buspirone in elderly subjects. *J Clin Pharm* 1989; **29**: 72–8.
7. Ruckdeschel H. Group psychotherapy in the nursing home. In *Professional Psychology in Long Term Care*. New York: Hatherleigh, 2000: 347.
8. Beck AT, Emery G. *Anxiety Disorders and Phobias: A Cognitive Perspective*. New York: Basic Books, 1985.
9. Ballenger JC, Davidson JRT, Lecrubier Y *et al*. Consensus statement on panic disorder from the International Consensus Group on Depression and Anxiety. *J Clin Psychiat* 1998; **59**(suppl 8): 47–54.
10. Sheehan DV, Ballenger JC, Jacobsen G. Treatment of endogenous anxiety with phobic, hysterical, and hypochondriacal symptoms. *Arch Gen Psychiat* 1980: **13**: 51.
11. Zitrin CM, Klein DF, Woerner MG, Ross DC. Treatment of phobias: I. Comparison of imipramine hydrochloride and placebo. *Arch Gen Psychiat* 1983; **40**: 115–38.
12. Hirschfeld RM. Sertraline in the treatment of anxiety disorders. *Depress Anxiety* 2000; **11**(4): 139–57.
13. Ballenger JC. *Drug Treatment of Panic Disorder and Agoraphobia*. 140th Annual Meeting of the American Psychiatric Association, Chicago: Symposium No. 200, 1987: 59.
14. Tesar G, Rosenbaum JF, Pollack M *et al*. Clonazepam vs. alprazolam in the treatment of panic disorder: interim analysis of data from a prospective, double-blind, placebo-controlled trial. *J Clin Psychiat* 1987; **48**: 16–19.
15. Hartley LR, Uugapen S, Davie K, Spencer DJ. The effect of β-adrenergic blocking drugs on speakers' performance and memory. *Br J Psychiat* 1983; **142**: 512–17.
16. Brantigan CO, Brantigan TA, Joseph N. Effect of β-blockade and β-simulation on stage fright. *Am J Med* 1982; **72**: 88–94.
17. Wlazlo Z, Schroeder-Hartwig K, Hand I *et al*. Exposure *in vivo* vs. social skills training for social phobia: long-term outcome and differential effects. *Behav Res Ther* 1990; **28**(3): 181–93.
18. Ost L-G. One-session treatment for specific phobias. *Behav Res Ther* 1989; **27**(1): 1–7.

103

Psychopharmacological Treatment of Anxiety

John L. Beyer and K. Ranga Krishnan

Duke University Medical Center, Durham, NC, USA

Even though the prevalence of anxiety disorders declines as people age, anxiety disorders still remain the most common psychiatric illness in the elderly[1]. This statistic represents not only the continuation of chronic anxiety disorders into later life for many people, but also the development of new anxiety disorders for others. Loneliness and fear of isolation, diminished sensory and general functional capacities, increased incidence of illness, financial limitations and the prospect of dying often generate considerable anxiety[2]. Elderly patients who recover from a mood disorder often develop persistent anxiety, especially in the morning. An estimated 10–20% of older patients experience clinically significant symptoms of anxiety[3]. Unfortunately, many individuals may never seek treatment, or their anxiety may not be recognized. The result has been a significant undertreatment of a very treatable illness.

This chapter reviews the pharmacologic treatment of anxiety disorders in the elderly. At this time, there is no "perfect" anxiolytic drug for treating the elderly[4,5]. Further, there are significant gaps in the research of anxiety disorders in the elderly, which makes the choice of treatment difficult[6]. This chapter will therefore begin with a review of general considerations a physician must make prior to selecting and starting pharmacologic treatment. A discussion of current pharmacologic options will follow. Classes of medication, rather than specific recommendations for each anxiety disorder, will be reviewed, since research has not clarified primary treatments for most anxiety disorders. Finally, guidelines for the evaluation and selection of pharmacologic treatments are suggested.

GENERAL CONSIDERATIONS

When to Treat

The decision to treat the anxious older patient with medication depends on the severity of the anxiety and the degree to which it interferes with the patient's functioning[7,8]. Anxiety may interfere with social and interpersonal activity in the older patient, resulting in a breakdown of support systems or coping skills. It may worsen cognitive function by decreasing a patient's concentration. Anxiety may also exacerbate physical illnesses or may be an unrecognized consequence of a medical disorder. Anxiety has been related to blood pressure variability and, by extension, to increased cardiovascular risk[9]. The DSM-IV has identified several subtypes of anxiety disorders (Table 103.1) for the general adult population. They are based on the presence of a cluster of symptoms with a characteristic course and treatment. However, anxiety may also present as a symptom of another disorder.

Therefore, the first task is to assess the impact of the anxiety symptoms on social and emotional functioning or the severity of a coexisting physical illness.

Differential Diagnosis

The diagnosis of anxiety, as either a disorder or a symptom, is not always apparent. This is especially true in the elderly patient. Elderly patients are often less willing to discuss "anxiety", but may report "anxiety-equivalent" complaints and physical illnesses. Thus a patient may deny being "anxious", but admit to being "jittery", "sick", "uneasy", "flustered", "hot", "restless", "ill", "achy", "agitated" or "bad". Alternatively, the patient may verbalize physical symptoms, such as being "sick to my stomach", or having "heart pain" or "insomnia". These complaints may obscure the true diagnosis or complicate another. The physician must therefore be attuned to what the patient is actually saying.

Further complicating the differential diagnosis is the fact that anxiety may present as a primary disorder (panic disorder, generalized anxiety disorder, obsessive–compulsive disorder, etc.) or a symptom of another primary diagnosis (such as depression, thyroid disease, cardiovascular disease or dementia). There are many conditions that may cause anxiety as a symptom (see Table 103.2); thus, differentiating the source or sources may be difficult. Common medical disorders associated with anxiety as a symptom in the elderly include chronic obstructive pulmonary disease, coronary artery disease, early dementia, major depressive episodes, and medication interactions or withdrawal. Environmental stressors, bereavement or anniversary reactions and experience of medical illness or hospitalizations are also commonly associated with anxiety in late life[10]. Non-prescription medications (especially caffeine-containing products, certain cold

Table 103.1 DSM-IV anxiety disorders

Panic disorder without agoraphobia
Panic disorder with agoraphobia
Agoraphobia without a history of panic disorder
Specific phobia
Social phobia
Obsessive–compulsive disorder (OCD)
Post-traumatic stress disorder (PTSD)
Acute stress disorder
Generalized anxiety disorder (GAD)
Anxiety disorder due to . . . *[a general medical condition]*
Substance-induced anxiety disorder
Anxiety disorder, NOS

Table 103.2 Medical disorders associated with anxiety as a symptom

Cardiopulmonary
  Asthma
  Chronic obstructive pulmonary disease
  Hypoxic states
  Angina pectoris
  Mitral valve prolapse
  Cardiac arrhythmias
  Congestive heart failure
  Cerebral arteriosclerosis
  Hypertension
  Pulmonary embolism

Neurologic
  Partial complex seizures
  Early dementia
  Delirium
  Post-concussion syndrome
  Cerebral neoplasm
  Huntington's disease
  Multiple sclerosis
  Vestibular dysfunction

Endocrine
  Carcinoid syndrome
  Cushing's syndrome
  Hypoglycemia; hyperinsulinism
  Hypo- or hyperthyroidism
  Hypo- or hyperparathyroidism
  Menopause
  Pheochromocytoma
  Premenstrual syndrome

Medications
  Anticholinergic medications
  Caffeine
  Cocaine
  Steroids
  Sympathomimetics
  Alcohol
  Narcotics
  Sedative–hypnotics

and flu medications, alcohol or nicotine withdrawal, and certain herbal remedies) may contribute to anxiety symptoms.

Adult Studies

Research in the treatment of anxiety disorders for elderly patients is limited. A recent summary of the National Institute of Mental Health Workshop on Late-life Anxiety[6] has highlighted this problem, noting three significant research gaps: (a) little consensus on the "best" approach to measure and count anxiety symptoms, syndromes or disorders in late life; (b) insufficient numbers of studies that examine anxiety among older adults; and (c) limited knowledge of the differences in "early" and "later" onset of various anxiety disorders. These limitations become especially significant in treatment recommendations for elderly patients with anxiety. A recent review of the literature[5] indicated that there are very few controlled clinical trials of medication or psychosocial interventions for anxiety disorders in the elderly. Many of the findings take the form of case reports, case series or open studies. Therefore, treatment decisions for elderly patients are usually extrapolated from the clinical studies of younger mixed-age adult populations and personal clinical experience. For the most part, there is little reason to doubt the applicability of the studies to the elderly patient, yet the clinician should be aware of the limitations of the research, and sensitive to the developing research in this area.

Special Adaptations for the Geriatric Patient

Before prescribing anti-anxiety agents for the elderly, the physician should be aware of the several age-related physiologic changes that may alter drug pharmacokinetics and contribute to increased risk of adverse reactions. These include changes in drug absorption, drug distribution, protein binding, cardiac output, hepatic metabolism and renal clearance[11–13]. In addition, changes in neurotransmitter and receptor function in the central nervous system (CNS) may make a patient more sensitive to psychotropic drugs[14]. In general, the usual starting dose of psychotropic drugs for geriatric patients is roughly one-half of the starting dose for younger adult patients.

PSYCHOPHARMACOLOGIC DRUGS

During the past three decades, a variety of agents have been used for the treatment of anxiety and anxiety disorders with varying degrees of success. These include benzodiazepines, buspirone, tricyclic antidepressants (TCAs), monoamine oxidase inhibitors (MAOIs), serotonin selective reuptake inhibitors (SSRIs), newer mixed-action antidepressants, antipsychotic neuroleptics, β-blockers and antihistamines. Despite the multiple medications available, none are completely safe or completely satisfactory in the treatment of anxiety. Zimmer and Gershon's[15] conclusion that the "ideal geriatric anxiolytic" has yet to be developed still holds true today. Therefore, effective methods of treating anxiety disorders are especially dependent upon thoughtful, comprehensive and accurate assessment of psychiatric, social and medical status, as well as a thorough knowledge of the patient's drug history and medication options.

BENZODIAZEPINES

Since the 1960s, the benzodiazepine class of compounds has been the mainstay of drug treatment for patients with situational anxiety, GAD and panic disorder[16]. They are also frequently prescribed for other indications, such as insomnia, relaxation prior to certain medical procedures, seizures, or agitation in demented patients. In the last two decades, increased attention has been given to the prescription pattern of benzodiazepines in the elderly. Benzodiazepines were prescribed at a much higher rate among elderly patients than in the general population[17]. Epidemiologic data suggest that benzodiazepines may be overused in the general elderly population[18]. This is significant because of the potential toxicity and side effects of benzodiazepines, especially common in the elderly.

Despite their multiple uses, benzodiazepines are usually classified in two groups: anxiolytics and sedative–hypnotics. Currently, seven benzodiazepines are available for the treatment of anxiety. Listed in their order of introduction, they are chlordiazepoxide, diazepam, oxazepam, clorazepate, lorazepam, alprazolam and clonazepam[19]. Prazepam and halazepam, two benzodiazepines previously used for the treatment of anxiety, are no longer available in the USA. The most common sedative–hypnotics are triazolam, temazepam and flurazepam. Commonly used benzodiazepines in the elderly are listed in Table 103.3.

Table 103.3 Commonly used benzodiazepines in the elderly

Generic name	Trade name	Onset of action	Indication	Half-life (h)	Metabolism	Active metabolites	Geriatric dose (mg/day)	Route of administration
Short to intermediate half-life								
Triazolam	Halcion	Fast	Hypnotic	2–5	Conjugation	None	0.125–0.5	Oral
Oxazepam	Serax	Intermediate to slow	Anxiolytic	5–15	Conjugation	None	5–30	Oral
Alprazolam	Xanax	Intermediate	Anxiolytic	6–15	Oxidation	Yes	0.125–3.0	Oral
Lorazepam	Ativan	Intermediate	Anxiolytic	10–20	Conjugation	None	0.5–3	Oral, IV, IM
Temazepam	Restoril	Intermediate to slow	Hypnotic	12–24	Conjugation	None	15–30	Oral
Long half-life								
Chlordiazepoxide	Librium	Intermediate	Anxiolytic	8–30	Oxidation	Yes	5–30	Oral, IV, IM
Diazepam	Valium	Fastest	Anxiolytic	26–53	Oxidation	Yes	2–10	Oral, IV, IM
Clorazepate	Tranxene	Fast	Anxiolytic	30–200	Oxidation	Yes	7.5–15	Oral
Flurazepam	Dalmane	Fast	Hypnotic	64–150	Oxidation	Yes	15	Oral
Klonopin	Clonazepam	Intermediate	Anxiolytic	30–40	Oxidation	Yes	0.25–3.0	Oral

Pharmacokinetics

Benzodiazepines undergo two kinds of biotransformation: oxidation and glucuronide conjugation. Oxidative transformation occurs slowly, giving the drugs a long half-life and producing many active metabolites. Conjugative transformation differs from oxidative transformation in that it occurs rapidly and the metabolic products are pharmacologically inactive. As a general rule, benzodiazepines that are inactivated by conjugation reactions appear to be less likely to interact with other medications. For example, cimetidine has been found to inhibit the metabolism of benzodiazepines that require oxidation, but not benzodiazepines inactivated by conjugation (such as lorazepam or oxazepam). Table 103.4 lists several important drug interactions with benzodiazepines.

Elimination half-lives of benzodiazepines are variable in the elderly. Usually the effects of ultrashort, short and intermediate half-life benzodiazepines do not carry over to the next day when they are used as a sedative[20]. Ultrashort benzodiazepines are generally used to treat insomnia rather than daytime anxiety. They can cause rebound insomnia after abrupt discontinuation. Safety concerns about triazolam (i.e. after being noted to cause confusion, agitation and hallucinations) have led to its ban in several European countries[18]. Benzodiazepines with long half-lives can significantly contribute to increased risk of falls and hip fracture in elderly patients[21].

The onset of action after a single dose is primarily dependent upon the drug's absorption rate. Most benzodiazepines are highly lipophilic. Benzodiazepines that are more lipid-soluble have a faster onset of action because they are absorbed and diffused into central synapses more rapidly[22,23]. This rapid onset of action can produce euphoria and thereby enhance abuse potential.

Efficacy

Benzodiazepines are effective for generalized anxiety disorder (GAD). Clonazepam has been shown effective for social phobia. Clonazepam and alprazolam are effective in panic disorder. Efficacy and use in post-traumatic stress disorder (PTSD) is limited. A paradoxical reaction has been documented when some patients with PTSD are treated with benzodiazepines. None of the benzodiazepines appear effective for obsessive–compulsive disorder (OCD).

Dependence and Withdrawal

True physiologic dependence, resulting in a withdrawal and abstinence syndrome, develops to benzodiazepines usually after 3–4 months of daily use[14]. Withdrawal symptoms are likely to be more severe with abruptly discontinued therapy, and with patients receiving short half-life benzodiazepines, or higher daily doses. The symptoms of withdrawal include tachycardia, orthostasis, intention tremors, diaphoresis, hyper-reflexia, anxiety, insomnia, nightmares, malaise, anorexia, headache, muscle pain and twitching, tinnitus, hyperacusis, photophobia, metallic taste, strange smells and, in more severe cases, hyperthermia, nausea, vomiting, delirium, seizures and psychosis.

Table 103.4 Drug interactions with the benzodiazepines

Drug	Effect
Alcohol	Increased CNS sedation
Neuroleptics	Increased CNS sedation
Narcotics	Increased CNS sedation
Antihistamines	Increased CNS sedation
MAO Inhibitors	Increased CNS sedation
Cimetidine	Increased elimination half-life and decreased clearance of alprazolam, diazepam and chlordiazepoxide
Isoniazid	Decreased metabolism of diazepam
Rifampin	Increased metabolism of diazepam
Antacids	Decreased absorption of clorazepate and chlordiazepoxide
Digoxin	Increased digoxin levels
Levodopa	Decreased control of parkinsonism by levodopa
Fluvoxamine	Increased levels of alprazolam

Side Effects

Although benzodiazepines have been shown to be effective in younger populations, systematic studies in the elderly are lacking. Judicious use is therefore important, since they may have several significant side effects. Adverse drug reactions to the benzodiazepines are almost twice as common in patients over the age of 70 years compared with those aged 40 years or less[24].

Benzodiazepines do tend to produce greater effects on the central nervous system of the elderly than in younger patients[12,13]. This is due partly to increased target-organ sensitivity and partly to altered pharmacokinetics in the elderly (i.e. duration of half-life and peak blood level)[7]. The most common benzodiazepine side effect is a dose-dependent CNS depression. Symptoms include fatigue, drowsiness, sedation, muscle weakness, blurred vision, nystagmus, dysarthria, ataxia and impaired psychomotor and cognitive performance[12,25,26]. The impairment of motor coordination causes drivers taking benzodiazepines to be five times more likely of being involved in a serious road accident[27]. Cognitive impairment can be severe enough to present as a pseudodementia in susceptible elderly patients.

Benzodiazepines may also cause a paradoxical reaction of restlessness, confusion, irritability and even aggression. Outbursts of anger in elderly patients receiving benzodiazepines may indicate the need to consider an alternative medicine. There are also published case reports of benzodiazepines inducing a secondary mania[28,29]. Benzodiazepines may cause mild respiratory depression in patients with chronic obstructive lung disease. Mixing benzodiazepines with other CNS depressants such as alcohol can lead to severe intoxication or (potentially lethal) respiratory depression.

Selection

In general, benzodiazepines are equivalent in terms of overall efficacy[30]. The selection of a particular benzodiazepine is primarily based upon the patient's particular problem and the medication properties (route of metabolism, length of half-life, onset of action, and presence of active metabolites)[31]. In general, the following guidelines should be considered when using a benzodiazepine:

1. Benzodiazepines that undergo conjugation to water-soluble glucuronides prior to excretion in the urine (e.g. temazepam, lorazepam, oxazepam) have no active metabolites and their pharmacokinetics are not significantly changed by the aging process[32]. They are probably the wisest choice for elderly patients with severely impaired hepatic function.
2. Short (but not ultrashort) half-life drugs are preferable to long half-life medications, since they appear less likely to increase the risk for hip fractures[21].
3. Accumulation of benzodiazepines is directly related to the amount of fat. Therefore, the obese or severely medically frail patients may be at increased risk.
4. Avoid benzodiazepine use in patients dependent on alcohol or other drugs.
5. Begin with lower doses and titrate upwards gradually ("start low and go slow").
6. Try to limit the length of use to 3–4 months. Taper benzodiazepines over a 4–8 week period.

Buspirone

Buspirone (Buspar) is a novel anti-anxiety agent unrelated to the benzodiazepines in chemical structure or pharmacologic characteristics. Its mechanism of action is probably related to its high affinity for the serotonin type 5-HT$_{1A}$ receptor, which causes reduced serotoninergic activity. In addition, it enhances brain dopaminergic and noradrenergic activity[33,34].

Efficacy

Buspirone is effective in the treatment of generalized anxiety disorder in the elderly. It is well tolerated and as effective as the benzodiazepines[35–38]. However, buspirone does not appear to be effective in the treatment of panic disorder[39]. Some researchers suggest that buspirone may be helpful in mixed anxiety/depression symptoms. It may also be effective as an adjunct treatment for OCD. Its use in PTSD and social phobia appears to be limited.

Administration

Therapeutic doses are in the range 20–60 mg daily; however, buspirone's short half-life (averaging 2–3 h) requires that it be given three times a day (usually with meals). Studies have demonstrated that buspirone may remain effective for at least 6 weeks, although longer efficacy is presumed.

Two major disadvantages of buspirone are the requirement for multiple daily dosing and the lack of immediate effect. Buspirone may take 1–3 weeks at therapeutic dosing before the anxiolytic effect begins. Some researchers have also suggested that the efficacy of buspirone may be reduced in patients who have previously been treated with benzodiazepines[40]. Others suggest using a benzodiazepine for the first 1–2 weeks when initiating treatment with buspirone until it becomes effective.

Side Effects

Buspirone side effects include nausea, headache, nervousness, dizziness, lightheadedness and fatigue. Unlike the benzodiazepines, buspirone does not appear to cause psychomotor impairment, dependence, withdrawal or abuse[41]. Further, it does not interact with alcohol and other sedative drugs. Buspirone lacks hypnotic, anticonvulsant and muscle relaxant properties. Therefore, it may be of particular value in the treatment of patients unable to tolerate the sedative effects of benzodiazepines[42], or patients with a history of substance abuse.

Antidepressants

Tricyclic Antidepressants

Efficacy. Tricyclic antidepressants (TCAs) have been shown to be effective in treating mixed anxiety–depression states, panic disorder and generalized anxiety disorder in the elderly[43–46]. In the general adult population, TCAs are frequently used in PTSD and clomipramine has been approved by the FDA to treat OCD. However, the overall use of TCAs has decreased as other options (especially the SSRIs) have become available. This is primarily due to the significant side effects TCAs have at therapeutic doses that also increase the risk to physically ill patients and potentiates toxicity in overdose. Further, like all other medications used for the treatment of anxiety (except the benzodiazepines), TCAs usually require several weeks to show maximal benefit. Despite their shortcomings, tricyclic antidepressants remain an alternative treatment for GAD[47].

Side Effects. Common side effects may be mediated by α-adrenergic blockade, anticholinergic effects and antihistaminergic effects. The α-adrenergic blockade of TCAs may cause significant orthostatic hypotension or cardiac conduction irregularities. The elderly are particularly susceptible to injury from orthostatic falls. Patients with complete heart block should not be given TCAs because these medications can cause a prolonged QRS complex. Trazodone, a heterocyclic antidepressant, is sometimes used as a sedative or in the treatment of agitation for demented patients, but the side effects of postural hypotension may limit its use[20].

Anticholinergic side effects of TCAs are dry mouth, blurred vision, constipation, urinary retention and confusion or even psychosis. This may be particularly significant in patients with

Alzheimer's disease or other disorders that impair memory. The major antihistaminergic effect is sedation.

Guidelines for Use. Imipramine and amitriptyline have long been established in the adult population for use in various anxiety disorders. However, their tertiary amine structure tends to cause increased anticholinergic, adrenergic and sedative side effects. The secondary amines, nortriptyline and desipramine, are preferred for use in the elderly due to their less intense side effects. In general, anxiety disorders appear to respond at doses lower than those used in mood disorders. A baseline EKG is highly recommended prior to starting therapy, since TCAs can cause a prolonged QRS complex.

Monoamine Oxidase Inhibitors (MAOIs)

Monoamine oxidase inhibitors have been effective in treating mixed anxiety–depression and panic disorder but not pure generalized anxiety[44,45]. MAOIs are rarely used now because of their potential side effects (especially the drug–diet interactions) and the wider availability of newer antidepressant choices. Phenelzine and tranylcypromine are the MAOIs of choice for the elderly in the USA[8]. Interestingly, phenelzine was found to be more effective in the elderly than in younger patients[44], and just as well tolerated as nortriptyline[48]. The starting dose is 15 mg daily in the morning, increasing by 15 mg every few days to an average dose of 45–60 mg[49]. Moclobemide, a reversible MAOI available outside the USA, is effective in social phobia and panic disorder[50,51].

Orthostatic hypotension is the major side effect of MAOIs; however, the major concern is the possibility of an acute hypertensive crisis due to the drug and dietary interactions.

Selective Serotonin Reuptake Inhibitors (SSRIs)

Efficacy. The introduction of SSRIs has transformed the treatment of both depression and anxiety in the adult population. Five SSRIs are now available for use in the USA: fluoxetine, sertraline, paroxetine, fluvoxamine and citalopram. Since their introduction, certain SSRIs have obtained indications for the treatment of not only depression, but also panic disorder, bulimia, OCD and social phobia. They are also used in the treatment of PTSD and GAD. Still, as with the other medications, the treatment of geriatric patients is primarily extrapolated from studies of younger adults. Case reports, open trials and some controlled studies in elderly patients have been completed in the elderly population. Fluoxetine has been shown to be effective in treatment of geriatric depressed patients with agitation[20]. Fluvoxamine and fluoxetine have been shown to be effective in clinical trials for OCD that have included some elderly patients[52,53]. Case studies have shown sertraline, paroxetine, venlafaxine, fluoxetine and fluvoxamine effective in social phobias and anxiety[54–57].

Side Effects. All SSRIs can cause gastrointestinal effects (nausea and diarrhea), sexual arousal and performance changes, and a decrease in appetite and weight. The nausea and diarrhea are usually dose-dependent and resolve for most patients within the first week of treatment. An increasing concern has been SSRI-associated weight gain, seen with extended use. Paroxetine has been noted to have some anticholinergic activity that may be more apparent in elderly, sensitive patients. A significant potential side effect of SSRIs includes a tendency to stimulate patients, causing tremor and jitteriness.

Guidelines for Use. Since some SSRIs have been associated with "activation" and worsening of anxiety, some clinicians have suggested avoiding them as an initial choice for treatment[20]. Smith and colleagues[58] have recommended that SSRIs that have shorter half-lives and are less activating, such as paroxetine or sertraline, be used preferentially to fluoxetine. However, it should be noted that fluoxetine has been shown to be effective in treating anxiety symptoms associated with depression. Because of the interaction between cytochrome P-450 and drug metabolism, caution should be used when combining SSRIs with tricyclic antidepressants, antiarrhythmics, codeine, carbamazepine, benzodiazepines, and β-blockers or calcium channel blockers.

Newer Antidepressants

Nefazodone offers promise as a useful antidepressant for depressed elderly patients who have concomitant anxiety symptoms[20]. It has an acceptable level of daytime sedation for the elderly[59], but minimal anticholinergic and other side effects. Its more moderate serotonin reuptake inhibition may make it less likely to create agitation than the SSRIs[60]. Nefazodone does inhibit P-450 isoenzymes and is contraindicated for use with terfenadine, astemizole and cisapride. It will also increase the plasma levels of alprazolam, midazolam and triazolam.

Venlafaxine, a newer antidepressant that enhances both norepinephrine and serotonin activity, is increasingly being used to treat depression and anxiety in the general adult population[61]. It is approved for the treatment of GAD. Its side-effect profile is similar to the SSRIs. Small elevations in blood pressure may be seen at dosages above 200 mg/day.

Mirtazapine is the first of a new class of antidepressants, the noradrenergic and specific serotoninergic antidepressants (NaSSA). In trials for antidepressant treatment in the general adult population, mirtazapine has shown beneficial effects on the concomitant symptoms of anxiety and sleep disturbances[62]. It has few anticholinergic, adrenergic and serotonin-related adverse effects, but can be very sedating due to the antihistaminergic effects. There is no current data on its effectiveness in the elderly.

Neuroleptics

Neuroleptics are often useful for treating severe agitation associated with psychosis, delirium, and dementia[63]. The newer antipsychotics such as olanzapine and risperidone are especially being used in the treatment of refractory anxiety in the context of dementia. However, the use of neuroleptics for the treatment of subjective anxiety states, especially in the elderly, has never been demonstrated[7]. It is important to remember that neuroleptic drug side effects, such as sedation, extrapyramidal reactions, orthostatic hypotension, anticholinergic effects and tardive dyskinesia, can have potentially devastating consequences in older people. Even the newer antipsychotic agents have significant side-effect profiles. Therefore, neuroleptics should not play a significant role in the treatment of anxiety disorders in the elderly.

β-Blockers

The usefulness of β-blockers for treatment of anxiety in the elderly is unclear, since the data for the elderly are restricted to clinical case reports[31]. β-Blocking agents have been shown to be specifically beneficial in younger patients with predominantly somatic symptoms associated with generalized anxiety or anxiety related to stressful situations[64]. They may also have potential use in the treatment of aggression and agitation in patients with organic brain disease[65]. Although β-blockers decrease autonomically mediated symptoms such as diaphoresis, palpitation, tremor and gastrointestinal upset, they usually do not reduce the inner subjective effects[2,4].

Propranolol in small doses (e.g. 5–10 mg one to four times a day) may be effective in elderly patients[20]. These drugs should not be used in patients with chronic obstructive pulmonary disease, congestive heart failure, heart block, insulin-dependent diabetes, severe renal disease or peripheral vascular disease.

Antihistamines

Sedating antihistamines such as hydroxyzine and diphenhydramine hydrochloride are sometimes useful for anxiety or insomnia in the elderly. They have been rarely recommended because they are less effective than benzodiazepines, and their anticholinergic side effects are outweighed by their weak anxiolytic effects[4]. They may be used in patients with mild symptoms, in severe chronic obstructive pulmonary disease, addiction-prone personalities, alcoholics, or patients for whom more traditional drugs are not effective[66]. However, physicians must be aware that the elderly patient is much more susceptible to their anticholinergic properties, which may cause blurred vision, tachycardia, dry mouth, urinary urgency, constipation, restlessness, hallucinations and confusion. Antihistamines have no potential for inducing drug dependency or addiction.

GENERAL GUIDELINES

Despite the limited data on treatment of anxiety disorders in the elderly, the clinician can successfully treat patients with a conservative and thoughtful use of medications. The following guidelines have been adapted from Small[20].

1. Conduct a complete psychiatric evaluation. Listen specifically for expression of anxiety. Does this patient have anxiety that significantly affects their quality of life or functioning?
2. Consider the full differential diagnosis. Does the pattern of anxiety identify itself as a formal anxiety disorder, or as a symptom of another psychiatric or medical disorder? Geriatric psychiatry has been called "the specialty of co-morbidity". There may be several potential etiologies for anxiety symptoms that should be considered before initiating treatment.
3. Consider non-pharmacologic treatments first. Education and reassurance are invaluable in the treatment of anxiety, and may themselves be adequate treatments. Specifically address social stressors and evaluate the effectiveness of the support systems. Attention to family caregivers may facilitate the positive response to other treatment. Remember, the ability to benefit from therapy is not based on age.
4. Minimize polypharmacy. In the geriatric population (especially those in the nursing care facilities), the use of multiple medications is the rule rather than the exception. Most clinicians stress the importance of reviewing the medication list for potential areas of reduction, prior to adding new treatments. Reducing the number of medications may actually treat the anxiety symptoms[20].
5. When selecting an anxiolytic, consider the full presentation rather than just the anxiety when selecting an initial medication. For example, use an antidepressant if depressive symptoms are apparent. Avoid anticholinergic medications in patients with dementia. Avoid benzodiazepines when the patient's ability to ambulate is compromised.
6. As far as possible, make medication changes one at a time in order to clarify whether a complaint results from a medication side effect or an underlying illness.
7. "Start low and go slow".

REFERENCES

1. Blazer DG, George LK, Hughes DC. The epidemiology of anxiety disorders: an age comparison. In Salzman C, Lebowitz BD, eds, Anxiety in the Elderly: Treatment and Research. New York: Springer, 1991; 17–30.
2. Shader RI, Greenblatt DJ. Management of anxiety in the elderly: the balance between therapeutic and adverse effects. J Clin Psychiat 1987; 42: 107–13.
3. Hocking LB, Koenig HG. Anxiety in medically ill older patients: a review and update. Int J Psychiat Med 1995; 25: 221–38.
4. Barbee JG, McLaulin JB. Anxiety disorders: diagnosis and pharmacotherapy in the elderly. Psychiat Ann 1990; 20: 439–45.
5. Krasucki C, Howard R, Mann A. Anxiety and its treatment in the elderly. International Psychogeriat 1998; 11(1): 25–45.
6. Pearson JL. Summary of a National Institute of Mental Health workshop on late-life anxiety. Psychopharmac Bull 1998; 34(2): 127–38.
7. Salzman C. Pharmacologic treatment of the anxious elderly patient. In Salzman C, Lebowitz BD, eds, Anxiety in the Elderly: Treatment and Research. New York: Springer, 1991; 149–73.
8. Schneider L. Overview of generalized anxiety disorder in the elderly. J Clin Psychiat 1996; 57(suppl 7): 34–45.
9. Watkins LL, Grossman P, Krishnan R, Blumenthal JA. Anxiety reduces baroreflex cardiac control in older adults with major depression. Psychosom Med 1999; 61(3): 334–40.
10. Corbett L. Anxiety in the elderly: current concepts. In Fawcett J, ed., Anxiety and Anxiety in the Elderly in Contemporary Psychiatry. Chicago, IL: Pragmaton, 1983; 37–41.
11. Jenike MA. Anxiety disorders of old age. In Rall TW, Nies A, Taylor P, Jenike MA, eds, Geriatric Psychiatry and Psychopharmacology: A Clinical Approach. Chicago: Yearbook Medical Publishers, 1989; 248–71.
12. Thompson TL II, Moran MG, Nies AS. Psychotropic drug use in the elderly. N Engl J Med 1983; 308: 134–8.
13. Ouslander JG. Drug therapy in the elderly. Ann Intern Med 1981; 95: 711–22.
14. Salzman C. Practical considerations in the pharmacologic treatment of depression and anxiety in the elderly. J Clin Psychiat 1990; 51 (suppl 1): 40–43.
15. Zimmer B, Gershon S. The ideal late-life anxiolytic. In Salzman C, Lebowitz BD, eds, Anxiety in the Elderly: Treatment and Research. New York: Springer, 1991; 277–303.
16. Hayes PE, Dommisse CS. Current concepts in clinical therapeutics. Anxiety disorders, Part 1. Clin Pharm 1987; 6(2): 140–47.
17. American Psychiatric Association. Benzodiazepine Dependence, Toxicity, and Abuse. Washington, DC: American Psychiatric Association, 1990.
18. Shorr RI, Robin DW. Rational use of benzodiazepines in the elderly. Drugs Aging 1994; 4: 9–20.
19. Baldessarini RJ. Drugs and the treatment of psychiatric disorders. In Goodman-Gilman A, ed., The Pharmacological Basis of Therapeutics, 8th edn. Oxford: Pergamon, 1990.
20. Small GW. Recognizing and treating anxiety in the elderly. J Clin Psychiat 1997; 58(suppl 3): 41–7.
21. Ray WA, Griffin MR, Downey W. Benzodiazepines of long and short elimination half-life and the risk of hip fracture. J Am Med Assoc 1989; 262: 3303–6.
22. Dubovsky SL. Generalized anxiety disorder: new concepts and psychopharmacologic therapies. J Clin Psychiat 1990; 51(suppl 1): 3–10.
23. Greenblatt DJ, Shader RI, Abernethy DR. Current status of benzodiazepines, part 1. N Engl J Med 1983; 309: 354–8.
24. Boston Collaborative Drug Surveillance Program. Clinical depression of the central nervous system due to diazepam and chlordiazepoxide in relation to cigarette smoking and age. N Engl J Med 1973; 288(6): 277–80.

25. Pomara N, Stanley B, Block R *et al.* Adverse effects of single therapeutic doses of diazepam on performance in normal geriatric subjects: relationships to plasma concentrations. *Psychopharmacology* 1984; **27**: 273–81.

26. Nikaido AM, Ellinwood EH Jr, Heatherly DG, Dubow D. Differential CNS effects of diazepam in elderly adults. *Pharmacol Biochem Behav* 1987; **27**: 273–81.

27. Skegg DCG, Richards SM, Doll R *et al.* Minor tranquilizers and road accidents. *Br Med J* 1979; **1**(6168): 917–19.

28. Weilburg JB, Sachs G, Falk WE. Triazolam-induced brief episodes of secondary mania in a depressed patient. *J Clin Psychiat* 1987; **48**(12): 492–3.

29. Goodman WK, Charney DS. A case of alprazolam, but not lorazepam, inducing manic symptoms. *J Clin Psychiat* 1987; **48**(3): 117–18.

30. Gershon S, Eison AS. Anxiolytic profiles. *J Clin Psychiat* 1983; **44**(11, 2): 45–57.

31. Sadavoy J, LeClair JK. Treatment of anxiety disorders in late life. *Can J Psychiat* 1997; **42**(suppl 1): 28–34S.

33. Eison AS, Temple DL Jr. Buspirone: review of its pharmacology and current perspectives on its mechanism of action. *Am J Med* 1986; **80**(suppl 3B): 1–9.

34. Goa KL, Ward A. Buspirone: a preliminary review of its pharmacologic properties and therapeutic efficacy as an anxiolytic. *Drugs* 1986; **32**: 114–29.

35. Napoleillo MJ. An interim multicentre report on 677 anxious geriatric out-patients treated with buspirone. *Br J Clin Pract* 1986; **40**: 71–3.

36. Singh AN, Beer M. A dose range finding study of buspirone in geriatric patients with symptoms of anxiety. *J Clin Psychopharmacol* 1988; **8**: 67–8.

37. Robinson D, Napoliello MJ, Schenk J. The safety and usefulness of buspirone as an anxiolytic drug in elderly versus younger patients. *Clin Ther* 1988; **10**(6): 740–6.

38. Bohm C, Robinson DS, Gammans RE *et al.* Buspirone therapy in anxious elderly patients: a controlled clinical trial. *J Clin Psychopharmacol* 1990; **10**(suppl 3): 47–51S.

39. Sheehan DV, Raj AB, Sheehan KH, Soto S. Is buspirone effective for panic disorder? *J Clin Psychopharmacol* 1990; **10**(1): 3–11.

40. Schweizer E, Rickels K, Lucki I. Resistance to the anti-anxiety effect of buspirone inpatients with a history of benzodiazepine use. *N Engl J Med* 1986; **314**: 719–20.

41. Banazak DA. Anxiety disorders in elderly patients. *J Am Board Fam Pract* 1997; **10**(4): 280–9.

42. Steinberg JR. Anxiety in elderly patients. A comparison of azapirones and benzodiazepines. *Drugs Aging* 1994; **5**(5): 335–45.

43. Rifken A, Klein DF, Dillon D, Levitt M. Blockade by imipramine or desipramine of panic induced by sodium lactate. *Am J Psychiat* 1981; **138**: 676–7.

44. Crook T. Diagnosis and treatment of mixed anxiety–depression in the elderly. *J Clin Psychiat* 1982; **43**(9): 35–43.

45. Hershey LA, Kim KY. Diagnosis and treatment of anxiety in the elderly. *Rational Drug Ther* 1988; **22**(3): 1–6.

46. Hoehn-Saric R, McLeod DR, Zimmerli WD. Differential effects of alprazolam and imipramine in generalized anxiety disorder: somatic vs. psychic symptoms. *J Clin Psychiatry* 1988; **49**: 293–301.

47. Rickels K, Downing R, Schweizer E *et al.* Antidepressants for the treatment of generalized anxiety disorder: a placebo-controlled comparison of imipramine, trazodone, and diazepam. *Arch Gen Psychiat* 1993; **50**: 884–95.

48. Georgotas A, McCue RE, Hapworth W *et al.* Comparative efficacy and safety of MAOIs vs. TCAs in treating depression in the elderly. *Biol Psychiat* 1986; **21**: 1155–66.

49. Fyer AJ, Sandberg D. Pharmacologic treatment of panic disorder. In Francis AJ, Hales RE, eds, *Review of Psychiatry*. Washington, DC: American Psychiatric Press, 1988; 88–120.

50. Tiller JW, Bouwer C, Behnke K. Moclobemide for anxiety disorders: a focus on moclobemide for panic disorder. *Int Clin Psychopharmacol* 1997; **12**(suppl 6): S27–30.

51. Versiani M, Amrein R, Montgomery SA. Social phobia: long-term treatment outcome and prediction of response—a moclobemide study. *Int Clin Psychopharmacol* 1997; **12**(5): 239–54.

52. Feighner JP, Boyer WF, Meredith CH, Hendrickson G. An overview of fluoxetine in geriatric depression. *Br J Psychiat* 1988; **3**: 105–8.

53. Perse TL, Greist JH, Jefferson JW, Rosenfield R, Dar R. Fluvoxamine treatment of obsessive-compulsive disorder. *Am J Psychiat* 1987; **144**: 1543–8.

54. Katzelnick DJ, Greist JH, Jefferson JW, Kobak KA. Sertraline in social phobia: a controlled pilot study. *Neuropsychopharmacol* 1994; **10**(suppl 35): 260S.

55. Kelsey JE. Venlafaxine in social phobia. *Psychopharmacol Bull* 1994; **31**: 767–71.

56. Van Ameringen M, Mancini C, Streiner DL. Fluoxetine efficacy in social phobia. *J Clin Psychiat* 1993; **54**: 27–32.

57. van Vliet IM, den Boer JA, Westenberg HG. Psychopharmacological treatment of social phobia: A double-blind placebo controlled study with fluvoxamine. *Psychopharmacology Berl* 1994; **115**: 128–34.

58. Smith SL, Sherrill KA, Colenda CC. Assessing and treating anxiety in elderly persons. *Psychiat Serv* 1995; **46**(1): 36–42.

59. van Laar MW, van Willigenburg AP, Volkerts ER. Acute and subchronic effects of nefazodone and imipramine on highway driving, cognitive functions, and daytime sleepiness in healthy adult and elderly subjects. *J Clin Psychopharmacol* 1995; **15**: 30–40.

60. Fawcett J, Marcus RN, Anton SF *et al.* Response of anxiety and agitation symptoms during nefazodone treatment of major depression. *J Clin Psychiatry* 1995; **37**: 713–38.

61. Silverstone PH, Ravindran A. Once-daily venlafaxine extended release (XR) compared with fluoxetine in outpatients with depression and anxiety. Venlafaxine XR 360 study group. *J Clin Psychiat* 1999; **60**(1): 22–8.

62. Kasper S, Przschek-Rieder N, Tauscher J, Wolf R. A risk–benefit assessment of mirtazapine in the treatment of depression. *Drug Safety* 1997; **17**(4): 251–64.

63. Chou JCY, Sussman N. Neuroleptics in anxiety. *Psychiat Ann* 1988; **18**(3): 172–5.

64. Peet M. The treatment of anxiety with β-blocking drugs. *Postgrad Med J* 1988; **64**(suppl 2): 45–9.

65. Greendyke R, Kanter D, Schuster D *et al.* Propranolol treatment of assaultive patients with organic brain disease: a double-blind cross-over, placebo-controlled study. *J Nerv Ment Dis* 1986; **174**: 290–4.

66. Rickels K. Non-benzodiazepine anxiolytics: clinical usefulness. *J Clin Psychiat* 1983; **44**(11): 38–43.

67. Blazer DG. Generalized anxiety disorder and panic disorder in the elderly: a review. *Harvard Rev Psychiat* 1997; **5**(1): 18–27.

68. Petrie WM, Ban TA. Propranolol in organic agitation. *Lancet* 1981; **1**: 324.

69. Pohl R, Balon R, Yeragani VK, Gershon S. Serotoninergic anxiolytics in the treatment of panic disorder: A controlled study with buspirone. *Psychopathology* 1989; **22**(suppl 1): 60–7.

70. Sheikh JI, Salzman C. Anxiety in the elderly: course and treatment. *Psychiat Clin N Am* 1995; **18**(4): 871–83.

71. Steinberg J. Prescription drug impairment in the elderly. *Drug Ther* 1994; **199**(suppl): 83–100S.

72. Weiss KJ. Optimal management of anxiety in older patients. *Drugs Aging* 1996; **9**(3): 191–201.

104

Obsessive–compulsive Disorder

James Lindesay

University of Leicester, Leicester, UK

Although obsessive–compulsive disorder (OCD) is known to occur in old age, studies are few and information is limited. This may be because it is often not perceived as a disorder of late life. The mean age of onset is 20–25 years[1-3] and it is unusual for OCD to have its first onset after the age of 50 years. However, OCD is a chronic disorder if untreated, and a significant proportion of cases persist into old age, when they may present to services for the first time. It is important, therefore, that old age psychiatrists are aware of this disorder and of its management.

CLINICAL FEATURES

Diagnostic Criteria

OCD is characterized by intrusive, persistent obsessive thoughts, images or impulses and/or compulsive behaviours that are a significant source of distress, or interfere with the patient's personal or social functioning. The current diagnostic criteria, as set out in DSM-IV[4] and ICD-10[5], apply to all patients, irrespective of age. The limited evidence available indicates that the clinical features of OCD in elderly patients are very similar to those of younger adults. In their comparative study, Kohn *et al.*[6] found that concerns about symmetry, need-to-know and counting rituals were less common in elderly patients, and hand-washing and fear of having sinned were more common, but otherwise there were few differences in clinical features compared with younger OCD patients. Extreme ego-syntonic religiosity has been proposed as a variant of OCD that may be more common in older patients[7].

Differential Diagnosis

Unpleasant, intrusive thoughts and abnormal stereotyped behaviours occur in other mental disorders, and OCD is not diagnosed if their content is *exclusively* related to another disorder, e.g. guilty preoccupations in depression, worries in generalized anxiety, concern with illness in hypochondriasis, weight control in anorexia or avoidance in phobic disorders[4]. It should be borne in mind that conditions such as depression, generalized anxiety and substance abuse may be co-morbid with OCD. In elderly patients, increased anxious orderliness may be a prodrome of dementia; however, this behaviour is not resisted or associated with the tension that occurs in OCD. The compulsive behaviours of OCD resemble the stereotyped behaviours that occur in certain other disorders, such as Tourette's syndrome, Sydenham's chorea, encephalitis and partial complex seizures. Tourette's syndrome

and OCD commonly co-occur[8], and patients with OCD may have a history of Sydenham's chorea in childhood[9].

Despite its similar name, obsessional personality disorder is quite distinct from OCD. It is characterized not by obsessions and compulsions, but by a preoccupation with orderliness, perfection and control dating back to early adulthood[4]. In some individuals, there is an inability to discard personal possessions, which may present as the so-called "senile squalor" syndrome after a lifetime of accumulated rubbish.

Not all patients with OCD have insight into the irrationality and inappropriateness of their obsessions and compulsions. If the obsessional thoughts are held with delusional intensity, an additional diagnosis of delusional disorder may be warranted. The ruminative delusions and stereotypies of schizophrenia are usually not ego-dystonic, and therefore would not be regarded as OCD[4].

Clinical Assessment

An effective treatment plan for OCD requires a detailed clinical assessment. What exactly are the main problems? What, if anything, exacerbates or improves the symptoms? How long has the condition been present, and how has it evolved since its onset? What treatments, if any, have been tried in the past? What other symptoms or disorders are present? Any concomitant depression, mania, psychosis or alcohol dependency will require specific management before behavioural treatments for OCD can be effective. If the patient is cognitively impaired, this will have implications for the choice of treatment; for example, some behavioural strategies will not work if information cannot be retained or recalled. In elderly patients with OCD of recent onset, it is important to investigate carefully for any underlying cerebral disease. Late-onset cases are associated with frontal dysfunction[10], which may be caused by a variety of focal and generalized disorders, including cerebrovascular disease, tumours and primary neurodegenerative dementias. Late-onset OCD may also be the result of external factors, such as adverse life events and exposure to trauma, that weaken an elderly individual's resistance to long-standing subclinical obsessionality[11].

EPIDEMIOLOGY

Most of our knowledge about the epidemiology of OCD in old age derives from the US National Institute for Mental Health (NIMH) Epidemiologic Catchment Area (ECA) Program. Overall, the 1 year prevalence for those aged 65 years and older was

Principles and Practice of Geriatric Psychiatry, 2nd edn. Edited by J. R. M. Copeland, M. T. Abou-Saleh and D. G. Blazer
©2002 John Wiley & Sons, Ltd

0.85% (men 0.75%, women 0.93%), as opposed to 1.65% for the sample as a whole[12]. A more detailed analysis of the elderly population at the Eastern Baltimore site found prevalence rates of 1.3% for those aged 65–74 years and 0.6% in those aged 75+[13]. Following the second wave of the ECA, annual incidence rates were estimated. In males aged 65+, the incidence rate of OCD was one-third of that for males of all ages, but in females there was a non-significant upturn in the incidence rate after age 65[14]. In common with a number of other psychiatric disorders, the lifetime prevalence of OCD decreased with age in this study. The reason for this is unclear, but it may be the result of cohort effects, differential mortality or age-specific differences in symptom ascertainment and recall.

AETIOLOGY

Genetic factors play an important role in the aetiology of OCD; it occurs in 40–50% of parents, 19–39% of siblings and 16% of children of probands with the disorder[15]. Just what is inherited is not clear; other anxiety disorders are also more common in the families of OCD probands[16]. Most of the evidence from clinical, neuropsychological and neuroimaging studies implicates the basal ganglia and their connections with the thalamus and the cerebral cortex in the aetiology of OCD[17]. Specifically, it has been proposed that there is dysfunction in a neuronal circuit involving the orbitofrontal cortex, the basal ganglia, the substantia nigra and the ventrolateral pallidum[18]. The specific response of OCD to serotonin (5-HT) reuptake-inhibiting drugs (see below) suggests that serotonergic neuronal systems are involved, directly or indirectly. In the cognitive-behavioural model of OCD, obsessions and compulsions result from pathological, anxiety-provoking over-control of normal intrusive cognitions[19].

TREATMENT

There are no randomized, controlled trials of treatment of OCD in elderly patients. Accordingly, the guidelines that follow are based upon case reports and extrapolations from studies in younger adults[20].

Non-pharmacological Treatments

Behavioural therapy, in the form of exposure and response-prevention (ERP), is well described as an effective intervention for OCD in younger adults[21]. This involves exposing the patient to the feared situation, and helping him/her to resist the urge to perform the compulsive behaviours that would normally follow this exposure[22]. ERP is least effective in those who have obsessional thoughts and covert rituals unaccompanied by compulsive behaviour. In these patients, a cognitive approach directed at modifying the misinterpretation of intrusive thoughts is more appropriate[23]. There have been a number of case-reports of effective behavioural interventions with elderly OCD patients[19,24–27], but most are difficult to interpret because of the concomitant administration of medication. In the case described by Calamari et al.[27], significant improvement following ERP was maintained without medication at 8 month follow-up.

Freud proposed that obsessional symptoms were a regression to a pregenital anal–sadistic phase of development. However, despite this and subsequent psychodynamic formulations of the disorder, there is no evidence that psychodynamic psychotherapy is an effective treatment for OCD at any age.

Pharmacological Treatments

Studies in younger adults indicate that 30–60% of patients with OCD show improvement on appropriate medication, and that drug treatment appears to be more effective for obsessional thoughts than for compulsive behaviours. In practice, drug treatment and behavioural therapy are often given in combination.

The theory that OCD is a disorder of serotoninergic function is based upon the empirical observation that it can be effectively treated by drugs that inhibit serotonin reuptake. Clomipramine is the most extensively studied drug treatment for OCD, and its effectiveness has been established in a number of double-blind placebo-controlled trials in younger adults[28]. However, the lack of receptor sensitivity means that it has significant anticholinergic and antihistaminergic side effects that limit its usefulness in elderly patients[29]. In this age group, the drug of first choice is one of the specific serotonin reuptake inhibitors (SSRIs). Fluoxetine, paroxetine and fluvoxamine are currently licensed in the UK for the treatment of OCD, although none of the trials supporting this indication specifically involved elderly patients. The effective dose for the treatment of OCD with these drugs tends to be higher than that required to treat depression, and the time taken to respond is typically much longer: 10–18 weeks. Studies suggest that long-term therapy is required, as discontinuation of medication leads to relapse of symptoms.

There is little evidence for the effectiveness of other drug treatments in OCD. There are some case reports suggesting that monoamine oxidase inhibitors (MAOIs) may be useful in patients with concomitant panic or severe anxiety. Anxiolytic drugs may also help with the anxiety associated with OCD, but do not appear to have any effect on the core symptoms. A possible exception is buspirone, which may augment the effect of fluoxetine[30,31]. Lithium augmentation of fluoxetine has also been reported as effective in one elderly case[32].

Physical Treatments

There is very little evidence to suggest that ECT is effective in the treatment of OCD in patients who are not also depressed[33]. Some good results have been reported for stereotactic neurosurgical procedures in patients with severe and treatment-refractory illness, including elderly subjects[20], but since negative outcomes are rarely described, this evidence is difficult to interpret.

CONCLUSIONS

OCD may present for the first time in old age, and many elderly patients with chronic illness will not have been exposed to the full range of pharmacological and cognitive-behavioural treatments that are now available. It is important that old age psychiatry services are aware of these treatments and develop some experience in their delivery. There is some evidence that they are effective in elderly patients, but further research is needed. Patients with a new onset of OCD in late life need careful assessment to exclude underlying organic brain disease.

REFERENCES

1. Rachman SJ, Hodgson RJ. *Obsessions and Compulsions*. Englewood Cliffs, NJ: Prentice Hall.
2. Thyer BA, Parrish RT, Curtis GC et al. Ages of onset of DSM-III anxiety disorders. *Comp Psychiat* 1985; **26**: 113–22.

3. Rasmussen SA, Tsuang MT. Epidemiology and clinical features of obsessive-compulsive disorder. In Jenike MA, Baer L, Minichiello WE, eds, *Obsessive Compulsive Disorders: Theory and Management*. Littleton, MA: PSG.

4. American Psychiatric Association. *Diagnostic and Statistical Manual of Mental Disorders*, 4th edn. Washington, DC: American Psychiatric Association, 1994.

5. World Health Organization. *International Classification of Diseases (10th Revision)*. Geneva: World Health Organization, 1992.

6. Kohn R, Westlake RJ, Rasmussen SA *et al*. Clinical features of obsessive-compulsive disorder in elderly patients. *Am J Geriat Psychiat* 1997; **5**: 211–15.

7. Fallon BA, Liebowitz MR, Hollander E *et al*. The pharmacotherapy of moral or religious scrupulosity. *J Clin Psychiat* 1990; **51**: 517–21.

8. Pauls D, Leckman J. The inheritance of Gilles de la Tourette's syndrome and associated behaviours: evidence for autosomal dominant transmission. *N Engl J Med* 1986; **315**: 993.

9. Swedo S, Rapaport J, Cheslow D *et al*. High prevalence of obsessive-compulsive disorder symptoms in patients with Sydenham's chorea. *Am J Psychiat* 1989; **146**: 246–9.

10. Philpot M, Banerjee S. Late onset obsessive-compulsive disorder (OCD): an organic disorder? In *Abstracts of the 7th International Psychogeriatric Association Congress*, Sydney, 1995: 124.

11. Colvin C, Boddington SJA. Behaviour therapy for obsessive compulsive disorder in a 78-year-old woman. *Int J Geriat Psychiat* 1997; **12**: 488–91.

12. Karno M, Golding JM. Obsessive-compulsive disorder. In Robins LN, Regier DA, eds, *Psychiatric Disorders in America*. New York: Free Press, 1991: 204–19.

13. Kramer M, German PS, Anthony J *et al*. Patterns of mental disorders among the elderly residents of Eastern Baltimore. *J Am Geriat Soc* 1985; **33**: 236–45.

14. Eaton WW, Kramer M, Anthony J *et al*. The incidence of specific DIS/DSM-III mental disorders: data from the NIMH Epidemiologic Catchment Area program. *Acta Psychiat Scand* 1989; **67**: 414–28.

15. Marks IM. Genetics of fear and anxiety disorders. *Br J Psychiat* 1986; **149**: 406–18.

16. Black DW, Noyes R, Goldstein RB, Blim N. A family study of obsessive-compulsive disorder. *Arch Gen Psychiat* 1992; **49**: 362–8.

17. Piggott TA, Myers KR, Williams DA. Obsessive-compulsive disorder: a neuropsychiatric perspective. In Rapee RM, ed., *Current Controversies in the Anxiety Disorders*. New York: Guilford, 1996: 134–60.

18. Insel TR. Neurobiology of obsessive compulsive disorder: a review. *Int Clin Psychopharmacol* 1992; **7**(suppl 1): 31–3.

19. Salkovskis PM. Cognitive-behavioural approaches to the understanding of obsessional problems. In Rapee RM, ed., *Current Controversies in the Anxiety Disorders*. New York: Guilford, 1996: 103–33.

20. Jenike MA, Baer L, Minichiello WE. *Obsessive Compulsive Disorders: Theory and Management*, 2nd edn. Chicago, IL: Yearbook Medical Publishers, 1990.

21. Marks IM, Lelliot P, Basoglu M, Noshirvani H. Clomipramine, self-exposure and therapist aided exposure for obsessive-compulsive rituals: I. *Br J Psychiat* 1988; **136**: 1–25.

22. Salkovskis PM, Kirk J. Obsessional disorders. In Hawton K, Salkovskis PM, Kirk J, Clark DM, eds, *Cognitive Behaviour Therapy for Psychiatric Problems: A Practical Guide*. Oxford: Oxford University Press, 1989: 129–68.

23. Salkovskis PM, Warwick HMC. Cognitive therapy of obsessive-compulsive disorder: treating treatment failures. *Behav Psychother* 1985; **13**: 243–55.

24. Rowen VC, Holborn SW, Walker JR and Siddiqui AR. A rapid multi-component treatment for an obsessive-compulsive disorder. *J Behav Ther Exp Psychiat* 1984; **15**: 347–52.

25. Junginger J, Ditto B. Multitreatment of obsessive compulsive checking in a geriatric patient. *Behav Modif* 1984; **8**: 379–90.

26. Austin LS, Zealberg JJ, Lydiard RB. Three cases of pharmacotherapy of obsessive-compulsive disorder in the elderly. *J Nerv Ment Dis* 1991; **179**: 634–5.

27. Calamari JE, Faber SD, Hitsman BL, Poppe CJ. Treatment of obsessive-compulsive disorder in the elderly: a review and case example. *J Behav Ther Exp Psychiat* 1994; **25**: 95–104.

28. Thoren P, Äsberg M, Cronholm B *et al*. Clomipramine treatment of obsessive-compulsive disorder: a clinical controlled trial. *Arch Gen Psychiat* 1980; **37**: 1281.

29. Jackson CW. Obsessive-compulsive disorder in elderly patients. *Drugs Aging* 1995; **7**: 438–48.

30. Markovitz PJ, Stagno SJ, Calabrese JR. Buspirone augmentation of fluoxetine in obsessive-compulsive disorder. Abstract No. 379, *Biological Psychiatry Annual Meeting*, San Francisco, CA, 1989.

31. Jenike MA, Baer L, Ballantine HT *et al*. Cingulotomy for refractory obsessive-compulsive disorder: a long-term follow-up of 33 patients. *Arch Gen Psychiat* 1991; **48**: 548–55.

32. Bajulaiye R, Addonizio G. Obsessive compulsive disorder arising in a 75-year-old woman. *Int J Geriat Psychiat* 1992; **7**: 139–42.

33. Mellman LA, Grossman JM. Successful treatment of obsessive-compulsive disorder with ECT. *Am J Psychiat* 1984; **141**: 596–7.

105

Hypochondriacal Disorder

Andree Allen[1] and Ewald W. Busse[2]

[1]*Dorothea Dix Hospital, Raleigh, NC, USA,*
and [2]*Duke University Medical Center, Durham, NC, USA*

The term "hypochondriasis" has its origins in the ancient Greek language. Anatomically, the hypochondrium refers to that part of the body between the ribs and the xiphoid cartilage. The ancient Greeks believed that this part of the body, especially the spleen, was the seat of morbid anxiety about one's health, depression, bad mood and simulated disease[1,2]. This old theory has not withstood the passage of time, but the term "hypochondriasis" has survived and is part of our modern diagnostic nomenclature[3–5]. Hypochondriasis has joined the ranks of syndromes known as somatoform disorder in DSM-IV, with the following diagnostic criteria:

1. The predominant disturbance is preoccupation with the fear of having or the belief that one has a serious disease based on the individual's interpretation of physical signs or sensations as evidence of physical illness (do not include misinterpretation of physical symptoms of panic attack).
2. Appropriate physical evaluation does not support the diagnosis of any physical disorder that can account for the physical signs or sensations or the individual's unwarranted interpretation of them, and the symptoms in (1) are not only the symptoms of panic attacks.
3. The fear of having, or the belief that one has, a disease persists despite medical reassurance.
4. The duration of the disturbance is at least 6 months.
5. The belief in (1) above is not a fixed delusion, as in delusional disorder, somatic type.

There are issues regarding hypochondriasis as a diagnostic entity. Some clinicians and the *International Classification of Diseases* regard it as a specific non-psychotic psychiatric disorder, while others hold that it is a syndrome (a collection of similar symptoms that occur together but are of multiple etiology). It is evident that hypochondriacal symptoms may be part of another disorder, such as a mood disorder or a defense mechanism, as well as a character trait. Starcevic[6] has dissected the hypochondriacal syndrome into potentially useful constructs that represent a stepwise progression. The "hypochondriacal core", as the preoccupation with bodily sensations and functioning, gives rise to a state of "somatic uncertainty", an insecurity feeling resulting in intense anxiety which is poorly tolerated by the individual. This leads to the "disease suspicion", which represents the fear of having a disease. "Hypochondriacal behaviors" ensue as the patient obsessively seeks a medical work-up to uncover the cause of his/her symptoms and is generally dissatisfied, as it is found that there is either an absence of physical disease or that the symptoms are out of proportion to the pathology. Starcevic points out that the hypochondriacal syndrome is a heterogeneous entity with varying degrees of bodily preoccupation, fear, suspicion and a variety of complaints.

Hypochondriasis, with its state of uncertainty, may be seen as a feature of an anxiety disorder. It may be part of a mood disorder, such as a masked depression, where the patient will deny feeling depressed but respond to antidepressant medication. Starcevic[6] makes the point that hypochondriasis may be incorporated into a long-standing, maladaptive pattern of functioning and that many personality disorders may have a hypochondriacal manifestation. There is a fine line to be crossed when the disease suspicion turns into "disease conviction" and the syndrome is no longer hypochondriasis, but a psychotic disorder, such as paranoid delusional disorder, paranoid schizophrenia or major depression with psychotic features.

In his 1987 review article on the subject matter, Lipowski[7] considers that predisposing factors such as genetics, developmental learning, personality and sociocultural environment play a role in hypochondriasis. Swedish investigators have gathered data from adoption studies in regard to familial somatization patterns. The subjects of their studies were drawn from 912 women born out of wedlock in Stockholm, Sweden, during 1930–1949. Between 1965 and 1973, the medical records of 859 subjects were reviewed for duration and number of sick leaves, chief complaint and diagnosis[8–10]; 144 were found to be somatizers. This study suggests that somatization is more common in adopted women than in non-adopted women. This raises the issue of genetic predisposition to somatization, as adoptees are known to have a higher percentage of biological parents with alcoholism and criminality compared to non-adoptees. There may be a complex interaction between the type of somatizers, alcoholism and antisocial behavior and sex differences. The interaction between biological predisposition and environmental influences requires additional attention.

Theories that conceptualize the genesis of hypochondriasis to learned behavior from childhood sound intuitively correct[11]. Children who grow up in families where a serious or chronic illness is present, or who are exposed to a hypochondriacal relative, may well learn a way to obtain attention, sympathy and support, or get the message that physical complaints are acceptable, while complaints of emotional distress are not. Children suffering from physical disorders may get anxious attention from parents. They may also learn that being sick is to avoid unpleasant duties. Somatization may serve as a way

Principles and Practice of Geriatric Psychiatry, 2nd edn. Edited by J. R. M. Copeland, M. T. Abou-Saleh and D. G. Blazer
©2002 John Wiley & Sons, Ltd

to deal with adverse social situations and to maintain self-esteem.

Kanner[2] felt that hypochondriacal attitudes in children often reflected school problems or "unhappiness at home". He observed that some mothers focused on their child's somatic functioning rather than their own, thus teaching the child to somatize. This improper maladaptive coping pattern may well continue in adulthood. While it is possible that these early childhood influences shape the child into a hypochondriacal character, it may not necessarily follow. There may be innate personality characteristics that predispose to somatization. Barsky and Klerman[5] pointed out that there are individuals who "amplify body sensations", focus on them, misinterpret them and reach the conclusions that they may indicate disease. Costa and McCrae[12] point out that somatizers tend to score highly on measures of neuroticism.

Predisposing factors appear by no means to be solely affected by stressful life events in childhood. In his studies on elderly hypochondriacs, Busse[13] has noted that contributing factors include recurrent exposure to criticism where there is no possibility of escape, reduction in economic status, loss of spouse and friends, isolation due to socioeconomic factors and deterioration in marital satisfaction.

As Lipowski[7] notes, sociocultural factors, such as linguistic habits, health beliefs and inhibition of expression, may play a role in somatization.

EPIDEMIOLOGY

While hypochondriasis is seen throughout the life cycle, it is the most frequent somatoform disorder in the elderly. One epidemiologic study[14] shows that 15% of the elderly in the community over the age of 65 reported perceiving that their physical health was poorer than their actual health status. Other investigators[15] have collected data on adults, but not necessarily exclusively in the elderly. Kellner and Sheffield[15] found that 60–80% of physically healthy individuals in the community had at least one physical complaint in 1 week. In their review of the prevalence of "functional complaints" in primary health care, Barsky and Klerman[5] show that a large proportion of patients (30–80%) who present to the doctor's office do not have evidence of significant physical disease. In their report of the Piedmont Epidemiologic Catchment Area (ECA) study, Swartz et al.[16] suggested that somatization symptoms are more prevalent in the rural than in the urban community, that somatization increases with age up to age 65, then tends to drop off, but still remains higher in the elderly over 65 than the age group 18–44. Interestingly, between the ages of 45 and 64, an increase in somatic symptoms is associated with separation, divorce and widowhood. Longitudinal studies of elderly persons living in the community revealed that hypochondriacal episodes are often transient, lasting a few months to several years. The hypochondriacal reaction is often a maladaptive response to social stress[17]. Another study[18] concludes that hypochondriasis is less a direct function of stressful life events than of the underlying personality, i.e. a characteristic way of perceiving life events. Patients with transient hypochondriacal reactions are common in a general medical clinic. A recent report[19] notes that, among outpatients confronted with a medical illness, those who are sensitive to somatic sensations and those with personality disorders are more likely to develop hypochondriasis.

TREATMENT CONSIDERATIONS

A number of psychotherapeutic approaches, including individual and group therapy[20], have been used in the treatment of hypochondriacal patients. Frequently, individual psychotherapeutic approaches have been based on the treatment methods for depression in those beyond the age of 60 years. This is understandable, because depression is not an unusual feature of hypochondriasis. However, many approaches have certain features in common such as the recognition of the hypochondriac's hostility toward the medical profession and the need to deal effectively with this hostility. Another is avoiding confrontation, specifically the insistence by the therapist that no pathology is present[17,21]. This is of particular importance to the geriatrician, as hypochondriasis is complicated by the existence of physical disabilities and degenerative disease in the majority of elderly persons.

Hospitalization for extensive medical evaluation is to be avoided[13] as the experience often increases the hypochondriac's conviction that a "missed" serious illness is likely and adds to the resistance to psychotherapy. Medications may be useful and often do have a transient placebo effect. Drugs should be selected with considerable care to avoid the complications of side effects and addictive qualities.

REFERENCES

1. *Dorland's Illustrated Medical Dictionary*, 26th edn. New York: WB Saunders, 1981: 638.
2. Kanner L. The minor psychoses. In Kanner L, *Child Psychiatry*. Springfield, IL: Charles C. Thomas, 1935; 448–83.
3. American Psychiatric Association. *Diagnostic and Statistical Manual of Mental Disorders*, 4th edn. (DSM-IV). Washington, DC: APA. 1994.
4. World Health Organization. *International Classification of Diseases*, 9th Revision (ICD-9). Geneva: WHO, 1978.
5. Barsky A, Klerman GL. Overview: hypochondriasis, bodily complaints and somatic styles. *Am J Psychiat* 1983; **140**: 273–83.
6. Starcevic V. Diagnosis of hypochondriasis: a promenade through the psychiatric nosology. *Am J Psychother* 1988; **42**(2): 197–211.
7. Lipowski ZJ. Somatization: the experience and communication of psychological distress as somatic symptoms. *Psychother Psychosom* 1987; **47**: 160–7.
8. Bohman M, Cloninger CR, von Knorring AL, Sigvardsson S. An adoption study of somatoform disorders III. Cross-fostering analysis and genetic relationship to alcoholism and criminality. *Arch Gen Psychiat* 1984; **41**(9): 872–8.
9. Cloninger CR, Sigvardsson S, von Knorring AL, Bohman M. An adoption study of somatoform disorders II. Identification of two discrete somatoform disorders. *Arch Gen Psychiat* 1984; **41**(9): 863–71.
10. Sigvardsson S, von Knorring AL, Bohman M, Cloninger CR. An adoption study of somatoform disorders I. The relationship of somatization to psychiatric disability. *Arch Gen Psychiat* 1984; **41**(9): 853–9.
11. Parker G, Lipscombe P. The relevance of early parental experiences to adult dependency, hypochondriasis and utilization of primary physicians. *Br J Med Psychol* 1980; **53**: 355–63.
12. Costa PT, McCrae RR. Hypochondriasis, neuroticism, and aging. *Am Psychol* 1985; **40**: 19–28.
13. Busse EW. Treating hypochondriasis in the elderly. *Generations* 1986; **10**(3): 30–3.
14. Blazer DG, Houpt JL. Perception of poor health in the healthy older adult. *J Am Geriat Soc* 1979; **27**(4): 330–4.
15. Kellner R, Sheffield BR. Psychotherapeutic strategies in hypochondriasis: a clinical study. *Am J Psychiat* 1982; **36**: 146–59.

16. Swartz M, Landerman R, Blazer D *et al.* Somatization symptoms in the community: a rural/urban comparison. *Psychosomatics* 1989; **30**(1): 44–53.

17. Busse EW. Hypochondriasis in the elderly. *Comp Ther* 1987; **13**(5): 37–42.

18. Brink TL, Janakes C, Martinez N. Geriatric hypochondriasis, situational factors. *J Am Geriat Soc* 1981; **29**(1): 37–9.

19. Barsky AJ, Wyshak G, Klerman GL. Transient hypochondriasis. *Arch Gen Psychiat* 1990; **47**(8): 746–52.

20. Barsky AJ, Geringer E, Wool CA. A cognitive educational treatment for hypochondriasis. *Gen Hosp Psychiat* 1988; **10**: 322–7.

21. Brown HN, Vaillant GE. Hypochondriasis. *Arch Intern Med* 1981; **141**: 723–6.

106

Other Neurotic Disorders

Jerome J. Schulte and David Bienenfeld

Wright State University, School of Medicine, OH, USA

REACTION TO SEVERE STRESS, AND ADJUSTMENT DISORDERS

Before World War II it was generally held that psychiatric patients were constitutionally different from "normals". During World War II it was observed that previously asymptomatic individuals experiencing unusual environmental stress sometimes suffered from transient psychiatric difficulties. This observation led to a reclassification of psychiatric disorders to allow for behavioral and emotional symptoms in people who would return to their premorbid state with the removal of the unusual environmental precipitant[1]. DSM-I and ICD-6 classified these transient difficulties as "gross stress reaction" and "adult situational reaction"; DSM-II and ICD-8 classified them as "transient situational disturbances". ICD-9 introduced the categories of "acute reaction to stress" and "adjustment disorder". ICD-10 defines "acute stress reaction", "post-traumatic stress disorder" and "adjustment disorder"; although DSM-III-R recognized only the latter two of these, DSM-IV recognizes all three.

ACUTE STRESS REACTION

Clinical Features

According to ICD-10, acute stress reaction is a transient disturbance, occurring in persons without apparent mental disorder, in response to exceptional physical and/or mental stress and subsiding in hours or days. The diagnosis should not be made for an exacerbation of symptoms of a diagnosable psychiatric disorder already present, except for accentuation of personality traits. Previous history of another psychiatric disorder does not invalidate this diagnosis. An immediate, clear connection between the stressor and the onset of symptoms should be seen.

Symptoms of this disorder show a mixed and changing picture, with no one symptom predominating for long. They appear within minutes of the stress and resolve rapidly when the stressor is removed or, if the stress remains, symptoms decrease after 24–48 h and are minimal after 3 days.

Typical symptoms include an initial state of "daze", constriction of consciousness, narrowing of attention, decreased comprehension of stimuli and disorientation. Withdrawal, agitation or overactivity may follow. Autonomic signs of panic (tachycardia, sweating, flushing) are common. Amnesia for the traumatic present may also be present. In the elderly, organic factors and life stage events can be predisposing factors to acute stress reaction[2]. The multiple bereavements which are not uncommon in late life can be the precipitants for acute stress reaction.

DSM-IV differs somewhat from ICD-10 in its diagnostic classification of acute stress disorder. Unlike ICD-10, which requires that symptoms appear within minutes of the stress and diminish to minimal intensity after 3 days, DSM-IV requires symptoms to last a minimum of 2 days and allows for persistence up to 4 weeks. DSM-IV also includes dissociative symptoms not included under ICD-10: a subjective sense of numbing, detachment or absence of emotional responsiveness; derealization and depersonalization. Another DSM-IV requirement is that the traumatic event is persistently re-experienced in at least one of the following ways: recurrent images, thoughts, dreams, illusions, flashback episodes, or a sense of reliving the experience; or distress on exposure to reminders of the traumatic event. DSM-IV also requires marked avoidance of stimuli that arouse recollections of the trauma[3].

Differential Diagnosis

The differential diagnosis includes post-traumatic stress disorder (PTSD) and adjustment disorder. PTSD (see below) occurs after a latency period of weeks or longer, while the symptoms of acute stress reaction begin immediately after the traumatic event. The repetitive, intrusive imagery characteristic of PTSD is not usually a feature of the ICD-10 diagnosis of acute stress reaction. DSM-IV, however, does include repetitive intrusive imagery among the features of acute stress disorder. If psychotic symptoms follow an extreme stress, acute (brief) psychotic disorder should be considered. Adjustment disorders are less severe, and longer lasting, than acute stress reactions. Events that precipitate adjustment disorders are also less intense than those responsible for acute stress reactions.

Therapy

By definition, the symptoms of acute stress reaction are time-limited and will resolve without specific therapeutic intervention. Treatment may be requested, however, for intolerable tension or insomnia. For tension, short-term use of benzodiazepines with simple metabolic pathways and short half-lives, such as lorazepam or oxazepam, are safest in the elderly. For insomnia, temazepam or the non-benzodiazepine sedative hypnotic zolpiden[4] are justified. Families and patients may be reassured that the acute response does not indicate a psychotic decompensation, and that the prognosis for rapid recovery is favorable. Acutely, and in the aftermath of the traumatic event, it is useful to help the patient gain mastery over the trauma[5] by using a brief treatment model, consisting of fostering abreaction and integration of the event as quickly as possible, with the expectation that the trauma victim will return to full functioning. Abreaction can be fostered through individual or group psychotherapy[6].

POST-TRAUMATIC STRESS DISORDER

Post-traumatic stress disorder (PTSD) first appeared in DSM-III but was based on older concepts tied to the history of warfare. Da Costa wrote of "irritable heart" following the American Civil War. In World War I the disorder was known as "shell shock". Early twentieth century psychoanalytic theory called it "traumatic neurosis" and in World War II it was known as "traumatic war neurosis" or "combat neurosis". In DSM-I it was renamed "gross stress reaction", a reaction to great stress in a normal personality. During the peace time between World War II and Vietnam, the category was omitted from DSM-II[7]. ICD-9 defined catastrophic stress and combat fatigue as two diagnoses under the category of acute reaction to stress.

DSM-III defined intrusive re-experience of the trauma, together with emotional numbing, as the central features of PTSD. DSM-III-R placed more emphasis on the avoidance of stimuli associated with the trauma and less on numbing. DSM-IV changed the definition of the trauma to an event where a person experienced, witnessed or was confronted with threatened death or serious injury or threat to physical integrity of self or others. Here, the response to the trauma involves intense fear, helplessness or horror. Also, where DSM-III-R required either numbing or avoidance behavior, DSM-IV requires both[3].

ICD-10 criteria more closely resemble those of DSM-III, highlighting the restriction of emotional responsiveness. In ICD-10 the late chronic sequelae of devastating stress, i.e. those manifesting decades after the stressful experience, should be classified under enduring personality change after catastrophic experience[2].

Clinical Features

The ICD-10 diagnosis of PTSD requires evidence of trauma, or a response to a stressful event or situation of exceptionally threatening or catastrophic nature, likely to cause pervasive distress in anyone. The central symptoms are repetitive and intrusive recollections (flashbacks) or re-enactment of the event in memories, daytime imagery or dreams. The onset follows the trauma with a latency period of a few weeks to months (rarely exceeding 6 months). There may also be a sense of "numbness" and emotional blunting, and avoidance of activities and situations reminiscent of trauma.

Anxiety, depression, suicidal ideation and insomnia are also common in many PTSD patients, particularly with advancing age[7]. PTSD is also associated with alcohol and drug abuse, possibly reflecting attempts to cope with PTSD symptoms. Dissociative symptoms, commonly described in younger PTSD victims, become less prevalent with increasing age[8,9].

It remains a subject of debate what factors, if any, predispose individuals to the development of the post-traumatic stress syndrome. Some traumata, particularly the concentration camp experience, are so severe that symptoms are almost universal in survivors. Because retrospective assessment of function before the traumatic event is always colored by the response to the event, correlations are difficult to draw and empirical analyses have been inconclusive[10]. Certain personality traits (e.g. compulsive, asthenic) and a previous history of neurotic illness may possibly lower the threshold for manifestation of the disorder[2].

PTSD can also develop from bereavement. A recent study surveyed surviving spouses 2 months after their spouses' deaths;

10% of those whose spouses died after a chronic illness met criteria for PTSD; 9% of those whose spouses died unexpectedly met PTSD criteria; and 36% of those whose spouses died from "unnatural" causes (suicide or accident) had PTSD[11]. PTSD can also occur when patients have suffered the "trauma" of having a stroke (9.8%)[12] and upon learning that they have breast cancer (3%)[13].

Although PTSD symptoms can persist for many years, with increased frequency of symptoms towards the end of life[14], the typical course is one of fluctuating symptoms[15] in many cases. One study, examining current PTSD symptoms in elderly World War II and Korean War prisoners of war (POWs), suggested that severity of exposure to trauma and lack of post-military social support were moderately predictive of PTSD. In this study, 53% of POWs met criteria for lifetime PTSD, with 29% meeting criteria for current PTSD, but for those POWs most severely traumatized, the lifetime PTSD rates were 83%, with current PTSD at 59%[16].

There are two types of PTSD to which the elderly seem susceptible: delayed-onset PTSD and chronic PTSD. In delayed-onset PTSD, patients may exhibit signs of the disorder decades after the trauma, and in chronic PTSD symptoms have been persistent since the time of the trauma.

Delayed-onset PTSD is a reactivation of an old PTSD, with many years relatively free of symptoms, or the first onset of symptoms years after the trauma. In some elderly World War II veterans, media coverage commemorating the 50th anniversary of the end of the war triggered PTSD symptoms[17]. Commonly, guilt, distorted memory, emotional numbing, estrangement and feelings of detachment, are seen[18]. Patients in this group can present with physical symptoms of cardiovascular, gastrointestinal and musculoskeletal diseases[10]. Generally, the onset of severe symptoms can be linked to a profound recent life event, such as death of a wife, job retirement or loss of physical integrity from illness[18]. Most often, the contemporary precipitant reawakens emotions and perceptions from the original trauma. Holocaust survivors and prisoners of war have been noted to begin displaying symptoms of PTSD after admission to nursing homes, where they re-experience a loss of freedom and autonomy. World War II veterans found the loss of physical integrity due to somatic illness particularly upsetting, since it evoked memories of a traumatic period when their physical integrity was in jeopardy[9].

Differential Diagnosis

Although adjustment disorders also occur in response to life events, these events are in the normal range of human experience, unlike the extraordinary traumata responsible for PTSD. Specific features of numbing and flashbacks do not occur, and adjustment disorders, by definition, do not last more than 6 months. Acute stress reaction is characterized by a more variable clinical picture that resolves within days.

While anxiety and depression are common features of PTSD, generalized anxiety disorder and phobic disorder have anxiety as a more specific and central symptom. Major depression is marked by deep and persistent mood disturbance, usually with loss of reactivity; dysthymia results in chronic, indolent dysphoria. None of these disorders includes the specific symptom of intrusive recollections.

Therapy

The signs and symptoms of post-traumatic stress disorder include distorted expectations and perceptions, mood disturbances, psychophysiological symptoms and social withdrawal. Thus, common sense dictates, and empirical data confirm, that multi-modal treatment is most advisable. Psychosocial intervention and pharmacotherapy each has its place. At all ages, the psychotherapy of PTSD starts with the retelling of the story of the events before, during and after the traumatic episode. The goal is to integrate the experience with the person's life history; the method is to frame the events from the perspective of the intact self, rather than leave them relegated to the weakened self of the past. It is particularly important in older patients, given the chronological distance from the event, to differentiate objective properties of the trauma from the fantasy attributions it accumulates over time[19].

Group therapy has been found to be particularly useful. Matching patients by age and by setting of trauma enhances feelings of understanding and group identification[20]. The focus of the group is on recurring memories, and benefits patients by relieving long-held guilt through objective evaluation of the traumatic incident, as well as enhancing their ability to tolerate life stressors[18,21,22].

Antidepressants can offer symptomatic relief by diminishing dysphoria, intrusive thoughts, insomnia and nightmares. In particular, selective serotonin reuptake inhibitors (SSRIs) can be effective, especially in reducing avoidant symptoms[24,25]. β-Adrenergic blocking agents have been used in younger PTSD patients for relief of symptoms of autonomic arousal, tremors and startle reactions[26]. Older patients, however, are less likely to display a clinical profile of hyperarousal, and are more susceptible to the cardiovascular complications and organic mood disorders associated with adrenergic blockade. Benzodiazepines should be avoided as much as possible, since they can cause paradoxical excitation and frequently induce subtle cognitive impairment in aging individuals[27].

ADJUSTMENT DISORDER

The diagnosis of adjustment disorder refers to a state of subjective distress or emotional disturbance, interfering with social functioning or performance, arising in a period of adaptation to a significant life change or subsequent to a stressful life event. It is assumed that the condition would not have arisen without the stressor. In ICD-10, onset is usually within 1 month of the stressor; in DSM-IV, it can be within 3 months of the stressor. In both ICD-10 and DSM-IV, duration of symptoms does not exceed 6 months, except in the case where the stressor is chronic (e.g. a chronic general medical condition) or the stressor has enduring consequences (e.g. the financial and emotional difficulties resulting from a divorce)[3].

Clinical Features

Symptoms of adjustment disorder may include: depressed mood, anxiety, worry, impairment in performance of daily routines and inability to cope or plan ahead. Adjustment disorders can be specified as brief depressive reaction, prolonged depressive reaction, adjustment disorder with predominant disturbance of other emotions, adjustment disorder with predominant disturbance of conduct, or adjustment disorder with mixed disturbance of emotions and conduct.

The precipitating events for adjustment disorders can affect social network or values, and may involve the individual, his group or community. Common events causing such symptoms in older patients include physical illness or injury, placement in a nursing home and retirement. The events, while subjectively profoundly meaningful, are of considerably smaller magnitude than those precipitating acute stress reaction and PTSD. Individual predisposition and vulnerability to these stressful life

events thus plays a greater role in the occurrence of adjustment disorders. Poor pre-stressor social and coexisting physical problems[28], current dementia[29] and a history of a past psychiatric disorder[30] all increase vulnerability to adjustment disorders.

Therapy

The cornerstone of treatment for adjustment disorders is focal psychotherapy. Based on a psychodynamic understanding of emotions and behavior, focal therapy identifies the most specific nidus of current distress and views it in the context of the patient's core conflicts or deficits. The therapy is of relatively brief duration, usually 6–20 sessions. The major techniques employed are clarification and confrontation[31].

Quite frequently, the precipitating event can be framed as a narcissistic threat or injury. In psychotherapy, the patient will come to view the therapist as a self-object, looking for restoration of the self-esteem provided by the lost function, role or friend. The therapist helps restore the wholeness of self by allowing the patient to modify his/her expectations of him/herself and environment[32].

DISSOCIATIVE AND CONVERSION DISORDERS

In the last three decades of the nineteenth century, dissociation was studied extensively by Janet and conversion by Freud. DSM-I incorporated the concepts of dissociation and conversion into its classification scheme. Conversion reaction was assigned to hysterical neurosis, and amnesia was placed in the category of dissociative reaction. In DSM-II they were united under the heading of hysterical neurosis, but divided into conversion type and dissociative type. In DSM-III, DSM-III-R and DSM-IV the two conditions were renamed and separated once again. Hysteria, conversion type, became conversion disorder and was assigned to somatoform disorders. Hysteria, dissociative type, was expanded into the dissociative disorders[33]. ICD-10, however, continues to contain both under the heading of dissociative disorders.

DISSOCIATIVE AMNESIA

Dissociative amnesia is characterized by loss of memory, usually of important recent events, that is too great to be explained by ordinary forgetfulness or fatigue; and amnesia, either partial or complete, for recent events that are of a traumatic or stressful nature. The amnesia is usually partial and selective. The extent and completeness of the amnesia varies from day to day and between inquirers, but a persistent common core cannot be recalled in the waking state. Complete, generalized amnesia is rare and is usually part of a dissociative fugue. Affective states in amnesia are varied but severe depression is rare. Perplexity, distress and varying degrees of attention-seeking behavior may be evident, but calm acceptance is also sometimes striking. Purposeless local wandering may occur, but is rarely accompanied by self-neglect and rarely lasts more than a day or two. Often in dissociative amnesia, new learning is preserved[34]. Disturbing external circumstances causing despair or anxiety may predispose an individual, but a single event is usually at the center of the syndrome.

Dissociative amnesia is uncommonly reported in the elderly, but has been seen in World War I combat soldiers[35] and soldiers in other conflicts. In most patients the amnesia is short-lived, 75% of cases lasting between 24 h and 5 days[36]. Its features resemble those of more frequently observed disorders. Organic amnesia is usually anterograde[34]. In postconcussional syndromes there may be a combination of hysterical and organic amnesia that can be difficult to untangle. In dementia, memory loss is seen in the context of global cognitive impairment, which is stable over a period of weeks to months. The syndrome of pseudodementia also features variable memory impairment, but affective disturbance, usually severe depression, is evident[37].

DISSOCIATIVE FUGUE

Fugue exhibits all the features of dissociative amnesia, plus an apparently purposeful journey away from home or place of work during which self-care is maintained. A new identity is assumed and organized travel may be undertaken to places previously known and of possible emotional significance. Although there is retrograde amnesia during the fugue, behavior during fugue is normal.

A severe precipitating stress is almost universal as a precipitant of dissociative fugue. Times of marital discord, financial difficulty, major role change or personal loss may precede the fugue. Depressed mood is frequently present before fugue symptoms are displayed[34].

Fugue is rare in elderly people. Because its features, with the exception of travel, are identical to those of dissociative amnesia, it has been proposed that the two disorders be considered as one.

Treatment

Therapy for dissociative amnesia and dissociative fugue is virtually identical. Patients usually seek treatment after the amnestic period has ended. They desire help in recovering memory of events during the fugue. Hypnosis and short-acting barbiturates have been used to reconstitute repressed memories, although typically they return spontaneously. Psychodynamic psychotherapy has been used to facilitate resolution of conflicts that lead to fugue states. This treatment may decrease the vulnerability of the patient to dissociate in future times of stress[38].

DISSOCIATIVE DISORDERS OF MOVEMENT AND SENSATION (CONVERSION DISORDERS)

In conversion disorder, there is a loss or alteration in movements or sensations (usually cutaneous) in a patient presenting as having a physical disorder. No somatic condition can be found, however, that explains the symptoms. Instead, the symptoms represent the patient's concept of the physical disorder, which may be at variance with physiological or anatomical principles. Here, mental state and social situation suggest that disability resulting from the loss of function is helping the patient to escape an unpleasant conflict, or helps the patient to express dependency or resentment indirectly. Conflicts may be evident to others, but the patient often denies their presence and attributes distress to the physical symptoms or the resulting disability.

In making the diagnosis it is essential that: (a) evidence of a physical disorder is absent; and (b) sufficient knowledge of the psychological and social setting and personal relationships of the patient allows a convincing formulation of the reasons for the disorder.

Predisposing factors to conversion disorder are premorbid abnormalities of personal relationships and personality. Also, close relatives or friends may have suffered from physical illness with symptoms resembling the patient's. A few patients establish a repetitive pattern of reaction to stress by production of these disorders, which can continue into middle and old age[2].

The most important differential diagnosis is the group of somatoform disorders (although DSM-IV classifies conversion disorder as a somatoform disorder instead of a dissociative disorder). In the latter, the patient's presentation centers around persistent requests for medical attention and pervasive concern with the perceived medical disorder; patients with conversion disorder are much more likely to take their presumed illnesses in stride. Conversion disorders generally begin in adolescence and young adulthood, and occur in single or recurrent episodes with substantial remission. Somatoform disorders may not increase in prevalence with increasing age, but they tend to assume the quality of a pervasive character style with little remission.

Most conversion disorders remit with non-specific, supportive interventions. Hypnosis, anxiolytics and behavioral relaxation exercises may be helpful. Also, psychotherapy aimed at helping the patient recognize and cope with the psychosocial stress that provoked the symptom can be impressively beneficial if the patient can be engaged in a cooperative alliance of therapeutic curiosity.

The prognosis of conversion disorder is generally good, since conversion symptoms are of short duration with abrupt onset and resolution. A few become chronic, and some recur, most commonly when the precipitating stress is chronic or recurrent, when there is other psychopathology or when there is marked secondary gain.

NEURASTHENIA (FATIGUE SYNDROME)

Historical Perspective

George Beard introduced the term 'neurasthenia' in 1869. He viewed neurasthenia as a physical illness due to loss of nerve strength. Janet differentiated psychasthenia from neurasthenia. Freud similarly separated anxiety neurosis, a "psychoneurosis", from neurasthenia, an "actual neurosis" he attributed to misdirected libidinal energy.

In World War I, the syndrome was defined by the term "shell-shock"; in World War II, "operational fatigue". Although it remains in ICD-10, the diagnosis of neurasthenia was deleted from DSM-III and replaced by dysthymia. In the USA the symptom cluster known as chronic fatigue syndrome is almost identical to the current ICD classification of neurasthenia[39-41].

Clinical Features

Neurasthenia is characterized by persistent, distressing complaints of fatigue after mental effort, or complaints of bodily weakness and exhaustion after minimal physical effort, along with at least two of the following: muscular aches and pains, dizziness, tension headaches, sleep disturbance, inability to relax, irritability or dyspepsia. If autonomic or depressive symptoms are present, they cannot be sufficiently persistent and severe to fulfill the criteria for any more specific disorder[2].

Differential Diagnosis

Differential diagnosis includes primarily major depression and somatoform disorders. In the elderly it is especially important to rule out depression, since somatic complaints and fatigue are common presentations of depressive disorders in late life. Physical symptoms with no demonstrable organic pathology are the essential features of somatoform disorders. However, these complaints do not include the specific physical symptoms of fatigue or exhaustion found in neurasthenia.

Therapy

Specific treatment for neurasthenia has not been established. Given the high likelihood, particularly in old age, that the neurasthenic picture is a manifestation of a mood disorder, treatment with antidepressant medication and psychotherapy, as for depressive conditions, is generally warranted.

REFERENCES

1. Ginsberg GL. Adjustment and impulse control disorders. In Kaplan HI, Sadock BJ, eds, *Comprehensive Textbook of Psychiatry*, vol. IV. Baltimore, MD: Williams and Wilkins, 1985; 1097–105.
2. World Health Organization. Mental and behavioural disorders. *Tenth Revision of the International Classification of Diseases and Related Health Problems* (ICD-10), chapter V. Geneva: World Health Organization, 1992.
3. American Psychiatric Association. *Diagnostic and Statistical Manual of Mental Disorders*, 4th edn (DSM-IV). Washington, DC: APA, 1994.
4. Stoudemire A. Epidemiology and psychopharmacology of anxiety in medical patients. *J Clin Psychiat* 1996; **57**(suppl 7): 64–72.
5. Pasnau RO, Fawzy FI. Stress and psychiatry. In Kaplan HI, Sadock BJ, eds, *Comprehensive Textbook of Psychiatry*, vol. V. Baltimore, MD: Williams and Wilkins, 1989; 1231–9.
6. Davidson JR. Post-traumatic stress disorder and acute stress disorder. In Kaplan HI, Sadock BJ, eds, *Comprehensive Textbook of Psychiatry*, vol. VI. Baltimore, MD: Williams and Wilkins, 1995; 1227–36.
7. McCartney JR, Severson K. Sexual violence, post-traumatic stress disorder and dementia. *J Am Geriat Soc* 1997; **45**: 76–8.
8. Davidson J, Kudler H. Symptom and comorbidity patterns in World War II and Vietnam veterans with posttraumatic stress disorder. *J Comp Psychiat* 1990; **3**(2): 162–70.
9. Lipton M, Schaffer W. Physical symptoms related to post-traumatic stress disorder in an aging population. *Military Med* 1988; **156**: 316.
10. Kinzie DJ. Post-traumatic stress disorder. In Kaplan HI, Sadock BJ, eds, *Comprehensive Textbook of Psychiatry*, vol. V. Baltimore, MD: Williams and Wilkins, 1989; 1000–8.
11. Zisook S, Chentsova-Dutton Y, Shuchter SR. PTSD following bereavement. *Ann Clin Psychiat* 1998; **10**(4): 157–63.
12. Sembi S, Tarrier N, O'Neill P *et al.* Does post-traumatic stress disorder occur after stroke: a preliminary study. *Int J Geriat Psychiat* 1988; **13**: 315–22.
13. Green BL, Rowland JH, Krupnick JL *et al.* Prevalence of posttraumatic stress disorder in women with breast cancer. *Psychosomatics* 1998; **39**: 102–11.
14. Hamilton JD, Workman RH. Persistence of combat-related posttraumatic stress symptoms for 75 years. *J Traum Stress* 1998; **11**(4): 763–8.
15. Tennant C, Fairley MJ, Dent OF *et al.* Declining prevalence of psychiatric disorder in older former prisoners of war. *J Nerv Ment Dis* 1997; **185**: 686–9.
16. Engdahl B, Dikel TN, Eberly R, Blank A. Posttraumatic stress disorder in a community group of former prisoners of war: a normative response to severe trauma. *Am J Psychiat* 1997; **154**: 1576–81.
17. Hilton C. Media triggers of post-traumatic stress disorder 50 years after the Second World War. *Int J Geriat Psychiat* 1997; **12**: 862–7.
18. Lipton M, Schaffer W. Post-traumatic stress disorder in the older veteran. *Military Med* 1986; **151**: 522–4.
19. Horowitz MJ. Posttraumatic stress disorder. In Karasu TB, ed., *Treatment of Psychiatric Disorders*. Washington, DC: American Psychiatric Association, 1989; 2065–83.
20. Fried H, Waxman H. Stockholm's Cafe 84: a unique day program for Jewish survivors of concentration camps. *Gerontologist* 1988; **28**: 253–5.
21. Snell FI, Padin-Rivera E. Group treatment for older veterans with post-traumatic stress disorder. *J Psychosoc Nurs* 1997; **35**(2): 10–16.
22. Muller U, Barash-Kishon R. Psychodynamic-supportive group therapy model for elderly holocaust survivors. *Int J Group Psychother* 1998; **48**(4): 461–75.
23. Falcon S, Ryan C, Chamberlain K *et al.* Tricyclics: possible treatment for post-traumatic stress disorder. *J Clin Psychiat* 1985; **46**: 385–8.
24. Sadavoy J. Survivors: a review of the late-life effects of prior psychological trauma. *Am J Geriat Psychiat* 1997; **5**(4): 287–301.
25. Davidson J, Roth S, Neewman E. Treatment of post-traumatic stress disorder with fluoxetine. *J Traum Stress* 1991; **4**: 419–23.
26. Van der Kolk BA. Psychopharmacologic issues in posttraumatic stress disorder. *Hosp Commun Psychiat* 1983; **34**: 683–91.
27. Salzman C. Principles of psychopharmacology. In Bienenfeld D, ed., *Verwoerdt's Clinical Geropsychiatry*, 3rd edn. Baltimore, MD: Williams and Wilkins, 1990; 234–49.
28. Lazaro L, Marcos T, Valdes M. Affective disorders, social support, and health status in geriatric patients in a general hospital. *Gen Hosp Psychiat* 1995; **17**: 299–304.
29. Orrell M, Bebbington P. Life events and senile dementia: affective symptoms. *Br J Psychiat* 1995; **166**: 613–20.
30. Oxman TE, Barrett JE, Freeman DH, Manheimer E. Frequency and correlates of adjustment disorder related to cardiac surgery in older patients. *Psychosomatics* 1994; **35**: 557–68.
31. Wheeler BG, Bienenfeld D. Principles of individual psychotherapy. In Bienenfeld D, ed., *Verwoerdt's Clinical Geropsychiatry*, 3rd edn. Baltimore, MD: Williams and Wilkins, 1990; 204–22.
32. Lazarus LW. Self-psychology: its application to brief psychotherapy with the elderly. *J Geriat Psychiat* 1988; **21**: 109–25.
33. Nemiah JC. Dissociative disorders. In Kaplan HI, Sadock BJ, eds, *Comprehensive Textbook of Psychiatry*, vol. IV. Baltimore, MD: Williams and Wilkins, 1985; 942–57.
34. Kopelman MD. Amnesia: organic and psychogenic. *Br J Psychiat* 1987; **150**: 428–42.
35. Van der Hart O, Brown P, Graafland M. Trauma-induced dissociative amnesia in World War I combat soldiers. *Aust NZ J Psychiat* 1999; **33**: 37–46.
36. Coons PM. The dissociative disorders: rarely considered and underdiagnosed. *Psychiat Clin N Am* 1998; **21**(3): 637–48.
37. Wells CE. Pseudodementia. *Am J Psychiat* 1979; **136**: 895–900.
38. Reither AM, Stoudemire A. Psychogenic fugue states: a review. *South Med J* 1988; **81**: 568–71.
39. Greenberg DB. Neurasthenia in the 1980s. *Psychosomatics* 1990; **31**: 129–37.
40. Fukuda K, Straus SE, Hickie I *et al.* The chronic fatigue syndrome: comprehensive approach to its definition and study. *Ann Intern Med* 1994; **121**: 953–9.
41. Demitrack MA. Chronic fatigue syndrome and fibromyalgia: dilemmas in diagnosis and clinical management. *Psychiat Clin N Am* 1998; **21**(3): 671–92.

Part I

Personality Disorders

Personality Disorders: Aetiology and Genetics

Victor Molinari[1], Tom Siebert[2] and Marvin Swartz[2]

[1]*VAMC Psychology Service, Houston, TX, USA,* [2]*Duke University Medical Center, Durham, NC, USA*

According to DSM-IV[1], "A Personality Disorder is an enduring pattern of inner experience and behavior that deviates markedly from the expectations of the individual's culture, is pervasive and inflexible, has an onset in adolescence or early adulthood, is stable over time, and leads to distress or impairment" (p. 629). Since the first edition of this chapter was published, there has been an ever-expanding body of knowledge about personality disorder (PD) in older adults. Notably, there has even been the publication of the first book[2] solely devoted to PD in older adults. However, as we shall see, there remain many unanswered questions spawned by thorny conceptual and methodological quandaries in this controversial area.

PD in older adults is an important area of study for a number of reasons. First, since PD affects the way an older adult copes with life, individuals with specific PDs may be less able to successfully negotiate age-related losses (e.g. obsessive–compulsive, dependent) or the interpersonal compromises necessary for peaceful institutional living (e.g. borderline, narcissistic). Second, PD can influence the presentation of Axis I symptomatology, frequently generating complicated assessment dilemmas. For example, disruptive behavior in the nursing home may camouflage the fact that the person is suffering from a depression that is exacerbating premorbid antisocial personality features. Third, just as for young adults, the presence of PD should modify treatment strategies and prognosis of co-morbid Axis I disorders in certain geriatric settings.

This chapter will summarize what is known about the etiology, genetics, epidemiology, assessment, prognosis and research implications of PD in older adults.

AETIOLOGY AND GENETICS

Reviewing PD necessitates some understanding of the complexity of the terms "personality disorder" and "personality", as well as their classification. Personality can be conceived as two interactive elements, representing "nature" and "nurture": temperament, a reflection of a genetically determined, constitutional disposition; and character, made up of learned attributes, which begin coalescing in early childhood, reflecting culture, norms and upbringing. Studies have focused on each of these elements in order to clarify the etiology of personality and PD, but these investigative efforts have been rendered more complicated by different measurement approaches.

Concerning PD among the elderly, it is helpful to focus on dimensional aspects of personality as well as the categorical diagnosis of PD. Because of the numerous biological changes that occur with aging, a major question for the geriatric clinician concerns the stability of personality traits throughout the aging process.

Most researchers agree that there is no uniform, stereotypic change in personality traits in late life. Cross-sectional and longitudinal investigations of personality across the life cycle[3] report the general stability of individuals' major traits. However, it is also clear that certain adults do change for the better or worse[4], perhaps due to some of the unique challenges they face over the lifespan.

Late-life theorists have made important contributions to conceptualizing those challenges that promote personality development. Erikson's[5] crisis of "integrity vs. despair" marks the culmination of his psychosocial framework. The challenge of this final stage is the individual's acceptance of the integrity of his/her self; failure results in a fear of death and an inability to find meaning in the life cycle. Erikson felt that the successful resolution of this stage depends on an adequate resolution of previous crises. From the point of view of personality, failure here may also trigger global dissatisfaction and lowered self-esteem. Erikson's developmental stages, intended for a practitioner audience, were not rigorously defined and were based on clinical and theoretical considerations rather than research data.

Levinson *et al.*'s[6] developmental scheme is based on their research on the life cycle. They view development as a series of eras and cross-era transitions. Older adults are seen from the point of view of the late adult transition and late adulthood. The late adult transition (age 60–65) is marked by major changes in role structure, physiology and intrapsychic challenges. It is possible that adaptation to these challenges provokes changes in personality structure (i.e. a decrease in authoritarianism; locus of satisfaction shifting from the self to others). Haan and Day[7] traced the relative prominence of different personal dimensions (such as information processing, inter-personal reaction, manner of self-presentation and responses to socialization) throughout the life cycle from adolescence onwards. Although most dimensions were stable, some changed in an orderly manner with age. Still others changed in a stage-wise manner. The authors believed that their results fitted an Eriksonian developmental model with an essential "sameness" of major personality functions, punctuated by times of regress before progress and longer periods of orderly change.

The investigation of constitutional factors that contribute to PD is affected by a number of methodological difficulties. Few studies have looked specifically at DSM Axis II criteria; many have looked at other variables, such as neuroticism and sociability, which cannot be compared well with PD as defined by DSM.

The most intensive studies of familial factors have been conducted on those with antisocial PD. Crowe[8] summarized data from twin studies in strong support of a heritable component

Principles and Practice of Geriatric Psychiatry, 2nd edn. Edited by J. R. M. Copeland, M. T. Abou-Saleh and D. G. Blazer

for antisocial PD. The mean concordance rate for monozygotic twins for the disorder was double that of dizygotic twins (68% vs. 33%). Adoption studies[9,10] have also found "temperamental" factors to be a major determinant for antisocial PD. Family studies find increased rates of substance abuse, antisocial PD and other psychopathology in first-degree relatives of felons, many with the diagnosis of antisocial PD[11].

Schizotypal PD has been well examined from a genetic perspective and owes much of its appearance as a diagnosis to that association. Schizotypal PD has a significant heritable relationship to schizophrenia. Kendler et al.[12] were unable to find an equivalent environmental association. Torgersen[13] confirmed the genetic link between schizoid and paranoid features of schizophrenia and schizotypal PD.

The final disorder that has yielded studies on heritability is borderline PD. A credible familial association has been found between borderline PD, affective disorders and other PD[14]. Previous associations between "borderline states" and the schizophrenic spectrum have been difficult to interpret because of differing definitions of "borderline states" and the relationships of these definitions to current DSM-IV criteria for borderline PD. Individuals with a history of impulsive or affective instability, which more closely fit present borderline PD criteria, may not have a greater prevalence of schizophrenia in their relatives[14].

In summary, there is clear evidence of heritability for some PD but much that remains unexamined. As Clarkin, Speilman and Klausner[15] note in their conceptual overview of PD in the elderly, the research on the relationship of genetic factors to PD is sparse, and speculations concerning the neurobiology of PD remains premature. The remaining "nurture" factors also comprise a significant component, but have yet to be clarified.

Neurobiological studies have been very rare. EEG slow-wave activity has been associated with antisocial PD. Borderline patients have a significantly higher percentage of marginal EEG abnormalities than controls[16]. They also show changes in cerebrospinal 5-hydroxyindole-acetic acid (5-HIAA), a measure of serotonin activity that is correlated negatively with measures of aggressivity. Finally, schizotypal and borderline PD have been linked with low platelet monoamine oxidase (MAO) activity[17,18]. Individuals with schizotypal PD may also show impaired smooth pursuit eye movement.[19,20].

ASSESSMENT

Assessment of PD requires an examination of variables that may be difficult to measure, especially in older adults. There are, for instance, problems in obtaining a reliable diagnosis. Since all the standardized instruments used to measure PD have been developed for a younger population, these devices thereby require more administration time for older adults (since they have longer personal histories). Consequently, there is no "gold standard" of diagnosis for PD in older adults. Molinari et al.[21] studied geropsychiatric inpatients with depression, and found general discordance between patient self-report, family informant ratings, social worker evaluations, and consensus case conference categorical diagnosis of PD. It appears that there are varied perceptions of an individual's personality, all of which should be taken into account for a comprehensive evaluation of Axis II pathology.

From a clinical perspective, PD is quite common in medical practice, yet infrequently recognized. Mental health professionals are loathe to diagnose PD, particularly in old age, due to concerns over pejorative bias, pessimistic belief in Axis II changes, managed care reimbursement biases, and focus on medical or Axis I pathology (particularly cognitive impairment) in old age. Often the PD patient presents with unrealistic expectations,

complaints and demands, and an inappropriate interpersonal stance. Essential features of PD, regardless of age, will include: maladaptive behavior as a lifestyle; inflexibility in managing interpersonal situations; multiple physical, social and interpersonal problems; and externalization of these problems in the absence of psychosis[22]. Yet these same features are sometimes accepted, erroneously, as part of the aging process. In a geriatric setting, somatic presentations of PD are common, which can complicate "teasing out" true co-morbid medical/cognitive problems from personality dysfunction. Patients with PD frequently present with chief complaints of "bad nerves", sleeplessness, non-specific requests for help and pain syndromes. In addition, Axis I disorders can confound appropriate diagnosis and confuse the long-term picture. For example, evidence suggests that older depressives are significantly more likely to have lifetime personality dysfunction than controls[23,24]. Therefore, it behooves the clinician to ascertain whether a pattern of historically maladaptive personality traits exist in the older patient with depression. Treatment of the depression may very well result in a symptom picture reflecting a baseline PD, rather than a depression in partial remission.

EPIDEMIOLOGY

Some early anecdotal reports suggested that personality characteristics become uniformly less harsh with age[25,26]. Other clinicians working with older adults believed that the "high-energy" PDs (e.g. Cluster B) mellow, while the "low-energy" PDs (e.g. Cluster C) may be aggravated by the aging process[27-29]. DSM-IV[1] states that, "Some PDs tend to become less obvious or remit with age, whereas this appears to be less true for some other types" (p. 632). This statement underscores some of the more recent empirical work in this area, and contrasts with the more benign general appraisals of DSM-III[30] and DSM-III-R[31], which merely note that PD becomes "less obvious" with age. Early research yielded wide variability in PD prevalence rates due to inadequate definitions of PD, non-standardized measures, and different samples of older adults. With the introduction of DSM-III and the development of instruments tied to DSM-III criteria, some consistent findings have emerged. This section on epidemiology will therefore largely focus on studies using standardized measures, and will be divided into community, institutional, outpatient and depression studies.

Community Settings

In community settings, two studies[26,32] compared young and older adults utilizing the Coolidge Axis II Inventory. Coolidge et al.[26], found a greater need for organization and more restricted affect in older adults, while Segal et al.[32] found that older adults were significantly higher on obsessive–compulsive and schizoid PD, but lower on the antisocial, borderline, histrionic, narcissistic and paranoid scales. Ames and Molinari[33] used the Structured Interview for Disorders of Personality scale (SIDP-R) and detected a trend of less PD in older adults, with significantly fewer older adults meeting the criteria for more than one PD. Cohen et al.[34] used the Structured Psychiatric Examination and found that those over the age of 55 were less likely (6.6% vs. 10.5%) to have PD, due to a three-fold decrease of Cluster B PD in older adults. These data documenting personality "mellowing" in older adult community samples are in stark contrast to the results of a more recent study by Segal et al.[35], who found that a high number (63%) of very old ($X = 76.2$ years) community-dwelling adults met PD criteria by self-report. However, this study was potentially flawed by failure to take into account the cognitive and sensory status of this aged sample, many of whom may have misunderstood the questions or exhibited executive deficit-related personality alterations.

Institutional Settings

Early PD prevalence rates in nursing home settings were reported to be 12–15%[36,37], while for geropsychiatric inpatients, PD estimates were more variable (7–55%). In a large sample of hospitalized male veterans, Molinari et al.[38] conducted a cross-sectional investigation of personality changes across different age groups for those clinically diagnosed with PD. Older adults with PD were more responsible and less impulsive, paranoid, energetic and antisocial than young adults diagnosed with PD. Kunik et al.[39] studied 547 older psychiatric inpatients, and found that a consensus case conference diagnosis of PD varied widely, depending upon the specific co-morbid Axis I diagnosis (e.g. 6% for patients with an organic mental disorder, but 24% for those with depression). Only two studies of geropsychiatric institutionalized patients utilized standardized instruments. Molinari et al.[40] used the SIDP-R and found that older adults had PD rates similar to those of a young adult comparison sample; however, older adults were less likely to meet criteria for more than one PD, and clinical diagnoses yielded fewer PDs than the SIDP-R. Likewise, Coolidge et al.[41] used the Coolidge Axis II Inventory and found similarly high PD rates among young (66%) and old (58%) chronically mentally ill patients, but the younger group was more likely to be specifically diagnosed with antisocial, borderline, and schizotypal PD.

Outpatient Settings

The findings from the lone study conducted with a structured PD scale in a geropsychiatric outpatient setting are consistent with the latter inpatient studies. Molinari and Marmion[42] found that older adults were less likely to meet the criteria for more than one PD than younger adults, and clinical diagnosis again yielded fewer PDs than the SIDP-R.

Depression

One area of intense study has been the relationship between PD and depression in older adults. Kunik et al.[24] studied 154 depressed older inpatients and identified 24% with co-morbid PD, while Molinari and Marmion[43] determined that 63% of depressed geropsychiatric outpatients met PD criteria. Thompson et al.[44] found that 33% of depressed older adults who were being treated with psychotherapy in a geropsychiatric outpatient clinic met DSM-III PD criteria. In a study investigating the relationship between PD and functioning in acutely depressed older psychiatric patients, Axis II pathology was found to be associated with greater disability and more impaired social and interpersonal functioning[45]. In their review of the literature on PD in older adults, Agronin and Maletta[46] posit that PD in late life may be intrinsically related to Axis I pathology, particularly major depressive disorder.

Summary of Epidemiological Studies

In an attempt to lend clarity to the burgeoning literature on PD in older adults, Abrams and Horowitz[47] conducted a meta-analysis of the most methodologically sophisticated epidemiological studies. They inferred a PD prevalence rate of 10% (with a range of 6–33%) for those over the age of 50, and concluded that, "at this time the literature neither supports nor contradicts previous suggestions of an age effect". However, these authors remark that the bulk of the evidence supports, at least for certain PDs, a decline in frequency and intensity with age. The cause for this decline is one of the most controversial and debated topics in the literature on PD in older adults. Four main reasons have been postulated.

First, there is a general mellowing of the "high-energy" Cluster B PDs due to biological (reduced testosterone in males) and developmental changes (those with PD finally master a single interpersonal strategy to manage stresses). This accounts for the consistent result that older adults are less likely to meet the criteria for more than one PD, and is also supported by the recent study of Segal et al.[32], who discovered lower levels of dysfunctional coping styles in older adults.

Second, the decline in "high-energy" PD relates to the greater mortality rates of those with Cluster B PD in their younger years. Older adults with PD are thereby a selective sample of less extreme PD "survivors". Third, PD is generally underdiagnosed, particularly in older adults, where cognitive and medical causes are emphasized or personality disturbance (avoidance, dependency, lability) is viewed as normal[48].

Fourth, the decline in PD with age is a methodological artifact, since some DSM criteria are age-insensitive. For example, occupational and vocational impairment are often irrelevant to older adults. From this point of view, there really is no true decline in PD rates with age, just a change in form that is inadequately assessed. These so-called "geriatric variants"[49] reflect the more subclinical, non-specific or age-relevant PD traits that account for PD NOS (not otherwise specified) to be diagnosed with particular high frequency in older adults. The construction of a new geriatric nosology has been proposed to accommodate the late life changes in Axis II pathology[46,47,49]. Such re-classification will need to: (a) reconsider the diagnostic requirement that maladaptive PD behavior be rooted so early in young adulthood; (b) routinely address Axis II pathology in the context of more acute Axis I symptomatology; and (c) integrate age-related developmental, medical (Axis III) and psychosocial/environmental stressors (Axis IV) with Axis II manifestations[46].

PROGNOSIS

Unfortunately, only a few seemingly contradictory studies have investigated the prognosis of PD in late life. In two separate studies of geropsychiatric outpatients, PD was found to be a poor prognostic sign for the psychotherapeutic treatment of depression[44,50]. However, Molinari[51] examined the 1 year relapse rates for 100 male geropsychiatric inpatients and found no significant differences for those diagnosed with and without PD. Consistent with Kunik et al.'s[24] finding that PD diagnosis had no impact on the acute response of inpatient treatment for depression with older adults, no differences were found in relapse rates for a subgroup of depressed inpatients with and without PD[51]. It appears that in inpatient geropsychiatric settings, Axis I symptomatology overrides Axis II pathology as an outcome predictor, probably related to the complex combination of medical, cognitive and psychiatric symptoms often observed in those older patients needing acute care.

RESEARCH IMPLICATIONS

Base rates mandating prohibitively large sample sizes render it difficult to make valid statements concerning age-related changes for most individual PDs. To expand our current inadequate knowledge base, research should concentrate on PD clusters and PD with older adults must be conducted using reliable scales tied to DSM-IV criteria across varied settings (e.g. medical, nursing home, psychiatric inpatient, psychiatric outpatient) populations (e.g. old-old, females, multicultural) and methodologies (e.g. longitudinal, cross-sectional). The inclusion of age-graded criteria for Axis II and perhaps also Axis I should be investigated. At the very least, since all the PD scales currently in use have been developed for younger adults and have yielded generally modest reliability ratings for most PD categories, validity studies must be conducted specifically with older adults[48]. Such studies must take into account the effect of cognitive status and medical problems on the responses of older adults. In this way, research concerning the psychological/developmental history of individuals with PD will generate valuable prognostic and treatment data. Research should also explore those PD features underlying late onset Axis I disorders. Hopefully, more sophisticated methodologies will probe the relative and combined merits of pharmacotherapy and different types/modes of psychotherapy (e.g. cognitive–behavioral vs. interpersonal; group vs. individual). Heuristic models of the interrelationship between the underlying neuropsychiatric and biological substrate of temperament, genetic factors and psychosocial changes in personality with aging must be generated. Finally, the ethical and clinical issues involved in the management of "difficult personality-disordered" patients in hospital, rehabilitation and nursing home sites should be explored, so that the needs of individuals can be balanced with those of families, staff and patient/resident peers[52–54].

SUMMARY

Over the last decade, there has been an increasing amount of research on PD in older adults using structured scales tied to DSM criteria. Major findings are:

1. Although still common in older adults, Cluster B pathology is less prevalent than in the young adult population; Cluster C pathology may be relatively more prominent in older adults.
2. Older adults are less likely to receive more than one PD diagnosis, suggesting that they may finally develop one main coping strategy to fulfill their interpersonal needs.
3. There may be an age-related mellowing of the "high-energy" personality characteristic of individuals with PD, and/or there are "geriatric variants" of PD not tapped by DSM.
4. There is a positive association between depression and PD diagnosis.
5. PD in older adults is prognostically useful in outpatient settings, where the Axis I symptomatology is less severe.
6. There are poor concordance rates of PD diagnosis between clinical examination, structured interviews and self-reports, suggesting the need for data collection from a variety of sources.

Although age-related changes in PD expression are probably in the less volatile and impulsive direction, novel PD manifestations can still create a significant burden in stressful caregiving contexts for family members, friends, healthcare professionals and administrators of institutions attempting to support a flawed but vulnerable older adult. Future research guided by conceptual advances promises to yield exciting progress in assessment and treatment.

ACKNOWLEDGEMENT

The author acknowledges the thoughtful review of a draft of this chapter by Dr Dan Segal.

REFERENCES

1. American Psychiatric Association. *Diagnostic and Statistical Manual of Mental Disorders*, 4th edn. Washington, DC: APA, 1994.
2. Rosowsky E, Abrams L, Zweig R, eds, *Personality Disorders in Older Adults: Emerging Issues in Diagnosis and Treatment*. Mahwah, NJ: Erlbaum, 1999.
3. Costa PT, McCrae RR. Stability and change in personality from adolescence through adulthood. In Halverson CF, Kohnstamm GA, Martin RP, eds, *The Developing Structure of Temperament and Personality from Infancy to Adulthood*. Hillsdale, NJ: Erlbaum, 1994; 139–50.
4. Vaillant G. *Adaptation to Life*. Boston, MA: Little, Brown, 1977.
5. Erikson EH. *The Life Cycle*. International Encyclopedia of the Social Sciences. New York: Macmillan, 1968.
6. Levinson DJ, Darrow CN, Klein EB *et al. The Seasons of a Man's Life*. New York: Alfred A. Knopf, 1978.
7. Haan H, Day D. A longitudinal study of change and sameness in personality development: adolescence to later adulthood. *Int J Aging Hum Dev* 1974; **5**: 1–39.
8. Crowe R. Antisocial personality disorder. In Tarter R, ed., *The Child at Psychiatric Risk*. New York: Oxford University Press, 1983.
9. Crowe R. An adoption study of antisocial personality. *Arch Gen Psychiat* 1974; **31**: 785–91.
10. Cadoret R, Cain C. Sex differences in the predictors of antisocial behavior in adoptees. *Arch Gen Psychiat* 1980; **137**: 1171–5.
11. Guze S. *Criminality and Psychiatric Disorders*. New York: Oxford University Press 1976.
12. Kendler KS, Gruenberg AM, Strauss JS. An independent analysis of the Copenhagen sample of the Danish Adoption Study. *Arch Gen Psychiat* 1981; **38**: 982–4.
13. Torgersen S. Genetic and nosological aspects of schizotypal and borderline personality disorders. *Arch Gen Psychiat* 1984; **41**: 546–54.
14. Siever LJ. Genetic factors in borderline personalities. In Grinspoon L, ed., *Psychiatry Update: The American Psychiatric Association Annual Review*, vol. 1. Washington, DC: APA, 1982.
15. Clarkin JF, Spielman LA, Klausner E. Conceptual overview of personality disorders in the elderly. In Rosowsky E, Abrams L, Zweig R, eds, *Personality Disorders in Older Adults: Emerging Issues in Diagnosis and Treatment*. Mahwah, NJ: Erlbaum, 1999; 3–15.
16. Cowdry RW, Pickar D, Davies R. Limbic dysfunction in the borderline syndrome. New Research Abstracts No. NR32. Presented at the 133rd Annual Meeting of the American Psychiatric Association, San Francisco, CA, 1980.
17. Baron M, Levitt M, Perlman R. Low platelet monoamine oxidase activity: a possible biochemical correlate of borderline schizophrenia. *Psychiat Res* 1980; **3**: 329–35.
18. Davidson JRT, McLeod MN, Turnbull CD *et al.* Platelet monoamine oxidase activity and the classification of depression. *Arch Gen Psychiat* 1980; **37**: 771–3.
19. Holzman PS, Proctor LR, Levy DL. Eye tracking dysfunctions in schizophrenic patients and their relatives. *Arch Gen Psychiat* 1974; **31**: 143–51.
20. Holzman PS, Kringler E, Levy DL, Haberman SJ. Deviant eye tracking in twins discordant for psychosis. *Arch Gen Psychiat* 1980; **37**: 627–31.
21. Molinari V, Kunik M, Mulsant B, Rifai H. The relationship between patient, informant, social worker, and consensus diagnoses of personality disorders in elderly depressed inpatients. *Am J Geriat Psychiat* 1998; **6**(2): 136–44.
22. Mahorney S. Personality disorders. In Walker JL, ed., *Essentials of Clinical Psychiatry*. Philadelphia, PA: J. B. Lippincott, 1985; 209–26.
23. Abrams RC, Alexopoulos GS, Young RC. Geriatric depression and DSM-III-R personality disorder criteria. *J Am Geriat Soc* 1987; **35**: 383–6.
24. Kunik ME, Mulsant BH, Rifai AH *et al.* Personality disorders in elderly inpatients with major depression. *Am J Geriat Psychiat* 1993; **1**: 38–45.
25. Hyer L, Harrison W. Late life personality model: diagnosis and treatment. In Brink TL, ed., *Clinical Gerontology: A Guide to Assessment and Treatment*. New York: Haworth, 1986; 399–415.
26. Coolidge FL, Burns EM, Nathan JH, Mull CE. Personality disorders in the elderly. *Clin Gerontol* 1992; **12**: 41–55.

27. Verwoerdt A. *Clinical Geropsychiatry*. Baltimore, MD: Williams & Wilkins, 1976; 85–8.

28. Sadavoy J, Fogel B. Personality disorders in old age. In Birren J, Sloane RB, Cohen G, eds, *Handbook of Mental Health and Aging*. San Diego, CA: Academic Press, 1992; 433–62.

29. Tyrer P, Seivewright H. Studies of outcome. In Tyrer P, ed., *Personality Disorders: Diagnosis, Management and Course*. London: Wright, 1988; 119–36.

30. American Psychiatric Association. *Diagnostic and Statistical Manual of Mental Disorders*, 3rd edn. Washington, DC: APA Press, 1980.

31. American Psychiatric Association. *Diagnostic and Statistical Manual of Mental Disorders*, 3rd edn, Revised. Washington, DC: APA Press, 1987.

32. Segal DL, Hook JN, Coolidge FL. Personality dysfunction, coping styles, and clinical symptoms in younger and older adults. *J Clin Geropsychol* (in press).

33. Ames A, Molinari V. Prevalence of personality disorders in community-living elderly. *J Geriat Psychiat Neurol* 1994; **7**(3): 189–94.

34. Cohen BJ, Nestadt G, Samuels JF *et al*. Personality disorders in late life: a community study. *Br J Psychiat* 1994; **165**: 493–9.

35. Segal DL, Hersen M, Kabacoff RI *et al*. Personality disorders and depression in community-dwelling older adults. *J Ment Health Aging* 1998; **4**(1): 171–82.

36. Teeter RB, Garetz FK, Miller WR, Heiland WF. Psychiatric disturbances of aged patients in skilled nursing homes. *Am J Psychiat* 1976; **133**: 1430–4.

37. Margo JL, Robinson JR, Corea S. Referrals to a psychiatric service from old people's homes. *Br J Psychiat* 1988; **136**: 396–401.

38. Molinari V, Kunik M, Snow-Turek L *et al*. Age-related differences in inpatients with personality disorder: a cross-sectional study. *J Clin Geropsychol* 1999; **5**(3): 191–202.

39. Kunik ME, Mulsant BH, Rifai AH *et al*. Diagnostic rate of co-morbid PD in elderly psychiatric inpatients. *Am J Psychiat* 1993; **151**(4): 603–5.

40. Molinari V, Ames A, Essa M. Prevalence of personality disorders in two geropsychiatric inpatient units. *J Geriat Psychiat Neurol* 1994; **7**(4): 209–15.

41. Coolidge FL, Segal D, Pointer JC *et al*. Personality disorders in older inpatients with chronic mental illness. *J Clin Geropsychol* 2000; **6**(1): 63–71.

42. Molinari V, Marmion J. Personality disorders in geropsychiatric outpatients. *Psychol Rep* 1993; **73**: 256–8.

43. Molinari V, Marmion J. The relationship between affective disorders and Axis II diagnoses in geropsychiatric patients. *J Geriat Psychiat Neurol* 1995; **8**(2): 61–5.

44. Thompson LW, Gallagher D, Czirr R. Personality disorder and outcome in the treatment of late-life depression. *J Geriat Psychiat* 1988; **21**: 133–46.

45. Abrams RC, Spielman LA, Alexopoulos GS, Klausner E. Personality disorder symptoms and functioning in elderly depressed patients. *Am J Geriat Psychiat* 1998; **6**(1): 24–30.

46. Agronin ME, Maletta G. Personality disorders in late life: understanding and overcoming the gap in research. *Am J Geriat Psychiat* 2000; **8**(1): 4–18.

47. Abrams RC, Horowitz SV. Personality disorders after age 50: a meta-analysis. *J Personality Disord* 1996; **10**(3): 271–81.

48. Segal DL, Coolidge FL. Personality disorders. In Bellack AS, Hersen M, eds, *Comprehensive Clinical Psychology: Clinical Geropsychology*, vol. 7. New York: Pergamon, 1998; 267–89.

49. Rosowsky E, Gurian B. Impact of borderline personality disorder in late life on systems of care. *Hosp Commun Psychiat* 1992; **43**: 386–9.

50. Vine RG, Steingart AB. Personality disorder in the elderly depressed. *Can J Psychiat* 1994; **39**: 392–8.

51. Molinari V. Personality disorders and relapse rates among geropsychiatric inpatients. *Clin Gerontol* 1994; **14**(2): 49–52.

52. Workman RH, Molinari V, McCullough L *et al*. An ethical framework for understanding patients with comorbid dementia and impulsive personality disorders: diagnosing and managing disorders of autonomy. *J Law Ethics Aging* 1997; **3**(2): 79–90.

53. Nahas Z, Molinari V, Kunik M. Premorbid personality of dementia patients and caregiver burden. *Clin Gerontol* 1997; **17**(2): 72–6.

54. Molinari V. Ethical issues in the clinical management of older adults with personality disorders. In Rosowsky E, Abrams L, Zweig R, eds, *Personality Disorders in Older Adults: Emerging Issues in Diagnosis and Treatment*. Mahwah, NJ: Erlbaum, 1999; 275–87.

108

Theoretical and Management Issues

Robert C. Abrams

The New York Hospital–Cornell Medical Center, New York, USA

The elaboration by DSM-III[1] of a domain of pathological personality typologies into the well-known Axis II personality disorders has stimulated an outpouring of clinical research. While most of this research has reaffirmed the usefulness of the personality disorder concept, substantial theoretical and methodological problems persist. For example, there is considerable heterogeneity of symptoms within individual disorders and overlap among different disorders[2]. It can be argued that the Axis II personality disorders to some degree lack both convergent and discriminant properties. Moreover, the theoretical underpinning of personality disorders is far from clear. Are these entities derived from interactions of heritable traits, as suggested by Cloningen[3], or are they based on a pathological intrapsychic organization, as suggested by Kernberg[4]? Alternatively, are personality disorders better understood in interpersonal or learning-behavior contexts? It has proved possible to apply each of these theoretical models; personality disorders are, by definition, relatively enduring patterns of dysfunctional behavior that permeate the entire person, are not due to a single abnormality and lead to pain and suffering of people in the patient's world, sometimes more than in the patient him/herself. It is thus not surprising that a variety of explanatory models have been used in efforts to understand these disorders.

Very little attention, however, has been directed to the existence of personality disorders in the elderly and their clinical management, despite the considerable interest in long-term follow-up studies of borderline personality disorder patients[5,6]. In part, this neglect may reflect the original perspective of DSM-III and DSM-III-R[7], that personality disorders are largely attenuated by middle- and old age. Probably another reason is the ongoing uncertainty about how best to assess personality in the elderly. Aging imposes complexities on the already difficult study of personality, adding the confounding factors of brain changes, environment and time. Finally, concepts of normal and pathological adult personality functioning may not be relevant to old age.

In this chapter the topic of personality disorders in old age will be approached first with a discussion of age-related personality change, followed by a review of methodological and clinical issues, including comments on the assessment of DSM personality disorder criteria in the elderly. It will conclude with a discussion of treatment and management.

THE AGING PERSONALITY: DO PEOPLE ACTUALLY CHANGE?

Although the aging personality has been the subject of extensive speculation[8–10], there has been no closure on the question of whether, or in what ways, people change in their dealings with the world; it is still not known whether change or persistence predominates over time. The literature in this area to date can be divided along theoretical and methodological lines into dimensional, categorical and psychoanalytic–developmental models, each with a different set of assumptions.

Using mostly dimensional approaches, conceived as continua of stable traits along which all individuals lie, the psychological literature suggests a picture of progressive changes in motivations and values over the adult years. For example, there appear to be steady increases from early to middle adulthood in self-confidence, independence, humanitarian concerns and personal rigidity[8–9]. Large-scale investigations of medical patients and normal subjects have been carried out using the Minnesota Multiphasic Personality Inventory (MMPI)[11,12]; older adult medical patients tended to score higher on scales measuring introversion, concern with health, immaturity and depression than younger adult medical patients. A decline in criminality with advancing age has also been well documented[13]. Together, these data suggest that traits related to a quiet, inner-directed attitude most typify the aging personality. The MMPI data in particular seem to lend support to the concept of disengagement, or gradual withdrawal from productive activity, as the pre-eminent social-psychological model for age-related personality changes[14]. The reduction in sociopathy and attenuation of hostile aggressive traits have also been highly consistent MMPI findings[1,12].

However, such dimensionally-modeled studies have not pointed conclusively to the existence or direction of age-related personality changes. For example, the MMPI data referred to above are based on large-scale cross-sectional studies involving thousands of medical patients and normal adult subjects, but have not been confirmed in longitudinal studies; the longitudinal MMPI studies have instead emphasized the stability of personality profiles of the individuals over time[15,16]. Similarly, dimensional scores on the Eysenck Personality Inventory Psychoticism (P), Extraversion (E) and Neuroticism (N) subscales show substantial persistence over 30 year periods[7].

Categorical models, such as the DSM-IV Axis II personality disorders, are operationally defined typologies of personality psychopathology, or clinical phenotypes. These models have been relatively little used to examine the aging personality. At the present time, for example, there is scarce cross-sectional information on DSM-IV personality disorders in the older age groups and virtually no longitudinal studies of personality disorder patients that track outcome as far as senescence. However, based upon cross-sectional regression analysis of the relationships of different personality disorder traits with age, Tyrer[18] has suggested that personality disorders can be divided into mature and immature categories. The mature disorders include obsessive–compulsive, schizotypal, schizoid and paranoid; these personality disorders show more stability and less variation with age than others. Schizotypal personality disorder, for example, would be expected to behave more like schizophrenia from the longitudinal perspective because of its spectrum and genetic relationships to the Axis I disorder[5-8]. The immature or flamboyant personality disorders include the borderline, antisocial, narcissistic, histrionic and passive–aggressive categories; these personality disorders may be more evident in younger individuals and may have earlier onset than mature personality disorders. In this scheme, mature personality disorders consist primarily of the Cluster A (odd–eccentric) disorders plus obsessive–compulsive disorder from Cluster C (anxious–fearful); immature personality disorders consist primarily of Cluster B (dramatic–emotional) disorders, plus passive–aggressive disorder from Cluster C.

Other authors, notably McGlashan[5] and Stone[6], have commented, on the basis of follow-up data, that the florid borderline symptomatology seen at index admissions substantially declines by the second decade of follow-up. Both male and female patients appear to advance occupationally and globally, as well as symptomatically, with time[5]. Tyrer[18] also reviewed data suggesting that patients with personality disorders have higher mortality by suicide than other psychiatric patients for a period of 5 years from diagnosis, after which differences in suicide rates between personality disorders and other psychiatric patients become negligible. These mortality data have been interpreted by Tyrer to support a maturation hypothesis, especially for antisocial and other immature personality disorders, in which impulsiveness and suicide become less likely over time. There are also suggestions that mature personality disorders are more frequent in the geriatric population than immature disorders[19,20].

Thus, it is possible to speculate about a "flattening" over time of at least some specific types of personality disorder symptomatology, which might explain why geriatric patients seem to have diffuse Axis II symptomatology, with relatively fewer full diagnoses of personality disorder[19,20]. In the case of borderline personality disorder, the assumption that symptoms are enduring and inflexible has been challenged; this disorder might now be viewed as a state of delayed maturation that improves with time, rather than as a set of chronic defects. However, even in borderline personality disorder, the improvement may not be uniform across different spheres of functioning. McGlashan[5] has suggested that borderline patients may improve considerably in occupational or instrumental functioning, yet never develop satisfactory personal relationships.

Moreover, aging does not necessarily imply linear reduction in severity of the immature personality disorders. An epidemiological study of personality disorders conducted by Reich et al.[21] found the dramatic cluster to be described by a reverse J-shaped curve, in which core traits decline to age 60, then take a slight upturn. Geriatric clinical experience also suggests that there are some individuals who have relatively mild personality dysfunction in young and middle adulthood, but in old age develop a marked and persistent worsening of these trends[22]. Thus, late-onset or emergent personality disorders are possible. Alternatively, individuals with lifelong personality dysfunction can have an affective denouement; they may be more likely to develop depression in old age, as some data suggest[19,20].

A recent body of contributions from psychoanalytic theorists and clinicians has been leading to a developmental theory of the second half of life[23]. Freud's early ideas about the declining plasticity of the personality[24], based on experience in clinical psychoanalysis, have given way to the notion that psychosocial development is continuous throughout life. Successful disengagement from active working and parental roles, and acceptance of the inevitability of death, are several of the proposed developmental tasks of aging. For example, awareness of one's eventual death has been thought to be marked by universal apprehension and, in some individuals, by phobias, paranoia and fear of sleep, attributed to a hypothesized "death anxiety"[25]. Jacques[26] has proposed that characterologically healthier individuals have mastered the anxiety associated with awareness of death at a relatively earlier age than those with personality dysfunction, who might be blocked from acknowledging the inevitability of death until overwhelmed by it. Recently, there has been a renewed interest in psychotherapeutic work with the elderly, most proponents of which argue that change and growth is possible[25-27]. In the view of Neugarten[28] and Costa[29,30], personality is the critical factor in adaptation to old age.

ASSESSING THE AGING PERSONALITY

Overview of Methodological Issues

Assessing personality in the elderly is a daunting task. Each of the three basic approaches cited above carries not only its own set of assumptions but its own limitations as well. The dimensional scales have restricted clinical relevance and yield abstract, somewhat reductionistic information about the individual. On the other hand, categorical diagnoses have been criticized as culture-bound and arbitrary[3], failing to "cut nature at its joints". DSM criteria, in particular, may be age-biased. Axis II criteria frequently appear to be addressing the concerns of a modal young adult, one who is expected to be establishing career and life-partner choices. If personality disorders "become less obvious in middle or old age", this may occur because Axis II does not relevantly assess the present-day experiences and behaviors of aging persons. Age bias could easily result in an underestimation of pathology, whereby symptoms are dismissed as "normative" for age. Overestimation of pathology is also possible, for example with dependency phenomena, where the realistic needs of an older person might be inappropriately viewed as symptomatic.

Psychoanalytic approaches have contributed to the study of personality and aging by encouraging the formulation of developmental theories for the second half of life. However, personality investigation of this type is focused on the individual patient, and its validity is ultimately predicated on a thorough knowledge of a few individuals; McHugh and Slavney have termed this "meaningful construct" validity[31]. While such models may explain how a patient's unique vulnerabilities and life circumstances interact to produce symptoms, large-scale empirical replication is impossible.

State–Trait Problems and Co-morbidity

Whichever theoretical–methodological model is used, the finding of age effects in personality study is frequently subject to the suspicion that they are not in fact true age effects, but rather reflect dysthymic, post-depressive or organic contaminants. This is the state–trait confound, a term that usually refers to the exaggerated self-report of some personality traits owing to the depressed state[32,33]. For example, recovered elderly depressives have been found to have more lifetime personality dysfunction than other elderly subjects[19], and in another study, twice as many recovered elderly depressives met full criteria for DSM-III-R personality diagnoses than did normal controls[20]. While recovery from depression in these studies was carefully documented, and no personality testing was carried out during symptomatic periods, it is impossible to completely rule out depressive influences in clinical personality assessment. The problem is especially evident in geriatric populations, in which some forms of chronic depression seem to be closely related to personality disorders. Dysthymia, a low-grade depressive syndrome appearing in as much as 15% of the geriatric population[34,35], could equally well be deemed an affective disorder with prominent character pathology, or a personality disorder with secondary affective symptomatology; there may in fact be subgroups of each, defined by response to antidepressant drugs[36].

Another chronic depressive disorder often seen in the geriatric population, also associated with significant personality psychopathology, is "double depression". Post[37] used the term "depressive invalidism" to describe "double depression" in the elderly, referring to a group of geriatric patients having severe recurrent depression with incomplete remissions. Finally, the term "masked depression" has been used to describe a depression syndrome, believed to be more common after mid-life, in which cognitive or somatic symptoms are more prominent than sadness, tearfulness, or other affective manifestations[38]. Masked depression may not only present as a mixed personality disorder in geriatric patients, but has also been associated with a number of dysfunctional premorbid personality traits[39,40].

In addition to these chronic depressive entities, anxiety states and disorders also have considerable co-morbidity with personality disorders and have been shown to strongly influence personality assessment[41,42]. Co-morbidity of personality dysfunction and Axis I disorders covers a wide range in geriatric patients and, as with younger patients, the relationship may take different forms. Personality disorders may variously predispose to Axis I disorders, may represent subclinical prodromes of Axis I disorders, may have a pathoplastic or interactional effect with depression or schizophrenia, or may appear as a complication or "scar" of an Axis I condition[43].

The Problem of Organicity

Behavioral change can occur in the context of organic brain pathology or with the use of a variety of medications, situations common in geriatric populations. However, it is not clear whether such behavior should be regarded as dysfunctional personality change or organic pathology. The approach of DSM-III-R was to categorize demented patients' symptoms concerned with the quality of affect and its regulation as an "Organic Personality Syndrome", while reserving the more purely cognitive symptomatology for the diagnosis of dementia. Spitzer et al.[44] proposed in the work-group stage of the development of DSM-IV that the term "organic" be eliminated. In this proposal, dementia, delirium, and amnestic disorder would be listed together in a "Cognitive Impairment Disorders" category, while the other "organic" disorders, including personality, mood and anxiety, would be viewed as "secondary". This proposal was adopted, in principle if not in detail, by the final DSM-IV[63], with its use of category "Personality Change Due To . . .". The nosological reclassification of organic personality disorder to secondary personality disorder emphasizes the personality aspect by listing this entity according to phenomenology rather than etiology. Implicit in the concept of "secondary" personality phenomena is an acknowledgement that personality is subject to change caused by exogenous factors or brain pathology. However, a secondary personality disorder might still be relatively enduring and pervasive, have an interpersonal focus, and lead to significant behavioral impairment; all general criteria for the diagnosis of personality disorder would be met, except for that of early onset.

Self-report vs. Informant Data

Another technical difficulty in personality study common to all theoretical viewpoints is the discrepancy between self-report and informant data[21]. For this reason, reliance upon self-report may be a particularly flawed clinical or research strategy. Among some elderly persons, including control subjects for psychiatric research, an attitude of unrealistic optimism has been observed[45]. This tendency to recast the past in positive terms can be viewed either as a pathological refusal to acknowledge earlier disappointments and failures, or as a healthier attempt to reintegrate and reconcile the same experiences[46]. The state influences of depression, as noted earlier, would argue in favor of informant corroboration of self-report personality data. Similarly, even the subtle cognitive impairment of early dementing illness would seriously reduce the value of self-report personality data. But who should be the informant? Adults who knew an elderly subject as a young child may no longer be alive, and adult children have not necessarily witnessed their parents' young adulthood; even then, their childhood memories might present a distorted picture. Probably it is necessary to have multiple informants, including, where possible, siblings and contemporaries of lifelong acquaintance, in order to provide the most meaningful long-range information about personality functioning.

Time-frame Considerations

Since personality is by definition concerned with established traits, or relatively enduring aspects of motivational or interpersonal behavior, over what periods of time should changes persist in order to be deemed new traits? In the clinical context, all versions of the DSM are vague on this point, stipulating that criteria for personality disorders should reflect current (past year) and long-term functioning, but not clearly requiring that symptoms be present continuously from adolescence to old age in order to qualify for a personality disorder diagnosis[7]. Also, there is no real provision for past personality disorders, those that have been present throughout much of adult life but are attenuated in old age, or for late-onset personality disorders, those first appearing or meeting full criteria in middle age or later. Recently developed standardized instruments for Axis II diagnoses may eventually produce better information on the natural course of personality disorders and the prevalence of past and late-onset disorders[46]. For the moment, it is left to the clinician to select an appropriate time frame for making a personality disorder diagnosis and to determine whether current behavior reflects personality functioning, affective state, organic brain changes, adjustment reaction to age-related life events, or a combination of these factors[47].

Outcome Measures

Assuming that a suitable set of dimensions, categories or developmental milestones can be selected for personality investigation in the elderly, against what outcomes might they be expected to co-vary? Satisfaction with life, a sense of global well-being and health concerns have seemed to some authors to be the most important outcome dimensions to evaluate in older people, because they are indicators of the quality of life[48-50]. Longitudinal investigation suggests that, overall, well-being tends to be stable over time, probably because the frequency and intensity of both positive and negative emotions decline with age[48]. However, associations between specific personality dimensions or categories and life satisfaction in old age have not been established. At the other end of the adjustment spectrum, it has already been noted that depressed elderly patients have had abundant lifetime personality psychopathology[19,20]. In a sample of completed suicides over age 60 years, 45% were estimated to have an Axis II disorder based on interviews with close relatives[51]. Nevertheless, it is not always intuitively clear what constitutes adaptive or maladaptive personality functioning in old age. For example, a relatively greater degree of risk-taking or sensation-seeking traits could be viewed as adaptive in a 20-year-old than in an elderly person; the older individual should optimally have some sensation-seeking behavior but could obviously be placed in situations of unreasonable risk without some reduction of sensation-seeking intensity. Interestingly, recovered elderly depressives have been found to have a greater preference for environmental stimulation, as suggested by higher scores on the Sensation-Seeking Scale[52,53] than normal elderly controls[53], implying a complex interaction among aging, trait preference for environmental stimulation, and affective illness.

Assessment of DSM Criteria in Geriatric Patients: Clinical Notes

The diagnosis of personality disorders requires evidence of symptomatic behavior, both currently and in the past; when examining the current period of old age for evidence of personality disorder criteria, it is necessary to interpret those criteria in a geriatric context. For example, in the odd–eccentric (Cluster A) personality disorders, including paranoid, schizoid and schizotypal personality disorders, suspiciousness of exploitation or harm (a criterion of paranoid personality disorder) or social and sexual isolation (a criterion of schizoid personality disorder) should be carefully weighed against realistic dangers and social limitations faced by the older person. For this, an informant who knows the patient well is often required.

Cluster B, the dramatic–emotional personality disorders (antisocial, borderline, histrionic and narcissistic), are assigned to geriatric patients especially infrequently, possibly because they are truly "immature" syndromes that prove unstable over long periods of time, and probably also because much latitude is necessary to fit the criteria to the experiences of geriatric patients. For example, evaluation for the borderline criterion of "idealization" should include consideration of such behavior when directed toward caregivers in a hospital or nursing home. Similarly, "self-damaging impulsiveness" need not be limited to reckless driving or sexual activity, as suggested by DSM-III-R, and "frantic efforts to avoid real or imagined abandonment" should not be confused with reactions to age-related losses or institutionalization. Thus, criteria such as "self-damaging impulsiveness" might be broadened to include the geriatric context, while other criteria, such as "frantic efforts to avoid abandonment", should be narrowed to account for the impact of realistic events.

Interpretive flexibility is also needed to assign Cluster C personality disorder diagnoses to elderly patients. Reactions and attitudes toward caregivers provide an appropriate context for many elderly patients in which to interpret Cluster C criteria, particularly those for passive–aggressive and dependent disorders. However, medical illness can transiently exacerbate dependency phenomena. For all of these disorders, it seems most appropriate to err on the side of conservatism or specificity in diagnosis. Obviously, the clinician can be most confident of the assessment when antecedents of criteria are traceable to the past, but there remains an obligation to determine what is or is not pathological in the older person's present reality.

TREATMENT OF ELDERLY PATIENTS WITH PERSONALITY DISORDERS

There is virtually no research data to guide the comprehensive treatment of elderly patients with personality disorders. However, based upon classic and recent writings in this area[23,25–27] and treatment reports in younger age groups, it is possible to set forth some general principles of management.

Co-morbid Axis I Disorders

It has already been noted that the depressed state may influence the assessment of personality disorders. It may also be true that, especially in the elderly, personality disorders exert their most clinically meaningful effects in the setting of major depressive disorder. For example, earlier onset of depression as well as greater severity and frequency of depressive episodes, have been found in elderly patients with personality disorders[2,38]. Personality disorder symptoms also appear to affect elderly patients' attitudes and behaviors toward antidepressant treatment. Personality-disordered patients have difficulty in establishing positive therapeutic alliances with psychotherapists and general physicians, a factor which in turn promotes poor adherence to either psychopharmacological or psychotherapeutic treatments. Finally, while personality dysfunction may not lengthen the depressive episode itself, in interaction with residual depressive symptoms, it appears to prolong depression-related declines in global functioning and quality of life[59].

Thus, it may be reasonable to address co-morbid Axis I conditions, particularly affective or anxiety disorders, before planning any treatment efforts directed specifically toward the personality component. In conditions such as dysthymia, where personality dysfunction and affective symptomatology at times seem to merge, it may also prove useful to defer long-term treatment planning and psychosocial decision-making until somatic treatments have reached maximum efficacy. Likewise, medical conditions that might affect the course of personality symptomatology should be fully evaluated.

Pharmacotherapy

Pharmacotherapy for geriatric personality disorder patients has not been investigated *per se* and remains an underdeveloped area. In younger age groups, there exists an older literature for borderline personality disorder, in which psychotic-spectrum symptomatology was shown to be more effectively treated by neuroleptic medication than placebo[54], and amitriptyline was usually more effective than placebo but no more effective than haloperidol in antidepressant effect[55]. MAO inhibitors[56], lithium[57] and carbamazepine[58] were proposed to have limited usefulness for specific traits or symptoms. More recently, there have been some studies in mixed-age populations showing modest effects of particular medications or medication classes on the symptomatology of the three Axis II clusters. For example, haloperidol and thiothixene have been found to be useful in the treatment of patients with schizotypal or other Cluster A personality disorders, especially the transient paranoia, agitation or rages associated with these disorders[60]; the selective serotonin reuptake inhibitors (SSRIs), fluoxetine and sertraline have shown some promise in treating impulsive, self-injurious and depressive behaviors associated with Cluster B personality disorders[61], and fluoxetine and MAOIs have been found to decrease the kind of avoidant behaviors found in individuals with Cluster C personality disorders[62].

Psychotherapy

Unless there is a co-morbid Axis I disorder that requires psychopharmacological intervention, the treatment of geriatric personality disorders is largely a psychotherapeutic endeavor. As described by Sadavoy[27], a major difference between the psychotherapy of older and younger patients is the time frame covered. Transference issues continue to be directed from childhood sources and early[8] parental relationships, but they will often contain an overlay from experience later in life. Usually the initial focus should be on the patient's present reality and presenting problems, secondarily on historical material and on the relationship with the therapist. Then, as it unfolds, more time and effort can be devoted to clarifying and perhaps analyzing distortions in the patient's attitudes and behaviors toward the therapist. Some patients, not necessarily the highest-functioning ones, will be able to focus usefully on the relationship with the therapist to a greater degree than others. In either case, special attention must be paid to the potential for transference issues to become painful and paralyzing for both patient and therapist. Ideally, discussion of the therapeutic relationship can provide a point of shared reality, which patient and therapist can examine together. Issues from the past then emerge more naturally, in an unforced and relevant fashion. Patients probably do have a need to mourn past losses, a process that can be fostered in psychotherapy, but it should be remembered that such mourning is not done globally or in a predictable sequence[27].

Another factor complicating psychotherapy in the elderly is that overall treatment plans often involve family, caregivers or institutional representatives. Important persons in the patient's social sphere must be engaged in treatment strategies because of the interpersonal field in which personality psychopathology, especially the Cluster B disorders, is expressed; also, older people with disabilities may function less autonomously. This creates potential boundary problems for the therapist, as well as concerns about confidentiality; these must be spelled out to the patient and an understanding reached between the patient and therapist on exactly what information may be transmitted to others and under what circumstances this will be done. Once this is accomplished, creative use can be made of family and institutional supports.

Whatever the approach taken in psychotherapy, limited and realistic goals should be set, based upon a collaterally informed picture of the patient's long-term functioning. A psychotherapy relationship cannot reasonably be expected to resolve the psychological deficits, and the consequences of those deficits of the elderly personality disorder patient—a lifetime of failed relationships, missed opportunities and unused talents. Nevertheless, it can be hoped that for some individuals, the loss of narcissistic gratifications associated with physical beauty and vocational competence can actually foster psychotherapeutic work. Patients may find themselves in old age to be motivated for self-examination as never before. The impetus provided by aging and the press of reality may render the older patient amenable to a process of growth and change.

REFERENCES

1. American Psychiatric Association. *Diagnostic and Statistical Manual of Mental Disorders*, 3rd edn. Washington, DC: APA, 1980.
2. Widiger TA, Frances A. The DSM-III personality disorders: perspectives from psychology. *Arch Gen Psychiat* 1985; **42**: 615–23.
3. Cloninger CR. A systematic method of clinical description and classification of personality variants. *Arch Gen Psychiat* 1987; **44**: 573–88.
4. Kernberg OF. *Borderline Conditions and Pathological Narcissism*. New York: Jason Aronson, 1986; 3–49.
5. McGlashan TH. The Chestnut Lodge follow-up study. III. Long-term outcome of borderline personalities. *Arch Gen Psychiat* 1986; **43**: 20–30.
6. Stone MH. Long-term outcome in borderline adolescents. In Shagass C, ed., *Proceedings of the IVth Congress on Biological Psychiatry*. New York: Elsevier, 1985; 61.
7. American Psychiatric Association. *Diagnostic and Statistical Manual of Mental Disorders*, 3rd edn, Revised. Washington, DC: APA, 1987.
8. Bee HL. Changes in personality, motivations, and values over the adult years. In Bee HL, ed., *The Journey of Adulthood*. New York: Macmillan, 1986.
9. Schaie KW. *Longitudinal Studies of Adult Psychological Development*. New York: Guilford, 1983.
10. Gynther MD. Aging and personality. In Butcher JN, ed., *New Developments in the Use of the MMPI*. Minneapolis, MN: University of Minnesota Press, 1979.
11. Swenson WM, Pearson JS, Osborne D. *An MMPI Source Book: Basic Item, Scale, and Pattern Data on 50 000 Medical Patients*. Minneapolis, MN: University of Minnesota Press, 1973.
12. Dahlstrom WG, Welsh GS, Dahlstrom LE. *An MMPI Handbook, vol. 1. Clinical Interpretation*. Minneapolis, MN: University of Minnesota Press, 1972.
13. Woodruff RA, Guze SE, Clayton PJ. The medical and psychiatric implications of antisocial personality (sociopathy). *Dis Nerv Syst* 1971; **32**: 712–14.
14. Cumming E, Henry WE. *Growing Old*. New York: Basic Books, 1961.
15. Leon GR, Gillum B, Gillum R et al. Personality stability and change over a 30-year period—middle age to old age. *J Consult Clin Psychol* 1979; **4**: 401–7.
16. Golden JS, Mandel N, Glueck BC, Feder Z. A summary description of fifty "normal" white males. *Am J Psychiat* 1962; **119**: 48–56.
17. Eysenck EJ, Eysenck MW. *Personality and Individual Differences*. New York: Plenum, 1985.
18. Tyrer P. *Personality Disorders: Diagnosis, Management and Course*. London: Wright, 1988.
19. Abrams RC, Alexopoulos GS, Young RC. Geriatric depression and DSM-III-R personality disorder criteria. *J Am Geriat Soc* 1987; **35**: 383–6.
20. Schneider LS, Zemansky M, Pollock V et al. Personality dysfunction in recovered depressed elderly subjects. Abstracts of the Annual Meeting of the Gerontological Society of America, Washington, DC, 1987.
21. Reich J, Nduaguba M, Yates W. Age and sex distribution of DSM-III personality cluster traits in a community population. *Comp Psychiat* 1988; **29**: 298–303.
22. Abrams RC. The aging personality (editorial). *Int J Geriat Psychiat* 1991; **6**: 1–3.
23. Colarusso CA, Nemiroff RA. Clinical implications of adult developmental theory. *Am J Psychiat* 1987; **144**: 1263–70.
24. Freud S. On psychotherapy (1906). In Riviere J, ed., *Collected Papers*, vol. I. London: Hogarth, 1942.
25. Meerlo JA. Transference and resistance in geriatric psychotherapy. In Steury S, Blank ML, eds, *Readings in Psychotherapy With Older People*. Washington, DC: US Department of Health and Human Services, 1981.
26. Jacques E. Death and mid-life crisis. In Ruitenbeck HM, ed., *Death: Interpretations*. New York: Delta, 1969.
27. Sadavoy J. Character disorders in the elderly: an overview. In Sadavoy J, Leszcz M, eds, *Treating the Elderly with Psychotherapy: The Scope for Change in Later Life*. New York: International Universities Press, 1987.
28. Neugarten P. Personality and aging. In Birren JE, Schaie KW, eds, *Handbook of the Psychology of Aging*. New York: Van Nostrand Reinhold, 1977.
29. Costa PJ, McCrae RR. Still stable after all these years: personality as a key to some issues in adulthood and old age. In Battes PB, ed., *Lifespan Development and Behavior*, vol 3. New York: Academic Press, 1980; 65–102.
30. Costa PJ, McCrae RR, Norris AH. Personal adjustment to aging: longitudinal prediction from neuroticism and extraversion. *J Gerontol* 1981; **36**: 78–85.
31. McHugh PR, Slavney PR. *The Perspectives of Psychiatry*. Baltimore, MD: Johns Hopkins University Press, 1983.

32. Coppen A, Metcalfe M. Effect of a depressive illness on MPI scores. *Br J Psychiat* 1965; **111**: 236–9.

33. Kerr TA, Schapira K, Roth M *et al.* The relationship between the Maudsley Personality Inventory and the course of affective disorders. *Br J Psychiat* 1970; **116**: 11–19.

34. Blazer D, Williams CD. Epidemiology of dysphoria and depression in an elderly population. *Br J Psychiat* 1980; **137**: 439–44.

35. Moore JT. Dysthymia in the elderly. *J Affect Disord* 1985; **I**(suppl): 515–21.

36. Akiskal HS. Dysthymic disorder: psychopathology of proposed chronic depressive subtypes. *Am J Psychiat* 1983; **140**: 141.

37. Post F. The management and nature of depressive illness in late life: A follow-through study. *Br J Psychiat* 1971; **21**: 393–404.

38. Kielholz P. Masked depressions and depressive equivalents. In Kielholz P, ed., *Masked Depression: An International Symposium*. Berne, Switzerland: Hans Huber, 1973.

39. Jacobowsky B. Psychosomatic equivalents of endogenous depression. *Acta Psychiat Scand* 1961; **162**: 253–60.

40. Lesse S. The multivariant masks of depression. *Am J Psychiat* 1968; **124**(suppl 1): 35–40.

41. Reich J, Noyes R, Coryell W *et al.* The effect of state anxiety on personality measurement. *Am J Psychiat* 1986; **45**: 977–86.

42. Reich J, Noyes R, Hirschfeld R *et al.* State and personality in depressed and panic patients. *Am J Psychiat* 1987; **144**: 181–7.

43. Hirschfeld RMA, Klerman GL, Clayton RJ *et al.* Assessing personality: effects of the depressive state on trait measurement. *Am J Psychiat* 1983; **140**: 695–9.

44. Spitzer R, Williams J, First M *et al.* A proposal for DSM-IV: solving the organic/non-organic problem. *J Neuropsychiat* 1989; **1**: 126–7.

45. Drinka PJ, Drinka TJK. Are elderly volunteers normal? *J Am Geriat Soc* 1988; **36**: 482–3 (letter).

46. Erikson EH, Erikson JM, Kivnick HQ. *Vital Involvement in Old Age*. New York: WW Norton, 1986.

47. Loranger AW, Susman VL, Oldham JM *et al.* The Personality Disorder Examination: a preliminary report. *J Personality Disord* 1987; **1**: 1–13.

48. Costa PT, Zonderman AN, McCrae RR *et al.* Longitudinal analyses of psychological well-being in a national sample: stability of mean bands. *J Gerontol* 1987; **42**: 50–5.

49. Malatesta CZ. Affective development over the lifespan: Involution or growth? *Merrill-Palmer Qu* 1981; **27**: 143–73.

50. Schulz R. Emotion and affect. In Birren JE, Schaie KW, eds, *Handbook of the Psychology of Aging*, 1st edn. New York: Van Nostrand Reinhold, 1985.

51. Loebel JP. Completed suicide in the elderly. Abstracts of the Third Annual Meeting and Symposium of the American Association for Geriatric Psychiatry, San Diego, CA, 1990.

52. Zuckerman M, Eysenck S, Eysenck HJ. Sensation-seeking in England and America: cross-cultural, age and sex comparisons. *J Consult Clin Psychol* 1978; **46**: 139–49.

53. Young RC, Abrams RC, Alexopoulos GS *et al.* Sensation-Seeking Scale scores in treated geriatric depressives and controls. *Biol Psychiat* 1989; **26**: 643–6.

54. Goldberg SC, Schulz SC, Schulz PM *et al.* Borderline and schizotypal personality disorders treated with low-dose thiothixene vs. placebo. *Arch Gen Psychiat* 1986; **43**: 680–6.

55. Soloff PH, George A, Nathan RS *et al.* Amitriptyline vs. haloperidol in borderlines. Paper presented at the 140th Annual Meeting of the American Psychiatric Association, Chicago, IL, May 12, 1987.

56. Liebowitz MR, Klein DF. Inter-relationship of hysteroid dysphoria and borderline personality disorder. *Psychiat Clin N Am* 1981; **4**: 67–89.

57. Shader RI, Jackson AH, Dodes LM. The anti-aggressive effects of lithium in man. *Psychopharmacologia* 1974; **40**: 17–24.

58. Cowdry RW, Gardner DL. Pharmacotherapy of borderline personality disorder: alprazolam, carbamazepine, trifluoperazine, tranylcypromine. *Arch Gen Psychiat* 1988; **45**: 111–19.

59. Abrams RC, Alexopoulos GS, Speilman LA *et al.* Personality disorder symptoms predict declines in global functioning and quality of life in elderly depressed patients. *Am J Geriat Psychiat* 2001; **9**: 67–71.

60. Goldberg SC, Schulz SC, Schulz PM *et al.* Borderline and schizotypal personality disorders treated with low-dose thiothixene vs. placebo. *Arch Gen Psychiat* 1986; **43**: 680–6.

61. Kavoussi RJ, Liv J, Cocarro EF. An open trial of sertraline in personality disorder patients with impulsive aggression. *J Clin Psychiat* 1994; **55**: 137–41.

62. Versiani M, Nardi AE, Mundim FD, Alves AB. Pharmacotherapy of social phobia: a controlled study with meclobemide and phenelzine. *Br J Psychiat* 1992; **161**: 353–60.

63. American Psychiatric Association. *Diagnostic and Statistical Manual of Mental Disorders*, 4th edn. Washington, DC: APA, 1994.

Part J

Mental and Behavioural Disorders
due to Psychoactive Substances

109

Alcohol Abuse in the Elderly

Helen H. Kyomen[1] and Benjamin Liptzin[2]

[1]*McLean Hospital, Belmont, MA, and* [2]*Baystate Medical Center, Springfield, MA, USA*

Alcohol abuse in the elderly may be defined as the persistent and intended use of ethyl alcohol despite the problems caused by its use[1,2]. In the elderly, alcohol abuse usually presents clinically as self-neglect, falls, confusion, lability, depression, unusual behavior, injuries, diarrhea, malnutrition, myopathy, incontinence or hypothermia[3,4]. In fact, the elderly person with alcohol abuse problems may be hospitalized for any one of these problems. During the course of the hospitalization, one may uncover signs of characteristic addictive use of ethyl alcohol, with: (a) tolerance; (b) withdrawal symptoms; (c) loss of control of use; (d) social decline; and (e) mental and physical decline[5]. Alcohol abuse in the elderly is an under-recognized problem that has become increasingly important due to the growing numbers of elderly people[6-10]. Prevalence estimates of alcohol-related problems are in the range 1–6% in community-dwelling elderly, 7–22% in medically hospitalized elderly, and 28–44% in elderly psychiatric inpatients[1,4]. In one study of older primary care outpatients, 15% of men and 12% of women regularly drank in excess of limits recommended by the National Institute of Alcohol Abuse and Alcoholism (>7 drinks/week for women and >14 drinks/week for men)[11].

EFFECTS OF ALCOHOL IN THE ELDERLY

Older people are at greater risk and more vulnerable to the toxic effects of alcohol for three main reasons:

1. A smaller volume of alcohol is required to produce the same effects as in a younger person. The elderly have a decreased volume of distribution due to decreased muscle mass, a greater proportion of fat and a smaller water compartment. These all result in a higher blood alcohol level than in a younger adult for the same amount of alcohol consumed[12-16]. This suggests that the elderly person's brain, liver, cardiac and other organ systems are subjected to a greater toxic effect from a given amount of alcohol. In a younger person, larger amounts of alcohol consumption may be necessary before detrimental effects from alcohol abuse become grossly evident. An elderly person may reach this threshold for hazardous use of alcohol after drinking a relatively small amount[17].

2. The general decrease in the capacity to withstand stress and maintain homeostasis, as well as a higher risk for medical illness and disability in elderly people, can magnify the effects of alcohol abuse in the elderly.

3. Some organ systems may be especially susceptible to alcohol in the elderly. For example, the central nervous system appears to be more sensitive to alcohol in the older person[18-21], and bone fractures are much more frequent among elderly who use alcohol than in those who do not[22].

The interaction of these three main factors places the elderly alcohol-using person at greater risk for multiple impairments resulting from the use of alcohol.

There are many possible detrimental effects from alcohol abuse in the elderly. Among them are the following:

1. Driving ability can be adversely affected with the consumption of minimal amounts of alcohol. Relatively small amounts of alcohol can lead to confusion, visuospatial impairment, problem-solving deficits and motor impairment in the elderly[23-25], which can inhibit the continuous attention and quick responses needed for driving. If the elderly person also has cognitive or sensory deficits, then the additional insults from alcohol use may make driving considerably more dangerous[17,20].

2. Cognitive impairments suggesting dementia may be caused by alcohol abuse[26,27]. Although some cognitive impairment can result from even social drinking, chronic alcohol consumption has been shown to cause marked cognitive deficits, with associated cortical atrophy and ventricular dilatation on brain scan[19,28,29]. Some researchers have suggested that alcoholism contributes to accelerated mental aging, but this is still controversial[19,30].

3. Elderly alcoholics have a higher prevalence of alcohol-related medical conditions than the elderly population at large. Such conditions include alcoholic liver disease, alcoholic cardiomyopathy, hypertension, chronic obstructive pulmonary disease, neurologic diseases (including cognitive brain syndromes and peripheral neuropathy), malnutrition, osteopenia, psoriasis, peptic ulcer disease and various cancers[22,31-36].

4. Alcohol use can adversely affect the elimination of some drugs and add to the toxicity of others. This places an elderly person with medical illness or disability who is taking prescription medication at great risk for having subtherapeutic or adverse effects from the medication[37,38]. The magnitude of this problem is evident when one considers that the elderly receive 25% of all drugs prescribed in the USA, while comprising only approximately 12% of the population[6,39,40,41].

5. The depressant effects of alcohol on the central nervous system may mimic or contribute to depression in the elderly[42,43]. Some elderly with depressed mood may resort to drinking in order to "self-medicate" themselves. This may alleviate the depressive symptoms initially, but later lead to an increase in depression, anxiety, sleep disturbances and impotence[40,44].

6. Alcohol can contribute to malnutrition in the elderly. Malnutrition can result from the interaction of the following factors[45,46]:

   (a) Food intake can be hindered if the elderly alcoholic develops depressed mood, becomes apathetic and experiences loss of appetite. If the elderly alcoholic's impaired ambulation results in a reduced capacity to obtain food, or if limited financial resources are used to purchase alcohol instead of food, dietary intake may be restricted further.

(b) The effect of alcohol on the gastrointestinal tract is to produce malabsorption of fats, fat-soluble vitamins, calcium, magnesium, iron and zinc. The active transport of B vitamins is also impaired.

(c) Alcohol can contribute to increased losses of magnesium, phosphate, potassium and zinc through the urine. If vomiting and diarrhea occur, there may be increased loss of sodium, potassium and chloride.

(d) Alcohol use increases the requirements for folate and pyridoxine.

7. Alcohol use contributes to accidents and injuries that may lead to fractures or subdural hematomas. A study of accidental drowning in Denmark found that between one-third and one-half of adult drownings were related to alcohol intake[47].

8. Alcohol use disorder has been associated with higher mortality in a study of older public housing residents[48].

9. Alcoholism can disrupt the elderly alcoholic's family structure and cohesiveness and may even lead to family violence. This can result in dysfunctional family relationships, with consequent increased difficulty in treatment of the alcohol-related problems.

Despite the many unfavorable effects of alcohol abuse in the elderly, researchers have also reported positive aspects of alcohol use. Moderate alcohol consumption has been associated with a decreased risk of ischemic stroke in elderly subjects[49]. A study of elderly Australians found that alcohol intake was associated with a significant increase in life expectancy[50].

CHARACTERISTICS OF ELDERLY ALCOHOL ABUSERS

Elderly alcohol abusers differ from younger alcohol abusers in a number of ways. Alcohol abuse in the elderly is often associated with a clustering of events, which are common in late life. These include such occurrences as job retirement, widowhood, the deaths of close friends and relatives, more medical illness and disability in oneself and one's peers, and perceived loss of a meaningful role or function. Some authors consider late-onset alcoholism to be "reactive alcoholism", where the dependence on alcohol is initiated by a need to alleviate the stresses of undergoing multiple losses. However, the extent to which alcohol abuse in the elderly is precipitated by stress from these losses is unclear. Some researchers have found little change in alcohol consumption or drinking behavior due to life stressors[51,52].

The time of onset of alcohol abuse may also significantly differentiate the younger alcoholic from the older one. Early-onset alcoholics have a greater amount of psychopathology and family history of alcoholism than late-onset alcoholics. Early-onset alcoholics are characterized by being male relatives of alcoholic men with histories of violence with and without alcohol, legal problems due to alcohol use, and illegal substance abuse. Late-onset alcoholics are characterized by having isolated alcohol-induced problems with health, marital relationships or self-care, and much reduced histories of arrests, violence or other substance abuse. Many elderly people with alcohol problems fall into the late-onset alcoholic group. These findings suggest that the etiology and predisposition of a person to an alcohol use disorder may differ by onset age. If this is so, the treatments and interventions for an alcohol use disorder may also differ with age of onset and need to be individualized accordingly[53,54].

Individual feelings towards alcohol use are affected by the cultural and historical attitudes one grows up with. For example, the experience of the American elderly alcoholic may differ from that of younger alcoholics in that the elderly alcoholic and his peers may have been exposed to the turmoil of the Prohibition era. The moral issues highlighted in this historical period may influence the willingness that some elderly may have in recognizing and accepting a diagnosis of, and treatment for, alcoholism.

THE RECOGNITION OF ALCOHOL ABUSE IN THE ELDERLY

Alcohol abuse in the elderly often comes to the attention of health professionals through presentation with a non-specific medical or psychiatric symptom, such as self-neglect, falls, confusion, lability, depression, unusual behavior, injuries, diarrhea, malnutrition, myopathy, incontinence or hypothermia. In cases where alcohol abuse is suspected, alcohol dependency must be considered. Alcohol dependency is suggested when there are: (a) tolerance; (b) withdrawal symptoms; (c) loss of control of use; (d) social decline; and (e) mental and physical decline.

Tolerance to alcohol may be assessed by establishing a reliable history of the patient's drinking pattern. Corroboration from family members and others close to the patient may be crucial. Tolerance is suggested if the patient exhibits a quantity and frequency of drinking which is increased over his baseline pattern of drinking. A patient with tolerance to alcohol will require a greater quantity of alcohol to achieve the same amount of inebriation that a lower quantity had been able to achieve previously. Tolerance is strongly suggested if there has been at least a 50% increase in the amount of alcohol required to attain a given effect, a blood alcohol level of 150 mg without intoxication, or the equivalent use of one-fifth gallon (750 mg) of alcohol or more in 1 day by a 180 pound person[55].

Withdrawal symptoms occur when a patient who is tolerant to alcohol experiences a rapid decrease in blood alcohol concentration. Symptoms of the alcohol withdrawal syndrome include tachycardia, with a pulse of greater than 110 beats/min, tachypnea, hypertension, low-grade fever, sweating, nausea, vomiting, hand tremors and increased anxiety. In some cases, the patient may develop seizures or delirium tremens with confusion, agitation and visual hallucinations. An elderly patient undergoing withdrawal may experience one or all of these symptoms[55,56].

Loss of control means that the patient is no longer able consistently to choose the amount of alcohol he/she will consume in a given situation. He/she may also experience blackouts and behave and feel in unpredictable ways[55].

Social decline in the elderly alcoholic is assessed from a baseline of age-appropriate behaviors[55]. Many elderly people no longer hold a steady job, do not drive or hold a driver's license, and have lost many of their close friends and associates with whom they used to socialize. Thus, it may not be as appropriate to assess for social decline by investigating these areas of the elderly patient's life as it would be in a younger patient. However, it is relevant and revealing to ask elderly people whether they are in contact with their children or grandchildren, and to what extent. It is also useful to find out whether the patient's relatives express any concern about the patient's alcohol use. Investigating the patient's functioning with respect to his/her hobbies or other enjoyed activities can also be useful.

Physical, psychological and laboratory findings may also uncover problems with alcohol use[55]. Addictive alcohol use can lead to malnutrition, gastrointestinal upset and bleeding, delirium, falls, depression, hypertension and neglect of self. Recurrent diseases of the stomach, pancreas or liver may also be caused by excessive alcohol abuse. These medical conditions often bring the elderly alcoholic to clinical attention. Laboratory results of macrocytosis, elevated mean corpuscular volume, and increased liver enzyme levels, especially γ-glutamyl transpeptidase, may correlate with alcohol abuse in the elderly. Blood alcohol levels, and urine or breath tests for alcohol, may be used to confirm alcohol intoxication.

Assessment of tolerance, withdrawal, loss of control, social decline and mental and physical decline are useful clinical parameters to recognize and diagnose alcohol addiction. Several screening instruments have been devised to help clinicians recognize alcoholism. These scales typically assess the quantity and frequency of drinking, social and legal problems resulting from alcohol abuse, health problems related to excessive alcohol use, symptoms of addictive drinking, and/or self-recognition of alcohol-related problems[57-59]. Many of these instruments have been validated for younger populations, but not specifically for the elderly. The validity of the CAGE screen for alcoholism in the elderly has been examined empirically[60]. "CAGE" is a mnemonic for the questions: Have you ever felt a need to Cut down on drinking? Have you ever felt Annoyed by others inquiring about your drinking? Have you ever felt Guilty about drinking? Do you ever use alcohol for an Eye-opener? If two or more of these questions are answered positively, a need for more extensive evaluation for alcohol abuse is indicated. Another more detailed screen is the Michigan Alcoholism Screening Test–Geriatric Version (MAST-G)[61]. In addition, the original MAST, scored with weighted (MAST) and unit scoring (UMAST), and two shorter versions, the Brief MAST (BMAST) and Short MAST (SMAST), have been tested in the elderly[62]. Researchers found that the MAST and UMAST gave excellent sensitivity and specificity for alcohol abuse in the study population of 52 hospitalized elderly male alcoholics, matched with 33 non-alcoholic controls. The MAST and UMAST may be useful screening instruments to help recognize alcoholism in the elderly.

THE TREATMENT OF ALCOHOL ABUSE IN THE ELDERLY

Once the diagnosis of alcohol abuse is confirmed, the first step in treatment is a thorough evaluation to identify any other coexisting medical or psychiatric problems. Treatment for these problems must be initiated at the same time as the patient is detoxified. Providing adequate nutrition and hydration is especially important in the elderly alcoholic, due to increased nutritional problems and impaired thirst mechanisms in the elderly. Benzodiazepines are generally avoided in the detoxification of elderly alcoholics, due to their potential for causing delirium. However, if significant withdrawal symptoms occur, benzodiazepines should be administered[56,63,64]. Elderly patients may experience more severe withdrawals from alcohol and require higher doses of benzodiazepines than younger patients. In general, detoxification with benzodiazepines with a short half-life is recommended in the elderly. However, these medications may not provide adequate anticonvulsant effect and the use of longer-acting benzodiazepines may be necessary[56].

Once the elderly alcoholic patient is detoxified, adequate relapse prevention and rehabilitative treatment is crucial for the patient to maintain sobriety. The elderly alcoholic must first come to an acceptance of his/her alcohol abuse problem. Family members or others who are close to the patient may be able to help the patient break through the denial regarding alcohol abuse seen in many alcohol abusers. Family members may also be instrumental in motivating the patient to stop drinking. Patient and family education about the effects of alcohol must be provided, and the need to abstain from alcohol must be stressed. A behavioral and self-management treatment module has resulted in marked success

in treating alcohol use problems in the elderly[65]. This module educates the elderly alcoholic about drinking behavior, the acquisition of self-management skills, and the re-establishment of social networks.

The elderly alcoholic patient's recovery and rehabilitation is an ongoing process. The patient needs to learn to readjust to life without alcohol. The patient's family and close relatives and friends can help him/her in this endeavor by supporting sobriety in the patient and incorporating the non-drinking patient into their lives without the presence of alcohol. Family members may have been "enabling" the patient to drink, and they need to be made aware of these patterns of behavior and change them through family education and family therapy. If the elderly alcohol abuser is a parent and the enablers are his children, the role reversal that is inherent in the children's setting limits on their parents may make this task especially difficult. Group therapy may help the patient adjust to a non-alcoholic lifestyle. In this setting, he/she can develop non-alcohol-related social skills and learn to bond with others in safe surroundings, free of the context of alcohol. If elderly alcoholics can be treated in age-specific groups, they may remain in treatment significantly longer and be more likely to complete treatment than those treated in mixed-age groups[65]. Involvement in Alcoholics Anonymous with people with whom the patient feels comfortable and can consider his/her peers is important, especially if he/she has no close relatives or friends. The relationships with others that can be formed in these settings can provide a replacement for the alcohol to which the patient was bonded previously. Family involvement with the patient in Alcoholics Anonymous and in other affiliated groups such as Alanon, Alateen or Alatot is also important, as alcoholism adversely affects family members who also need support, education and treatment.

Use of alcohol-deterrent medications, such as naltrexone or disulfiram, may serve as adjunctive treatments. These drugs may help motivated alcohol abusers to reduce the quantity of alcohol used or the number of drinking days. However, these medications generally are not effective unless prescribed and monitored as part of an overall, multidisciplinary treatment and relapse prevention plan. Opioid receptor antagonists, such as naltrexone or related compounds, may be less toxic than disulfiram in elderly patients[66-68].

The cultural aspects of alcohol abuse intervention are also worthy of consideration. The above recommendations for treatment are a description of treatment conceptualizations in the USA. These interventions may need to be modified for other countries. In instituting any type of treatment or intervention, it is important to consider the context of the problem being addressed and the context into which the treatment or intervention will be instituted. The consumption of alcohol can take on a variety of cultural meanings. To some groups, ethanol is a food or is associated with religious rituals. For others, it is a means to relax and calm one's nerves. For still others, alcohol is considered to be a sinful intoxicant used by those of weak moral fiber. To intervene most effectively with an aged person for whom alcohol consumption has become a problem, it is important to understand what meaning the use of the alcohol has for him as an individual, a family member and as part of the greater society, including his cultural group. The contextual meaning of the change in alcohol use must likewise be considered. To understand these contextual meanings most effectively, the clinician must be aware of what his/her inherent assumptions may be about these contextual meanings and try not to confound with his/her own biases his/her understanding of the situation. Members of the patient's contextual and cultural groups may be very helpful in providing meaningful insights into these understandings. Once these cultural factors are understood, interventions to reduce the problematic alcohol consumption to the desired outcome of abstinence or perhaps of less harmful alcohol use, can be creatively formulated and instituted more effectively and efficiently.

CONCLUSION

In summary, alcohol abuse in the elderly is a significant problem that needs to be addressed aggressively. Recognition and diagnosis of alcohol abuse may be more difficult in the elderly. The biological and psychosocial losses and decline that are often used to identify alcoholism in younger people can occur in many elderly who do not abuse alcohol. The clinical presentation of an elderly alcoholic is often with a medical condition that may be masked by other medical diagnoses. For these reasons, the clinician must be especially alert to the possible presence of alcohol abuse in this age group. If alcohol abuse is identified, the clinician must then be prepared to direct or initiate treatment in a culturally appropriate, sensitive, flexible and creative manner that is geared to the elderly individual and his/her family and significant others.

REFERENCES

1. Council on Scientific Affairs, American Medical Association. Alcoholism in the elderly. *J Am Med Assoc* 1996; **275**: 797–801.
2. Goldstein MZ, Pataki A, Webb MT. Alcoholism among elderly persons. *Psychiat Serv* 1996; **47**: 941–3.
3. Lieber CS. Medical disorders of alcoholism. *N Engl J Med* 1995; **333**: 1058–65.
4. Fink A, Hays RD, Moore AA, Beck JC. Alcohol-related problems in older persons. *Arch Intern Med* 1996; **156**: 1150–6.
5. American Psychiatric Association. *Diagnostic and Statistical Manual of Mental Disorders*, 4th edn. Washington, DC: APA, 1994.
6. Taeuber C. Sixty-five plus in America. In *Current Population Reports*. Series P-23, No. 178. Washington, DC: US Government Printing Office, 1992.
7. Widner S, Zeichner A. Alcohol abuse in the elderly. *Clin Gerontol* 1991; **11**: 3–18.
8. Gurnack AM, Hoffman NG. Elderly alcohol misuse. *Int J Addict* 1992; **27**: 869–78.
9. Liberto JG, Oslin DW, Ruskin PE. Alcoholism in older persons: a review of the literature. *Hosp Comm Psychiat* 1992; **43**: 975–84.
10. Bode M, Haupt M. Alcoholism in the elderly. A review of diagnosis, therapy and psychological effects. *Fortschr Neurol Psychiat* 1998; **66**: 450–8.
11. Adams WL, Barry KL, Fleming MF. Screening for problem drinking in older primary care patients. *J Am Med Assoc* 1996; **276**: 1964–7.
12. Vestal RE, McGuire EA, Tobin JD *et al*. Aging and ethanol metabolism. *Clin Pharmacol Ther* 1977; **21**: 343–54.
13. Dufour MC, Archer L, Gordis E. Alcohol and the elderly. *Clin Geriat Med* 1992; **8**: 127–41.
14. Ozdemir V, Fourie J, Busto U, Naranjo CA. Pharmacokinetic changes in the elderly. Do they contribute to drug abuse and dependence? *Clin Pharmacokinet* 1996; **31**: 372–85.
15. Davies BT, Bowen CK. Total body water and peak alcohol concentration: a comparative study of young, middle-age, and older females. *Alcohol Clin Exp Res* 1999; **23**: 969–75.
16. Adams WL. Alcohol and the health of aging men. *Med Clin N Am* 1999; **83**: 1195–211.
17. Moore AA, Morton SC, Beck JC *et al*. A new paradigm for alcohol use in older persons. *Med Care* 1999; **37**: 165–79.
18. Smith DM, Atkinson RM. Alcoholism and dementia. *Int J Addict* 1995; **30**: 1843–69.
19. Akiyama H, Meyer JS, Mortel KF *et al*. Normal human aging: factors contributing to cerebral atrophy. *J Neurol Sci* 1997; **152**: 39–49.
20. Neiman J. Alcohol as a risk factor for brain damage: neurologic aspects. *Alcohol Clin Exp Res* 1998; **22**(7 suppl): 346–51S.

21. Oslin D, Atkinson RM, Smith DM, Hendrie H. Alcohol-related dementia: proposed clinical criteria. *Int J Geriat Psychiat* 1998; **13**: 203–12.
22. Bikle DD, Stesin A, Halloran B *et al*. Alcohol-induced bone disease: relationship to age and parathyroid hormone levels. *Alcohol Clin Exp Res* 1993; **17**: 690–5.
23. Oscar-Berman M, Bonner RT. Matching and delayed matching to sample performance as measures of visual processing, selective attention, and memory in aging and alcoholic individuals. *Neuropsychologia* 1985; **23**: 639–51.
24. Oscar-Berman M, Hutner N, Bonner RT. Visual and auditory spatial and nonspatial delayed-response reformance by Korsakoff and non-Korsakoff alcoholic and aging individuals. *Behav Neurosci* 1992; **106**: 613–22.
25. Oscar-Berman M. A comparative neuropsychological approach to alcoholism and the brain. *Alcohol Alcoholism* 1994; **2**(suppl): 281–9.
26. DeFranco C, Tarbox AR, McLaughlin EJ. Cognitive deficits as a function of years of alcohol abuse. *Am J Drug Alcohol Abuse* 1985; **11**: 279–93.
27. Oscar-Berman M, Ellis RJ. Cognitive deficits related to memory impairments in alcoholism. *Recent Dev Alcohol* 1987; **5**: 59–80.
28. Bergman H, Borg S, Hindmarsh T *et al*. Computed tomography of the brain and neuropsychological assessment of male alcoholic patients and a random sample from the general male population. *Acta Psychiatr Scand* 1980; **286**(suppl): 77–88.
29. Pfefferbaum A, Sullivan EV, Rosenbloom MJ *et al*. Increase in brain cerebrospinal fluid volume is greater in older than in younger alcoholic patients: a replication study and CT/MRI comparison. *Psychiat Res* 1993; **50**: 257–74.
30. Holden KL, McLaughlin EJ, Reilly EL, Overall JE. Accelerated mental aging in alcoholic patients. *J Clin Psychol* 1988; **44**: 286–92.
31. Piano MR, Schwertz DW. Alcoholic heart disease: a review. *Heart Lung* 1994; **23**: 3–17.
32. Fletcher A, Bulpitt C. Epidemiology of hypertension in the elderly. *J Hypertens* 1994; **12**(suppl): S3–5.
33. Butterworth RF. Pathophysiology of alcoholic brain damage: synergistic effects of ethanol, thiamine deficiency and alcoholic liver disease. *Metab Brain Dis* 1995; **10**: 1–8.
34. Lieber CS. Medical disorders of alcoholism. *N Engl J Med* 1995; **333**: 1058–65.
35. Felson DT, Zhang Y, Hannan MT *et al*. Alcohol intake and bone mineral density in elderly men and women. The Framingham Study. *Am J Epidemiol* 1995; **142**: 485–92.
36. Patel VB, Why HJ, Richardson PJ, Preedy VR. The effects of alcohol on the heart. *Adverse Drug React Toxicol Rev* 1997; **16**: 15–43.
37. Adams WL. Interactions between alcohol and other drugs. *Int J Addict* 1995; **30**: 1903–23.
38. Adams WL. Potential for adverse drug-alcohol interactions among retirement community residents. *J Am Geriat Soc* 1995; **43**: 1021–5.
39. Basen MM. The elderly and drugs: problem overview and program strategy. *Publ Health Rep* 1977; **92**: 43–8.
40. Abrams RC, Alexopoulos GS. Substance abuse in the elderly: alcohol and prescription drugs. *Hosp Comm Psychiat* 1987; **38**: 1285–7.
41. Chrischilles EA, Foley DJ, Wallace RB *et al*. Use of medications by persons 65 and over: data from the established populations for epidemiologic studies of the elderly. *J Gerontol* 1992; **47**: M137–44.
42. Saunders PA, Copeland JR, Dewey ME *et al*. Heavy drinking as a risk factor for depression and dementia in elderly men. *Br J Psychiat* 1991; **159**: 213–16.
43. Gomberg ES. Older women and alcohol: use and abuse. *Recent Dev Alcohol* 1995; **12**: 61–79.
44. Neubauer DN. Sleep problems in the elderly. *Am Fam Physician* 1999; **59**: 2551–60.
45. Gambert SR. Alcohol abuse: medical effects of heavy drinking in late life. *Geriatrics* 1997; **52**: 30–7.
46. Lieber CS. Hepatic and other medical disorders of alcoholism: from pathogenesis to treatment. *J Stud Alcohol* 1998; **59**: 9–25.
47. Steensberg J. Epidemiology of accidental drowning in Denmark. *Accident Anal Prevent* 1998; **30**: 755–62.
48. Black BS, Rabins PV, McGuire MH. Alcohol use disorder is a risk factor for mortality among older public housing residents. *Int Psychogeriat* 1998; **10**: 309–27.

49. Sacco RL, Elkind M, Boden-Albala B *et al*. The protective effect of moderate alcohol consumption on ischemic stroke. *J Am Med Assoc* 1999; **281**: 53–60.

50. Simons LA, McCallum J, Friedlander Y, Simons J. Alcohol intake and survival in the elderly: a 77 month follow-up in the Dubbo study. *Aust NZ J Med* 1996; **26**: 662–70.

51. Ekerdt DJ, DeLabry LO, Glynn RJ, Davis RW. Change in drinking behaviors with retirement: findings from the normative aging study. *J Stud Alcohol* 1989; **50**: 347–53.

52. Welte JW, Mirand AL. Drinking, problem drinking and life stressors in the elderly general population. *J Stud Alcohol* 1995; **56**: 67–73.

53. Schonfeld LS, Dupree LW. Antecedents of drinking for early- and late-life onset elderly alcohol abusers. *J Stud Alcohol* 1991; **52**: 587–92.

54. Liberto JG, Oslin DW. Early vs. late onset of alcoholism in the elderly. *Int J Addict* 1995; **30**: 1799–818.

55. Beresford TP, Blow FC, Brower KJ *et al*. Alcoholism and aging in the general hospital. *Psychosomatics* 1988; **29**: 61–72.

56. Liskow BI, Rindk C, Campbell J, DeSouza C. Alcohol withdrawal in the elderly. *J Stud Alcohol* 1989; **50**: 414–21.

57. Graham K. Identifying and measuring alcohol abuse among the elderly: serious problems with existing instrumentation. *J Stud Alcohol* 1986; **47**: 322–6.

58. Jones TV, Lindsey BA, Yount P *et al*. Alcoholism screening questionnaires: are they valid in elderly medical outpatients? *J Gen Intern Med* 1993; **8**: 674–8.

59. Morton JL, Jones TV, Manganaro MA. Performance of alcohol screening questionnaires in elderly veterans. *Am J Med* 1996; **101**: 153–9.

60. Buchsbaum DG, Buchanan RG, Welsh J *et al*. Screening for drinking disorders in the elderly using the CAGE questionnaire. *J Am Geriat Soc* 1992; **40**: 662–5.

61. Blow FC. Michigan Alcoholism Screening Test-Geriatric Version (MAST-G): a new elderly specific screening instrument. Presented at the 38th Annual Meeting of the American Society on Aging, 15 March 1992, San Diego, CA.

62. Willenbring ML, Christensen KJ, Spring WD, Rasmussen R. Alcoholism screening in the elderly. *J Am Geriat Soc* 1987; **35**: 864–9.

63. Brower KJ, Mudd S, Blow FC *et al*. Severity and treatment of alcohol withdrawal in elderly vs. younger patients. *Alcohol Clin Exp Res* 1994; **18**: 196–201.

64. Kraemer KL, Conigliaro J, Saitz R. Managing alcohol withdrawal in the elderly. *Drugs Aging* 1999; **14**: 409–25.

65. Kofoed LL, Tolson RL, Atkinson RM *et al*. Treatment compliance of older alcoholics: an elder specific approach is superior to "mainstreaming". *J Stud Alcohol* 1987; **48**: 47–51.

66. Oslin D, Liberto JG, O'Brien J *et al*. Naltrexone as an adjunctive treatment for older patients with alcohol dependence. *Am J Geriat Psychiat* 1997; **5**: 324–32.

67. Chick J. Safety issues concerning the use of disulfiram in treating alcohol dependence. *Drug Safety* 1999; **20**: 427–35.

68. Swift RM. Drug therapy for alcohol dependence. *N Engl J Med* 1999; **340**: 1482–90.

Epidemiology of Alcohol Problems and Drinking Patterns

Celia F. Hybels and Dan G. Blazer

Duke University Medical Center, Durham, NC, USA

A key finding from the Epidemiologic Catchment Area (ECA) community studies of adults 18 or older conducted in the USA two decades ago was the high prevalence of alcohol use and dependence, as defined by DSM-III criteria[1,2]. The lifetime prevalence of alcohol abuse/dependence in the ECA sample was 13.8%. Gender differences were significant. Among men, the lifetime prevalence was 23.8%, while among women the prevalence was only 4.6%. Age differences in lifetime prevalence were noted for both males and females. The lifetime prevalence of alcohol abuse/dependence for men in the ECA was lowest in those 65 or older (14%) compared to 21% in those ages 45–64, 28% in those ages 30–44 and 27% in those ages 18–29. The 1 month prevalence among men 65 or older was 1.93%. A similar decreasing prevalence with age was seen in women, with a lifetime prevalence of 1.49% in women 65 or older and a 1 month prevalence of less than 1% (0.4%).

While the proportion of elderly with defined alcohol abuse or dependence may appear low, alcohol consumption at any level may potentially be problematic in older adults. Because of decreased lean body mass and smaller volume of distribution, higher peak ethanol concentrations per dose are found in older compared to younger subjects[3]. Also, even in small amounts, alcohol may exacerbate or mask symptoms of illness. Finally, many elderly are users of both prescription and over-the-counter medications that may interact with alcohol[4]. As the numbers of elderly will increase significantly over the next several decades (as the post-World War II generation ages) and alcohol use rates are not likely to decrease, alcohol use in older adults is an important public health concern. In addition, females are increasing their rate of alcohol use and make up a larger proportion of the elderly, potentially resulting in increased prevalence overall[5].

Recent reviews have focused on the epidemiology of alcohol use among older adults[6–11]. These reviewers have concluded that alcohol use in older adults in excess of recommended limits is an important clinical issue. Chermack *et al.*[12] examined the relationship between alcohol consumption patterns and the presence of DSM-III-R alcohol symptoms among 443 current drinkers, 55 years of age or older, and found that both average daily consumption and days of heavy drinking in the past year independently predicted symptom status. Consumption levels for men and women were only different for problem drinkers. The authors suggest that their results support the recommendation that moderate consumption levels should be lower for older than for younger adults, with a recommendation not to exceed one drink/day.

The prevalence of any alcohol use and the prevalence of heavy drinking among elders, as well as the factors and outcomes associated with drinking, are addressed below.

PREVALENCE OF ALCOHOL USE

The prevalence of alcohol use has been shown in cross-sectional studies to decline with age[13–17]. Early studies in the USA noted this age difference[13,14]. In 1968, Cahalan and Cisin[13] conducted a national survey of drinking practices in the USA using a representative sample of 2746 persons aged 21 +, and reported the prevalence of alcohol use declined with age. Among adults aged 60 +, 65% of the males and 44% of the females drank alcohol within the past year. The prevalence was lower than that observed in younger males (84% in men aged 21–29 and 86% in men 30–39) and in younger females (70% in women 21–29 and 72% in women 30–39). In a probability study of adults living in western New York, conducted 25 years ago, the prevalence of alcohol use was lower in persons aged 60 or older than in those under 60, and the proportion of adults with alcohol-related problems was much less in those 60 +. The proportion of moderate and heavy drinkers was also lower among those aged 60 + than in those younger. Only 7% of those aged 60 + were heavy drinkers, compared to 24% of those aged 50–59 and 30% of those aged 18–49[14].

Recent studies have confirmed these earlier findings. The prevalence of alcohol use in the past year among persons aged 55 + participating in the National Longitudinal Alcohol Epidemiologic Survey was 29.5%, and there was an inverse relationship between alcohol use and increasing age[15]. In the 1988 Alcohol Supplement of the National Health Interview Survey (NHIS), the prevalence of alcohol use, defined as 12 or more drinks in the past year, was 60.9% in those aged 18–29, 58.3% in those 30–44, 47.3% in those 45–64 and 30.4% in those 65 +. The prevalence of lifetime abstainers in those aged 65 + was 30.8%, compared to only 17.9% in those 45–64 and 13.1% in those 30–44. The prevalence of lifetime infrequent drinking and former drinking also increased with age[16]. Ruchlin used data from the 1990 Health Promotion and Disease Prevention supplement to the National Health Interview Survey to examine prevalence of alcohol consumption in adults aged 55 +. A total of 46% reported that they had consumed alcohol during the past year. The study found a continuous decline across age groups, from 52.9% of those aged 55–64 categorized as current drinkers within the past year, compared to 24.7% of those aged 85 +. Of the sample aged

Principles and Practice of Geriatric Psychiatry, 2nd edn. Edited by J. R. M. Copeland, M. T. Abou-Saleh and D. G. Blazer

55+, 17% reported that they had consumed alcohol every day in the past 2 weeks. In controlled regression analyses, more people aged 65–74 drank every day, compared to those 55–64 (OR = 1.36), but people aged 75+ drank less than those 55–64. Males and Whites used alcohol more frequently and were more likely to be heavy drinkers than females and non-Whites. The lower one's perceived health status, the lower the odds of drinking every day. Believing excessive drinking increases the chances of getting cirrhosis of the liver decreased the odds of moderate and heavy drinking[17].

There are various explanations why the prevalence of alcohol use is lower in the elderly. Selective survival may be a factor, in that persons who drink are less likely to survive to older ages. Cohort effects are also possible. Persons who grew up in the era of Prohibition and economic depression prior to World War II may have had lower alcohol use throughout their lives[5]. Studies have also shown that some elderly decrease their use of alcohol as they grow older. Barnes found half of the subjects aged 60+ who were current abstainers reported that they were former drinkers, with "bad health" most often given as a reason for giving up drinking[14]. Busby et al.[18] investigated alcohol use in a community-based sample of adults aged 70+ in New Zealand. Both frequency and quantity of intake decreased with age. A total of 60.1% of the men and 30.3% of the women said they drank less compared to middle age, and only 7.4% of the men and 11.1% of the women said they drank more. The main reasons cited for decreased use of alcohol were change in health and fewer social opportunities, with reasons cited for increased intake being more time and money[18]. Similarly, a significant proportion of male current drinkers, but not abusers, selected from medical admissions aged 65+ in the UK reported heavier drinking in the past. The most frequent reasons given for reduction in intake were onset of ill-health (36%), loss of social contact (28%) and financial difficulties (19%)[19].

Using data from the Normative Aging Study, Glynn et al.[20] studied generational effects on alcohol consumption in a sample of 1859 male adult volunteers interviewed at baseline and 9 years later. Older men drank less than younger men at both assessments, yet there was no tendency for men to decrease their consumption levels over time. Each older cohort had a lower prevalence of problems with drinking than the next youngest cohort. The authors suggested that their results show that aging is not as important as generational changes in prevalence[20]. In contrast, Adams et al. followed a cohort of 270 healthy community-dwelling elderly aged 60+ over 7 years[21]. At baseline, the investigators found a decline in the percentage of drinkers with increasing age[22]. In the 7 year follow-up, there was a 2%/year decline in the percentage of subjects consuming any alcohol, but mean alcohol intake did not change for those who continued to drink, except among heavy drinkers, suggesting an age-related decline rather than a cohort effect[21]. Smart and Adlaf[23] pooled data from four cross-sectional surveys of adults in Ontario and found no dramatic changes in alcohol use between 1976 and 1984 among persons aged 60+. Elderly respondents were more likely to report abstention from drinking than those younger (40% of those aged 60+ compared to 15% of those 30–59 and 13% of those 18–29). Of the elderly respondents, 17% reported consuming five or more drinks in a single sitting, a much lower prevalence than among those 30–59 (44%) and those 18–29 (60%)[23].

Regardless of a decline with age, the prevalence of alcohol use in the elderly remains high. Meyers et al. found, in their study of the drinking behavior of 928 residents of Boston aged 60+, that 53% were abstainers, 26% had less than one drink/day, 16% one to two drinks/day and 6% two or more drinks/day[24]. In a sample of 270 healthy men and women aged 65–89 living in the southwestern USA, 48% of the participants reported in their 3 day diet record they had consumed alcohol, with 66% reporting that they consumed alcohol at least monthly[22].

The prevalence of alcohol use in the recently conducted multi-site Established Populations for Epidemiologic Studies of the Elderly (EPESE) studies of persons aged 65+ varied by site. In East Boston, 70.5% of the sample drank alcohol in the past year and 54.7% had used alcohol in the past month. Similar findings were reported from New Haven; 65.8% had used alcohol in the past year and 51.9% in the past month. The proportions were lower in Iowa and North Carolina. In the Iowa sample, 46.3% had used alcohol in the past year, while 31.2% had done so in the past month. In the North Carolina EPESE, 33.4% had used alcohol in the past year and 24.6% in the past month. Men were more likely to report use of alcohol in the past month than were women[25,26].

Samples from clinical populations have found similar proportions of high use. In one of the first studies done in the UK, Bridgewater et al. interviewed 101 patients aged 60+ from a general practice and found that 92% of the men and 77% of the women used alcohol[27]. Iliffe et al. studied 241 patients from general practice aged 75+ and found that 51% of the men and 22% of the women reporting using alcohol in the past 3 months[28]. Using data from the Liverpool Longitudinal Study of Continuing Health in the Community, Saunders et al.[29] reported, among 1070 men and women aged 65+ randomly selected from patient rosters, that 10.5% admitted to drinking more or less every day (17.7% men and 6.1% women). At the 3 year follow-up, one-fifth of the subjects were regular drinkers, drinking on at least one occasion per week[29]. Among a sample of 132 general hospital patients aged 65+ in Leiden, The Netherlands, the prevalence of alcoholism was 9% (13% among men and 7% among women)[30]. Callahan and Tierney[31] found the prevalence of alcoholism to be 10.6% among 3954 primary care patients aged 60+. Patients with alcoholism were more likely to be younger, have fewer years of education, and be male, Black, smokers and malnourished[31]. In a sample of 539 medical admissions aged 65+ in the UK, the prevalence of alcohol abuse was 7.8%. An additional 29.7% of the sample who were neither abstainers nor occasional drinkers nor alcohol abusers drank regularly; 42.9% of the men and 15.9% of the women[19].

In summary, research studies conducted in both community and clinical samples over the last several decades have consistently shown that alcohol use among older adults is not uncommon, and that over half of community-dwelling older males may consume alcohol on a regular basis. While the prevalence of use may be lower than that seen in younger populations, it is still not clear whether this is a cohort or an age effect.

PREVALENCE OF HEAVY DRINKING

Estimates of the prevalence of heavy use are also quite high in the elderly. Cahalan and Cisin reported from their community sample that 20% of the males and 2% of the females aged 60+ were classified as heavy drinkers[13]. Meyers et al.[24] found in their sample of Boston residents 60 or older that 1% were self-reported problem drinkers. All problem drinkers had long-term drinking problems and were less likely to be satisfied with their social relationships. While the proportion of problem drinkers was lower in those aged 75+ compared to those aged 60–75, the proportion of drinkers who report problems was similar for both groups[24]. Mirand and Welte studied a sample of community-dwelling adults aged 60+ in Erie County, New York, and found the prevalence of heavy drinking was 6%[32]. In their sample of 270 healthy male and female volunteers aged 65+, Goodwin et al. found that 17% drank more than 30 g alcohol/day on average[22]. In the EPESE, the percentage of persons who drank two or more ounces of absolute alcohol/day was 8.4% in East Boston, 6.6% in New Haven, 5.4% in Iowa, and 7.2% in North Carolina[25,26].

The prevalence of heavy drinking in clinical samples is similar. Adams et al. screened 5065 patients aged 60+ seen in primary care and found 15% of the men and 12% of the women regularly drank in excess of recommended limits; 9% of the men and 2% of the women reported regularly consuming more than 21 drinks per week[33]. Bridgewater et al. reported that the prevalence of heavy drinking was 27% in men and 9% in women in their sample of 101 patients from general practice[27]. In their Liverpool study, Saunders et al. found a total of 6.1% of the men and 2.4% of the year 3 subjects regularly exceeded safe consumption limits. These figures translate into 19.5% of the men and 19.6% of the women being regular drinkers who were exceeding sensible limits. They observed a decline with age in the proportion of subjects who were regular drinkers[29]. Bristow and Clare interviewed 650 medical and geriatric admissions over 65 and found 9% of the men but few (0%) of the females drank in excess of recommended safety limits. Another 10% had cut down, primarily because of medical reasons. Compared to the non-drinkers and light drinkers, the heavy drinkers were more likely to smoke, not to be married, and to have some impairment of mobility[34]. Iliffe et al. found 3.6% of the men in their sample and 3.2% of the women admitted consuming more than 21 and 14 units of alcohol per week, amounts in excess of recommended safe limits for males and females. Neither drinking status nor total weekly alcohol consumption was associated with age, cognitive impairment, depression, falls or inpatient or outpatient care[28].

Although the overall prevalence is low, heavy drinking among older adults is of much concern, with perhaps as much as 20% of users drinking in excess of recommended limits.

IDENTIFICATION OF PROBLEM DRINKING IN THE ELDERLY

Physicians may have difficulty recognizing alcoholism in elderly subjects. First, screening instruments used in younger populations may not be reliable for older adults. Adams et al. compared responses to a beverage-specific self-administered questionnaire about the quantity and frequency of alcohol use and episodes of binge drinking to the widely used CAGE questionnaire (Cut down, Annoyed by criticism, Guilty about drinking, Eye-opener drinks)[35] in 5065 primary care patients aged 60+ and found the CAGE performed poorly in detecting heavy or binge drinkers[33]. Lutrell et al. similarly concluded the sensitivity of standardized screening instruments was low in patients aged 65+ admitted as emergencies[36]. In addition, many of these screening instruments inquire about frequency and quantity of alcohol use. Many elderly may drink daily but in smaller amounts. These small quantities, however, may cause problems because of interactions with medications and chronic illness[4].

Second, criteria for alcoholism often include problems with social and/or occupational functioning. However, many older adults are less likely to be married or employed, and therefore less likely to report marital or job problems. Older drinkers may be more likely to maintain a "low profile" and not cause public disturbances resulting in legal problems[5].

Finally, physicians may fail to diagnose alcoholism in the elderly, perhaps because they often fail to obtain alcohol histories[37] or because they confuse perceived symptoms of aging with symptoms of alcoholism[5]. Curtis et al. screened all new admissions to the medical service at the Johns Hopkins Hospital for alcoholism using the CAGE[35] and the Short Michigan Alcohol Screening Test (SMAST)[38]. The prevalence of alcoholism was 27% in patients under age 60 and 21% in patients 60+. These age differences were not significant. However, 60% of screen-positive younger patients were identified as having alcoholism by their house officers, compared to only 37% of those aged 60+. Elderly patients with alcoholism were less likely to be diagnosed if they were White, female or had completed high school[39].

In a similar study, Adams et al. screened patients aged 65+ who came to the emergency department for alcoholism. Using their criteria of either CAGE-positive or self-reported drinking problem and alcohol use within the past year, they found the current prevalence of alcohol abuse was 14%, with a high prevalence (22%) among those presenting with gastrointestinal problems. Physicians, however, detected only 21% of current alcohol abusers[40]. In a study conducted in The Netherlands, scores on the Dutch version of the Munich Alcoholism Test[41] and medical records were obtained from 132 patients aged 65+ staying at University Hospital Leiden. Two-thirds of the alcoholic patients were recognized by the attending physician[30]. Finally, medical staff identified only 33 of 99 problem drinkers among inpatients aged 65+ in three hospitals in New South Wales[42].

These studies consistently show that older problem drinkers may be more difficult to identify as a result of poor screening instruments, failure of clinicians to consider problem drinking as a possible contributing diagnosis, and difficulty in separating problems caused by alcohol from those caused by other diseases.

FACTORS ASSOCIATED WITH ALCOHOL USE IN THE ELDERLY

Among the elderly, alcohol use has been shown to be associated with male gender[17,22,31–33,43], higher income[22], more education[22,33], lower socioeconomic status[32], being married[33] and current or former smoking[32–34]. Other studies have found alcohol use associated with less education[31]. Goodwin et al. found no differences in social support between elderly drinkers and non-drinkers and no relationship between alcohol intake and emotional status[22].

Two factors often associated with alcoholism in late life are depression and impairments in cognitive functioning. Saunders et al., using data from their Liverpool study, reported 44% of men 65 or older with a history of heavy drinking were given current psychiatric diagnoses, compared with 12% of the men without a history of heavy drinking. The most common diagnoses were depression and dementia. The association between drinking history and current psychiatric morbidity was not explained by current drinking habits[44]. Finlayson et al.[45] studied 216 patients aged 65+ admitted to the hospital for treatment of alcoholism. Patients with late-onset alcoholism (aged 60+) reported a higher frequency of life events associated with problem drinking compared to those with earlier onset. The most common co-morbid psychiatric disorders were tobacco dependence (67%), organic brain syndrome (25%), atypical or mixed organic brain syndrome (19%) and affective disorder (12%); 14% of the patients had a drug abuse or dependence problem, all using legally prescribed drugs[45]. Similarly, Speckens et al. found that alcoholics used more psychotropic drugs compared to non-alcoholics and suffered more often from organic brain disease[30].

Iliffe et al., however, found among patients aged 75+ that current drinking was not related to age, depression or mental status score[28]. Goodwin et al. found that those elderly who consumed alcohol performed better on the cognitive functioning tests, but no relationship was found between past alcohol consumption and present cognitive performance. The authors concluded that alcohol may not impair cognitive functioning in the elderly[22]. In a study of adults aged 70–75 in Italy, self-reported alcohol consumption was associated with male gender, better mood, less cognitive and functional impairment, better health, not living alone and being married, while CAGE-positive alcoholism was associated with male gender, poorer cognitive function and income dissatisfaction. The groups did not overlap much, suggesting some positive aspects of alcohol use, and that self-reported consumption (they used the top 10% of quantity) may not necessarily be associated with alcoholism[46].

Mangion et al. found that men aged 65+ classified as alcohol abusers were more independently mobile than those not abusing alcohol, suggesting greater physical fitness[19]. Bristow and Clare, however, found that in an elderly inpatient sample, drinking in excess was associated with impairment in mobility[34].

Mirand and Welte studied the relationship between health-orientated lifestyle and heavy drinking among the elderly in Erie County, New York, and reported that the prevalence of heavy drinking was 6%. Heavy drinking was positively associated with being male, having suburban residency and currently smoking, and negatively associated with SES, rural residency and degree of health orientation. Age and level of active lifestyle were not related to drinking[32].

Molgaard et al. found racial differences among 65+ subjects in drinking level, both before and after age 40. Among Whites, 73.8% reported drinking after age 40, compared to 48.6% of Blacks and 44.3% of Mexican-Americans. A higher proportion of Whites than Blacks or Mexican-Americans reported more minimal drinking before and after age 40. However, there were no statistically significant differences for severe drinking among the groups[47].

ONSET OF PROBLEM DRINKING IN THE ELDERLY

Recent research has focused on the age-of-onset among elderly problem drinkers. Specifically, in several studies two groups have emerged. First, there are elderly who have had problems with alcohol most of their adult life and have survived to old age, generally referred to as "early-onset problem drinkers". There are also elderly who may or may not have consumed alcohol earlier in their lives, but who do not become problem drinkers until later in their adult life. This group is generally referred to as late-onset problem drinkers and the incidence of problem drinking has been hypothesized to be a result of a stressor.

Atkinson et al. studied the age of onset among 132 60+ men admitted into an outpatient treatment program and found onset after age 60 in 15% of the sample and in 29% of the sample aged 65+. Later-onset alcohol problems were milder and associated with greater psychological stability. Treatment variables were better predictors of treatment outcome than age of onset[48].

Brennen and Moos reported that late middle-aged problem drinkers reported more negative life events, chronic stressors, and social resource deficits than did non-problem drinkers[49]. However, in their same population, Brennen and Moos[50] studied men and women aged 55–65 and compared age-related loss events, overall negative life events and chronic stressors reported by late-onset, early-onset and non-problem drinkers. Late-onset problem drinkers consumed less alcohol than early-onset ones, reported fewer alcohol-related problems, functioned better, and had fewer stressors than early-onset drinkers. They did not find evidence for an association between age-related loss events and the onset of late-life drinking patterns. Similarly, Barnes found that neither widowhood nor retirement was related to heavy drinking. Heavy drinking was twice as prevalent among those subjects aged 60+ who were employed compared to unemployed[14].

Brennen et al.[51] found gender differences among late-middle-aged and older problem drinkers. Specifically, women with drinking problems consumed less alcohol, had fewer drinking problems, and reported more recent onset of drinking problems than did male problem drinkers. The female problem drinkers also used more psychoactive medications, were more depressed

and were less likely to seek treatment. Osterling and Berglund studied gender differences in first-time admitted alcoholics aged 60+ to a treatment center in Sweden and found that age of onset of problem drinking occurred significantly later in females compared to males. During the period 1988–1992, sex ratios indicated a significant convergence of female patients compared with a decade earlier. The authors make it clear that it is not known whether this represents an increase in problem drinking in elderly females, or whether females feel more free to seek treatment than a decade earlier[52]. Hurt et al.[53] studied 216 patients aged 65+ admitted to an alcoholism treatment program. Early-onset alcoholism was present in 59% of the men and 51% of the women, while late-onset alcoholism was present in 39% of the men and 46% of the women (time of onset was not available for 2%). Few differences were noted between the two groups[53].

Moos et al.[54] followed their cohort of problem drinkers aged 55–65 for 1 year. Remitted problem drinkers were those who did not experience any problems in the 1 year follow-up period. At baseline, the to-be-remitted problem drinkers consumed less alcohol, reported fewer drinking problems, had friends who approved less of their drinking, and were likely to seek help from mental health practitioners. In addition, late-onset problem drinkers were more likely to remit over the 1 year period.

OUTCOMES ASSOCIATED WITH PROBLEM DRINKING IN THE ELDERLY

Some medical disorders have been found to be more prevalent in elderly with a history of alcohol use or current use. Hurt et al.[53] described 216 elderly patients aged 65+ treated for alcoholism in an inpatient treatment program. The frequency of serious medical disorders among this group was higher than what would be expected for the overall population aged 65+. Hypertension was less frequent among these patients, while alcoholic liver disease, chronic obstructive pulmonary disease, peptic ulcer disease and psoriasis were more prevalent among the alcoholic group. The frequencies of ischemic heart disease, cerebrovascular disease and diabetes mellitus were about the same as would be found in the general elderly population[53]. Bristow and Clare found, in their inpatient sample, that excess drinking was associated with more non-malignant respiratory disease and less ischemic heart disease[34].

Increased hospitalizations have also been linked with alcohol use in the elderly. Callahan and Tierney reported from their sample of patients aged 60+ that patients with alcoholism were more likely to be hospitalized (21.5% vs. 16.9%) ($p = 0.02$) within the year following the interview, compared to those without alcoholism[31]. Using 1989 hospital claims data, the prevalence of alcohol-related hospitalizations among people aged 65+ in the USA was 54.7 per 10 000 population for men and 14.8 per 10 000 for women, a proportion of hospitalizations among the elderly similar to that seen for myocardial infarction[55].

Alcoholism has also been linked with mortality in the elderly. Callahan and Tierney found in their sample of elderly patients that those with alcoholism were more likely to die within 2 years than those without evidence of alcoholism, 10.6% compared to 6.3% ($p = 0.001$), controlling for age, gender, race, education and smoking history[31]. In their study of inpatients treated for alcoholism, Hurt et al. followed 60 of their patients for an average of 5.2 years (range 2–11 years). A total of 32% of the alcoholic patients had died by follow-up. Of those who died, 47% of the deaths could be attributed to the patient's alcoholism[53]. Colsher and Wallace, using data from the Iowa 65+ Rural Health Study, found that 10.4% of the men had self-reported histories of having been previously heavier drinkers. Three-year mortality was higher among this group, compared to those men without a history of heavy drinking[56]. Mellstrom *et al.* examined a cohort of 468 70-year-old Swedish men in 1971–1972, and reinterviewed them 5 years post-baseline (1976–1977) ($n = 342$) when they were 75 years old. In addition, they interviewed a control group of 70-year-old men in 1976–1977. Registration at the Temperance Board (recidivists) was used to measure previous alcohol abuse or large-scale consumption. Morbidity from diabetes and chronic bronchitis was higher in the recidivists, as was the overall 5 year mortality rate. Impaired functioning and a high consumption of institutional care were also more frequent among the recidivists[57].

Other researchers have also found impairments in functioning in those elderly with a history of alcohol use. Colsher and Wallace found that men with a history of heavy drinking had more illness, poorer self-perceived health, more physician visits, more depressive symptoms, lower levels of life satisfaction and smaller social networks compared to non-heavy drinkers and non-drinkers. The authors concluded that a history of heavy drinking was predictive of impairments in physical, psychological and social health and functioning among elderly men[56].

Some studies have found a protective effect of moderate alcohol use in the elderly. Scherr *et al.*, using the EPESE data from three sites, found that low to moderate alcohol consumption was associated with lowered 5 year total mortality as well as cardiovascular mortality in two of the sites, East Boston and New Haven. In Iowa, there were no differences in mortality by alcohol consumption. There was no association with cancer mortality found at any of the three sites. Patients with a baseline history of heart attack, stroke or cancer were excluded from their analyses[58]. LaCroix *et al.* found, by following three of the EPESE cohorts of elderly aged 65+ for 4 years, that risk of losing mobility, defined as the ability to climb up and down stairs and walk a half a mile, was associated with not consuming alcohol, compared with small to moderate amounts of alcohol consumption[59]. Galanis *et al.* recently conducted a longitudinal study of drinking and cognitive performance in elderly Japanese-American men and found lower scores on cognitive functioning tests in non-drinkers and heavy drinkers (more than 60 ounces of alcohol/month). Compared with non-drinkers, the risk of a lower score (more errors) on a cognitive functioning test was lowered by 22–40% among men who consumed 1–60 ounces of alcohol/month[60].

Finally, in a sample of 216 inpatients treated for alcoholism, the treatment outcome was favorable (i.e. the patient was either abstinent since treatment or abstinent with three or fewer minor slips) for 28% of the cohort of 60 patients, showing that the elderly alcoholic can be successfully treated[53].

SUMMARY

In summary, alcohol use, including drinking in excess, among older adults is prevalent, particularly among males. Because of interactions with chronic disease and use of prescribed medications, the use of alcohol among elderly individuals is an important health concern. Based on current use, the prevalence of alcohol use in future generations may be even higher. Screening and questioning for alcohol problems should be routine, since effective treatments are available. Drinking within recommended guidelines could potentially affect the proportion of alcohol-related illness, hospitalizations and mortality seen in the population.

REFERENCES

1. American Psychiatric Association. DSM-III: *Diagnostic and Statistical Manual of Mental Disorders*, 3rd edn. Washington, DC: APA, 1980.

2. Helzer JE, Burnam A, McEvoy LT. Alcohol abuse and dependence. In Robins LN, Regier DA, eds, *Psychiatric Disorders in America: The Epidemiologic Catchment Area Study*. New York: Macmillan, 1991: 81–115.

3. Vestal RE, McGuire EA, Tobin JD *et al.* Aging and ethanol metabolism. *Clin Pharmacol Ther* 1977; **21**: 343–54.

4. Schuckit MA, Pastor PA. The elderly as a unique population: alcoholism. *Alcohol Clin Exp Res* 1978; **2**: 31–8.

5. Blazer DG, Pennybacker MR. Epidemiology of alcoholism in the elderly. In Hartford JT, Samorajski T, eds, *Alcoholism in the Elderly*. New York: Raven, 1984: 25–33.

6. Adams WL, Cox NS. Epidemiology of problem drinking among elderly people. *Int J Addict* 1995; **30**: 1693–716.

7. Crome IB. Alcohol problems in the older person. *J R Soc Med* 1997; **90**: 16–22.

8. Dufour M, Fuller RK. Alcohol in the elderly. *Ann Rev Med* 1995; **46**: 123–32.

9. Johnson I. Alcohol problems in old age: a review of recent epidemiologic research. *Int J Geriat Psychiat* 2000; **15**: 575–81.

10. Lakhani N. Alcohol use amongst community-dwelling elderly people: a review of the literature. *J Adv Nurs* 1997; **25**: 1227–232.

11. Liberto JG, Oslin DW, Ruskin PE. Alcoholism in older persons: a review of the literature. *Hosp Commun Psychiat* 1992; **43**: 975–84.

12. Chermack ST, Blow FC, Hill EM, Mudd SA. The relationship between alcohol symptoms and consumption among older drinkers. *Alcohol Clin Exp Res* 1996; **20**: 1153–8.

13. Cahalan D, Cisin IH. American drinking practices: summary of findings from a national probability sample. *Qu J Stud Alcohol* 1968; **29**: 130–51.

14. Barnes GM. Alcohol use among older persons: findings from a western New York State general population survey. *J Am Geriat Soc* 1979; **27**: 244–50.

15. Grant BF. Prevalence and correlates of alcohol use and DSM-IV alcohol dependence in the United States: results of the National Longitudinal Alcohol Epidemiologic Survey. *J Stud Alcohol* 1997; **58**: 464–73.

16. Grant BF. Alcohol consumption, alcohol abuse and alcohol dependence: the United States as an example. *Addiction* 1994; **89**: 1357–65.

17. Ruchlin HS. Prevalence and correlates of alcohol use among older adults. *Prevent Med* 1997; **26**: 651–7.

18. Busby WJ, Campbell AJ, Borrie MJ, Spears GFS. Alcohol use in a community-based sample of subjects aged 70 years and older. *J Am Geriat Soc* 1988; **36**: 301–5.

19. Mangion DM, Platt JS, Syam V. Alcohol and acute medical admission of elderly people. *Age Ageing* 1992; **21**: 362–7.

20. Glynn RJ, Bouchard GR, LoCastro JS, Laird NM. Aging and generational effects on drinking behaviors in men: results from the Normative Aging Study. *Am J Publ Health* 1985; **75**: 1413–19.

21. Adams WL, Garry PJ, Rhyne R *et al.* Alcohol intake in the healthy elderly: changes with age in a cross-sectional and longitudinal study. *J Am Geriat Soc* 1990; **38**: 211–16.

22. Goodwin JS, Sanchez CJ, Thomas P *et al.* Alcohol intake in a healthy elderly population. *Am J Publ Health* 1987; **77**: 173–7.

23. Smart RG, Adlaf EM. Alcohol and drug use among the elderly: trends in use and characteristics of users. *Can J Publ Health* 1988; **79**: 236–42.

24. Meyers AR, Hingson R, Mucatel M, Goldman E. Social and psychologic correlates of problem drinking in old age. *J Am Geriat Soc* 1982; **30**: 452–6.

25. Cornoni-Huntley J, Brock D, Ostfeld A *et al. Established Populations for Epidemiologic Studies of the Elderly: Resource Data Book*. Bethesda, MD: National Institute on Aging, 1986.

26. Cornoni-Huntley J, Blazer D, Lafferty M *et al. Established Populations for Epidemiologic Studies of the Elderly: Resource Data Book*. Washington, DC: National Institute on Aging, 1990.

27. Bridgewater R, Leigh S, James OFW, Potter JF. Alcohol consumption and dependence in elderly patients in an urban community. *Br Med J* 1987; **295**: 884–5.

28. Iliffe S, Haines A, Booroff A *et al.* Alcohol consumption by elderly people: a general practice survey. *Age Ageing* 1991; **20**: 120–3.

29. Saunders PA, Copeland JRM, Dewey ME *et al.* Alcohol use and abuse in the elderly: findings from the Liverpool Longitudinal Study

of Continuing Health in the Community. *Int J Geriat Psychiat* 1989; **4**: 103–8.

30. Speckens AEM, Heeren TJ, Roojmans HGM. Alcohol abuse among elderly patients in a general hospital as identified by the Munich Alcoholism Test. *Acta Psychiat Scand* 1991; **83**: 460–2.

31. Callahan CM, Tierney WM. Health services use and mortality among older primary care patients with alcoholism. *J Am Geriat Soc* 1995; **43**: 1378–83.

32. Mirand AL, Welte JW. Alcohol consumption among the elderly in a general population, Erie County, New York. *Am J Publ Health* 1996; **86**: 978–84.

33. Adams WL, Barry KL, Fleming MF. Screening for problem drinking in older primary care patients. *J Am Med Assoc* 1996; **276**: 1964–7.

34. Bristow MF, Clare AW. Prevalence and characteristics of at-risk drinkers among elderly acute medical inpatients. *Br J Addict* 1992; **87**: 291–4.

35. Mayfield D, McLeod G, Hall P. The CAGE questionnaire: validation of a new alcoholism screening instrument. *Am J Psychiat* 1974; **131**: 1121.

36. Luttrell S, Watkin V, Livingston G *et al*. Screening for alcohol misuse in older people. *Int J Geriat Psychiat* 1997; **12**: 1151–4.

37. Naik PC, Jones RG. Alcohol histories taken from elderly people on admission. *Br Med J* 1994; **308**: 248.

38. Selzer ML, Vinokur A, Rooijen L. A self-administered Short Michigan Alcoholism Screening Test (SMAST). *J Stud Alcohol* 1975; **36**: 117.

39. Curtis JR, Geller G, Stokes EJ *et al*. Characteristics, diagnosis, and treatment of alcoholism in elderly patients. *J Am Geriat Soc* 1989; **37**: 310–16.

40. Adams WL, Magruder-Habib K, Trued S, Broome HL. Alcohol abuse in elderly emergency department patients. *J Am Geriat Soc* 1992; **40**: 1236–40.

41. Feuerlein W, Ringer C, Kufner H, Antons K. Diagnosis of alcoholism: the Munich Alcoholism Test (MALT). *Curr Alcohol* 1979; **7**: 137–47.

42. McInnes E, Powell J. Drug and alcohol referrals: are elderly substance abuse diagnoses referrals being missed? *Br Med J* 1994; **308**: 444–6.

43. Graham K, Carver V, Brett PJ. Alcohol and drug use by older women: results of a national survey. *Can J Aging* 1995; **14**: 769–91.

44. Saunders PA, Copeland JRM, Dewey ME *et al*. Heavy drinking as a risk factor for depression and dementia in elderly men: findings from the Liverpool Longitudinal Community Study. *Br J Psychiat* 1991; **159**: 213–16.

45. Finlayson RE, Hurt RD, Davis LJ, Morse RM. Alcoholism in elderly persons: a study of the psychiatric and psychosocial features of 216 inpatients. *Mayo Clin Proc* 1988; **63**: 761–8.

46. Geroldi C, Rozzini R, Frisoni GB, Trabucchi M. Assessment of alcohol consumption and alcoholism in the elderly. *Alcohol* 1994; **11**: 513–16.

47. Molgaard CA, Nakamura CM, Stanford EP *et al*. Prevalence of alcohol consumption among older persons. *J Commun Health* 1990; **15**: 239–45.

48. Atkinson RM. Aging and alcohol use disorders: diagnostic issues in the elderly. *Int Psychogeriat* 1990; **2**: 55–72.

49. Brennen PL, Moos RH. Life stressors, social resources, and late-life problem drinking. *Psychol Aging* 1990; **5**: 491–501.

50. Brennen PL, Moos RH. Functioning, life context, and help-seeking among late-onset problem drinkers: comparisons with nonproblem and early-onset problem drinkers. *Br J Addict* 1991; **86**: 1139–50.

51. Brennen PL, Moos RH, Kim JY. Gender differences in the individual characteristics and life contexts of late-middle-aged and older problem drinkers. *Addiction* 1993; **88**: 781–90.

52. Osterling A, Berglund M. Elderly first time admitted alcoholics: a descriptive study on gender differences in a clinical population. *Alcohol Clin Exp Res* 1994; **18**: 1317–21.

53. Hurt RD, Finlayson RE, Morse RM, Davis LJ. Alcoholism in elderly persons: medical aspects and prognosis of 216 patients. *Mayo Clin Proc* 1988; **63**: 753–60.

54. Moos RH, Brennen PL, Moos BS. Short-term processes of remission and nonremission among late-life problem drinkers. *Alcohol Clin Exp Res* 1991; **15**: 948–55.

55. Adams WL, Yuan Z, Barboriak JJ, Rimm AA. Alcohol-related hospitalizations of elderly people: prevalence and geographic variation in the United States. *J Am Med Assoc* 1993; **270**: 1222–5.

56. Colsher PL, Wallace RB. Elderly men with histories of heavy drinking: correlates and consequences. *J Stud Alcohol* 1990; **51**: 528–35.

57. Mellstrom D, Rundgren A, Svanborg A. Previous alcohol consumption and its consequences for ageing, morbidity and mortality in men aged 70–75. *Age Ageing* 1981; **10**: 277–86.

58. Scherr PA, LaCroix AZ, Wallace RB *et al*. Light to moderate alcohol consumption and mortality in the elderly. *J Am Geriat Soc* 1992; **40**: 651–7.

59. LaCroix AZ, Guralnick JM, Berkman LF *et al*. Maintaining mobility in late life. II. Smoking, alcohol consumption, physical activity, and body mass index. *Am J Epidemiol* 1993; **137**: 858–69.

60. Galanis DJ, Joseph C, Masaki KH *et al*. A longitudinal study of drinking and cognitive performance in elderly Japanese-American men: the Honolulu–Asia Aging Study. *Am J Publ Health* 2000; **90**: 1254–9.

111

Drug Misuse in the Elderly

Paul Bown, A. H. Ghodse and M. T. Abou-Saleh

St George's Hospital Medical School, London, UK

Substance misuse occurs mainly in young adults, with most of research focusing on this group. However, increasing age brings with it multiple pathologies and polypharmacy, with the attendant risks of dependence upon medication. There is evidence to support a growing trend to increased alcohol consumption in the over-65s, especially among women, while a generation of lifetime drug users are now entering old age[1]. The need for awareness of the possibility of the existence of such a hidden disorder has never been greater in this age group. The Persian physician Avicenna described four ages of man: an age of growth, an age of prime, an age of decline and an age of decrepit old age[2]. Those aged 65+ will include individuals in any of the latter three ages. Most research in the field has examined substance misuse by those in the declining stage.

USE, ABUSE AND HARMFUL USE

When considering drug use among the elderly it is helpful to consider substances of misuse in three broad categories: medications, both prescribed and non-prescribed; socially sanctioned psychoactive substances; and illicit substances. Religious, cultural and legal differences result in the same substances, e.g. alcohol or cannabis, being differently categorized around the world. For example, alcohol may fall within each of the three categories[3]. Some of the consequences of drug misuse are determined by the status of the drug rather than the physical effects of the drug. Difficulties in obtaining a drug supply and financing that use may account for as much harm as the physical effects of the drugs themselves in younger adults. Among the elderly, drugs from the medicines category are over-represented in cases of misuse when compared to other age groups. This reflects the increased access to medicines among this group, allied to the physical and social barriers that make accessing other drugs harder for this group.

At an intuitive level the clinician may balk at categorizing patients with poor compliance with misusers of non-therapeutic drugs. The aetiology, social perception and treatment approaches of the two groups differ markedly. This chapter will focus on drug misusers who display "harmful use". This is defined as:

> A pattern of psychoactive drug use that causes damage to health, either mental or physical[8].

This definition allows consideration of individuals suffering damage as a result of drug use, irrespective of the nature or the source of the drug of abuse. It excludes cases where omission of a psychoactive medication may be harmful, e.g. in cases of underuse of antidepressants.

Harmful use may be related to a single episode of drug misuse resulting in harm, such as a fall while intoxicated. More often it is a chronic condition associated with a dependence syndrome. "Dependence syndrome" describes the cluster of cognitive, behavioural and physical phenomena that are observed when use of a substance becomes a greater priority for the individual than other previously more valued activities. It is characterized by:

- A compulsion to take the substance.
- Difficulties in controlling the substance use in terms of timing and levels of use.
- Withdrawal symptoms on discontinuation of the substance, with relief of these symptoms on reinstatement of use.
- Tolerance or neuroadaptation, where increasing amounts of the substance are required to achieve effects previously possible at lower doses.
- Progressive neglect of alternative activities, due to prioritization of drug-related behaviour.
- Persistant use of the substance in spite of evidence of harmful consequences.

Presence of three or more of the above features simultaneously in the last year supports a definite diagnosis of dependence syndrome, using World Health Organization criteria[9].

PHARMACOKINETICS

Ageing is associated with a series of physiological changes that significantly alter the fraction of an ingested drug available for a psychoactive effect. Drug absorption shows little variation with age, despite changes in gastrointestinal motility and acidity, reduced absorption surface and slowed gastric emptying. However, once absorbed, the volume of distribution in an elderly subject is likely to have changed.

Ageing results in an increase in percentage body fat and a fall in total body water. Hydrophilic drugs, such as alcohol, are distributed in body water, such that with increasing age the volume of distribution falls and the peak concentration for a given dose may rise by 20%[10], resulting in lower levels of intake giving the same intoxicant effect. Conversely, lipophilic drugs, such as benzodiazepines and other psychotropics, that are stored in fatty tissue will remain in the body for longer but at lower peak concentrations. A fall in plasma albumin in old age results in increased bioavailability of protein-bound drugs, such as warfarin and diazepam.

Drug elimination occurs primarily through direct excretion or metabolism. Both routes are reduced in the elderly. Glomerular filtration rates fall steadily in old age, leading to the accumulation of renally excreted drugs. This may be compounded by renal damage due to drug misuse, e.g. analgesic abuse[11]. Hepatic metabolism is impaired due to a loss of liver mass and a reduced blood flow, which may also be compounded by toxic drug effects, such as alcohol leading to fatty liver. The efficiency of microsomal oxidation also falls with age, leading to reduced drug excretion of hepatically metabolized drugs[12]. The combination of these effects may greatly alter pharmacokinetics in the elderly. For example, Klotz estimated the half-life of diazepam in the very elderly to be over 3 days, compared with 20 h in a younger subject[13].

Multiple drug use increases the difficulty of prediction of the behaviour pattern of an individual substance, due to competition for binding sites and metabolic pathways. Polypharmacy may have different effects, depending on whether it is acute or chronic. Alcohol will inhibit microsomal enzyme activity in acute use, while prolonged administration will induce the same enzymes. Hence, alcohol will acutely raise concentrations of benzodiazepines, while lowering them if used chronically[14].

Pharmacodynamics also alter in the elderly. Sensitivity to drugs, particularly those acting on the central nervous system, tends to increase, while drug receptor populations also change with increased age. The particular effect of the changes depends in part upon whether the receptor involved is facilitatory or inhibitory.

As a consequence of all these variables, the prediction of a drug's effects in the elderly, based on observation of its effects on younger adults, is foolhardy. Similarly rigid application of recommended "safe levels" of substance use, such as those issued by the Department of Health in the UK, may result in false reassurance to clinicians and patients with a consequent failure to identify cases of harmful use in the elderly.

CONCLUSION

The terms "old age" and "substance misuse" are both terms that have a wide range of meaning to different readers. The current literature is based primarily upon chronological age banding of individuals, as opposed to banding by overall health, possibly a more valid measure. Definitions of substance misuse are similarly varied. Often in transgenerational studies definitions of caseness are set at a level to prevent false-positive reports for younger adults. In older age groups, where less of a substance may have a greater effect, there is the possibility of missing cases if such standards are applied. The greater likelihood of drug interactions in the elderly should be considered when determining the dependency potential of any given drug or medication.

PREVALENCE AND CORRELATES

The elderly may display harmful use of any psychoactive substance. Misuse of alcohol, opioids, cannabinoids, sedatives, stimulants, hallucinogens and tobacco are all reported among the elderly. However, access to a potential substance of abuse is key to determining what an individual may misuse. Alcohol is obtainable with ease in most industrialized nations and is a socially acceptable and accessible psychoactive drug. Amongst the elderly, ill-health is common. Sedatives, hypnotics and analgesics are easily accessible through prescription and consequently, along with alcohol, are responsible for the majority of cases of harmful use. Over-the-counter medication is also easily obtained and may be misused. Illicit drugs are usually only available in potentially dangerous environments from individuals who may pose a significant risk to vulnerable older adults. Illicit drug use is not commonly observed in the elderly.

BENZODIAZEPINES

Benzodiazepines replaced barbiturates as the mainstay of pharmacological interventions in both anxiety and sleep disturbance. They maintain their relative dominance in this field despite the recent development of newer drugs with reportedly less addictive potential. Benzodiazepines accumulate more readily in the elderly due to changes in body composition, leading to a greater volume of distribution for lipophilic drugs. Chronic use may contribute to toxic effects, including cognitive impairment, poor attention and anterograde amnesia, cerebellar signs such as ataxia, dysarthria, tremor, impaired coordination and drowsiness[39]. Increased falls and hip fractures are associated with benzodiazepine use[40], whilst withdrawal may be accompanied by rebound insomnia, agitation, convulsions and an acute confusional state. If benzodiazepines are required then short-term use of low doses of short- or medium-acting drugs is advised. There is no "safe" period of use but tolerance and dependence levels increase with prolonged use[41].

Prevalence of Benzodiazepine Use

Establishing levels of benzodiazepine use is subject to the same difficulties as establishing alcohol use except where it is a prescription medication, when some idea of identity and demographic characteristics of the potential user should be available. In areas where benzodiazepines are available over the counter, the nature of users and misusers is harder to establish. National prescription audits can reflect trends in use but are unhelpful when considering particular population subgroups. Prescribing of benzodiazepines in England and Wales has fallen from 20.6 million prescriptions in 1987 to 13.9 million in 1996[42], a fall of 32%. In England in 1996, 55% of prescriptions for benzodiazepines were issued to patients over the age of 60. Many of these prescriptions were issued to long-term users. A recent community follow-up study of 5000 over-65s in Manchester[43] revealed that 10% were using benzodiazepines on first assessment and that of these some 70% were taking a benzodiazepine 2 years later. A further 4 year follow-up revealed that 69% of these were still on benzodiazepines. Patients entering the study on benzodiazepines had a 52% chance of taking benzodiazepines throughout the 4 year period. Women were twice as likely to be taking a benzodiazepine as men at any stage in the study. In the USA, a study found 6.3% of a large sample of over-65s used a hypnotic, one-third of these daily and nine-tenths for at least 1 year[44]. Five year follow-up found 46.6% still using hypnotics, but with a switch away from barbiturates and longer-acting benzodiazepines towards short-acting ones[45].

Use of benzodiazepines in institutional samples has traditionally been higher and associated with female gender, greater age, bereavement and poor health[46]. In the USA it has been shown that one-fifth of nursing-home residents were taking potentially addictive drugs on a daily basis. The medication in question is usually a benzodiazepine[47]. Studies from other countries reveal similarly high levels of benzodiazepine use among institutionalized older adults[48]. The level of morbidity among institutional residents is likely to be higher than community-dwelling elders. It is unclear whether this morbidity is sufficient to explain a doubling in levels of use of benzodiazepines in this group. While chronic pain may require treatment with dependence-inducing medication, there are few indications for long-term benzodiazepine use. It has been argued that the regular use of benzodiazepines in institutions is a form of behavioural control, used more for the benefit of staff and others than these users. In many cases, the individual may be incapable of giving valid consent to taking such medication. The use of medication in such circumstances may be considered benzodiazepine misuse by some and as elder abuse by others[49].

Correlates

Psychiatric Morbidity

Significantly high rates of psychiatric disorder have been described among elderly benzodiazepine users[50]. Among elders using short-acting benzodiazepines as hypnotics, one-third reach caseness for depression, while a further one-third have a diagnosable anxiety disorder. Amongst users of anxiolytic benzodiazepines, half are depressed and one-fifth are anxious in spite of treatment. These results are not evidence of a causative relationship, although the most likely indications for initiation of such medication by a prescriber are likely to be presentation with such symptoms. As with alcohol misusers, one-third of elders requiring inpatient treatment for benzodiazepine misuse are of late onset, while two-thirds have graduated from misusing benzodiazepines or other drugs whilst younger[51]. The incidence of co-morbid alcohol abuse has not been consistently shown to be significantly greater among benzodiazepine misusers[51,52]. An all-age study found that DSM-III-R Axis I co-morbidity existed in all cases of a sample of benzodiazepine dependent users in Spain[53]. The commonest diagnoses were insomnia, anxiety disorders and affective disorders. Obsessive–compulsive, histrionic and dependent personality disorders were found in half the cases and physical problems in one-third of cases.

Gender and Age

Benzodiazepine use is over-represented among women of all ages. The likelihood of use of a benzodiazepine increases with age. There is little evidence that this gender divide narrows on reaching old age. Legislative approaches and prescribing guidelines have made some inroads into the over-representation of prescribing to the elderly[53]. Increasing public awareness of the side effects of benzodiazepines and an increase in advocacy services for the elderly are likely to have a similar effect.

Other Prescribed and Over-the-counter Medication

As indicated earlier, the elderly routinely receive a wide variety of medications, the majority of which may be misused. A quarter to half of the elderly experience chronic pain. In acute use the dependency potential of analgesics is believed to be around 0.1%. In chronic conditions the situation is somewhat different. Ten per cent of over-64s are on prescribed analgesics at any one time, with at least an equal number using over-the-counter medication. Edwards and Salib[54] found 3% of a community sample of over-65s to have been using mild opiate analgesics for a period of at least 1 year; 40% of this group were deemed to fulfil the criteria for dependence upon these drugs, with dependence levels as high as two-thirds among users of co-proxamol.

In addition to the dependence caused by these drugs, physical harm may also result, e.g. nephropathy may be caused by the use of paracetamol, salicylates and pyrazole derivatives, while renal impairment occurs with non-steroidal anti-inflammatory drug use[55]. Chronic nephropathy may also be caused by the excessive ingestion of analgesic mixtures combining two or more anti-pyretic analgesics, along with codeine or caffeine (both independently capable of causing addiction). Such acute and chronic effects are more likely amongst the elderly, where relative drug levels are higher and less biological reserve exists. Similar physical complications may arise from the misuse of other medications, the commonest being laxatives and cough mixtures.

ILLICIT DRUG MISUSE

Little is known about levels of illicit drug use among the over-65s, although the general perception is that it has been less of a problem than the misuse of prescribed medication. In the Epidemiological Catchment Area Study (ECA), only 0.1% of elders met the criteria for drug abuse for an illicit substance in the previous month[56]. Lifetime prevalence was 1.6% for over-65s. This may change as younger generations with a pattern of recreational drug use reach old age. In the UK, few cases of illicit drug use among the over-65s have found their way into the literature; one exception is a series of seven elderly reported to have initiated injecting heroin in later life. They attributed their behaviour to a combination of loneliness and depression[57]. In the USA, in a recent study of a Veterans' Administration old age psychiatry inpatient facility, 3% of the patients were found to have a primary drug misuse disorder involving prescribed medication, while 1% were addicted to illicit substances[58]. Also in the USA, attendance at methadone maintenance clinics by the elderly is reported to be rising, although over-60s still form 2% of those attending[59]. Similarly, a number of elders are reported to continue their use of cannabis into late life[47]. Anecdotal evidence also points to some individuals initiating the use of cannabis in later life in a search for its reputed therapeutic benefit in conditions such as disseminated sclerosis.

On balance, it appears that illicit drug use is less of a problem in the elderly than the abuse of legally sanctioned drugs. It remains to be seen whether individuals currently abusing illicit substances in younger age groups carry this behaviour over into old age. The nature of the subject has not lent itself to prospective studies as yet. One might expect greater levels of illicit drug use in future generations of older adults, although difficulties associated with obtaining a supply of such drugs with increasing infirmity are likely to account for some cessation in use. It is also tempting to speculate that those abusing illicit drugs as younger adults may switch to misusing prescribed medication in later life.

POLYSUBSTANCE MISUSE

The elderly have access to a variety of drugs of misuse. In many cases they may misuse one drug without misusing others. This is often the case with prescribed medication, where one medication is overused while compliance with the prescription is maintained for the others. Where non-prescribed substances become involved, the possibility of abuse of more than one substance is elevated. Finlayson[50] found 15% of over-65s requiring inpatient detoxification from alcohol were also dependent upon a second substance, usually a hypnotic, anxiolytic or analgesic.

The phenomenon of cross-tolerance must also be considered. Psychoactive substances may have a cumulative effect, due to either a shared outcome effect or to different drugs acting as interchangeable substitutes for one another (cross-tolerance). Cross-tolerance exists within each class of drug, such that the clinician should always consider the total benzodiazepine, barbiturate or opioid dose, using class-specific equivalence charts[60]. Cross-tolerance for some drugs may also occur outside of the class, most notably for alcohol, chlormethiazole and benzodiazepines. While this phenomenon is widely exploited for detoxification, failure to consider the possibility of its existence may lead to overlooking cases of dependence.

Conclusion

The abuse of alcohol and of prescribed medication remain the most prevalent substance misuse problems. There is little clear evidence of great changes in individuals' addictive behaviour patterns with increasing age. When one considers the prevalence of substance misuse among younger cohorts, it would appear that, as the population ages, not only will the absolute numbers of elderly with a substance misuse problem increase but the proportion of the elderly population with such a problem will increase too.

TREATMENT

Treatment of substance misuse is a multistage process involving the integrated use of physical, psychological and social interventions. These interventions should, where possible, run concurrently as opposed to consecutively and must be provided in a form that is acceptable to the individual and sensitive to the specific needs of the elderly. Amongst this client group, individuals rarely present complaining directly of a substance misuse disorder but may present with associated physical problems, or a problem may be detected during routine consultation with health professionals or carers.

The first step of treatment is the identification of cases. This requires clinical observation allied to sensitive yet persistent enquiry. The routine use of standardized screening tools may help to focus clinical impression more accurately. Once identified as potential candidates for treatment, the patient's attitude towards his/her substance misuse requires examination. Exploration of the risks and a discussion of potential avenues for change may help to establish or reinforce the motivation to change. Drugs that cause significant physical dependence may necessitate detoxification regimens, while co-morbid conditions such as depression that perpetuate the disorder need to be adequately treated. Social issues, such as housing and a social network that comprises mainly of substance misusers, may perpetuate the problem and need to be examined for opportunities to change. The individual requires psychological rehabilitation to address the issues that may have contributed to the uncontrolled use of substances and to provide future coping strategies to prevent a relapse into substance misuse. While these approaches apply to all substances of misuse, the majority of research has focused on alcohol misuse.

DETECTION

Self-presentation by elders may be limited by a number of factors[61]. Practical issues, such as accessibility of treatment centres to disabled individuals, large print information sources for the visually impaired and the availability of domiciliary treatment, are fundamental. Elders may not realize that they are ill, or may not realize that the medical profession identifies substance misuse as an illness and will offer help. Traditional forms of service promotion may fail to reach the elderly, while a service staffed by young professionals may seem intimidating or inappropriate for someone much older, particularly if his/her substance misuse is associated with a high degree of shame as is often the case in this group.

If self-presentation is unlikely, then the number of professional caregiver contacts that the elderly have provides a further opportunity for education of individuals about the problem and potential sources of help. This resource appears underdeveloped at present, with a need for better training for carers in identification of at-risk individuals and in appropriate actions once misusers are identified[62]. Currently, evidence suggests that carers are often unaware of sources of help and frequently are in collusion with alcohol misuse, citing reasons such as the elder "has not got long to live" or that "it's his only pleasure"[63]. Studies have found that many agencies providing care for the elderly have no written policy to guide their employees when encountering a client with an alcohol problem. Greenwood[64] argues that substance misusers, and the elderly in particular, suffer as the result of stigmatization, as their disorder is perceived as self-inflicted and with a poor outcome prognostically. This stigmatization may contribute to difficulties in communication and empathy on the part of some caregivers, including doctors. This stigma may be reflected in a clinician's reluctance to become involved by acknowledging a problem. For other carers, their own previous experiences with elderly substance misusers, both professional and personal, may lead to attempts to justify the behaviour, resulting in a similar loss of objectivity.

BENZODIAZEPINE USE DETECTION

Prevention and early recognition form the basis of management of benzodiazepine and other drug misuse among the elderly. Appropriate prescribing of sedatives for time-limited periods should be accompanied with vigilance for drug-seeking behaviours. Such behaviours include early requests for repeat prescriptions or requests for increased doses and should be regarded with suspicion. The elderly may also receive medication from multiple sources, particularly where they are under the care of prescribing hospital specialists as well as their primary prescribers. Careful exchange of clinical information is vital in such settings. For those abusing over-the-counter medication, chance presentation or the intervention of a pharmacist present the best hope of detection.

No screening tools have been validated to detect cases of elder benzodiazepine use. While urine screening provides a reliable means of establishing the presence or absence of drug metabolites, its clinical utility is limited by the unacceptability of the test to many who may be offended by the suggestion that they have a substance misuse problem. Second, urine screening is usually qualitative rather than quantitative. For those abusing a prescribed drug, the mere presence or absence of the drug is clinically uninformative. Individual variation in pharmacokinetics makes qualitative testing unreliable. With these considerations in mind, the need for dependence-inducing drug prescriptions should be regularly reviewed and co-morbid contributory conditions, such as depression, should be actively treated. Changes in legislation on prescribing practice may reduce the opportunity for drug misuse[71].

INITIATING TREATMENT

There are no published data about the level of uptake of offers of help once elders abusing substances are identified. Motivational interviewing and education as to the risks of alcohol use, along with the benefits of even a small reduction in levels of alcohol intake, may persuade some elders to change. Unfortunately, the pessimistic attitudes held by many professionals and carers towards the likelihood of successful resolution of the problem are frequently also held by the individual too. A fatalistic resignation to a life of substance misuse is often reported, particularly by long-term users, while more recent-onset users may express greater motivation for treatment[72].

Once long-term use of benzodiazepines is established, dose reduction can be difficult to achieve. Withdrawal insomnia and rebound anxiety make patient motivation difficult to achieve. Where abstinence is desired, a conversion to a medium-acting benzodiazepine and a gradual reduction in dosage over the course of months is advisable. Rapid detoxification is associated with breakthrough withdrawal symptoms and may be complicated by convulsions. If a rapid withdrawal is necessary, it is best conducted in an inpatient setting if severe dependency is suspected. As with alcohol, the withdrawal period for the elderly is more likely to be complicated by confusion than in younger adults.

In cases where abstinence is not achievable or desirable, a minimization of dose and adoption of a non-daily pattern of use are reasonable targets. Psychological techniques, such as relaxation training and educative initiatives in the areas of sleep hygiene and correct medication use, may also prove valuable. Cormack[81] demonstrated that writing to benzodiazepine users in primary care urging them to reduce their medication use resulted in a fall in total use by one-third over the next 6 months.

Treatment of other forms of drug misuse in the elderly is underresearched. Anticipation of problems and safe prescribing remain paramount in treatment and prevention. Misuse of analgesics may require formal detoxification if opioids are involved or physical dependence has developed. More often the patient requires information to allow him/her to make an informed choice about drug use and an alternative form of treatment for his/her condition. Still less information is available on the treatment of illicit drug use in the elderly. At present there is no evidence to suggest that an approach other than that used for younger adults should be adopted, although adaptations of such treatments should involve lower doses of medication and the adoption of a less directly confrontational approach.

PSYCHOLOGICAL INTERVENTIONS

Once a patient is detoxified, rehabilitation is necessary to address the issues behind his/her substance use and to foster coping strategies for the future. Few studies have examined the particular needs of the elderly in a rehabilitation setting. Janik and Dunham report on comparative outcomes for over 3000 over-60-year-olds and younger entrants into alcohol treatment programmes[82]. Outcome measured in terms of alcohol intake, therapist assessment and alcohol problems after 6 months showed no differences between the groups.

Outcomes from programmes designed specifically with the elderly in mind may be more appropriate for consideration. Some success has been claimed for models encouraging the development of social networks with self-management skills[83]. Kofoed[84], in a small study, reported that retention in outpatient treatment of older adults was greater in an age-specific treatment group that focused on socialization and minimal confrontation (a mainstay of many programmes), compared with older patients in a mixed-age treatment group. At 1 year follow-up the effect was lost. Variations of the Alcoholics Anonymous 12-step model tailored to the needs of elders have been reported upon[85] in the USA, with varying degrees of success. Models low on confrontation, traditionally regarded as fundamental to overcoming denial on the part of the patient, appear to be supported by the work of Kashner[86], who found that 1 year follow-up of elders in a confrontational programme revealed half the levels of abstinence as compared with a group in a programme where self-esteem, tolerance and peer relationships were promoted. Behavioural approaches, including cue identification and avoidance, have also been reported to be of clinical benefit[83]. A programme focusing on cognitive techniques, such as cognitive restructuring, assertion training and self-monitoring of drinking, resulted in 75% of those completing the programme sticking to their treatment goals at 1 year follow-up. The evidence suggests that a range of therapeutic techniques may be beneficial for the elderly and that local provision may depend upon the skills available to the treating agency. It is suggested that even if an elder's only therapeutic programme is not available, a better therapeutic outcome may occur from a more homogeneous group, where the opportunity for identification and vicarious learning is enhanced.

The above studies all relate to the outcome of alcohol treatment programmes. Even less age-specific studies are available to guide the clinician in the provision of aftercare to the elderly nonalcoholic drug user. An avoidance of drugs that have a dependence potential is advisable if practical. Adequate rehabilitation and continuing support of the individual are indicated. This may be provided through generic old age psychiatry services or through specialist drug services, depending upon which service appears best able to cater for the specific needs of the user. The choice of service provider should reflect the lifestyle of the patient, as opposed to being a decision based solely on chronological as opposed to biological age. Further services may also be available in the form of mutual support groups similar to those available for alcohol. The adoption of a cognitively-based programme low on confrontation and designed to foster strong social support appears optimal, as shown in work in the field of alcohol.

Conclusion

Substance misuse and old age psychiatry have long been unpopular choices for specialization. Both fields are known for providing challenging patients with differing priorities to those of the clinician. Research in either field is hampered by the difficulty in obtaining reliable clinical data on conditions for which few empirical measures exist. The field of old age substance misuse has suffered to some extent in clinical practice, where patients do not fit neatly into either service and welcomed by neither.

It is, however, clear that there exists a significant morbidity due to drug use in the elderly. The problem may be iatrogenic and autogenic in origin. Increased life expectancy and the cohort effect of generations of recreational drug users reaching old age are likely to intensify the problem. Adequate research to identify atrisk individuals and the provision of appropriate and accessible treatment services for the elderly drug misuser remain one of the major challenges to health care providers at the start of the new millennium.

REFERENCES

1. Patterson TL, Jeste DV. The potential impact of the baby-boom generation on substance abuse among elderly persons. *Psychiat Serv* 1999; **50**: 1184–8.
2. Grimley-Evans J. Geriatric medicine (geriatrics). In Walton J, Barondess JA, Lock S, eds, *The Oxford Medical Companion*. Oxford: Oxford University Press, 1994: 321–6.
3. Murphy JT, Harwood A, Gotz M, House AO. Prescribing alcohol in a general hospital: not everything in black and white makes sense. *J R Coll Physicians Lond* 1998; **32**: 358–9.
4. Pascarelli EF. Drug abuse and the elderly. In Lowinson JH, Ruiz P, eds, *Substance Abuse: Clinical Problems and Perspectives*. Baltimore, MD: Williams and Wilkins 1981: 752–7.
5. Breeze J. Hollister impression. *Br J Nurs* 1993; **3**: 905–8.
6. Blenkiron P. The elderly and their medication: understanding compliance in family practice. *Postgrad Med* 1996; **72**: 671–6.
7. Eisdorfer C, Basen MB. Drug misuse in the elderly. In Dupont RL, Goldstein A, O'Donnell J, eds, *Handbook on Drug Abuse*. Washington, DC: National Institute on Drug Abuse, 1979: 271–6.
8. United Nations International Drug Control Programme. *World Drug Report*. Oxford: Oxford University Press, 1997: 9–14.
9. World Health Organization. *The ICD-10 Classification of Mental and Behavioural Disorders*. Geneva: WHO, 1992: 75–7.

10. Dunne FJ, Schipperheijn JAM. Alcohol and the elderly; need for greater awareness. *Br Med J* 1989; **298**: 1660–1.
11. Ghodse AH. Substance misuse leading to renal damage. *Prescrib J* 1993; **33**: 151–3.
12. Sheehan O, Feely J. Prescribing considerations in elderly patients. *Prescriber* 1999; 5 Dec: 75–82.
13. Klotz U, Avant GR, Hoyumpa A et al. The effects of age and liver disease on the disposition and elimination of diazepam in adult men. *J Clin Invest* 1975; **55**: 437–59.
14. Lisi DM. Alcoholism in the elderly. *Arch Intern Med* 1997; **157**: 242–3.
15. Oscar-Berman M, Bonner RT. Matching and delayed matching to sample performance as measures of visual processing, selective attention and memory in aging and alcoholic individuals. *Neuropsychologia* 1985; **23**: 639–51.
16. Iber FL. Alcoholism and associated malnutrition in the elderly. *Prog Clin Biol Res* 1990; **326**: 157–73.
17. Grant BF, Harford TC, Chou P. Prevalence of DSM-III-R alcohol abuse and dependence. United States 1988. *Alcohol Health Res World* 1991; **15**: 91–6.
18. Holzer CE, Robins LN, Myers JK et al. Antecedents and correlates of alcohol abuse and dependence in the elderly. In Maddox G, Robins LN, Rosenberg N, eds, *Nature and Extent of Alcohol Problems in the Elderly*. Research Monograph No. 14, Rockville, MD: National Institute of Drug Abuse, DHSS, US Government Printing Office, 1984.
19. Saunders PA, Copeland JRM, Dewey ML. Alcohol use and abuse in the elderly. Findings of the Liverpool longitudinal community study. *Int J Geriat Psychiat* 1989; **4**: 103–8.
20. Bridgewater S, Leigh S, James OFW, Potter JF. Alcohol consumption and dependence in elderly patients in an urban community. *Br Med J* 1988; **295**: 884–5.
21. Bristow MF, Clare AW. Prevalence and characteristics of at-risk drinkers among elderly acute medical patients. *Br J Addict* 1992; **87**: 291–4.
22. Ganry O, Joly JP, Queval MP, Dubreuil A. Prevalence of alcohol problems among elderly patients in a university hospital. *Addiction* 2000; **95**: 107–13.
23. Mears HJ, Spice C. Screening for problem drinking in the elderly: a study in the elderly mentally ill. *Int J Geriat Psychiat* 1993; **8**: 319–26.
24. Office for National Statistics. *Living in Britain: Results from the 1996 General Household Survey*. London: Stationery Office, 1998.
25. Glynn RJ, Bouchard GR, Cocastro JS, Laird NM. Aging and generational effects on changing behaviours in men: results of the normative aging study. *Am J Publ Health* 1985; **75**: 1413–19.
26. Temple MT, Leino EV. Long-term outcomes of drinking: a 20 year longitudinal study of men. *Br J Addict* 1989; **84**: 889–99.
27. Schonfeld L, Dupree LW. Alcohol abuse among older adults. *Rev Clin Gerontol* 1994; **4**: 217–25.
28. Roisin AJ, Glatt MM. Alcohol excess in the elderly. *Q J Stud Alcohol* 1971; **32**: 53–9.
29. Jennison KM. The impact of stressful life events and social support on drinking older adults: a general population survey. *Int J Aging Hum Dev* 1992; **35**: 99–123.
30. Byrne GJ, Raphael B, Arnold E. Alcohol consumption and psychological distress in recently widowed older men. *Aust NZ J Psychiat* 1999; **33**: 740–7.
31. Grant BF, Harford TC. Co-morbidity between DSM-IV alcohol use and major depression: results of a national survey. *Drug Alcohol Depend* 1995; **39**: 197–206.
32. Schukit MA. Alcoholism and affective disorder: diagnostic confusion. In Goodwin DW, Ericson CK, eds, *Alcoholism and Affective Disorders*. New York: Spectrum, 1979: 1–9.
33. Vaillant GE. Is alcoholism more often the cause or the result of depression? *Harvard Rev Psychiat* 1003; **1**: 94–9.
34. Schutte KK, Brennan PL, Moos RH. Predicting the development of late-life late-onset drinking problems: a 7-year prospective study. *Alcohol Clin Exp Res* 1998; **22**: 1349–58.
35. Goodman C, Ward M. *Alcoholic Problems in Old Age*. London: Staccato, 1989: 19–23.
36. Simoni-Wastila L. The use of abusable prescription drugs: the role of gender. *J Women's Health Gender-based Med* 2000; **9**: 289–97.
37. Jones D. Characteristics of elderly people taking psychotropic medication. *Drugs Aging* 1992; **2**: 389–94.
38. Fichter M, Witzke W, Hippius H. Psychotropic drug use in a representative community sample: the Upper Bavarian Study. *Acta Psychiat Scand* 1989; **80**: 68–77.
39. World Health Organization. *Programme on Substance Abuse. Rational Use of Benzodiazepines*. Geneva: WHO, 1996.
40. McCree D. The appropriate use of sedatives and hypnotics in geriatric insomnia. *Am Pharmacol* 1989; **5**: 49–53.
41. Grantham P. Benzodiazepine abuse. *Br J Hosp Med* 1987: **37**: 292–300.
42. Milburn A. House of Commons Written Answers, *Hansard* 6th May 1998: 423.
43. Taylor S, McCracken CFM, Wilson KCM, Copeland JRM. Extent and appropriateness of benzodiazepine use. Results from an elderly urban community. *Br J Psychiat* 1998; **173**: 433–8.
44. Stewart R, May E, Hale W, Marks R. Psychotropic drug use in an ambulatory elderly population. *Gerontology* 1982; **28**: 328–35.
45. Stewart R, May E, Moore M, Hale W. Changing patterns of psychotropic drug use in the elderly: a five year update. *Drug Intell Clin Pharmacol* 1989; **23**: 610–13.
46. Morgan K. Sedative–hypnotic drug use and aging. *Arch Gerontol Geriat* 1983; **2**: 181–99.
47. Solomon K, Manepalli J, Ireland GA, Mahon GM. Alcoholism and prescription drug abuse in the elderly: St. Louis University grand rounds. *J Am Geriat Soc* 1993; **41**: 57–69.
48. Opedal K, Schjott J, Eide E. Use of hypnotics among patients in geriatric institutions. *Int J Geriat Psychiat* 1998; **13**: 846–51.
49. Pillemer K. Maltreatment of patients in nursing homes: overview and research agenda. *J Health Soc Behav* 1988; **29**: 227–38.
50. Finlayson RE, Davis JL. Prescription drug dependence in the elderly population: demographics and clinical features in 100 out-patients. *Mayo Clin Proc* 1994; **69**: 1137–45.
51. van Balkom AJ, Beekman AT, de Beurs E et al. Co-morbidity of the anxiety disorders in a community-based older population in The Netherlands. *Acta Psychiat Scand* 2000; **101**: 37–45.
52. Martinez-Cano H, de Iceta Ibanez de Gauna M, Vela-Bueno A, Wittchen HU. DSM-III-R co-morbidity in benzodiazepine dependence. *Addiction* 1999; **94**: 97–107.
53. Brahms D. Benzodiazepine overprescribing: successful initiative in New York State. *Lancet* 1990; **336**: 1372–4.
54. Edwards I, Salib E. "Silent dependence syndrome" in old age. *Int J Geriat Psychiat* 1999; **14**: 72–4.
55. Elseviers MM, De Broe ME. Analgesic abuse in the elderly. Renal sequelae and management. *Drugs Aging* 1998; **12**: 391–400.
56. Regier DA, Boyd JH, Burke JD. One-month prevalence of mental disorders in the United States. *Arch Gen Psychiat* 1988; **45**: 977–86.
57. Frances J. Pain killer. *Commun Care* 1994; Dec: 15–21.
58. Edgell RC, Kunik ME, Molinari VA et al. Non-alcohol-related use disorders in geropsychiatric patients. *J Geriat Psychiat Neurol* 2000; **13**: 33–7.
59. Pascarelli EF. Drug abuse and the elderly. In Lowinson JH, Ruiz P, eds, *Substance Abuse: Clinical Problems and Perspectives*. Baltimore, MD: Williams and Wilkins, 1981: 752–7.
60. Taylor D, McConnell D, McConne H, Abel K. *Bethlem and Maudsley Prescribing Guidelines*. London: Martin Dunitz, London, 2000.
61. Goodman C, Ward M. *Alcoholic Problems in Old Age*. London: Staccato, 1989: 19–23.
62. Wesson J. *The Vintage Years*. Birmingham: Aquarius, 1992: 9.
63. Herring R, Thom B. The role of home carers: findings from a study of alcohol and older people. *Health Care Later Life* 1998; **3**: 199–211.
64. Greenwood J. Stigma: substance misuse in older people. *Geriat Med* 2000; **30**(4): 43–5.
65. Willenbring ML, Chrristensen KJ, Spring WD, Rasmussen R. Alcoholism screening in the elderly. *J Am Geriat Soc* 1987; **35**: 864–9.
66. Buchsbaum DG, Buchannan RG, Welsh J et al. Screening for drinking disorders in the elderly using the CAGE questionnaire. *J Am Geriat Soc* 1992; **40**: 662–5.
67. Adams WL, Barry KL, Fleming MF. Screening for problem drinking in older primary care patients. *J Am Med Assoc* 1996; **276**: 1964–7.
68. Naik PC, Jones RG. Alcohol histories taken from elderly people on admission. *Br Med J* 1994; **308**: 248.
69. McInnes E, Powell J. Drug and alcohol referrals: are elderly substance abuse diagnoses and referrals being missed? *Br Med J* 1994; **308**: 444–8.

70. Reid MC, Anderson PA. Geriatric substance use disorders. *Med Clin N Am* 1997; **81**: 999–1016.

71. Brahms D. Benzodiazepine overprescribing: successful initiative in New York State. *Lancet* 1990; **336**: 1372–4.

72. Schonfeld L, Dupree LW. Alcohol abuse among older adults. *Rev Clin Gerontol* 1994; **4**: 217–25.

73. Liskow BI, Rinck C, Campbell J, DeSouza C. Alcohol withdrawal in the elderly. *J Studies Alc* 1989; **50**: 414–21.

74. Brower KJ, Mudd S, Blow FC. Severity of treatment of alcohol withdrawal in elderly versus younger patients. *Alcohol Clin Exp Res* 1994; **18**: 196–202.

75. Kraemer KL, Mayo-Smith MF, Calkins DR. Impact of age on the severity, course, and complications of alcohol withdrawal. *Arch Int Med* 1997; **157**: 2234–41.

76. Kraemer KL, Conigliaro J, Saitz R. Managing alcohol withdrawal in the elderly. *Drugs Aging* 1999; **14**: 409–25.

77. Goldstein MZ, Pataki A, Webb MT. Alcoholism among elderly persons. *Psychiat Serv* 1996; **47**: 942–3.

78. Reid MC, Tinetti ME, Brown CJ. Physician awareness of alcohol use disorders among older patients. [see comments; comment in: *J Gen Intern Med* 1998; **13**: 781–2] *J Gen Intern Med* 1998; **13**: 729–34.

79. Atkinson R. Depression, alcoholism and aging: a review. *Int J Geriat Psychiat* 1999; **14**: 905–10.

80. Kristenson H, Ohlin H, Hulten-Nosslin MJ. Identification and intervention of heavy drinking in middle-aged men: results and follow-up of 24–60 months of long-term study with randomised controls. *Alcohol Clin Exp Res* 1983; **7**: 203–10.

81. Cormack M, Sweeney KG, Hughes-Jones H. Evaluation of an easy and cost effective strategy for reducing benzodiazepine use in general practice. *Br J Gen Pract* 1994; **44**: 5–8.

82. Janik SW, Dunham RG. A nationwide examination of the need for specific alcoholism treatment programs for the elderly. *J Stud Alcohol*, 1983; **44**: 307–15.

83. Dupree LW, Broskowski H, Schonfeld L. The gerontology alcohol project: a behavioural treatment program for elderly alcohol abusers. *Gerontologist* 1984; **24**: 510–16.

84. Kofoed LL, Tolson RL, Atkinson RM. Treatment compliance of older alcoholics: an elder-specific approach is superior to "mainstreaming". *J Stud Alcohol* 1987; **48**: 47–53.

85. Schonfeld L, Dupree LW. Antecedents of drinking for early- and late-onset elderly alcohol abusers. *J Stud Alcohol* 1991; **52**: 587–91.

86. Kashner TM, Rodell DE, Ogden SR *et al*. Outcomes and costs of two VA inpatient programs for older alcoholics. *Hosp Commun Psychiat* 1992; **43**: 985–9.

Benzodiazepine Use and Abuse in the Community: Liverpool Studies

Kenneth C. M. Wilson and Pat Mottram

St Catherine's Hospital, Birkenhead, UK

Benzodiazepine use in older people is associated with increased falls[1] and psychomotor changes, leading to the recommendation that they should rarely be prescribed[2]. Despite the fact that they may play an important role in the treatment of some psychiatric conditions[3], it is evident that they should be used with caution in this age group.

Recent epidemiological studies in Liverpool clearly demonstrate cause for concern. Between 1982 and 1983 we examined the prevalence of mental illness and the use of drugs in a random sample of 1070 community residents aged 65 + [4]. A similar study was conducted on a larger age- and gender-stratified sample ($n = 5222$) of the same age group between the years 1989 and 1991[5]. The Geriatric Mental State Examination was used in both studies. The instrument also collects data concerning prescribed and non-prescribed drug use over the month preceding the interview.

The results of the two studies have been compared in some detail[6]. The overall prevalence of benzodiazepine use was 12.8 (CI: 10.8–14.8) in 1982–1983 and 10.8 (CI: 9.9–11.6) 10 years later, indicating no significant change in drug use prevalence. Over the 3 years of the later study, 2.5% of non-users started taking benzodiazepines. Over two-thirds of all users were still taking benzodiazepines 3 years later. Analyses by mental state demonstrated that the largest proportion of people receiving benzodiazepines were depressed. People aged 80 + were three times more likely to be users than those aged 65–70. Both depression and anxiety were risk factors. Subsequent analyses of the data[7] examined the use of benzodiazepines in the context of depression. It is evident that nearly twice as many depressed older people were users of benzodiazepines than antidepressants. This may be explained by the increased emphasis on agitation, initial insomnia[8] and the relative under-reporting of depressed mood in older depressed people[9].

The findings of these studies should be viewed with some caution in view of the relatively long period between interviews in each study. It is self-evident that users may be intermittent in their use of benzodiazepines and other medications. However, the larger study incorporated questions concerning compliance. Data were available from 203/208 benzodiazepine users at their last interview. Of these, 89.6% stated that they were taking drugs as prescribed, 4.4% occasionally missed a dose and 5.4% often missed a dose. Only one stated that he/she had stopped taking the prescribed medication.

The findings of these studies imply that approximately 10% of older community residents are prescribed and taking benzodiazepines. Benzodiazepines are frequently prescribed to the very old and depressed, the majority of whom remain depressed for a significant period of time. Once commenced on benzodiazepines the majority take them for at least 3 years. There does not appear to be any change in prescribing habits across the interim period of 10 years.

REFERENCES

1. Neutel C, Hirdes J, Maxwell C *et al*. New evidence on benzodiazepines and falls: the time factor. *Age Ageing* 1996; **25**: 273–8.

2. Beers MH, Ouslander JG, Rollingher I *et al*. Explicit criteria for determining inappropriate medication use in nursing homes. *Arch Intern Med* 1991; **151**: 1825–32.

3. Shader I, Greenblat D. Use of benzodiazepines in anxiety disorders. *N Engl J Med* **328**: 1398–405.

4. Sullivan C, Copeland J, Dewey M *et al*. Benzodiazepine use amongst the elderly: findings of the Liverpool community survey. *Int J Geriat Psychiat* 1988; **3**: 289–92.

5. Saunders PA, Copeland J, Dewey M *et al*. The prevalence of dementia, depression and neurosis in later life: the Liverpool MRC–ALPHA study. *Int J Epidemiol* 1993; **22**: 838–47.

6. Taylor S, McCracken C, Wilson K, Copeland J. Extent and appropriateness of benzodiazepine use. Results from an elderly urban community. *Br J Psychiat* 1998; **173**: 433–8.

7. Wilson K, Copeland J, Taylor S *et al*. Natural history of pharmacotherpay of older depressed community residents: the MRC–ALPHA study. *Br J Psychiat* 1999; **175**: 439–43.

8. Brown R, Sweeny J, Loutsch E *et al*. Involutional melancholia revisited. *Am J Psychiat* 1984; **137**: 439–44.

9. Copeland J, Davidson I, Dewey M *et al*. Alzheimer's disease, other dementias, depression and pseudodementia: prevalence, incidence and three year outcome in Liverpool. *Br J Psychiat* 1993; **3**: 95–8.

Part K

Learning and Behavioural Disorders

112

Old Age and Learning Disability

Oyepeju Raji and Sheila Hollins

St George's Hospital Medical School, London, UK

The age structure of people with learning disabilities is changing and more are surviving into old age, indicating considerable achievements in health and social development.

Historically, there was little provision for the needs of older persons with learning disability. The reason for this was that such persons had a short lifespan and many died before reaching old age, for reasons such as inadequate medical treatment and the life-threatening complications associated with their condition. During recent years, the provision of formal care for adults with learning disabilities has changed from a largely institutional service to an increasingly community-based one. This has affected the collection of health statistics. Hospital populations provided the main source of data in the past. Although registers of need are a statutory requirement for children in the UK, there is no similar requirement for adults with disabilities. However, many local authorities do maintain learning disabilities registers, and include a wider range of service users than those who would previously have been long-stay hospital patients.

SOCIAL BACKGROUND

In the mid- to late 1800s, "mentally defectives" (including people with learning disabilities and those with mental illness) were kept away from society and were housed in asylums. One reason for the institutionalization of mildly learning-disabled people can be found in the social turmoil of the early 1900s. Young adults were placed in institutions to curb their sexuality, as it was thought that their offspring would have intellectual limitations and would themselves have low-IQ children, and that eventually the national IQ would fall. After the menopause, many of the women were allowed out on licence, working as ladies' maids, for example, and returning to the asylum when the problem of old age meant they were of no further use. Many were of normal intelligence, brought into institutions because of adverse social circumstances and detained there. After World War II, life expectancy began to improve within the institutions with better medical care and more positive lifestyles[2,3]. Mildly disabled older adults were highly valued as a substantial work force in the institution.

In 1959, a review of the Mental Health Act allowed patients an informal status and many became voluntary patients and discharged themselves, made their way into the world and were lost to helping agencies and statistics. Others stayed on in institutions, probably because of infirmity or institutionalization. Many of these will have been discharged as elderly individuals in the wave of community care in the 1980s, promoted by the philosophy of normalization and governmental encouragement. Wolf and Wright[3] found that younger, more able people were more readily discharged into the community and the older and more disabled population remained in institutions.

CAUSES OF DEATH

People with learning disabilities are living longer overall but the level of disability is correlated with longevity and this association is more marked in the earlier years. Improved standards of care, higher expectations and more positive attitudes to treatment for serious illness have contributed to increasing longevity. Prolonged survival is now the norm, even for the most severely disabled children. In people with Down's syndrome, for example, heart disease is now treated surgically if indicated and overall medical care is much improved. The overall increased longevity means that disorders such as dementia and cancer have become more prevalent. There is a tendency for profoundly learning-disabled people to be more seriously physically disabled and to have more health problems. Even with better care, the life expectancy of profoundly and multiply disabled people is still reduced. The mortality rate for people with learning disabilities is higher compared with the general population. Carter and Jancar[4,5] studied a hospital population and found marked changes in the causes of death over a 50 year period. Prior to 1955, tuberculosis was a major cause of death, and after 1955 non-tubercular respiratory infection accounted for 46% of all deaths examined. Other identified causes were myocardial infarction, cerebrovascular accidents, pulmonary embolism and status epilepticus, which accounted for 15%. Epilepsy is both more prevalent and more likely to occur in a poorly controlled form with significantly increased mortality[2]. Hollins et al.[6] reported that death certificates were not a reliable source of data about cause of death and that learning disabilities were rarely mentioned, with respiratory disease being the major cause of death, suggesting a failure to recognize underlying medical conditions. Those with mild disabilities have lifespans close to those of the general population, dying from cardiovascular, neoplastic and terminal infections, similar to those of elderly people of originally normal intelligence[7].

FREQUENCY OF DEMENTIA IN PEOPLE WITH LEARNING DISABILITY

Epidemiological studies, whether cross-sectional or longitudinal, are often difficult to do. The assessment of the premorbid state is affected by limited educational opportunities, social deprivation and the low expectations of many people with learning disabilities. The true intellectual functioning of the person with a learning

Principles and Practice of Geriatric Psychiatry, 2nd edn. Edited by J. R. M. Copeland, M. T. Abou-Saleh and D. G. Blazer
©2002 John Wiley & Sons, Ltd

disability at baseline is often difficult to measure[1]. Studies suggest that dementia is about as common in the learning-disabled population as in the general population and has the same range of clinical phenomena, provided that each patient's unique intellectual baseline is allowed for[8]. Cooper[9] surveyed a population of elderly people with learning disabilities and found that 22% had dementia; however, the small number precluded analysis of subtypes. An earlier survey by Reid et al.[15] found a prevalence of 13.6%. Tait[10] found a prevalence of dementia similar to that in the general population.

THE MEDICAL CONTRIBUTION TO THE DIAGNOSIS OF DEMENTIA

Dementia can only be diagnosed after a careful history is taken and an examination made, the premorbid and presenting personalities assessed and other reasons for deterioration excluded. Long-standing visual and hearing problems are common in people with learning disabilities and may only be discovered as sensory deficits increase and further affect functioning[11]. Hypothyroidism, deterioration caused by inappropriate medication, communication disorders and psychiatric illness, both organic and functional, may all cause pseudodementia. Depression is often precipitated by loss of caregivers or familiar environments and may present, in addition, as behavioural and personality change. Symptoms such as incontinence may be related to the inappropriate architecture of the residence or to shortage of staff.

A detailed clinical examination will highlight dental and chiropody needs, general medical disorders and complications of long-standing disability. Consideration can be given to the need for aids and appliances to minimize the deficits and ease the burden for carers. People with learning disabilities rarely have access to health education or health promotion, so that screening for anaemia, hypertension, glaucoma or carcinoma of breast or cervix will hardly ever have been done.

The examination of someone with learning disabilities who may have superimposed dementia may therefore offer the opportunity to put right some of the deficiencies of older-style services, identify current social dilemmas, diagnose dementia in the context of long-standing deficits and consider, with the caregivers and the multidisciplinary team, how needs can be met[12].

Thorough assessment will provide information on the following:

1. The developmental intellectual disability.
2. Other long-standing disabilities and comorbid conditions.
3. Long-standing psychiatric illness and behaviour disorder.
4. Illness and disability superimposed and due to ageing.
5. Psychiatric illness associated with old age.
6. Dementia, if present.
7. The skills and needs of the person.
8. Recent life experiences.
9. The patient's wishes and those of the caregiver for residential and social care.

DEMENTIA AND DOWN'S SYNDROME

The association between ageing in adults with Down's syndrome and the development of dementia attracts interest from both researchers and clinicians. There is now a substantial literature on the genetic link between Down's syndrome and Alzheimer's disease. Several studies, using a variety of diagnostic criteria, have reported increasing age-specific prevalence rates for Alzheimer's disease in people with Down's syndrome. However, whilst the prevalence rates vary across studies, in no study has the rate reached 100%, which might be expected given the neuropathological data[13]. Dementia is often accompanied by epilepsy, loss of skills (which perhaps were not well developed in the first place) and transient behaviour problems, together with personality changes.

Families who have cared for their relative with Down's syndrome to the point where they develop dementia need support, information and the chance to talk to someone who understands the natural history of Alzheimer's disease. They may feel guilty and confused. An understanding of their confusion is required, and support is needed as they accept the diagnosis of dementia and its inevitable outcome. They may need to consider changes to their lifestyle and to look to the wider network for longer-term care and support.

WHAT OF SERVICES?

One of the most challenging ways to think about service development is through the proper consideration of the philosophy of normalization, which states that services that are highly valued and normative should be used by those who are at risk of being devalued. The difficulty is that both "the elderly" and "people with learning disabilities" are potentially devalued groups; both services tend to be underfunded and considered to be bottomless pits of needs.

The major debate is whether to use the services the rest of the population use, i.e. the geriatric or psychogeriatric services, to continue with learning disability services (improved as necessary), or to develop something new. Probably the best solution is to consider services for each individual, facilitating access to what is available and campaigning for what is not.

In England, national policy requires local authorities to offer person-centred planning to all people with learning disabilities. People living at home with elderly family carers are a priority group for receiving services and supports based on what is important for them as individuals and for receiving a regularly updated health action plan[16].

REHABILITATION INTO THE COMMUNITY

The closure of long-stay mental handicap hospitals in the UK has created new social and medical dilemmas[10]. Some people have been in hospital for many years, and moving into the community presents many difficulties, with geriatric needs superseding developmental needs. Some hospitals have remained to accommodate this small group, but many hospitals have closed completely and people moved to community residential provision. Many elderly people with learning disabilities have their only network of friends on the campus of the hospital, and it is important to try and maintain this. They are usually out of touch with relatives and a return to the county or borough of origin is not always meaningful or in their best interest. With careful introduction, these people may usually be accommodated in community services and may be far more competent than typical geriatric patients[14]. Because their life experience is so different, it may be better to care for them in an establishment able to take several residents from the same hospital.

CARE IN THE FAMILY HOME

The elderly person with learning disability may be cared for by an ageing parent with a similar dependency level. The fragile world of a person with learning disability has often been prematurely closed because of the declining abilities of the caregiver. With the death of remaining carers, the experience of multiple loss may precipitate depression as part of the bereavement response[17]. A small group home may then provide a substitute for the family home. With foresight and planning, some people may stay in their own home, with up to 24 hours support if needed.

THE PERSON WITH MULTIPLE DISABILITIES

Learning disability is known to be associated with an increased prevalence of coexisting diagnoses that also affect life expectancy, with the result that those with multiple disabilities and super-imposed problems of old age are few in number. There are challenges in management which may require a combination of learning disability, psychiatric and geriatric expertise. Some hospitals have developed special units to accommodate this small group, but new services are community-based and provide a multispecialty and multidisciplinary format. Private and voluntary agencies have often led the way.

DAY CARE

Accommodation and care varying from minimal to total are only part of the needs to be met. Daily activities and social contacts will need to be provided, and this may be difficult if the person has relocated in an area where he/she is not known. Because of shortage of places in social education centres (the core provision for adults with learning disability in the community), adults with learning disabilities usually retire by 65 years and then have only the occasional part-time arrangement in day centres for the elderly, clubs, adult education institutes and religious activities. As the number of elderly people with learning disabilities in the community increases, person-centred approaches to planning individual arrangements will be more important.

COMMUNITY TEAMS

Most areas in the UK have multidisciplinary community teams for people with learning disabilities and the trend is for these specialist staff to facilitate access to assessment and management within mainstream geriatric and psychogeriatric services. The opportunities of working together are great, thereby ensuring that dividing lines in health care do not detract from whole-person medicine.

TERMINAL CARE

Elderly people with learning disabilities may die at home, in oncology or general medical wards or in a hospice. The combined community services may be needed and include the terminal care team. Chaplains, moving from long-stay hospitals into ecumenical teams in the community, may be called to minister, together with community nurses and community team members, to ensure a dignified and good death.

CONCLUSION

The majority of elderly people with learning disability now live in the community and are more likely to outlive their parents and share the experience of becoming old with the rest of the population. This is an opportunity to meet their several needs successfully and not to repeat the errors of segregation that have littered learning disability services throughout the industrial world. There is need for more research at a clinical and planning level to underpin creative services, and up-to-date knowledge available for those who do the caring and for those who help the carers.

REFERENCES

1. DiGiovanni L. The elderly retarded: a little-known group. *Gerontologist* 1978; **18**: 202–66.
2. McLoughlin IJ. A study of mortality experiences in a mental handicap hospital. *Br J Psychiat* 1988; **153**: 645–9.
3. Wolf LC, Wright RE. Changes in life expectancy of mentally retarded persons in Canadian institutions: a 12 year comparison. *J Ment Defic Res* 1987; **31**: 41–59.
4. Carter G, Jancar J. Mortality in the mentally handicapped—a 50 year survey at the Stoke Park Group of Hospitals (1930–1980). *J Ment Defic Res* 1983; **27**: 143–56.
5. Carter G, Jancar J. Sudden deaths in the mentally handicapped. *Psychol Med* 1984; **14**: 691–5.
6. Hollins S, Attard MT, Von Fraunhofer N *et al.* Mortality in people with learning disability: risks, causes, and death certification findings in London. *Dev Med Child Neurol* 1998; **40**: 50–6.
7. Jancar J, Eastman RD, Carter G. Hypercholesterolaemia in cancer and other causes of death in the mentally handicapped. *Br J Psychiat* 1984; **145**: 59–61.
8. Reid AH, Aungle PG. Dementia in ageing mental defectives: a clinical psychiatric study. *J Ment Defic Res* 1974; **18**: 15–23.
9. Cooper S-A. Psychiatric symptoms of dementia among elderly people with learning disabilities. *Int J Geriat Psychiat* 1997; **12**: 662–6.
10. Tait D. Mortality and dementia among ageing defectives. *J Ment Defic Res* 1983; **27**: 133–42.
11. Cooke LB. Hearing loss in ageing mentally handicapped persons. *Aust NZ J Dev Disabil* 1989; **12**: 321–7.
12. Linter C. Aspects of ageing in mental handicap. *Br J Ment Subnorm* 1986; **32**: 114–18.
13. Crayton L, Oliver C, Holland A, Bradbury J, Hall S. The neuropsychological assessment of age-related cognitive deficits in adults with Down's syndrome. *J Appl Res in Intellectual Disabilities* 1998; **11**: 255–72.
14. Cotten PD, Sison GFP, Start S. Comparing elderly mentally retarded and non mentally retarded individuals: Who are they? What are their needs? *Gerontologist* 1981; **21**: 359–65.
15. Reid AH, Maloney AFJ, Aungle PG. Dementia in ageing mental defectives: a clinical and neuropathological study. *J Ment Defic Res* 1978; **22**: 233.
16. *Valuing People: A New Strategy for Learning Disability for the 21st Century.* Department of Health 2001; 49–50.
17. Hollins S, Esterhuyzen A. Bereavement and grief in adults with learning disabilities. *Br J Psychiat* 1987; **170**: 497–501.

Elderly Offenders

Janet M. Parrott

Bracton Centre, Oxleas NHS Trust, UK

EXTENT AND PATTERN OF CRIMINAL BEHAVIOUR IN THE ELDERLY

Criminal behaviour is most common during youth and declines sharply with increasing age. Older people are responsible for only a small part of the total amount of recorded crime and it is likely that they also make a limited contribution to the "dark figure" of unrecorded offences. The lower proportion of males in the elderly population, their retired status and the absence of the risk-taking attitudes of youth may be of relevance. A review of the criminal statistics for England and Wales indicates that the elderly's share of most offence categories is less than 1% of the total for all ages. Shoplifting is the most common indictable offence to involve the elderly and this is the only offence category where older women make a significant contribution[1]. The elderly's share of sex offences (other than rape) is higher than for other indictable offences, varying between 5% and 9% of each category in England and Wales. Schichor[2] notes a similar 5% figure for the elderly's contribution to overall sex offences in the USA. Offences involving children are most common. In Craissati and McClurg's study of a consecutive series of 356 men from two London boroughs convicted of sex offences or released on parole (1993–2001), 22 men (6.1%) were aged 60 or over, 19 men were convicted of offences against children, two against adults and one of possession of prohibited material involving children[3,4]. The elderly contribute very little to the total number of those convicted of burglary, robbery and drug offences.

Violent behaviour in the elderly leading to conviction is extremely rare. Essex Police District recorded reports of violent incidents in only three people aged 65+ during a 14-month period[5]. In 1998–1999, 3.9% of homicides (19 cases) in England and Wales involved those aged 60+; six of these were convicted of Section 2 manslaughter (diminished responsibility), comprising 31.6% of the elderly group. In comparison, 6.8% of homicide cases where the perpetrators were under 60 resulted in a Section 2 manslaughter verdict, supporting the more prominent role of psychiatric disorder in the older offenders[1].

Kratcoski and Walker[6] studied 82 cases of homicide committed by those aged 60+ in the USA and concluded that elderly homicides were more likely to involve a spouse or other relative as victim than the non-elderly; 81% of the offenders were male, and 15% of the elderly offenders committed suicide, the victim being the wife in each instance.

Hucker and Ben Aron[7] compared 16 elderly violent offenders with a group of young violent offenders and with another group of non-violent elderly sex offenders, all selected by referral to a psychiatric clinic in a case note study; 69% of the elderly violent group were diagnosed as having either an organic brain syndrome or a functional psychosis, compared with only 19% of the non-violent elderly and none of the younger group. Paranoid symptoms were prominent in the elderly violent group, irrespective of diagnosis.

MENTAL ABNORMALITY AND OFFENDING IN OLD AGE

The most common associations of criminal behaviour in the elderly are alcohol abuse[8], homelessness and psychiatric illness[9]. In an early paper on this topic, Norwood East[10] suggested, on the basis of his clinical experience in prisons, that the possibility of psychiatric disorder should always be considered in those who offended for the first time in old age. Particular attention has also been drawn to first-offender shoplifters[11], although the contribution this disturbed group make to the whole is unknown.

In a study of 153 referrals aged 60+ to the community services branch of Essex police[12], 97 had been apprehended for shoplifting. The prevalence of psychiatric disorder in the 50 people interviewed was higher than in other community samples; 38% of those charged with shoplifting were identified as cases, with 9/11 cases belonging to AGECAT organic and depressive syndrome groups[13]. In a study of men remanded in custody, Taylor and Parrott[9] found that nearly 3% of men were aged 55+. Half of these men had active symptoms of psychiatric disorder and half some form of physical disorder—twice the rates of those under 55. The commonest psychiatric problems were alcoholism (27%) and major functional psychosis (37%). Less than a quarter of the over-65s had a permanent address, suggesting that homelessness was an important determinant of custodial remand. Twenty-four of 1062 restricted patients admitted to hospital in 1998 in England and Wales were aged 60+; nine of these patients had been convicted of homicide, six of other violent offences and two of sexual offences[14].

CLINICAL ASPECTS OF OFFENDING IN THE ELDERLY

Affective Disorder

Roth[15] noted that the rare violent acts committed by aged men often arise in a setting of depressive illness with suicidal ideation. Depressive homicide most often involves a man killing his wife. The killing is generally viewed by the patient as at least partly altruistic, on account of thoughts that she would be unable to cope without him, although a dynamic formulation may indicate unacknowledged hostility. It is common for the act to be followed by suicide. Knight described several cases, noting that there is generally no history of previous violence or discord[16].

The disinhibition and irritability of mania may also lead to aggressive behaviour, although serious violence is uncommon. Both types of mood disorder may be associated with shoplifting, on account of poor concentration, diminished concern about social rules or associated dynamic factors. In relation to shoplifting, an emotional disturbance following a life crisis but falling short of depressive illness may form the background to the offence. It should also be borne in mind that the trauma of arrest itself in an elderly person with no previous symptoms may lead to psychiatric sequelae, including suicidal ideation.

Case History 1: Depressive Homicide

A 68-year-old man with previous episodes of depressive illness developed depressed mood and agitation over several weeks. There was no history of violence and he was known as a quiet kindly man. He became preoccupied with two themes, first that the water supply in his house was infected and had caused his wife's psoriasis, and second with guilt regarding a minor sexual misdemeanour that had occurred during his teens. His wife asked him to just try and do the shopping, something he found particularly difficult when depressed. He experienced the sudden thought that if he killed her, the action would have the dual benefit of releasing his wife from her misery and ensuring that he received a life sentence, a fitting punishment for the sexual misdemeanour. He strangled her and rang the police. He was bailed to hospital and later placed on probation, with a condition of psychiatric treatment.

Case History 2: Shoplifting and Depression

A 75-year-old retired plasterer with no previous convictions received the news that his son-in-law was having an affair. He himself had endured a stressful marriage for a lifetime. He became depressed in mood and overwhelmed by intrusive, angry thoughts towards his son-in-law. His sleep became disturbed and his powers of concentration diminished. While shopping he was observed to pick up a paint brush and slip it into his jacket. He then clambered over a barrier to leave the store. The shop refused to stop proceedings, but the Court dismissed the charge on hearing psychiatric evidence. The emotional crisis subsided with time and a period of supportive counselling.

Schizophrenia

The most common offence associated with schizophrenia in those that are homeless is shoplifting. However, both violent offences and arson may occur, on account of paranoid ideation.

Case History 3: Violence Associated with Paranoid Delusions

A 75-year-old man was arrested following his approaching a group in his local pub, grabbing one person by the neck and cutting his lower throat with a carving knife. The publican reported that the elderly man was a moderate drinker and that he had been expressing abnormal ideas over the previous year. He had had a partial pneumonectomy for lung cancer 3 years prior to the offence. At interview he said that neighbours watched him all the time, made derogatory remarks about him and had a laser machine which they used on his body. On the day of the offence, he said he had heard one of the group of men say "He stinks", and

concluded that they were associated with those acting against him. He returned home for a knife and said later he only wished to frighten the victim. No evidence of recurrence of his lung cancer was found at that stage. Following treatment with antipsychotic medication, he no longer complained of abnormal experiences, although he retained some delusional ideas. He became relaxed and content in contrast to his agitated state prior to treatment and said that he had no desire to revenge himself on the people involved in the paranoid ideation. He pleaded guilty to wounding with intent and was placed on a hospital order under Section 37 of the Mental Health Act (1983), with restrictions on discharge under Section 41. There were no management problems, although he remained in hospital until his death with metastases 18 months later.

Dementia

Assaultative behaviour in dementia is not uncommon, although within a family or institutional setting the behaviour is unlikely to form the basis of a formal charge. Disinhibition, misinterpretation and the pressures of close living with others may be contributory factors. Petrie et al.[17] studied a series of 222 consecutive admissions to a psychogeriatric unit in the USA and noted that 139 had shown verbal aggression or violence, 18 incidents involving the use of knives or guns; 39 of these patients were suffering from senile dementia and the remainder from functional psychoses. Disinhibited sexual behaviour or fire-setting may also reflect the loss of cortical inhibiting factors in dementia.

Persistent theft from shops may be linked with absent-mindedness in the early stages of illness or with a more general deterioration in social behaviour at a later stage. Mendez described a case of persistent stealing in a 71-year-old man with dementia who constantly picked up small items with no explanation for his actions[18].

Alcoholism

In addition to alcohol-related offences, such as driving while intoxicated, problem drinking may be associated with theft, criminal damage, violent or sex offences. Many cases involve a variety of factors, e.g. about one-third of elderly homicide offenders in a series studying coroners' files had been drinking at the time of the killing[6].

ASSESSMENT OF THE ELDERLY OFFENDER

A careful assessment of mental and physical health and of the person's social circumstances and the quality of relationships within this is necessary. Particular note should be taken of the use of alcohol and of prescribed or proprietary medication. Where the charge is more serious, full details of the allegation should be obtained from witness statements and informants.

In assessing a defendant's fitness to plead, consideration is particularly given to the defendant's ability to understand the nature of the charge and the significance of his plea and to follow the process of the trial. In some cases, discontinuation of proceedings may be more appropriate.

THE ELDERLY WITHIN THE CRIMINAL JUSTICE SYSTEM

Appropriate assessment that would identify those offenders requiring social and psychiatric intervention is often lacking, although there has been a greater emphasis on diversion from the criminal justice system in recent years. Cautioning is as common a disposal as conviction in England and Wales for all but the most serious crimes in those aged 60+[5]. In addition, many shops have adopted policies of not reporting shoplifting in those of retirement age, preferring to ban persistent offenders from their premises. In the USA a number of schemes have been developed to deal with the older offender, both pre-trial and after sentencing[17].

In the Essex cohort of 153 elderly offenders studied by Needham-Bennett et al.[12], 97 (65%) were cautioned and in 42 (28%) there was no further action. The police, however, referred only half of those later identified as psychiatric cases to welfare agencies, suggesting that closer links between the police and community psychiatric teams for the elderly might facilitate the identification of unmet mental health needs at an early stage.

The elderly serving sentences comprise both those imprisoned for the first time in old age and those who have grown old in prison. About 1% of the prison population in the UK is aged 60+ and about 5% in the USA. The number of sentenced prisoners in the UK aged 60+ has increased in recent years, from 333 in 1988 to 1055 in 1998, although there has not been a similar increase in the elderly remand population[1]. A case history-based study in the USA of 25 new elderly offenders, most of whom were imprisoned for sex offences or homicide[19], drew attention to their initial reaction to imprisonment, often being characterized by family conflict, depression, suicidal thoughts and a fear of dying in prison[19]. The physical health of older prisoners is also important, with about half of older prisoners having a long-standing illness or disability[20]. The prison system makes scant provision for vulnerable groups and older prisoners may experience particular difficulties in adjustment on release.

REFERENCES

1. Home Office. Research and Statistics Directorate, London, UK.
2. Schichor D. Patterns of elderly law breaking in urban, suburban and rural areas: what do arrest statistics tell us? In Wilbanks W, Kein P, eds, *Elderly Criminals*. New York: University Press of America, 1984.
3. Craissati J, McClurg G. The Challenge Project: perpetrators of child sexual abuse in south east London. *Child Abuse Neglect* 1996; **20**(11): 1067–77.
4. Craissati J (personal communication).
5. Markham GR. A community service for elderly offenders. *Geriat Med* 1981; **11**(2): 63–6.
6. Kratcoski PC, Walker DB. Homicide among the elderly: analysis of the victim/assailant relationship. In McCarthy B, Langworthy RH, eds, *Older Offenders*. New York: Praeger, 1988.
7. Hucker SJ, Ben Aron MH. Psychiatric aspects of crime in old age. In Newman ES, Newman DJ, Gewirtz ML, eds, *Elderly Criminals*. Cambridge, MA: Oelgeschlager, Gunn and Hain, 1984.
8. Akers RL, La Greca AJ. Alcohol, contact with the legal system and illegal behaviour among the elderly. In McCarthy B, Langworthy RH, eds, *Older Offenders*. New York: Praeger, 1988.
9. Taylor PJ, Parrott JM. Elderly offenders. A study of age-related factors among custodially remanded prisoners. *Br J Psychiat* 1988; **152**: 340–6.
10. East WN. Senescence and senility. *J Ment Sci* 1944; **90**: 836–49.
11. March GS, Zimmer B, Stein E. Clinical perspectives on elderly first offender shoplifters. *Hosp Comm Psychiat* 1988; **39**: 648–51.
12. Needham-Bennett H, Parrott J, MacDonald AJD. Psychiatric disorder and policing the elderly offender. *Crim Behav Ment Health* 1996; **6**: 241–51.
13. Copeland J, Dewey M, Griffiths-Jones H. Computerised psychiatric diagnostic system and case nomenclature for elderly subjects. GMS and AGECAT. *Psychol Med* 1986; **16**: 89–99.
14. *Home Office Statistical Bulletin*, Issue 7/00, Mar 2000.
15. Roth M. Cerebral and mental disorders of old age as causes of antisocial behaviour. In de Reuck AUS, Porter R, eds, *CIBA Foundation Symposium: The Mentally Abnormal Offender*. London: Churchill, 1968.
16. Knight B. Geriatric homicide—or the Darby and Joan syndrome. *Geriat Med* 1983; **13**(4): 297–300.
17. Petrie WM, Lawson EC, Hollender MH. Violence in geriatric patients. *J Am Med Assoc* 1982; **284**: 443–4.
18. Mendez MF. Pathological stealing in dementia. *J Am Geriat Soc* 1988; **36**(9): 825–6.
19. Aday R. Ageing in prison: a case study of new elderly offenders. *Int J Offender Ther Comp Criminol* 1994; **38**(1): 80–91.
20. Bridgwood A, Malbon G. *Survey of the Physical Health of Prisoners 1994*. London: OPCS, HMSO, 1994.

Sleep and Ageing:
Disorders and Management

Helen Chiu

Chinese University of Hong Kong, People's Republic of China

Sleep complaints are very common in the elderly, with up to 40% being affected by insomnia. Further, a disproportionately large number of prescriptions of sedative–hypnotics are given to elderly people. Sleep disturbances in the elderly may be the result of physiological changes with the ageing process, poor sleep hygiene, medical and psychiatric conditions (particularly depression) leading to secondary sleep disturbance, and primary sleep disorders[1].

A number of changes in sleep characteristics and architecture occurs with ageing. In general, the older person takes more time to fall asleep, has more awakenings and less efficient sleep, as well as more napping in the daytime. Moreover, the older person tends to go to bed early and rise early, reflecting a phase-advanced rhythm of the sleep–wake pattern. In addition, there is a decrease in slow wave sleep and rapid eye movement (REM) sleep but an increase in light sleep, i.e. stages 1 and 2 of NREM sleep[1–3].

Inadequate sleep hygiene includes poor sleep habits and engaging in sleep-incompatible behaviour[4]. Excessive time in bed, irregular hour of going to bed, lack of exercise, excessive caffeine intake, alcohol withdrawal and noisy environment are all factors that might influence sleep.

Numerous medical conditions can lead to sleep disturbances, especially when pain is a significant feature. In the elderly, dementia is a common cause of sleep disturbance. In Alzheimer's disease, there is a decrease in slow-wave sleep and REM sleep, with increased fragmentation of sleep. A disrupted sleep–wake cycle is frequently found. Agitation and confusion in the evening and at night (sundowning) may also occur in some patients[5].

As for primary sleep disorders, sleep apnoea, REM sleep behaviour disorder and periodic leg movement during sleep (PLMS) are the ones with increased prevalence in the elderly, and will be dealt with in this chapter.

SLEEP APNOEA

A period of apnoea is defined by a cessation of breathing for 10 s or more, whereas a hypopnoea period is a 50% reduction in the respiratory depth for 10 seconds or more. Sleep apnoea is characterized by recurrent episodes of apnoea and hypopnoea during sleep, and is usually associated with oxygen desaturation in the blood[6].

There are two main types of sleep apnoea, obstructive and central. Obstructive sleep apnoea is the more common form. Cardinal features are loud snoring and excessive daytime sleepiness. Associated features include headache, insomnia, apnoea observed during sleep, excessive movements during sleep, cognitive impairment, personality changes and enuresis. Physical problems include systemic hypertension, pulmonary hypertension and cor pulmonale[6], which might explain why sleep apnoea is associated with an increased mortality due to cardiovascular events.

The exact prevalence of sleep apnoea is unknown but it is estimated that about 2–4% of the general population meet minimal criteria for obstructive sleep apnoea[7]. Its frequency increases with age, reaching a maximum between 50 and 70 years of age, and there is a male predominance. In the elderly, prevalence rates of 26–73% have been reported in various studies[8]. This shows that disordered breathing is a common problem in the elderly. However, a major unresolved issue is whether sleep apnoea is a less pathological condition in the elderly. Studies in clinical populations have shown that disturbed respiration during sleep in the elderly has minimal association with mortality and morbidity, while epidemiologic studies in the elderly have suggested otherwise[2]. Pending further studies to clarify the issue, older people with symptomatic sleep apnoea probably should be treated in the same way as younger patients.

In the management of sleep apnoea, general measures include weight reduction and avoidance of alcohol and benzodiazepines before bedtime. In the majority of patients with sleep apnoea, continuous positive airway pressure (CPAP) during sleep is the treatment of choice. Surgical treatment may be indicated for patients with specific upper airway abnormality who have failed CPAP therapy or did not want CPAP for various reasons, such as frequent travelling[9].

REM SLEEP BEHAVIOUR DISORDER (RSBD)

This is a recently described parasomnia[10]. Presenting features are usually excessive motor activity during sleep, which may lead to repeated injuries to the patients or their bed-partners. Patients may talk or shout aloud in sleep, accompanied by vigorous limb movements, walking, falling out of bed, or carrying out various activities in their dreams. After awakening, patients may recall dreams that coincide with their motor activities. This suggests that the motor activity in sleep is a form of dream enactment. Some patients resort to various measures to protect themselves from injury, like tying themselves to the bed or putting a mattress on the floor. In addition, the nature of their dreams may change over the years, becoming very vivid and action-packed[11]. The diagnosis of RSBD should be considered in elderly people presenting with sleep-related injury or violence.

Principles and Practice of Geriatric Psychiatry, 2nd edn. Edited by J. R. M. Copeland, M. T. Abou-Saleh and D. G. Blazer
©2002 John Wiley & Sons, Ltd

There are very few studies on the prevalence of RSBD. A study in the general population by telephone interview found that 0.5% had probable RSBD[12]. Another study on a community sample of elderly reported a rate of 0.4%[13]. RSBD tends to occur predominantly in the elderly, and males are more affected. In general, the awareness of this condition is low among the public as well as clinicians, and misdiagnosis is common.

RSBD occurs in transient or chronic form[11]. The transient form may be induced by drugs as well as alcohol withdrawal. The chronic form is either idiopathic or associated with neurological disorders in up to 50% of cases, such as dementia, Parkinson's disease, multiple system atrophy and vascular or neoplastic lesions of the central nervous system. In particular, there is a strong association with Parkinson's disease and dementia with Lewy bodies[14,15].

The exact aetiology and pathophysiology of RSBD is unclear. In normal people, there is generalized muscle paralysis during REM sleep, sparing only the diaphragm and extraocular muscles. In RSBD there is a disruption of this pattern and patients can thus move and act out their dreams[11].

Management of RSBD includes drug treatment with clonazepam, which is effective in up to 90% of cases, as well as safety measures to protect the patients from injuries[16].

PERIODIC LEG MOVEMENT IN SLEEP

Previously known as nocturnal myoclonus, PLMS consists of stereotyped, periodic jerky movements of the lower limbs, usually occurring in light sleep. Symptoms include leg jerks, insomnia, daytime sleepiness and sometimes cold feet[17]. PLMS is associated with restless legs syndrome (RLS), which is characterized by the presence of unpleasant sensation in the lower limbs occurring when the patient lies down in bed, frequently leading to insomnia. However, PLMS can occur independently of RLS.

PLMS may occur as an isolated finding, but has been observed in a number of pathological conditions, such as chronic myelopathies and peripheral neuropathies, uraemia and sleep apnoea[18].

PLMS is very common in the elderly; studies have reported rates up to 45%[17]. Nevertheless, the relationship of PLMS and insomnia is still a matter of debate. It has been suggested that PLMS may be coincidental with sleep–wake disorders, rather than being a cause of it; indeed, many elderly with PLMS are completely asymptomatic.

Mild cases of PLMS may not need any treatment. For more severe cases, options of drug treatment include benzodiazepines (particularly clonazepam), L-dopa, bromocriptine and opiates[18].

REFERENCES

1. Vitiello MV. Sleep disorders and aging: understanding the causes. *J Gerontol* 1997; **52A**: M189–91.
2. Bliwise DL. Normal aging. In Kryger MH, Roth T, Dement W, eds, *Principles and Practice of Sleep Medicine*, 2nd edn. Philadelphia, PA: W.B. Saunders, 1994; 26–39.
3. Jagus CE, Benbow SM. Sleep disorders in the elderly. *Adv Psychiat Treatm* 1999; **5**: 30–8.
4. Becker PM, Jameison AO. Common sleep disorders in the elderly: diagnosis and treatment. *Geriatrics* 1991; **47**: 41–52.
5. Bliwise DL. Dementia. In Kryger MH, Roth T, Dement W, eds, *Principles and Practice of Sleep Medicine*, 2nd edn. Philadelphia, PA: W.B. Saunders, 1994; 790–800.
6. Parkes JD. Sleep apnoea and other respiratory disorders during sleep. In Parkes JD, ed., *Sleep and Its Disorders*. London: W.B. Saunders, 1985: 335–403.
7. Strohl KP. Obstructive sleep apnea syndrome. In Pocota JS, Mitler MM, eds, *Sleep Disorders: Diagnosis and Treatment*. Clifton, NJ: Humana, 1998: 117–35.
8. Fleury B. Sleep apnoea syndrome in the elderly. *Sleep* 1992; **15**: S39–41.
9. Powell NB, Guilleminault C, Riley R. Surgical treatment for obstructive sleep apnoea. In Kryger MH, Roth T, Dement W, eds, *Principles and Practice of Sleep Medicine*, 2nd edn. Philadelphia, PA: W.B. Saunders, 1994: 706–21.
10. Schenck CH, Bundlie SR, Ettinger MG *et al*. Chronic behavioural disorders of human REM sleep: a new category of parasomnia. *Sleep* 1986; **9**: 293–308.
11. Mahowald MW, Schenck CH. REM-sleep behaviour disorder. In Thorpy MJ, ed., *Handbook of Sleep Disorders*. New York: Marcel Dekker, 1990: 567–93.
12. Ohayon MM, Caulet M, Priest R. Violent behavior during sleep. *J Clin Psychiat* 1997; **58**: 369–76.
13. Chiu HFK, Wing YK, Lam LCW *et al*. Sleep-related injury in the elderly—an epidemiological study in Hong Kong. *Sleep* 2000; **23**: 513–17.
14. Schenck C, Mahawold M. Delayed emergence of a parkinsonian disorder in 38% of 29 older males initially diagnosed with idiopathic REM sleep behavior disorder. *Neurology* 1996; **46**: 388–93.
15. Boeve BF, Silber MH, Ferman TJ *et al*. REM sleep behavior disorder and degenerative dementia: an association likely reflecting Lewy body disease. *Neurology* 1998; **51**: 363–70.
16. Chiu HFK, Wing YK. REM sleep behaviour disorder—an overview. *Int J Clin Pract* 1997; **51**: 451–4.
17. Ancoli-Israel S, Kripke DF, Klauber MR *et al*. Periodic limb movements in sleep in community-dwelling elderly. *Sleep* 1991; **14**: 496–500.
18. Montplaisir J, Godbout R, Pelletier G, Warnes H. Restless legs syndrome and periodic leg movements during sleep. In Kryger MH, Roth T, Dement W, eds, *Principles and Practice of Sleep Medicine*, 2nd edn. Philadelphia, PA: W.B. Saunders, 1994: 589–97.

Rating Scale for Aggressive Behaviour in the Elderly

L. C. W. Lam

The Chinese University of Hong Kong, People's Republic of China

Aggressive behaviour is one of the commonest causes for psychogeriatric admissions. It is highly correlated with carers' distress and rejection, as well as a decision for long-term institutional care[1-2]. To rationally evaluate the effectiveness of intervention strategies for aggressive behaviour, it would be very important to identify suitable assessment tools. The Rating Scale for Aggressive Behavior in the Elderly (RAGE) is specifically designed for the assessment of this aspect of behavioural problems in psychogeriatric institutional settings[3].

The RAGE is a 21-item rating scale administered by trained professionals, usually the nursing staff in the setting. The items include different dimensions of aggression (verbal, agitation and physical aggression), with no pre-defined diagnostic specifications. Aggressive behaviour is defined in the RAGE as "an overt act, involving the delivery of noxious stimuli to another organism, object or self, which is clearly not accidental". The scale is observer-rated and the staff is requested to complete the questionnaire based on observation in the ward over a 3 day period.

Patel and Hope[1] reported that the RAGE demonstrated good psychometric properties, with satisfactory reliability and validity. Comparison of RAGE with two other commonly used scales for aggression, the Cohen–Mansfield Agitation Inventory and the Brief Agitation Inventory, revealed that the three scales all highly intercorrelated, with meaningful constructs[4].

Studies using RAGE to measure aggressive behaviour in institutional settings revealed that about half of the elderly in psychogeriatric wards had positive ratings in aggressive episodes over a 3 day observation period. It was found that elderly schizophrenic patients, when compared with the demented elderly, were more frequently rated as overall aggressive, albeit with the same total scores in the RAGE[5]. The scores on the RAGE were found to be higher in moderate degree of dementia, and were also reported to be associated with activity disturbance and the presence of psychotic features[6].

Table 1. Items in the RAGE

Item	Ratings
Demanding	0–3
Shouted	0–3
Swore	0–3
Disobeyed ward rules	0–3
Uncooperative	0–3
Irritable	0–3
Sarcastic	0–3
Impatient	0–3
Threatened to harm	0–3
Antisocial acts	0–3
Pushed others	0–3
Destroyed property	0–3
Angry with self	0–3
Attempted to kick	0–3
Attempted to hit	0–3
Attempted to bite	0–3
Used object to hurt others	0–3
Self-inflicted injury	0–3
Injury to others	0–3
Sedation or restraint	0–3
Overall aggressiveness	0–3

REFERENCES

1. Patel V, Hope RA. A rating scale for aggressive behavior in the elderly—the RAGE. *Psychol Med* 1992; **22**: 211–21.
2. Patel V, Hope RA. Aggressive behavior in elderly psychiatric inpatients. *Acta Psychiat Scand* 1992; **85**: 131–5.
3. Patel V, Hope RA. Aggressive behavior in elderly people with dementia: a review. *Int J Geriat Psychiat* 1993; **8**: 457–72.
4. Shah A, Evans H, Parkash N. Evaluation of three aggression/agitation behavior rating scales for use on an acute admission and assessment psychogeriatric ward. *Int J Geriat Psychiat* 1998; **13**: 415–20.
5. Lam LC, Chiu HF, Ng J. Aggressive behavior in the Chinese elderly—validation of the Chinese version of the rating scale for aggressive behavior in the elderly (RAGE) in hospital and nursing home settings. *Int J Geriat Psychiat* 1997; **12**: 678–81.
6. Gormley N, Rizwan MR, Lovestone S. Clinical predictors of aggressive behavior in Alzheimer's disease. *Int J Geriat Psychiat* 1998; **13**: 109–15.

114

Sexual Disorders

J. M. Kellett

St George's Hospital Medical School, London, UK

THE CAUSE OF ERECTILE FAILURE

Although levels of free testosterone fall with age. this does not relate to levels of sexual activity[1,2], which correlate closely with age itself. Three hypotheses for the decline remain (although whether loss of interest leads to erectile failure or vice versa is in doubt); these are: (a) that increasing atheroma causes a failure of vasodilation sufficient to cause an erection; (b) that degenerative changes in the autonomic system are the cause; and (c) that levels of self-confidence decline with age, leading to psychogenic failure. Clinical impressions do not support the latter hypothesis, and a study of 28 men with erectile failure over age 65 compared to 25 aged-matched men who were potent showed no differences in their GHQ[3].

Feldman *et al.*[4] compared measures of health in 1290 males aged 40–70 in Massachusetts and found erectile failure to be increased with heart disease, diabetes, hypertension, depression and anger, and decreased by high-density cholesterol and by levels of dihydroepiandrosterone, a breakdown product of testosterone, but not by levels of testosterone itself. They did not measure neuronal ageing. Rowland *et al.*[5] found that penile sensitivity was related to erectile response. In our study[3] reported above, we found that only a measure of autonomic neuronal integrity (pilocarpine-induced sweating) distinguished the two groups fully. This might suggest that most elderly men with erectile failure would respond to corporeal vasodilators, which would be less effective if the cause was atheroma. The subject is well covered by Schiavi[6].

TREATMENT

Counselling allows the couple to express their fears and inhibitions, whilst the therapist can educate them about the normal changes of ageing. Elderly men, for example, often overestimate the importance of penetration, compared to petting, in the pleasure they give to their partner. Physical remedies are more widely used and include vacuum pumps[7], intracavernosal[8] and intraurethral[9] administration of alprostadil, oral sildenafil[10], which prolongs the action of cavernosal nitric oxide, and oxpentifylline for vasculogenic failure. Dopaminergic drugs can restore libido, if fear of prostatic cancer contraindicates testosterone. Disorders of female arousal are reduced by HRT and also respond to sildenafil[11].

REFERENCES

1. Davidson J, Chen J, Crapo L *et al*. Hormonal changes and sexual function in aging men. *J Clin Endocrinol Metab* 1983; **57**: 71–7.
2. Schiavi R, Schreiner-Engel P, White D, Mandell J. The relationship between pituitary–gonadal function and sexual behaviour in healthy aging men. *Psychosom Med* 1991; **53**: 363–74.
3. Bandl J, Ford R, Kellett J. Is erectile failure in the elderly caused by psychological factors? Paper presented to the inaugural meeting of BEDS, London, 1996.
4. Feldman H, Goldstein I, Hatzichristou D *et al*. Impotence and its medical and psychosocial correlates: results of the Massachusetts male aging study. *J Urol* 1994; **151**: 54–61.
5. Rowland D, Greenleaf W, Dorfman L, Davidson J. Aging and sexual function in men. *Arch Sex Behav* 1993; **22**: 545–57.
6. Schiavi R. *Aging and Sexual Function*. Cambridge: Cambridge University Press, 1999.
7. Cooper AJ. Preliminary experience with a vacuum constrictor device (VCD) as a treatment for impotence. *J Psychosom Res* 1987; **31**: 413–18.
8. Linet OI, Ogrine FG. Efficacy and safety of intracavernosal alprostadil in men with erectile dysfunction. *N Engl J Med* 1996; **334**: 873.
9. Padma-Nathan H, Hellstrom WJ, Kaiser FE *et al*. Treatment of men with erectile dysfunction with transurethral alprostadil. *N Engl J Med* 1998; **336**: 1–7.
10. Booleli M, Gepi-Attee S, Gingell C *et al*. Sildenafil, a novel effective oral therapy for male erectile dysfunction. *Br J Urol* 1996; **78**: 257–61.
11. Riley A. Personal communication, 1998.

Principles and Practice of Geriatric Psychiatry, 2nd edn. Edited by J. R. M. Copeland, M. T. Abou-Saleh and D. G. Blazer

115

Phenomenology of Wandering

A. Habib and G. T. Grossberg

St Louis University, MO, USA

With current increases in the elderly population, dementia and its related behavioral disturbances are receiving much more attention. Wandering is one of the common, often treatment-resistant behavioral concomitants of progressive dementia. Most research on wandering has focused on nursing home- or dementia clinic-based samples. In these samples, wandering occurs in up to 65% of patients at some point in the disease process[1-7].

DEFINITION AND PHENOMENOLOGY

There has been much debate about the appropriate definition of wandering, as well as its phenomenology. A major difficulty in wandering research has been the lack of a uniform definition and of reliable assessment instruments. Wandering was initially defined as "aimless movement"[8,9]. More recent definitions have viewed wandering not only as aimless, but also as having purposeful intent[10,11]. Wandering has further been classified, on the basis of phenomenology, as benign or problematic[8]. A benign wanderer is a patient who roams aimlessly and is easily redirectable, whereas a problem wanderer is one who is disruptive to family, staff or other residents and includes the individual who is resistant to redirection. Attempts have made to quantify wandering behavior into two broad categories, continuous and sporadic. "Continuous wanderers" are defined as ambulating more than 50% of their wakeful time, while "sporadic wanderers" move about for less than half of their wakeful time.

A common theme that is consistently supported in the literature is that wandering is primarily influenced by a continuity of behaviors from earlier premorbid times[12]. Recent research[13] has also focused on the relationship of premorbid personality and wandering. Overall, wandering is viewed as having a beneficial effect for the wanderer by fulfilling a particular need. De Leon *et al.*[18] showed that wanderers had poorer parietal lobe functioning than subjects with similar degrees of cognitive impairment. However, in a multisite, random sample of 163 ambulatory, cognitively impaired subjects, wanderers showed significantly greater impairment in basic skills (orientation, memory and concentration) and in the higher-order skills of language, abstract thinking, judgement and spatial skills[14]. In Monsour and Robb's[12] sample of wanderers, 36/44 subjects had dementia or Alzheimer's disease; eight had cerebral vascular accidents or arteriosclerosis. Although wanderers may have more cognitive decline, they often exhibit an intact social facade, which masks their deficits[15]. Snyder *et al.* also identifies that wanderers had a higher number of psychosocial needs than non-wanderers on the Human Development Inventory (HDI).

Table 115.1 Why patients wander

Trying to find "home"
Trying to find bathroom
Are hungry
Are in pain
Acute medical or environmental trigger, stress, or loss
Drug side effect or withdrawal
Are bored

Triggers of Wandering

Table 115.1 lists some common reasons why patients wander. They may be trying to find "home" or their room, whereas some are merely driven by the urge to void and are trying to find a bathroom. Some patients may be scavenging for food because they are hungry. Wandering behavior may be due to pain, e.g. arthritis or other painful medical states, which the patient cannot communicate. If the wandering behavior is of abrupt onset, one needs to ask if an acute stress or loss, whether a medical (e.g. an infection) or environmental (e.g. death of a roommate or family member) factor has triggered the wandering behavior. At times, wandering may be due to boredom.

TREATMENT

Table 115.2 highlights general treatment approaches to wandering behavior. The management of wandering behavior can be classified into three groups according to the potential etiology of the wandering behavior: (a) medical; (b) psychosocial; and (c) environmental.

The most important cause of wandering to exclude is an acute or chronic underlying medical problem, for example, an abrupt arrhythmia. Also, could the need to be on the move be a side effect of medications? Akathisia with neuroleptics or agitation with

Table 115.2 Treatment of wandering: general approaches

Eliminate physical/chemical restraints
Wander-safe indoor and outdoor areas
Eliminate distracting light and noise from environment
Use of electronic elopement prevention devices and patient identification bracelets
Proper staffing
Staff education and training
Philosophy of rehabilitation

Principles and Practice of Geriatric Psychiatry, 2nd edn. Edited by J. R. M. Copeland, M. T. Abou-Saleh and D. G. Blazer
©2002 John Wiley & Sons, Ltd

fluoxetine are examples. Perhaps a withdrawal syndrome, such as from alcohol or benzodiazepines, may be implicated. Pain as a trigger for wandering always needs to be considered.

In the nursing home, proper staffing, appropriate staff training with regard to causes and management of wandering behavior, coupled with supervised structured activities, such as music therapy and simple crafts, are important. Use of planned activities and distraction techniques may be helpful.

One of the key elements in managing wandering behaviors is to provide an appropriate and safe environment where wandering behavior can be tolerated. This should ideally include specially designed indoor and outdoor roaming areas that lack safety hazards or distracting elements. Innovative ideas include a "reduced stimulation unit"[11,16] and a "wanderer's lounge program"[17]. It is vital that wandering behavior is not dealt with via the use of physical restraints or the heavy use of sedatives or tranquilizers. Patients often fight such measures, resulting in more significant problem behaviors.

A major concern for family or institutional caregivers is that the wandering patient may elope and come to physical harm, e.g. run into automobile traffic. The use of "Wander-Guard"-type devices on doors and a special identification bracelet, labeled "cognitively impaired—if lost, please call (phone number of facility)" may help.

CONCLUSIONS

Wandering exacts a heavy toll on family and professional caregivers. For the wanderer, issues of safety are of paramount concern. To ease the burden on caregivers, it is important to try to ascertain *why* the patient is wandering. This will usually give clues to appropriate management. Unfortunately, wandering patients usually cannot communicate why they are wandering because of their cognitive impairment. Consequently, caregivers need to place themselves in the patient's shoes to come up with the answers.

REFERENCES

1. National Center for Health Statistics. *The National Nursing Home Survey: 1977 Summary for the United States*. Washington, DC: US Department of Health Education and Welfare.
2. Warshaw G, Moore J, Friedman W *et al*. Functional disability in the hospitalized elderly. *J Am Med Assoc* 1982; **248**(7): 847–50.
3. Kramer JR. Education and consultation on mental health in LTC facilities: problems, pitfalls, and solutions, a process approach to staff training and consultations. *J Geriat Psychiat* 1977; **10**(2): 197–213.
4. Goldfarb AI. Prevalence of psychiatric disorders in metropolitan old age and nursing homes. *J Am Geriat Soc* 1984; **10**: 77–84.
5. Teeker RB, Garetz FK, Miller WR *et al*. Psychiatric disturbances of aged patients in skilled nursing homes. *Am J Psychiat* 1976; **133**(12): 1430–4.
6. Zimmer JG, Watson N, Trent A. Behavioral problems among patients in skilled nursing facilities. *Am J Publ Health* 1984; **76**: 118.
7. Rovner BW, Kafonek S, Flipp L *et al*. Prevalence of mental illness in a community nursing home. *Am J Psychiat* 1986; **143**: 1446–9.
8. Grossberg G. Forms of wandering. In Copeland JRM, Abou-Saleh MT, Blazer DG, eds, *Principles and Practice of Geriatric Psychiatry*. Chichester: Wiley, 1994; 139–40.
9. Snyder L, Rupprecht P, Pyrek J *et al*. Wandering. *Gerontologist* 1978; **18**(3): 272–80.
10. Coons H. Wandering. *Am J Alzheimer's Care Rel Disord Res* 1988: January/February: 31–42.
11. Schwab M, Rader J, Doan J. Relieving the anxiety and fear in dementia. *J Gerontol Nurs* 1985; **11**: 8–12.
12. Monsour N, Robb S. Wandering behavior in old age: a psychosocial study. *Social Work* 1982; **27**: 411–16.
13. Thomas D. Wandering: a proposed definition. *J Gerontol Nurs* 1995; September: 35–41.
14. Algase DL. Wandering: Assessment and intervention. 1999: 163–75.
15. Dawson P, Reid D. Behavioral dimensions of patients at risk of wandering. *Gerontologist* 1987; **27**(1): 104–7.
16. Sawyer JC, Mendlovitz AA. A management program for ambulatory institutionalized patients with Alzheimer's disease and related disorders. Paper presented at the Annual Conference of the Gerontological Society, Boston, 1982.
17. McGrowder-Lin R. A wanderer's lounge program for nursing home residents with Alzheimer's disease. *Gerontologist* 1988; **28**(5): 607–9.
18. De Leon MJ, Potegal M, Gurland B. Wandering's parietal signs in senile dementia of Alzheimer's type. *Neuropsychobiology* 1984; **11**: 155–7.
19. Algase DL. A century of progress: today's strategies for responding to wandering behavior. *J Gerontol Nurs* 1992; **18**(11): 28–34.
20. Rader J, Doan J, Schwab S. How to decrease wandering, a form of agenda behavior. *Geriat Nurs* 1985; July/August: 196–9.

Part L

The Presentation of Mental Illness
in Elderly Persons in Different Cultures

Part I

Problems of Assessing Psychiatric Symptoms and Illness in Different Cultures

Melanie Abas

University of Auckland, New Zealand

Increasingly, psychiatrists must have the skills to assess and deliver care for people from different cultures. Many areas can only be touched on here, and several of the references stem from the cross-cultural literature in younger adults. The context is very broad, covering industrialized countries with multicultural populations and less-industrialized countries. It is worth noting that, due to a range of barriers, many people from different cultures have, of course, very poor access to psychiatric assessment and care[1–4].

COMMUNICATION AND CULTURAL AWARENESS

While health staff often come from different cultures than their patients[5], they are usually working within at least a familiar framework and landscape. With someone from a very different culture, the ability to assess appearance, behaviour and symptoms will be limited. The practitioner must work harder to gather the information to make an accurate assessment and to develop rapport and trust. Awareness of one's lack of information of one's own cultural "encumbrances" and of potential strong feelings about each other's cultures is crucial[6]. Training and consultation with a wide circle of people from the relevant culture is needed. Ask the patient early on about his/her background and, for migrants, his/her place of origin and experience in the new setting. Listening, asking open questions, acknowledging family expectations and a willingness to discuss issues such as racism and social needs are all vital. Within reasonable professional boundaries, the psychiatrist should be willing to respond to some questions about him/herself. For example, with older Jamaican migrants, culture-specific care providers stressed that making "a connection" with the doctor would facilitate the assessment and acceptance of care[7]. Show sensitivity but do not neglect important areas on "cultural" grounds, such as alcohol intake in Muslims. Apparent persecutory ideas must be explored and may reflect an appropriate response to injustice.

Language barriers should be addressed through the employment of ethnically close bilingual workers, otherwise use a competent interpreting and advocacy service[8]. Using relatives or other staff to interpret should be limited to emergencies. Requiring patients to speak in their second language can distort the clinical picture[6]. Aspects of non-verbal communication may also differ, such as avoidance of direct eye-to-eye contact in some Asian and Pacific cultures.

DIFFERENT PRESENTATIONS OF EMOTIONAL DISTRESS

People from all cultures experience both somatic and psychological symptoms when emotionally distressed[9]. One reason for a more somatic presentation may be that this is seen as a more appropriate focus for medical consultation by some cultures. Second, there may be a continuum of experience and interpretation, with the more "somatizing" cultures at one end and the more "psychologizing"[10,11] at the other. Thirdly, a large number of "somatic" complaints are actually metaphors for mental distress. Many of these relate to heart discomfort (e.g. a heart that is "sinking" or "uncomfortable")[12–14] and to abdominal sensation[15,16].

Culture-bound syndromes usually represent cultural explanations for recognizable psychoses or neuroses[13]. For example, Dhat, a belief that semen is leaking from the body in urine, is a complaint in India. It may be a presenting feature, and is used as an explanation for weakness due to depression or organic disease.

DEPRESSION

There has been much debate about the existence of depression as a universal cross-cultural category[10,17]. It is reasonably established that depressive disorders exist across cultures and are strongly related to local constructs[15,18,19]. However, symptoms vary (e.g. depressed older Jamaicans and African-Americans describe feeling "low", "bad" or "fed-up")[20,21]; multiple somatic symptoms or metaphors may be presented; and some cultures may emphasize their explanation (e.g. social or spiritual) for their symptoms[22]. The validity of screening scales may vary, e.g. a lower cut-off point for the Geriatric Depression Scale has been recommended for older African-Caribbeans, African-Americans and Mexican-Americans[23,24]. Symptom profiles in depressed cases may also differ considerably across cultures, as shown even across European centres in older people[34]. Depression at community level also appears to be highly correlated with anxiety[25]. The implications are that: (a) it is important to enquire about the *full* range of affective and neurotic symptoms; and (b) a wide definition of mood disorders is likely to be most useful in the clinical setting.

Principles and Practice of Geriatric Psychiatry, 2nd edn. Edited by J. R. M. Copeland, M. T. Abou-Saleh and D. G. Blazer

FUNCTIONAL PSYCHOSES

Psychotic symptoms and signs appear similar in form across a wide variety of settings[26], although the content, e.g. of delusions, will be influenced by culture. Also, of course, the patient and his family's explanation for the illness will depend on their cultural framework[27]. Hence, someone from Zambia may explain his/her schizophrenia as he/she might explain a stroke, depression or a burglary—as due to bewitchment or to having angered a spirit.

Culturally-supported dissociative states and altered states of consciousness can be misleading[6]. Pseudohallucinatory phenomena have been described in non-psychotic depression, anxiety and distress states[13,28].

An apparently unusual idea, such as believing oneself to be bewitched, is only a delusion if it is out of keeping with the beliefs of others in the culture. This must be checked by asking someone with appropriate knowledge. If faced with the patient alone, ask how he/she came to believe this, and if others close to him/her agree. If a traditional healer told him/her so, and his/her peers agree, then it is at least likely that this is a culturally sanctioned belief. Another error is to assume that a belief is culturally normal when it is actually abnormal.

DEMENTIA

DSM-IV criteria[29] for dementia require the demonstration of cognitive impairment of sufficient severity to interfere with the activities of daily living. However, cultures vary in the extent to which they expect older people to take responsibility, e.g. for domestic activities. Also, impairment from physical conditions is commoner in socially disadvantaged people and will be difficult to distinguish from that due to dementia, requiring greater emphasis on physical examination and tests[6,30]. Many cognitive tests include items affected by education (e.g. requiring reading, writing or arithmetic skills) and/or which may have little relevance in certain cultures (e.g. "Who is the President?", "Take 7 from 100"). When testing those unfamiliar with such approaches, be courteous, encouraging (without "helping"), give explicit instructions and some dummy tasks to allay anxiety[30]. Rather than doggedly adhering to the original version of instruments, it is appropriate either to make rational adaptations (as described for the MMSE[35]) or to develop new instruments[31]. Novel adaptations will, of course, require translation, back-translation and pre-testing[33]. Suitable informants should be screened for any decline in function of their close contact[32]. The Community Screening Instrument for Dementia[31,33] combines culture-fair cognitive testing with a structured informant interview. This approach should become more routinely applied, both in primary and secondary care.

REFERENCES

1. Bahl V. Access to health care for Black and ethnic minority elderly people: general principles. In Hopkins A, Bahl V, eds, *Access to Health Care for People from Black and Ethnic Minorities*. London: Royal College of Physicians of London, 1993; 93–7.
2. Baker F. Ethnic minority elders: a mental health research agenda. *Hosp Commun Psychiat* 1992; **43**: 337–8, 342.
3. Bhugra D, Lippett R, Cole E. Pathways into care: an explanation of the factors that may affect minority ethnic groups. In Bhugra D, Bahl V, eds, *Ethnicity: An Agenda for Mental Health*. London: Royal College of Psychiatrists, 1999; 29–39.
4. Desjarlais R, Eisenberg L, Good B, Kleinman A. *World Mental Health: Problems and Priorities in Low-income Countries*. Oxford: Oxford University Press, 1995; 207–27.
5. Laugharne R. Evidence-based medicine, user involvement and the post-modern paradigm. *Psychiat Bull* 1999; **23**: 641–3.
6. Westermeyer J. Clinical considerations in cross-cultural diagnosis. *Hosp Commun Psychiat* 1987; **38**(2): 160–5.
7. Abas M. Functional disorders in ethnic minority elders. In Holmes C, Howard R, eds, *Advances in Old Age Psychiatry: Chromosomes to Community Care*. Petersfield: Wrightson Biomedical, 1997; 234–45.
8. Jayaratnam R. The need for cultural awareness. In Hopkins A, Bahl V, eds, *Access to Health Care for People from Black and Ethnic Minorities*. London: Royal College of Physicians of London, 1993; 11–20.
9. Helman CG. *Culture, Health and Illness*, 2nd edn. Bristol: Wright, 1990.
10. Kleinman A. Anthropology and psychiatry. *Br J Psychiat* 1987; **151**: 447–54.
11. Leff J. *Psychiatry Around the Globe*, 2nd edn. London: Gaskell, 1988; 43–53.
12. Good B. The heart of what's the matter: the semantics of illness in Iran. *Culture Med Psychiat* 1977; **1**: 25–58.
13. Rack P. *Race, Culture and Mental Disorder*. London: Tavistock, 1982.
14. Yanping Z, Leyi X, Qijie S. Styles of verbal expression of emotional and physical experiences: a study of depressed patients and normal controls in China. *Culture Med Psychiat* 1986; **10**: 231–43.
15. Abas M, Broadhead J. Depression and anxiety among women in an urban setting in Zimbabwe. *Psychol Med* 1997; **27**: 59–71.
16. Cheetham W, Cheetham R. Concepts of mental illness amongst the Xhosa people in South Africa. *Aust NZ J Psychiat* 1976; **10**: 39–45.
17. Marsella A, Sartorius N, Jablensky A, Fenton F. Cross-cultural studies of depression. In Kleinman A, Good B, eds, *Culture and Depression*. Berkeley, CA: University of California Press, 1985; 299–324.
18. Beiser M, Cargo M, Woodbury M. A comparison of psychiatric disorder in different cultures: depressive typologies in south-east Asian refugees and resident Canadians. *Int J Methods Psychiat* 1994; **4**: 157–72.
19. Patel V. *Culture and Common Mental Disorders in Sub-Saharan Africa: Studies in Primary Care in Zimbabwe*. Hove: Psychology Press, 1998.
20. Abas M, Phillips C, Richards M et al. Initial development of the new culture specific screen for emotional distress in older Caribbean people. *Int J Geriat Psychiat* 1996; **12**: 1097–103.
21. Baker F, Wiley D, Velli C, et al. Depressive symptoms in African-American medical patients. *Int J Geriat Psychiat* 1995; **10**: 9–14.
22. Patel V. Spiritual distress: an idiom of psychosocial distress amongst Shona speakers in Harare. *Acta Psychiat Scand* 1995; **92**: 103–7.
23. Abas M, Phillips C, Carter J et al. Culturally sensitive validation of screening questionnaires for depression in older African-Caribbean people living in south London. *Br J Psychiat* 1998; **173**: 249–254.
24. Baker F, Espino D, Robinson B, Stewart B. Assessing depressive symptoms in African-American and Mexican-American elders. *Clin Gerontol* **14**(1): 15–29.
25. Jacob K, Everitt B, Patel V. The comparison of latent variable models of non-psychotic morbidity in four culturally different populations. *Psychol Med* 1998; **28**: 145–52.
26. World Health Organization. *The International Pilot Study of Schizophrenia*, vol 1. Geneva: WHO, 1973.
27. Fabrega H. Psychiatric stigma in non-Western societies. *Comp Psychiat* 1991; **32**: 534–51.
28. Patel V, Simunyu E, Gwanzura F et al. The Shona Symptom Questionnaire: the development of an indigenous measure of non-psychotic mental disorder in Harare. *Acta Psychiat Scand* 1997; **95**: 469–75.
29. American Psychiatric Association. *Diagnostic and Statistical Manual of Mental Disorders (DSM-IV)*, 4th edn. Washington, DC: APA, 1994.
30. Chandra V, Ganguli M, Ratcliff G et al. Studies of the epidemiology of dementia: comparisons between developed and developing countries. *Aging Clin Exp Res* 1994; **6**: 307–21.
31. Hall K, Hendrie H, Brittain H, Norton J. The development of a dementia screening interview in two distinct languages. *Int J Methods Psychiat Res* 1995; **3**: 1–28.

32. Jorm A, Scott R, Cullen J, MacKinnon A. Performance of the Informant Questionnaire on Cognitive Decline in the Elderly (IQCODE) as a screening test for dementia. *Psychol Med* 1991; **21**: 758–90.

33. Hall K, Ogunniyi AO, Hendrie H *et al*. A cross-cultural community-based study of dementias: methods and performance of the survey instrument in Indianapolis, USA, and Ibadan, Nigeria. *Int J Methods Psychiat Res* 1996; **6**: 129–42.

34. Copeland J, Beekman A, Dewey M *et al*. Cross-cultural comparison of depressive symptoms in Europe does not support stereotypes of ageing. *Br J Psychiat* 1999; **174**: 322–38.

35. Ganguli M, Ratcliff G, Chandra V *et al*. A Hindi version of the MMSE: the development of a cognitive screening instrument for a largely illiterate rural elderly population in India. *Int J Geriat Psychiat* 1995; **10**: 367–77.

Depression in the Indian Subcontinent

Vikram Patel

London School of Hygiene and Tropical Medicine, London, UK, and The Sangath Society, Goa

Common mental disorders, such as depression in late life, are not well understood or acknowledged by either the community or the medical profession in India, for three important reasons. First, recognition of common mental disorders as a psychiatric problem in general is relatively poor. Most patients present with somatic symptoms. While many patients and health providers acknowledge the non-organic basis of these symptoms, neither group is comfortable with labels that imply a relationship to psychiatry. Indeed, terms such as "depression" and "anxiety", when used to define diagnostic categories of psychiatric disorder, have no conceptual equivalent in any Indian language. Ethnographic studies have shown that symptoms of depression are attributed to tension, family conflict and lack of family affection, rather than being seen as a biomedical psychiatric problem[1]. The second reason for low recognition is that the relative proportion of elders is less than 5% for most Indian communities. This is bound to change in the future, with falling birth-rates and rising longevity leading to predictions that, over 20 years, this oldest sector of the population will exceed 100 million. The implications are grave, for India has no systematic social welfare system for the aged, and is faced with the gradual breakdown of traditional extended family systems that have formed the bulwark for the care of the disabled and chronically ill[1]. The third reason is:

> the fatalistic attitude toward aging in India, which mandates that elderly persons accept their physical and mental condition as a normal part of old age. Not only are elderly persons with mental illnesses rarely brought to a physician, but those with treatable medical conditions also often receive no medical attention[2].

There are few epidemiological studies of common mental disorders in elders in India and no published studies, to date, that have used structured psychiatric interviews. Prevalence rates for depression in a community sample of elders have varied from 6% in southern India[3] to over 50% in rural West Bengal[4]. The common presenting complaints are tiredness, sleep complaints, aches, tingling-numbness in the hands and palpitations. On enquiry, however, most depressed elders will admit to cognitive and emotional symptoms typical of depression. The hallmark cognitive feature is anhedonia, or loss of interest. Suicidal feelings and agitation are also common[3]. The suicide rate in the 50+ age group (12/100 000) is nearly twice the national average (7/100 000). Co-morbidity with physical ill-health is common; by some estimates, more than 90% of elders with a psychiatric disorder also have some physical disorder[3]. Risk factors for depression include low education, poverty, social isolation and family discord.

The latter is on the rise as a result of the breakdown of traditional community structures resulting from the massive migration of the younger productive members of families to urban areas and reduced economic activity in rural areas. The commonest treatments in primary care are symptomatic. Thus, benzodiazepines for insomnia and vitamins and "tonics" for tiredness are amongst the commonest prescriptions for common mental disorders in general health care, while antidepressants or psychotherapy are rarely offered[5].

The rising rates of recognized risk factors, relatively low recognition of depression and even lower rates of appropriate interventions should cause considerable concern to public health policy and planning in India. One major limitation in influencing policy and practice is the lack of systematic evidence of the epidemiology of depression, and the efficacy and cost-effectiveness of treatments for depression, in elders in India. Research into the mental health needs of elders in India is clearly an important area for future psychiatric research. Health education should aim to educate health workers and the community to recognize that anhedonia and insomnia are not the expected price of growing old, but the result of a common, disabling and treatable illness. Removing stigma may require integrating the subject of depression into training programs for community and general health workers, and collaborating with non-governmental organizations that are pioneering programs to empower the elderly, support families with a mentally ill elder and provide health care sensitive to their needs. Working with the existing manpower and health and social service infrastructure is likely to be more successful in meeting the mental health needs of elders in India than developing specialized psychogeriatric services throughout the country.

REFERENCES

1. Patel V, Prince M. Ageing and mental health in developing countries: Who cares? Qualitative studies from Goa. *Psych Med* 2001; **31**: 29–38.
2. Chandra V. Cross-cultural perspectives: India. *Int Psychogeriat*, 1996; **8**(suppl 3): 479–81.
3. Venkoba Rao A. Psychiatry of old age in India. *Int Rev Psychiat* 1993; **5**: 165–70.
4. Nandi PS, Banerjee G, Mukherjee S. A study of psychiatric morbidity in an elderly population in a rural communty in West Bengal. *Ind J Psychiat* 1997; **39**: 122–9.
5. Patel V, Pereira J, Fernandes J, Mann A. Poverty, psychological disorder and disability in primary care attenders in Goa, India. *Br J Psychiat* 1998; **172**: 533–6.

Dementia in the Indian Subcontinent

S. Rajkumar[1], M. Ganguli[2] and D. V. Jeste[3]

[1]*University of Newcastle, NSW, Australia,* [2]*University of Pittsburgh, PA, USA, and*
[3]*University of San Diego, and VA San Diego Healthcare System, CA, USA*

Of India's population of nearly one billion, 50 million are aged 65 years or older and constitute a major potential high-risk group for dementia, yet pathological studies of dementia in India suggest that Alzheimer's disease (AD) is rare or unrecognized in most clinic populations. The few published epidemiological studies of dementia from India suggest potential regional differences in prevalence, which may be partly attributable to literacy or urban/rural residence. Differences across studies may also reflect methodological difficulties and differences. Psychometric and other screening instruments must be standardized in different Indian languages for elderly populations with widely varying levels of literacy, education and urbanization. Older individuals frequently have inadequately corrected sensory impairments, which can interfere with testing. They may have little interest in current national or world events, and thus appear to be impaired, and may not know their dates of birth. Cognitive deficits may be under-recognized and under-reported by family members, out of respect for, as well as reflecting low expectations of, the elderly. Prevalence rates of dementia from different studies in India[1-5] have ranged from a low of 1.36% to a high of 3.5% among those aged 65+. These low rates were found despite the use of highly standardized instruments for case detection, e.g. the GMS–AGECAT program and the community version of the GMS at the Madras site of a WHO multicenter study[4].

Lower prevalence may be due to shorter life expectancy, with selective survival of those not at risk for dementia, and also to shorter duration or survival with the disease. Survival may be underestimated if the manifestations of dementia are detected late or attributed in their earlier stages to normal aging. Plausible risk factors yet to be explored in Indian populations include head trauma, thyroid disease and illiteracy. Potential protective factors might range from family caregiving to low-fat diets. Tolerance of memory loss in old age, as well as lack of financial resources, may delay acceptance of treatment across the majority of Indian communities. Although prevalence is low, dementia may still pose a major public health challenge given the vastly growing population, the minimal existing infrastructure and the transitions in family structure in these regions.

REFERENCES

1. Rajkumar S, Kumar S. Prevalence of dementia in the community: a rural–urban comparison from Madras, India. *Aust J Ageing* 1996; **15**: 9–13.
2. Rajkumar S, Kumar S, Thara R. Prevalence of dementia in a rural setting: a report from India. *Int J Geriat Psychiat* 1997; **12**: 702–7.
3. Shaji S, Promodu K, Abraham T *et al.* An epidemiological study of dementia in a rural community in Kerala, India. *Br J Psychiat* 1996; **168**: 745–9.
4. Copeland JRM, Dewey ME. The computer assisted systems. In Hoveguimian S *et al.*, eds, *Classification and Diagnosis of Alzheimer's Disease. An International Perspective.* Hogrefe and Huber, 1989: 87–94.
5. Chandra V, Ganguli M, Pandav R *et al.* Prevalence of Alzheimer's disease and other dementias in rural India: the Indo-US Study. *Neurology* 1998; **51**: 1000–8.

Principles and Practice of Geriatric Psychiatry, 2nd edn. Edited by J. R. M. Copeland, M. T. Abou-Saleh and D. G. Blazer
©2002 John Wiley & Sons, Ltd

117

Dementia and Depression in Africa

Olusegun Baiyewu

University of Ibadan, Ibadan, Nigeria

Africa is a multicultural, multiracial society, consisting mainly of Negroid people, although Arabs predominate in the north and white settlers constitute a minority in the south. There are no policies and programmes for old age in most countries of Africa, and the majority of elderly people live in often neglected rural areas. Most older Africans are impoverished, have little or no education and depend on their children for sustenance. Provision for their medical care is grossly inadequate. In this chapter the situation of the elderly in Nigeria will be used as a prototype for Africa.

Only about 3% of Nigerians are aged 65 years and older[1]. The thrust of healthcare policy is towards communicable diseases in children, and geriatrics and geriatric psychiatry are both in their infancy. About the only policy document regarding old age care states that nursing homes will be discouraged, while home visits to older citizens will be encouraged and day care centres will be established. Federal, state and local governments are expected to share responsibilities for the care of older citizens[2]; however, as with most policies, there is a big gap between conception and implementation.

RESEARCH

Although geriatric research is limited, a number of studies have looked into dementia and depression. Because of the low level of education, most questionnaires designed in Western societies will require modification before application to older persons in Africa, especially in those that measure cognitive functions. Role expectations of older persons are also different, e.g. they are not expected to do household chores in the multigenerational living arrangements which are popular.

Dementia

Initial publications on dementia in Africa were about hospital patients, Lambo[3] in Nigeria and Ben-Arie *et al.*[4] in coloured older persons in South Africa. An earlier community study on dementia created the impression that Alzheimer's disease (AD) was rare or non-existent in Nigerians[5]. This conclusion is probably related to methodological issues in the study.

A major community-based study comparing older African-Americans in Indianapolis with older Nigerians in Ibadan has been ongoing since 1992. Prevalence rates of both dementia and AD were significantly higher in Indianapolis compared with Ibadan, 4.82% vs. 2.29% for dementia and 3.69% vs. 1.41% for AD[6]. More importantly, there was a progressive increase in the prevalence rates of both dementia and AD with increasing age after 65 years. Another important finding was that the Apoe4 allele, which has been reported to be associated with AD in most studies, was found to be unrelated to AD in Nigerians[7]. Important risk factors for dementia in Nigerians included age and female sex only; other well-known risk factors were not identified[15]. Behavioural disorder symptoms were found both in Nigerians and African-Americans but it was felt that Nigerians are generally more tolerant of behavioural disorder symptoms in their demented family members, who are often not treated[8].

In another major community survey of people aged 60+ in Egypt, Farrag *et al.*[9] reported a prevalence rate of 4.5% for all dementias, 2.2% for AD and 0.9% for multi-infarct dementia. In that study also the rate of dementia doubled every 5 years.

Depression

Lambo[3] diagnosed more depression in hospital older male patients compared to older females; Baiyewu *et al.*[10] reported that 5.4% of older Nigerians were depressed in a community survey with a preponderance of males. Recently, Sokoya[11] also showed that 5.4% of older primary care attendees were depressed, using AGECAT criteria[12]. Depression was related to low income but there was no gender difference. Depression was not often recognized and treated.

Nursing Homes

Nursing homes are very few in Nigeria, as in other African countries. However, in a study of psychiatric disorders in two Lagos nursing homes, using AGECAT and DSM-III-R[13] diagnoses, 48% of patients had dementia and 17% had depression[14]. Although the sample size was small and it is difficult to generalize, the figures are close to those reported in centres in Western societies, which may portend that the problem will become more evident in future as the number of older persons increases.

FUTURE TRENDS

There have been two major community studies on dementia in Africa; the study among the Arabs of Egypt gave prevalence rates twice as high as for Nigerians. There is an urgent need to have more studies on psychiatric disorders among older persons in Africa. Such studies will be informative on rates, patterns of illness and risk factors, as well as assisting in policy formulation.

Principles and Practice of Geriatric Psychiatry, 2nd edn. Edited by J. R. M. Copeland, M. T. Abou-Saleh and D. G. Blazer
©2002 John Wiley & Sons, Ltd

REFERENCES

1. National Population Commission of Nigeria. *Census 1991—National Summary*. National Population Commission, 1994.
2. Federal Ministry of Social Welfare. *Social Policy for Nigeria*. Eleme Enugu, Nigeria: DSC Unit, 1989.
3. Lambo TA. Psychiatric disorder in the aged epidemiology and preventive measures. *W Afr Med J* 1966; **15**: 121–4.
4. Ben-Arie O, Swartz L, Teggin AF, Elk R. The coloured elderly in Cape Town—a psychosocial, psychiatric and medical community survey. *S Afr Med J* 1986; **64**: 1056–61.
5. Ogunniyi AO, Osuntokun BO, Lekwauwa UG, Falope ZF. Rarity of dementia as measured by the DSM-III-R in an urban community in Nigeria. *E Afr Med J* 1992; **69**: 64–8.
6. Hendrie HC, Osuntokun BO, Hall KS *et al*. Prevalence of Alzheimer's disease and dementia in two communities: Nigerian-Africans and African-Americans. *Am J Psychiat* 1995; **152**: 1485–92.
7. Osuntokun BO, Sahota A, Ogunniyi AO *et al*. Lack of association between the e4 allele of APOE and Alzheimer's disease in a community study of elderly Nigerians. *Ann Neurol* 1995; **38**: 463–5.
8. Hendrie HC, Baiyewu O, Eldermire D, Prince C. Behavioural disorders in dementia: cross-cultural perspectives: Caribbean, Native American and Yoruba. *Int Psychogeriat* 1996; **8**: 483–6.
9. Farrag A, Farwiz HM, Khedr EH *et al*. Prevalence of Alzheimer's disease and other dementing disorders: Assiut–Upper Egypt study. *Dement Geriat Cogn Disord* 1998; **9**(6): 323–8.
10. Baiyewu O, Adeyemi JD, Ikuesan BA *et al*. Dementia and depression in Nigerian elderly community residents. *Nigerian Med J* (in press).
11. Sokoya OO. Depression and its correlates among geriatric care attenders. Dissertation submitted to the West African College of Physicians, 1999.
12. Copeland JRM, Dewey ME, Griffiths-Jones HM. Computerised Psychiatric Diagnostic System and case nomenclature for elderly subjects: GMS and AGECAT. *Psychol Med* 1986; **16**: 89–99.
13. American Psychiatric Association. *Diagnostic and Statistical Manual of Mental Disorders*, 3rd edn, Revised. Washington, DC: APA, 1987.
14. Baiyewu O, Adeyemi JD, Ogunniyi A. Psychiatric disorders in Nigerian nursing home residents. *Int J Geriat Psychiat* 1997; **12**: 1146–50.
15. Hall KS, Gureje O, Gao S *et al*. Risk factors in Alzheimer's disease: a comparative study of two communities. *Aust NZ J Psychiat* 1998; **280**: 698–706.

118

Mental Illness in South America

Sergio Luís Blay

Federal University of São Paulo, Brazil

This chapter will present some features of psychogeriatrics in Latin America. With this aim in mind, the situation with regard to epidemiology, risk factors, recognition of symptoms, the influence of culture and the state of development of services will be outlined.

EPIDEMIOLOGY

Depression

Estimates of the frequency of depression symptoms vary widely from 8 to 46.2% (see Table 118.1). Such a variation depends heavily on the instruments used, cut-off points and severity of the symptoms. Using higher cut-off points, Cornejo and Lazlo[1] obtained a prevalence of 8%. Eisirik[2], using the DSM-III-R checklist, found a prevalence of 4.7% for major depression in an urban sample. Women presented higher rates, 5.8% vs. 2% for men.

Dementia

The prevalence of organic brain syndromes varies (4.3–29.7%). The study of Veras and Coutinho[3] investigated three subdistricts of the city of Rio de Janeiro. The figures varied dramatically: 5.9 in Copacabana subdistrict to 29.7 in Santa Cruz. Several socio-economic variables accounted for such differences.

Cognitive impairment ranged from 10.5% to 29%. The study conducted by Xavier[4] relied on the oldest sample (80+) and investigated the age-associated cognitive decline through a neuropsychological battery (19.7%). Silberman et al.[5] have found the highest figure (29%) in a small urban community sample.

Herrera et al.[6] conducted a survey using a three-stage design in the city of Catanduva in the state of São Paulo. The MMSE was used as a screening instrument. All the suspected cases were further investigated by a specialist, using a set of evaluations. All subjects with a diagnosis of dementia went through a complete laboratory examination; 1660 subjects aged 65+ were interviewed. The prevalence of dementia was 7.1%. In the series of 118 cases, as many as 64 cases (54.1%) were diagnosed as having Alzheimer's disease, 11 (9.3%) vascular dementia and 17 (14.4%) an association of vascular dementia and Alzheimer's disease. The prevalence of dementia was age-associated: 1.3% in the age group 65–69; 3.4%, 70–74; 6.7%, 75–79; 17%, 80–84; and 36.9%, 85+. Education was an important protective variable against dementia. The prevalence rates can be seen in Table 118.2.

Table 118.1 Prevalence of depression symptoms in Latin America

Ref.	Age	Instrument	Sample size	Prevalence (%)
16	65+	Zung SRDS	26	46.2
1	68+	Brink GDS	433	8 (severe depression)
3	60+	Short care	738	20.9–36.8
5	60+	MADRAS	62	30
2	60+	MADRAS	344	21.5
—		DSM-III-R		4.7 (major depression)

Prevalence of Mental Disorders

Ramos et al.[7] conducted a household survey using a multidimensional functional assessment questionnaire (OARS methodology); 1062 elderly aged 60+ living in three subdistricts of the city of São Paulo, Brazil, were interviewed. Among other data 27% of the subjects were considered psychiatric cases, as assessed by the mental health screening questionnaire included in the methodology. Eizirik[2], using the SRQ as a screening instrument, observed that 10.2% of subjects were considered positive psychiatric cases in a sample of 344 individuals aged 60+.

Alcoholism

Community studies are mainly focused on adult samples. Data concerning elderly populations are usually restricted to a small number of elderly persons. Yamamoto et al.[8], studying an unselected sample in Lima, Peru (n=815), screened seven men (43.75%) out of 29 subjects aged 65+ for lifetime alcohol abuse or dependence.

RISK FACTORS

The Latin-American literature is not extensive in this respect. Epidemiological data[6] have indicated that dementia of the Alzheimer's type occurs somewhat more often in women, in a proportion of 2:1. Sadigursky and Oliveira[9] investigated the association between religious practice and depression on women aged 60+ attending a geriatric clinic. This case-controlled study examined 90 women. They found that the regular practice of religious activities had a protective effect on depression (7.4%) compared with less interested in religious activities (44.4%).

Principles and Practice of Geriatric Psychiatry, 2nd edn. Edited by J. R. M. Copeland, M. T. Abou-Saleh and D. G. Blazer
©2002 John Wiley & Sons, Ltd

Table 118.2 Prevalence of dementia in Latin America

Reference	Age	Instrument	Sample size	Prevalence (%)
Organic brain syndromes				
18	55+	QMPA	139	4.3
	65+		44	6.8
12	65+	FHT	91	5.5
3	60+	Short care	738	5.9–29.7
Cognitive impairment				
5	60+	MMSE	62	29
2	60+	MMSE	344	24.7
4	80+	Battery	77	19.7
17	60+			10.5
Dementia				
6	65+	MMSE	1660	7.1

Studies of adaptation to high altitudes have led investigators to examine whether altitude itself is associated with mental problems in late life. Countries like Peru or Bolivia have a peculiar geography suitable for these type of studies. They have communities living both at sea level and at 4000 m above sea level. Alarcón et al.[10] examined 93 subjects aged 60+ living in Lima (150 m) and 140 in Cusco (3400 m). Among other findings, they verified that the frequency of symptoms of anxiety and cognitive decline was greater at high altitudes than at sea-level.

RECOGNITION OF SYMPTOMS AND THE INFLUENCE OF CULTURE

An ethnographic study conducted in north-western Brazil examined the meaning of sadness in this low-income population. This qualitative study, which included retired subjects aged 60 years, found three main semantic clusters for sadness: an inner set, the body set and the interaction set[11].

Cross-cultural comparisons between unselected samples of elderly in two urban populations, Mannheim, Germany, and São Paulo, Brazil, using similar instruments, found similar symptom profiles in both cities. Some disparities between the samples are thought to be real and to relate to sociocultural differences as well as the greater stresses of daily life in São Paulo[12].

STATE OF THE DEVELOPMENT OF SERVICES

The pattern of service utilization in Latin-America by older patients with mental health problems is not well known. Few studies have investigated the ability of primary care services to meet the demand[13] and to determine different potential users' expectations and needs[14]. It is reasonable to suppose that important inter-regional differences exist in the delivery of care. In some places the only source of available psychiatric treatment is the hospital, generating a misuse of psychiatric resources[15].

REFERENCES

1. Cornejo W, Lazo M. La depresión en ancianos del Ande. *Rev Hosp Psiquiat Habana* 1988; **XXVIII**(1): 7–18.
2. Eizirik CL. Rede social, estado mental e contratransferência: estudo de uma amostra de velhos da região urbana de Porto Alegre. PhD Thesis, University of Porto Alegre, 1997.
3. Veras RP, Coutinho E. Estudo de prevalência de depressão e síndrome cerebral orgânica na população de idosos, Brasil. *Rev Saúde Públ* 1991; **25**(3): 209–17.
4. Xavier FMF. Prevalência de declínio cognitivo associado ao envelhecimento em uma população de idosos com mais de 80 anos residentes na comunidade. MS Thesis, University of São Paulo, 1999.
5. Silberman C, Souza C, Wilhems F et al. Cognitive deficit and depressive symptoms in a community group of elderly people: a preliminary study. *Rev Saúde Públ* 1995; **29**(6): 444–50.
6. Herrera E, Jr, Caramelli P, Nitrini R. Estudo epidemiológico populacional de demência na cidade de Catanduva; Estado de São Paulo, Brasil. *Rev Psiquiat Clín* 1998; **25**(2): 70–3.
7. Ramos LR, Rosa TEC, Oliveira ZM et al. Perfil do idoso em área metropolitana na região sudeste do Brasil: resultados do inquérito domiciliar. *Ref Saúde Públ* 1993; **27**(2): 87–94.
8. Yamamoto J, Arturo Silva J, Sasao T et al. Alcoholism in Peru. *Am J Psychiat* 1993; **150**: 1059–62.
9. Sadigursky D, Oliveira MR. Estudo de caso controle de associação entre prática religiosa e depressão em mulheres idosas. *Rev Baiana Enfermag* 1993; **6**(2): 89–102.
10. Alarcón I, Dante G, Gustavo G. Aspectos psicologicos del anciano que reside a nivel del mar y en la altura. *Acta Andina* 1993; **2**(2): 201–13.
11. Costa LAF, Pereira AM. Expressão da tristeza em camada popular urbana de Salvador, Bahia, Brasil. *Cadern Saúde Públ* 1995; **11**(3): 448–55.
12. Blay SL, Bickel H, Cooper B. Mental illness in a cross-national perspective. Results from a Brazilian and a German community survey among the elderly. *Soc Psychiat Psychiat Epidemiol* 1991; **26**: 245–51.
13. Carvalho MS, d'Orsy E, Prates EC et al. Demanda ambulatorial de três serviços da rede pública do município do Rio de Janeiro, Brasil. *Cadern Saúde Públ* 1994; **10**(1): 17–29.
14. Gattinar BC, Ibacache, Puente CT et al. Percepción de la comunidad acerca de la calidad de los servicios de salud públicos en los Distritos Norte e Ichilo, Bolivia. *Cadern Saúde Públ* 1995; **11**(3): 425–38.
15. Lancman S. Instituições psiquiátricas e comunidades: um estudo de demanda em saúde mental no Estado de São Paulo, Brasil. *Cadern Saúde Públ* 1997; **13**(1): 93–102.
16. Eblen A, Vivas V, Garcia J. Prevalencia del sindrome depressivo y su relación com factores socioeconomicos en una muestra de la poblacion de la ciudad de Valencia, Estado Carabobo, Venezuela. *Acta Cient Venezolana* 1990; **41**: 250–54.
17. Mangone CA. Cross-cultural perspectives. Argentina. *Int Psychogeriat* 1996; **8**(suppl 3): 473–8.
18. de Almeida Filho N. Family variables and child mental disorders in a Third World urban area (Bahia, Brazil). *Soc Psychiatry* 1984; **19**: 23–30.

Part M

The Practice of
Psychogeriatric Medicine

MI   The British Model of the Organization of Services

MII   The North American Model
        of the Organization of Services

MIII   Liaison with Medical and Surgical Teams

MIV   Rehabilitation and General Care

MV   Prevention of the Mental Disorders of Old Age

MVI   Education

Psychiatry of the Elderly—the WPA/WHO Consensus Statements

Cornelius Katona

Royal Free and UCL Medical School, London, UK

Between 1997 and 1999, under the Chairmanship of the late Professor Jean Wertheimer, the World Psychiatric Association, Section of Geriatric Psychiatry, published a series of consensus statements in collaboration with the World Health Organization Division of Mental Health. A wide range of non-governmental organizations (NGOs) participated.

The first Consensus Statement[1] defined the scope of the specialty, emphasizing that this has become necessary because of increasing longevity (most markedly in the developing world); the relatively high prevalence of both functional mental disorders and the dementias in old age; and the need to adopt a multidisciplinary approach, while defining professional roles within the team. The scope of psychiatry of the elderly is "the psychiatry of 'retired' people", and includes the full range of mental illnesses, including affective disorders, psychoses, substance abuse, the dementias and the mental health problems of "graduates" whose mental health problems continue into old age. The specialty also needs to address psychological, physical and social aspects of mental health problems in older people and the biosociocultural changes associated with ageing.

The characteristics of a successful psychiatry service for the elderly are summarized as community orientation, a multidisciplinary approach, an emphasis on abilities as well as deficits, and a core aim to improve quality of life rather than simply to alleviate symptoms. The main objectives of treatment are the restoration of health, improvement of quality of life, the minimization of disability, the preservation of autonomy, and addressing the needs of family and other carers as well as those of the individual patient. The high relapse rate of functional psychiatric problems in old age necessitates close follow-up after successful initial treatment.

Priorities within any new specialist service include teaching psychiatry of the elderly to primary healthcare workers; training existing mental health professionals in special mental health problems of the elderly, and establishing at least one multidisciplinary resource/expertise centre.

The second Consensus Statement[2] identified general principles that should underpin any quality specialist psychiatry of the elderly service:

- Good health and optimal quality of life are fundamental human rights irrespective of age or mental disorder
- All people have right of access to appropriate services
- Recognized needs should, within resource constraints, be met appropriately and ethically
- This can only be achieved through health and social measures adapted to local needs
- Older people with mental health problems and carers should be involved, individually and collectively, in care planning
- Governments should recognize the crucial role of non-governmental organisations and work with them.

The specific qualities of a good service are that it should be Comprehensive, Accessible, Responsive, Individualized, Transdisciplinary, Accountable and Systemic (CARITAS), and should attempt to both prevent mental health problems from arising and identify them early when they do arise. As well as offering comprehensive assessment and acute management, the service should provide continuing care and support to patients and carers and address spiritual and leisure needs as well as medical needs.

The third Consensus Statement[3] focused on education. Targets for educational initiatives include: health and social care professionals at undergraduate, postgraduate and continuing education levels; health and social service managers; other care workers; family and other informal carers; voluntary workers; public policy makers; and the general public. Although such a wide range of target groups inevitably start with different needs and different starting levels of knowledge, a generic core curriculum can be derived from the learning needs of health professionals. Essential curriculum elements include:

- Processes of ageing in individuals.
- The demography, economics and politics of ageing societies.
- The epidemiology, pathology, clinical features, assessment, diagnosis, treatment and management of the mental disorders of old age.
- Physical disorders and impairments of function that commonly occur in old age.
- The special significance in old age of the interdependence of mental, physical and social factors.
- Principles of health promotion and the preventive psychiatry of old age.
- Ethical and legal issues relevant to older people.
- Principles of planning, provision and evaluation of services in different settings.
- Needs of carers and approaches to their support.
- End-of-life issues.
- Principles and practice of multidisciplinary teamwork.
- Interviewing and communication skills.
- Fostering of positive attitudes and insight into the reasons for negative attitudes.

Principles and Practice of Geriatric Psychiatry, 2nd edn. Edited by J. R. M. Copeland, M. T. Abou-Saleh and D. G. Blazer
©2002 John Wiley & Sons, Ltd

REFERENCES

1. World Health Organization. Psychiatry of the elderly: a consensus statement. Document No. WHO/MNH/MND/96.7. Geneva: WHO, 1996.

2. World Health Organization. Organization of care in psychiatry of the elderly: a technical consensus statement. Document No. WHO/MNH/MND/97. Geneva: WHO, 1997.
3. World Health Organization. Education in psychiatry of the elderly: a technical consensus statement. Document No. WHO/MNH/MND/98.4. Geneva: WHO, 1998.

120

Development of Health and Social Services in the UK in the Twentieth Century

John P. Wattis

University of Huddersfield, Huddersfield, UK

IMPERIAL BEGINNINGS: THE POOR LAW AND THE ASYLUM

In Britain, the twentieth century dawned in a blaze of imperial glory. Three years earlier, Queen Victoria's diamond jubilee had been celebrated across the globe with a splendid procession in London itself. The mood of the nation was confident, even optimistic, and world-domination was accepted almost as a birthright of the British people. Britain had survived the rigours of the Industrial Revolution and had come up fighting. Yet, at this time, public health measures were rudimentary and confined largely to the establishment (in 1848) of sanitary authorities with medical officers of health to oversee sewers and water supplies. The poor law was still in force and poor law institutions were made deliberately unpleasant. This followed the principle of "lesser eligibility", set out in 1834, which stated that those receiving poor law assistance should not be as "eligible" (well provided for) as an "independent labourer of the lowest class"[1]. For the poor sick this had been ameliorated, to some extent, by the setting up of poor law infirmaries in 1868, but there was still a vast gulf between these institutions and the voluntary hospitals, which were supported by rich philanthropists. Retirement pensions, even retirement itself, were things of the future and there was an association between poverty, ill-health and old age which was recognized by an 1895 Royal Commission on the aged poor.

Mentally ill people were still incarcerated in large county asylums. In 1808, partly as a response to the appalling conditions in some private "madhouses", local magistrates had been given the power to set up asylums and in 1845 this provision had been made mandatory.

From 1900 onwards, developments have been influenced by major world events, political philosophy, public opinion and the power of pressure groups. The Boer War, starting in 1899, revealed the poor physical fitness and ill-health of many young men. Improvements in midwifery and child care were soon legislated for, with school meals starting in 1906 and the notification of live births, health visiting and the school medical service soon following. In 1908 the first national scheme for old age pensions was set up to try to alleviate poverty amongst old people. It was non-contributory and means-tested. Initially, recipients also had to be "of good character"!

The Royal Commission on the Poor Laws and the Relief of Distress in 1909 considered most of the issues of domiciliary and hospital medical care. A minority report condemned the poor law institutions as a public scandal, with the infirmaries understaffed and lacking skilled medical input[2]. Out of hospital, the poor law doctors had no contact with local authority public health services, the voluntary dispensaries were overcrowded and ineffective and the medical clubs, financed by workers' subscriptions, underpaid their doctors and did not cater for the chronic sick or dependants. The writers of this report dismissed the idea of a medical insurance system.

Yet, in 1911, the establishment of such a system marked an important development in the evolution of general practice in the UK. The medical profession fought for, and won, independence and capitation fees rather than a salaried service, and administration by insurance-based panels rather than local authorities[3]. Higher income groups, families and hospital care were excluded but the scheme was nevertheless a qualified success.

THE MINISTRY OF HEALTH: BETWEEN THE WARS

In 1918 the Ministry of Health for England and Wales was formed and the Minister quickly appointed a consultative council, which in 1920 produced a report described by Pater[2] as "nothing less than the outline of a national health service" (p. 7). Their scheme might well have avoided some of the split between general practitioners and hospital doctors that has been one of the problems of the National Health Service (NHS) as it was eventually implemented.

Control of the workhouses passed to local authorities in 1930, the beginning of the end for the poor law. After a post-war cash crisis, the voluntary hospitals continued, becoming more specialized in acute care and leaving the chronic sick and infectious diseases to the local authorities. A number of reports pressed for a more coordinated hospital system and for universal health insurance. Knowledge was advancing. In 1935 Warren[4,5] began her work in developing geriatric medicine and, a few years later, pioneers began to write of the issues concerning old people with mental illness[6-8].

Before the Second World War, the Emergency Medical Service (EMS) was set up to cope with expected severe civilian casualties from the bombing of cities. On the declaration of war, 140 000 people, many of them elderly, were discharged from hospital over 2 days[9]. The EMS also coordinated the work of the voluntary and local authority hospitals, providing the framework for the future NHS Regional Hospital Boards. Physicians and surgeons from the elitist voluntary hospitals came face to face with the conditions of the poor law institutions.

Principles and Practice of Geriatric Psychiatry, 2nd edn. Edited by J. R. M. Copeland, M. T. Abou-Saleh and D. G. Blazer
©2002 John Wiley & Sons, Ltd

THE POST-WAR NATIONAL HEALTH SERVICE

The last of the series of British Medical Association (BMA) reports pressing for reform in 1942 coincided with the Beveridge report and was followed in 1944 by the NHS White Paper, enacted in 1946 and effective in 1948.

The National Health Service, as then set up, was tripartite. Primary care services—general practitioners, opticians, dentists and pharmacists—were answerable to local executive committees; maternity, child welfare, health visiting, health education, immunization and ambulances remained the responsibility of the local authority; and hospitals were administered by Regional Hospital Boards with teaching hospitals retaining boards of governors directly answerable to the Ministry of Health. One of the assumptions when the NHS was set up was that increasing health in the population would cause health expenditure to level off. It never did, and in 1956 the Guillebaud Committee, appointed to find ways of avoiding a rising charge upon the exchequer, concluded that there was no evidence of inefficiency or extravagance in the NHS. In fact, the committee was concerned about a lack of capital expenditure (a concern again of relevance more recently). In 1962, this problem was addressed in the Hospital Plan.

Meanwhile, in the mental health field, the idea of community care was gaining ground. Tinker[10] attributed this to five factors. First, there was a general dissatisfaction with institutional care and a search for alternatives. Some of the experiments in the "therapeutic community" work of the Second World War had challenged the accepted authoritarian culture of the mental hospital[11]. In addition, the advent of electroconvulsive therapy (ECT), antipsychotics and effective antidepressants facilitated the move away from custodial care to medical treatment at home or in ordinary hospitals. Next, there were beginning to be practical problems in running residential establishments, including staff recruitment. Then there was concern about the cost of institutional care and, finally, a recognition that mentally ill people were entitled to live in as normal a way as permitted by modern treatments. The 1959 Mental Health Act liberalized the treatment of mentally ill people and opened the way for a move away from the old psychiatric hospitals to the new concept of psychiatric units attached to the district general hospitals of the 1962 Hospital Plan.

The large institutions were, in any case, rocked by a series of scandals about the mistreatment of patients. This resulted in the establishment of the Hospital Advisory Service (later the Health Advisory Service), effectively an inspectorate to monitor standards and spread good practice.

In general practice, a financial allowance for practices in deprived areas combined with other factors to promote the rapid development of local health centres and group practices from the mid-1960s. Local authorities produced their own health and welfare plans but there was poor coordination with the hospital authorities and the general practitioners' executive committees. Within the local authorities, the Seebohm report (1968) was followed by the Social Services Act, which required the setting up of social services departments. The Department of Health and Social Security was created in 1968 by the amalgamation of the Ministries of Health and Social Security, a merger that lasted for some 20 years.

Reforms

In 1974, for the first time since its inception, the NHS itself was reorganized. The chief elements of this reorganization were the separation out of health and social services functions, the integration of all health functions under one management and the establishment of area health authorities, generally co-terminous with local authorities, to facilitate joint planning. Community Health Councils were also created to represent the views of consumers. Unfortunately, the reformed service did not work well. There were too many layers of responsibility and taking decisions seemed to be delayed whilst information and responsibility were passed up and down the tree. There was an increase in clerical and administrative staff without a corresponding increase in managerial efficiency. During this period, important government reports were produced, including *Better Services for the Mentally Ill*[12] and *A Happier Old Age*[13].

In 1982 the Area Health Authorities were abolished and new district health authorities combined the functions of the old areas and districts. In some areas, co-terminosity with local government was lost. A new government was determined to cut public expenditure and the rate of growth of the NHS slowed. Following the Griffiths report[14], a general management structure was established within the NHS and Family Practitioner Committees became independent. Government payment for continuing care was channelled to the private sector and social services and hospital provision for this group of patients/residents was either reduced or failed to keep pace with demographic changes[15].

Psychiatric services were coping with the implementation of the 1983 Mental Health Act, which set up time-consuming quasi-judicial procedures for reviewing patients who were detained in hospital under compulsory orders. The new Act also set up a Mental Health Act Commission to review treatment of detained patients and to advise on certain types of treatment.

MARKET FORCES: A RADICAL DEPARTURE?

Then came the most radical reform of the NHS attempted to that date, a reform not just of the service but of the basic philosophy of "service" underlying it. Some suspected that it was the beginning of the end for the National Health Service. The 1990 National Health Service and Community Care Act introduced the concept of an "Internal Market". The new health authorities became planners and purchasers of health care at "arm's length" from the providers, which were initially directly managed units (DMUs), and became semi-independent Trusts. The health authorities were provided with a budget for the local population and placed contracts for care with Trusts or the private and voluntary sector in order to obtain the best "value for money". Quality was, at least in theory, specified in the contract and monitored.

Competition and other features of business life were "introduced" into the NHS, not least by setting up groups of "fundholding" general practitioners, who were enabled to make their own contracts for secondary care. Some of the changes were potentially positive, such as the setting up of Trust Boards to manage local services and an emphasis on sound financial regulation through corporate governance. Unfortunately, the bottom line was very clearly financial and in many cases clinical services were sacrificed to balance the books.

These proposals were pushed through in the teeth of strong opposition from staff and groups representing the consumer. Honigsbaum[16] analysed the situation in 1990 and concluded that if patient care suffered, then "the nation may decide that the restraints imposed are not worth the savings they produce. Today, as in 1911 and 1948, it is the public interest that will predominate". The medical profession were excluded from the plans for this reorganization. Klein concluded that, if a new political settlement were not reached between the government and the profession, it seemed unlikely that the NHS would survive long into the twenty-first century[17].

A NEW NHS?

In fact, perhaps partly because of public disatisfaction with what was happening to the NHS, the government was not re-elected and a radical reforming Labour government came to power. The engines of privatization and the internal market were reversed and new reforms were produced. In December 1997 a White Paper, *The new NHS: Modern, Dependable*[18], outlined a comprehensive new vision for the NHS. Two of the main planks of the new policy were the setting up of primary care groups (PCGs) to replace the fundholding/non-fundholding split and the introduction of comprehensive quality controls to ensure high standards and equity in access across the country. PCGs are local groupings of general practices that are involved in the commissioning of local community and secondary services and may eventually become Primary Care NHS Trusts, providing community services and commissioning secondary services. More recently still, the concept has been developed of "Care Trusts which could provide primary care and some secondary services, such as mental health services". The quality framework involves a three-layer approach[19]. Clear standards of service will be set by National Service Frameworks and a National Institute for Clinical Excellence (NICE), which will evaluate new treatments. An SF for Older People was published in 2001[20]. The first of eight standards was "rooting out age discrimination". The seventh concerned mental health and included NICE guidelines for anti-dementia drugs. The new NSF made it clear that standards in the Mental Health NSF already published applied to older people. Local delivery of services will be made dependable by a combination of lifelong learning[21] linked to professional self-regulation and clinical governance. Clinical governance[22] places obligations on Chief Executives of NHS Trusts to make arrangements to monitor and continuously improve the quality of health care they provide. Finally, all this will be underpinned by the national monitoring of standards involving a National Performance Framework, an inspectorate (the Commission for Health Improvement) and a National Patient and User Survey. This ambitious vision sets a massive agenda for change and demands radical shifts in the management and clinical cultures of the NHS of a magnitude that will not easily be achieved[23]. Without adequate resources, these well-intentioned reforms may well overload the capacity for change of both managers and clinicians working in the NHS.

Primary care groups (in England) result in a much greater influence for general practitioners and other primary care workers in the commissioning of secondary services. Their boards are dominated by primary care workers. When they become Primary Care Trusts, good corporate governance demands a board structure with executive and non-executive directors, more analogous to the boards of existing Hospital and Community Trusts. This will result in general practitioners effectively losing their quasi-independent status. The Trusts are likely to be direct providers of many community services currently provided by Community or Community and Mental Health Trusts. In Scotland, where different arrangements pertain, mental health is part of primary care groups, but they do not control the budgets of secondary care Trusts in the same way as in England. In Wales the arrangements are closer to those in England. In England and Wales it seems likely that, in the larger cities at least, "stand-alone" Mental Health Trusts will be the order of the day. For old age psychiatry, this probably means that the managerial separation between old age psychiatry and geriatric medicine will be perpetuated. Unless imaginative and pragmatic solutions are found, this could result in many demarcation problems. However, a new culture of collaboration rather than competition and a government apparently committed to encouraging "joined-up" thinking and working means that these difficulties may be overcome.

The funding of the NHS is probably even more important than its organization in determining the future of health care in the UK. It was the squeeze on NHS development in the 1980s that provoked the medical profession to campaign for more development money. In the light of international comparisons, both of spending on health care and the age structure of the population, this campaign seemed fully justified. The previous reorganization increased management costs and reduced the morale of many in the NHS. So far, although the new government has promised more capital investment in the NHS, it has continued to support the controversial Private Finance Initiative (PFI) as a main strand of funding, which reduces the Public Sector Borrowing Requirement. There is concern that PFI will result in a reduction in bed numbers and diversion of money away from services to support repayments to private providers in respect of capital developments. If more money for services comes with the new reorganization, then the potential for positive change exists. If it does not, then the new reforms, like the Internal Market before them, are doomed to failure. Another problem with introducing improvements is the shortage of trained staff. The government has recognized the need to train more doctors and nurses, but it will take time to turn this recognition into staff-delivering services.

OTHER INNOVATIONS

The direct reforms of the NHS have been accompanied by a Royal Commission to review long-term care. The report of this Commission[24] controversially suggested that the personal care and residential elements of continuing care should be separately funded. Personal care should be paid for from general taxation, whilst living and housing expenses should continue to be means-tested and subject to co-payment. The government has yet to make an unequivocal positive response to this. Standards in psychiatric services for old people continue to improve generally but it remains to be seen whether the latest reforms will ensure that quality is universally high and that funding is adequate.

REFERENCES

1. Brocklehurst JC. *Textbook of Geriatric Medicine and Gerontology*. Edinburgh: Churchill Livingstone, 1978: 747.
2. Pater JE. *The Making of the National Health Service*. London: King Edward's Hospital Fund for London, 1981: 2–4, 7.
3. Ham C. *Health Policy in Britain*. London: Macmillan, 1985: 11–12, 24–5, 180–3.
4. Warren MW. A case for treating chronic sick in blocks in a general hospital. *Br Med J* 1943; **i**: 822–3.
5. Warren MW. Care of the chronic aged sick. *Lancet* 1946; **i**: 841–3.
6. Post F. Some problems arising from a study of mental patients over the age of 60 years. *J Ment Sci* 1944; **90**: 554–65.
7. Lewis A. Ageing and senility: a major problem of psychiatry. *J Ment Sci* 1946; **92**: 150–70.
8. Affleck J. Psychiatric disorders among the chronic sick in hospital. *J Ment Sci* 1948; **94**: 33–5.
9. Means R, Smith R. *The Development of Welfare Services for Elderly People*. London: Croom Helm, 1985: 25.
10. Tinker A. *The Elderly in Modern Society*. London: Longman, 1984: 37–8.
11. Martin DV. *Adventure in Psychiatry*. London: Cassirer, 1974.
12. DHSS. *Better Services for the Mentally Ill*. London: HMSO, 1975.
13. DHSS. *A Happier Old Age*. London: HMSO, 1978.
14. DHSS. *NHS Management Inquiry* ("The Griffiths Report"). London: HMSO, 1983.

15. Grundy E, Arie T. The falling rate of provision of residential care for the elderly. *Br Med J* 1982; **284**: 799–802.

16. Honigsbaum F. The evolution of the NHS. *Br Med J* 1990; **301**: 694–9.

17. Klein R. The state and the profession: the politics of the double bed. *Br Med J* 1990; **301**: 700–2.

18. *The New NHS: Modern—Dependable.* Cm3807. London: The Stationery Office, 1997.

19. Department of Health. *A First Class Service: Quality in the New NHS.* London: Department of Health, 1998.

20. Department of Health National Service Framework for Older People. London: Department of Health, 2001.

21. Wattis J, McGinnis P. Clinical governance and continuing professional development. *Adv Psychiat Treat* 1999; **5**: 233–9.

22. Department of Health. *Clinical Governance: Quality in the New NHS.* London: Department of Health, 1999; 1–25.

23. Wattis J, McGinnis P. Clinical governance: making it work. *Clinician Managem* 1999; **8**: 12–18.

24. The Royal Commission on Long-term Care. *With Respect to Old Age: a Report.* London: The Stationery Office, 1999.

The Pattern of Psychogeriatric Services

John P. Wattis

Leeds Community and Mental Health Services, Leeds, UK

HISTORIC BACKGROUND

The roots of the National Health Service (NHS) and the development of psychogeriatric services in the UK are discussed in the previous chapter. The evolution of psychogeriatric services has been guided by professional knowledge and opinion, by the politics of the health and social services, by financial constraints and, occasionally, by public opinion. From the inception of the NHS, which effectively antedated the beginning of provision of specialist psychogeriatric services until the 1990s, there was a consensus about how developments in services should occur in response to changing demography and epidemiology as well as advances in medical knowledge.

This consensus was threatened in the UK by the imposition of the ideology of "market forces". Much long-stay hospital accommodation was effectively "privatized" by decisions to support patients in private nursing and residential homes from state funds and to close down as many long-stay NHS beds as possible. The ideology of market forces was briefly applied to local authority provision of community care. Since April 1991, psychiatric patients with social needs have been subject to a "care-planning procedure" in which all parties, including social services, have to agree. In April 1993 the full implementation of the Community Care Act made local social services departments responsible for purchasing continuing nursing and residential home care, largely from the private sector and with a limited budget.

In the late 1990s, a government came to power that did not share the vision of market forces as the best way to regulate the NHS. This government emphasized *equity* and *quality* and returned to a modified vision of the NHS as a centrally regulated nationalized service industry. It is not certain that the opposition shares this vision, and so there is a danger of the NHS remaining a "political football". For the time being, though, despite the distractions provided by problems in under-resourced psychiatric services for working-age adults, it seems likely that the conditions in the NHS will again be more favourable to the growth of old age psychiatry services, which are essentially a collaborative rather than a competitive enterprise.

THEORETICAL BASIS FOR PSYCHOGERIATRIC SERVICES

The pioneers of specialist psychiatric services for old people were motivated by the increasing need for psychiatric services for the age group, consequent upon increased life expectancy, the growing knowledge base about psychiatric disorders amongst old people, and the success of geriatric medicine. The special needs of older people were not always recognized by the generic services. Diagnostic problems included the differential diagnosis of dementia, the association of apparent cognitive impairment with some cases of depressive illness, and the non-specific presentation of disease in old people. The multiple pathology suffered by old people led to a need for new patterns of multidisciplinary working and for close liaison with physicians in geriatric medicine and social services[1-3]. As in the early days of geriatric medicine, assessment and treatment in the community were emphasized not only because of "blocked beds" but also because a more realistic picture of the patient's health problems usually emerged. More recently, advances in psychosocial care[4], interest in the spiritual needs of old people[5] and the advent of new classes of antidepressant, antipsychotic and antidementia drugs (discussed elsewhere in this volume), have all had their impact on the organization and delivery of psychiatric services.

CARE OR TREATMENT—PRIMARY OR SECONDARY?

One of the key theoretical issues for the future development of community services is likely to be the distinction between care and treatment. "Care" is a word with many connotations. Some are positive but, in the medical world at least, some are negative. For example, "care" is seen as what is provided when there is no possibility of effective treatment, as in the "prescription" of "tender loving care" for the terminally ill person. "Care" tends to be relegated to untrained (although not necessarily unskilled) workers employed by Social Services, whereas "treatment" is the province of highly trained personnel employed by the Health Service. The move to "Care in the Community" may serve to reclassify older mentally ill people as not needing medical treatment, and this will have to be resisted vigorously.

This situation is further complicated by the tendency of some health planners to equate primary care with *low cost and community care*, and secondary care with *high cost and hospital care*. Old age psychiatry services straddle the hospital–community divide and provide essentially secondary services, largely in a community setting. The new term, "intermediate care", describes well some of these community services, but some who use the term believe that community psychiatric nursing services should be part of "primary care", when in fact they work most effectively as part of secondary community care.

KEY COMPONENTS OF PSYCHOGERIATRIC SERVICES

Catchment Area and Comprehensiveness

Virtually all psychogeriatric services in the UK work to a defined geographical catchment area and the vast majority aim to provide a comprehensive psychiatric service to all people over the age of 65 years[6,7]. Many services are now also trying to provide for people with early-onset dementia, although often without any dedicated resources[7].

The Multidisciplinary Team

For some this is an outmoded concept, for others an ideal that cannot be obtained, but for many psychogeriatricians it is an essential context for all their endeavours. Most multidisciplinary teams for the elderly incorporate *community nurses*, a *social worker*, one or more *occupational therapists*, a *physiotherapist*, and often a *psychologist*. Various patterns of working have evolved and been described but they have in common an attempt to involve all disciplines in formulating treatment plans for the patient.

Home Assessment

This lies at the heart of most psychogeriatric services. Surveys[6,7] have shown that around two-thirds of referrals were seen at home by a doctor, one-fifth by other members of the team and one-tenth in outpatient clinics. Just over one in 10 were seen as liaison referrals, although in some services this rises to a quarter or even one-third, perhaps partly depending on the admission policies of local geriatric services. Less than one in 20 were admitted direct without prior assessment.

Community Treatment

The rate of acute admissions was only one-third of the rate of referrals, reflecting the fact that most home assessments do not result in admission but in treatment in the community. Home visits by community nurses are probably the commonest form of treatment in the community, although home visits by doctors and other members of the multidisciplinary team also play an important part.

Day Hospitals

In 1985, there were about 1.2 day hospital places/1000 elderly people, and this had not changed significantly by the mid-1990s. Some services and Health Regions had relatively more and others less. The use of day hospitals varied from area to area, depending on the resource availability locally. Anecdotal evidence suggests that government guidelines overestimate the need for dementia places. In many but not all cases of dementia, the need is for *care* rather than *treatment* and so a proportion of this day provision can be provided by Social Services or voluntary agencies. Here, however, issues will have to be addressed as to what kind of care is of most benefit to older people with dementia and their relatives, neighbours and friends. Elderly people with functional illness often have problems with psychiatric or psychological management that demand the *treatment* resources of a true day hospital.

Acute Inpatient Beds

The national rate of provision in 1985 was around 1/1000 elderly served, and again did not vary much over the next 10 years. This may be insufficient to cope with the increasing demands caused by demographic changes and the relative loss of long-stay beds but a great deal depends on the community services available, since there is potential for considerable "marginal shift" between community and inpatient resources. One study showed that around a quarter of acute psychiatric beds for all age groups were occupied by elderly people with depressive illness, and in many areas anecdotal evidence suggests that a greater proportion of acute psychiatric beds are being used for functional illness, principally depression. As with day hospital places, it appears that the old guidelines may have overestimated the needs for dementia assessment beds and underestimated the needs for patients with depressive illness and other functional illnesses. Because of the high prevalence of physical illnesses in mentally ill old people, it is recommended that acute beds should be on a general hospital site. Some services are now beginning to differentiate the assessment and management of behavioural problems in demented people, which can be carried out in the community or in community-based units, from the management of patients with depression, who often have major associated physical illness or disability (and may need ECT) and are therefore better managed on an acute hospital site. The same may apply to atypical dementia patients requiring high levels of investigation or to patients with dementia and delirium. This last group may be best helped on geriatric medical wards.

Long-stay Beds

The provision in 1985 was around 3.4 beds/1000 elderly. Since then a large number of beds appear to have been closed, with patients discharged to the private sector, where developments have been funded through the Social Security budget. In 1996 the number had reduced to around 1.1 beds/1000 elderly. Since provision is largely (but not exclusively) for those with severe dementia, whose main need is for care rather than treatment, this development appears to demand a cautious welcome. Patients are generally being cared for in smaller units. However, there must be reservations. The smaller units are harder to inspect and they are not necessarily in the patients' communities of origin, since planning permission and housing costs enter into the commercial equation. They are subject to capricious changes in the market, including government refusal to pay the "going rate". They are not under specialist medical management and there is some evidence that this management may be one of the factors that reduces the rate of decline in demented elderly people, a factor which, if confirmed, might also have relevance in the day care setting. The switch to private care has been engineered for political reasons and its impact is yet to be fully assessed. Psychogeriatric services will need to retain a proportion of their long-stay beds for rehabilitation, for treatment of old people with resistant functional illnesses (especially depression) and for treatment of behavioural disturbances amongst demented people. A survey of old age psychiatrists[8] showed the majority in favour of around 1.5 long-stay (including respite) beds/1000 elderly in community NHS units, with national rather than local eligibility criteria. The use of such beds for respite care to support carers in the community is now well established, and there is a potential for developing community units as centres of excellence for dementia care, as well as bases for multi-disciplinary community teams.

GUIDELINES

The first guidelines for provision of psychiatric services for old people came in a Department of Health circular in 1972[9]. The government White Paper, *Better Services for the Mentally Ill*[10], in 1975, suggested that services for old people should often be provided by a psychiatrist with "a special interest" and incorporated guidelines for bed and day hospital provision for the "elderly severely mentally infirm". Subsequently, the Royal College of Psychiatrists produced guidelines intended to help College representatives reviewing job descriptions for new or replacement consultants. These were endorsed by the Health Advisory Service in its report, *The Rising Tide*[11], and by the joint Royal College of Physicians and Psychiatrists report, *Care of Elderly People with Mental Illness*[12]. The second joint report[13] adopted a more multidisciplinary approach and described the different types of mental illness in old age as well as appealing for equity and "national reference frameworks", which corresponded closely to the concept of "National Service Frameworks" introduced by the new government[14]. It cited "indicative service levels".

REALITY AND GUIDELINES

Although in the UK, old age psychiatry is now recognized as a specialty by the Department of Health, we are still awaiting the collection of routine statistics. Initial manpower statistics appear to be grossly inaccurate. The most comprehensive data available are from the 1985 survey, updated by the 1996 survey, which unfortunately did not achieve such wide coverage. There are also now agreed international standards for old age psychiatry services[15] and an international survey has established that basic levels of service exist in 12 countries worldwide[16].

SPECIALIST SERVICES OR NOT?

In view of the documented rapid expansion of services over the years, this question may seem superfluous. However, it was possible as a result of the 1985 survey to compare services where psychogeriatricians work half-time or more in the specialty with those where the consultant commitment to the elderly is less than half-time[17]. Specialist services had generally higher staffing ratios (with the exception of non-consultant medical staff), a higher proportion of acute beds on general hospital sites and a greater proportion of long-stay beds within the area served. These last two could be regarded as surrogate indicators of quality of care. In addition, the specialist psychiatrists were more likely to look after all mental illness in old age—the recommended pattern of service—to engage in teaching and to show an interest in research.

CONCLUSION

Psychogeriatrics has "come of age" in the UK. Provision, although geographically patchy and relatively under-resourced, still provides one model for future developments. This model, fostered in the National Health Service with its principles of equality of access, payment from general taxation and central planning, survived the major changes of the 1990 "reforms" and should thrive under the regime of equity and quality proposed by the present UK government, always provided that old age psychiatrists show adequate leadership and that governments furnish adequate resources.

REFERENCES

1. Arie T. Morale and planning of psychogeriatric services. *Br Med J* 1971; **iii**: 166–70.
2. Arie T, Dunn T. A "do-it-yourself" psychiatric–geriatric joint patient unit. *Lancet* 1973; **ii**: 1313–16.
3. Royal College of Psychiatrists, British Geriatric Society. Guidelines for collaboration between geriatric physicians and psychiatrists in the care of the elderly. *Bull R Coll Psychiat* 1979; **11**: 168–9.
4. Kitwood T. *Dementia Reconsidered: the Person Comes First*. Buckingham: Open University Press, 1997.
5. Koenig HG. *Aging and God*. Binghampton, NY: Howarth Pastoral, 1994.
6. Wattis JP. Geographical variations in the provision of psychiatric services for old people. *Age Ageing* 1988; **17**: 171–80.
7. Wattis J, Macdonald A, Newton P. Old age psychiatry: a specialty in transition—results of the 1996 survey. *Psychiat Bull* 1999; **23**: 331–5.
8. Wattis J, Macdonald A, Newton R. Old age psychiatrists' views on continuing inpatient care. *Psychiat Bull* 1998; **22**: 621–4.
9. Department of Health and Social Security. *Services for Mental Illness Related to Old Age, HM(72)71*. London: DHSS, 1972.
10. Department of Health and Social Security. *Better Services for the Mentally Ill*. London: DHSS, 1975.
11. National Health Service. *Rising Tide: Developing Services for Mental Illness in Old Age*. Sutton, Surrey: NHS Health Advisory Service, 1982.
12. *Care of Elderly People with Mental Illness: Specialist Services and Medical Training*. London: Royal College of Physicians of London and the Royal College of Psychiatrists, 1989.
13. *Care of Older People with Mental Illness*. CR69. London: The Royal College of Psychiatrists and The Royal College of Physicians of London, 1999.
14. Department of Health. *A First Class Service: Quality in the New NHS*. London: Department of Health, 1998.
15. World Health Organization and World Psychiatric Association. *Organization of Care in Psychiatry of the Elderly*. Geneva: WHO, 1997.
16. Reifler BV, Cohen W. Practice of geriatric psychiatry and mental health services for the elderly: results of an international survey. *Int Psychogeriat* 1998; **10**: 351–7.
17. Wattis JP. A comparison of specialised and non-specialised psychiatric services for old people. *Int J Geriat Psychiat* 1989; **4**: 59–62.

Organization of Services for the Elderly with Mental Disorders

Edmond Chiu

University of Melbourne, Victoria, Australia

In 1997, the Section of Geriatric Psychiatry (now Section of Old Age Psychiatry), World Psychiatric Association, with the participation of the Division of Mental Health and Prevention of Substance Abuse, World Health Organization, met at Lausanne to develop a Consensus Statement[1] on the *Organization of Care in Psychiatry of the Elderly*. Under the very able leadership of the late Jean Wertheimer of Lausanne, a multidisciplinary group of leaders in the field produced such a statement. This chapter briefly abstracts and highlights the central issues contained in this document with my personal annotations and explanations in italics.

GENERAL PRINCIPLES

Any organization of care must be founded in firm principles of human rights of the elderly with mental disorders. The historical discrimination towards the mentally ill should be actively fought and the destigmatization of mental illness must be conducted in the context of the unalienable human rights of each individual.

- Good health and life of good quality are fundamental human rights. This applies equally to people of all age groups and to people with mental disorders.
- All people have the right of access to a range of services that can respond to their health and social needs. These needs should be met appropriately for the cultural setting and in accordance with scientific knowledge and ethical requirements.
- Governments have a responsibility to improve and maintain the general and mental health of older people and to support their families and carers by the provision of health and social measures adapted to the specific needs of the local community.
- Older people with mental health problems and their families and carers have the right to participate individually and collectively in the planning and implementation of their health care.
- Services should be designed for the promotion of mental health in old age as well as for the assessment, diagnosis and management of the full range of mental disorders and disabilities encountered by older people.
- Governments need to recognize the crucial role of non-governmental agencies and work in partnership with them.
- Preparing for increasing life expectancy and ensuing health risks calls for significant social innovations at the individual and societal level, which must be founded on a knowledge base drawn from contributions by, and collaboration among, the medical, behavioural, psychological, biological and social sciences.
- In developing countries it may be difficult to provide resources for the provision of care. This, however, does not invalidate the aims of helping the elderly by the application of the principles listed above and the specific principles that follow.

SPECIFIC PRINCIPLES

The acronym CARITAS was deliberately chosen as a cogent reminder that "care and love" underpin these principles. The word "systemic" in some service contexts may be replaced by the word "seamless", representing a service organization that does not permit each individual to fall between gaps.

Good quality care for older people with mental health problems is: Comprehensive, Accessible, Responsive, Individualized, Transdisciplinary, Accountable, and Systemic (CARITAS).

- A *comprehensive* service should take into account all aspects of the patient's physical, psychological and social needs and wishes and be patient-centred.
- An *accessible* service is user-friendly and readily available, minimizing the geographical, cultural, financial, political and linguistic obstacles to obtaining care.
- A *responsive* service is one that listens to and understands the problems brought to its attention and acts promptly and appropriately.
- An *individualized* service focuses on each person with a mental health problem in his/her family and community context. The planning of care must be tailored for, and acceptable to, the individual and the family, and should aim wherever possible to maintain and support the person within his/her home environment.
- A *trans-disciplinary* approach goes beyond traditional professional boundaries to optimize the contributions of people with a range of personal and professional skills. Such an approach also facilitates collaboration with voluntary and other agencies to provide a comprehensive range of community-orientated services.
- An *accountable* service is one that accepts responsibility for assuring the quality of the service it delivers and monitors this in partnership with patients and their families. Such a service must be ethically and culturally sensitive.
- A *systemic* approach flexibly integrates all available services to ensure continuity of care and coordinates all levels of service providers, including local, provincial and national governments and community organizations.

COMPONENTS OF SERVICE

The concept of "surround with care" as represented by Figure 1, of concentric cycles, provides the concept of service delivery to have as its core the patients and their family carers. By enveloping them with seamless service organization with "permeable" boundaries represented by "dotted lines" in the figure, they are totally supported, and with changing circumstances can move from one service component to another without hindrance.

The described components of service, A–H, when put into place effectively, will meet the international best practice expected by this Consensus Statement.

The components of services can be summarized in Figure 1, which portrays the concept that individual patients, together with family and carers, are surrounded by the care service; these are flexibly interlocking, overlapping and integrated to provide a unified system for continuing care and best possible quality of life. Structural obstacles are minimized, as represented by the dotted lines of the figure, enabling the smooth movement of the patient from one service component to another as changing circumstances require. This section describes the components that can be put into place to address the care needs described in the previous section.

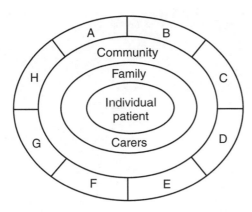

Figure 1 Surround with care

The following components ideally should be the responsibility of specialized teams of trained healthcare professionals working in psychiatry of the elderly. Where there is a scarcity of trained staff and resources, it will be necessary to use *ad hoc* solutions in order to provide the necessary components—while trying to develop services fully.

1. *Community Mental Health Teams (CMHTs) for Older People.* The lead in organizing the following components of the service should ideally be taken by multidisciplinary specialist teams working on psychiatry of the elderly. The CMHT may consist of doctors, psychiatric nurses, psychologists, social workers, therapists and secretaries. Referral to the CMHT is usually from primary care. One of the main responsibilities of the CMHT is the specialist assessment, investigation and the treatment of people in their home setting. In situations where such personnel are not available, the responsibility may be taken by general psychiatric or geriatric medicine teams.

2. *Inpatient services.* Acute inpatient units need to provide specialist assessment and treatment for the full range of mental disorders. This may in some cases include rehabilitation before return to the community.

3. *Day hospitals.* This is an acute service which offers assessment and treatment to older people who can be maintained at home, supported by the multidisciplinary team. The day hospital team could include doctors, nurses and therapy staff. Transport may need to be available.

4. *Outpatient services.* These provide assessment, diagnosis and treatment for people fit enough to live in the community and get to and from the hospital base. Outpatient services should be close to the inpatient and day-patient units. They may involve subspecialty clinics (e.g. memory or mood disorder clinics) and mobile clinics.

5. *Hospital respite care.* Hospital beds may be used to provide a respite service for people with chronic and severe mental illness and associated difficult behavioural problems, in order to give their carers a break and enable care at home to continue as long as possible.

6. *Continuing hospital care.* Care for life in a hospital setting may be required for people with chronic and severe mental illness and associated difficult behavioural problems. Such care should be provided in as relaxed and homely an environment as possible, with carers encouraged to participate.

7. *Liaison services.* Consultations and/or liaison services should be provided between facilities for elderly people with mental disorders and those serving general and geriatric medicine, general psychiatry, residential facilities and social agencies. This relationship should be of a reciprocal nature.

8. *Primary care.* The primary care team has the initial responsibility for identifying, assessing and managing mental health problems in older people. The decision to refer to the CMHT is usually made in primary care.

9. *Community and social support services.* These are services (both formal and informal) to enable the elderly person to remain at home, including a range of activities (home care, day care, residential care, respite care, self-help groups, etc.) provided by voluntary or government/social services.
   (a) *Respite facilities.* A range of short-term, time-limited, in-the-home and out-of-the-home services (residential services, other carers, day programmes) to support the carers.
   (b) *Residential care.* For those patients whose physical, psychological and/or social dependencies make living at home no longer possible, a spectrum of residential facilities should be provided. These range from supported accommodation with low-level supervision, medium-level care facilities, to full nursing facilities. These should be organized to achieve the best possible quality of life.

10. *Prevention.* The mental health team for the elderly should engage in the prevention of relapse of disorders by careful follow-up. They should also identify the risk factors for mental disorders in the elderly (e.g. hypertension, alcohol and substance abuse) and ensure these are effectively managed by appropriate medical, social strategies. Within each service, preventive activities need to be coordinated in collaboration with relevant public health and other healthcare professionals. These may include educational activities to improve early identification of mental health problems by carers, families and primary care personnel in the community.

CONCLUSION

While it may be seen to be less than realistic for some economically less-advantaged countries to achieve this best-practice ideal, nevertheless, both the WPA and WHO would recommend that such an ideal be both aspirational and inspirational. The paragraph:

> In developing countries it may be difficult to provide resources for the provision of care. This, however, does not invalidate the aims of helping the elderly by the application of the principles listed above and the specific principles that follow

in the General Principles section is reiterated here as a reminder that all available resources should be deployed within limited resources. For the "developed" countries that fail to meet these ideals, the WPA and WHO strongly urge their governments, policy makers and healthcare professionals to strive towards satisfying and exceeding the described principles and components of service.

As development of services is always a dynamic process, it is hoped that, in the future, this consensus statement will be reviewed and extended to incorporate improvements and innovations.

The central philosophy is that all elderly people with mental disorders should be provided with the best quality of life and the best quality of care in recognition of their esteemed status as Elders in our society.

REFERENCES

1. World Health Organization and World Psychiatric Association. *Organization of Care in Psychiatry of the Elderly—a Technical Consensus Statement.* WHO/MSA/MNH/MND/97.1. Geneva: WHO, 1997.
2. Jolley D, Arie T. Developments in psychogeriatric services. In Arie T, ed., *Recent Advances in Psychogeriatrics*, No. 2. Edinburgh: Churchill Livingstone, 1992.

122

The Multidisciplinary Team

Henry Rosenvinge

Moorgreen Hospital, Southampton, UK

Teamwork in the animal kingdom is a behaviour that enables survival. One example of its success is the male emperor penguin, who incubates his precious single egg balanced on his feet for 60 days through the total darkness of the Antarctic winter. This deed is achieved by the emperors huddling together and shuffling around in a constant movement, providing ever-changing relief from the gale-force wind[1].

The ability to behave in such a team has evolved through generations of practice. In care of the elderly in human populations there has been no such tradition and, for those suffering from psychiatric illness, the need for effective teamwork was never more urgent. The problem list presented by the functionally or organically ill elderly patient is often disconcertingly long and complex. The psychiatric disorder cannot be isolated from physical health problems, neither can the patient's functioning be assessed outside the context of his/her own domestic and social situation. Thus, in attempting to treat the patient it is necessary to combine the skills of psychiatric and geriatric medicine, together with those of nursing, clinical psychology, remedial therapy and social work. In many situations, input from the Housing Department, voluntary agencies and the local chaplaincy will be required. The creation of community care packages defined by the UK Government White Paper, *Caring for People in the Next Decade and Beyond*, highlighted the development of teamwork in case management[2]. The UK Government has extended this strategy to include carers as partners of professionals in the planning and delivery of care[3]. Teamwork in the management of the detained patient, particularly in respect of discharge planning and aftercare, are recommended as good practice by the Department of Health[4].

No one profession can attempt to provide all the various skills necessary in the management of every case. It is the relationship between the different professions that is so important. The concept of the multidisciplinary team can be described as a group of members of different professions whose working skills, when combined for the needs of the patient, aim to exceed in quality the simple summation of their individual abilities. Teamwork adds that extra vital ingredient, which needs further exploration.

The multidisciplinary team should be restricted in size to those personnel actively involved in management of cases and in close geographical proximity, to enable face-to-face contact between workers. However, the team should not exist in isolation from other services. The services that collaborate most successfully internally have been shown to not necessarily work best with other agencies[5]. Between different agencies there should be formal liaison and agreed policies over borderline cases and service demarcations.

FEATURES OF SUCCESSFUL MULTIDISCIPLINARY TEAMWORK

Communication

The Personal Social Service Council, in its review of community care, found that failures in communication and negotiation with other agencies led to ignorance of the roles and skills of other professional groups. The organization of care was less good in the more complex situations. As a result, wrong courses of action were taken by some professionals, including inappropriate admissions to both hospital and residential care. The need for joint planning was stressed, particularly between professionals of the different agencies at the operational level[6]. Effective communication is grafted onto the rootstock of mutual trust and respect for the individual roles and skills of other team members. Autonomous decisions, unnecessary duplication of work and stereotyping of one professional by another are thus avoided.

It is important that communication within the multidisciplinary team is afforded formal expression in regular meetings. Too much "corridor" decision making can lead to mistrust. Regular attendance by all personnel complements the identity and strength of the team. This results in the creation of a suitable arena for the airing of grievances and resolving of disputes. Teamwork involves allowing the patient and carer to participate in the process. The therapeutic team could include the patient[7], although the current climate of consumerism in care might be perceived as threatening by some workers.

Leadership

Traditionally, the leadership role in health care is assumed by the senior doctor; this in part reflects society's expectations and faith in the medical profession. Treatment directives may be instigated by the initial medical assessment and form the basis for the leadership role in the clinical team. The dominant role of the doctor in the healthcare team may have a stabilizing effect on the team's structure and prevent leadership struggles by other members[8]. Too hierarchical a structure, though, will result in too many decisions made by one person. More democratic teams will develop more flexible work practices and collective decision making. The doctor may in fact be the least qualified in management and leadership skills within the team. Moreover, the reason why multidisciplinary teams can work so badly is frequently the scant regard paid to them by the medical profession. Non-medical leadership of the multidisciplinary team can work, particularly if the issue of responsibility for

Principles and Practice of Geriatric Psychiatry, 2nd edn. Edited by J. R. M. Copeland, M. T. Abou-Saleh and D. G. Blazer
©2002 John Wiley & Sons, Ltd

decisions is satisfactorily addressed. A major DHSS document is clear that a consultant may not be held responsible for negligence on the part of others, simply because he is the "Responsible Medical Officer". It states he is not accountable like a military commander; "the multidisciplinary team has no commander in this sense"[9]. There is, however, a tendency to equate responsibility with out-of-hours accessibility, especially during a crisis.

It is important to remember that the key worker may not be the same person responsible for providing alternative care in the event of a crisis; e.g. the community mental health nurse (CMHN) may be the link with the elderly person at risk, but is unable to access directly residential care facilities should they be needed urgently.

For whoever dons the mantle of leader, skills in communication are a vital requirement, as is the ability to create a feeling of mutual trust and respect in order to maximize members' strengths and create compromise between individual members to fit in with overall team goals. Much of the motivation for the team will depend on the qualities of leadership. The creation of realistic goals gives a sense of purpose and a framework. Obviously, resource constraints are a major barrier to this process. It is important to distinguish the demands of budget holding from clinical management, and where the multidisciplinary leader is also the budget holder, the team members will need to learn the wider issues in the face of restrictions caused by tight fiscal control. They will need to feel the leader's commitment and sincerity in the care of their clients or patients.

Audit

The Department of Health encouraged medical audit as a means of improving service delivery and management[10]. Care of the elderly psychiatrically ill requires more complex assessment than pure medical audit, and the multidisciplinary team is in the key position to instigate clinical audit because of its potential for knocking down interprofessional barriers and prejudice. Multidisciplinary audit can be attempted if the process is viewed from a positive and non-defensive position. Good and bad practices in liaison will be easily revealed, particularly if the patients' and carers' views are included in outcome measures. The team should be in a constant state of evolution and be able to incorporate new ideas. This sense of objectivity and self-assessment will be created by a positive clinical audit programme and will itself become part of the quality of the successful team.

Morale

Clearly, morale is dependent on the key issues—leadership, communication, achievement of goals and self-assessment, described above. Other ingredients need adding to the recipe. Morale relies heavily on personal support and encouragement within the team. Through time, most team members experience stresses and problems, which may affect their judgement and possibly their self-esteem. This support may be available discreetly or offered more formally through staff groups and supervision. Whatever its form, its value is its ready accessibility and confidentiality.

The ability of the team members to see the funny side of a situation is often a vital component in the maintenance of morale. Involvement in non-clinical activities, such as fundraising or games matches against other units, may have positive effects on morale—even in defeat. In essence, it is important to create in team members a sense of personal value and ownership of their team. In the current climate of health service reorganization and cost–benefit assessment, the sharing of successes in patient treatment can contribute greatly to good morale.

FUTURE DEVELOPMENT OF THE MULTIDISCIPLINARY APPROACH

The introduction of goal-orientated multidisciplinary methods of treatment require changes in structures of healthcare organization[11]. Sadly, the move towards care management detailed in *Caring for People in the Next Decade and Beyond*[2] has not been complemented by sufficient funding to meet the requisite planning, training and research needs. Either the resources are not available to get multidisciplinary teams properly established, or there is insufficient funding to achieve even modest treatment goals. It is disputes over limited funding that can lead to the break-up of collaboration between agencies and effective teamwork.

Planning

The last decade has, however, seen an encouraging trend in the sophistication of expertise within the psychogeriatric team, producing greater quality of care of the elderly psychiatrically ill. The CMHN has developed roles in early case assessment and liaison with associated professionals. Because of the high profile in the locality, the CMHN has forged links with many agencies, e.g. district nurses, specialist housing, residential care facilities, and facilities for the treatment of alcoholism. Together with the increasingly skilled work with dementia sufferers, functionally ill patients and carers, the CMHN now brings to the multidisciplinary team a more vital and complex role. The social worker is still not given sufficient time to use her training in casework from the all too demanding accommodation-finding role. Historically, the champion of patients' rights, the social worker, may now access independent advocacy schemes. The roles of the occupational therapist and physiotherapist have been further strengthened by their involvement in community assessment liaison. The clinical psychologist finds much demand within the team, not only for assessment of areas of cognitive deficit in the patient, but also increasingly for the treatment of functional disorder, e.g. cognitive therapy and the evaluation of staff management methods and attitudes. There remains a paucity of training places in clinical psychology.

The shifting nature of the multidisciplinary team approach is further advanced by the recognition of the increasing role the voluntary sector can offer, both informally, using volunteers as befrienders of the patient, and more formally by such organizations as Age Concern and the Alzheimer's Disease Society, providing essential services such as day care. The role of the coordinator of such services can play an important part within the multidisciplinary team[12].

The expanding therapeutic team must recognize the problems that may arise when a new worker comes to fill a specific role carried out more generally by other workers, e.g. a social worker being appointed where previously much informal casework was conducted by the CMHN. Members of smaller teams may appear to have less distinct professional roles. Concentration on individual strengths, not weaknesses, will enable expansion of the team to take place.

Training

It is not clear that such growth in individual professional expertise in care of the elderly psychiatrically ill has been matched by the requisite training in multidisciplinary teamwork skills, particularly in undergraduate medical education. The General Medical Council, in its publication, *Teaching Tomorrow's Doctors*, has recognized this shortfall[13]. Attitudes and techniques in cooperation with other disciplines will need to be explored in order to escape from the purely medical model of treatment.

Case studies have been described as being well suited for teaching, in an interesting and understandable way, the complexities in the field of geriatric medicine, where an increased degree of integration with other services is required[14]. This must also be true in geriatric psychiatry. By the careful selection of cases to illustrate psychological, medical and social issues, the trainee should be stimulated rather than confused. This is an ideal opportunity for multidisciplinary teaching, enabling the learner to understand the different professional roles. The aim should be to show that complex cases might be manageable by the establishment of treatment goals, even if they are necessarily limited. Cultural, ethical and legal issues can be shown to have an important influence on the equation. Teaching by the use of case studies can be a good focus for multidisciplinary learning for groups of trainees from different professional backgrounds.

Planned community visiting sessions with the CMHN or social worker are highly valued by undergraduates of all relevant professions at Southampton University Medical School.

Doctors in higher training to be consultants in the field of old age psychiatry demand experience in multidisciplinary teamwork and should have flexibility in their programmes to permit in-depth exploration of the roles of the different members of the team. A variety of multidisciplinary teams should be observed, including those in other psychogeriatric units.

Individual professional training must be mirrored by developments encompassing different professional groups. A training model has been devised to overcome the organizational isolation of agencies serving mutual elderly clients with mental health problems in Philadelphia[15]. Training issues were explored at a conference on interdisciplinary issues in mental health and ageing, where interprofessional cooperation was reaffirmed and strengthened[16]. There is a rising swell of workshops on collaborative care in the management of the elderly psychiatrically ill, much of it promoted by initiatives from the voluntary sector and much of it relevant to the training needs of the multidisciplinary team.

Research

Objective research in the workings of the multidisciplinary team has received little attention in the case of the elderly psychiatrically ill. A review of the role and effect of this teamwork in the management of delirium in dementia found insufficient data for the development of evidence-based guidelines[17]. A difficulty is that evaluation has been mainly restricted to descriptive terms using, for example, in-depth individual case studies. In this area in particular, clinical audit and operational research are almost indistinguishable. Outcome measures, however, using quantity and timing of liaison, do not measure the essential components of the workings of the team—the quality of the relationships and the ability to respond as a whole to the needs of the patient. Study is still required into the methods of evaluating the effect of the quality of these relationships, particularly within the field of old age psychiatry.

REFERENCES

1. Attenborough D. *The Life of Birds*. London: BBC Domino, 1998: 288–92.
2. Department of Health, Department of Social Security. *Caring for People in the Next Decade and Beyond*. London: HMSO, 1989.
3. Department of Health. *Caring about Carers—A National Strategy for Carers*. London: HMSO, 1999.
4. Department of Health and Welsh Office. *Code of Practice*. London: The Stationery Office, 1999.
5. Wright J, Ball C, Coleman P. Collaboration in Care. Age Concern/ Institute of Gerontology Research Paper 2. London: Age Concern, 1988.
6. Personal Social Services Council, DHSS. *Collaboration in Community Care—a Discussion Document*. London: HMSO, 1988.
7. Schoenberg E, ed. *A Hospital Looks at Itself*. Oxford: Bruno Cassirer, 1972: 41–50.
8. Bakheit AMO. Effective teamwork in rehabilitation. *Int J Rehab Res* 1996; **19**: 301–6.
9. Department of Health and Social Security. *Organizational and Management Problems of Mental Illness Hospitals* (*the Nodder Report*). Paragraph 6.17. London: DHSS, 1980.
10. Department of Health. *Working for Patients*. London: HMSO, 1989.
11. Draper RJ. The chronically mentally ill: planning a future. *Psychiat J Univ Ottawa* 1989; **14**(3): 463–6.
12. Rosenvinge H, Guion J, Dawson J. A sitting service for the elderly confused. *Health Trends* 1986; **18**(2): 47.
13. General Medical Council. *Tomorrow's Doctors' Recommendations on Undergraduate Medical Education*. London: GMC, 1993.
14. Nahemow L, Ponsada L. *Geriatric Diagnostics—a Case Study Approach*. New York: Springer, 1983: 41.
15. Persky T, Taylor A, Simson S. The Network Trilogy Project. Linking aging, mental health and health agencies. *Gerontol Geriat Ed* 1989; **9**(3): 79–88.
16. Rickards LD. Conference on Interdisciplinary Issues in Mental Health and Aging. Workshop issues and recommendations. *Gerontol Geriat Ed* 1989; **9**(3): 61–7.
17. Britton A, Russell R. *Multidisciplinary Team Interventions in the Management of Delirium in Patients with Chronic Cognitive Impairment—a Review of the Evidence of Effectiveness*. In the Cochrane Library. Oxford: Update Software, 1998.

123

Community Care: the Background

Colin Godber

Moorgreen Hospital, Southampton, UK

The specialty of old age psychiatry in Britain grew out of the failure of orthodox, institutionally-based psychiatry to meet the needs of the growing number of elderly people with dementia. Its success stemmed from its proactive community-based approach, an emphasis on the support of family and other carers and the demonstration of the positive outcomes obtainable through better recognition and energetic treatment of much of the functional illness of old age[1]. Crucial to that approach and the effectiveness of the elderly mental health service itself has been the development of partnerships across health and social services, support to informal carers and the increasing range of care staff working directly with patients. Just as it has led the rest of psychiatry in assertive outreach, it has often taken over from the increasingly hospital-centred geriatric medicine as a catalyst and advocate for community care for older people. This chapter will look at some of the components and contributors to that care, as well as some of the wider organizational and political factors that have influenced it.

PRIMARY HEALTH CARE

General practice has always been the cornerstone of the National Health Service (NHS) in Britain, providing continuity of individual and family care and acting as gatekeeper to secondary care. Aggregation into group practices paved the way to the establishment of the primary healthcare team (PHCT), with its core membership of general practitioner (GP), practice nurse, district nurse and health visitor, and later a looser attachment or sessional input from community mental health nurses (CMHNs), podiatrists, physiotherapists, counsellors and specialists from secondary care. The PHCT provides the bulk of domiciliary health care and surveillance of those at risk and the main day-to-day link with social services, housing and other local agencies supporting disabled people in their homes.

With the aim of strengthening the locality and primary care focus of the NHS, the incoming Labour government[2] has aggregated groups of PHCTs covering "natural" localities of 50–150 000 population into primary care groups (PCGs). Health-care budgets for these localities have been devolved to PCGs, who are responsible for increasing the equity and quality of primary care within local populations, for assessing their health needs and for commissioning secondary care services. There is also the option/expectation that PCGs will progress to fuller autonomy as primary care trusts (PCTs). These will be empowered to take over the management, for instance, of community hospitals and appropriate secondary care services and will be expected to develop closer partnerships with local social services. It is likely, therefore, that PCTs will take on a much more comprehensive role in the provision of community care within the Health Service. Parallel legislation[3,4] will also facilitate partnership with local authority services by enabling them to pool and ring-fence budgets to promote joint services, long advocated by proponents of community care.

INFORMAL CARERS

By far the largest contribution to domiciliary care, particularly for those with dementia, is of course that of family members and friends. The main carer is usually a spouse or partner, although care by daughters, sons and daughters-in-law remains substantial, despite greater geographical mobility, changing employment patterns and the steadily falling ratio of middle-aged to elderly people. Input from neighbours can also be vital and some areas have well-developed community networks. The House of Commons Social Services Select Committee[5] estimated the "replacement cost" of informal carers for the disabled in Britain (over three-quarters of a million "on their feet" for more than 50 h week) as well above the total expenditure on all statutory care. The government recently acknowledged the importance of carers and the load they carry and announced a strategy to ensure that their needs will be properly assessed and that they become eligible for extra financial support[6].

BACK-UP FROM GERIATRIC PSYCHIATRY

Partnership with family carers is fundamental to the practice of old age psychiatry, especially in the context of dementia. Initial assessment should include the extent of informal care, the health and attitude of the carers and the prospects for sustaining such care in the future, given adequate help. Carers need the support of a key worker with a good knowledge of the "system" who can help them access appropriate services and allowances and the practical and psychological value of carer support groups. Important aspects of that key working are its continuity, attention to the health and morale of the carers and prompt arrangement of further assessment, intervention and respite when the need arises.

For those with psychiatric illness, and particularly dementia, the key worker will usually be the CMHN, working closely with colleagues in primary health care and social services teams. CMHNs also have an important support and educational role, with the increasing number of untrained voluntary and paid carers working with patients in their homes, day centres and residential care. They will also draw on the range of skills and

Principles and Practice of Geriatric Psychiatry, 2nd edn. Edited by J. R. M. Copeland, M. T. Abou-Saleh and D. G. Blazer

resources of the specialist team itself for further assessment, treatment, respite or crisis intervention. A great deal of the work of the elderly mental health service takes place in the patient's home. Ours, for example (catering for an elderly population of 60 000), has 20 CMHNs, all with large case-loads and between them clocking up about 20 000 patient contacts a year. This is complemented by outreach from other members of the service (e.g. 8000 medical community contacts), two day hospitals and deployment of staff to support day centres specializing in the care of the elderly patients with mental health problems. An original bed complement of 250 (mainly long-stay) has reconfigured to 40 continuing-care and 90 short-stay beds, 35 of the latter for functional illness. This has necessitated extensive outreach and support to residential and nursing homes but has released funds to redeploy into community developments, such as the establishment[7] of a sitting service to offer home respite to carers for demented patients. This has now diversified into other areas of community support for elderly people with mental health problems as a thriving provider in the new mixed economy of community care.

SOCIAL CARE IN THE COMMUNITY

Progress in community care in Britain has been hampered by the very different way in which health and social services are organized and financed and the frequent lack of co-terminosity in their local boundaries. The NHS is funded from taxation and is predominantly free at the point of delivery. It has strong central direction and is coordinated locally by (unelected) district health authorities. Social and housing services are run by (elected) local authorities, which receive block allocations from central government but also have to raise much of their revenue through local taxation and by means-tested charging of services to clients. Local authorities were traditionally the main providers of domiciliary and residential support for disabled people.

The 1970s saw many initiatives in specialized supported housing for older people[8–10] and in individualized and sometimes intensive domiciliary services to support, in their own homes, frail elderly people who might otherwise have required residential care. Evaluation of these and subsequent projects usually showed them to be valued by clients and generally cost-effective at low and moderate levels of disability, but decreasingly so (and at times very expensive) for those with heavier dependency[10,11]. Because they generally rely on intermittent carer input or on the client summoning assistance, they tend to be less effective for patients with advancing dementia than for those with a purely physical disability.

Generalization of these initiatives in community care was seriously hampered by the economic problems of the 1970s and early 1980s. The incoming Thatcher government found things reaching crisis point but was unwilling to give the necessary support to local authorities to expand domiciliary based care. Instead, it changed the regulations governing social security benefits[12] to allow these to be used to pay fees in private residential and nursing homes, with no provision for needs assessment. This led to a huge expansion (from £10 million to over £1 billion a year during the 1980s) in this sector, but none in domiciliary provision, which was not eligible for this source of funding. This wasteful and retrograde trend was castigated by the Audit Commission[13], which drew attention to the contrasting effectiveness and popularity of the Kent Community Care scheme[14,15]. This had been using care management to assess the needs of frail elderly people in the community and to put together packages of domiciliary care, drawing on a range of neighbourhood resources. This was enabling many people who would otherwise have needed residential care to remain in their own homes, despite a budget ceiling well below the cost of the residential placement.

To establish a transition to this model, the Audit Commission proposed a ring-fencing of all public expenditure on community and institutionally-based continuing care (including all residential, nursing home and NHS continuing care) to be administered by a single district care agency on a care management basis. These proposals were endorsed by the government's management guru[16], who also stressed the need to ring-fence the budgets for all continuing care and to ensure adequate transitional funding to secure ample early investment in domiciliary-based options. The resulting White Paper[17] unfortunately ignored these two crucial points. The result gave Social Services departments the responsibility for care management (including the purchase of long-term nursing home care) but without arrangements for any transfer of funds released within the NHS if it closed equivalent continuing-care beds.

Implementation of the Act since 1993 has therefore brought about a modified resurgence of community care for older people in Britain. Social services departments were encouraged to focus on the assessment and care management functions and to stimulate a mixed economy of domiciliary care providers, from whom they purchase packages tailored to the needs of clients. It is very gratifying to see one's patients getting individualized support packages, combining informal, social and healthcare elements and often assembled at short notice in the event of a crisis. Aware of the growing pressure on acute hospital beds, some health and social services departments have also collaborated to develop domiciliary and intermediate care options to reduce the need for hospital admission and facilitate early discharge[18]. The advent of PCGs should certainly stimulate that sort of approach. Unfortunately, because the means-testing rules make residential care cheaper for social services than the domiciliary equivalent for anyone with moderate care needs, the cost ceiling applied by most departments to domiciliary packages for individual clients is a long way below the level of residential home fees. This rules out such care for many people for whom it would otherwise have continued to be cost-effective, particularly those with dementia.

POLITICAL AND ECONOMIC FACTORS

Lack of investment has been the main cause of our slow progress with community care for older people in Britain. The politicians have generally been seduced into thinking that it is a cheap option, but at times of economic hardship domiciliary provision has always been the first target for cuts. In the 1980s spending on care of the elderly increased greatly but in the wrong direction and it is taking a long time for the pendulum to swing back. The separate organization and funding of health and social care have created perverse incentives, which have been exploited to preserve an inadequately funded NHS by narrowing its focus to the care of acute illness. This constriction of the range of free NHS care has led to artificial and increasingly absurd demarcations between health and social care, which undermines efficient and effective partnership and has thrown an increasing share of the cost onto patients themselves. Failure to ring-fence the NHS continuing care within the community care budget has allowed the closure of 60 000 beds since 1990 (with savings redeployed to support other NHS priorities), while social services have had to pick up the load with an increase in their nursing home purchasing from 100 000 to 180 000 beds—a cost shift to social services and (through means testing) to patients and families of over £300 million a year. Not surprisingly, this has encroached on investment in domiciliary care, which only increased by 56% in the first 5 years of implementation of the community care legislation[18].

This shrinkage in the role of the NHS in continuing care and rehabilitation and the barrier to effective services created by the artificial distinction between health and social care[19] has been widely criticized[18,20,21]. There is growing consensus that things will only get properly "joined up" when the funding rules for health and social care are harmonized and the nettle of the cost of our ageing population is properly grasped by the politicians. The Royal Commission[23] set up by the government recommended that all care (as opposed to board and lodging and general living) costs should be publicly funded from general taxation, eliciting little response as yet from a government still wedded to reducing taxation and maintaining means testing. The earlier Joseph Rowntree Enquiry[22] reached similar conclusions on the care costs but favoured a hypothecated, prospective, compulsory health/social care insurance levied on payrolls as a way of enabling each generation to fund its own care in old age. If the government finally accepts one or other of these options, the millennium could usher in an exciting new phase in community care.

REFERENCES

1. Arie T, Isaacs AD. The development of psychiatric services for the elderly in Britain. In Isaacs AD, Post F, eds, *Studies in Geriatric Psychiatry*. Chichester: Wiley, 1978: 241–61.
2. Department of Health. *The New NHS: Modern and Dependable*. London: HMSO, 1997.
3. Department of Health. *Partnership in Action*. London: HMSO, 1998.
4. Department of Health. Health Act, 1999. London: The Stationery Office, 1999.
5. House of Commons. *Community Care: Carers*. Social Services Select Committee Report. London: HMSO, 1990.
6. Department of Health. *Caring About Carers: a National Strategy for Carers*. London: DOH, 1999.
7. Rosenvinge HP, Dawson J, Guion J. Sitting service for the elderly confused. *Health Trends* 1986; **18**: 47.
8. Godber C. Kinloss Court: an experiment in sheltered housing and collaboration. *Social Work Service* 1978; **15**: 42–5.
9. Lewis RJ. Flying Warden answers 80-year-old's Monday call. *Mod Geriat* 1979; **3**: 26–33.
10. Tinker A. *An Evaluation of Very Sheltered Housing*. London: HMSO, 1989.
11. Challis D, Chesterman J, Darton R, Trasker K. Case management in the care of the aged: the provision in difficult care settings. In Bournat G et al., eds, *Community Care: a Reader*. Milton Keynes: Macmillan/Open University, 1993.
12. DHSS. *Resource and Single Payment Amendment Regulations*. Regulation 9, Supplementary Benefit Requirement. Circular 7/143, 1980.
13. Audit Commission. *Making a Reality of Community Care*. London: HMSO, 1986.
14. Davies B, Challis D. *Matching Resources to Needs in Community Care*. Aldershot: Gower, 1986.
15. Challis D, Darton R, Johnson L et al. *Case Management and Health Care of Older People: The Darlington Community Care Project*. Aldershot: Arena, 1995.
16. Griffiths R. *Community Care: Agenda for Action*. London: HMSO, 1988.
17. Secretaries of State for Health, Social Security, Wales and Scotland. *Caring for People*. Cm 849. London: HMSO, 1989.
18. Calviou A, Hockley J, Schofield. *An Evaluation of Marlow EPICS*. South Buckinghamshire NHS Trust and Buckingham County Council Social Services, 1997.
19. Department of Health. *NHS Responsibilities for Meeting Continuing Health Care Needs*. HSG(95)8, LAC(95)5. London: HMSO, 1995.
20. House of Commons. *NHS Responsibility for Meeting Continuing Health Care Needs*. Health Select Committee, Session 1995–96, First Report, Volume 1.
21. Audit Commission. *The Coming of Age: Improving Care Services for Older People*. London: HMSO, 1997.
22. Joseph Rowntree Foundation Enquiry. *Meeting the Cost of Continuing Care: Report and Recommendations*. York: Joseph Rowntree Foundation, 1996.
23. Royal Commission on Long Term Care. *With Respect to Old Age: Long-term Care—Rights and Responsibilities*. Cm 4192, 1,11/1,11/3. London: The Stationery Office, 1999.
24. *National Health Service and Community Care Act*. London: HMSO, 1990.

Health Care of the Elderly: the Nottingham Model

Tom Arie

University of Nottingham, UK

The Nottingham University Department of Health Care of the Elderly was designed as a collaboration in which physicians, psychiatrists, gerontologists and other health workers are equal partners. It is neither a department of psychiatry with geriatricians on its staff, nor vice versa: it is an integrated joint enterprise. It was the model for 20 years. Following the retirement of the foundation professor, the university restructured the Department but the service ethos continues, as does the joint teaching programme. Described here is the Joint Department as it was, and as it became well known, from 1977 to 1997.

Diagrams may put things best. Figure 1 shows the structure, and makes the important point that although the department is unified, its services are differentiated. Physicians do medical work, psychiatrists psychiatry. There is cross-training, and above all constant formal and informal collaboration and support, both in the hospital and in assessing and keeping people going at home.

The aim is to make easily available what patients need. Thus, a patient of the psychiatric service has as easy access to physicians and their facilities as if he/she were their patient, and vice versa. In this way it is possible to offer responses that match the pattern of morbidity characteristic of the very old, namely that it is mixed and often unpredictably changeable. There are no demarcation disputes, and there is no waiting list. Things were very different when the department was established in 1977.

INTEGRATION

The services are based in two general teaching hospitals. In University Hospital the professorial unit has a medical and a psychiatric ward side-by-side. There are close links with the rest of the health specialties and professions, both inside and outside the hospital. For instance, trainees rotate from general medicine,

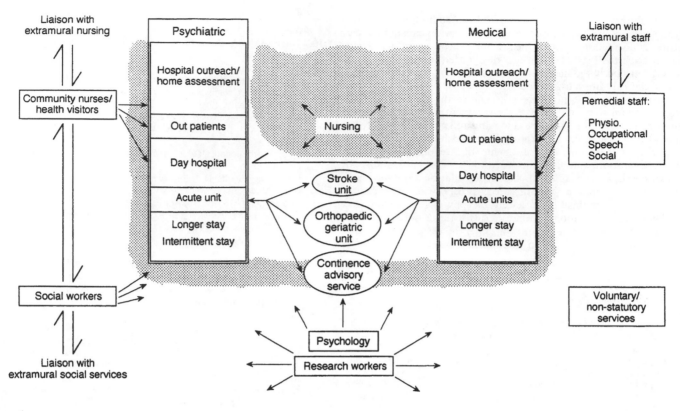

Figure 1

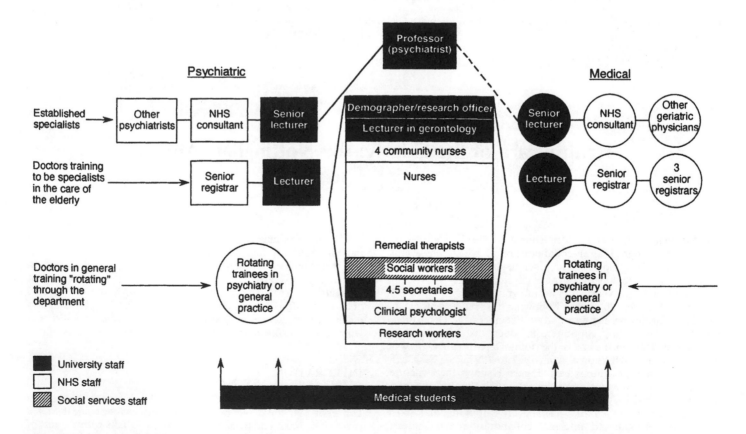

Figure 2

psychiatry and general practice (Figure 2), and there is pairing with medical and surgical firms. The department is embedded in the local medical community, and particularly values its links with the parent disciplines of medicine and psychiatry and its closeness to primary care. All referrals to the psychiatric side of the department are initially seen at home by a senior psychiatrist, usually together with a medical student, and any other team members or community staff who are involved and able to be present, and if possible the family doctor is present too. In practice, most visits are by psychiatrist and medical student. On the medical side of the department a home assessment service is freely available, but the majority of patients are seen in the clinic, or admitted as emergencies. Community nurses, working outwards from the hospital, are part of both the medical and psychiatric services.

EDUCATION AND RESEARCH

All Nottingham medical students spend a month full-time in the department. Teaching is a joint effort between all staff, of whatever specialty, medical and non-medical. The course comprises: a clinical clerkship, inside and outside the hospital; a planned course of teaching; and a personal project under supervision. With about 150 students a year, there is a heavy teaching load. The course is well received and many students come back as postgraduate trainees. Rotating trainees come to acquire better skills (and, we hope, greater job satisfaction) in dealing with old people in whatever field they decide eventually to work. Only the senior registrars are being trained to become specialists in old age.

Research thrives on collaboration and transcends boundaries of departments: we have long been collaborating with other departments, and within a mixed department research collaboration comes easily. Major projects include longitudinal studies of well-being of old people at home—the Activity and Ageing Study—and participation in the Medical Research Council study of Cognitive Function and Ageing (CFAS). Most projects have involved staff from both of the main branches of the department.

CONCLUSION

What has been called "the Nottingham Model" works well, and is a satisfying way in which to work. There have naturally been day-to-day problems, some general, others parochial, but none that have divided the department along specialty lines. Above all, patients do not fall between stools and bucks do not get passed.

REFERENCES

1. Arie T. Combined Geriatrics and Psychogeriatrics: a new model. *Geriatr Med* 20th Anniversary Issue, April 1990: 24–7 (on which this Special Article is based, with permission).
2. Arie T. Education in the care of the elderly. *Bull NY Acad Med* 1985; **61**(6): 492–500.
3. Bendall MJ. The interface between geriatrics and psychogeriatrics. *Curr Med Lit Geriat* 1988; **1**(1): 2–7.

124

The Development of Day Hospitals and Day Care

Rosie Jenkins and D. J. Jolley

Penn Hospital, Wolverhampton, UK

ORIGINS

Day hospitals are said to be among the few notable creations that psychiatry has given to medicine[1]. The concept that older people could be given treatment, rehabilitation and care without resorting to "inpatient" status within hospitals or related "institutions" was accepted enthusiastically in the UK from the late 1960s. "Partial hospitalization" (usually day hospital care, but sometimes night care, relief admission programmes, rotating care or shared bed schemes), linked to active community services, has been a feature of the services provided for the elderly, not only by psychiatrists but also geriatric physicians. Non-medical agencies, such as social services departments and voluntary bodies, have also participated. Interestingly, and perhaps significantly, the private sector has been much less enthusiastic for partial hospitalization schemes. This appears to be true for other countries.

ATTRACTIONS

The attractions of day care are most obvious for the patient, who is enabled to maintain his/her home routines and contact with his/her supports, whilst taking advantage of professional expertise in treatment during certain parts of the day. Family members or carers may have mixed perceptions: their burden of anxiety and responsibility for the ill or disabled patient is relieved only episodically and only in part; yet many are pleased with this opportunity to continue to contribute to care and for therapy with the guidance of professionals. The resources of the day hospital add to the resources of family life[2]. For the health care agency (the National Health Service), day hospital development has been attractive for its flexibility and apparent cheapness. It may not, however, represent a cheap option. Its importance to health care systems lies in its influence on the effectiveness and smooth running of inpatient and other domiciliary or extramural and partial hospitalization projects. These are increasingly likely to be cooperative ventures with other care-providing agencies, such as social services[3].

SPREAD WITHIN THE UK

At the end of the 1960s, the Department of Health was prompted by a pressing need to review the services it was providing to the increasing numbers of older people suffering from dementia and other major psychiatric disorders. This revealed a woeful situation, with relatively few beds, badly supported and in inappropriate locations, frequently operating with waiting lists, that saw patients dying before admission[4].

A review of provision based on the 1971 census was to establish the baseline for inpatient services[5] and health authorities were encouraged to create day hospital places in equal numbers, often starting from zero[6]. As little guidance was given in respect of the development of these day hospitals, a wide variety of interpretations arose from practitioners and planners trying to produce the best possible facilities. Between 1976–1986 the total number of day hospital places for the mentally ill increased by 50%. Provision for the elderly ranged from 129 places/10 000 in East Anglia to 693/10 000 in the North West[7]. Wide variations persist between areas in respect of day hospital places available to the elderly populations served, and the Royal College of Psychiatry's recommendations of one place for every 500 (or fewer) of the elderly population[8] is not yet seen everywhere, for a variety of financial and other reasons.

STRUCTURES

The cheapest option for developing day hospital provision was to place the facility in a disused part of a mental hospital, and risk the deficiencies of the parent hospital transferring to the new unit. Interestingly, the effect tended to be positive, for both the new venture and the existing facilities for this patient group, and illustrates a potential of such care—the link with inpatient services benefits the day care unit, its attenders and their carers, and encourages wards to provide care more relevant to population needs. Alternatively, developments took advantage of existing premises, designed for other purposes but away from the mental hospital and often in the area to be served[9]. "Travelling" day hospitals used a network of such premises, staff moving between the locations to provide care on different days[10], a useful system for rural communities.

The ideal would be purpose-built units, probably on health authority land and sited conveniently in the catchment area. No bed provision is required and staff are not employed when the unit is closed. These developments can also create a positive image for a vital, if unfashionable, service by raising its community profile.

Such "stand-alone" day hospitals run the risk of being seen as distant from the inpatient services, and may detract from the reputation of the latter, especially as they are often seen as more thrusting and challenging. This can hinder cooperative efforts, such as when a patient requires a period of short-term, rotating or prolonged inpatient care[11]. Probably the best model places day hospital and inpatient facilities within the same unit, with several

Principles and Practice of Geriatric Psychiatry, 2nd edn. Edited by J. R. M. Copeland, M. T. Abou-Saleh and D. G. Blazer

such units of modest size at strategic sites throughout the community to be served (Figure 124.1).

FUNCTIONS

A day hospital may aim to provide one or more of a series of care options for the elderly attender. It may offer assessment and treatment otherwise requiring admission, facilitate early discharge from inpatient care, provide rehabilitation, or help attenders deskilled or disabled by long experience of illness. Additionally, it may provide continuing support for patients with established disabilities (with or without a known vulnerability to major decompensations), arguably in itself a rehabilitative regimen attempting to prevent further deterioration and also providing carer support. In practice, many day hospitals perform mixed functions and may not have formally determined aims. The experience of others can serve to inform the process of defining such objectives.

Bergmann et al.'s[12] general hospital-based day hospital in Newcastle functioned as an assessment and early treatment unit, without initial home visits and very much in the manner of a tertiary referral facility for other teams working out of existing mental hospitals. Alongside was a small ward with a similar

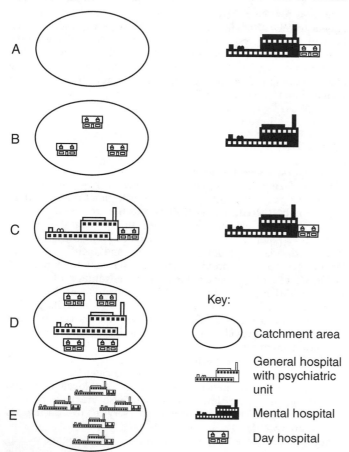

Figure 124.1 Models of day hospital provision. (A) Large mental hospital geographically distant from catchment area served, starting day care on site. (B) Mental hospital supported by stand-alone day hospitals within catchment area. (C) Mental hospital beginning to give way to district hospital unit, both sites with inpatient and day hospital facilities. (D) General hospital with psychiatric unit supported by stand-alone day hospitals. (E) General hospital with day hospital unit and supported by several units within the catchment area, each offering inpatient and day hospital care.

Key:

⬭ Catchment area

General hospital with psychiatric unit

Mental hospital

Day hospital

function, and the team also undertook liaison work—probably representing the best use for this day hospital within the city's then mental health provision. Even so, and despite a highly skilled and single-minded team, the successful pursuit of "assessment only" is difficult to sustain. Bergmann reported that the day hospital's advice, after assessment, was taken or acted upon in disappointingly few cases. Whitehead[13] also stressed the assessment and treatment potential of the day hospital, designating it perhaps the key element in a community-orientated old age service. He was, however, providing a comprehensive range of services within one team, with home-based assessment and treatment available before a decision regarding the use of the day hospital or a small inpatient unit. His unsatisfactory experience of poor-quality mental hospital wards determined his philosophy that recourse to inpatient care would be taken for very few patients.

Such models of care are attractive, but were influenced by other factors: for Bergmann, longer-term care was available elsewhere, and Whitehead had a supportive nursing home sector sympathetic to his vision[14]. Other authors have been uncomfortable with day hospitals that appear to function mostly to delay entry into long-term care[15,16]: however, for some individuals and their carers, this may be the very help they want, and should be evaluated in this light.

Arie[17] identified two groups of patients benefiting from long-term day hospital attendance: dementia sufferers living with carers wanting them to remain at home, but who needed help and some respite from the carer role; and patients with relapsing illnesses complicated by persisting "neurotic" symptoms when well. The latter were almost all women living alone. Others working in well-sited and well-equipped day hospitals have confirmed these images of the successful long-term patient. Here, the male:female ratio of dementia sufferers was often equal, and some attended from rest homes. There was also an intermediate group, suffering from mood disorder or neurotic symptoms associated with quite severe physical disability (from stroke, parkinsonism, arthritis, chest or heart conditions), having nursing needs as great as those of dementia sufferers, but with psychological needs akin to other "functional" patients[11].

The "mix" of day hospital attenders can be crucial. Individuals severely damaged by dementia benefit from simple, structured and repetitive activities that are unhelpful and unrewarding to their cognitively intact peers. Where dementia has caused a decline in physical abilities, basic group physiotherapy techniques can be beneficial, whereas other patients with complex physical and psychological needs may only thrive with individually tailored personal care interventions. Mixing patients with widely differing cognitive abilities can be unacceptable to both the better and the less able. Potential tensions can be reduced by using different areas of the unit for different purposes, or by having day-specific activities. Where several local day hospitals coexist, they may develop specialized roles[11].

Most practitioners with day hospitals available for their patients are enthusiastic about their potential, but there have been few robust evaluations of the efficacy of day hospitals. Philpott's review[18] cautiously concluded that day hospitals remained experimental care delivery systems. Creed and colleagues, after reviewing studies of day hospital care[19], evaluated day hospital activities in the north-west of England[20]. They confirmed that day hospitals are able to provide alternative care for many patients but that not all such facilities can, or want to, provide the same service[21]. Longer periods of treatment may be offset by greater efficacy in preventing relapse and maintaining independence[22].

The costs of day hospital care are probably lower than those for inpatient care. MacDonald et al.[23] undertook an extensive study of outcomes in matched groups of elderly people with mild to moderate dementia in four care settings in London. They found no significant differences in mortality or in changes on dementia scores. They concluded that non-hospital day centres offered the best value.

Panella *et al.*[24] found that only 69 of 314 elderly demented patients likely to benefit from day hospital programmes in Burke, USA, took advantage of them. For these, the costs were estimated to be considerably lower than nursing home care and the programme was acceptable to patients and carers. Zeeli and Isaacs[25], despite describing a geriatric day hospital where 75% of attenders' time was spent in active therapy and transport problems were non-existent, still showed only half the patients completing planned treatment. Only one-third achieved staff-determined objectives or felt improved by 3 months.

Transport problems, along with changes in health or social circumstances, were often associated with costly lost days of care in the comprehensive review performed by Eagle *et al.*[26], but the work confirmed the positive effects of day hospital care on the physical and emotional health of elderly attenders.

The Audit Commission[27] has confirmed the expense of day care when linked to domiciliary support services to the moderately disabled—it can exceed the cost of residential care, and the cost of informal care is all but impossible to calculate. This does not mean it is not preferable to other forms of care.

Donaldson, Wright and Maynard[28] emphasized the need to consider several measures when assessing day hospital care. These included the costs of all services used over a designated period, with clinical, social and psychological measures at set intervals related to treatment and follow-up, and carer and patient satisfaction scores. As yet, few if any studies have examined all these aspects of care, although a work in progress by Read and her colleagues in a joint day care/day hospital project in Wolverhampton is designed along very similar lines to those suggested by Donaldson's team[29]. This evaluation is also attempting to place such care in context with other care and services available. More comprehensive assessments of the efficacy of all available complementary facilities individually and within systems are necessary to tease out the particular effects of day hospitals. These would include measures of the morale and self-image of professional carers in the sectors and their views and attitudes towards other complementary services, patients and their carers. These considerations reflect the complexities of the processes of care delivery to the elderly mentally ill, and the relationships between "consumers" and "providers".

CONCLUSION

Day hospitals for the elderly mentally ill have become established services, especially within the UK. There is little reason to doubt that they fulfil a useful and acceptable function. Providing something of this nature has both energized and encouraged developments in many areas. Refinements of practice occur over time as individual day hospitals modify what they do in the context of a changing awareness of their own potentials and weaknesses, and in relation to changes in other services available to the potential client or patient group. Formal research evaluations continue and may better inform such evolutionary developments and future planning. It remains important to be aware of the limitations of such evaluative research and it would be quite wrong to stop good ideas being put into practice on the "quasi-scientific" basis that "its cost-effectiveness cannot be demonstrated".

REFERENCES

1. Farndale J. *The Day Hospital Movement in Great Britain.* Oxford: Pergamon, 1961.

2. Hodgson SP. Day hospital for dementia: a safety net for a high-wire act? In Reed J, Lomas S, eds, *Psychiatric Services in the Community: Developments and Innovations.* London: Croom Helm, 1984; 191–6.

3. Currie A, McAllister-Williams RH, Jaques A. A comparison study of day hospital and day centre attenders. *Health Bull* 1995; **53**(6): 365–72.

4. Carse J, Panton N, Watt A. A district mental health service: the Worthing experiment. *Lancet* 1958; **i**: 39–42.

5. Jolley D. Hospital in-patient provision for patients with dementia. *Br Med J* 1977; 1335–6.

6. Department of Health and Social Security. *Services for Mental Disorder Related to Old Age.* Circular HM(72)71. London: HMSO.

7. Department of Health and Social Security. *Mental Health Statistics for England, 1986: Booklet 9: Mental Illness Hospitals and Units: Facilities and Services.* London: Government Statistical Service, 1986.

8. Joint Working Party of Royal College of Psychiatrists and Royal College of Physicians. *The Care of Older People with Mental Illness: Specialist Services and Medical Training.* Council Report CR69. London: Royal College of Psychiatrists and Royal College of Physicians, 1998.

9. Baker AA, Byrne RJ. Another style of psychogeriatric service. *Br J Psychiat* 1977; **130**: 123–6.

10. Hettiaratchy P. The UK's travelling day hospital. *Age Int* 1985; Summer: 10–11.

11. Jolley S, Jolley D. Psychiatric disorders in old age. In Bennett D, Freeman H, eds, *Community Psychiatry.* Edinburgh: Churchill Livingstone, 1991; 268–96.

12. Bergmann K, Foster EM, Justice AW, Matthews V. Management of the elderly demented patient in the community. *Br J Psychiat* 1978; **132**: 442–9.

13. Whitehead T. *In the Service of Old Age*, 2nd edn. Aylesbury: HM and M, 1971.

14. Whitehead T. Mental infirmity: the cottage hospital approach. *Geriat Med* 1983; February: 99–103.

15. Green JG, Timbury GC. A geriatric psychiatry day hospital service: a five year review. *Age Ageing* 1979; **8**: 49–53.

16. Peace SM. *Caring from Day to Day.* London: Mind, 1980.

17. Arie T. Day care in geriatric psychiatry. *Gerontol Clin* 1975; **17**: 31–9.

18. Philpott RM. Organisation of services and training. *Curr Opin Psychiat* 1989; **2**: 555–60.

19. Creed F, Black D, Anthony P. Day hospital and community treatment for acute psychiatric illness. *Br J Psychiat* 1989; **154**: 300–10.

20. Creed F, Black D, Anthony P *et al.* Randomized controlled trial comparing day and inpatient psychiatric treatment. *Br Med J* 1990; **300**: 1033–7.

21. Creed F, Black D, Anthony P *et al.* Randomised controlled trial of day and in-patient treatment 2: comparison of two hospitals. *Br J Psychiat* 1991; **158**: 183–9.

22. Wimo A, Mattson B, Adolfsson R *et al.* Dementia day care and its effects on symptoms and institutionalization—a controlled Swedish study. *Scand J Prim Health Care* 1993; **11**(2): 117–23.

23. MacDonald AJD, Mann AH, Jenkins R *et al.* An attempt to determine the impact of four different types of care upon the elderly in London by the study of matched groups. *Psychol Med* 1982; **12**: 193–200.

24. Panella JJ, Lilliston BA, Brush D, McDowell FH. Day care for dementia patients. *J Am Geriat Soc* 1984; **32**: 883–4.

25. Zeeli D, Isaacs B. The efficiency and effectiveness of geriatric day hospitals. *Postgrad Med J* 1988; **64**: 683–6.

26. Eagle DJ, Guyatt G, Patterson C, Turpie I. Day hospitals, cost and effectiveness. *Gerontologist* 1988; **27**(6): 735–40.

27. Audit Commission. *Making a Reality of Community Care.* London: HMSO, 1986.

28. Donaldson C, Wright K, Maynard A. Determining value for money in day hospital care for the elderly. *Age Ageing* 1986; **15**: 1–7.

29. Read K, Hossack A, Jenkins R. The Blakenhall Model: evaluating the effectiveness of a new approach to day care for the older people with mental health needs (work in progress).

125

Day Care

John M. Eagles and Jill Warrington

Royal Cornhill Hospital, Aberdeen, UK

The first psychiatric day hospitals in the UK opened in the late 1940s and their numbers have continued to grow over the five subsequent decades. In geriatric psychiatry, as in geriatric medicine, the proliferation of day care facilities came rather later, with large expansions of such services since the 1960s. A similar proliferation of day care facilities for the elderly with psychiatric difficulties has occurred in other parts of the world[1-3], with parallel expansions in both the health and social care sectors[4]. Since their inception, day care facilities, in all their many and disparate forms, have come to be viewed as essential components of most comprehensive old age psychiatry services. This chapter will seek to follow a brief description of day care facilities with a discussion of their aims and effectiveness, concluding with some current issues and possible future directions for day care services.

MODELS OF DAY CARE

Models of day care for the elderly mentally ill are extremely diverse. Indeed, given the relative lack of critical evaluation of such services, this is perhaps to be expected. This diversity is enhanced by the range of bodies funding and running day care services, including local authorities, the health service, voluntary agencies and the private sector.

Day hospitals and day centres are often described as distinctly differing facilities (as they will be in this chapter for the sake of clarity), although in reality the two types of facility more probably form part of a continuum. Day hospitals tend to be funded solely through health service budgets and to be staffed by health service professionals. Day hospitals will often be linked geographically with a hospital site and will thus have access to a full range of physical treatment and investigative facilities. The programmes at day hospitals are often intensive[5], with reality orientation, formalized social interaction, occupational therapy, physical activities and frequent meetings with the patients' families. Day centres, by contrast, are funded more usually by local authorities and/or voluntary agencies, and have a much lower proportion of health service professionals on their staff. Day centres are optimally sited in the community, close to the patient's home. The programmes at day centres tend to be less intensive and "medicalized", with greater emphasis on informal socialization and diversionary activities. Almost self-evidently, day centres are significantly cheaper to run than are day hospitals.

There is debate as to the optimal "mix" of patients/clients in day care facilities. Most day hospitals do mix the demented and the functionally ill elderly, although the latter group would usually form only 10–20% of the total. Since the first day hospitals were established, the numbers of functionally ill patients have probably declined, not through explicit policy decisions but as a result of increasing pressure from the growing number of demented elderly patients[6]. Some regions tend to incorporate the functionally ill elderly into general adult day hospitals, feeling that this affords such patients an environment that can be more accurately tailored to their needs. Chodosh *et al.*[7] describe a day care programme that mixes physically infirm with demented patients, but these authors reflect that their mentally infirm attenders would probably be better suited to a separate programme, in view of their shortened attention spans. In areas of low population density, taking services out to the patients, through travelling day hospitals, can be a very useful innovation[8,9]. In more rural areas, especially since underutilization of expensive custom-built facilities can have an adverse influence upon cost-effectiveness[10], it may be appropriate to integrate demented patients requiring day care into small community-based inpatient units[11].

AIMS OF DAY CARE

While it is fair to say that there is a general lack of clarity and agreement as to the aims of day care for the elderly, certain themes would be common to most patients in most settings. These would include relief from loneliness and boredom and the provision of stimulation and social support[12], while the aims of day hospitals will usually be broader and more ambitious.

As noted above, the substantial majority of elderly day hospital attenders suffer primarily from dementing illness. Most day hospitals, therefore, are geared more towards the needs of the demented than of the functionally ill elderly, whose day care requirements have thus received rather less attention. Cited roles of day hospitals for the functionally ill include assessment, continuation of treatment after hospital care, monitoring and encouraging compliance with medication, and focused group activities dealing with issues such as bereavement.

For the demented elderly, many aims of day hospital care have been described and these would include: assessment, providing an alternative to institutional care, treatment of cognitive and non-cognitive symptoms of dementia, relieving stress on caregivers, determining whether institutional care is required and what the optimal form thereof will comprise, easing the transition from home to institutional care, shortening hospital stays, acting as centres of expertise from which skills can be "exported", enhancing the morale of old age staff who rotate through day hospitals, and providing a focus for liaison with other care providers. The issue of whether these aims are effectively fulfilled will be discussed below.

Principles and Practice of Geriatric Psychiatry, 2nd edn. Edited by J. R. M. Copeland, M. T. Abou-Saleh and D. G. Blazer

It may sometimes be the case that the role of a day care facility is more reactive than proactive, and one pragmatic view is that the shape of day care develops partly to plug gaps in local services[13]. It may be worth noting also that the literature about the aims and benefits of day care is written almost exclusively by health care professionals about patients; certainly among younger patient groups, the most valued aspects of day care may not accord at all closely with those that might be highlighted by staff[14].

EFFECTIVENESS OF DAY CARE

There has been no evaluative research on the effectiveness of day care for the functionally ill elderly. If one can validly extrapolate from findings in younger patients, then compliance with medication can be enhanced by focused interventions with day hospital attenders[15]. Similarly, extending findings from the demented elderly might suggest that the often very stressful activity of caring for a depressed or psychotic relative would be relieved by the patient entering day care.

While it remains an under-researched area, there has been more evaluation of the effects of day care attendance among the demented elderly, although many of the hypothesized functions of day care have not been meaningfully scrutinized. For example, while many old age services regard assessment as a pivotal role of their day hospitals[9,16,17], another view is that this can be conducted just as well as an outpatient and/or in the patient's home[10]. There are no data to support either standpoint.

Reports of specific cognitive or non-cognitive benefits of day care among demented patients have not been consistent or confirmed, and tend to be based on anecdote[18]. Where ratings of change are made by carers, then such ratings may be influenced by improvements in the carers' well-being as a result of their dependants' day care attendance. If day care is indeed specifically beneficial to patients, then the improvements may be more subtle than can be measured with existing rating measures, and Donaghy[19] has noted that a validated quality of life measure for the demented elderly would constitute a significant advance. It is perhaps noteworthy that professionals now working with the demented elderly predict that day care would enhance their own quality of life should they develop dementia[20].

While day hospitals developed largely as an alleged alternative to long-term inpatient or other institutional care,[17] this hypothesized role may be outdated and there is little evidence that they fulfil this function. Patients admitted into long-stay care following day hospital attendance have been found to be no more disabled, cognitively or behaviourally, than those who had no experience of day care[21], suggesting that there was no delay in institutionalization. New day care facilities in an area do not appear to change the requirements for long-stay care[16]. It may be, however, that day care can shorten stays in acute inpatient facilities by acting as something of a "half-way house" between hospital and home while community links are re-established[17]. Mintzer et al.[22] in South Carolina, found that there was equal improvement in the agitation of demented patients who had a short admission followed by home assessment plus "partial hospitalization" and those who experienced a lengthier hospital stay.

The strongest evidence for the effectiveness of day care is in improving the well-being of carers. Earlier studies, such as that by Gilleard[23], tended to be naturalistic but demonstrated improvements in the psychological well-being of carers after their dependant commenced day care attendance. These improvements were not related to changes in the problems presented by their dependant and seemed to derive, therefore, from "time out" from the stresses of the care-giving role. More recently, quite well-designed controlled studies have been conducted. In Australia, Wells et al.[2] conducted a "before and after" day care comparison of supporters, and also a comparison of supporters receiving and those waiting for day care. They found no differences in caregivers' well-being but reflected that the average period of relief (11.9 hours/week) may have been insufficient to confer benefits. In a recent large study, Zarit et al.[24] found that supporters of demented day care attenders (minimum of 2 days/week) felt less overloaded, strained, depressed and angry than did supporters whose dependant had no access to day care. The issue of what the "effective dose" of day care might be to enhance carers' well-being remains a fairly open question[18].

COST-EFFECTIVENESS OF DAY CARE

Given the relative dearth of evaluative studies on the effectiveness of day care, it is unsurprising that cost-effectiveness is also an understudied area. With regard to the dementing elderly, the Scottish Chief Scientist Working Party[25] concluded, in 1988, that "the available research indicates that virtually nothing is known about the economics of day hospitals", and since then little useful information has accrued[18]. The study by Mintzer et al.[22] mentioned above, did conclude that their use of "partial hospitalization" was clearly a cost-effective method of instigating and continuing treatment for agitated patients with dementia. In Sweden, Wimo et al.[3] compared 55 demented patients in day care with 45 waiting list controls and noted a statistically non-significant trend suggesting that day care may be more cost-effective than other types of service provision. In their review of 16 adult day centres across the USA, Reifler et al.[26] considered that one of the keys to cost efficiency was improved utilization, which related to meeting "customer demands", such as the need for transport and opening for a longer day between 7.30 a.m. and 6 p.m. Perhaps specific to health and social care systems in the USA, these authors make other suggestions as to how the financial viability of day care facilities can be enhanced.

DAY HOSPITALS OR DAY CENTRES?

Studies of demented attenders at day hospitals and at day centres tend to find that those at the former are rather more demented and more behaviourally disturbed, but that the similarities are more striking than the differences between the two groups of attenders[27-29]. This gives rise to the view that a proportion of demented attenders at day hospitals could have their needs met more cost-effectively at day centres, as has also been suggested for younger adults attending day hospitals in north-west England[30]. This view is strengthened by findings that supporters of the demented elderly attending day hospitals do not derive more psychological benefit than those whose dependant goes to a day centre[28,31,32]. Comparisons against day centres of other suggested functions of day hospitals, such as assessment and treatment of non-cognitive symptoms, have not been conducted. Furthermore, no randomized trials of day hospital vs. day centre care have been conducted among demented subjects, and while such studies would be difficult to conduct, they are likely to be feasible, given that they are possible among the physically disabled elderly[33].

PROBLEMS AND ISSUES IN DAY CARE

As has been indicated above, there is a considerable need to address the issue of the effectiveness and the cost-effectiveness of different day care programmes and of the specific components of these programmes, even although this is an undeniably complex task. Other common issues in day care will be touched upon below.

Within busy day care settings, it is often difficult to ensure continuity of care for those attending. This potential problem can be ameliorated by the appointment for each client of a "key worker", whose role is to coordinate the programme for that individual. This process can be facilitated by a "problem list", with a corresponding list of proposed action for each problem area. The key worker can also play a crucial role in helping to coordinate other community services: Peach and Pathy[34] have shown that day hospital attendance can be coupled with a reduction in other social supports without deleterious effects upon the patient. The key worker can also maintain links with other members of the multidisciplinary team who are involved in the patient's care.

Levin et al.[31] have highlighted the underprovision of day care facilities, with a minority of demented individuals in the community having access to such facilities. While selection of demented patients for day care seems somewhat arbitrary[28], it might be considered reasonable to prioritize day hospital places for those with complex needs, where assessment, problem identification and management may lead to improvement in the patient or allow for easier caregiving. Day hospital assessment may be especially helpful in the assessment of patients who live alone, where adequate information cannot be gathered through home or outpatient assessment. In the absence of complex needs and where the main aims are stimulation for the patient and respite for the caregiver, then lower-cost day centre care may suffice. Linked to this issue is the question of how many days per week a patient should attend. Research is required into whether day care should seek to provide a lot of respite for a few selected carers or a little respite for many more carers.

The vast majority of day care programmes operate during normal working hours. It is likely that supporters would be even more appreciative of time for themselves in the evenings and at weekends[31,35].

SUMMARY AND FUTURE DIRECTIONS

Few mental health practitioners would dispute that "day care, whatever its source, is a key component of comprehensive services to elderly persons and their families"[31]. However, in this increasingly cost-conscious age, such an assertion will not ensure continuation and expansion of day care services without adequate evaluation of their efficacy and cost-effectiveness. Day care services will probably become progressively aligned with other community resources for the elderly and it will surely be helpful if there is increased integration of health service day hospitals and social services day centres. Unless benefit can be demonstrated from the intensive involvement of mental health professionals, particularly nursing staff, then it is likely that there will be a progressive move toward staffing day care programmes predominantly with (cheaper) untrained personnel. In addition to studies of efficacy, there is a need to investigate further the selection of patients for day care, the most appropriate hours for programmes to operate and the optimal degree of respite that should be offered to supporters of the demented elderly.

REFERENCES

1. Teresi JA, Holmes D, Koren MJ et al. Prevalence estimates of cognitive impairment in medical model adult day health care programs. Soc Psychiat Psychiat Epidemiol 1998; 33: 283–90.
2. Wells YD, Jorm AF, Jordan F, Lefroy R. Effects on care-givers of special day care programmes for dementia sufferers. Aust NZ J Psychiat 1990; 24: 82–90.
3. Wimo A, Mattsson B, Krakau I et al. Cost-effectiveness analysis of day care for patients with dementia disorders. Health Econ 1994; 3: 395–404.
4. Warrington J, Eagles JM. Day care for the elderly mentally ill: diurnal confusion? Health Bull (Edinb) 1995; 53: 99–104.
5. Panella JJ, Lilliston BA, Brush D, McDowell FH. Day care for dementia patients: an analysis of a four-year program. J Am Geriat Soc 1984; 32: 883–6.
6. Greene JG, Timbury GC. A geriatric psychiatry day hospital service: a 5 year review. Age Ageing 1979; 8: 49–53.
7. Chodosh HL, Zeffert B, Muro ES. Treatment of dementia in a medical day care program. J Am Geriat Soc 1986; 34: 881–6.
8. Wilkinson DG. The psychogeriatrician's view: management of chronic disability in the community. J Neurol Neurosurg Psychiat 1992; 55(suppl): 41–4.
9. Rosenvinge HP. The role of the psychogeriatric day hospital. Psychiat Bull 1994; 18: 733–6.
10. Fasey C. The day hospital in old age psychiatry: the case against. Int J Geriat Psychiat 1994; 9: 519–23.
11. Ebmeier KP, Besson JAO, Blackwood GW et al. Continuing care of the demented elderly in Inverurie. Health Bull (Edinb) 1988; 46: 32–41.
12. Vaughan PJ. Developments in psychiatric day care. Br J Psychiat 1985; 147: 1–4.
13. Murphy E. The day hospital debate. Int J Geriat Psychiat 1994; 9: 517–18.
14. Riordan D, Appleby L. What do day hospital attenders really want? A survey of patient preferences. Psychiat Bull 1995; 19: 623–6.
15. Cramer JA, Rosenheck R. Enhancing medication compliance for people with serious mental illness. J Nerv Ment Dis 1999; 187: 53–5.
16. Ballinger BR. The effects of opening a geriatric psychiatry day hospital. Acta Psychiat Scand 1984; 70: 400–3.
17. Howard R. Day hospitals: the case in favour. Int J Geriat Psychiat 1994; 9: 525–9.
18. Zarit SH, Gaugler JE, Jarrott SE. Useful services for families: research findings and directions. Int J Geriat Psychiat 1999; 14: 165–77.
19. Donaghy M. Commentary on "Useful services for families". Int J Geriat Psychiat 1999; 14: 180–1.
20. Reifler BV. What I want if I get Alzheimer's disease. Arch Fam Med 1995; 4: 395–6.
21. Eagles JM, Gilleard CJ. The functions and effectiveness of a day hospital for the demented elderly. Health Bull (Edinb) 1984; 42: 87–91.
22. Mintzer JE, Colenda C, Waid LR et al. Effectiveness of a continuum of care using brief and partial hospitalisation for agitated dementia patients. Psychiat Serv 1997; 48: 1435–9.
23. Gilleard CJ. Influence of emotional distress among supporters on the outcome of psychogeriatric day care. Br J Psychiat 1987; 150: 219–23.
24. Zarit SH, Stephens MAP, Townsend A, Greene R. Stress reduction for family caregivers: effects of adult day care use. J Gerontol B Psychol Sci Soc Sci 1998; 53B: S267–77.
25. Chief Scientist Working Party. Report of the Working Party on Care of the Dementing Elderly: a review of published research and recommendations for future research priorities. Health Bull (Edinb) 1988; 46: 127–38.
26. Reifler BV, Henry RS, Rushing J et al. Financial performance among adult day centers: results of a national demonstration program. J Am Geriatr Soc 1997; 45: 146–53.
27. Currie A, McAllister-Williams RH, Jacques A. A comparison study of day hospital and day centre attenders. Health Bull (Edinb) 1995; 53: 365–72.
28. Warrington J, Eagles JM. A comparison of cognitively impaired attenders and their coresident carers at day hospitals and day centres in Aberdeen. Int J Geriat Psychiat 1996; 11: 251–6.
29. Collier EH, Baldwin RC. The day hospital debate—a contribution. Int J Geriat Psychiat 1999; 14: 587–91.
30. Mbaya P, Creed F, Tomenson B. The different uses of day hospitals. Acta Psychiat Scand 1998; 98: 283–7.
31. Levin E, Sinclair 1, Gorbach P. Families, Services and Confusion in Old Age. Aldershot: Gower, 1989.
32. MacDonald AJD, Mann AH, Jenkins R et al. An attempt to determine the impact of four types of care upon the elderly in London by the study of matched groups. Psychol Med 1982; 12: 193–200.
33. Burch S, Longbottom J, McKay M et al. A randomized controlled trial of day hospital and day centre therapy. Clin Rehabil 1999; 13: 105–12.
34. Peach H, Pathy MS. Social support of patients attending a geriatric day hospital. J Epidemiol Comm Health 1978; 32: 215–18.
35. Jones IG, Munbodh R. An evaluation of a day hospital for the demented elderly. Health Bull (Edinb) 1982; 40: 10–15.

126

New Technology and the Care of Cognitively Impaired Older People

Andrew J. Sixsmith

University of Liverpool, UK

Recent years have seen a rapid growth in research and development of new technologies to improve services and enhance the independence and quality of life of older people. The actual and potential role of new technologies has been recognized by the UK Royal Commission on Long-term Care[1], by the European Commission in their COST-A5 initiative on "Ageing and Technology" and TIDE R&D programme on "Telematics for Disabled and Elderly People". A wide range of products is being developed[2-4], using new technologies within robotics, telecommunications and information processing. In this chapter, telecare concepts and applications are discussed in terms of their potential benefits for cognitively impaired older people.

TELECARE CONCEPTS AND APPLICATIONS

"Telemedicine" is now well established worldwide and refers to the use of electronic information and communication technologies to link medical practitioners and patients[5]. This could include applications to support a wide range of medical practices, such as diagnostics, patient monitoring, therapy, rehabilitation and health education. "Telecare" is a more recent concept[6,7] and refers to the use of new technology to deliver and facilitate health and social care support services in the community.

New technology is likely to play a significant role in the community support of older people for several reasons[8]. Increasing numbers of older people have forced health and social services to look at more cost-effective approaches to care and support. Health and social care policy argues that most older people want to stay in their own homes and the improved services and enhanced levels of safety and security afforded by telecare systems may have the potential to help very disabled people to do so. Manufacturers and service providers have recognized the market potential for meeting the demand from older people and their carers for new products and related services. A number of telecare applications are available or being developed within several application areas.

Health and Social Care Information Systems

These are used to provide healthcare professionals and clients with health information. These can include simple operator-based systems, interactive websites and self-navigating information services using terminals in surgeries[6].

Client Support

Telecare can include telephone-based services to sophisticated medical systems utilizing state of the art telecommunications. These can be used to provide emergency response, counselling, training, information and client and carer support[9,10].

Client Records and Care Planning

Huston[11] argues that medical records are a weak link within telemedicine and telecare and outlines a model for a comprehensive medical records system. The EU-funded ITHACA project aims to provide a standard IT-based system for the assessment and planning of client care.

Assessment

Home-based technology can provide patient data that can be used for assessment and the specification of treatment and care. Doughty and Costa[12] outline a system to assess the ability of elderly people to live alone in the community, using sensors to provide electronic measures of activities that indicate functional performance after discharge from hospital.

Teleconsultation

This refers to the use of technology to facilitate communication between a healthcare professional and client. For example, Whitten *et al.*[13] report the use of a cable television interactive video system to deliver home health services from "telenursing cockpits".

Patient Monitoring

The most widespread technologies are community alarms or personal response systems[14], which allow a person to raise an alarm at a central control facility by pressing a button on his/her telephone or on a pendant worn around the neck. Recent work[15,16] has been aimed at developing a second generation of systems that use sensors in the home and artificial intelligence to automatically detect emergencies, even when a person is unable to raise an alarm him/herself.

Smart Housing

Smart housing helps frail or disabled people to live independently in their own homes by making the home environment more manageable. Remote control by dwellers, carers or care professionals and "intelligence" built into home systems means that some of the tasks of everyday living can be performed automatically. These include systems for controlling room temperature, home security, cookers, curtains, windows and so on.

TELECARE AND DEMENTIA

Despite considerable research and development activity in all the above areas, very little research has specifically focused on the needs of older people with cognitive impairments, and this remains a neglected area[17,18]. For example, only two of 32 projects, funded under the final phase of TIDE[3], made a reference to this client group, while none of the 127 R&D projects within the European Commission's Health Telematics programme[5] specifically mentioned people with cognitive impairments. This situation perhaps reflects assumptions made by engineers and designers about the abilities of cognitively impaired people to use and benefit from technologies. However, there may be considerable scope for new technologies for this client group within a number of key areas[19].

Supervision and Surveillance

A major concern in supporting demented older people at home is the potential safety risk involved, and the use of automatic alarms to highlight dangerous situations has received increasing attention from technologists and academics[18,20]. For example, wandering behaviour may pose a significant risk for an individual, as he/she may get lost or be unable to cope with the potential dangers of the outside world. However, restraint may be an undesirable or unethical option for wanderers. Simple sensors can be installed to determine whether a person has left a room or building and send a message to a carer or service provider. "Tagging" devices may be useful in locating people outside the immediate home environment.

Environmental Control

The home environment can be a dangerous place for cognitively impaired people. For example, they may leave cookers and heaters unattended, while gas and electricity are potentially lethal if misused. "Smart housing" technologies may be particularly useful for people with dementia, automatically shutting off devices or allowing remote control by carers or service providers. Smart housing could also use sensors linked to computers to control household appliances, devices, lighting and heating, depending on the movements and activities of the cognitively impaired person.

Quality of Life Care

The telecare applications discussed above generally focus on safety and security. However, there may be opportunities for more positive uses of technology to enhance the lives of people with dementia. For example, using technology to identify when a person is restless and bored and then initiating a familiar or enjoyable activity, such as playing familiar music or videos. Aromatherapy rooms could emit relaxing aromas to alleviate stress, while video telecommunications could help to reduce social isolation.

Carer Support

Carer support is a key aspect of care in the community. Using telecommunications to carry out more routine tasks, such as shopping or going to the bank or post office, may provide them with more free time, relieving the "burden" of care. Access to information advice and counselling is also important.

Reminder Devices

New technology could also provide "reminder devices" to support independent living. For instance, the TIDE-funded TASC project[3] aims to provide cognitively impaired people with suitable decision support software to help in carrying out household activities, social participation, communication and vocational tasks.

ETHICAL ISSUES

The discussion so far has highlighted the benefits of telecare. However, Sixsmith[16] argues that new technology can be a double-edged sword and that a number of potential problems need to be addressed:

- Will telecare increase the range of care options or will it just limit choice in a different way?
- Will the technology be intrusive, leading to an inevitable loss of privacy and dignity?
- Will the use of telecommunications mean the loss of human contact in the mental health care of older people?
- Will the introduction of new technology simply reflect marketing strategies, rather than the real needs of older people?
- Will financial savings made through the use of technology be reinvested in products and services or would it be another cost-cutting exercise?
- Will new technology just be used as another form of restraint to control the lives and activities of people with dementia?

CONCLUSION

This chapter has highlighted a number of potential areas for the development and application of new technology to support the independent living of cognitively impaired older people. However, it is clear that considerable research and development work is required if ideas are to become a reality. Moreover, there needs to be a shift in emphasis within research and development to reflect the specific needs of cognitively impaired people as well as those people with physical impairments (e.g. mobility, sensory, motor, control and manipulation). For physically impaired people, the underlying basis for technological development and design is to remove the environmental barriers that turn a person's impairment into a disability. In contrast, cognitively impaired people may have impaired abilities to understand their environment, formulate plans, carry out actions, communicate or remember what they have done or where they are. This has a number of implications for the development and implementation of telecare for this client group.

First, the inability to use a technology may be a serious limitation. Researchers and product designers will need to develop innovative ways of allowing cognitively impaired people to interact with the range of telecare systems, e.g. voice and visual interfaces, rather than traditional interfaces (keypads, etc.).

Second, the use of "smart" technologies may be a particularly useful approach for cognitively impaired people who are unable to articulate their needs and desires. The idea of smart or "proactive" technologies involves the use of sensors and artificial intelligence to interpret a person's observable/physical behaviours and to anticipate his/her needs from these. For example, agitated behaviour patterns may indicate that a person is hungry or wishes to go to the toilet. The telecare system could then initiate some appropriate human or machine response, e.g. send a message to a carer or provide behavioural cues to the person him/herself. The information generated by these kinds of systems has the potential to provide a much more flexible, person-centred care regimen.

Finally, it is important that the implementation and application of new technologies are grounded in a thorough understanding of the individual within his/her social and care networks[17]. The needs and abilities of the person may vary considerably. People in the early stages of dementia may be able to cope reasonably well with only limited care, while others may require considerable help and support. Important individual factors to consider are level and stage of cognitive impairment, ability to carry out the activities of daily living, and problematic and emotional factors, such as anxiety and tendency to "wander". The informal and formal care networks will also determine the kinds of technological interventions that are needed. Again, this will vary from individual to individual, depending on factors such as availability of informal carer, physical proximity, carer network and capacity to provide care. The application of new technology needs to be tailored in order to complement the person's abilities and capacities and to provide help and support to care providers.

REFERENCES

1. Royal Commission on Long-term Care. With respect to old age. Cm 4192-I. The Stationery Office, 1999.
2. Bouma H, Graafmans J. *Gerontechnology*. Amsterdam: IOS Press, 1992.
3. European Commission. *Telematics Applications Programme, Disabled and Elderly Sector: Project Summaries*. Brussels: EC, 1996; DGXIII-C5.
4. Cullen K, Robinson S. *Telecommunications for Older and Disabled people in Europe*. Amsterdam: IOS, 1997.
5. European Commission. *97 Healthcare Telematics. vol 1, General Overview*. Health Telematics Unit, BU 29 3/56, Brussels: EC, 1997; DGXIIIC4.
6. Curry R, Norris A. *A Review and Assessment of Telecare Activity in the UK and Recommendations for Development*. Southampton: New College, University of Southampton, 1997.
7. Tinker A, Wright F, McCreadie C, Askham J, Hancock R, Holmans A. Alternative models of care for older people. Report by Royal Commission on Long Term Care. CM4192-II/2. London: The Stationery Office, 1999.
8. Sixsmith AJ. New technology and community care. *Health Soc Care* 1994; **2**: 367–78.
9. Erkert T. High quality television links for home based support for the elderly. *J Telemed Telecare* 1997; **3**(suppl 1): 26–8.
10. Strawn B, Hester S, Warren S. Telecare: a social support intervention for family caregivers of dementia victims. *Clinical Gerontologist* 1998; **18**(3): 66–9.
11. Huston J. A telemedical record model. *J Telemed Telecare* 1997; suppl 1: 86–8.
12. Doughty K, Costa J. Continuous automated assessment of the elderly. *J Telemed Telecare* 1997; **3**(suppl 1): 23–5.
13. Whitten P, Mair F, Collins B. Home telenursing: patients' perceptions of uses and benefits. *J Telemed Telecare* 1997; **3**(suppl 1): 67–9.
14. Tinker A. Alarms and telephones in personal response: research from the UK. *Int J Technol Ageing* 1991; **4**(1): 21–5.
15. Doughty K, Cameron K, Garner P. Three generations of telecare for the elderly. *J Telemed Telecare* 1996; **2**(2): 71–80.
16. Sixsmith AJ. Telecare at home. In Walker A, ed., *European Home and Community Care 1998/99*. London: Campden, 1998: 141–2.
17. Pieper R, Riederer E. Home care for the elderly with dementia. In Graafmans J, Taipale V, Charness N, eds, *Gerontechnology: A Sustainable Investment in the Future*. Amsterdam: IOS, 1998; 324–30.
18. Sweep M, van Berlo A, Stoop H. Technology for dementing persons; a relief for informal carers. In Graafmans J, Taipale V, Charness N, eds, *Gerontechnology: A Sustainable Investment in the Future*. Amsterdam; IOS, 1998: 331–6.
19. Sidsel Bjørneby S, Päivi Topo P, Holthe T. *Technology, Ethics and Dementia: A Guidebook on How to Apply Technology in Dementia Care*. Oslo: Norwegian Centre for Dementia Research ISBN 82-91054-62-2, 1999.
20. Leikas J, Salo J, Poramo R. Security alarm system supports independent living of demented persons. In Graafmans J, Taipale V, Charness N, eds, *Gerontechnology: A Sustainable Investment in the Future*. Amsterdam: IOS, 1998; 402–5.

127

The United States System of Care

Christopher C. Colenda[1], Stephen J. Bartels[2] and Gary L. Gottlieb[3]

[1]*Michigan State University, East Lansing, MI,* [2]*Dartmouth Medical School, Hanover, NH,*
and [3]*Harvard University School of Medicine, Boston, MA, USA*

OVERVIEW

In the first edition of this book Fogel characterized the US system of health care for older adults with late-life mental disorders as a "non-system of care", plagued by irrational incentives and multiple access barriers[1]. This description highlighted a system that encouraged entrepreneurial activities among practitioners and health systems, was best at delivering specialized high-quality hospital-based care, and was constrained by perverse funding mechanisms that incentivized hospital-based and institutional care (nursing homes) but disincentivized outpatient and home-based care. While the individual elements of a comprehensive continuum of care could be found, services were described as fragmented, inadequate and poorly financed. As we move from one century into the next, considerable attention has been focused on the rapid changes occurring in health care and the changes that will need to occur in order to accommodate an aging population.

Has mental health care kept pace with these developments? Has much changed since Fogel's original assessment? Since the original report, the USA has struggled with the need to slow the growth of rising medical expenditures. The efforts to reduce global medical expenditures have centered on the application of managed care principles and practices and government cutbacks. The emphasis has been on cost reduction, not system's integration. In this chapter we will provide an update and overview of the current system of mental health care for older persons in the USA, with a specific emphasis on the organization and financing of services. The following components and trends will be addressed: (a) The structure and organization of mental health services for the elderly; (b) fee-for-service financing of mental health services for the elderly; (c) mental health managed care for older adults; and (d) emerging and future trends in integrated services and financing.

THE STRUCTURE AND ORGANIZATION OF MENTAL HEALTH SERVICES FOR THE ELDERLY

In an ideal system, the organization, financing and delivery of mental health services to the elderly would be a seamless continuum involving acute and continuing services across inpatient, outpatient and long-term care service settings, and networked with the general medical sector. Since mental disorders are a leading risk factor for institutionalization, improving the provision of mental health services in community settings is a major focus of public policy[2]. The following section summarizes current mental health service settings and highlights several demonstration projects designed to provide integrated care for the frail elderly.

Psychiatric Service Settings

Primary Care

Initial access to care for older adults is usually through the primary care sector, especially for older adults without a history of severe and persistent mental illness (SPMI). Many older persons prefer to receive treatment in primary care, and this service sector offers the advantages of proximity, affordability and coordination of medical and psychiatric co-morbidity[3]. Many older adults may present to primary care physicians (PCPs) with symptoms of mental distress, difficult to classify in current psychiatric classification systems[4]. The most prevalent disorders in the primary care sector are depression, anxiety, anxiety symptoms, dementia syndromes and misuse of prescription medications and alcohol use. Adequate detection, treatment and referral to the specialty mental health sector remain problematic, and have been attributed to such issues as: stigma; low priority of mental health issues in patients with serious medical disorders; inadequate referral resources; complexity of patient needs (psychiatric, medical and social); and lack of time and expertise in dealing with psychiatric problems[5]. Additionally, PCPs tend to approach psychiatric disorders using a medical model, which encourages over-reliance on medications for common disorders[6].

Despite the problems identified, PCPs will continue to be important mental health service providers. Thus, training in geriatric psychiatry and research that focuses on how to improve PCP effectiveness remains an important challenge for the coming decades[4,7]. PCPs will also be important mental health care providers for geriatric minority populations with late-life mental disorders in coming years[8].

Outpatient Psychiatric Service Settings

The proportion of psychiatrists reporting large geriatric case loads has steadily increased over the last two decades[9,10], a trend paralleled by other mental health providers, such as psychologists and social workers. More services are being delivered, in large part due to consumer demand, better treatments, an increased recognition of how untreated late-life mental illness contributes to excess disability, and more favorable Medicare reimbursement policies.

Principles and Practice of Geriatric Psychiatry, 2nd edn. Edited by J. R. M. Copeland, M. T. Abou-Saleh and D. G. Blazer
©2002 John Wiley & Sons, Ltd

Through the American Psychiatric Association's Practice Research Network (PRN), we are just now able to describe a nationally representative profile of patient characteristics and treatments received from psychiatrists[11]. Similar practice-based research for other mental health disciplines has yet to be launched, and only recently have data been reported that describes the demographic and treatment characteristics of patients aged 65+ treated by psychiatrists[12]. Generally speaking, PRN psychiatrists provide a full array of diagnostic and treatment services for older patients. PRN provides descriptive baseline data. About 51% of patients aged 65+ in the PRN have a primary diagnosis of an affective disorder, followed by cognitive disorders (20%) and schizophrenia (19%). Older adults have more medical co-morbidities and lower initial global assessment of functioning scores. About 49% of older patients were seen in outpatient settings, followed by hospital settings (32%) and nursing home settings (16%). Over 50% of patients receive both pharmacotherapy and psychotherapy, and 40% of older patients receive pharmacotherapy alone. Only 2% receive psychotherapy alone. Of patients receiving medications, over 60% of older patients received antidepressants, 40% antipsychotics and 48% benzodiazepine medications.

Data are lacking on how well psychiatrists or other mental health clinicians employ best practices or adhere to existing treatment guidelines for older adults. Future research will be needed to answer these types of questions and establish the effectiveness of treatments for subpopulations of elderly patients, such as minorities, those living in different environments and those with significant medical–psychiatric co-morbidity.

Community Mental Health Centers

Older patients with severe and persistent mental illness (SPMI) pose significant challenges for the US system of care. These individuals have long-term care needs, have limited financial resources, and secular trends in managed care, home- and community-based alternatives to institutional care are being promoted as the major venue for mental health services[13]. About 2% of persons aged 55+ in the USA have SPMI, which is expected to double over the next 30 years[14]. The downsizing and closure of state hospitals over the last few decades has resulted in trans-institutionalization of SPMI patients into nursing homes and other less restrictive environments, such as boarding care homes, assisted living and other forms of community-based living arrangements. Currently, over 89% of all institutionalized older adults with SPMI reside in nursing homes[15]. It is unlikely that nursing homes will be a principal resource for care of older patients with SPMI, as further effects of nursing home reform (OBRA-87) and managed Medicaid are reinforced by patient preference[14].

Mental health services for the elderly SPMI population has been provided largely through community mental health centers (CMHCs). The CMHCs have not been particularly attuned to, or capable of, accommodating the unique and complex needs of the elderly, and they may not be capable of coordinating medical–psychiatric treatments[16]. Older persons with severe mental illness also receive services from home health agencies that provide limited mental health care and, to a lesser extent, from the general medical sector[14]. As with patients with less severe mental illness, older patients with SPMI require close collaboration among providers in the general and specialty mental health sectors. Promising models of integrated care include co-location of medical and mental health providers, multidisciplinary treatment teams and cross-training of medical–psychiatric providers. These programs must also include social support services to maintain function and improve quality of life, integrative case management

services, home-based residential family support services, caregiver training and psychosocial rehabilitation[14]. Managed care may be the vehicle to promote such service integration because of the possibility of pooling resources from federal, state and local funding agencies. Appropriate risk adjustment mechanisms to account for the psychiatric medical and social service complexity of these patients will be required for programs to be successful.

Nursing Homes

In 1997 almost 1.5 million elderly resided in nursing homes. One-half of these people were aged 85+ and three-quarters were women[17]. Nursing homes have supplanted state hospitals as the major loci of institutionally-based long-term care for older adults with psychiatric disorders. Surveys of nursing home residents show uniformly high prevalence rates of dementia (46–78%)[18–20], and clinically significant depression (20–40%)[21]. Early in the trans-institutionalization movement, nursing homes became the repository of many SPMI patients. Current trends, however, find many older SPMI patients live in community settings[14].

OBRA-87 legislation, also known as the Nursing Home Reform Act of 1987, was enacted in response to inappropriate and inadequate care for mental illnesses in nursing homes. The legislation restricted the inappropriate use of restraints, physical and pharmacologic, and required pre-admission screening for all persons suspected of having a serious mental illness. Screening was designed to improve treatment and psychosocial assessment for nursing home residents with mental disorders. In 1998, the Institute of Medicine (IOM) convened a follow-up analysis examining the effectiveness of the original legislation. From a psychiatric services perspective, the results have been mixed[22]. Pharmacoepidemiologic evidence has shown a downward trend in the use of psychotropic medications, and interventional trials designed to reduce physical–chemical restraints in nursing homes demonstrated that educational efforts complementing consultation by skilled mental health professionals had the best results[23,24]. Physician prescribing practices have also changed. A new generation of psychotropic medications are now commonly being prescribed that have fewer side effects and are better tolerated by frail nursing home residents[25]. Multidisciplinary treatment guidelines have been developed to deal with difficult psychiatric and behavioral problems, such as depression and agitation, in dementia patients. Less certain outcomes of OBRA-87 include unnecessary tensions between the legitimate use of medications and federal/state survey procedures; collection of uniform information on nursing home residents that do not have sufficient flexibility to measure quality-of-life outcomes or quality indicators; logistic barriers for medically necessary psychiatric services; and the unintended effect of establishing incentives for the inappropriate provision of some mental health services, e.g. psychotherapy services for severely demented patients[22].

Important components in state-of-the-art mental health services in nursing homes include "intrinsic" and "extrinsic" mental health services[22]. Intrinsic services refer to the biopsychosocial elements of daily patient care activities and range from the nursing home environment to individual attitudes of professional staff, which are tied to respect, dignity and empathetic interpersonal exchanges. In addition, intrinsic services may include specialized settings and discrete units that provide behaviorally orientated services with highly trained staff. Dementia care units, "special care units" and psychiatric nursing home units are examples of specialized intrinsic services that are relevant to the treatment of older persons with mental disorders. Extrinsic services are linked to the ability of nursing home residents to gain access to specialized psychiatric services in a timely, efficient and sensitive manner. Extrinsic services generally refer to specialized mental health services that are provided from outside the facility through a consulting or other contractual arrangements. A variety of consulting models of mental health services to nursing homes have been described and optimally include components of assessment and evaluation, with a strong emphasis on collaborating with the treating medical physician and on educating nursing staff[26]. However, surveys of nursing home directors indicate that there is considerable unmet need for psychiatric consultation services, especially addressing non-pharmacologic management and staff training. However, incentives are lacking for adequate service provision by psychiatrists in nursing homes and there are substantial challenges to identifying the most effective interventions and services[27]. Appropriate institutional and patient outcome measures need to be developed that can identify the most cost-effective intrinsic and extrinsic mental health services for nursing homes.

Acute Inpatient Hospitalization

Geriatric patients with late-life mental disorders requiring acute inpatient hospitalization are principally and appropriately cared for in secondary and tertiary care hospitals[1]. Inpatient units within general hospitals have access to subspecialist consultation and diagnostic technology required to provide accurate diagnosis and treatment recommendations. Over the last 15 years, there has been a substantial increase in the rate of admissions of geriatric patients to nine federal general hospitals. Specialized medical psychiatry units have increased the levels of sophisticated treatment for patients with severe mood disorders, mood disorders complicated by psychotic features, and those elder patients with mixed medical and psychiatric disorders[1]. Inpatient services offer multidisciplinary interventions, including psychiatric services, family evaluation and therapy, social service evaluations and, in ideal situations, coordinated aftercare services.

FINANCING MENTAL HEALTH CARE: THE UNDERPINNINGS OF THE CURRENT STRUCTURE OF THE US SYSTEM OF CARE

Ideally, health systems follow the rule that "form follows function". In the US system of care, a more cautious approach might be "form follows finance". In this respect, the character and dimensions of mental health services for older adults in the USA has flowed directly from the structure, incentives and limitations of the system of financing and reimbursement. In this section we will describe these recent developments in fee-for-service financing of mental health services for older adults, followed by a discussion of current trends in managed care. For geriatric patients with late-life mental disorders, Medicare is the principal payment source for acute psychiatric services in the USA. Aside from out-of-pocket expenses, state-managed Medicaid, a blended Federal and state insurance program for the poor, is the primary source of payment for institutional and long-term care services. Hence, we will concentrate on an overview of Medicare and Medicaid as the two principal sources of payment for mental healthcare services provided to older persons in the USA.

Traditional Fee-for-service Medicare

Medicare, the federally funded health insurance program, is the primary payer of acute general health and psychiatric care services for the elderly, people with chronic disabilities and people with chronic renal failure. In 1997, approximately 39 million individuals were covered by Medicare, of whom about 33.6 million were aged 65+. Total Medicare expenditures in 1997 were almost $207 billion and accounted for more than 11% of the US federal budget[28]. Medicare's nearly universal coverage for the elderly is important because of the impact of adverse risk selection on insurance premium costs. Adverse risk selection refers to the attraction of high-cost consumers to insurance plans that offer coverage for high-cost conditions. In this respect, insurance plans that cover high-risk populations (e.g. the elderly, with multiple co-morbidities and chronic conditions) are likely to assume disproportionate risk compared to insurers covering services of younger populations with low use of expensive services such as acute hospitalizations and long-term care. In other words, the actuarial risk for high medical service utilization among the elderly is high. Thus, if Medicare were privatized and premiums reflected actual utilization, costs would be prohibitive for most older adults. This effect would be exaggerated for elders, as 11% of them live in poverty and another 6.4% are between poverty and 125% of the poverty level[28,29].

Traditional Medicare is similar to typical indemnity insurance products featuring retrospective fee-for-service (FFS) payment, deductibles and co-insurance, but it does not have limits on annual personal spending. It also does not fully cover medical equipment costs, and fails to cover prescription medicines and the costs of long-term care[28]. Cost sharing and uncovered benefits have created the private "supplemental insurance" market, the premiums for which constitute the largest source of personal spending for community-dwelling beneficiaries[28]. Supplemental policies may have inpatient and outpatient mental health benefits, designed to cover co-payments and deductibles. They do not alter basic coverage limits.

The proportion of Medicare expenditures devoted to mental health is relatively small, however. For example, in 1996 Medicare expended about $9.8 billion for mental health services, up from just under $5.1 billion in 1994[30,31]. Most Medicare expenditures for mental health services are for Part A services, and less than one-half of 1% are for older adults in non-institutional settings[32,33].

Medicare's Benefit Design for Mental Health Services: Fee-for-service and Managed Care Arrangements

Traditional FFS Medicare has two components; part A, which covers inpatient psychiatric hospital care (up to 190 days life-time maximum in free-standing psychiatric hospitals and unlimited days in general hospital psychiatric units) and outpatient care in some hospital-based clinics and other hospital technical fees[34]; part B covers medically necessary physician, partial hospitalization and related ancillary services. Psychotherapy services provided by psychiatrists, non-psychiatric physicians, psychologists and other mental health providers, as well as outpatient electroconvulsive therapy are subject to a 50% co-payment, while medical management services are subject to a 20% co-payment[34].

Since the enactment of the Medicare legislation in 1965, reimbursement policies have been a financial barrier to accessing needed mental health services for the elderly and disabled, especially for outpatient services. Until reforms were enacted in the late 1980s, Medicare's inpatient coverage was similar to private insurance, while outpatient service coverage was de minimus[35]. For example, Medicare reimburses inpatient services carefully, less a 1 day deductible for the first 60 days; it requires a 25% co-payment for days 61–90 and a 50% co-payment for days 90–150[34]. In contrast, in 1966–88 Medicare covered outpatient mental health services up to a maximum of $500, subject to a 50% co-payment, e.g. Medicare only paid $250. In 1984, limitations on medically-based psychiatric services for Alzheimer's disease were not subject to the $500 and 50% cap. The Omnibus Budget

Reconciliation Acts of 1987 and 1989 (OBRA-87 and OBRA-89, respectively) changed reimbursement for outpatient psychotherapy services. OBRA-87 raised the $500 cap for psychotherapy reimbursement to $2200, but retained the 50% co-payment, effectively paying only $1100. OBRA-87 exempted medical management of psychotropic medications from the limit, in addition to reducing the co-payment to 20%. Partial hospitalization services were authorized. OBRA-89 removed the cap on outpatient mental health services, although the 50% co-payment was retained[35].

Changes in benefit design contributed to increasing expenditures for mental health services by 136% between 1987–1992[36]. Correspondingly, service utilization increased, thus correcting the historic underutilization of mental health services by the elderly, e.g. mental health service users rose 76%, and the number of services per beneficiary over age 65 years rose 15%[36]. Difficult to estimate, however, are expenditures for mental health services delivered by physicians in general medical settings, which reflect actual treatment services for psychiatric conditions not coded by providers or treatment services for psychiatric conditions misdiagnosed as general medical disorders.

Although increases in expenditures for mental health services provided to older persons over the last decade suggest that progress has been made in better meeting the need, it is important to note that most of the services remain biased towards costly inpatient care. In 1994 about 12.7% of Medicare claimants had a MH/SA disorder based on primary diagnosis and/or procedure codes[37]. Cano et al.[38] estimated that in 1995 Medicare beneficiaries aged 65+ with a primary psychiatric diagnosis accounted for 325 000 hospital and skilled nursing facility stays and accounted for approximately $1.8 billion or 53% of all acute psychiatric payments made by Medicare. The majority of admissions were to psychiatric units in general hospitals (42%), followed by general hospital admissions (29%), psychiatric hospitals (15%), and skilled nursing facilities (14%). Overall, the burden of mental disorders in the elderly is substantial; Smyer and Shea[39] estimated that the total direct costs for mental illness for individuals aged 65+ were $17.3 billion.

Medicaid

Medicaid is the primary public insurer for acute care for medically indigent populations and for long-term care in the USA. Medicaid is a joint federal and state program, with an individual state contributing up to 50% of costs. Variability in benefit design among states makes it difficult to generalize about the effects of Medicaid on care nationally[14]. For example, states differ on eligibility criteria (this applies to people eligible for both Medicare and Medicaid), on the scope of coverage for inpatient and outpatient mental health services, pharmacy benefits, co-payment arrangements for enrollees, pre-authorization rules for inpatient and outpatient services, and managed care arrangements. Common to Medicaid programs, however, is a 20–30% reduction in reimbursement schedules compared to regional market rates[14].

Figure 127.1 summarizes national Medicaid expenditures in 1995. Excluding administrative expenses and disproportionate share allocations to hospitals serving large numbers of poor people, Medicaid spent about $132 billion in 1995 on about 34.8 million recipients, of whom only 11% were aged 65+. However, this latter group accounted for about 30% of all expenditures. About 19% of Medicaid expenditures were spent on nursing facilities, 6% on home health services, and only 2% on mental health services[40]. It is difficult to determine what proportion of the $7.1 billion in Medicaid expenditures for mental health services in 1994 was for older adults[31]. Medicaid spent approximately

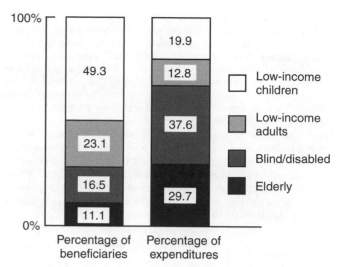

Figure 127.1 Distribution of Medicaid beneficiaries and expenditures in 1995: $132.3 billion for 34.8 million recipients. Adapted from MedPac

$10 129 per elderly beneficiary, and 75% of this amount was allocated to long-term care services[40].

Mental Health Managed Care for Older Adults

Over the last decade, managed care has had stunning impact on private commercial and public financing and delivery of mental services in the USA. While universal definitions of managed care have not been agreed upon, for the purposes of this chapter, managed care is defined as systems of care that integrate the financing and delivery of appropriate healthcare services to health plan enrollees by means of provider network arrangements. Managed care organizations (MCOs) furnish comprehensive healthcare services; set standards for the selection of providers; use formal and ongoing quality improvement and utilization review programs; and place emphasis on preventive services in order to avoid more costly medical care services. MCOs use incentives to use health plan providers and services in order to limit out-of-network providers[41]. Recall this definition of managed care later in the chapter, when we discuss demonstration projects designed to integrate geriatric healthcare services for the frail elderly.

To a large extent, managed care has succeeded in reducing healthcare expenditures in both the general health sector and specialty mental health sector, especially for private commercial health plans. For example, under the Federal Prospective Payment System (PPS) to hospitals, inflation in global operating costs per hospital case declined from a yearly average of 9.5% during 1985–1990, to a yearly average of −0.5% during 1993–1997[42]. The rate of growth of global physician expenditures has also declined. Using the Medicare Economic Index (MEI), which measures various inputs used to produce physicians' services, such as earnings, staff salaries, supplies, etc., MEI increases in 1985–1992 averaged 3.1%/year, but have declined to 2.1%/year since 1992[43]. In the non-Medicare specialty mental health sector, cost reductions have also occurred. The Hay Group Management Corporation and the National Association of Psychiatric Hospital Systems (NAPHS) recently reported that the value of behavioral healthcare expenditures for commercial insurance plans (nongovernmental insurance) decreased in 1988–1997 by 54.1%, compared to 7.4% for general healthcare costs[44]. As a proportion of total healthcare benefit costs, behavioral health benefits decreased from 6.1% in 1988 to 3.1% in 1997. The disproportionate reduction in behavioral health benefit expenditures can be attributed to both impositions on utilization patterns (24.6% decline in outpatient utilization) and benefit design (57% of plans imposed day limits on inpatient care, and 48% placed outpatient visit limits by 1997)[44].

Medicare Managed Care and the Balanced Budget Act of 1997

Encouraged by the private sector's success in managed care, coupled with rising healthcare costs, federal initiatives have stimulated the growth of Medicare managed care, especially since the enactment of Public Law 105-33, the Balanced Budget Act of 1997 (BBA-97). According to the Department of Health and Human Services' Health Care Financing Administration (HCFA), about 6.1 million Medicare beneficiaries were enrolled in Medicare risk-managed care plans by December, 1998[45]. The enrollment growth has slowed in 1998–1999 and Health Maintenance Organizations (HMOs) holding nearly 100 risk contracts have indicated that they will withdraw from Medicare managed care in 1999 (about 409 000 enrollees) because of payment rates and regulatory burdens[45]. Medicare predicts that about 44.5 million Medicare beneficiaries will be in managed care programs by 2008[46].

Several managed care options existed for Medicare patients prior to the BBA-97. These included Medicare risk contracting (MRC) plans, point of service options (POS), social HMOs or demonstration projects called programs of all-inclusive care for the elderly (PACE). Social HMOs or PACE programs are demonstration projects that combine Medicare and Medicaid funding into one funding base, providing a continuum of healthcare services, including inpatient, outpatient and long-term care[5]. The BBA-97 created the Medicare + Choice program, a new Part C of Medicare. Medicare + Choice expanded these options to include medical savings accounts, POS options that allow patients to select from a broader panel of practitioners outside of the HMO network, religious fraternal benefits plans, and other coordinated care plans meeting a set of established standards[46].

MRC plans are the most frequent type of Medicare managed care arrangement. A MRC plan receives a set payment per month per patient, based on a county level adjusted average per capita cost (AAPCC), as determined by HCFA. The BBA-97 made significant changes in the payment methodology to MRC plans that have had historically high AAPCC payment rates. Beginning in 2000, the risk adjustment methodology used to pay many HMOs also changed, further reducing HMO payment rates[47]. To remain solvent, MRC plans must ensure that their costs do not exceed the AAPCC payments. Concerns over the payment methodology have forced some plans to leave the market, while others have reduced benefits and increased co-payments and premiums.

By law, MRCs must offer basic Medicare benefits, including mental health benefits. In order to entice Medicare beneficiaries into joining Medicare HMOs, many plans offer enhanced supplemental benefits, such as prescription drug benefits, dental coverage, optical or hearing services[47]. Neither HCFA nor the managed care industry has established policies or procedures for how mental health services should be delivered to the elderly. Largely undefined, or using criteria from commercial managed care plans, are medical necessity criteria, co-payment policies, credentialing standards for providers, hospital network standards, geographic access rules, referral mechanisms and quality improvement mechanisms[5]. Case management guidelines, coordinated care for patients with medical–psychiatric co-morbidity, dementia care and long-term care policies (beyond the 90 day rule for skilled nursing home care) have not yet been clarified. These plans may also fail to risk-adjust for chronicity and medical–psychiatric co-morbidity of late-life mental disorders, such as Alzheimer's disease or recurrent major depression[35].

Managed Medicaid

Over the last several years, many states have created Medicaid managed care arrangements. As of 1996, about 38.6% of all Medicaid beneficiaries were under Medicaid managed care arrangement, and increased 12% during 1995–1996[40]. The move to Medicaid managed care has been encouraged by program waivers from the Federal Government under Section 1915(b) and Section 1115 of the Social Security Act[40]. Section 1915(b) allowed states to mandate enrollment into managed care programs. Section 1115(a) allowed the US Secretary of Health and Human Services to approve time-limited demonstration projects that test and evaluate innovative approaches to delivery and financing of health care. Section 1115(a) also allowed some states to expand Medicaid eligibility for acute care services; however, it has been used to enroll Medicaid beneficiaries into prepaid managed care programs[40]. The impact of these new financial arrangements on access to mental health and long-term care services by older persons is yet to be determined. The degree to which state-run Medicaid programs will reallocate resources away from long-term care programs used by elders towards children and low-income families is also unclear.

Mental Health Managed Care Arrangements: The "Carved-out" vs. "Carved-in" Debate

Most Medicare MRC plans "carve out" the mental health benefit package, similar to what they do for commercial patient populations. Mental health "carve-outs" refer to the practice of setting aside funds for mental health benefits and then contracting with a vendor, who is responsible for managing all mental health services. Benefits of carve-out mechanisms include protection of the HMO from expenditures above the contracted percentage of premium paid to the carve-out vendor, reduction of HMO staffing and space needs, patient confidentiality and mental health professional input for difficult cases. Proponents of carve-outs purport that these financial arrangements for mental health services are superior because vendors are able to manage costs and services through superior technical knowledge, skills and service delivery networks[58]. "Carve-out" approaches to Medicare managed care may not be the best approach for older adults because of medical–psychiatric co-morbidities. These arrangements may not provide coordinated psychiatric and primary care services[48]; may restrict physician involvement through profiling and paneling[49]; may increase access barriers to care[50]; and may limit the quantity of needed services[51]. Carve-out arrangements may pose problems with demonstrating cost offset for mental health services, especially for those patients with significant medical–psychiatric co-morbidity[14]. A study of dominant carve-outs providing service to MRC payers demonstrated little or no requirement for specialty-trained providers or evidence of experience in caring for the elderly[52].

Some argue that mental health benefits for older adults should be "carved-in", e.g. where mental health services are included as part of the general health benefit. Advocates argue that this benefit design better integrates mental and physical care, decreases access barriers due to stigma, and produces cost offsets in general healthcare expenditures because of the high medical–psychiatric co-morbidity among older adults[14]. Other benefits include better collaboration among psychiatric and physical health providers, as

Table 127.1 Selected features of managed care programs for the frail elderly: PACE, social health maintenance organizations (S/HMOs), and EverCare programs

Characteristic	PACE	S/HMO	EverCare
Setting	Community setting	Community setting	Nursing home
Start-up	1971, On Lok Program 1990, PACE	1985, first generation of S/HMO 1997, second generation of S/HMO	1994
Number of active programs in 1999	25	First generation, 3 Second generation, 1	Six demonstration projects
Focus	Integrate delivery and financing of acute and long-term care for frail elderly	First generation: test models of integrating acute and long-term care, and social services in a capitated HMO setting Second generation: required improvements in service, and benefit design including: geriatric assessments, multidisciplinary teams, expanded case management services for individuals at risk for disability	Enrolls permanent nursing home residents into managed care programs with a focus on providing Medicare covered outpatient services in order to reduce hospital and emergency room use
Eligibility requirements	Eligible enrollees must meet state nursing home eligibility requirements	Initially limited to frail beneficiaries aged 65+	Nursing home residents
Benefit structure	Acute and long-term care benefits covered through Medicare, Medicaid and private capitation payments. Prescription drugs are covered	All Medicare benefits, expanded benefits (similar to typical Medicare Risk Contracts), and long-term care benefits. Prescription drugs are covered	Similar to Medicare Risk Contract but no prescription drug benefit
Enhanced mental health services	Not addressed	Not addressed	Not addressed

Adapted from MedPac[56].

well as improved psychiatric services for those older patients who receive most of their mental health service from primary care providers. Carved-in benefit designs are not without hazards. Functional integration of mental and general health services are far from guaranteed, and mental health services are likely to receive low priority in these types of managed care arrangements. Comprehensive services for mental health, e.g. parity, may not occur, and payment methodology that adequately risk-adjusts for the more seriously ill patients are not well developed, thus placing a health plan at risk for substantial financial loss[14,53].

EMERGING AND FUTURE TRENDS IN INTEGRATED SERVICES AND FINANCING

While recent legislative changes in Medicare and Medicaid have incentivized some efforts toward the goal of a seamless continuum of care for the most frail and vulnerable geriatric patient populations, much work remains. Promising demonstration projects have emerged, such as out-of-pocket-financed community-based dementia respite care programs[54]. While Medicare's psychiatric and mental health benefit has been liberalized over the last 13 years, parity between mental health and general health care benefit coverage has not occurred. Nevertheless, the BBA-97 expanded three demonstration projects designed to care for those frail Medicare beneficiaries who need more long-term chronic and acute care. Programs include the program of all-inclusive care for the elderly (PACE)[55], social health maintenance organizations (S/HMOs) and the Evercare Demonstration Projects care[56]. These programs were not specifically designed for older adults with late-life mental disorders; however, because the frail elderly are at increased risk for psychiatric illness, mental health services will be part of the package of services.

Table 127.1 summarizes the select features with PACE, S/HMOs and the Evercare programs. PACE is a community-based program that is designed to delay or prevent the use of hospital or nursing home care by providing a comprehensive range of preventive, acute and long-term care services in community settings. The first generation of S/HMOs was designed to test the integration of financing and service delivery of a full range of acute and long-term care services through capitated HMOs. The second-generation S/HMOs have expanded programming, including such services as geriatric assessment, case management services and a multidisciplinary team approach to care. EverCare is a program that enrolls permanent nursing home residents into managed care programs and provides "in-place" primary care services to nursing home residents[56]. Primary care services include both acute and preventive services, provided within the nursing home setting.

All three programs use managed care financing, case management principles, and provide a wider array of medical and social services. Enrollees in the S/HMOs have similar demographic characteristics to those beneficiaries enrolled in Medicare, but PACE and Evercare enrollees are significantly older, and a higher proportion of them are Medicaid-eligible. Unfortunately, none of these demonstration projects have specific requirements for the provision of mental health services, although the profile of beneficiaries expected to enroll in these programs would have considerable psychiatric co-morbidity. Program evaluations for the PACE Program and S/HMOs have demonstrated mixed outcomes. For both PACE and S/HMO, enrollee satisfaction was generally high[56], although enrollees in the S/HMO with physical impairments were usually less satisfied[57]. Psychiatric outcomes have not been measured to date.

SUMMARY

The last half of the twentieth century included an explosion in the size of both the older-adult population and the US healthcare system. Since the introduction of Medicare and Medicaid in the

1960s, older adults have had universal access to acute health care and their demand for services has driven the development of a highly capitalized, technologically advanced but severely fragmented system. This interaction has contributed to the extension of life expectancy, a probable improvement in life quality for many, and staggering growth of expenditure. The last two decades have been consumed by efforts to contain and reduce costs, despite continued technology growth that has had marginal effect on efficiency. Throughout this period, mental health has been, at best, a poor stepchild. While enjoying advances in science and recognition of its importance, the care of older people with late-life mental disorders has evolved services that reflect modest reimbursement schemes while attempting to meet a minimal subset of population needs. The provision of mental health services for the elderly is inextricably linked to primary care and, for the frail elderly, must attend to the problems of medical–psychiatric co-morbidity. Recent reforms in the organization and financing of health care are beginning to address co-morbidity issues through integrated acute and long-term care delivery systems, such as PACE, S/HMOs and the Evercare programs. State Medicaid managed care initiatives are also creating opportunities to reallocate support to the development of home- and community-based alternative models of care, with the goal of supporting least restrictive and less costly long-term care services. Demonstration projects must examine behavioral outcomes and analyze their effects on general health, mental health, functional capacity and quality of life. Yet to be determined is the impact of these types of programs on increasing access to medically necessary mental health services.

At the dawn of the new millennium and in the face of extraordinary projected population growth of those aged 65+, opportunity must be seized from innovation. The shift of some insurance risk to providers from payers and the government may be perilous, but it is the first opportunity to align incentives to benefit the populations we serve.

REFERENCES

1. Fogel BS. The United States' system of care. In Copeland JRM, Abou-Saleh MT, Blazer DG, eds, *Principles and Practices of Geriatric Psychiatry*, 1st edn. Chichester: Wiley 1994; 923–31.
2. Katz IR, Parmelee PA. Overview. In *Depression in Long-term and Residential Care*. Rubinstein RL, Lawton MP, eds, New York: Springer, 1997; 1–28.
3. Department of Health and Human Services. Older adults and mental health. In *Mental Health: A Report of the Surgeon General*. Rockville, MD: DHHS, 1999; 335–401.
4. Gallo JJ, Lebowitz BD. The epidemiology of common late-life mental disorders in the community: themes for the new century. *Psychiat Serv* 1999; **50**: 1158–66.
5. Colenda CC, Banazak D, Mickus M. Mental health services in managed care: quality questions remain. *Geriatrics* 1998; **53**(8): 49–63.
6. Gallo JJ, Ryan SD, Ford DE. Attitudes, knowledge and behavior of family physicians regarding depression in late life. *Arch Fam Med* 1999; **8**: 249–56.
7. Colenda CC. Essential curriculum in geriatric psychiatry for general internal medicine residency and geriatric medicine fellowship programs: opportunities to improve clinical competency. *Am J Med* 1994; **97**(suppl 4a): 15–18S.
8. Cooper-Patrick L, Gallo JJ, Powe NR et al. Mental health service utilization by African-Americans and Whites: the Baltimore Epidemiologic Catchment Area follow-up. *Med Care* 1999; **37**(10): 1034–45.
9. Colenda CC, Goldstein MZ, Pincus H et al. Changing characteristics of psychiatrists who treat geriatric patients. *Am J Geriat Psychiat* 1995; **3**: 330–8.
10. Colenda CC, Pincus H, Tanielian TL et al. Update of geriatric psychiatry practices among American psychiatrists. Analysis of the 1996 National Survey of Psychiatric Practice. *Am J Geriat Psychiat* 1999; **7**: 279–88.
11. Pincus H, Zarin DA, Tanielian TL, Marcus SC. Psychiatric patients and treatments: findings from the American Psychiatric Association Practice Research Network. *Arch Gen Psychiat* 1999; **56**(5): 441–9.
12. Colenda CC, Mickus M, Marcus SC et al. Comparison of adult and geriatric practice patterns: findings from the American Psychiatric Association's Practice Research Network. New Orleans: Abstracts of the Psychiatric Services Institute, October 31, 1999.
13. Meeks S, Murrell SA. Mental illness in late life: socioeconomic conditions, psychiatric symptoms, and adjustment of long-term sufferers. *Psychol Aging* 1997; **12**: 298–308.
14. Bartels SJ, Levine KJ, Shea D. Community-based long-term care for older persons with severe and persistent mental illness in an era of managed care. *Psychiat Serv* 1999; **50**: 1189–97.
15. Burns BJ. Mental health services research on the hospitalized and institutionalized CMI elderly. In Lebowitz BD, Light E, eds, *The Elderly with Chronic Mental Illness*. New York: Springer, 1991; 207–15.
16. Light E, Lebowitz BD, Bailey F. CMHCs and elderly services: an analysis of direct and indirect services and service delivery sites. *Commun Ment Health J* 1986; **22**: 294–302.
17. Kramarow E, Lentzner H, Rooks R et al. Health and Aging Chartbook. *Health, United States, 1999*. Hyattsville, MD: National Center for Health Statistics, 1999; 11.
18. Rovner BW, Karonek S, Filipp L. Prevalence of mental illness in a community nursing home. *Am J Psychiat* 1986; **143**: 1446–9.
19. Tariot PN, Podgorski CA, Blazina L, Leibovici A. Mental disorders in the nursing home: another perspective. *Am J Psychiat* 1993; **150**: 1063–9.
20. Class CA, Unverzagt FW, Gao SJ et al. Psychiatric disorders in African-American nursing home residents. *Am J Psychiat* 1996; **153**: 1063–9.
21. Parmalee PA, Katz IR, Lawton MP. Depression among institutionalized aged: assessment and prevalence estimation. *J Gerontol* 1989; **44**: M22–9.
22. Colenda CC, Streim J, Greene JA et al. The impact of OBRA '87 on psychiatric services in nursing homes. Joint testimony of the American Psychiatric Association and the American Association for Geriatric Psychiatry. *Am J Geriat Psychiat* 1999; **7**(1): 12–17.
23. Evans LK, Strumpf NE, Allen-Taylor SL et al. A clinical trial to reduce restraints in nursing homes. *J Am Geriat Soc* 1997; **45**: 675–81.
24. Lance MS, Giambanco V, Buchalter EN. A ten-year review of the effect of OBRA-87 on psychotropic prescribing practices in an academic nursing home. *Psychiat Serv* 1996; **47**: 951–5.
25. Lasser RA, Sunderland T. Neuropsychotropic medication use in nursing home residents. *J Am Geriat Soc* 1998; **46**: 202–7.
26. Gupta S, Goldstein MZ. Psychiatric consultation to nursing homes. *Psychiat Serv* 1999; **50**(12): 1547–50.
27. Reichman WE, Coyne AC, Borson S et al. Psychiatric consultation in the nursing home: a survey of six states. *Am J Geriat Psychiat* 1998; **6**(4): 320–7.
28. MedPac. A framework for considering Medicare payment policy issues. In *Medicare Payment Advisory Commission Report to Congress: Medicare Payment Policy*. Washington, DC: MedPac, 1999; 3–24.
29. MedPac. Beneficiaries' financial liability and Medicare's effectiveness in reducing personal spending. In *Medicare Payment Advisory Commission: Report to Congress; Selected Medicare Issues*. Washington, DC: MedPac, 1999; 3–15.
30. Department of Health and Human Services. Organizing and financing mental health services. In *Mental Health: A Report of the Surgeon General*. Rockville, MD: DHHS, 1999; 405–33.
31. Witkin MJ, Atay JE, Manderscheid RW. Highlights of organized mental health services in 1994 and major national and state trends. In Manderscheid RW, Henderson MJ, eds, *Mental Health United States, 1998*. Publication No. (SMA) 99-3285. Washington, DC: Department of Health and Human Services, 1998; 143–75.
32. Shea D. Economic and financial issues in mental health and aging. *Publ Policy Aging Rep* 1998; **9**(1): 7–12.
33. Sherman J. *Medicare's Mental Health Benefits: Coverage Utilization and Expenditures, 1992*. Washington, DC: American Association of Retired Persons, Public Policy Institute, 1992.

34. Manderscheid RW, Henderson MJ (eds). Appendix A: description of health plans. In *Mental Health United States, 1998*. Publication No. (SMA) 99-3285. Washington, DC: Department of Health and Human Services, 1998; 247–50.

35. Bartels SJ, Colenda CC. Mental health services for Alzheimer's disease: current trends in reimbursement and public policy, and the future under managed care. *Am J Geriat Psychiat* 1998; **6**: S85–100.

36. Rosenbach M, Ammering C. Trends in Part B mental health utilization and expenditures: 1987–1992. *Health Care Financing Rev* 1997; **18**(3): 19–42.

37. Larson MJ, Farrelly MC, Hodgkin D *et al*. Payments and use of services for mental health, alcohol, and other drug abuse disorders: estimates from Medicare, Medicaid and private health plans. In Manderscheid RW, Henderson MJ, eds, *Mental Health United States, 1998*. Publication Number: (SMA) 99-3285. Washington, DC: Department of Health and Human Services, 1998; 124–41.

38. Cano C, Hennessy K, Warren J, Lubitz J. Medicare Part A utilization and expenditures for psychiatric services, 1995. *Health Care Financing Rev* 1997; **18**(3): 177–94.

39. Smyer MA, Shea DG. Mental health among the elderly. In Vitt LA, Sigenthaler JK, eds, *Encyclopedia of Financial Gerontology*. Westport, CT: Greenwood, 1996; 365–71.

40. Physician Payment Review Commission. Medicaid: spending trends and the move to managed care. In *Physician Payment Review Commission: Annual Report to Congress, 1997*. Washington, DC: PPRC, 1997; 412–48.

41. Health Insurance Association of America. Introduction to Managed Care. In *Managed Care: Integrating the Delivery and Financing of Health Care*. Washington, DC: Health Insurance Association of America, 1996; 1–13.

42. MedPac. Updating and reforming prospective payment for hospital inpatient care. In *Medicare Payment Advisory Commission: Report to Congress, Medicare Payment Policy*. Washington, DC: MedPac, 1999; 49–67.

43. MedPac. Continuing reform of Medicare payments to physicians. In *Medicare Payment Advisory Commission: Report to Congress; Medicare Payment Policy*. Washington, DC: MedPac, 1999; 117–28.

44. Hay Group Management. *Health Care Plan Design and Cost Trends: 1988–1997*. Washington, DC: National Association of Psychiatric Health Systems, 1998; 1–2.

45. MedPac. Medicare+choice: a program in transition. In *Medicare Payment Advisory Commission: Report to Congress; Medicare Payment Policy*. Washington, DC: MedPac, 1999; 27–46.

46. Medicare Managed Care. Face Sheet. The Kaiser Family Foundation. http://www.kff.org/content/archive/2052/mngcare.html

47. Langwell K, Topoleski C, Sherman D. *Analysis of Benefits Offered by Medicare HMOs, 1999: Complexities and Implications*. Menlo Park, CA: Henry J. Kaiser Foundation, 1999; 1.

48. Wells KB, Astrachan BM, Tischler GL, Unutzer J. Issues and approaches in evaluating managed mental health care. *Milbank Qu* 1995; **73**(1): 57–75.

49. Wells KB. Cost containment and mental health outcomes: Experiences from US studies. *Br J Psychiat* 1995; **166**(suppl 27): 43–51.

50. Dana RH, Conner MG, Allen J. Quality of care and cost-containment in managed mental health: policy, education, research, advocacy. *Psychol Rep* 1996; **79**: 1395–1422.

51. Physician Payment Review Commission. Revising the method for determining Medicare capitated payments. In *Physician Payment Review Commission: Annual Report to Congress, 1997*. Washington, DC: PPRC, 1997; 53–75.

52. Gottlieb GL. *Managed Behavioral Healthcare Standards, Guidelines, and Competencies for Older Adults with Mental Illness*. Rockville, MD: Center for Mental Health Services (SAMSHA), 1998.

53. Frank RG, McGuire TG, Bae JP, Rupp A. Solutions for adverse selection in behavioral healthcare. *Health Care Financing Review* 1997; **18**: 109–22.

54. Reifler BV, Cox NJ, Jones BN *et al*. Service use and financial performance in a replication program on adult day centers. *Am J Geriat Psychiat* 1999; **7**(2): 98–109.

55. Eng C, Pedulla J, Eleazer GP *et al*. Program of all-inclusive care for the elderly (PACE): an innovative model of integrated care and financing. *J Am Geriat Soc* 1997; **45**(2): 223–32.

56. MedPac. Managed care for frail Medicare beneficiaries: payment method and program standards. In *Medicare Payment Advisory Commission: Report to Congress; Selected Medicare Issues*. Washington, DC: MedPac, 1999; 79–104.

57. Newcomer R, Harrington C, Preston S. Satisfaction in the social/health maintenance organization: a comparison of members, disenrollees, and those in fee-for-service. In Luft H, ed., *HMOs and the Elderly*. Ann Arbor, MI: Health Administration Press, 1994; 111–39.

58. Bartels SJ, Levine KJ. Meeting the needs of older adults with severe and persistent mental illness: public policy in an era of managed care and long-term care reform. *Publ Policy Aging Rep* 1998; **9**(1): 1, 3–6.

59. Lee W, Eng C, Fox N, Etienne M. PACE: a model for integrated care of frail older patients. Program of all-inclusive care for the elderly. *Geriatrics* 1998; **53**(6): 62, 65–6, 69, 73.

Community-based Psychiatric Ambulatory Care: the Private Practice Model in the USA

Elliott M. Stein and Gary S. Moak

Private Practice in Miami Beach, FL, USA

In the USA, ambulatory or outpatient psychiatric care of individuals in later life is provided in a variety of public and private office settings. These include publicly-financed community mental health centers, hospital-sponsored outpatient clinics or services, the offices of psychiatrists (and other mental health professionals) in private practice, health maintenance organizations (HMOs, both privately and government-funded), and others. This chapter will focus on practical aspects of providing psychiatric treatment to older Americans in office-based psychiatric private practices. We will not discuss the details of treatment in these settings, but rather the "mechanics" of the process. An important focus of community-based psychiatric ambulatory care is the need to create relationships with other community services and providers of care and assistance. This provides both a framework and a means by which many of the services are provided. Some of the barriers and obstacles to care will also be reviewed.

In providing community-based ambulatory care, the psychiatrists must have a comprehensive and patient-centered focus, following the patient to provide whatever psychiatric treatments are needed in whatever setting. While there are some geriatric psychiatrists who limit their activities to specific treatment locations, such as in offices or in-hospital programs, this type of care may require the patient to be seen and treated sequentially in many places and circumstances.

INFLUENCES ON PRIVATE PRACTICE

For the purposes of this chapter, we will define private practitioners as independently employed or self-employed psychiatrists who work alone or in small groups. These practitioners provide treatment to patients who individually seek their help, and who pay for services received, primarily with Medicare health insurance benefits. Notwithstanding the large-scale reorganization occurring in the American healthcare system, private practice remains the widespread model of medical practice in the USA. In many ways it has served as a starting point for the pattern of care provided in the other settings mentioned above. Many of the techniques discussed below are applicable to other models of treatment. Older patients seek care from private practitioners or other mental health providers with varying degrees of utilization and satisfaction[1,2].

The private practice of medicine in the USA has evolved as a cottage industry within an historically unsystematized, free-enterprise, fee-for-service climate. Changing lifestyle preferences and demographics among young physicians are having some impact on this pattern. From its inception in 1965, the Medicare system has had a built-in prejudice against the provision of outpatient psychiatric services. There remains a discriminatory 50% patient co-payment requirement for all psychiatric treatment services delivered outside of an acute care hospital setting (unlike all other covered medical services, for which the patient co-payment is 20%). This has constrained provision of these services to the elderly. Over the past 5–10 years, however, much greater influence has been felt from a multitude of outside forces, at times impeding geriatric psychiatry practice[3,4], but in some cases expanding it. These forces (to list a few) include: efforts by the federal government to rein in Medicare spending[5,6]; the penetration of health maintenance organizations (HMOs) into Medicare; the advent of federal nursing home reform regulations; the growing presence of healthcare agency accrediting bodies, such as the Joint Commission for the Accreditation of Healthcare Organizations (JCAHO) and the National Council of Quality Assurance (NCQA); the creation by the American Board of Psychiatry and Neurology of subspecialty board examinations in geriatric psychiatry; social attitudes (e.g. public attitudes about medical care and doctors, as well as about mental illness and psychiatric care); the influences of physician attitudes[7] and medical malpractice litigation[8]; the availability of newer psychopharmacologic agents (including their increased acceptance by the public and their increased utilization by primary care physicians); patient finances; and folklore and "common sense" of both the professional and the general population. Geography also is a factor, as there is significant regional variation among practitioners and communities in different areas of the country. Adaptation of geriatric assessment and treatment principles has been slow, for the most part, in private medical practice. Nevertheless, successful practitioners need a working knowledge of these forces in order to function. As a relatively new field in the USA, there are few established examples of psychogeriatric care that have proven generally applicable. In fact, the fee-for-service system in the USA has thus far been a relative failure in geriatrics, since it has not incorporated many of the accepted principles of geriatric care[9].

The incursion of managed care HMOs into the Medicare system held out promise to change this state of affairs. HMOs, in theory, employ methodologies such as integrated delivery systems, screening, prevention and case management that are ideally suited to geriatrics[10]. Their track record has been disappointing, however, and their approach to managing mental health care has been largely ineffective for the elderly. Managed care companies often "carve out" the management of mental health services by subcontracting it to managed behavioral healthcare companies with specialized expertise in mental health benefits management[11]. Such companies rarely have any expertise in geriatrics, and do not appreciate its differences from general adult psychiatry[12]. These companies have often ageist attitudes built into their coverage utilization guidelines, and inappropriately limit treatment or completely deny it, especially involving members with Alzheimer's disease, which they do not view as a covered psychiatric disorder. To the extent that managed care has penetrated Medicare, this practice has made the practice of geriatric psychiatry unnecessarily burdensome for many American psychiatrists.

PRIVATE PRACTICE AS A BUSINESS

Another important factor in discussing this type of psychiatric practice is the awareness that it is a business, and that the patients are customers. As such, it behooves the psychiatrist to organize the practice and to provide services in ways that answer the needs of these customers. The psychiatrist may help the patient to define these needs, provide information about them, alter them, or aid them in various ways. The psychiatrist may need to refuse patients' requests when professional judgment dictates this. American consumers, especially the adult children of geriatric patients, are becoming increasingly distrustful of the healthcare system and doctors. If the psychiatrist does not do a good job or does not adequately address at least some of the patient's needs (and/or their adult child's needs), the psychiatrist may lose that patient's business. Thus, it is clear that the interaction between them is an exchange of service for payment. By providing a comprehensive service, as mentioned above, the psychiatrist may provide more services in more locations, which is often very satisfying and helpful to patients. At the same time, the business opportunities for income are maximized. In a community-based private practice, people are often referred to the individual doctor, rather than to a hospital, a university or a public clinic where they may be assigned a doctor. Patients may be referred because of the doctor's quality of service, reputation or relationships with the referring party. These qualities therefore become significant aspects of the psychiatrist's success in business as well as clinical practice.

Important factors in satisfying the patient/customer include:

1. *Cost*: reasonable fees and/or helpfulness and knowledgeability in filling out insurance claims.
2. *Accessibility*: convenient and comfortable office location and surroundings.
3. *Availability*: the availability of the psychiatrist to go to the patient if needed (e.g. to consult at a medical hospital if the patient is admitted by another physician for a physical ailment, or to see the patient at home, in a nursing home, or an assisted living facility) is very important. The convenience of the geriatric psychiatrist going to where the patient lives, rather than the patient coming to the doctor's office, is very attractive to family caregivers responsible for transportation. The viability of this form of practice, in private practice, depends upon arrangements with facilities that ensure an adequate volume of patient visits for each trip to the facility.
4. *Scheduling*: flexibility to see patients at convenient times without excessively long delays in scheduling appointments. This is crucial, since many frail patients are brought by their adult children who work.
5. *Communications:* the ability to contact the psychiatrist quickly and easily at need (e.g. by telephone by the patient and, when appropriate, by the patient's family). This includes the willingness of the psychiatrist to return such phone calls quickly, and the friendliness and accuracy of the psychiatrist's secretary or answering service. It also includes the ability and willingness of the psychiatrist to speak to the patient (and family) about his/her symptoms, illnesses and treatments in a clear and patient manner.
6. *Concern*: the feeling that the therapist has a genuine interest and concern for the patient. This feeling of concern extends to the patient's interactions with the office staff. This is an especially vital factor for the older population[13].
7. *Confidence*: patients need to feel that the psychiatrist knows what the patient's problem is and has an idea about what can be done. The doctor does not need to define answers, but must indicate a grasp of the situation and some ideas for an approach to it. This helps to provide a structure to what is often a strange and frightening experience. Empathy with the patient's distress is very helpful in this, as is reassurance to the patient that his/hers is not the worst case the doctor has ever seen (a common fantasy).

There are only limited data available on income and workload for geriatric psychiatrists as a group. For all psychiatrists, 1998 median annual gross income was $171 490 (a 3.5% increase from 1997) and annual net income was $118 630 (a 4.33% increase from 1997). This was the second lowest income of the 20 largest specialties (above general practitioners) surveyed by Medical Economics that year. The rate of inflation in the year 1997–1998 was 1.6%. Comparable 1998 income data for all US physicians show an annual gross income of $256 290 (down 0.7% from 1997) and a net income of $163 940 (up 2.2%); for non-surgical specialties the gross income was $227 300 (up 1.7%) and the net income was $147 140 (up 2.4%)[14]. When these data are compared to the median annual net income for psychiatrists in the USA in 1989, which was $103 570 (the fourth lowest of 15 office-based specialties surveyed that year; the only doctors who made less were general practitioners, family physicians and pediatricians)[15], we find that the income of psychiatrists had risen 14.5% in that period. The median net income for all fields of medicine rose just under 25% during the same period, while the cumulative inflation rate added up to 35%.

Although most American psychiatrists see few or no geriatric patients, this trend is changing somewhat. There were over 5400 out of the over 36 000 members of the American Psychiatric Association who expressed an interest in geriatrics during their 1997–1998 Professional Activities (Biographical) Survey[16]. The membership of the American Association for Geriatric Psychiatry has grown to over 1800[17] and interest among general psychiatrists is increasing. In 1991, the American Board of Psychiatry and Neurology first administered a Board Certifying subspecialty examination in geriatric psychiatry. As of September 2000, there were 2508 individuals who have passed this examination[18].

In 1996, 18% of American general psychiatrists had geriatric caseloads exceeding 20% of their practices[19]. Overall, in this 1996 survey of 970 responders, an average of $14.0 \pm 17.7\%$ of their psychiatric patients were aged 65 +[19], compared to 8.4% found in a 1987 study[20]. When psychiatrists who provide a higher proportion of geriatric services (more than 20% of their case load—HGPs) were compared to those who were low-volume providers with the elderly (less than 20% of their workload—LPGs), it was found that the HPGs spent proportionately less time in their offices (although still spending most of their time there), more time in hospitals and significantly more time in nursing homes, than LPGs[19]. In view of relatively low numbers of psychiatrists with a specific interest treating the elderly, when the medical and general communities know that a particular psychiatrist is a geriatric specialist, there is usually no shortage of patients needing these services.

OFFICE PLANNING AND DESIGN[21,22]

Establishing a practice to treat older patients requires some attention be paid to the setting in which such treatment will occur and to factors that might act as barriers to treatment. Offices that can only be reached by climbing stairs, or those with varying levels into which one must step up or down, are difficult and potentially hazardous. Long corridors that must be traversed are similarly problematic. Chairs should be available that are sturdy and have armrests and firm seats, high enough for ease in sitting or rising. Adequate lighting, readable signs and patient information literature should be planned with poor vision in mind. Area carpets, spring-hinged doors and other possible hazards should also be considered.

Mobility and transportation problems are another potential obstacle to treatment. Selection of an office location in a rural community, or in an area with poor public transportation or poor handicapped access, may be factors. Treatment may be interrupted during the winter months if the cold interferes with the patient's ability to get to the office. Some communities have senior transportation services, which will take people with limited mobility to physicians if reservations are made 24–48 hours in advance. Some hospitals may transport patients to and from the hospital or to physicians' offices located in adjoined buildings. Offices may also be located in senior retirement buildings or communities.

THE BEGINNING OF THE RELATIONSHIP

Older patients seek out, are referred to or are brought to the psychiatrist's office for care. An initial "gatekeeper" function may occur by means of inquiries (usually by telephone) into the reasons for the request to be seen, the age of the prospective patient, the referring source, the status of insurance coverage or other financial information. Such inquiries may lead a particular practitioner who prefers to specialize in geriatrics to decline to accept an adolescent as a patient, or to suggest that a patient being seen by another psychiatrist first discusses the idea of transferring with the current therapist, or to refer the patient to a geriatric psychiatrist in a geographically more convenient location.

A prospective patient, once given an appointment, should be told about additional information the psychiatrist would like to have available at the time of the first visit (e.g. the names of the patient's other treating physicians, current medications being taken, information about past psychiatrists, psychiatric medications, hospitalizations, etc.). If the referring source is a physician, family member or a member of the staff of a senior-living facility, information from them as to the nature of the problem referral may be requested.

THE RANGE OF SERVICES

Among the most important services a psychogeriatric specialist can provide are diagnostic services. Too often, inadequate or erroneous evaluation leads to inadequate or erroneous treatment. A knowledge of physiology, psychology and the illnesses of late life, a comprehensive approach to history taking, assessment and testing and the ability to formulate an appropriate treatment plan form the basis of a unique contribution by geriatric specialists[23,24]. In fact, the ability to provide such a comprehensive evaluation and treatment perspective may be a primary reason why patients and referral sources seek the assistance of a geriatric psychiatrist.

An important aspect of the coordinated treatment plan is the collection of past information. With the patient's permission, contact is established with the patient's family, other physicians and therapists. Past records, diagnoses, psychological testing reports, doctors' treatments, psychotherapy records, laboratory and radiological reports are collected. While not revealing confidential information, these contacts also benefit the patient by making the patient's other physician and support system aware of your activities with the patient. This increases the likelihood that you will be notified of future problems that may occur and that other medical treatments will be coordinated with you by other physicians. In the absence of such relationships, physicians may call a different psychiatrist to provide treatment, due to lack of awareness of your involvement.

As has been reviewed elsewhere[22,25,26], including sections of this volume, older individuals can be suitable candidates for many of the therapeutic modalities provided to younger patients, including individual, group and family psychotherapies, which utilize insight-orientated, cognitive, behavioral and other techniques. Some approaches, such as reminiscence or life-review therapy[27], have more specific applicability to the aging person. Modification of family therapy may be necessary, e.g. to address the role of adult children in assisting in the care of a demented or otherwise impaired parent.

Unfortunately, the federal government has been increasingly scrutinizing and denying payment for psychotherapy services for Medicare beneficiaries, including many elderly patients. Under the Clinton Administration's program "Operation Restore Trust", an effort to reduce fraud and waste in the Medicare and Medicaid programs, many psychotherapy services came to be viewed as unnecessary or fraudulent, particularly those provided to demented patients or in nursing homes[28,29].

Psychopharmacologic treatment of the elderly often requires alteration in the selection, dosing and scheduling of medication because of changes in absorption, distribution, metabolism, receptor sensitivity and excretion[30,31]. Once again, the geriatric psychiatrist may be sought out in recognition of this expertise by the patient and others involved in the patient's care. Pharmaco-economic trends in the USA create additional conflicts for geriatric psychiatrists in private practice. First, many patients who have Medicare have no prescription drug benefits (although this was an important political issue in the US presidential election of 2000). Pharmaceutical costs are escalating rapidly in the US compared to many other countries. Patients may have coverage for the physician visit but not the drugs the physician prescribes[32]. Those beneficiaries who have opted for managed care plans may have some drug benefits. However, treatment options are often limited by restrictive formularies designed with cost containment in mind, but often without any consideration of the greater sensitivity of elderly plan members to medication side effects. Nursing homes have also adopted formularies to contain their costs, even in the absence of significant managed care penetration. Consultant pharmacists are employed by the homes to monitor physician prescribing, with respect not only to federal regulations but also to formulary requirements. Psychiatrists in private practice are thus often under pressure to prescribe less costly drugs or to run the risk of receiving fewer referrals from primary care physicians or nursing homes.

Sometimes assistance provided may be primarily educational, such as telling the patient or his/her family about the nature of the aging process or the symptoms, prognosis and treatment of an illness. Treatment may be primarily informational, directing patients and carers to appropriate senior housing, services for the blind or hearing-impaired, continuing education programs or volunteer work. At times treatment may be directive, e.g. telling a patient to get a physical examination, buy a hearing aid or give up driving, or telling a family member to seek the assistance of respite services to provide some relief in caring for a cognitively impaired person, or to advise that the parent or sibling should no longer live alone. The community-based psychiatrist must develop expert knowledge of the available community resources, as well as relationships with the providers of them.

The initial psychiatric diagnostic evaluation of the patient also is the time of the patient's actual evaluation of the doctor. The practitioner must address the overt and covert concerns, the anxieties and fantasies about the nature of geriatric psychiatry, the reasons why the patient is there and the treatments that will be instituted. Although these anxieties are not unique to this model, the need to address them is. Unlike treatment limited to one location or modality or situation, this relationship will be multifactorial and ongoing. Furthermore, a privately operating care provider is likely to represent an entry contact point into mental health care. If the patient and the associated significant family members are not put at ease, their questions answered and concerns addressed, the contact may quickly end.

Older patients are often novices regarding mental illness and its treatment. They are often fearful of being thought "crazy" or of being "put away". Structuring the beginning of the initial interview can help relieve their anxiety. You may start with 10–15 min of specific questions, such as address, age, date of birth, concrete information on marriages, children, parents, siblings, education, employment, interests, etc. This can also give you a lot of information in a short time, helping to give a more complete picture of the patient. Simultaneously, you are assessing aspects of mental status and memory.

Treatment of the older patient includes the time when the patient is away from the office. The patient is helped when assured of the doctor's continued interest and care. This can often be done using relatively simple techniques: (a) providing specific information tells the patient that you know what is going to happen, e.g. "This medicine is going to take 2–3 weeks to build up in your system. You may experience some side effects during that period but you will not experience the benefit for 2–3 weeks. You need to be patient during that time"; (b) assuring access and inviting communication, e.g. "My telephone number is a 24 hour number. If you have any problems or need to reach me, you can call any time". Patients rarely do call outside of office hours after being told this, but they feel very reassured; (c) specific instructions for behavior and for contacts, e.g. instead of saying, "Call me if you have any problems", saying "Call me next Tuesday", assures the patient that you want to hear from him/her. It also reduces the number of calls he/she might otherwise make before next Tuesday.

FAMILY INVOLVEMENT

Families are often interested and involved in the psychiatric care of elders. Relatives and friends can be important sources of information to the doctor. Interactions may include mediation and other interventions into the family system, re-interpretation and re-framing of past and present events, support, reassurance and education. Attention to family issues is especially important in treatment of patients with dementing disorders[33,34].

Because of the increased interrelationships and involvements some families have in an older patient's status and treatment, it is often vital to maintain contact and a positive rapport with the family. Also, patients will often request this. Conversely, when family members feel unnecessarily excluded or denied access to information, they can influence or disrupt the treatment entirely. This is not to imply that therapeutic confidentiality is not maintained; families generally understand this. They do, however, want to know that appropriate help is being provided. Such reassurance can have a positive therapeutic effect on the patient, as a reflection of the family's confidence in the doctor. It can also

have the practical influence/effect of helping to keep the patient in treatment.

In situations where there are no immediate relatives, non-kinship, support networks become increasingly important[35]. The therapist may at times utilize the assistance of family surrogates in gathering information and in helping the patient. Where such networks are weak or absent, assisting the patient in their creation can be of great benefit.

RELATIONSHIPS WITH OTHER PHYSICIANS

In the absence of the formalized organization of a university environment or the planned hierarchy of a hospital or corporate structure, the geriatric psychiatrist in private practice must create or seek out relationships with other practitioners. This can be done through involvement in professional societies, participation in the activities of the community's hospitals and through non-medical social contacts. Eventually, further relationships will also be created by patients who seek psychiatric services and request that contact be established with their other treating physicians. Collegial relationships thus created can provide advice and assistance, help in monitoring the status of patients between visits to the psychiatrist and provide sources of referrals for new patients.

RELATIONSHIPS WITH OTHER PSYCHIATRISTS

As with other physicians in general, private practitioners must create a network of relationships with other psychiatrists in the area, both near and far. Those at some distance, or whose special areas of interest or expertise differ, can be sources of referrals. Other psychiatrists may receive inquiries or have patients referred to them whom they are unable to treat; they may then direct them to you. Psychiatrists who practice in closer proximity may also be sources of new patient referrals, especially when their treatment interests differ from yours. Furthermore, a certain percentage of patients, especially those with chronic or recurring illness, may be "doctor-shoppers" and spontaneously, or by referral, change from one practitioner to another over a period of time. Developing good rapport with other local psychiatrists helps in providing better care to these patients by sharing understanding of their needs, pathology and past successful treatments and by helping to avoid duplication of previously attempted unsuccessful treatments.

Formal or informal groupings of private psychiatrists may gather for continuing education and study, to help with supervision, second opinions or "risk-management" of difficult cases, or to share tasks, such as psychiatric coverage for a local hospital's emergency room. When a private practitioner takes a break, to go on vacation or to a conference, it may be one or more of these local psychiatrists who is asked to be available to take care of emergencies or to provide ongoing services to patients who are hospitalized at the time. Often such favors are done reciprocally as a courtesy.

RELATIONSHIPS WITH OTHER PROFESSIONALS

Other professional care providers with whom privately practicing geriatric psychiatrists and their patients come into contact include psychologists, social workers, nurses, speech therapists, occupational therapists, hospital administrators and the operators of nursing homes and congregate-living facilities. Knowledge of these and other community resources is essential for the geriatric psychiatrist. At times the best treatment offered to a patient may be a referral to one of them. Needless to say, each of these can provide valuable services. As they get to know the geriatric psychiatrist, they can also be valuable resources, e.g. they can be excellent sources of information about a patient's status and functioning when the patient is not in the doctor's office. They may allow the psychiatrist to provide more and better service to patients by helping to monitor, care for and carry out treatments with the patient. They can alert the doctor when problems are developing, often earlier than the patient might have, and can assist in the management of a crisis by supporting and reassuring the patient. These individuals are sources of referral to the practitioner. They will also speak to others in the community of their experiences and contacts with the practitioner. This is an important facet of how a professional reputation is made.

RELATIONS WITH HOSPITALS

Each psychiatric program within a hospital can have its own rules, regulations, standards, patterns of practice and pattern of relations with community-based practitioners. Some hospital facilities employ psychiatrists on staff; others may not. Some programs are organized more in accord with the direction given by the hospital and the hospital-based staff. Others encourage more involvement in program planning by the community staff physicians. Some facilities are sites for training programs and have psychiatric residents who provide services. There are some geriatric facilities within free-standing psychiatric hospitals and others that are geriatric units within medical hospitals; some are located in private, for-profit hospitals, or in non-profit or public or charitably-funded institutions, or in university-affiliated programs. While the rules, staffing patterns and required paper forms may vary from hospital to hospital, these variations are, for the most part, not so onerous as to be unworkable or impossible to deal with for the community-based practitioner. In some of these settings, the community-based practitioner may be able to influence the nature of the hospital's policies and treatment program by participation in psychiatric departmental meetings and activities.

The differences among hospitals requires some flexibility on the part of the doctor, but also may allow the possibility of tailoring referrals to the hospital most appropriate to the patient. For a variety of reasons, different hospital units acquire different patient populations and characteristics. Some programs are age-segregated, with specifically designated geriatric psychiatry wards. Others are age-integrated, with younger and older patients sharing and participating in the treatment program together. Some programs may be more suitable for cognitively intact, physically healthy older people suffering from affective or anxiety disorders or relationship dysfunctions.

THE POSSIBILITY OF INPATIENT HOSPITAL TREATMENT[36]

At the time of the initial visit or at some subsequent time in the course of the treatment of an older patient, the psychiatrist may recommend inpatient hospital treatment. The process begins with an assessment of whether the hospitalization is something that would be beneficial and therapeutic but non-emergent, or is an urgently needed admission due to imminent danger to the patient or others. Immediately after this decision, the psychiatrist must decide whether the patient is capable of consenting to this plan. Depending upon the hospitals and resources available in the community, these assessments may lead to a decision to use a particular inpatient facility. For example, there may be one that can admit people on an involuntary basis, or care for people who

are potentially suicidal or aggressive. Similar choices may result from the ability of a specific hospital's psychiatric ward to care for elderly patients who have concurrent severe medical problems, or who are wanderers, or who need the hospital's specific therapeutic approach. Other factors that affect the choice of inpatient service include locations of past hospitalizations, the hospitals used by the patient's other treating physicians, proximity to the patient and the patient's family to allow for visitation and, importantly, whether a particular hospital has a room available for the patient at the time it is needed, and whether the admission can or can not be delayed until a bed becomes available. In some cases, where room is not available locally or at the time needed or where local facilities are not appropriate, referral for hospitalization may have to be made to a psychiatrist or facility elsewhere.

ADMISSION TO HOSPITALS

Various hospitals and psychiatric facilities within hospitals may have different procedures for arranging admissions. Typically, the psychiatrist communicates with a designated person or office to make the reservation for admission. Information that must be provided at this point varies but usually consists of the patient's name, age and admitting diagnosis. Some facilities may also wish information regarding the geriatric patient's ability to function in activities of daily living, mobility, signs and symptoms of the patient that warrant admission, a preliminary treatment plan, or the likelihood of the patient being a danger to self or others.

When the patient is admitted, each hospital's usual procedure begins. Administrators and nurses fill out forms. The patient is shown to a room, belongings are put away and the staff makes the patient acquainted with the facility and program of activities. At about the same time, the private psychiatrist is notified that the patient has arrived. If not already given, initial orders are requested. When the psychiatrist is not available to come to the hospital immediately, orders might be given by telephone to the ward nurse, addressing such needs as diet, monitoring of vital signs, laboratory tests, ward therapies and medications to be started, etc.

IN-HOSPITAL TREATMENT[36,37]

In-hospital treatments for the elderly can include the full spectrum of therapeutic approaches devised for psychiatric patients in general, although these might vary depending upon the resources and philosophy of the facility and the specific instructions of the doctor. The psychiatrist may personally provide individual psychotherapy, family therapy, psychotherapeutic medication management, electroconvulsive therapy, or other treatments, as well as ongoing diagnostic evaluation. Many older patients also benefit from group, occupational, recreational and ward milieu therapies, physical therapy, speech therapy or reality-orientation/memory-stimulating techniques. Often, the community psychiatrist is not directly involved in these treatments; the hospital's staff members provide them as part of the hospital's program and report back to the doctor regarding the patient's progress. Nurses, social workers and other staff members also inform the psychiatrist about the patient's status, symptoms, behavior and reactions to treatment as observed during the day. Coordination, mutual understanding of achievable goals, cooperation and respect between the psychiatrist and the hospital administration and staff facilitate the psychiatrist's functioning and the treatment of the patient. It is vital that a good working relationship be achieved. If it is not, the doctor can be undermined in numerous ways.

Working in the hospital requires flexibility on the part of doctors and staff. The staff must accommodate to various physicians and their styles of treatment. The doctors must adapt to the hospital and its program, including its staffing pattern, its treatment approach and its physical plant. Patients may be seen at times under less than ideal conditions, including differing circumstances, locations, times and schedules (e.g. seeing a patient in a semi-private room, planning hospital rounds to not conflict with group therapy programs, visiting patients only to find that they are in physical therapy or getting X-rays).

POST-HOSPITAL TREATMENT

Planning for hospital follow-up begins during the hospital stay. The physician can direct the social service worker regarding possible directions and options for such problems as living situation changes, needs for at-home services, assistance or care, possible adult congregate-living facility or nursing home placement[38]. The social worker can investigate these and coordinate planning with the physician, patient and patient's family. Other post-discharge options the doctor can order include visiting nurses, physical therapy and other home health treatments or referral to a senior day center or a partial hospitalization day program[39,40]. The patient's needs, desires, finances and therapeutic considerations (including the options for follow-up treatment with the psychiatrist) are important factors in these choices. Similarly, the available, involved members of the family may have opinions or suggestions. They may also direct the psychiatrist's attention toward additional problems or issues they feel are significant.

An important part of discharge planning is the re-engagement of the patient in outpatient treatment in the psychiatrist's office. An appointment can be given at the time of discharge or the patient may be instructed to make an appointment within a specified period of time. The psychiatrist makes certain that needed hospital records, including discharge summary, list of discharge medications, copies of laboratory and radiograph reports and medical consultation reports, are sent to the office. This enhances completeness and continuity of care.

In addition to other usual psychotherapeutic issues that can be discussed in the post-hospital treatment, it is important to include a review of the patient's reactions to the hospital, the symptoms that necessitated the admission and the patient's progress there. Also, it is important to watch for post-hospital regressions and symptom recurrences, as the patient returns to his/her usual surroundings or to a new environment. Medication compliance and monitoring is another post-discharge task that requires attention, especially if the medication is new, if it is causing some side effects or if it requires special care in its use (e.g. special diet or times of administration).

CONCLUSION

Community-based ambulatory psychiatric care is a relatively young and growing avenue for the treatment of older adults in the USA. There have been relatively few specific models of private psychogeriatric care described to date. Aspects of the treatment of younger adults in the community are being applied to the care of seniors; however, modifications are important in order to more fully address the special problems and needs of this population.

REFERENCES

1. Stein SR, Linn MW, Edelstein J, Stein EM. Elderly patient's satisfaction with care under HMO vs. private systems. *South Med J* 1989; **82**(12): 3–8.
2. Thomas C, Kelman HR. Health services use among elderly under alternative health services delivery systems. *J Commun Health* 1990; **152**: 77–92.
3. Gottlieb GL. Financial issues. In Sadovoy J, Lazarus LW, Jarvik LF, eds, *Comprehensive Review of Geriatric Psychiatry*. Washington, DC: American Psychiatric Press, 1991: 667–86.
4. Goldman HH. Financing the mental health system. *Psychiat Ann* 1987; **17**(9): 580–5.
5. Goldman HH, Cohen GD, Davis M. Expanded Medicare outpatient coverage for Alzheimer's disease and related disorders. *Hosp Commun Psychiat* 1985; **36**: 939–42.
6. Hsiao WC, Braun P, Becker E *et al. A National Study of Resource-based Relative Value Scales for Physician Services*. Final Report. Boston: Dept. of Health Policy and Management, Harvard School of Public Health, 1988: 27–43.
7. Ford C, Sbordone R. Attitudes of Psychiatrists Toward Elderly Patients. *Am J Psychiat* 1980; **137**: 571–5.
8. Klein JL, Macbeth JE, Nonek J. *Legal Issues in the Private Practice of Psychiatry*. Washington, DC: American Psychiatric Press, 1984.
9. Lachs MS, Ruchlin HS. Is managed care good or bad for geriatric medicine? *J Am Geriat Soc* 1997; **45**: 1123–7.
10. Lachs MS, Wagner EH. The promise and performance of HMOs in improving outcomes in older adults. *J Am Geriat Soc* 1996; **44**: 1251–7.
11. Bartels SJ, Colenda CC. Mental health services for Alzheimer's disease. Current trends in reimbursement and public policy, and the future under managed care. *Am J Geriat Psychiat* 1998; **6**: 85–100.
12. Bachman SS. Managed mental health care for elders: the role of the carve-out. *Publ Policy Aging Rep* 1998; **9**: 14–16.
13. Logsdon L. *Establishing a Psychiatric Private Practice*. Washington, DC: American Psychiatric Press, 1985.
14. Goldberg J. Doctor's earnings: You call this progress? *Med Econ* 1999; **18**: 172.
15. Clark L. Pressure grows on psychiatrists' earnings. *Med Econ* 1991; **68**(7): 60–70.
16. Unpublished data, courtesy of American Psychiatric Association, 2000.
17. Unpublished data, courtesy of American Association for Geriatric Psychiatry, 2000.
18. Unpublished data, courtesy of American Board of Psychiatry and Neurology, 2000.
19. Colenda CC, Pincus H, Tanielian TL *et al.* Update of geriatric psychiatry practices among American psychiatrists. *Am J Geriat Psychiat* 1999; **7**: 279–88.
20. Loran LM, Taintor Z, Mirza M. Patient characteristics and treatment modalities. In Koran LM, ed., *The Nation's Psychiatrists*. Washington, DC: American Psychiatric Association, 1987: 109.
21. Stein EM. Some practical considerations in the private practice of psychogeriatrics. *Clin Gerontol* 1983; **2**(1): 56–8.
22. Stein EM. Geriatric psychiatry in office and clinic. *J Appl Gerontol* 1983; **2**: 102–11.
23. Blazer D. The psychiatric interview of the geriatric patient. In Busse EW, Blazer D, eds, *Geriatric Psychiatry*. Washington, DC: American Psychiatric Press, 1989: 263–84.
24. Blazer D, Busse EW, Craighead WE, Evans D. Use of the laboratory in the diagnostic workup of the older adult. In Busse EW, Blazer D, eds, *Geriatric Psychiatry*. Washington, DC: American Psychiatric Press, 1989: 285–312.
25. Lazarus L. Psychotherapy. In Busse EW, Blazer D, eds, *The Ambulatory Care Setting in Geriatric Psychiatry*. Washington, DC: American Psychiatric Press, 1989: 567–91.
26. Nemiroff RA, Colarusso CA. *The Race Against Time—Psychotherapy and Psychoanalysis in the Second Half of Life*. New York: Plenum, 1985.
27. Butler RN, Lewis MI. *Aging and Mental Health: Positive Psychosocial Approaches*. St Louis, MO: C.V. Mosby, 1973.
28. Mental Health Services in Nursing Facilities. Department of Health and Human Services Office of Inspector General, June Gibbs Brown, Inspector General, May 1996. OEI-02-91-00860.
29. *Ten-state Review of Outpatient Psychiatric Services at Acute Care Hospitals*. Department of Health and Human Services, Office of Inspector General June Gibbs Brown, Inspector General. March 2000, A-01-99-00507.

30. Young RC, Meyers BS. Psychopharmacology. In Sadovoy J, Lazarus LW, Jarvik LF, eds, *Comprehensive Reviews of Geriatric Psychiatry*. Washington, DC: American Psychiatric Press, 1991: 435–68.

31. Davidson J. The Pharmacologic Treatment of Psychiatric Disorders. In Busse EW, Blazer D, eds, *The Elderly in Geriatric Psychiatry*. Washington, DC: American Psychiatric Press, 1989: 515–42.

32. Moriarty PL. Prescription benefits, pharmacoeconomics, and Alzheimer's disease: implications for geriatric health care. *Clin Geriat* 1999; **7**: 33–47.

33. Cohen D, Eisdorfer C. *The Loss of Self*. New York: Norton, 1986.

34. Mace NL, Rabins PV. *The 36 Hour Day*. Baltimore, MD: Johns Hopkins University Press, 1981.

35. Stein EM. Normal aging—psychological and social cultural aspects. In Lazarus W, ed., *Essentials of Geriatric Psychiatry*. New York: Springer, 1988: 1–24.

36. Whanger AD. Inpatient treatment of the older psychiatric patient. In Busse EW, Blazer D, eds, *Geriatric Psychiatry*. Washington, DC: American Psychiatric Press, 1989: 593–634.

37. Tourigny-Rivard MF. Acute care inpatient treatment. In Sadovoy J, Lazarus LW, Jarvik LF, eds, *Comprehensive Review of Geriatric Psychiatry*. Washington, DC: American Psychiatric Press, 1991: 583–602.

38. Curlik SM, Frazier D, Katz IR. Psychiatric aspects of long-term care. In Sadovoy J, Lazarus LW, Jarvik LF, eds, *Comprehensive Review of Geriatric Psychiatry*. Washington, DC: American Psychiatric Press, 1991: 547–64.

39. Rosie JS. Partial hospitalization: a review of recent literature. *Hosp Commun Psychiat* 1987; **38**(12): 1291–9.

40. Steingart A. Day programs. In Sadovoy J, Lazarus LW, Jarvik LF, eds, *Comprehensive Review of Geriatric Psychiatry*. Washington, DC: American Psychiatric Press, 1991: 603–12.

The Psychiatrist's Role in Linking Community Services

Deirdre Johnston, Kimberly A. Sherrill and Burton V. Reifler

Wake Forest University School of Medicine, Winston-Salem, NC, USA

In addressing the mental health needs of older adults in the USA, psychiatrists are faced with a number of significant challenges. One of them remains sheer demand: the number of patients needing services still outstrips the availability of psychiatrists, especially those with specialized geriatric training. A second challenge is that of collaborating effectively with the primary care sector who, as will be described in some detail later, provide mental health care for the vast majority of the elderly. Third is the challenge of understanding and working effectively with a wide range of non-physician providers of services to older adults. These and other difficulties will likely become more pressing as the demographic trends towards an older society are accompanied by increasing financial restrictions.

Many psychiatrists are responding to these challenges by enlarging their role from that of generalist clinicians to geriatric-specific educators, academicians and researchers, as well as sources of expertise for innovative community-based programs. We will begin by documenting the need for services, alluded to above, and follow with examples of how those role changes are being manifested in important new programs and initiatives. We conclude with comments on future directions for the psychiatrist's role in the process of change, and a discussion of some of the premises underlying the current system of mental health care for the elderly.

THE NEED FOR MENTAL HEALTH SERVICES AMONG THE COMMUNITY-BASED ELDERLY

One way to estimate the current need for mental health services among the community-dwelling elderly is to take the prevalence rates of mental illness and subtract the portion of those already receiving services. In terms of prevalence rates, the elderly appear to have rates of mental disorders about the same as those of younger adults[1]. One of the more conservative estimated prevalence rates for lifetime psychiatric disorders, 12.3%[2], comes from the Epidemiological Catchment Area (ECA) study, while another recent community-based study documents a higher rate of 31%[1].

Using specific and fairly restrictive criteria, Shapiro *et al.*[3] estimated from ECA data that some 7.8% of those aged 65+ need mental health services. If the ECA study results can be generalized to the population as a whole, and given that the vast majority (99.6%) of the nation's 29.8 million adults aged 65+ reside in the community rather than in institutional settings (US Census Bureau statistics, 1987), then some 2.3 million community-residing elderly may be said to need mental health care.

Many of those needing services are not seeing a mental health professional. In Goldstrom *et al.*'s Bunker Hill study[1], among patients aged 65+ with a psychiatric disorder, only 42% had at least one visit to a mental health professional, compared to 68% among the 18–44 age group ($p < 0.01$) and 53% among the 44–64 age group ($p < 0.01$). Shapiro *et al.* calculated that 5.7% of the total population of elderly need, but are not receiving, mental health services. About one-third of those needing mental health services are being seen by the specialty mental health sector, another one-third receive care only from general medical care providers, and the other one-third receive no care[2]. Recent evidence suggests that considerable barriers still exist in the public sector that prevent the elderly from receiving specialized psychiatric care[4]. The elderly have tended to be slow to report psychiatric symptoms compared to younger adults[5].

The fact that so many patients with *mental* health needs are being seen by the *general* medical sector (the "*de facto* mental health system")[6] is important for several reasons. Numerous studies document that primary care practitioners overlook psychiatric disorders in their patients[7,8], and, even when treating patients for mental disorders, tend to do so inadequately[9]. It has also been suggested that physicians may misinterpret somatic markers of depression as being due to physical illness[10]. In the USA, an increasing number of older adults are enrolled in managed care plans, which usually require that the primary care physician treat most uncomplicated illnesses, limiting access to specialist care. Recent evidence suggests significant differences in the treatment of older people with depression enrolled in health maintenance organizations (HMOs) compared with younger depressed patients. Older patients received fewer mental health specialty visits, fewer prescriptions for SSRI antidepressants, and were more likely to be prescribed benzodiazepines[11]. As the managed care model expands nationwide, the evidence remains that the depressed elderly are underserved[12]. Thus, there is a great need to train primary providers in the detection and treatment of mental disorders. Also, geriatric patients with mental disorders make twice as many office visits to their primary care providers as do those without a mental disorder[1]. If those patients received adequate treatment, then according to the so-called "cost-offset" hypothesis, the improvement in mental health would result in substantial decreased utilization of other health care services, thus "offsetting" the expense of providing mental health care[13,14]. Investigators estimate that treatment for mental disorders is accompanied by an overall 20% decrease in the use of general

Principles and Practice of Geriatric Psychiatry, 2nd edn. Edited by J. R. M. Copeland, M. T. Abou-Saleh and D. G. Blazer

healthcare services, especially for inpatient care[15,16]. In a climate of fiscal restrictions, such information lends needed support to the value of adequate mental health care.

CLINICIANS AS GERIATRIC SPECIALISTS

The tremendous need for expertise in caring for geriatric patients has been part of the impetus for the evolution of geriatric psychiatry into fully-fledged subspecialty status. The American Association of Geriatric Psychiatry was founded in 1978. Recognition as a subspecialty came with the administration of the first examination for added qualifications in Geriatric Psychiatry in April 1991 by the American Board of Psychiatry and Neurology. By 1999, 2360 psychiatrists had passed the examination and there were 39 ACGME-accredited geriatric psychiatry fellowship programs nationwide.

Becoming a geriatric specialist in psychiatry involves assuming a unique constellation of familiar roles, rather than some distinctive singular role. Diversity is the hallmark of the team membership roles geriatric psychiatrists are called upon to assume. Examples of that diversity include coordinating clinical care, taking part in community initiatives and participating at various levels in educational activities.

CLINICAL ROLES

Clinical care has evolved to a model that is much more comprehensive than before, with an emphasis on multidisciplinary assessment. One successful model for a geriatric assessment clinic originating in Seattle[17] included a psychiatrist, an internist and a social worker. The assessment took three to four clinic visits, one for each of the following: (a) a psychiatric evaluation; (b) a medical evaluation; (c) a home visit; and (d) a family conference at the conclusion of the evaluation, for discussion of results and recommendations. When the patient suffered from cognitive impairment, the model often included neuropsychiatric assessment.

The Seattle clinic demonstrates the emergence of a common theme that has become the standard for comprehensive geriatric assessment: a focus on the patient's psychosocial context. Families of geriatric patients have attracted much interest since the emergence of the subspecialty of geriatric psychiatry, because of the critical role they play in the care of demented elderly patients. While attention to families has always been characteristic of certain areas within psychiatry, notably child psychiatry, until the notion of comprehensive geriatric assessment was developed, families of psychiatrically ill geriatric patients were considered ancillary, rather than integral to patient care. A major catalyst behind this broadened perspective has been a large body of research, which demonstrates the vital role of psychosocial issues for the health and well-being of older adults[18,19]. In recent years, research has focused on the mental health of caregivers and caregiver factors influencing service utilization and institutionalization[20,21].

Other innovative programs have been described, e.g. Bienenfeld reported on a liaison service to nursing homes[22] and Reifler et al. described an outreach program for mentally impaired older adults in Seattle[23]. However, although it is by now well established that there is a high prevalence of psychiatric morbidity in nursing homes, there remains a great need for psychiatric consultation in this setting. Legislation limits the prescription of psychotropics in US nursing homes in order to prevent the use of "chemical restraint", and pharmacists conduct periodic reviews to ensure compliance with these rules. One innovation that may enhance psychiatric involvement in the care of nursing home patients is video teleconsultation, which enables the psychiatrist to interview patients at remote locations, usually with the nurse in attendance on the patient. Research to date suggests that this can be an effective and economically viable medium[24].

COMMUNITY ROLES

Social service agencies, nursing homes, local Alzheimer's Associations, home healthcare organizations, hospice care and other organizations that coordinate services for the elderly are eager for psychiatric expertise. Collaboration also allows geriatric psychiatrists to become well acquainted with available resources and to learn when to refer to such organizations. An incentive for the development of innovative community-based programs is the increasing cost of long-term care.

One example of innovative community-based care that has begun to involve geriatric psychiatrists is the adult day center (ADC) movement. The idea of ADCs actually evolved from the mental healthcare system, where day programs had been utilized for some of the more seriously ill psychiatric patients who needed greater support than could be provided by periodic outpatient clinic visits. Adaptation of that notion to the needs of geriatric patients began to appear in the mid-1970s and early 1980s, and the movement mushroomed from only 15 documented ADCs in 1975 to over 4000 by 1998[25].

The Robert Wood Johnson foundation initiated a national demonstration project (the Dementia Care and Respite Services Program) in the late 1980s to promote further growth of dementia-specific ADCs. One of the primary goals of the project was to determine whether centers could become financially viable through charging for their services. Centers had struggled with unstable financial bases, which depended on their ability to obtain grant support or contributions or to utilize transient state and federal funds. The 4 year program began funding for 19 model ADCs in 1988[26]. The "Partners in Caregiving" initiative, which included the initial 19 sites and a subsequent demonstration program involving 50 sites across the USA, showed that adult day care centers could care for individuals with all degrees of dementia, from mild to severe, while remaining financially viable by meeting over 80% of their expenses through out-of-pocket payments and Medicaid[25].

Other community-based models involving psychiatrists have developed. Robinson[27] reviewed four of them, including: (a) the Channeling Demonstration, a federally-funded initiative awarded to 12 states, designed to serve severely impaired elderly people at risk of being institutionalized and to test two types of case management; (b) the Social/Health Maintenance Organization (S/HMO), a concept developed by Brandeis University, which is a managed care system of health and long-term care; (c) the On Lok Senior Services Program, a consolidated group of medical and support services based in San Francisco; and (d) Life Care Communities, which include some 600 continuing care communities nationwide, as well as the case-management delivery system called "Life Care at Home". The Channeling Demonstration, while it did not save money, did improve quality of life for clients and caregivers. The S/HMO model achieved its goal of integrating the funding and social services of long-term care, but did not succeed in integrating medical and social services or utilizing geriatric specialists[28]. An updated series of HMOs ("S/HMO II") has begun, which have pledged to incorporate professionals with expertise in geriatrics into the range of services provided. The On Lok model, now known as the Program of All-inclusive Care for the Elderly (PACE), has been replicated in dozens of cities around the USA, with almost 3000 enrollees nationwide. Participants average 80 years of age, and have seven or eight medical conditions. All of their health care is provided by a PACE interdisciplinary team. Outcome studies are under way. So far, the program has been shown to lower hospital and nursing home utilization costs, and most of the patients fared as well as or better than predicted, based on their baseline clinical status[29].

EDUCATIONAL ROLES

Many psychiatrists have responded to the acute need for geriatric-specific services and education in the community by conducting workshops and seminars for professional groups and providing consultation for various organizations. However, a response that provides for community needs for a long-term perspective is to teach geriatrics to medical students. A 1978 Institute of Medicine report urged medical schools to incorporate teaching related to aging in both the basic and clinical sciences. In 1993, the Institute of Medicine Committee on Strengthening the Geriatric Content of Medical Training convened to assess the status of geriatric training and to develop recommendations on strategies for improving the training of physicians in geriatrics[30]. It found a decline in the number of applicants for funded fellowship programs in geriatric-related specialties. It also found that the number of geriatric faculties in all specialties nationwide was insufficient (and in psychiatry by 1221 positions) to meet the training needs of all undergraduate medical students and residents. In response to this report, the John A. Hartford Foundation initiated a project to "Integrate Geriatrics into the Subspecialties of Internal Medicine". Recognizing that the majority of the teaching of medical students and residents is performed by those in the medical subspecialties, this initiative was designed with the goal of raising awareness and competence of the medical subspecialist in the care of the elderly.

This 6 year, $3.5 million project has sought to identify leading subspecialists, to redirect their attention to the subtleties of geriatric aspects of their discipline, and to ascertain opportunities for teaching and research within those aspects. The primary vehicle for this is the Geriatric Education Retreat (GER), a 5 day gathering of leaders in the subspecialty and geriatricians[31]. As a result of this project, nearly every national medical organization has added a symposium to their annual meeting, focusing on geriatric aspects of the discipline; fellowship training curriculum is being developed within half of the identified subspecialties; the residency Review Committee of Internal Medicine has added the requirement that all fellows must have substantial experience with patients aged 70+, and the American Board of Internal Medicine has recently adopted a "cross-content" blueprint for all examinations, which includes internal medicine. An essential curriculum in geriatric psychiatry for general internal medicine residents and geriatric medicine fellows has been described[32]. The Foundation has provided an extension grant to convene a GER for the specialties of Neurology and Psychiatry with the goals of "gerontologizing" the practicing neurologist and psychiatrist and infiltrating the curriculum of the residency and fellowship programs with the knowledge needed to provide competent geriatric care.

CONCLUSIONS

Several important areas of need, and examples of efforts to respond to them, have been discussed briefly in this chapter. In summary, although progress has been made in training general psychiatrists and other specialists in the care of the elderly, there remains a need for psychiatrists to improve their ability to diagnose and treat psychiatric disorders in the elderly; to participate in improved training in geropsychiatry for primary care physicians as well as for other mental health professionals; to participate in developing innovative new models of service delivery; and finally to be willing to enter research and academic careers with a focus on geriatrics[33].

Goldman and Frank[34] noted that addressing the needs listed above are particularly difficult, given the emphasis on cost-containment and efficiency prevalent today, in contrast to the mood of equity and access to care that was characteristic of the 1960s. Indeed, critics of the current approach to geriatric psychiatry state that the system is problem-driven, evolving in a way that is reactive to economic, political and social forces. They argue that a prevention-driven system is needed, which springs from more proactive efforts, anticipating needs and attempting to respond to them in light of available resources.

Several premises that underlie mental health care for the elderly in the USA were set forth by Burns and Taube[2] and may help to explain the rationale behind the evolution of our current system: (a) there is a preference for providing care in the community instead of institutions; (b) there is a belief in the value of managed care approaches, such as the use of case managers and primary care physicians as gatekeepers to the mental health system, and organizations such as HMOs and preferred provider organizations; (c) there is a preference for service provision general providers instead of specialists when feasible; and (d) there is a belief that care should be comprehensive, continuous and of high quality.

There are, of course, many other needs that are beyond the scope of this chapter, such as those dealing with economics, health policy and political considerations. Nevertheless, there is a great potential for positive change if the basic problem areas listed above can be satisfactorily addressed.

REFERENCES

1. Goldstrom ID, Burns BJ, Kessler LG et al. Mental health services use by elderly adults in a primary care setting. *J Gerontol* 1987; **42**: 147–53.
2. Burns BJ, Taube CA. Mental health services in general medical care and in nursing homes. In Fogel BS, Furino A, Gottlieb GL, eds, *Mental Health Policy for Older Americans: Protecting Minds at Risk*. Washington, DC: American Psychiatric Press, 1990: 63–84.
3. Shapiro S, Skinner EA, German PS et al. Need and demand for mental health services in an urban community: an exploration based on household interviews. In Barrett J, Rose RM, eds, *Mental Disorders in the Community: Progress and Challenge*. New York: Guilford, 1986.
4. Swartz MS, Wagner HR, Swanson JW et al. Administrative update: utilization of services. 1. Comparing the use of public and private mental health services: the enduring barriers of race and age. *Commun Ment Health J* 1998; **34**(2): 133–4.
5. Centers for Disease Control and Prevention. Reported frequent mental distress among adults—United States, 1993–1996. *J Am Med Assoc* 1998; **279**(22): 1772–3.
6. Regier DA, Goldberg ID, Taube CA. The *de facto* US mental health services system: a public health perspective. *Arch Gen Psychiat* 1978; **35**: 685–93.
7. Jencks SF. Recognition of mental distress and diagnosis of mental disorder in primary care. *J Am Med Assoc* 1985; **253**: 1903–7.
8. Rapp SR, Parisi SA, Walsh D, Wallace CE. Detecting depression in elderly medical inpatients. *J Clin Consult Psychol* 1988; **56**: 509–13.
9. Kamerow DB, Pincus HA, McDonald DI. Alcohol abuse, other drug abuse, and mental disorders in medical practice: prevalence, costs, recognition, and treatment. *J Am Med Assoc* 1986; **255**: 2054–7.
10. Heithoff K. Does the ECA underestimate the prevalence of late-life depression? *J Am Geriat Soc* 1995; **43**: 2–6.
11. Bartels SJ, Horn S, Sharkey P, Levine K. Treatment of depression in older primary care patients in health maintenance organizations. *Int J Psychiat Med* 1997; **27**(3): 215–31.
12. Unutzer J, Katon W, Russo J et al. Patterns of care for depressed older adults in a large-staff model HMO. *Am J Geriat Psychiat* 1999; **7**(3): 235–43.

13. Levitan SJ, Kornfield DS. Clinical and cost benefits of liaison psychiatry. *Am J Psychiat* 1981; **138**: 790–3.

14. Strain JJ, Hammer JS, Lyons JS *et al*. Cost offset from the psychiatric intervention liaison for elderly hip fracture patients. *Psychosom Med* 1989; **51**(abstr): 261.

15. Johns KR, Vishi TR. Impact of alcohol, drug abuse and mental health treatment on medical care utilization: a review of the research literature. *Med Care* 1979; **17**(suppl): 1–82.

16. Mumford E, Schlesinger HJ, Glass GV *et al*. A new look at evidence about reduced cost of medical utilization following mental health treatment. *Am J Psychiat* 1984; **141**: 1145–58.

17. Reifler BV, Eisdorfer C. A clinic for the impaired elderly and their families. *Am J Psychiat* 1980; **137**: 1399–403.

18. Cohen JD, Brody JA. The epidemiological importance of psychosocial factors in longevity. *Am J Epidemiol* 1981; **114**: 451–61.

19. Blazer DG. Depression in Late Life. St Louis, MI: C. V. Mosby, 1982: 105.

20. Cochrane JJ, Goering PN, Rogers JM. The mental health of caregivers in Ontario: an epidemiological survey. *Am J Publ Health* 1997; **87**(12): 2002–7.

21. Zarit S, Gaugler J, Jarrott S. Useful services for families: research findings and directions. *Int J Geriat Psychiat* 1999; **14**(3): 165–77.

22. Bienenfield D, Wheeler BG. Psychiatric services to nursing homes: a liaison model. *Hosp Commun Psychiat* 1989; **40**: 793–4.

23. Reifler BV, Kethley A, O'Neill P *et al*. Five-year experience of a community outreach program for the elderly. *Am J Psychiat* 1982; **139**: 220–3.

24. Jones B. Telemedicine and long-term care. *Nurs Home Econ 3* 1996; **3**: 17–19.

25. Reifler BV, Cox N, Jones B *et al*. Service use and financial performance in a replication program on adult day centers. *Am J Geriat Psychiat* 1999; **7**: 98–109.

26. Sherrill KA, Reifler BV, Henry R. *Respite Care for Dementia Caregivers: Findings from the Robert Wood Johnson Foundation Projects*. New York: Springer (in press).

27. Robinson GK. The psychiatric component of long-term care models. In Fogel BS, Furino A, Gottlieb GL, eds, *Mental Health Policy for Older Americans: Protecting Minds at Risk*. Washington, DC: American Psychiatric Press, 1990: 157–76.

28. Harrington C, Lynch M, Newcomer R. Medical services in social health maintenance organizations. *Gerontologist* 1993; **33**: 790–800.

29. Eng C, Pedulla J, Eleazer G *et al*. Program of all-inclusive care for the elderly (PACE): an innovative model of integrated geriatric care and financing. *J Am Geriat Soc* 1999; **45**: 223–32.

30. Institute of Medicine Committee on Strengthening Training in Geriatrics for Physicians. Washington, DC: National Academy Press, 1993.

31. Hazzard RW, Woolard N, Regenstreif DI. Integrating geriatrics into the subspecialties of internal medicine: the Hartford Foundation/American Geriatrics Society/Wake Forest University Bowman Gray School of Medicine initiative. *J Am Geriat Soc* 1997; **45**: 638–40.

32. Colenda C. Essential curriculum in geriatric psychiatry for general internal medicine residency and geriatric medicine fellowship programs. Proceedings of a Conference: Geriatrics Curriculum Development of Conference and Initiative. *Am J Med* 1994; **97**(4A): 15–18S.

33. Fogel BS, Gottlieb GL, Furino A. Present and future solutions. In Fogel BS, Furino A, Gottlieb GL, eds, *Mental Health for Older Americans: Protecting Minds at Risk*. Washington, DC: American Psychiatric Press, 1990: 257–77.

34. Goldman HH, Frank RG. Division of responsibility among payers. In Fogel BS, Furino A, Gottlieb GL, eds, *Mental Health for Older Americans: Protecting Minds at Risk*. Washington, DC: American Psychiatric Press, 1990: 85–95.

The Medical Psychiatry Inpatient Unit

David G. Folks[1] and F. Cleveland Kinney[2]

[1]*University of Nebraska College of Medicine, Omaha, NE, and*
[2]*University of Alabama School of Medicine, Birmingham, AL, USA*

Medical psychiatry inpatient units primarily serving older adults have increased in popularity and numbers in North America in recent years. Several model programs have been described with respect to structure and organization, clinical care and logistical advantages in the management of older psychiatric patients who suffer from significant medical and surgical problems. The literature also suggests that medical psychiatry inpatient units offer great advantages over traditional settings in the diagnosis and treatment of elderly patients with combined disorders. Older psychiatric patients with acute medical illness, chronic medical conditions, the negative physiologic and psychologic concomitants of ageing, the problems of polypharmacy, drug interaction and compliance, together with the need for a more comprehensive and effective clinical approach, have culminated in a number of refinements in these units. The senior author's own experience in developing, organizing, operating and continually evaluating a dynamic geriatric medical psychiatry program lends support to the importance and utility of this treatment modality. This chapter will review in detail the structure, organization and clinical characteristics and financing of a medical psychiatry inpatient unit.

STRUCTURE AND ORGANIZATION OF THE GERIATRIC MEDICAL PSYCHIATRY INPATIENT UNIT

The medical psychiatry inpatient unit is generally orientated towards the admission and treatment of patients with combined medical and psychiatric illnesses. An attempt is made to integrate medical and psychiatric care, utilizing a biopsychosocial or systems treatment approach. The unit itself may be influenced by the administrative structure of the facility, the orientation of the medical and psychiatric community, the priorities among the clinical and administrative leaders and/or the general resources and expectations of the population to be served. Young and Harsch[1] alluded to three guiding principles that must be met in order for a medical psychiatry unit to succeed. These are the following: (a) the provision of a distinct type of care; (b) an improved quality of care; and (c) more efficient care. Another primary consideration in North America is the need to demonstrate that added costs to third-party payers and hospitals will yield greater benefits for both the patient population and the medical facility. The financing of these units with respect to changes in the USA are to be addressed in this chapter.

The medical psychiatry inpatient unit maintains a distinctive patient population by virtue of admission criteria. Patient characteristics may also be determined by affiliation with various governmental or community agencies, or perhaps by other referring psychiatric facilities that are unable to provide care for medically ill psychogeriatric patients. Of course, healthier psychiatric patients may also benefit from the medical model adopted in a medical psychiatry unit. However, these units truly provide a therapeutic edge and hold promise for the successful clinical approach to a growing number of seriously medically ill or functionally compromised elderly psychiatric patients[2]. Furthermore, the work-up and treatment may potentially be performed without major increases in length of stay. Incidentally, these units are known to provide an excellent milieu for clinical training in psychiatry and other disciplines.

The ideal physical environment of a medical psychiatry inpatient unit ensures safety for delirious or behaviourally disturbed elderly patients, facilitates the rendering of medical services, and provides a pleasant environment suitable for relatively long hospital stays. The overall space requirements do not differ markedly, but do exceed the space ideal for general hospital or free-standing psychiatric units. Presumably, the facility contains essential equipment and structure that would not otherwise be found on a psychiatric unit; the level of care delivered could, therefore, not be provided, or provided as well, on the "typical" psychiatric unit. This inpatient approach is in contrast to the consultation–liaison model of managing medically ill psychiatry patients on existing medical/surgical wards.

Features of patient rooms in a medical psychiatry unit may vary depending on the individual characteristics of the patients. Essential safety features include shatterproof windows, break-away curtain rods, electrical outlets that disconnect in response to tampering and lockable water taps, especially with semi-private baths. Certainly, for medically acute patients, lighting for bedside examination, outlets for oxygen and suction and adjustable hospital beds are necessary. A voice-call light system, a facility for glucose monitoring and availability of cardiac telemetry are highly desirable. Medical psychiatry inpatient units are also expected to provide care for patients requiring intravenous fluids/therapy or nasogastric suction, who need total care in a bedridden or debilitated state, as well as oxygen support or clinical management of common medical conditions, e.g. diabetes, hypertension, angina, congestive heart failure, chronic pulmonary disease, electrolyte or fluid balance disturbances, and urinary tract or pulmonary infections. Patients with great acuity may be too labor-intensive, i.e. the ideal unit should be designed to strike a balance between the provision of basic medical care and the provision of intensive psychotherapeutic care. The ideal unit will also consist of patient rooms that are largely private, but some therapeutic benefits may be derived from semi-private rooms for patients who are withdrawn, or for cases in which a higher-functioning roommate can provide aid to another with respect to orientation and structure. All patient room entrances and bathroom facilities should be wheelchair-accessible. An emergency cord should be available in the bathroom and should be reachable from the floor by patients who may have fallen. The same architectural suicide prevention considerations found on general psychiatric units should be built into the medical psychiatry inpatient unit. Other needs include shower and patient-lifting devices, a bedside weight scale, suitable chairs, supply facilities/cart and, more controversially, mechanical (soft) restraints and effective methods of observation.

The unit ideally will include built-in handrails along the walls, television facilities for bedridden patients, and industrial-grade carpet to soften falls in the hallways and/or common or public areas but with vinyl to facilitate cleaning in patient rooms. Patient rooms are designed to maximize observation and minimize noise that may distract the staff. Finally, consideration must be given to whether a medical psychiatry unit will be locked, closed or controlled, and whether involuntary patients will be admitted. With adequate numbers of trained staff, it should not be necessary to have barriers to free movement. Where sufficient trained staff cannot be provided, some units have double-handed doors. The controlled unit, utilizing electronic beep or entry computer codes, ensures that wandering by cognitively impaired patients can be thoughtfully controlled. The locked or controlled-access unit provides both safety and containment. Separate areas are designed for activities and occupational or physical therapy.

The flow of staff and consultants tends to be great on a medical psychiatry unit; thus, workspace is an important consideration. Nursing units may be better divided into modular work stations with built-in cabinetry and shelving. The record and medication room can be separated by a locked door and the entire nursing station designed as an enclosed area with an observation/reception window made of safety glass. Sufficient storage space for medical equipment and supplies should also be considered. The care of complex, medical–psychiatric patients often requires frequent, small conferences among professionals of different disciplines and specialties in order to coordinate care. On-site professional offices for the medical director, social worker, head nurse and trainees afford privacy and a quiet environment for conferences and interviews. Preferably, physical therapy should be provided on-site if at all possible; a physical therapist permanently assigned to a medical psychiatric unit may incorporate psychiatric skills into the therapy treatments and may become an integral part of the treatment team. In addition to common areas for group dining, activities, educational programs, family meetings, group therapy and occupational therapy, additional space is necessary for staff meetings and conferences. An adequate staff lounge not only improves morale but also facilitates communication between the healthcare professionals and multidisciplinary personnel.

OPERATIONAL FEATURES OF THE GERIATRIC MEDICAL PSYCHIATRY INPATIENT UNIT

A multidisciplinary treatment team is generally assembled in order to address the complex needs of geriatric patients with combined disease. Each member contributes to the administration and operation of the unit, and each discipline contributes uniquely. A nurse clinical specialist with both medical and psychiatric experience may act as a milieu coordinator/supervisor for the nursing staff. Complex social work interventions require great expertise in family consultation, assessing hospital and community services and providing assistance in disposition. Consulting

psychologists with experience in neuropsychology, personality assessment and behaviour therapy are invaluable team members. The nursing staff should consist primarily of registered nurses combining medical–surgical and psychiatric skills. Practical nurses and nurses' aides can participate in the delivery of care and may also become adept in the clinical care of combined medical–psychiatric problems. Senior nurses with extensive psychiatric experience often contribute greatly to the management of behaviourally difficult patients. Irrespective of experience and background, nurses who enthusiastically support the model of combined medical–psychiatric care are ideal. Above all, the nursing staff must possess flexibility and resourcefulness combined with a practical and optimistic approach, in view of the constant changes in demands.

The usual format for the medical psychiatry inpatient unit in North America employs a model in which a psychiatrist or internist acts as an attending professional, experienced in directing a team and communicating with both mental health professionals and medical–surgical professionals. The medical director is responsible for gatekeeping, quality assurance, staff supervision, training, in-service education, trouble-shooting and the provision of consultation (directly or indirectly) in difficult cases. Liaison with community agencies, public affairs and assistance with legal and ethical problems in patient care are also required of the medical director. Administrative interfaces with the affiliated department, hospital, community mental health center and referring resources are essential. These interactions will vary according to the individual orientation and characteristics of the facility. Similarly, other third-party, legal and governmental interactions will vary accordingly.

CLINICAL AND PATIENT CHARACTERISTICS OF A GERIATRIC MEDICAL PSYCHIATRY UNIT

A variety of patient subtypes may be considered appropriate for an inpatient medical psychiatry unit. Three patient subtypes have been identified by Stoudemire and Fogel[3]: (a) patients with severe medical illness requiring daily medical coverage in addition to treatment of psychiatric illness; (b) psychiatrically disordered patients who require frequent but not daily medical attention from a surgeon or internist, e.g. diabetic or post-surgical cases; and (c) patients who merely require an initial consultation or periodic access or review/adjustment of medications by a medical consultant. Depression in the medically ill, chronic schizophrenia with concurrent physical disease, i.e. stroke, epilepsy, Parkinson's disease, head trauma, delirium, complications of dementia, or paroxysmal behaviour disorders, and a variety of other general medical illnesses with complex family or psychosocial issues, characterize appropriate cases for admission and treatment.

The average length of stay on a typical unit is generally approximately 7–21 days. Site-specific considerations pertaining to the selection of appropriate patients must be analyzed in order to determine specific inclusion and exclusion criteria. A well-defined priority system can then be established in order to determine which patients are admitted or provided with access to care. Regarding admission, patients on affiliated medical/surgical wards, and cases seen by the emergency or staff physicians, are typically given special consideration. Above all, patient acuity, dispositional resources and the staffing will determine the answers to many gate-keeping decisions. Moreover, the primary mission of these units remains the provision of psychiatric care to individuals who also have significant medical/surgical illness. Again, these patients are often *not* welcome in either traditional psychiatry or medical/surgical units. Finally, decisions regarding admission or transfer of inpatients from medical/surgical units may depend on the likelihood that the patient will receive true benefit, respond to psychiatric treatment or require close observation in order to achieve diagnostic or therapeutic results.

Patients with general medical problems associated with psychiatric disturbances are challenging with respect to clinical management. However, several studies have implied that patients treated on such a unit benefit with respect to improved quality of care and shorter length of stay[4]. Medical psychiatry units are also more likely, compared to traditional units, to benefit patients with functional or cognitive impairment. For example, patients with coexisting dementia and depression are much more effectively addressed in a shorter time frame, with resultant decrease in length of stays, compared to those patients treated on a general medical unit[5,6]. Moreover, treatment in the medical psychiatry unit with aggressive outpatient follow-up may obviate the need for nursing home placement[6]. Primary interventions on a medical psychiatry unit may include pharmacologic or somatic therapies, as well as ongoing efforts to optimize the patients' general medical/physiologic status. Coping with illness, issues relating to loss and self-esteem, feelings toward a caregiver and social changes are other important psychotherapeutic themes commonly addressed in a geriatric medical psychiatry unit. Medical emergencies, e.g. cardiac arrest or status epilepticus, must be considered and anticipated. Emergent symptoms of delirium may also need attention and in these cases, the legal doctrine of implied consent applies.

PROBLEMS, ADVANTAGES AND CAVEATS WITH GERIATRIC MEDICAL PSYCHIATRY INPATIENT UNITS

The quintessential factor that determines the success of a medical psychiatry inpatient unit is *nursing care*. Ideally, nurses recruited from medical/surgical units or critical care areas who are keenly interested in psychological dimensions of patient care, are considered best-suited to the medical psychiatry inpatient unit. Professional attire and more traditional uniforms often help to minimize confusion about the medical role of the unit. Non-psychiatric nurses may be useful in order to update and maintain medical skills of the staff, and serve to maintain familiarity with newer techniques of intravenous therapy, oxygen therapy, suction and skills in cardiac monitoring, respiratory care and postsurgical care. Because nursing is the critical element in the successful operation of these units, appropriate head nurses are invaluable and a difficult resource to obtain.

Reimbursement and financial integrity are long-standing issues with the medical psychiatry unit[7]. For example, in the USA, the Tax Equity and Fiscal Responsibility Act (TEFRA) of 1982 has determined payment for services in psychiatric units. The Balanced Budget Act (BBA) was passed by Congress in 1997 and has replaced the TEFRA of 1982. This has resulted in a reduction of approximately 7–8% in revenues for care provided in a psychiatric unit. However, patients with concurrent medical and psychiatric illness may add an average of 40% to the annual cost of health care when compared to patients without concurrent medical and psychiatric illness[8–10]. Thus, psychiatric programs in general hospitals catering to the medically ill psychiatrically disordered patient are progressively less able to meet financial goals, because of the costs of ancillary medical service utilization, and free-standing psychiatric hospitals are also unable to include these patients in their patient mix. On average, psychiatric facilities are already losing money when they treat patients with combined medical–psychiatric illness[11]. Further, under the Balanced Budget Act, facilities in the USA stand to lose an additional 12% or more on such cases.[12]

Medical psychiatry units in the USA that pride themselves on the ability to treat complicated geriatric patients with co-

morbid illness must consider the need to take immediate steps that will allow them to remain fiscally solvent. Further limits on admissions with no medical co-morbidity, or preference to patients with low psychiatric acuity, are the easiest solutions. However, these solutions do not allow the medical psychiatry inpatient unit to respond to the clinical needs of the complicated, high-cost co-morbid patient. A more satisfactory solution to this problem has been suggested by Goldberg and Kathol[11]. Specifically, a partnership among medical/surgical professionals, hospital administration and psychiatric departments is suggested. A model of providing full psychiatric care, yet billing to general medical reimbursers, is recommended, allowing higher reimbursement of *per diems* through medical service billings that are adequate to cover the costs of medical tests and procedures typically not included in psychiatric or behavioural health payments. Such service integration can be done in such a way that units can actually cover direct costs and make significant contributions to the indirect costs in healthcare systems, while improving care[13]. This is particularly true if general medical patients at high risk for, or demonstrating, psychiatric co-morbidity with high healthcare utilization are targeted for admission. When this is done, costs savings for such patients accomplished through shortened length of stay can be as much as $4000 per admission[11,13]. Thus, it is possible to capitalize on the relatively higher reimbursement available with general medical admissions—even under the DRG system, which is also affected by the BBA, while continuing to address psychiatric difficulties.

The interaction of medical and psychiatric illness requires a unit organized in the fashion previously outlined. As forementioned, this approach allows treatment that assists the patient in moving toward recovery, with the development of policies and standards that document quality, improved outcomes and better attention for patients treated with medical psychiatry morbidity[14]. Under this format, the psychiatric unit director or consultant becomes involved in creating and finding ways to enforce these standards and adequate reimbursement to cover costs is achievable. Clearly, general hospital units will not be able to afford to provide psychiatric care for the medically ill, and medical psychiatric units under pressure from the Balanced Budget Act in the USA will require reorganization in order to contend with the facets of the prospective payment system introduced in 1999. Without a medical psychiatry approach, medical psychiatry patients will be scattered about the hospital, with practices that will necessarily lead to poorer quality and higher costs in the average medical setting. Hospital administrations in the USA will find that the impact on medical length of stay will create worse financial liabilities for the DRG reimbursement. Administrators therefore must continuously monitor length of stay, admission diagnoses, and dispositional plans, while maintaining a favorable prospective payment format. Direct care costs, indirect operating costs, recovery of costs, costs offset with reduced utilization, as well as other indicators of cost effectiveness, should be considered in the overall economic equation.[2] Mumford et al.[15] have reported that treatment in a medical psychiatry inpatient unit may resolve problems that might otherwise become chronic and more expensive. Generally, however, units must deny admission to certain patient types whose care would exceed the permissible stay, and units must not become a way-station for problem patients. Without strict and clear guidelines, the medical psychiatry unit may become clogged and ultimately result in denial of care to a more appropriate patient. Cost-effectiveness studies are clearly needed to clarify many of these fiscal issues.

Kathol[13] is of the opinion that many advantages of a medical psychiatry unit depend heavily upon the medical director. Perhaps the most convenient model employs collaboration between the medical director and a liaison internist or psychiatrist who provides appropriate consultative care. Because the medical psychiatry unit as a treatment modality may increase the risk for loss of continuity of care or actual loss of follow-up, strategies for interim and longitudinal care should be carefully considered. A mechanism should be devised by the medical director for coordination of all clinical care following discharge. A distinct advantage of continuity of care after discharge from these units is the opportunity to assess the impact of psychological and psychosocial interventions among general medical populations.

CONCLUSION

The geriatric medical psychiatry inpatient unit could continue to be increasingly important as disproportionate growth occurs among the older population in North America (and Europe). An integrative model is essential in the delivery of care, preferably in a well-equipped setting that is organized to concentrate on the combined care of medical–psychiatric patients. These units are also quite useful in teaching and research programs, or in settings where large consultation–liaison psychiatry programs exist. Leadership provided by the medical director and head nurse, clearly articulated admission criteria and a well-organized multi-disciplinary approach are all essential ingredients for a successful operation. Finally, as economic, social and scientific factors converge and shape geriatric psychiatry, the medical inpatient unit may prove to be an optimal setting for intensive, inpatient geriatric treatment.

REFERENCES

1. Young LD, Harsch HH. Inpatient unit for combined physical and psychiatric disorders. *Psychosomatics* 1986; **27**: 53–60.
2. Goldberg RJ, Stoudemire A. The future of consultation–liaison and medical–psychiatric units in the era of managed care. *Gen Hosp Psychiat* 1995; **17**: 268–77.
3. Stoudemire A, Fogel BS. Organization and development of combined medical psychiatry unit: pt 1. In *Principles of Medical Psychiatry Units*. New York: Grune & Stratton, 1987; 677–83.
4. Folks DG. The role of the consultation liaison psychiatrist on the geriatric service. In Michels R, Cooper AM, Guze SB *et al.*, eds, *Psychiatry*. Philadelphia, PA: Lippincott-Raven, 1997.
5. Gertler R, Kopec-Schrader Em, Blackwell CJ. Evolution and evaluation of a medical-psychiatric unit. *Gen Hosp Psychiat* 1995; **17**: 26–81.
6. Kales HC, Blow FC, Dopeland LA *et al.* Health Care Utilization by older patients with coexisting dementia and depression. *Am J Psychiat* 1999; **156**: 550–6.
7. Fogel BS, Stoudemire A. Organization and development of combined medical-psychiatric units: pt II. *Psychosomatics* 1986; **27**: 417–28.
8. Unutzer J, Patrick DL, Simon G *et al.* Depressive symptoms and the cost of health services in HMO patients aged 65 years and older. A 4-year prospective study. *J Am Med Assoc* 1997; **277**(20): 1618–23.
9. Mayou R, Hawton K, Feldman E. What happens to medical patients with psychiatric disorder? *J Psychosom Res* 1988; **32**(4–5): 541–9.
10. Goetzel RZ, Anderson DR, Whitmer RW *et al.* The relationship between modifiable health risks and health care expenditures. *J Occup Environ Med* 1998; **40**(10): 843–54.
11. Goldberg RJ, Kathol R. Implications of the Balanced Budget Act of 1997 for general hospital psychiatry inpatient units providing medical and psychiatric services. *Gen Hosp Psychiat* 2000; **22**: 11–16.
12. Liu C-F, Cromwell J. *Impact of the Balanced Budget Act of 1997 on PPS-exempt Psychiatric Facilities*. Waltham, MA: Health Economics Research Inc., 1998.
13. Kathol RG. Integrated medicine and psychiatry treatment programs. *Med Psychiat* 1998; **1**: 10–16.
14. National Committee Quality Assurance. *1999 standards*, vol 7. 1999, 46.
15. Mumford E, Schlesinger HJ, Glass GV *et al.* A new look at evidence about reduced cost of medical utilization following mental health treatment. *Am J Psychiat* 1984; **141**: 1145–58.

130

The Psychiatrist in the Nursing Home

William E. Reichman

University of Medicine and Dentistry, Piscataway, NJ, USA

In the USA, nursing homes and other related long-term care facilities care for approximately 1.5 million persons annually. There are nearly 600 000 beds in these facilities across the country. While at any given time only 5% of the nation's elderly reside in these settings, up to 50% of citizens can expect to spend some portion of their lives there[1]. Over the past several years, many authors have described the impressive prevalence and vast array of psychiatric disorders complicating the care of nursing home residents. When dementia is included, rates of diagnosable mental illnesses have exceeded 80%[2–9]. The widespread use of psycho-active medications[10,11] and mechanical restraints[12,13] for the treatment of disturbed behavior in this setting has been well documented[5]. The National Medical Expenditures Survey in 1987 reported that 31% of nursing home residents had a non-dementia-related primary or secondary diagnosis of mental illness[14]. The principal psychiatric conditions that are especially noteworthy in the nursing home include dementia-associated behavioral complications, such as agitation[15], depression[16–18], anxiety[19–21], sleep impairment[22,23,29–31], psychosis[19,24–26] and substance abuse[27]. While the prominence of mental disorders in long-term care settings is now beyond dispute, in the USA, staffing patterns, staff expertise, environmental design and models of care delivery much more closely approximate subacute and chronic general medical care capabilities than thoughtfully conceived mental health services[9]. As a result, there is a great need to redesign the accessibility, structure and quality of psychiatric care in American nursing homes. Toward this end, this chapter will address the fundamentally important functions that may appropriately be provided by the psychiatrist in the nursing home setting.

THE ROLE OF THE PSYCHIATRIST

In the USA, contemporary training in general psychiatry emphasizes application of the biopsychosocial model to the understanding and treatment of mental disorders and behavioral symptomatology. This orientation is especially appropriate for accurately diagnosing and successfully treating the elderly nursing home resident, in whom there is often the co-morbid occurrence of physical, neurological, psychological and social contributors to disturbances of behavior. By virtue of their medical training, psychiatrists are uniquely qualified to integrate biological, psychological and social factors into a multidimensional treatment plan that reflects the full complexity of a given resident's behavioral symptomatology. Specifically, well-trained psychiatrists are potentially able to offer approaches to treatment that include recommendations for the appropriate use of a wide variety of psychoactive medications as well as psychological, behavioral

and milieu-orientated therapies. Unfortunately, little is presently known about the availability of psychiatrists to consult or manage residents in nursing homes in the USA. Additionally, a paucity of services research has been done to assist healthcare planners to better understand the character, quality and quantity of those professional functions that are provided by psychiatrists working within the nursing home milieu. In most settings, it appears that psychiatrists assume a purely consultative role, in which the primary physician (internist or family medicine practitioner) orders medication and is responsible for the course of treatment. In other settings, full responsibility for the management of the resident's psychiatric treatment resides more definitively with the psychiatrist. The factors that determine the relative intensity and scope of the psychiatrist's role vs. that of the primary physician in any given facility are largely unknown.

In a recently published study, Reichman *et al.*[28] examined the availability, characteristics and perceived adequacy of psychiatric consultation in nearly 900 nursing homes throughout the USA through a mailed survey to the directors of nursing of these facilities. Results indicated that 38% of nursing home residents were noted to be in need of a consultation by a psychiatrist. The frequency of these services was rated as "adequate" by only half of these homes. Nursing homes in urban and suburban regions reported better availability of psychiatric services than those located in rural areas. Nursing homes with larger bed capacities were also more likely to receive a higher frequency of services by a consulting psychiatrist. In examining the perceived adequacy of the psychiatrist's functions, these specialists were noted by two-thirds of the facilities as adequately providing diagnostic and psychopharmacologic recommendations. However, advice regarding non-medication approaches to treatment (e.g. psychotherapeutic, behavioral or milieu interventions), staff support, staff education, and attending to occasional conflict between the staff of the nursing home and resident families were reported as inadequately provided by consulting psychiatrists. Overall, the results of this study suggest that, in nursing homes in the USA, the perceived need for services provided by psychiatrists is significantly greater than the level actually provided. Additionally, it appears that the nursing directors of these settings would welcome an expanded treatment role for psychiatrists in the care of their residents with mental illness and behavioral disturbances.

While a substantial amount of research remains to be done to identify best practices for the delivery of psychiatric services in nursing homes, it is clear that the specialty of psychiatry has a vital role. In many facilities, the template of consultation–liaison psychiatry is most appropriately applied. In this framework, the psychiatrist attends to the specific mental health needs of an

Principles and Practice of Geriatric Psychiatry, 2nd edn. Edited by J. R. M. Copeland, M. T. Abou-Saleh and D. G. Blazer

individual resident, while also focusing on the needs of the nursing home staff. Resident-focused interventions provided by a psychiatrist in this context include diagnostic clarification and leadership in the assembly of a multidimensional treatment plan. For most nursing home residents suffering from mental disorders, the best outcomes likely result from optimal diagnostic accuracy and treatment that includes resident-focused psychotherapeutic or behavioral approaches, thoughtfully selected pharmacology, and specific modifications of the resident's milieu.

The liaison functions so vital to successful psychiatric care in the nursing home are varied. Clearly, the psychiatrist can be an essential resource to help staff to understand better the complex phenomenology and multifaceted treatment of dementia and mental illness in their work setting. The psychiatrist is also ably prepared to assist staff in effectively identifying and successfully managing their own job-related stress. Importantly, psychiatrists are often appropriately called upon to assist a nursing home's clinical or administrative staff in resolving conflict between the facility and a given resident's family members.

SUMMARY

In many respects, the contemporary nursing home, despite its staffing patterns and physical structure, is in large part a long-term psychiatric residential facility. Little research has been done to adequately inform the character of the best psychiatric clinical practices in this setting. However, existing data in the USA suggest that the need for formal psychiatric services in nursing homes is significant and largely under-met. By virtue of their interest and training, psychiatrists are well-suited to work as members of a multidisciplinary care team in the construction and implementation of a multidimensional treatment plan directed at a resident's mental disorder. Additionally, through the established role of liaison, the psychiatrist can do much to foster an improved sense of well-being among nursing home staff.

REFERENCES

1. German PS, Rovner BW et al. The role of mental morbidity in the nursing home experience. Gerontologist 1992; 32: 152–8.
2. Zimmer JG, Watson N, Treat A. Behavioral problems among patients in skilled nursing facilities. Am J Publ Health 1984; 74: 1118–21.
3. Rovner BW, Kafonek S, Filipp L et al. Prevalence of mental illness in a community nursing home. Am J Psychiatry 1986; 143: 1446.
4. Borson S, Liptzin B, Nininger J et al. Psychiatry in the nursing home. Am J Psychiat 1987; 144: 1412–18.
5. Rovner BW, German PS, Broadhead J et al. The prevalence and management of dementia and other psychiatric disorders in nursing homes. International Psychogeriatrics 1990; 2: 13–24.
6. Strahan GW. Prevalence of selected mental disorders in nursing and related care homes. In Manderscheid RW, Sonnenschein M, eds, Mental Health, United States. DHHS Publication No. (PHS) 90-3470. Rockville, MD: Agency for Health Care Policy and Research, 1990.
7. Rovner BW, Katz IR. Psychiatric disorders in the nursing home: a selective review of studies related to clinical care. Int J Geriat Psychiat 1993; 8: 75.
8. Smyer MA, Shea DG, Streit A. The provision and use of mental health services in nursing homes: results from the national medical expenditure survey. Am J Publ Health 1994; 84: 284–7.
9. Kim E, Rovner B. The nursing home as a psychiatric hospital. In Reichman WE, Katz PR, eds, Psychiatric Care in the Nursing Home. New York: Oxford University Press, 1996; 3–9.
10. Beardsley RS, Larson DB, Burns BJ et al. Prescribing of psychotropics in elderly nursing home patients. J Am Geriat Soc 1989; 37: 327–30.
11. Avorn J, Soumerai SB, Everitt DE et al. A randomized trial of a program to reduce the use of psychoactive drugs in nursing homes. N Engl J Med 1992; 327: 168.
12. Evans LK, Stumpf NE. Tying down the elderly: a review of the literature on physical restraint. J Am Geriat Soc 1989; 37: 65–74.
13. Tinetti ME, Liu WI, Marottoli RA et al. Mechanical restraint use among residents of skilled nursing facilities. J Am Med Assoc 1991; 265: 468–71.
14. Emerson Lombardo NB et al. Achieving Mental Health of Nursing Home Residents: Overcoming Barriers to Mental Health Care. Hebrew Rehabilitation Center for Aged, HCRA Research Training Institute, Boston, MA, and Mental Health Policy Resource Center, Washington, DC, 1996.
15. Cohen-Mansfield J, Marks M, Werner P. Agitation in elderly persons: an integrative report of findings in a nursing home. Int Psychogeriat 1992; 4(suppl 2): 221–40.
16. Ames D. Epidemiological studies of depression among the elderly in residential and nursing homes. Int J Geriat Psychiat 1991; 6: 347.
17. Rovner BW, German PS, Brant IJ et al. Depression and mortality in nursing homes. J Am Med Assoc 1991; 265: 993–6.
18. Katz IR, Parmelee PA, Streim JE. Depression in older patients in residential care: significance of dysphoria and dimensional assessment. Am J Geriat Psychiat 1995; 3: 161–9.
19. Junginger J, Phelan E, Cherr K et al. Prevalence of psychopathology in elderly persons in nursing homes and the community. Hosp Commun Psychiat 1993; 44: 381–3.
20. Parmelee PA, Katz IR, Lawton MP. Anxiety and its association with depression among institutionalized elderly. Am J Geriat Psychiat 1993; 1: 46–58.
21. Howell, T. Anxiety disorders. In Reichman WE, Katz PR, eds, Psychiatric Care in the Nursing Home. New York: Oxford University Press, 1996; 94–108.
22. Ancoli-Israel S, Klauber MR, Kripke DF et al. Sleep apnea in female nursing home patients: increased risk of mortality. Chest 1989; 96: 1054–8.
23. Bliwise DL, Bevier WC, Bliwise NG et al. Systematic 24-hour behavioral observations of sleep and wakefulness in a skilled nursing facility. Psychol Aging 1990; 5: 16–24.
24. Morriss RK, Rovner BW, Folstein MF, German PS. Delusions in newly admitted residents of nursing homes. Am J Psychiat 1990; 147: 299–302.
25. Chandler JD, Chandler JE. The prevalence of neuropsychiatric disorders in a nursing home population. J Geriat Psychiat Neurol 1988; 1: 71.
26. Reichman WE, Rabins, PV. Schizophrenia and other psychotic disorders. In Reichman WE, Katz PR, eds, Psychiatric Care in the Nursing Home. New York: Oxford University Press, 1996; 109–17.
27. Solomon K, Shackson JB. Substance abuse disorders. In Reichman WE, Katz PRT, eds, Psychiatric Care in the Nursing Home. New York: Oxford University Press, 1996; 165–87.
28. Reichman WE, Coyne AC, Borson S et al. Psychiatric consultation in the nursing home. A survey of six states. Am J Geriatr Psychiatry 1998; 6(4): 320–7.
29. Ancoli-Israel S, Parker L, Sinaee R et al. Sleep fragmentation in patients from a nursing home. J Gerontol Med Sci 1989; 44(1): M18–21.
30. Bliwise DL, Carroll JS, Dement WC. Predictors of observed sleep/wakefulness in residents in long-term care. J Gerontol Med Sci 1990; 45: M126–30.
31. Bliwise DL, Nino-Murcia G, Forno LS et al. Abundant REM sleep in a patient with Alzheimer's disease. Neurology 1990; 40: 1281–4.

Patient Autonomy vs. Duty of Care—
the Old Age Psychiatrist's Dilemma

Adrian Treloar

Memorial Hospital, London, UK

The twentieth century has seen huge transitions in medical and legal practice based upon changes in the philosophy underpinning the way in which doctors relate to patients. At its lowest points, the Nazi programmes of extermination and forced sterilization in the USA, Sweden and elsewhere have demonstrated the capacity of doctors for abuse of their patients[1]. In the UK poor-quality procedures around consent, and scandals such as patients being charged by carers for their weekly bath and other "privileges", have shown just how easy it is for the vulnerable to be abused. Arising from this has been a philosophical, legal and medical trend towards self-determination and autonomy. Advance directives have been promoted as a solution to the loss of autonomy. They have, however, been shown to have limitations. Indeed, one study found that the entire health gain from cardiac rehabilitation programmes was neutralized because patients in the study signed advance directives[2].

Old age psychiatry must, if it is honest, admit that it views autonomy as a limited concept. The use of legal tools such as the UK Mental Health Act to detain mentally ill patients, along with the widespread housing of demented people behind locked doors, even without a formal detention order[3], shows that autonomy does not rule undisputed. There is also evidence that the practice of administering medication covertly within foodstuffs is widespread in the UK[4]. How can we justify such acts? In a landmark judgement, the UK Law Lords held that the mentally incapacitated could be detained and treated in their best interests because it was their illness that primarily removed their autonomy and not the fact of their detention[5]. Doctors and others may therefore treat the mentally incapacitated against their wishes when the patients themselves will clearly benefit from such treatment.

This shows that old age psychiatrists have an inescapable and awesome responsibility to balance the principles of autonomy and good clinical care when they are in opposition. This balancing act must be open to scrutiny and requires that good clinical care of the patient is the focus. The twentieth century was too heavily littered with examples of patients' needs coming second to the intentions of others for it to be otherwise. In essence, to be trustworthy, doctors can never intend harm.

REFERENCES

1. Kevles DJ. Eugenics and human rights. *Br Med J* **319**: 435–8.
2. Treloar AJ. Advance directives: limitations upon their applicability in elderly care. *Int J Geriat Psychiat* 1999; **14**: 1039–43.
3. Shah A, Dickenson D. The Bournewood judgement and its implications for health and social services. *J Roy Soc Med* 1998; **91**: 349–51.
4. Valmana A, Rutherford J. Over a third of psychiatrists had given a drug surreptitiously or lied about a drug. *Br Med J* 1997; **314**: 300.
5. House of Lords. R v. Bournewood Community and Mental Health NHS Trust ex part L. Judgement, 25 June 1998.

131

Psychiatric Services in Long-term Care

Ira R. Katz[1,2], Kimberly S. Van Haitsma[3] and Joel E. Streim[1,2]

[1]University of Pennsylvania, [2]Philadelphia VA Medical Center and [3]Philadelphia Geriatric Center, Philadelphia, PA, USA

Older people require long-term care when they have care needs that go beyond what they and their families can provide. It can consist of subacute, step-down or convalescent care for individuals discharged from hospitals, rehabilitative services for those recovering from illness or injury, and hospice care for those with terminal illness, as well as life-long care for those with irreversible disability. Increasingly, the landscape of settings for long-term care is expanding to include home- and community-based programs. Even for those who require residential care, the options are expanding to include increasingly diverse forms of assisted living or personal care facilities, as well as nursing homes. Nevertheless, nursing homes remain the most important settings for long-term care, especially for those individuals who are oldest and most disabled. However, nursing homes are also evolving, with increasing numbers of patients admitted for short stays for subacute or rehabilitation care and a proliferation of special care units designed for patients with dementia.

According to recent government reports[1-4], there are approximately 1.6 million residents occupying 1.76 million beds in 16 840 American nursing homes. For persons who turned 65 in 1990, an estimated 43% will enter a nursing home at some time. Of this group, 55% will have a total lifetime use of at least 1 year, and 21% will have total lifetime use of 5 years or more. Although both the number of facilities and the number of beds increased almost 20% from the mid-1980s to the mid-1990s, they did not keep pace with the growth of the elderly population. The ratio of nursing home beds to the size of the population aged 75 years and over dropped 17% from 1987 to 1996—127–117 beds/1000 people. However, the occupancy rate declined from 92.3% in 1987 to 88.8% in 1996. Thus, the nursing home market is beginning to experience the combined effects of healthier aging and the availability of alternative approaches to long-term care.

US nursing homes are heterogeneous: 65.5% are for-profit vs. 27.9% non-profit, 6.6% are government-owned; 53.8% are owned by chains; and 13.6% are hospital-based. In 1997, 67.4% of nursing home costs were paid by Medicaid (approximately half of this paid by the federal government and half by the states), 9.4% by Medicare, and 23.3% from private funds or other payers. Federal payments account for the majority of expenditures for nursing home care and have been estimated in the late 1990s to be approximately $40 billion/year.

Among all US nursing home residents in 1996, the average age was 84.6; 9% were under 65, 12% 65–74, 30% 75–84 and 49% 85+; 71.6% of residents were women; 88.7% of residents were White, and 8.9% African-American; 13.9% required assistance with one or two activities of daily living tasks, and 83.3% with three or more; 88.2% required assistance with dressing, 96.5% with bathing, 59.7% with eating, 73.6% with transferring into or out of bed, 66.4% with mobility and 79.7% with toileting.

Compared to comparable findings from a decade earlier, the average age of residents increased by 0.9 years; the proportion aged 85+ increased from 49% to 56% for women and from 29% to 33% for men. Disability of residents also increased and the proportion of those requiring assistance in three or more activities of daily living was 15% higher in 1996 than 1987.

The psychiatric needs of nursing home residents are thus those of a population characterized by extreme old age and high levels of disability. Accordingly, the delivery of psychiatric services in the nursing home must be informed by knowledge of the clinical psychiatry of this population. However, mental health providers must also be aware of other factors that shape the delivery of care. These include the potential for use of the nursing home environment as a therapeutic agent, either in Special Care Units for dementia or in other programs, and the extensive federal regulations that govern clinical services in US nursing homes.

CLINICAL PSYCHIATRY IN THE NURSING HOME

According to recent reports from the Nursing Home Component of the Medical Expenditure Panel Survey (MEPS), approximately 48% of US nursing home residents have a diagnosis of a dementia[1]. However, this figure probably underestimates the actual prevalence. Other MEPS data demonstrate that approximately 70% of residents have memory problems, 73% orientation problems, and 80% impairments in decision-making capacity. It also estimates that approximately 30% of residents have behavioral problems; 11.8% are verbally abusive, 9.1% are physically abusive, 14.5% are socially inappropriate, 12.5% are resistive to care, and 9.4% wander. In addition to this high prevalence of cognitive impairment, the MEPS reports that approximately 20% of residents have a diagnosis of a depressive disorder. Comparing these figures with comparable data from a decade earlier suggests that the number of residents with diagnoses of dementia or depression has increased. However, the number of individuals with schizophrenia has declined, especially among the younger residents[5]. Findings from this national representative sample confirm earlier research reports about the high prevalence of psychiatric disorders in nursing home residents[6]. In particular, they support the validity and generalizability of estimates from research in a single facility that demonstrated that 80% of residents have a psychiatric diagnosis. Findings from this earlier research provided insight into the nature of the disorders; 67% of residents had dementia, with most having Alzheimer's disease; approximately 40% of those with dementia had other psychiatric syndromes as complications (psychosis 13.5%, depression 6.3%, and delirium 7.3%); and 12.8% had other psychiatric disorders, most

Principles and Practice of Geriatric Psychiatry, 2nd edn. Edited by J. R. M. Copeland, M. T. Abou-Saleh and D. G. Blazer
©2002 John Wiley & Sons, Ltd

commonly depression[7]. Among those with dementia, it was those with psychiatric complications who were most likely to exhibit behavioral problems.

The available findings suggest that, in spite of significant changes in American nursing homes over recent years, the high levels of psychiatric morbidity and the distribution of disorders has remained the same. There has, however, been significant progress in developing and validating treatments for psychiatric disorders in nursing homes. One particularly promising intervention for residents with dementia and behavioral problems combined augmented activities, guidelines for use of psychotropic medications, and educational rounds[8]. It was tested in a randomized clinical trial and found to be effective in reducing the prevalence of behavioral disorders and the use of both antipsychotic drugs and physical restraints. Another series of studies has shown that individualized consultations to staff nurses about the management of patients with dementia can reduce the use of physical restraints[9]. There has been little research on the effectiveness of specific psychotherapies for nursing home residents with depression. Although available findings are highly promising[10], research on individualized behavioral interventions for patients with behavioral and psychological symptoms of dementia have been limited to case series or small-scale controlled studies.

Psychotherapeutic medications are widely used in nursing homes. The US Health Care Financing Administration estimated that use of these agents increased during the 1990s from 21.7% in 1991 to 46.1% in 1997[3,4]. This reflected a 59.8% decrease in the use of antipsychotic medications from 33.7% to 16.1%, but a 97% increase in the use of antidepressants from 12.6% to 24.9%. These changes probably reflect a number of factors, including scientific developments, accumulating effects of professional education and specific federal regulations (as described below).

Two randomized clinical trials have demonstrated the efficacy of the atypical antipsychotic agent risperidone for the treatment of the psychotic and behavioral symptoms in residents with dementia[11,12]. The available findings suggest that it has both antipsychotic effects and independent effects on aggression or agitation. Longer-term follow-up studies suggest that it may cause less tardive dyskinesia than typical neuroleptics[13]. A randomized clinical trial of olanzepine vs. placebo has demonstrated similar efficacy[14] and additional findings on other atypical antipsychotic agents are expected in the near future. However, the controlled clinical trials on antipsychotic agents have evaluated only their acute effects, typically for periods of 6–12 weeks, and little is known about the effectiveness of antipsychotic drug treatment over longer periods of time. In fact, recent double-blind, placebo-controlled studies of neuroleptic discontinuation demonstrate that the majority of patients who have been receiving longer-term treatment with these agents can be withdrawn from them without ill-effects[15,16]. Two randomized clinical trials studies evaluated the efficacy of mood-stabilizing anticonvulsants for the treatment of agitation and aggression. One studied carbamazepine and found that it was effective for agitation, hostility and aggression but not for other symptoms, such as hallucinations or delusions[17]. Findings from staff reports demonstrated that treatment with active medication led to decreases in the nursing time required for patient care. Another recent study evaluated valproate vs. placebo and found evidence for efficacy[18].

There are now several acetylcholinesterase inhibitors approved for use in patients with mild to moderate Alzheimer's disease, and there have been questions about whether they are useful in treating nursing home residents with more advanced disease. One randomized clinical trial demonstrated that use of donepazil was associated with improvements in cognitive performance comparable to those observed in less impaired outpatients[19]. Although there have been suggestions that cholinesterase inhibitors may be useful in managing behavioral symptoms, this issue is unresolved at this time.

There have been two randomized clinical trials evaluating the effects of antidepressants in nursing home residents, both using the classical tricyclic nortriptyline. One of the studies was placebo-controlled[20]. Positive findings were used to confirm the validity of the diagnosis of major depression among nursing home residents in spite of potential confounds from medical, environmental and existential factors. Another finding from this study was that patients with major depression, low levels of serum albumin and high levels of self-care disability were less likely to respond to treatment; this led to the suggestion that patients with this clinical profile may benefit from early hospitalization and evaluation of the need for electroconvulsive therapy. The second study randomized patients to regular vs. low-dose nortriptyline and found significant plasma level response relationships in those patients who were cognitively intact, again confirming the validity of the diagnosis of depression[21]. However, the plasma level response relationship was significantly different in patients with dementia, suggesting that the depression of dementia may be a distinct disorder. There have been no randomized clinical trials of selective serotonin reuptake inhibitors (SSRIs) or related medications in nursing home residents, and available open-label studies have mixed results, especially with respect to the outcomes of treatment in nursing home residents with dementia[22–26]. In a related area, there is evidence from an older clinical trial that the stimulant medication methylphenidate may be useful in demented patients with symptoms of apathy and withdrawal[27].

The recent estimate that almost 25% of US nursing home residents are receiving an antidepressant medication reflects an extraordinary change in patterns for drug utilization, especially in light of findings indicating that a generation ago only 15% of residents with a known diagnosis of depression were receiving antidepressants[28]. Although significant components of current antidepressant usage may be for other putative indications, such as agitation, sleep or pain, it is important to note that reported utilization rates are comparable to estimates for the prevalence of depression. Research is needed to determine whether it is possible to demonstrate an impact of prescribing on the mental health of the population as a whole.

THE NURSING HOME AS A MENTAL HEALTH CARE ENVIRONMENT

In the past decade there has been a growing awareness of the importance of the psychosocial and mental health aspects of nursing home care and a number of conceptual models have been developed to focus on the person–environment interaction as the target for care practices. These have included "progressively lowered stress threshold"[29], "stimulation-retreat"[30], and "person-centered"[31–33] care. Other widely discussed concerns that reflect the increased awareness of the psychosocial aspects of nursing home care include quality of life[34], individualization of care[35], the importance of the patient's perspective[36,37], and autonomy[38,39].

Many of these concepts have been applied in the design and operation of special care units (SCUs) for residents with cognitive impairment. The popularity of these units has been phenomenal, with current estimates that 22% of nursing homes have designated SCUs for patients with dementia. Outcome studies evaluating special vs. traditional care have suggested positive effects in a variety of selected outcomes, such as the nature of the services provided, depression, family perception of quality of life and the rate of decline in mobility[40–43]. However, more rigorous randomized clinical trials have reported positive outcomes only in circumscribed areas, such as catastrophic reactions[44] and observed positive emotional responses[45].

While it is encouraging to find evidence that the outcomes of care in nursing homes may be modifiable, it is important to recognize that there are no effects that are consistent across studies. However, these mixed findings are not unexpected, given the tremendous variability in the definitions, structure and programs of SCUs as well as other methodological limitations, such as selection biases, attrition and measurement limitations. Therefore, many researchers have increasingly called for studies focused on the evaluation of specific interventions associated with improved comfort, health status and quality of life, in attempts to identify and evaluate the "active ingredients" of special care[37,46,47].

Many programs have been based upon modification of the physical environment to decrease behavioral difficulties and enhance positive quality of life in the nursing home. Promising programs that incorporate natural elements into the environment, include a bathing intervention that uses bird songs, pictures of nature and food during bathing to decrease agitated or aggressive behavior[48], and use of "white noise" machines emitting sounds of ocean waves or waterfalls[49]. The use of bright lights in the care environment has been shown to consolidate sleep and to reduce agitation, but only in those with disturbed sleep-wake cycles[50]. An intervention that decreased noise and light in the night-time environment did not, by itself, improve the quality of the residents' night-time sleep; however, when combined with a daytime program of increased physical activity, it did provide benefits[51,52].

Some programs have gained great popularity in the clinical community, but have not yet been evaluated in controlled studies. These include the "Eden Alternative", which attempts to increase biological diversity in the institutional setting by incorporating children, plants and animals into the day-to-day life of the nursing home[53], and horticultural interventions[54]. Another set of promising interventions are based upon spirituality or religiously-based programming[55,56]. Music therapies, in particular, have been studied more intensively and may be effective in increasing positive emotional and social engagement and decreasing problem behaviors[57].

Technological interventions have been used in the nursing home, either to provide enhanced surveillance to increase safety or to use modalities such as audio or videotapes as therapeutic tools. Only one of these therapeutic interventions has shown positive results after testing under controlled conditions—simulated presence therapy[58], in which residents with dementia are asked to listen to taped, simulated telephone conversations with family members, was superior to placebo in decreasing problem behaviors and increasing well-being.

Several studies have demonstrated efficacy in programs designed to promote functional independence in persons with dementia residing in the nursing home. One focused on altering "dependency support scripts" and found increased independent behavior on the part of residents[59]. Other studies have focused on evaluating programs designed to target specific functional capabilities. Several groups have found positive effects from programs that modify usual routines for morning care and dressing. One analyzed videotapes of dressing behaviors to develop care prescriptions, and found that these led to increased independence in dressing[60]. Another used a "skill elicitation" intervention and found that it significantly increased the amount of time participants were engaged in dressing and other ADLs, while simultaneously decreasing the frequency of disruptive behavior[61]. A third found that an "abilities-focused" program, teaching direct care staff to modify the moment-to-moment procedures used in morning care on the basis of knowledge of the residents' specific cognitive deficits, led to improvement in calm/functional behaviors, agitation and social functioning[62].

Other important factors affecting the psychosocial environment in nursing homes are those related to the caregiving staff. It is certified nursing assistants (CNAs) who serve as primary caregivers to a population characterized by ever-increasing levels of dementia, dependency and mental health disorders. There is no doubt that the increased demands on skills and time, together with the physically and emotionally demanding labor, require attention to selection, training, supervision, and a focus on the role of the CNA as a provider of psychosocial care. There are multiple sources of stress for these paraprofessionals, including individual self-related needs, off-the-job stressors, patient contact, and administrative and organizational factors. One study demonstrated that 57% of CNAs screen positive for clinically significant levels of distress[63]. However, the paraprofessional staff do not, as a rule, receive adequate support from the psychological and psychiatric community in addressing such issues as non-pharmacologic management techniques, assisting with family conflicts and coping with job-related stress[64].

Fortunately, there is evidence that training programs for CNAs can have positive outcomes for the CNAs, including increased interaction and sensitivity to resident cues, provision of more choice and praise, and increased behavioral management skills. Moreover, these can translate into improvements in residents' mood and functioning[65,66]. Another line of research has found that mental health outcomes can be affected by structural and organizational elements of nursing homes, such as chain status, size, staffing levels, turnover, staff selection, job assignments, job design and the adequacy of supplies; moreover, interventions modifying formal elements of staff management can have positive effects on staff behavior[67].

THE REGULATORY ENVIRONMENT IN US NURSING HOMES

Although nursing homes have historically been designed to care for patients with medical and surgical conditions, the vast majority of their residents have psychiatric disorders. The mismatch between resident needs and facility characteristics in US nursing homes has been associated with inadequate, inappropriate and even inhumane treatment[68]. During the 1980s, concerns expressed by advocacy and professional groups were reinforced by a report from the Institute of Medicine[69] documenting major problems in the quality of care provided in nursing homes. Specific issues included the undertreatment of depression and use of physical and chemical restraints to control behavioral symptoms in patients with dementia. Other concerns at that time were that elderly patients with chronic and severe psychiatric conditions were discharged from state hospitals and inappropriately placed in nursing homes at Medicaid expense, thereby denying them access to the active psychiatric treatment they needed, and shifting a substantial portion of the costs of their care from the states to the federal government.

Recognition of problems in the quality of care in US nursing homes, together with ongoing concerns about costs, prompted Congress to pass legislation, the Nursing Home Reform provisions of the Omnibus Budget Reconciliation Act (OBRA) of 1987[70], which has transformed nursing homes into one of the most highly regulated environments for healthcare delivery in the USA. To operationalize the laws enacted under OBRA '87, Congress directed the Health Care Financing Administration (HCFA), the agency that administers Medicare and Medicaid, to issue specific regulations that govern nearly all aspects of nursing home operations[71], and charged the states with the responsibility for conducting surveys to determine whether nursing facilities were in compliance. In response, HCFA developed a set of interpretive guidelines for state surveyors[72], which has been revised over the past 10 years to reflect changes in healthcare practice and policy. Mental health screening, evaluation, care planning and treatment are addressed under sections of the regulations related to resident assessment, resident rights, facility practices and quality of care.

The OBRA regulations require preadmission screening and annual resident review (PASARR) to prevent inappropriate nursing home admissions for patients with severe psychiatric disorders, and to ensure that those with acute psychiatric conditions are not placed in nursing homes before receiving the benefits of acute psychiatric treatment[73]. However, patients who have a primary diagnosis of dementia are considered eligible for nursing home admission regardless of psychiatric complications or co-morbid conditions. After admission to a nursing facility, all patients are required to undergo periodic comprehensive assessments using the Minimum Data Set (MDS), a standardized instrument that includes several areas relevant to mental health: mood, cognition, communication, behavior patterns, activities, functional status, psychosocial well-being, oral/nutritional status, co-morbid disease, medications and other treatments[74]. Responses on the MDS that indicate deficits or changes in the patient's health status serve as triggers for resident assessment protocols (RAPs), which are second-stage assessment tools that furnish prompts to help nursing staff recognize signs and symptoms that are indicators of potentially significant clinical problems, algorithms to direct further evaluations, and guidelines for treatment planning. RAP problem areas related to mental disorders and behavioral health include delirium, cognitive loss/dementia, psychosocial well-being, mood state, behavior problems, psychotropic drug use and physical restraints. The regulations hold facilities responsible for ensuring that the MDS is completed on time and the RAPs are followed.

The OBRA regulations also contain provisions that affect psychiatric treatment in the nursing home, prohibiting the use of physical restraints or psychotropic drugs when they are "administered for purposes of discipline or convenience and not required to treat the resident's medical symptoms" or promote improved functioning[71]. There are specific regulations concerning antipsychotic drugs, designed to ensure that residents receive these agents only when "necessary to treat a specific condition as diagnosed and documented in the clinical record". The regulations also require periodic "gradual dose reductions and behavioral interventions, unless clinically contraindicated, in an effort to discontinue these drugs". Syndromes such as delirium and dementia, when accompanied by agitated or psychotic features, are listed among the accepted indications for the use of these agents. However, use of these medications must be supported by documentation that there are specific target symptoms associated with resident distress, functional impairment or danger to self or others.

Regulations related to quality of care further require that each resident's drug regimen be free from unnecessary drugs, defined as any drug used in excessive dose (including duplicate therapy); for excessive duration; without adequate monitoring; without adequate indications for its use; or in the presence of adverse consequences indicating the need for dose reduction or discontinuation[71]. The interpretive guidelines that accompany these regulations specifically limit the use of antipsychotic drugs, antianxiety agents and sedative–hypnotics, but not antidepressants[72]. For each of these medications, the guidelines provide a list of acceptable indications as well as specific agents that may not be used; daily dose limits which, if exceeded, require documentation that the benefits justify the risks; requirements for monitoring treatment and adverse effects; and time frames for attempting dose reductions and discontinuation. These guidelines were updated in 1999 to reflect new clinical knowledge and accepted practice and to include newly approved drugs.

Beginning in July, 1999, HCFA introduced quality indicators (QIs) derived from the MDS to enable surveyors to compare individual facilities to others in the same state[75]. There are 24 QIs within 11 different domains, including behavioral/emotional problems, cognitive patterns and psychotropic drug use. Behavioral/emotional patterns cover the prevalence of behavioral symptoms affecting others (e.g. verbally or physically abusive, socially inappropriate or disruptive behavior); prevalence of symptoms of depression; and prevalence of depression without antidepressant therapy. The cognitive pattern domain examines the incidence of cognitive impairment when consecutive MDS assessments reveal new onset of impairments in short-term memory or decision-making ability. The psychotropic drug use domain includes the prevalence of antipsychotic use for patients without psychotic conditions, the prevalence of antianxiety/hypnotic use, and the prevalence of hypnotic use more than twice in the previous 7 days. QIs that are indirectly related to mental disorders and their treatment include the use of nine or more different medications, and the prevalence of falls, weight loss, daily physical restraints, and little or no activity. Whenever a review in any of these areas results in a deficiency citation, a plan of correction must be developed and approved.

SUMMARY

In spite of significant changes in American nursing homes over the past 10–15 years, the high prevalence rates for dementia and depression remain as persistent problems. Fortunately, there have been major advances in knowledge about the outcomes of psychiatric care for nursing home residents. Chapters in textbooks from a decade ago may have been eloquent about the need for mental health services, but they had little to say about their outcomes. Now, it is possible to review evidence for benefits of specific interventions. In addition to pharmacological and behavioral treatments that are designed to be delivered to individual patients, other interventions are designed for delivery to nursing units or to residential care facilities as a whole. Promising interventions in this domain include augmented activities, modifications of the physical environment, use of technologies to augment interpersonal interventions, modifications in patterns for the delivery of basic nursing care, staff education, and changes in administrative structures. All of these must be delivered in the context of a complex regulatory environment. Thus, the delivery of psychiatric services in nursing homes must attend to the needs of the individual patients and to the context in which they receive care. To be successful, it requires partnerships between mental health professionals, direct care staff and the facilities' administration.

REFERENCES

1. Krauss NA, Altman BM. *Characteristics of Nursing Home Residents— 1996. MEPS Research Findings No. 5*, AHCPR Pub. No. 99-0006. Rockville, MD: Agency for Health Care Policy and Research, 1998.

2. Rhoades J, Krauss N. *Nursing Home Trends, 1987 and 1996. MEPS Chartbook No. 3*, AHCPR Pub. No. 99-0032. Rockville, MD: Agency for Health Care Policy and Research, 1999.

3. Harrington C, Carrillo H, Thollaug SC, Summers PR. Nursing facilities, staffing, residents, and facility deficiencies, 1991–1997. Available at http://www.hcfa.gov/medicaid/nursfabk.pdf. Checked 9/07/00.

4. Health Care Financing Administration. A Report to Congress Study of Private Accreditation (Deeming) of Nursing Homes, Regulatory Incentives and Non-Regulatory Incentives, and Effectiveness of the Survey and Certification System. Available at http://www.hcfa.gov/medicaid/reports.htm. Checked 9/07/00.

5. Mechanic D. McAlpine DD. Use of nursing homes in the care of persons with severe mental illness: 1985 to 1995. *Psychiat Serv* 2000; **51**: 354–8.

6. Rovner BW, Katz IR. Psychiatric disorders in the nursing home: a selective review of studies related to clinical care. *Int J Geriat Psychiat* 1993; **8**: 75–87.

7. Rovner BW, German PS, Broadhead J *et al*. The prevalence and management of dementia and other psychiatric disorders in nursing homes. *Int Psychogeriat* 1990; **2**: 13–24.

8. Rovner BW, Steele CD, Shmuely Y, Folstein MF. A randomized trial of dementia care in nursing homes. *J Am Geriat Soc* 1996; **44**: 7–13.

9. Evans LK, Strumpf NE, Allen-Taylor SL *et al*. A clinical trial to reduce restraints in nursing homes. *J Am Geriat Soc* 1997; **45**: 675–81.

10. Allen-Burge R, Stevens AB, Burgio LD. Effective behavioral interventions for decreasing dementia-related challenging behavior in nursing homes. *Int J Geriat Psychiat* 1999; **14**: 213–28.

11. Katz IR, Jeste DV, Mintzer JE *et al*. Comparison of risperidone and placebo for psychosis and behavioral disturbances associated with dementia: a randomized, double-blind trial. *J Clin Psychiat* 1999; **60**: 107–15.

12. De Deyn PP, Rabheru K, Rasmussen A *et al*. A randomized trial of risperidone, placebo, and haloperidol for behavioral symptoms of dementia. *Neurology* 1999; **53**: 946–55.

13. Jeste DV, Okamoto A, Napolitano J *et al*. Low incidence of persistent tardive dyskinesia in elderly patients with dementia treated with risperidone. *Am J Psychiat* 2000; **157**: 1150–5.

14. Street JS, Tollefson GD, Tohen M *et al*. Olanzapine for psychotic conditions in the elderly. *Psychiat Ann* 2000; **30**: 191–6.

15. Cohen-Mansfield J, Lipson S, Werner P *et al*. Withdrawal of haloperidol, thioridazine, and lorazepam in the nursing home: a controlled, double-blind study. *Arch Intern Med* 1999; **159**: 1733–40.

16. Bridges-Parlet S, Knopman D, Steffes S. Withdrawal of neuroleptic medications from institutionalized dementia patients: results of a double-blind, baseline-treatment-controlled pilot study. *J Geriat Psychiat Neurol* 1997; **10**: 119–26.

17. Tariot PN, Erb R, Podgorski CA *et al*. Efficacy and tolerability of carbamazepine for agitation and aggression in dementia. *Am J Psychiat* 1998; **155**: 54–61.

18. Tariot PN, Schneider LS, Mintzer JE *et al*. Safety and tolerability of divalproex sodium in the treatment of signs and symptoms of mania associated with dementia: results of a double-blind, placebo-controlled trial. Presented at American Psychiatric Association New Research Symposium, 2000.

19 Tariot PN, Cummings JL, Katz IR *et al*. A randomized, double-blind, placebo-controlled study of the efficacy and safety of donepezil in patients with Alzheimer's disease in the nursing home setting (submitted manuscript).

20. Katz IR, Simpson GM, Curlik SM *et al*. Pharmacologic treatment of major depression for elderly patients in residential care settings. *J Clin Psychiat* 1990; **51**(suppl): 41–7.

21. Streim JE, Oslin DW, Katz IR *et al*. Drug treatment of depression in frail elderly nursing home residents. *Am J Geriat Psychiat* 2000; **8**: 150–9.

22. Oslin DW, Streim JE, Katz IR *et al*. Heuristic comparison of sertraline with nortriptyline for the treatment of depression in frail elderly patients. *Am J Geriat Psychiat* 2000; **8**: 141–9.

23 Trappler B, Cohen CI. Use of SSRIs in "very old" depressed nursing home residents. *Am J Geriat Psychiat* 1998; **6**: 83–9.

24. Trappler B, Cohen CI. Using fluoxetine in "very old" depressed nursing home residents. *Am J Geriat Psychiat* 1996; **4**: 258–62.

25. Magai C, Kennedy G, Cohen CI, Gomberg D. A controlled clinical trial of sertraline in the treatment of depression in nursing home patients with late-stage Alzheimer's disease. *Am J Geriat Psychiat* 2000; **8**: 66–74.

26. Rosen J, Mulsant BH, Pollock BG. Sertraline in the treatment of minor depression in nursing home residents: a pilot study. *Int J Geriat Psychiat* 2000; **15**: 177–80.

27. Kaplitz SE. Withdrawn, apathetic geriatric patients responsive to methylphenidate. *J Am Geriat Soc* 1975; **23**: 271–6.

28. Heston LL, Garrard J, Makris L *et al*. Inadequate treatment of depressed nursing home elderly. *J Am Geriat Soc* 1992; **40**: 1117–22.

29. Hall G, Gerdner L, Szygart-Stauffacher M, Buckwalter K. Principles of nonpharmacological management: caring for people with Alzheimer's disease using a conceptual model. *Psychiat Ann* 1995; **25**: 432–40.

30. Lawton MP, Van Haitsma KS, Klapper JA. Observed affect in nursing home residents. *J Gerontol Psychol Sci* 1996; **51**: P3–14.

31. Chestor R, Bender M. Brains, minds, and selves: changing conceptions of the losses involved in dementia. *B J Med Psychol* 1999; **72**: 203–16.

32. Kitwood T. *Dementia Reconsidered: The Person Comes First*. Buckingham: Open University Press, 1997.

33. Zeman S. Person-centered care for the patient with mid and late stage dementia. *Am J Alzheim Dis* 1999; **14**: 308–10.

34. Lawton MP. Quality of life in Alzheimer Disease. *Alzheim Dis Assoc Disord* 1994; **8**: 138–50.

35. Tornquist EM. *Individualized Dementia Care: Creative, Compassionate Approaches*. New York: Springer, 1996; 47–82.

36. Cotrell V, Schulz R. The perspective of the patient with Alzheimer's disease: a neglected dimension of dementia research. *Gerontologist* 1993; **33**: 205–11.

37. Kane R, Kane R, Ladd R. *The Heart of Long-term Care*. New York: Oxford University Press, 1998.

38. Cohen-Mansfield J, Werner P, Weinfield M, Braun J. Autonomy for nursing home residents: the role of regulations. *Behav Sci Law* 1995; **13**: 415–23.

39. Gamroth L, Semradek J, Tornquist E. *Enhancing Autonomy in Long-term Care: Concepts and Strategies*. New York: Springer.

40. Leon J, Ory M. Effectiveness of special care unit (SCU) placements in reducing physically aggressive behaviors in recently admitted dementia nursing home residents. *Am J Alzheim Dis* 1999; **14**: 270–7.

41. Frisoni G, Gozzetti A, Bignamini V *et al*. Special care units for dementia in nursing homes: a controlled study of effectiveness. *Arch Gerontol Geriat* 1998; **6**: 215–24.

42. Kutner N, Mistretta E, Barnhart H, Belodoff B. Family members' perceptions of quality of life change in dementia SCU residents. *J Appl Gerontol* 1999; **18**: 423–39.

43. Saxton J, Silverman M, Ricci E *et al*. Maintenance of mobility in residents of an Alzheimer's special care facility. *Int Psychogeriat* 1998; **10**: 213–24.

44. Swanson E, Maas M, Buckwalter K. Catastrophic reactions and other behaviors of Alzheimer's residents: special unit compared with traditional units. *Arch Psychiat Nurs* 1993; **7**: 292–9.

45. Lawton MP, Van Haitsma K, Klapper J *et al*. A stimulation-retreat special care unit for elders with dementing illness. *Int Psychogeriat* 1998; **10**: 379–95.

46. Marshall M, Archibald C. Long-stay care for people with dementia: recent innovations. *Rev Clin Gerontol* 1998; **8**: 331–43.

47. Sloane P, Lindeman D, Phillips C *et al*. Evaluating Alzheimer's special care units: reviewing the evidence and identifying potential sources of study bias. *Gerontologist* 1995; **35**: 103–11.

48. Whall A, Black M, Groh C *et al*. The effect of natural environments upon agitation and aggression in late stage dementia patients. *Am J Alzheim Dis* 1997; **12**: 216–20.

49. Burgio L, Scilley K, Hardin J *et al*. Environmental "white noise": an intervention for verbally agitated nursing home residents. *J Gerontol Psychol Sci* 1996; **51**: 364–73.

50. Lyketos C, Veiel L, Baker A, Steele C. A randomized controlled trial of bright light therapy for agitated behaviors in dementia patients residing in long-term care. *Int J Geriat Psychiat* 1999; **14**: 520–5.

51. Schnelle J, Atessi C, Al-Samarrai N *et al*. The nursing home at night: effects of an intervention on noise, light, and sleep. *J Am Geriat Soc* 1999; **47**: 430–8.

52. Alessi C, Yoon E, Schnelle J *et al*. A randomized trial of a combined physical activity and environmental intervention in nursing home residents: do sleep and agitation improve? *J Am Geriat Soc* 1999; **47**: 784–91.

53. Thomas W. *The Eden Alternative: Nature, Hope, and Nursing Homes*. Sherbourne, NY: Eden Alternative Foundation, 1994.

54. Ousset P, Nourhashemi F, Albarde J, Vellas P. Therapeutic gardens. *Arch Gerontol Geriat* 1998; **6**: 369–72.

55. Elliot H. Religion, spirituality, and dementia: pastoring to sufferers of Alzheimer's disease and other associated forms of dementia. *Disabil Rehab Int Multidisciplin J* 1997; **19**: 435–41.

56. Kirkland K, McIlveen H. Full circle: spiritual therapy for people with dementia. *Am J Alzheim Dis* 1999; **14**: 245–7.

57. Koger S, Chapin K, Brotons M. Is music treatment an effective intervention for dementia? A meta-analytic review of literature. *J Music Ther* 1999; **36**: 2–15.

58. Camberg L, Woods D, Ooi WL *et al.* Evaluation of simulated presence: a personalized approach to enhance well-being in persons with Alzheimer's Disease. *J Am Geriat Soc* 1999; **47**: 446–52.

59. Baltes M, Newmann E, Zank S. Maintenance and rehabilitation of independence in old age: an intervention program for staff. *Psychol Aging* 1994; **9**: 179–88.

60. Beck C, Heacock P, Mercer S *et al.* Improving dressing behavior in cognitively impaired nursing home residents. *Nurs Res* 1997; **46**: 126–32.

61. Rogers J, Holm M, Burgio L *et al.* Improving morning care routines of nursing home residents with dementia. *J Am Geriat Soc* 1999; **47**: 1049–57.

62. Wells DL, Dawson P, Sidani S *et al.* Effects of an abilities-focused program of morning care on residents who have dementia and on caregivers. *J Am Geriat Soc* 2000; **48**: 442–9.

63. Proctor R, Stratton-Powell H, Tarrier N, Burns A. The impact of training and support on stress among care staff in nursing and residential homes for the elderly. *J Ment Health* 1998, **7**. 59–70.

64. Reichman W, Coyne A, Borson S *et al.* Psychiatric consultation in the nursing home: a survey of six states. *Am J Geriat Psychiat* 1998; **6**: 320–7.

65. Beck C, Ortigara A, Mercer S, Shue V. Enabling and empowering certified nursing assistants for quality dementia care. *Int J Geriat Psychiat* 1999; **14**: 197–211.

66. Proctor R, Burns A, Powell HS *et al.* Behavioural management in nursing and residential homes: a randomised controlled trial. *Lancet* 1999; **354**: 26–9.

67. Stevens A, Burgio L, Bailey E *et al.* Teaching and maintaining behavior management skills with nursing assistants in a nursing home. *Gerontologist* 1998; **38**: 379–84.

68. Streim JE, Katz IR. Federal regulations and the care of patients with dementia in the nursing home. *Med Clin N Am* 1994; **78**: 895–909.

69. Institute of Medicine, Committee on Nursing Home Regulation. *Improving the Quality of Care in Nursing Homes*. Washington, DC: National Academy Press, 1986.

70. Omnibus Budget Reconciliation Act of 1987, Public Law, 100–203 (USA).

71. Health Care Financing Administration. Medicare and Medicaid: requirements for long-term care facilities, final regulations. *Fed Register* 1991; **56**: 48865–921.

72. Health Care Financing Administration. *State Operations Manual: Provider Certification, Transmittal No. 250*. Washington, DC: US Government Printing Office, 1992.

73. Health Care Financing Administration: Medicare and Medicaid programs: preadmission screening and annual resident review. Federal Register 1992; **57**;56450–504.

74. Health Care Financing Administration. Medicare and Medicaid: resident assessment in long-term care facilities. *Fed Register* 1992; **57**: 61614–733.

75. Clark TR (ed.). *Nursing Home Survey Procedures and Interpretive Guidelines. A Resource for the Consultant Pharmacist*, Section 3. Alexandria, VA: American Society of Consultant Pharmacists, 1999; 1–8.

Care in Private Psychiatric Hospitals

K. G. Meador[1], M. M. Harkleroad[2] and W. M. Petrie[2]

[1]Duke University, Durham, NC, and [2]Memory Disorders Center, Nashville, TN, USA

Psychiatric care and treatment for mental disorders in the elderly in a private psychiatric setting is fundamentally a public health issue. The location of treatment and the clinical services available are shaped by public policy, financial incentives and the emergence of managed care. With the implementation of the Medicare Part A Hospital Insurance Trust Fund, most acute inpatient psychiatric care and treatment for the elderly in the 1970s and 1980s occurred in special geropsychiatric units in general medical units and private psychiatric hospitals. Data reflect the trend of the shift from public sector inpatient care to private and general medical hospital inpatient units. State and county organizations providing mental health care decreased 7.6%, while private hospitals increased 95.5% and general medical hospitals with inpatient mental health services increased 21.6%. The relative percentage of mental health expenditures for state and county hospitals decreased from 48.5% in 1975 to 23.6% in 1994 for total mental health expenditures; while the percentage of expenditures for private psychiatric hospitals increased from 7.1% to 19.5% during that same time period. Outpatient and community-based programs, including partial hospital programs, increased as a relative percentage of total mental health expenditures from 1.8% in 1975 to 26.8% in 1994[1]. In addition to addressing concerns inherent to providing quality medical care, any discussion focused on the care of older persons must include content regarding the logistical and ethical dimensions of financial and familial responsibilities. In the context of an increasingly aged population, Henderson[2] challenges us with a public health agenda of: (a) developing "bold and innovative means for assisting families to care for a relative with dementia"; (b) improving the "contributions of general practice to the care of mental disorders in the elderly"; and (c) investigating the social environment of the mentally ill elderly and promoting more adaptive alternatives when feasible. These challenges are particularly pertinent in the private psychiatric facility, where the "financial disincentives and shortages of trained personnel"[3] common to the discipline of geropsychiatry are frequently amplified.

There are several factors that necessitate the private psychiatric community becoming more aggressive and innovative in the care of older persons, despite the substantial constraints and disincentives. The first is the void left by the inadequacies in the community mental health center and the shift from treatment in state and county hospital programs for this population[4]. Second, the overall demand for inpatient psychiatric treatment for the elderly has continued to grow as the number of elderly, especially those over 80, has grown dramatically[5]. A third factor leading to an increased demand for private psychiatric care is that internists and primary care physicians are frequently not trained in the behavioral management of geriatric patients, and there is a growing subspecialty of geriatric psychiatry which is generating paradigms for diagnosis and treatment of older persons with neuropsychiatric and behavioral disorders.

The World Health Organization has identified acute inpatient psychiatric care as an important component in the continuum of care for the elderly[6]. Although the USA and the American Psychiatric Association have not published specific practice guidelines for geriatric inpatient treatment, there are generally accepted principles of quality care and treatment of elderly individuals in inpatient settings. These principles of care include: preadmission screening and linkages with community providers of care; comprehensive assessment and care planning; multidisciplinary staff with specialized experience and interest in the elderly; ongoing staff training and education; therapeutic programming and care approaches sensitive to the needs of an aging population; environmental and physical design of program; individual, group and family therapy; discharge and aftercare planning. With the emergence of managed care and financial incentives for community care, there has been a lack of coordination and integration of mental health services, especially for the elderly with severe mood disorders, psychosis, and dementing illnesses with complicating psychiatric and behavioral disorders. These forces combine to magnify significant gaps in treatment for the most frail and psychiatrically needy elderly who need comprehensive psychiatric and medical treatment, most appropriately provided in an acute inpatient geropsychiatric treatment program. Keill[7] proposes that it is "still possible within the system and with proper incentives to provide an accessible, comprehensive network". He emphasizes that within this network there must be a continuity of care, which is defined by Bachrach[8] as "a process involving the orderly, uninterrupted movement of patients among the diverse elements of the service delivery system". In the context of these challenges and stipulations, we present an example of a geropsychiatry service in a private hospital through which such issues can be discussed.

DESCRIPTION OF PROGRAM

The Parthenon Pavilion at Centennial Medical Center in Nashville, Tennessee, is a 162 bed private proprietary psychiatric hospital that has developed a cost-effective model program for the delivery of acute inpatient geropsychiatric services. The hospital currently operates two 12 bed Alzheimer's disease and related disorders–memory disorders units and a 16 bed general

Principles and Practice of Geriatric Psychiatry, 2nd edn. Edited by J. R. M. Copeland, M. T. Abou-Saleh and D. G. Blazer
©2002 John Wiley & Sons, Ltd

geropsychiatry unit, which together function as a regional referral center for the treatment of the elderly with complex and concurrent psychiatric and medical problems. Parthenon Pavilion's geriatrics program opened in 1985 and the original memory disorders unit was developed in 1987. This program provides a structure for supporting continuity of care by organizing clinical services and concentrating resources around the diverse and specialized needs of patients with severe psychiatric disorders, often complicated by behavioral difficulties and/or serious medical problems. The hospital also includes a geriatric partial hospitalization program which adds another dimension to the continuum of psychiatric care for senior adults.

Clinical Process

The geriatrics program has developed a philosophy of treatment and a clinical services model that places an emphasis on interdisciplinary care, so as to provide psychiatric and medical management of treatable symptoms in order to reduce distress, disability and complications in the older patient. A second major tenet of the program's treatment philosophy is that the family and professional caregiver systems are helped by providing: (a) accurate diagnosis and education around the nature of disease processes in the context of the unique manifestations of a disease in a given individual; and (b) supportive assistance and practical guidance tailored to the care and management issues of a given patient and caregiver system. This clinical services model also places a high priority on providing consultative and clinical liaison services to families, agencies, nursing homes and residential facilities, to assure continuity of care and maintenance of the clinical goals established during hospitalization for patients after they are discharged from the program.

The importance of family involvement in such a program cannot be overstated. Hardwig[9] challenges the ethically simplistic notions of patient autonomy frequently espoused when he points out the integral role of the family in making medical decisions. This is especially relevant when working with older persons, due to the prevalence of cognitive impairment found in this group. When a patient becomes demented, family members must frequently assume decision making in medical situations. This may violate family taboos as well as established patterns of family interaction, which may require renegotiation. Family conferences, as a means for mediating the moral process of medical decision-making and planning for ongoing care, are an integral aspect of the clinical services offered by the Geriatric Program, and result in a consistently high level of family satisfaction.

Administrative and Team Function

The administrative structure of this program includes: the clinical director, who is a psychiatrist specializing in geropsychiatry; a program director who is a Master's-trained social worker; a nurse manager with experience in geriatric nursing; and access to a clinical nurse specialist with a Master's degree in psychiatric nursing. The clinical director provides leadership in program planning, program evaluation and quality assurance, while also being available to provide consultation to other attending psychiatrists as needed. The program director coordinates the day-to-day operation of the program and works closely with the clinical director and nurse manager in implementing the above-designated functions.

Each patient has an attending psychiatrist, who directs the treatment, meets with families in diagnostic feedback conferences, participates in clinical liaison activities with nursing homes and

other placement facilities and develops an aftercare plan, along with other disciplines represented on the staff[10]. The program is supported by a number of psychiatrists with added qualifications in geriatric psychiatry and considerable experience in the treatment of such patients. Although many private psychiatric facilities have limited professional staff with particular expertise in geriatrics, such persons are increasingly available, due to an increasing number of specialized training programs. The program is joined by a group of board-certified internists, who have special interest and expertise in evaluating and treating acute and chronic medical problems in the elderly. Upon admission, the internist conducts a comprehensive review of systems and physical examination on each patient. Throughout the hospitalization, the internist provides follow-up of existing or developing medical problems and, when necessary, participates in family conferences and team staffing. Medical subspecialists, such as neurologists and cardiologists, are consulted when clinically indicated and their availability is fostered by the fact that the hospital/program is part of a regional tertiary care medical center which also provides access to available technology, brain imaging, laboratory services and specialized neuropsychological testing as medically indicated.

Nursing care is delivered through a primary nursing system. Nurses are recruited who have strong medical/surgical background along with geropsychiatric interests[11]. Meeting these staffing demands remains challenging, particularly in an era when most hospitals are experiencing professional nursing shortages. Supportive nursing administration within the program and the promotion of educational opportunities have fostered a reduced staff turnover rate well below the 20% annual rate experienced nationally[12]. The program director and the nurse manager are involved in pre-admission screening and clinical liaison activities, along with providing inpatient clinical services to family and professional caregivers. The social workers coordinate discharge planning and aftercare follow-up, which is a vital linkage in maintaining continuity of care. Activity therapists conduct functional assessments and design appropriate activities for the units within the program, according to the level of function of the patients. They can provide feedback to families and professional caregivers regarding functional abilities and deficits, making recommendations for modifications in the patient's environment and activities to support remaining abilities. Staff education is conducted through a variety of means, including weekly teaching rounds conducted by the clinical director, monthly interdisciplinary staff education meetings, and special teaching modules designed by the clinical nurse specialist.

Physical and Environmental Features

The physical design of the geriatric program provides for separate units divided by a nursing station. Two are for patients with dementia and memory disorders; the other for the general geriatric population. Prior to the development of the specialty units, demented patients were integrated with non-demented patients and separate therapeutic activities and groups were planned for each population[13]. However, it ultimately was determined that separating the program into specialty units, serving cognitively impaired patients with Alzheimers's disease and related disorders and a general geropsychiatric unit provided the optimal arrangement both clinically and administratively. The memory disorders units are designed for security and have unit doors that can be locked. Such a unit is specifically designed and adapted for the particular needs of sensory and cognitively impaired persons. There is an emphasis on music, videotapes and appropriate sensory stimulation without overload. The general geropsychiatry unit and the memory disorders units are pod-shaped, with a day room outside the bedrooms, and have activity rooms that can be used for special activities as needed. The care environments are designed to be adaptive in nature and focus upon remaining rather than lost abilities.

Financial Considerations

A necessity in the private psychiatric hospital is to operate in a cost-effective manner, so that the program does not have a significantly negative financial impact on the hospital. One means of achieving this goal has been to establish a program-based preadmission screening and consultative service to assure that each person admitted to the program meets Medicare intensity and severity criteria for a psychiatric admission. The preadmission service also screens for persons primarily needing medical treatment or long-term care, and focuses on orientating the family and referral sources to the goals and limitations of inpatient psychiatric treatment. Consultative and crisis management assistance is provided when hospital treatment is either inappropriate or not immediately available.

Another means of maintaining cost-effective utilization of resources is to avoid inappropriately extended stays by assuring that discharge planning begins with the preadmission process and is an integral aspect of ongoing treatment. Length of patient stay is monitored through a case review-orientated quality assurance program, coordinated by the program director working in cooperation with the clinical director. Regular review of the length of stay and systematic documentation of reasons for continued hospitalization not only enhances the quality of care but also provides a peer-reviewed justification for continued stay when reviewed by regulatory agencies. A major challenge during the past decade has been the shift to Medicare Managed Care, an HMO, for cost containment and utilization. A goal of such programs is to achieve more cost-effective care and treatment and to prevent unnecessary hospitalization. However, aggressive cost containment can negatively affect access and quality of care for the elderly with severe mental disorders and dementia, complicated by co-morbid medical conditions. This effort has resulted in undertreatment and limited access to inpatient care. In addition, with psychiatric care "carved out" of medical benefits and financial incentives to limit care, the distinction between medical and psychiatric coverage in demented patients may have significant financial impact on third-party payers.

Summary

In summary, the key elements of the program used in the model emphasize: (a) preadmission assessment and screening in the context of consultative services; (b) treatment by an interdisciplinary team, which includes an attending psychiatrist, internist, primary nurse, social worker, activities therapist and other ancillary staff, each with a commitment to the particular needs of the older person; (c) individualized educational programs for families and professional caregivers to augment existing clinical services; (d) individualized behavioral approaches that incorporate written behavioral management plans as an adjunct or substitute for psychopharmacological approaches; (e) discharge and aftercare planning services, family conferences and post-hospitalization follow-up with families and institutional caregivers; (f) environmental and physical design; and (g) cost-effective inpatient treatment. Approaches for assuring continuity of care for individual patients with complicated behavioral and psychiatric symptoms have included written behavioral prescriptions for families and caregivers, demonstrations of appropriate caregiving techniques during hospitalization, and videotape demonstrations designed to serve as training tools for nursing

home staff members. In 1999, Parthenon Pavilion provided leadership and financing for a new initiative to focus on improved mental health care for older adults. The initiative represents an innovative approach to clinical collaboration among select organizations providing mental health services to the elderly. The clinical Senior Links mental health consortium included representatives from home health, the local mental health association and Alzheimer's association, a community mental center and senior center providing community-based mental health services, staff of Parthenon Pavilion, and geriatric partial hospital programs located in the community. This program serves as a potentially innovative approach to improve the delivery of mental health services for senior adults and provides a forum for focusing on improved access, assessment and treatment, aftercare coordination and education for the consortium members and the community.

CHALLENGES FOR THE FUTURE

The primary challenges facing private psychiatric hospitals serving the elderly include: (a) monitoring and modifying admission criteria as Medicare intensity and severity criteria continue to become more restrictive and prospective payment is implemented; (b) developing intervention strategies with family caregivers to avoid inappropriately extended stays for non-clinical reasons; (c) maintaining quality care in the context of financial disincentives, especially magnified by increased enrollment in Medicare managed care plans, and regulatory policies which impact negatively on hospitals serving geriatric patients with severe psychiatric illnesses frequently complicated by behavioral and medical problems; (d) maintaining quality staff in all disciplines, especially with the growing nursing shortages and shrinking revenues; (e) developing consultative and outreach services to respond to the growing trend for nursing homes to serve increased numbers of residents with mental disorders and severe dementia with psychiatric and behavioral disorders.

We face these challenges in a cultural and federal regulatory environment that is ambivalent at best in its support of Medicare. Medicare accounted for only 9% of the federal budget in the USA in 1989, but sustained 36% of all budgeting cutbacks. Of even greater consequence for the elderly with mental disorders is the fact that Medicare spends only 3% of its budget on mental health care[14]. The claims are made that "key business values, including attention to a guiding mission statement, the needs of consumers, accountability and marketing, have a positive impact on the quality of milieu treatment"[15], but these assertions are put forth in a consumer-market paradigm and the pitfalls of this approach have not been adequately assessed. Tischler[16] points out the lack of systematic studies that include qualitative intermediate or long-term outcomes of mental health care. Studies examining utilization review outcomes have included only service utilization and expenditures. The program model presented here is committed to perpetual quality improvement, but clinical quality and reimbursement issues are inextricably linked in the private setting and future excellence may be jeopardized if current trends continue.

REFERENCES

1. National Center for Health Statistics. *Health, United States, 2000. With Adolescent Health Chartbook.* Hyattsville, MD: National Center for Health Statistics, 2000.
2. Henderson AS. The social psychiatry of later life. *Br J Psychiat* 1990; **156**: 645–53.
3. Moak GS. Improving quality in psychogeriatric treatment. *Psychiat Clin N Am* 1990; **13**(1): 99–110.

4. Keill SL. Integration of psychiatric services into a comprehensive health care system for the aged. *Bull NY Acad Med* 1986; **62**: 182–7.

5. Fredman L, Haynes SG. An epidemiologic profile of the elderly. In Phillips HT, Gaylord SA, eds, *Aging and Public Health*. New York: Springer, 1985.

6. Skeet M. The influence of world trends upon health. *Curationis* 1983; **6**: 11–15.

7. Keill SL. Integration of psychiatric services into a comprehensive health care system for the aged. *Bull NY Acad Med* 1986; **62**: 182–7.

8. Bachrach LL. Continuity of care for chronic mental patients: a conceptual analysis. *Am J Psychiat* 1981; **138**: 1449–56.

9. Hardwig J. What about the family? *Hastings Center Rep* 1990; **20**: 5–10.

10. Gaitz CM. Multidisciplinary team care of the elderly: the role of the psychiatrist. *Gerontologist* 1987; **27**: 553–6.

11. Robinson L. The future of psychiatric/mental health nursing. *Nurs Clin No Am* 1986; **21**: 537–43.

12. Jones CB. Staff nurse turnover costs: part II. Measurements and results. *J Nurs Admin* 1990; **20**: 27–32.

13. Beehan P, Roman M, Wells CE. A comprehensive inpatient service. *Generations* 1986; **10**: 1–3.

14. Strickler MD. Hospitals take charge: survival tactics for the 90s. *Psychiat Hosp* 1990; **21**: 183–8.

15. Fleming IL. Business values and quality in psychiatric hospital treatment. *Psychiat Hosp* 1989; **20**: 115–23.

16. Tischler GL. Utilization management of mental health services by private third parties. *Am J Psychiat* 1990; **147**: 967–73.

133

Quality of Care and Quality of Life in Institutions for the Aged

M. Powell Lawton

Philadelphia Geriatric Center, PA, USA

Although the form and function of the institution for older people changed considerably over the second half of the twentieth century in the USA, UK and other countries, the central task endures—providing protective care for older people unable to care independently for themselves. At the beginning of this period there were still people in the system whose lack of independence was primarily financial. Physical ill-health and, later and into the present, mental and cognitive ill-health became the main reason for entry into an institution.

The details of how such care was delivered differed in major ways across countries, to the point where knowledgeable comparisons were possible only for highly specialized experts who had the time to become familiar with more than one system. The present chapter is written when such differences are still evident. It is thus necessary at the outset to acknowledge that any attempted generalization about institutions for the aged must be interpreted in the light of differing cross-national social and cultural traditions. Nonetheless, this chapter will assert that there are characteristics common across localities that are universally accepted as indicators of quality of care and quality of life in institutions for older people (sometimes referred to as "nursing homes", as in the USA).

After establishing the importance of the quality concept, this chapter will review issues in maintaining quality in this type of residential case. Some of the recent literature will be reviewed, followed by the presentation of a model for defining quality of care and quality of life now under development by Rosalie Kane, Robert Kane and the author.

WHY BE CONCERNED ABOUT QUALITY IN NURSING HOMES?

Quality has been an issue among US nursing homes from the beginning of such institutions. Governmental monitoring of quality has been a threat to for-profit entities because their profits might be threatened by external quality-monitoring efforts. Poor quality may also be found among governmentally sponsored and non-profit homes. Suffice it to say that there has always been a major gap between accepted standards and the actuality of care, sometimes to a shockingly unacceptable degree, in the USA.

Governmental regulation, although resisted by many elements of the nursing home network, has been the major device used to enhance the quality of nursing home care in the USA. The system now in place requires each state to hire and train professionals ("surveyors") to spend time at least every second year on site with staff, residents and archival records to assess each institution on a series of written standards.

The procedure for monitoring nursing home quality required by the US government is instructive in defining current standards. There are 185 such regulations, which are organized into 15 categories: resident rights; admission/discharge rights; resident behavior and institutional practices; quality of life; resident assessment; quality of care; nursing services; dietary services; physician services; rehabilitation services; dental services; pharmacy services; infection control; physical environment; and administration[1]. Classification problems are immediately apparent. All categories are aspects of quality of care, and many may also reflect quality of life. Both of these subcategories are defined for monitoring purposes in a much more limited way than seems appropriate to this author. In 1997 the 10 most prevalent deficiencies in US nursing homes were: food sanitation; resident assessment; care plans; accidents; pressure sores; quality of care; restraint use; housekeeping quality; dignity; and accident prevention[2].

Citation for deficiencies may result in fines, temporary suspension of reimbursement for care or, at worst, removal of a license and closing of the institution. Suspension of reimbursement or license rarely occurs; in fact, the problems of finding care for residents in the offending institution are viewed as more stressful than continued low-grade care. Regulation is quite different, of course, in the UK. For instance, until recently it was only privately-administered facilities that were subjected to outside regulation, on the theory that local authorities were, by definition, assuring adequate quality by the nature of their direct responsibility for care[3]. This separation has changed, however. It seems likely that the phenomena of diversification of sponsorship (especially into the for-profit sector) and the need for local authorities to lean more heavily on professionals for quality controls than on local monitoring will make the two countries' systems become more similar in the future.

DEFINING QUALITY OF CARE

The classic system view of the health-care institution denotes the structural, given characteristics as input, care and treatment as process, and the resultant effect on the patient as output[4]. It has been noted frequently that output is difficult to identify when the institution constitutes the last residence and the final outcome is death. In addition, research over the past couple of decades has demonstrated the dynamic character of the structure of institutions. Administrative, care-delivery and physical environmental changes in fashion, including remodeling and simple space-use changes designed to encourage desired behaviors, attest to the ability of most institutional elements to be shaped toward higher-quality care[5].

Thus the literature of quality of care has been characterized either by value-based assertions that particular processes were intrinsically associated with higher quality of care, or were statistically correlated with overall quality as assessed by experts. The Institute of Medicine (IOM) report on nursing home quality called for making direct assessments of performance outcomes in terms of clearly undesirable states, such as death rate, infection rate, decubitus rate, or malnutrition[6]. More recently, other indicators reported on the required periodic assessment contained in the Minimum Data Set of the US nursing home system (MDS) have included accidents, questionable medication use, restraint use, infections and other obviously undesirable outcomes[7,8].

DEFINING QUALITY OF LIFE

Clearly, poor-quality care will lower overall quality of life. A distinction between quality of care and quality of life is useful to make, however. In a rough sense, quality of life must include features of everyday life that enhance enjoyment and sense of hope or purpose above the average level. An individual's quality of life is a subjective assessment made by that person alone. Quality of life of an environment, such as a nursing home, is represented by institutional attributes that have a statistical probability of leading to higher individually perceived quality of life for its occupants. There is thus a dual perspective on quality of life, the individual–subjective and the environmental–objective[9].

If quality of life is to be monitored, both perspectives must be assessed. Ideally, positive features of residential care would be identified by their association with positive subjective responses by a majority of the consumers of such care. The importance of the consumer was recognized in the regulations that followed passage of the Nursing Home Reform section of 1987 legislation[10]. Nursing homes are required to solicit opinions on the quality of care and quality of life experienced by residents.

In practice, however, it is not possible to demonstrate a direct parallel between nursing home resident perspectives and features that represent quality in the institution. Until the state of the art of measuring both consumer evaluation and environmental attributes is further advanced, it is necessary to make many assumptions about what constitutes quality, based on the available literature. Thus, the assessment system must encompass a large array of both personal and environmental features.

A Conceptual Basis for the Search for Quality

Kane, Kane and Lawton[11] have found it convenient to organize quality into 11 domains: security; functional competence; comfort; dignity; autonomy; privacy; meaningful activity; social relationships; enjoyment; individuality; and spiritual well-being. These domains represent universal individual needs, whose satisfaction may be enhanced or blocked by the environment in which the person pursues the gratification of needs. In overview, an approach to assessment evaluates the extent to which residents' needs are fulfilled and the extent to which environmental features relevant to these needs are present. Although the actual design of the measures is still in process, their components may be viewed as a model that could be useful for later investigators.

Resident Needs

Many modes of consumer assessment have recently become available[12,13]. Our own approach queries residents systematically about their evaluation of how well the residential environment fits each need. All such direct approaches require ordinary comprehension of questions and the willingness to respond frankly. Because many people in residential care are cognitively impaired and others may be loath to express critical comments, other complementary or parallel sources of information must be sought.

Resident Needs as Perceived by Others

Caregiving staff and family members are an obvious source of information on some domains. Such characteristics as functional health, cognitive performance, participation in activities or depression may be rated by an outsider. Some intrinsically subjective domains are less amenable to these types of judgments, e.g. the degree to which dignity is experienced in nursing home life. An outsider may assess a resident's ongoing affect states but clearly is limited in access to the resident's actual happiness, sadness or other feeling states[14].

Direct Observation

On the other hand, systematic observation by research staff or quality-control staff may reveal very concrete instances of behavior relevant to quality of care and quality of life. An observer may be trained to be less susceptible to bias than the resident in terms of denying socially unacceptable behavior, and is capable of being instructed in the subtle indicators of quality that may be exhibited in settings such as morning care, mealtimes, activities or unprogrammed time. Examples from earlier research include systematic observation of the "behavior stream" or the non-verbal indicators of emotional state[14,15]. It is also possible to train experts in more global aspects of direct observation that focus on concepts rather than small behavioral acts. The Professional Environmental Assessment Protocol (PEAP)[16], for example, requires an environmentally trained professional to spend about an hour in a care area, after which global ratings are made on the environment's ability to foster orientation, safety and security, privacy, stimulation quality, regulation of stimulation, functional competence, personal control, and continuity of self[17]. One important way in which direct observation adds to the quality attainment process is that it allows for the input of expertise in judgments of quality. Not all goal-relevant information is evident to the consumer. Some of what is learned from observation is thus complementary to the resident's perspective.

Integrating the perspectives of residents, significant others and objectively-viewed phenomena is not a straightforward process. Although most experts would wish to give primacy to the views of residents themselves, around 20–40% are cognitively unable to express evaluations and preferences that might guide the enhancement of quality[18]. It might be argued that the most-capable 60% should be able to articulate a consumers' view that would also fit the cognitively impaired. We must recognize, however, that major impairments in cognitive and self-care ability may also translate into needs quite different from those who are intact. The perspectives of significant others and value-judgments based on observable behavior clearly add something to knowledge about quality. Yet we cannot automatically substitute them for the absent judgments of those who are too impaired to be questioned. At best, putting together the three perspectives is at present more an artistic endeavor than a scientific one. How one accounts for biases in perspectives or for the differential weighting of the several types of input into measuring quality are tasks for the future.

The Economic Perspective

This chapter cannot do justice to the economic ramifications of quality of care and quality of life. In general, increased quality comes at a cost. In the case of both the profit-seeking institution and the governmental or non-profit institution, there are obvious constraints on the extent to which higher quality can be financed. This observation helps identify another distinction between quality of care and quality of life. Quality of care, being a life-and-health issue, is capable of being defined in terms of minimally acceptable threshold levels. These levels can in turn be defined reasonably clearly and used as the basis for licensing or potential decertification.

CONCLUSION

It is a different issue whether what has been defined as quality of life can be audited and used legally to improve the quality of nursing homes. Surveyors could conceivably become equipped to diagnose quality-of-life deficiencies and cite them to the point of removal of licensure. This appears problematic because quality of life has so many subjective aspects. Surveyors would no doubt be reluctant to make such citations and political pressure from owners would minimize the legal clout of such citations. One possible outcome is that the present survey process will continue to be used to correct the most egregious lapses in minimum quality of care. Beyond the merely adequate quality of care attained by correcting basic deficiencies, improvement in quality of life up through the positive to excellent ranges may be a matter better controlled by the marketplace than by legal enforcement. Quality-of-life audits could lead toward intrafacility self-assessment, staff training and growth, articulating possible avenues for improvement on which administration and staff could work proactively. The greatest weakness of the market-place hypothesis, however, is that the present market is responsible primarily to the upper income range of client families. If market-driven improvement in quality of life is to occur, we should have to see greater equalization of opportunity and increasing competition for the patronage of government-subsidized residents as well as those who pay in full for their care. Despite such difficulties, we should leave room for the possibility that improved quality of life in nursing homes may emerge better with indigenous rather than legal motivation. In the UK, there is some hope that the cultural and ethical norms may support the general public and governmental view that quality of care and quality of life are both basic rights of all citizens. This motivation might over time become more effective than either legal regulation or market competition[19].

REFERENCES

1. US Department of Health and Human Services (HHS), Health Care Financing Administration. *State Operations Manual. Provider Certification*, nos 272, 273 and 274. Washington, DC: DHHS, 1995.
2. Harrington C, Carrillo H, Thollang SC, Summers PR. *Nursing Facilities, Staffing, Residents, and Facility Deficiencies.* San Francisco, CA: University of California Department of Social and Behavioral Sciences, 1997.
3. Peace SM. Caring in place. In Brechin A, Walmsley J, Katz J, Peace S, eds. *Care Matters: Concepts, Practice, and Research in Health and Social Care.* London: Sage, 1998.
4. Donabedian A. Evaluating the quality of medical care. *Milbank Memorial Fund Qu* 1966; **44**: 166–206.
5. Hiatt LG. *Nursing Home Renovation Designed for Reform.* Boston, MA: Butterworth Architecture, 1991.
6. Institute of Medicine. *Improving the Quality of Care in Nursing Homes.* Washington, DC: National Academy Press, 1986.
7. Morris JN, Hawes C, Fries BE. Designing the national resident assessment instrument for nursing homes. *Gerontologist* 1990; **30**: 293–302.
8. Zimmerman DR, Karon SL, Arling G et al. Development and testing of nursing home quality indicators. *Health Care Financ Rev* 1995; **16**: 107–36.
9. Lawton MP. A multidimensional view of quality of life. In Birren JE, Lubben JE, Rowe JC, Deutchman DE, eds, *The Concept and Measurement of Quality of Life in the Frail Elderly.* New York: Academic Press, 1991; 3–17.
10. Congress of the United States. Public Law 100–203 (Omnibus Budget Reconciliation Act of 1987). Washington, DC: US Congress, 1987.
11. Kane RA, Kane RL, Lawton MP. Measurement, indicators, and improvement of the quality of life in nursing homes. Contract with Health Care Financing Administration. Minneapolis, MN: Division of Health Care Services Research and Policy, University of Minnesota, 1999.
12. Applebaum RA, Straker JK, Geron SM. *Assessing Satisfaction in Health and Long-term Care.* New York: Springer, 2000.
13. Cohen-Mansfield J, Ejaz F, Werner P. *Consumer Surveys in Long-term Care.* New York: Springer, 1999.
14. Lawton MP, Van Haitsma K, Klapper J. Observed affect in nursing home residents with Alzheimer's disease. *J Gerontol Psychol Sci* 1996; **51B**: P3–14.
15. Van Haitsma K, Lawton MP, Kleban MH et al. Methodological aspects of the study of behavior in elders with dementing illness. *Alzheim Dis Assoc Disord* 1997; **11**: 228–38.
16. Weisman J, Lawton MP, Sloane PS et al. *The Professional Environmental Assessment Protocol.* Milwaukee, WI: School of Architecture University of Wisconsin at Milwaukee, 1996.
17. Lawton MP, Weisman G, Sloane P et al. A Professional Environmental Assessment Procedure for special care units for elders with dementing illness and its relationship to the Therapeutic Environment Screen Schedule. *Alzheim Dis Assoc Disord* 2000; **14**: 28–38.
18. Simmons SF, Schnelle JF, Uman GC et al. Selecting nursing home residents for satisfaction surveys. *Gerontologist* 1997; **37**: 543–50.
19. Peace S, Kellaher L, Willcocks D. *Re-evaluating Residential Care.* Buckingham: Open University Press, 1997.

134

Liaison with Medical and Surgical Teams

Sheila A. Mann

Clacton and District Hospital, Clacton-on-Sea, UK

In one of the early textbooks of geriatric medicine, Agate[1] wrote, "As a sign of acute physical illness in old age, mental change is more significant than a rise in temperature or pulse rate...". Not only is delirium (acute organic brain syndrome) more frequently found in old age than in earlier life, but the incidence of dementia rises sharply and affective disorders, particularly depression, remain common. Thus, someone presenting with medical or surgical problems may well have coincidental, as well as causal or resultant, psychiatric symptoms. It is hard, therefore, for physicians and surgeons to ignore the psychiatric problems of their patients.

PREVALENCE OF PSYCHIATRIC DISORDER IN NON-PSYCHIATRIC INPATIENTS

A number of investigators have surveyed psychiatric disorder present in patients in non-psychiatric beds. Lipowski[2] estimated that psychiatric disorder or distress of significant degree was present in 30% of the patients he studied. Bergmann and Eastham[3] published a series of 100 elderly patients admitted to an acute medical unit in the UK, whom they screened for psychiatric disorder. They found that 7% had a diagnosis of dementia, 16% delirium and 19% functional illness. Mezey and Kellett[4] summarized a series of UK studies and found prevalence of 5–51%.

Nowhere are such numbers of patients referred for a psychiatric opinion. Other studies have investigated consultation rates.

CONSULTATION RATES

Wallen[5] and her co-workers looked at consultation rates in short-term general hospitals in the USA, using a national sample of 327 hospitals. This was retrospective and adequate information was not recorded in 25% of the hospitals. Patients admitted specifically for a psychiatric illness were excluded. Less than 1% of those admitted were referred for psychiatric opinion. The highest rates were in hospitals attached to medical schools, those in urban areas and those in the north-eastern USA. Not surprisingly, these characteristics were highly correlated with each other.

Wallen and co-workers found that, in general, female patients and younger patients were more likely to be referred. Those referred were sicker, i.e. had been given more "medical" diagnoses, and had more complex problems. They therefore tended to use more resources. Ethnic origin was not a significant variable, but payment system was. Patients on Medicaid (government financed medical care for low-income persons) were more likely to be referred than those admitted under private insurance schemes.

In this, as in many earlier studies, all ages were considered together; in subsequent work, consultation rates for elderly patients were compared with those for younger patients. For instance, Popkin *et al.*[6] compared a series of 266 psychiatric consultations to patients aged 60+ with consultations to a younger group. They found that the consultation rate for patients under 60 was 2.85% and for those aged 60+ 1.99%, a highly significant difference. In no specialty service did the rate for those aged 60+ exceed that for younger patients. The diagnoses given by psychiatrists differed between older and younger patient groups: 46% of the older group were diagnosed as having organic mental disorder compared with 14% of the younger inpatients. The psychiatrists also recommended more psychotropic medication for the older patients, which could be explained by the high percentage of organic diagnoses, and more diagnostic tests, which could not. The psychiatrists assessing the elderly patients were not described as specialists in geriatric psychiatry.

In the UK, consultation rates were also studied. At Guy's Hospital, Anstee[7] looked at the pattern of referrals in 1968–1969—10 years after Fleminger and Mallett[8] had done so. He found that the referral rate had doubled from 0.7% to 1.4%. Of the 254 patients referred, 49 were elderly; 35 had been referred from medical and 13 from surgical wards. Also at Guy's Hospital, Poynton[9] compared referrals from August 1982 to November 1983, when there was no specialist psychogeriatric consultation service, with those from December 1983 to January 1985, when such a service had been introduced. The rate of referral rose from 0.64% to 1.40%, there being a greater rise in male referrals (0.34% to 0.96%) than in females (0.97% to 1.17%). In both periods, depression was the commonest single reason for referral. Anderson[10] reported a similar rise in referral rate following the setting up of a specialist consultation service in Liverpool. The rate rose from 0.7% to 1.96%; proportionately more referrals were for depression in the second period (p. 142).

WHY SUCH LOW REFERRAL RATES?

Goldberg[11] suggests that medical and surgical patients are referred for psychiatric opinion either because some cue alerts their doctor

---

Principles and Practice of Geriatric Psychiatry, 2nd edn. Edited by J. R. M. Copeland, M. T. Abou-Saleh and D. G. Blazer

that there is a psychiatric problem or because the symptoms cannot be accounted for by known organic disease. He has suggested five reasons for non-detection:

1. Many patients do not provide cues, although they will describe their problem if asked.
2. Patients often mention depression or anxiety at the beginning of the interview, together with somatic symptoms, but only the latter are selected for further questioning.
3. Medical histories are often taken in open wards, where lack of privacy does not encourage patients to mention psychiatric problems.
4. A known organic cause does not exclude a psychiatric disorder.
5. Even when a psychiatric disorder is suspected, many clinicians are not confident of their ability to make a psychiatric assessment.

Other reasons for non-detection/non-referral that have been postulated include the following:

1. Attitudes of physician and of patient/patients' relatives. Physicians may still cherish misconceptions that depression and cognitive impairment are an inevitable accompaniment of ageing or that psychiatric disorder is not amenable to treatment. Fauman[12] found that 19% of surgeons and 9% of physicians believed that psychiatric illness was incurable. Elderly patients and their relatives may have a greater fear of public exposure and stigma than younger ones, although this may be changing.
2. Alternatively, some physicians may have an increased tolerance of cognitive and behavioural disturbance in their elderly patients.
3. Cognitive impairment, or symptoms such as paranoia, may make it hard for patients to relate their symptoms.
4. Some doctors feel that organic mental disorder is not a psychiatric problem.
5. Psychogeriatric services may be inaccessible, either geographically or personally, i.e. if too much pressure on the psychogeriatrician delays liaison visits.
6. There may be fear that a psychiatric referral will lead to an increased length of stay, either for further investigation or for treatment.
7. Physicians may wish to treat their patients' psychiatric problems themselves. They appear particularly likely to wish to treat depression, anxiety, psychosomatic disorders and organic brain disease, and most unlikely to wish to treat suicide attempts or psychoses[12].

The commonest reasons for referral are generally for advice on management, including drugs, or assessment of cognitive state. Other reasons include delayed recovery, advice on the psychiatric side effects of drugs, help in the selection of patients for other procedures, "disposal" problems or because of a previous psychiatric history. Covert reasons may emerge, e.g. a history of conflict, either between members of the medical team or between team and patient, especially when the patient declines to follow medical advice. The psychiatrist may then be expected to act as mediator.

There is no doubt, also, that referral rates may depend on local or personal factors. In one hospital, a high referral rate was thought to be due to the siting of the psychiatrist's office next to the medical ward, resulting in many verbal referrals.

Benbow[13], reviewing the old age psychiatry service in the centre of a large conurbation, found that most referrals from hospital doctors (58%) came from physicians in geriatric medicine, the remainder from other physicians and surgeons. These referrals accounted for 35% of the department's work load.

OUTCOME

What is the effect of referral to the psychiatry of old age service? In terms of immediate outcomes, the most frequent consequences appear to be suggestions for further investigation, advice concerning psychotropic medication, social services, counselling or other brief psychotherapeutic intervention or behavioural approaches by ward staff. Few patients are judged to need transfer to a psychiatric bed—6.6%[14]; 9%[15].

Querido[16] found that there was a significant increase in the chance of recovery for patients looked after by a team consisting of a physician, a social worker and a psychiatrist, assessing all aspects of their care, compared with those treated in a conventional way. He found that predictions based on team assessments were more accurate than clinical forecasts based on the patients' physical illness.

Others have shown that psychiatric disorder present during an inpatient stay is associated with subsequent increased mortality rates; e.g. in open heart surgery[17] or from myocardial infarction[18,19]. Treatment might be expected to have a positive effect on the mortality rate. It has also been shown that psychiatric intervention can lessen length of stay[20,21].

Hawton[22], following up a cohort, examined during admission by Maguire et al.[23] after discharge, found that the presence of a psychiatric disorder during the initial admission was associated with higher subsequent mortality. He found that increased mortality rate was associated with age (not surprisingly) and the presence of psychiatric disorder. Excess mortality was not just due to more deaths in hospital or shortly after discharge, neither could it be explained by a higher percentage of patients with organic mental disorder; the mortality rate was also higher in patients with affective disorder.

Cooper[24] screened 626 patients aged 65–80 in an urban West German hospital and followed them up 1 year later. He found that the outcome—whether measured in terms of mortality, dependency or admission to continuing institutional care—was worse for those with organic mental disorder, 42% of whom had died at follow-up; 18% of those with functional illness, and the same percentage of those with "normal" mental states, had died. Functional illness appeared to correlate with increased dependency on others (42% needed help, as against 29% of "normals").

Feldman et al.[25] obtained similar findings: 49% of patients aged 70+ with organic mental disorder died within a year of assessment, compared with 20% of those without cognitive impairment.

Johnston et al.[26], in a prevalence study of psychiatric disorder in patients aged 65+ in non-psychiatric beds in a district general hospital, found that patients with significant psychiatric disorder had a greater length of stay. This appeared to be largely due to problems in placement.

Although some work has been done on the effects of intervention, less attention has been paid to financial aspects, either due to psychiatric intervention, or saved by it. This is becoming of vital importance to everyone in health care. Levitan and Kornfeld[27] studied outcome in a group of 24 patients undergoing surgery for fractured femur, where there was extensive liaison, and compared it with outcome in 26 patients treated in the same surroundings but without involvement of a psychogeriatrician. Mean length of stay for the first group was 30 days and for the control group 42 days, a significant difference. Twice as many liaison patients returned home, as opposed to discharge to institutional care.

A SPECIALIST PSYCHOGERIATRIC LIAISON SERVICE?

Evidence has been cited to show that there is much undetected psychiatric disorder in patients occupying non-psychiatric beds, that there is a higher mortality rate in patients with such disorder, and that psychiatric intervention can reduce length of stay. Even though it would be wrong to assume, as some psychiatrists do, that all patients with emotional disorder require specialist assessment, it is probable that a good deal of suffering on the part of patients and their relatives and carers could be avoided by early detection and treatment. There is therefore a case to be made for a liaison service to elderly, as well as to younger, patients: "Coordination of medical care with any psychosocial care is likely to result in a better outcome and more effective use of medical services"[25].

Two models of service have been described: a "consultation" service and a "liaison" service. In a "consultation" service, the psychiatrist will only see patients specifically referred. Because of pressure of work, many of these assessments take place outside normal working hours and therefore without direct contact with the referrer. As a rule, further investigation and management will be recommended and will be carried out by the referring team. There is frequently no further contact with the psychiatrist unless problems occur—"please get in touch with me again if necessary...".

In a liaison service, a member of the psychiatric team joins the medical or surgical team usually on a weekly basis, e.g. on a ward round. He/she will take an active role in the further management of the patient. In practice, geriatric medical services most frequently have an attached liaison psychiatrist and many services offer a mixed consultation/liaison model.

Swanwick et al.[28] compared the two models. They found no major differences in reason for referral, broad diagnostic category or in suggested intervention and follow-up. They did find that in the liaison model there was a higher percentage of accurate diagnoses made by referring physicians.

Concern has often been expressed that the introduction of such a service would lead to too great an increase in referrals for the capacity of the old age psychiatry unit. Swanwick et al.[28] found no evidence for an increased referral rate—in fact, in the liaison model there were fewer referrals relative to the number of beds.

In other services, an increased referral rate has been described. Scott et al.[29], after setting up a liaison service with a senior psychiatric trainee (a specialist registrar) attending geriatric medicine ward rounds, found a 100% increase in the referral rate initially. Referrals from medical teams increased, while those from surgical teams remained the same, at a small percentage. This, however, was counteracted by the benefits achieved. Like Swanwick, she found an increased accuracy in diagnosis, 28% of patients referred having a diagnosis of affective disorder as against 12% before the service was introduced.

Studies have generally found that, with an increased knowledge of psychiatric disorders and the potential beneficial effects of treatment, there are fewer inappropriate referrals and physicians treat more such disorders themselves. Scott[29] and Baheerathan and Shah[30], who also studied the introduction of a liaison service, found that the benefits of charge in referral pattern more than offset the cost of the liaison psychiatrist.

Most of the consultation/liaison work described has been carried out by psychiatrists. Collinson and Benbo[31] describe a successful liaison service using an experienced psychiatric nurse. Others, for example Camus et al.[32], advocate the benefits of a full multiprofessional psychiatric team working within the general hospital with patients in non-psychiatric beds.

Why should this not be part of an overall liaison service, which might have organizational advantages? What can specialist psychogeriatricians offer? This has been answered by Popkin et al.[6]; they will have special knowledge and awareness with respect to the evaluation of physical illnesses that give rise to psychiatric symptoms; they are practised in differentiating organic mental disorder from mood disorders; they have extensive knowledge of psychotropic medication and of the consequences of altered pharmacokinetics in elderly people; and they are well equipped to evaluate and address psychosocial factors, the family and social support. Some of the aims of a psychogeriatric liaison service are listed in Table 134.1.

What will be the problems of providing such a service? They are likely to include:

- The identification of need.
- Accessibility of interested psychogeriatricians.
- Acceptability to patients, relatives, physicians/surgeons and members of their teams.
- Fear of increased length of stay for diagnosis and/or treatment.
- The cost—and who should pay.

With respect to identification of need, much can be done in educational programmes with all (not only medical) staff. In fact, most psychiatric disorder will be suggested by an adequate medical and social history and examination, as is taught in undergraduate curricula. Often the importance of this is not appreciated, and time and other factors do not encourage it. Other staff—nurses, occupational therapists, physiotherapists and social workers—are well able to identify and describe psychiatric problems if they are taught what to look for. They are also able to initiate plans for discharge at an early stage, e.g. with orthopaedic patients, rather than waiting until surgical rehabilitation is complete. Psychiatric staff need to learn the needs of their colleagues on the general wards and how to assist them; in particular, the fear and distress that mental illness and behavioural disturbance arouse in those unaccustomed to them. It is thus imperative that psychogeriatricians be involved in planning in-service training.

The use of screening tests has been shown to increase detection rates. The subject has been discussed extensively in recent papers[26,33,34]. Geriatricians have found the abbreviated Mental Test Score[35] useful for cognitive impairment. The Mini-Mental State Examination[36] and the Clifton Assessment Procedures for the Elderly[37] have some advantages, the latter being rather long but more inclusive, the former quicker and therefore more acceptable. It is more difficult to single out tests for functional illness: brief versions of the General Health Questionnaire[38,39] or the Geriatric Depression Scale[40] have been shown to be useful.

Table 134.1 Aims of a psychogeriatric liaison service

- To increase awareness of the prevalence and benefits of treating psychiatric disorders in elderly people
- To stress availability of psychiatric advice
- To provide a well-published referral system
- To offer a prompt response
- To offer a clear, practical assessment and recommendations with explanation, and transfer if needed
- To adopt a helpful attitude to behavioural disturbance
- To provide follow-up as inpatient and after discharge, if necessary
- To run an acceptable educational programme
- To undertake an evaluation of service

```
PSYCHIATRY OF OLD AGE UNIT: REQUEST FOR
OPINION

Patient name:
Address:
General Practitioner:
Consultant:
Urgent: Yes/No
Date of birth:
Telephone No:
Hospital/Ward:
Known to: Social Worker? CPN? Other?
Reason for admission:
Reason for referral:
Relevant pathological findings:
Screening tests: Mobility? Vision? Hearing?
Living circumstances: Alone?
                      With carer?
                      Other?
Social problems?
Previous psychiatric history?
Any other relevant information?
Name of referrer:
Position:
Date:
```

Figure 134.1 Specimen referral form. CPN, community psychiatric nurse

The Brief Assessment Schedule[41] has been used to screen for both organic and functional disorder.

The majority of psychogeriatricians in the UK are aware of the importance of liaison; their accessibility varies. The organization of the service depends on local factors; many liaison services are based on linking a psychiatric team with one or more specialist firms. This has worked for much of adult psychiatry and has benefited both teams. It may conflict with the more usual pattern in psychiatry of old age services, where the team is responsible for residents of a defined catchment area and "follows" them throughout their care.

Those in other specialties need to know of the psychogeriatric liaison service. Notices in ward information packs and inclusion in induction courses for new staff are essential. Often the provision of a special referral sheet, such as that in Figure 134.1, helps both to remind and to focus on the information needed by the psychiatrist. There must be a means of telephone referral— preferably one number, with the psychiatric department sorting out the details of who should deal with the referral. As there must be an emergency service available out of hours, and this is usually provided by the duty psychiatrist, he, too, needs instruction.

Acceptability is usually best achieved by the results of an effective service. For instance, Bergmann and Eastham[3] stated that, with respect to affective disorder, when liaison work took place staff attitudes on medical wards changed, including "...a new enthusiasm and willingness to look for affective disorders in other patients and to try to obtain treatment for them whenever possible".

Similarly, fear concerning length of stay and cost can best be assuaged by explanation and discussion, and finally resolved in the light of successful practical experience.

REFERENCES

1. Agate J. *The Practice of Geriatrics*. London: William Heinemann Medical Books, 1970: 361.

2. Lipowski ZJ. Review of consultation psychiatry and psychosomatic medicine. 11. Clinical aspects. *Psychosom Med* 1967; **28**: 201–24.

3. Bergmann K, Eastham EJ. Psychogeriatric ascertainment and assessment for treatment in an acute medical ward setting. *Age Ageing* 1974; **3**: 174–88.

4. Mezey AG, Kellett JM. Reasons against referral to the psychiatrist. *Postgrad Med J* 1971; **47**: 315–19.

5. Wallen J, Pincus HA, Goldman HH, Marcus SE. Psychiatric consultations in short-term general hospitals. *Arch Gen Psychiat* 1987; **44**: 163–8.

6. Popkin MK, MacKenzie TB, Callies AL. Psychiatric consultation to geriatric medically ill inpatients in a university hospital. *Arch Gen Psychiat* 1984; **41**: 703–7.

7. Anstee BH. Pattern of referrals in a general hospital. *Br J Psychiat* 1972; **120**: 631–4.

8. Fleminger JJ, Mallett BL. Psychiatric referrals from medical and surgical wards. *J Ment Sci* 1962; **108**: 183–90.

9. Poynton AM. Psychiatric liaison referrals of elderly in-patients in a teaching hospital. *Br J Psychiat* 1988; **152**: 45–8.

10. Anderson DN, Philpott RM, Wilson KC. Psychogeriatric liaison referrals. *Br J Psychiat* 1988; **153**: 413.

11. Goldberg D. Identifying psychiatric illness among general medical patients. *Br Med J* 1985; **291**: 161–2.

12. Fauman MA. Psychiatric components of medical and surgical practice. II. Referral and treatment of psychiatric disorders. *Am J Psychiat* 1983; **140**: 760–3.

13. Benbow SH. Liaison referrals to a department of psychiatry for the elderly. *Int J Geriat Psychiat* 1987; **2**: 235–40.

14. Taylor G, Doody K. Psychiatric consultations in a Canadian general hospital. *Can J Psychiat* 1979; **24**: 717–21.

15. Mainprize E, Rodin G. Geriatric referrals to a psychiatric consultation liaison service. *Can J Psychiat* 1987; **32**: 5–9.

16. Querido J. An investigation into the clinical, social and mental factors determining the results of hospital treatment. *Br J Prevent Soc Med* 1959; **13**: 33–49.

17. Kimball CP. Psychological response to the experience of open heart surgery. 1. *Am J Psychiat* 1969; **126**: 348–59.

18. Bruhn JG, Chander B, Wolf S. A psychological study of survivors of myocardial infarction. *Psychosom Med* 1969; **31**: 8–19.

19. Silverstone P. Depression and outcome in myocardial infarction. *Br Med J* 1987; **294**: 219–220.

20. Mumford E, Schlesinger J, Glass GV. The effects of psychological intervention on recovery from surgery and heart attacks. An analysis of the literature. *Am J Publ Health* 1982; **72**: 141–52.

21. Pincus HA. Making the case for consultation–liaison psychiatry. Issues in cost-effectiveness analysis. *Gen Hosp Psychiat* 1984; **6**: 173–9.

22. Hawton K. The long-term outcome of psychiatric morbidity detected in general medical patients. *J Psychosom Res* 1981; **25**: 237–43.

23. Maguire GP, Julier DL, Hawton KE, Bancroft J. Psychiatric morbidity and referral on two general medical wards. *Br Med J* 1974; **i**: 268–70.

24. Cooper B. Psychiatric disorders among elderly patients admitted to general hospital wards. *J R Soc Med* 1987; **80**: 13–16.

25. Feldman E, Mayou R, Hawton K *et al.* Psychiatric disorder in medical in-patients. *Q J Med* 1987; **241**: 405–12.

26. Johnston M, Wakeling A, Graham N, Stokes F. Cognitive impairment, emotional disorder and length of stay of elderly patients in a district general hospital. *Br J Med Psychol* 1987; **60**: 133–9.

27. Levitan SJ, Kornfeld DS. Clinical and cost benefits of liaison psychiatry. *Am J Psychiat* 1981; **138**: 790–3.

28. Swanwick GRJ, Lee H, Clare AW, Law LDR. Consultation–liaison psychiatry: a comparison of two service models for geriatric patients. *Int J Geriat Psychiat* 1994; **9**(6): 495–9.

29. Scott J, Fairbairn A, Woodhouse K. Referrals to a psychogeriatric consultation/liaison service. *Int J Geriat Psychiat* 1988; **3**: 131–5.

30. Baheerathan M, Shah A. The impact of two changes in service delivery on a geriatric liaison service. *Int J Geriat Psychiat* 1999; **14**(9): 767–75.

31. Collinson Y, Benbow SM. The role of an old age psychiatry consultation liaison nurse. *Int J Geriat Psychiat* 1998; **13**(3): 159–63.

32. Camus V, De-Mendonca-Lima CA, Simeone I, Wertheimer J. Geriatric psychiatry liaison–consultation. The need for specific units in general hospitals. *Int J Geriat Psychiat* 1994; **11**: 933–5.

33. Mayou R, Hawton K. Psychiatric disorder in the general hospital. *Br J Psychiat* 1986; **149**: 172–90.
34. Pitt B. Depression in the physically ill. *Int J Geriat Psychiat* 1991; **6**: 363–70.
35. Hodkinson M. Evaluation of a mental test score for assessment of mental impairment in the elderly. *Age Ageing* 1972; **1**: 233–8.
36. Folstein MF, Folstein SE, McHugh PR. "Mini-Mental State". A practical method for grading the cognitive state of patients for the clinician. *J Psychiat Res* 1975; **12**: 189–98.
37. Pattie AH, Gilleard CJ. *Manual of the Clifton Assessment Procedures for the Elderly*. Sevenoaks: Hodder & Stoughton Educational, 1979.
38. Goldberg D. *The Detection of Psychiatric Illness by Questionnaire*, Maudsley Monograph 21. London: Oxford University Press, 1972.
39. Goldberg D. *Manual of the General Health Questionnaire*. Slough: National Foundation for Educational Research, 1978.
40. Yesavage JA, Brink TL, Rose TL *et al*. Development and validation of a geriatric depression screening scale: a preliminary report. *J Psychiat Res* 1983; **17**(1): 37–49.
41. Macdonald AJD, Mann AH, Jenkins R *et al*. An attempt to determine the impact of four types of care upon the elderly in London by the study of matched groups. *Psychol Med* 1982; **12**: 193–200.

135

Education and the Liaison Psychogeriatrician

D. N. Anderson

Mossley Hill Hospital, Liverpool, UK

The elderly are under-represented among referrals to psychiatry from general hospital wards in relation to younger patients and bed occupancy. Less than 3% of general elderly admissions are seen by a psychiatrist and only 20–25% of all liaison contacts are with older people, even though they occupy 40–50% of general hospital beds and 30–50% might be expected to have or develop a psychiatric problem[1]. This represents 3000–5000 cases/10 000 admissions and even if more were referred, only a fraction could realistically be seen by a psychogeriatrician[2].

The frequency of mental disorder in acute elderly medical admission populations is approximately twice that of the community[3,4]. Depression, dementia and delirium are the common syndromes. Psychiatric problems are much more common on medical and orthopaedic than general surgical wards[5–7]. The frequency of organic brain syndromes increases with age[8] but there is less evidence that depression is age related[9].

The identification of mental disorder by general clinicians is poor[10], particularly the detection of depression[11] and delirium[12,13]. Clinicians appear to detect the syndrome of dementia more reliably than cognitive symptoms[14] but with depression it is symptoms that are more often recognized than the syndrome[15]. The possible adverse effects of a co-morbid psychiatric disorder upon the outcome of a medical admission makes the recognition and treatment of these disorders important to both patient and clinical service[6,16,17].

A priority for the psychogeriatric consultation–liaison service has to be education (acting as it does at the interface between psychiatry and general departments) that encourages good practice and alters attitudes to mental illness in old age. With such morbidity it is essential to improve the ability of general staff to detect and prescribe appropriate treatment for the majority of simple disorders, while recognizing those cases that need the specialist psychiatric service[18]. Currently, the treatment of mental disorder by general staff, particularly for depression, appears poor[19].

There is indirect evidence that specialist consultation–liaison psychiatry for the elderly does influence the behaviour of general clinical staff toward psychiatric problems. The introduction of a consultation–liaison service is certainly associated with increased rate of referral[1,20–23]. This increase is most marked for depression[1,23], perhaps the most neglected and inappropriately managed condition, but close liaison produces a general improvement in the quality of referrals[23].

Research in the old age liaison field is in its infancy and has concentrated on quantifying levels of morbidity, examining referral rates and exposing clinicians' difficulties in recognizing psychiatric disorders. Preliminary work suggests that psychiatric involvement with older patients can have positive effects on outcome[24] but this may not be targeted at the most appropriate cases[18]. If the management of mental disorder in this context is to improve, then general services will need education. The process of education is complex and multifaceted and a new research direction would involve a closer examination of the enabling role of specialist consultation–liaison, identifying approaches and style of service with the greatest educational impact and the most effective methods of disseminating knowledge and expertise.

It is the management of non-referred cases that will ultimately prove the measure of success. As the ageing population grows, this research is timely and these important areas of study need to be explored.

REFERENCES

1. Anderson DN, Philpott RM. The changing pattern of referrals for psychogeriatric consultation in the general hospital: an eight year study. *Int J Geriat Psychiat* 1991; **6**: 801–7.
2. Anderson DN, Philpott RM, Wilson KCM. Psychogeriatric liaison referrals. *Br J Psychiat* 1988; **153**: 413.
3. Cooper B. Psychiatric disorders among elderly patients admitted to hospital medical wards. *J R Soc Med* 1987; **80**: 13–16.
4. Burn WK, Davies KN, McKenzie FR *et al*. The prevalence of psychiatric illness in acute geriatric admissions. *Int J Geriat Psychiat* 1993; **8**: 171–4.
5. Incalzi RA, Gemma A, Capparella O *et al*. Effects of hospitalisation on affective status of elderly patients. *Int Psychogeriat* 1991; **3**: 67–74.
6. Holmes J. Psychiatric illness and length of stay in elderly patients with hip fracture. *Int J Geriat Psychiat* 1996; **11**: 607–11.
7. Millar HR. Psychiatric morbidity in elderly surgical patients. *Br J Psychiat* 1981; **138**: 17–20.
8. Ames D, Tuckwell V. Psychiatric disorders among elderly patients in a general hospital. *Med J Aust* 1994; **160**: 671–5.
9. Fenton FR, Cole MG, Engelsmann F, Mansouri I. Depression in older medical inpatients. *Int J Geriat Psychiat* 1994; **9**: 279–84.
10. Bowler C, Boyle A, Branford M *et al*. Detection of psychiatric disorders in elderly medical inpatients. *Age Ageing* 1994; **23**: 307–11.
11. Koenig HG, Goli V, Shelp F *et al*. Major depression in hospitalised medically ill men. *Int J Geriat Psychiat* 1992; **7**: 23–34.
12. Gustafson Y, Brannstrom B, Norberg A *et al*. Under diagnosis and poor documentation of acute confusional states in elderly hip fracture patients. *J Am Geriat Soc* 1991; **39**: 760–5.
13. Francis J. Delirium in older patients. *J Am Geriat Soc* 1992; **40**: 829–38.
14. Harwood DMJ, Hope T, Jacoby R. Cognitive impairment in medical inpatients. II: Do physicians miss cognitive impairment? *Age Ageing* 1997; **26**: 37–9.
15. Jackson R, Baldwin B. Detecting depression in elderly medically ill patients: the use of the Geriatric Depression Scale compared with medical and nursing observations. *Age Ageing* 1993; **22**: 349–53.

Principles and Practice of Geriatric Psychiatry, 2nd edn. Edited by J. R. M. Copeland, M. T. Abou-Saleh and D. G. Blazer

16. Saravay SM, Lavin M. Psychiatric comorbidity and length of stay in the general hospital. *Psychosomatics* 1994; **35**: 233–52.

17. Francis J, Martin D, Mapoor WN. A prospective study of delirium in hospitalised elderly. *J Am Med Assoc* 1990; **263**: 1097–101.

18. Cole MG, Fenton F, Engelsmann F, Mansouri I. Effectiveness of geriatric psychiatry consultation in an acute care hospital: a randomised clinical trial. *J Am Geriat Soc* 1991; **39**: 1183–8.

19. Koenig HG, George LK, Meador KG. Use of antidepressants by non-psychiatrists in the treatment of medically ill hospitalised depressed elderly patients. *Am J Psychiat* 1997; **154**: 1369–75.

20. Pauser H, Bergstram B, Walinder J. Evaluation of 294 psychiatric consultations involving in-patients above 70 years of age in somatic departments in a university hospital. *Acta Psychiat Scand* 1987; **76**: 152–7.

21. Poynton AM. Psychiatric liaison referrals of elderly inpatients in a teaching hospital. *Br J Psychiat* 1988; **152**: 45–7.

22. Grossberg GT, Zimny GH, Nakra BRS. Geriatric psychiatry consultations in a university hospital. *Int Psychogeriat* 1990; **2**: 161–8.

23. Scott J, Fairbairn A, Woodhouse K. Referrals to a psychiatric consultation liaison service. *Int J Geriat Psychiat* 1988; **3**: 131–5.

24. Strain JJ, Lyons JS, Hammer JS *et al*. Cost offset from a psychiatric consultation–liaison intervention with elderly hip fracture patients. *Am J Psychiat* 1991; **148**: 1044–9.

136

Rehabilitation

Rob Jones

Queen's Medical Centre, Nottingham, UK

Rehabilitation of the older person with psychiatric disorder means restoring and maintaining the highest possible level of psychological, physical and social function despite the disabling effects of illness. More broadly, it also means preventing unnecessary handicap associated with illness, preventing unnecessary handicap secondary to maladaptive responses to illness, and combating the deadening effects of low expectations of older people amongst patients, families and society in general. Managing chronic disease and disability is the greatest challenge to modern medicine. Within this, the rehabilitation of many older people with psychiatric disorder looms large—although, of course, many old people with psychiatric disorders respond well to "curative" therapy and require little rehabilitation.

In fact, rehabilitation is a fundamental and inseparable part of old age psychiatry. Perhaps for this reason, as with rehabilitation in geriatric medicine[1], little has been written about the topic specifically. Some particular techniques, such as psychological approaches with the cognitively impaired, have been well described[2,3] but little evaluated[4], and evaluative research is much needed here.

SPECIAL PROBLEMS WITH PSYCHIATRIC DISORDER IN THE ELDERLY

"Old age" may span 30 years or more, posing quite different rehabilitation problems; but the most major concern is with the old-old. In this group, multiple disability is prominent, with the complicating danger of polypharmacy, and physical and mental ill-health interact in complex ways. With this frail population, disentangling the respective influences of ageing, previous personality and current ill-health can be exacting. Two-thirds of the UK's disabled population are older people and the true extent of handicap due to psychiatric disorder is probably still not established.

With depression, especially, there may be restriction of physical activity, threatening physical capacity and health. Depression associated with stroke disorder[5] or with Parkinson's disease[6] particularly illustrates both the connection between physical and psychiatric problems and the importance of physiotherapy in psychiatric rehabilitation.

Physical factors are frequently of great importance in dementia. A quiescent individual may become delirious and disturbed at night through heart failure, obstructive airways disease or even the uncomfortable effects of severe constipation. Settling such problems may transform the reality of care for a carer and seeking out such therapeutic opportunities is an important part of rehabilitation. Similarly, in dementia, physiotherapy to promote and maintain the best possible physical capacity is a key element.

Advice and practical aid to carers, such as with lifting and handling the physically disabled demented person, can be crucial.

A judicious mixture of the "therapeutic" (curative) and the "prosthetic" (supportive) approaches[7,8] is very necessary in old age psychiatry. Whilst much functional psychiatric disorder and delirium can be "cured", and this must be the aim, most older people with dementia need some degree of supportive care at some stage. The poor financial and housing state of many older people, together with the lack of children or spouses to help as carers for many of the old-old, are further complicating factors. Maximizing "participation" despite psychiatric disorder needs to be a major goal, maintaining as far as possible a role in the family, social contact, a range of activities and a minimization of loss of autonomy or institutionalization. This requires an approach that embraces psychiatric, medical, rehabilitation, nursing and social perspectives. Seeking active prevention of disability/reduced participation as a consequence of psychiatric disorder is a vital part of rehabilitation.

SPECIAL PRINCIPLES IN REHABILITATION OF THE OLDER PERSON WITH PSYCHIATRIC DISORDER

Table 136.1 summarizes the principles. The first principle is to make the home the focus of attention. That is where problems have arisen and where they will need to be overcome. Planning for rehabilitation should begin at the earliest moment; an initial assessment at home by a senior psychiatrist, or other experienced team member, is invaluable—even if "home" is an institution in the community. Home is also where the carers, and often any social services support staff involved, may readily be found. This contrasts with standard medical rehabilitation, where often no such opportunity exists.

Table 136.1 Principles of rehabilitation for the older person with psychiatric disorder

Focus on the home
Ensure comprehensive assessment
Encourage normal function
Treat the treatable
Analyse disabilities and chart progress
Clarify team goal with patient and carers early
Clarify team goal with support workers early
Teach what can be relearnt
Adapt the adaptable
Coordinate support and follow-up
Promote flexibility and ingenuity
Promote realistic optimism

Principles and Practice of Geriatric Psychiatry, 2nd edn. Edited by J. R. M. Copeland, M. T. Abou-Saleh and D. G. Blazer
©2002 John Wiley & Sons, Ltd

Frequently further assessment by, say, an occupational therapist, physiotherapist or another specialist team member may be necessary—and this can perhaps also be arranged at home. But avoiding disruptive admission should not be at the cost of meeting assessment needs. The day hospital and its team is often useful to complete such assessments.

Poor function or morbidity should never be accepted as immutable and still less as normal. Assessment should aim at a thorough understanding of social, physical and psychological function, as well as the previous pattern of personality and lifestyle. From this, diagnoses and specific treatment for the treatable should follow. But also analysis should show the extent of disability, how it is mediated and how it may be overcome. Problems should be clearly recorded, with proposed solutions and with regular review of progress[9,10]. From the earliest moment, independent function and improvement should be sensitively encouraged, especially with hospitalized patients.

As early as possible, the agreed goal of rehabilitative efforts needs to be clarified with the patient, with the relatives/carers, with the whole rehabilitation team and with any support workers needed in the community. Education, guidance and a rehabilitative "demonstration" may well be necessary to resolve conflicting views on the prospects for progress. Carers may need therapy or rehabilitation in their own right. Almost always the support of carers is essential, although some stoutly independent patients manage well without this.

A prognosis-based plan is useful. This means assessing: what are the problems and what are their causes? Prognostication will follow: will these get better or worse? To what degree? Over how long a period? From this a plan can flow consistent with what seem the most major likely developments of a problematic nature, over a foreseeable timescale and taking account of what is most remediable.

Sometimes, disability strongly distorts the previously stable power and dominance pattern in the family[11] so that, for instance, a forceful mother becomes dependent on a passive daughter. Relationships are always important and such phenomena can strongly influence outcome. They need to be understood and often complex ambivalence worked through[12]. Such factors are frequently important when carers seem reluctant to resume caring[13] and need to be carefully teased out when juggling with the various elements of risk and risk minimization in supporting a vulnerable person at home[14]. The patient's "crutch is not made of wood but of some other person's tolerance or patience"[15].

An agreed balance should be sought between the needs of carers and the patient's right and desire for continued comparative independence despite significant disability—bearing in mind the team's prime responsibility to the patient. In effect, carers should be "recruited" as rehabilitation therapists' "aides". But often they will need practical help and advice on rehabilitation techniques and, always, the reassurance of the services' continuing availability for support and sensitive expert response. Similar considerations apply with any support staff necessary to help the patient at home—principally social services staff in the UK. Their early involvement and integration into the assessment and rehabilitation process can be logistically difficult but generally is most effective. Good teamwork is of the essence. Clarity and consistency within the multidisciplinary specialist team are essential. Nurses and therapists, for instance, must communicate well, each complementing and enhancing the other's approach. Specialist and general practitioner must be in accord. The specialist team must carry the confidence of those who will work with the patient outside hospital. Table 136.2 lists many of the team members and resources requiring coordination for rehabilitation—inevitably there is great overlap[7]. Clear goals should be set, in accord with patient and carers, and clearly understood by all[16,17]. This is much easier said than done with the vulnerable frail elderly person; but vitally important is good communication.

Patients are taught what they can learn or relearn but often only modification of domestic equipment, provision of aids or modifications of the home will overcome their disability. More often still, problems are only overcome through support services—home-delivered meals or a home help/community care assistant—coming into the home. Ingenuity and diplomacy may be needed with an old person reluctant to accept such necessary support. The great majority of support is provided by relatives/carers and supporting the supporters is the main task. This may require day hospital therapy, day care or respite admissions. Maintaining confidence in the care service is vital.

At some stage with hospital patients, except in the most grossly deteriorated person, a home assessment is advisable with an occupational therapist or physiotherapist, or both, and perhaps with other team members. Hospital-based staff can be too pessimistic and, allowed to function in his/her familiar environment, even a significantly demented patient can sometimes perform surprisingly well. Often serial home assessments are helpful with increasing challenge, leading to overnight stays. Also, initial failure to manage satisfactorily should not preclude the possibility of later improvement with further therapy or support.

Above all, rehabilitation with older people requires flexibility allied to a realistic but constructively optimistic approach. Innovation and ingenuity are frequently necessary. The complex interaction between physical, social and psychological factors in older patients is further complicated by the likelihood that

Table 136.2 People and facilities to aid rehabilitation of the older person with psychiatric disorder

	Specialist psychiatric team	Social services and local authority services	Primary care team
People	Psychiatrists	Social workers	General practitioners
	Ready access to geriatricians	Domiciliary services manager	Practice nurse
	Hospital nurses	Home help/community care assistants	District nurse
	Community psychiatric nurses	Meals on Wheels	Health visitor
	Physiotherapist	Community OT	
	Occupational therapist (OT)	Support to voluntary sector	
	Clinical psychologist	Sitter services	
	Social worker	Carers' groups	
	(Speech therapist—sometimes)		
	(Dietician—sometimes)		
	Carers' groups		
Facilities	Assessment ward	Luncheon club (often voluntary)	Health centre
	Nursing home	Day centres (often voluntary)	
	Day hospital	Long-stay and short-stay residential care	
	Outpatients	Housing adaptation	
	Long-stay and respite care facilities	Sheltered housing	

circumstances, perhaps especially physical health, may change dramatically; this demands a flexible response. The solution, carefully constructed and successful on one day, may need major change on the next as the situation radically alters. For this reason, rehabilitation with older people is rarely completely finished and "maintenance" measures are often necessary. Careful planning of continuing care, follow-up and continuing availability as problems arise are essential features. The strength and determination of patients, relatives and support staff are considerably bolstered by the knowledge that this approach is backing them up.

REHABILITATION AND LONG-STAY CARE

Many patients, predominantly demented individuals, will require long-term care but rehabilitation must remain a strong theme. Such deteriorating multiply-disabled demented patients require 24 h care. They often exhibit difficult and disturbed behaviour and need heavy physical care. Providing the best quality of life, given often quite limited resources, is the aim and a major strategy is preventing unnecessary dependency and promoting the maximum retention of function. With descriptions[18] of the care of such patients in various settings, a frequent theme has been the availability of skilled and expert staff from the multidisciplinary team to help maintain good function. Evaluation of such long-term care programmes has proved complex and difficult[19,20].

There has been concern in the UK that such disabled patients will increasingly be excluded from hospital care for funding reasons, in favour of health authority contracted private nursing home care or simply standard care in private nursing homes[20–22]. In the USA (and many other countries), much long-term care of older people has long been provided in the private sector. But in the USA the Omnibus Budget Reconciliation Act (OBRA Act)[23] requires nursing homes to ascertain and meet any needs for therapy and treatment. In the UK the fear is that the drive in the best hospital care to provide a good quality of life may be replaced in private nursing homes by a desire for a quiet life; passivity and dependency (possibly resulting from unnecessary tranquillizing medication[24–26]) could be more acceptable than the patient's exercise of individuality, movement and self-expression.

Reports of high levels of depression in homes for older people[27–30] emphasize the worry about effective rehabilitation and care for older people with chronic psychiatric disorder. Any institution providing shelter is at risk of providing a relatively impoverished environment[15] and undue restriction of independence.

Bennett[15] called unnecessary social inactivity and dependence "the psychiatric equivalent of contractures". Hospitals (and social services) have provided much good practice. Accounts of good long-stay care for demented people emphasize the invaluable input of occupational therapy, physiotherapy and person-centred approaches[30,31]. Sensibly ensuring activity in a structured day and enriching the environment with, for example, music therapy, art therapy, drama therapy[32] or reminiscence therapy[33] are important wherever the setting.

Community psychiatric nurse (CPN) support (indeed, availability of all the specialist team to give support) to such homes can be feasible and helpful. But concern remains about how to monitor effectively and maintain standards in private long-stay care[20]. Ultimately, good care here depends on the commitment of sufficient appropriately trained staff to help disabled old people experience to the full their remaining scope for independence and capacity for joy.

ATTITUDES

Adverse feelings about older people have been noted by many[34]. Geriatricians have commented on unhelpful attitudes in health professionals of all kinds, including GPs[13]. Modern medical education is inculcating a better knowledge base for tomorrow's doctors and also better attitudes[35]. The educational potential of psychogeriatric services, not least exploiting the educational opportunity afforded by rehabilitation (and other concerns) with the most disabled, has been described[36]. Not only medical students[37], but all varieties of medical and other professional staff concerned with older people with mental health problems, and also carers and lay audiences, benefit from this educational effort. Public education especially is vital in engendering constructive attitudes in society, on which ultimately will depend all efforts towards care in the community and the political will to provide decent services.

REFERENCES

1. Nocon A, Baldwin S. *Effective Practice in Rehabilitation: The Evidence of Systematic Reviews*. London: King's Fund, 1992.
2. Holden U, Woods RT. *Positive Approaches to Dementia Care*, 3rd edn. Edinburgh: Churchill Livingstone, 1995.
3. Kitwood T. *Dementia Reconsidered: the Person Comes First*. Buckingham: Open University Press, 1997.
4. Woods RT. In Woods RT, ed., *Handbook of the Clinical Psychology of Ageing*. Chichester: Wiley, 1996; 575–600.
5. House A, Dennis M, Mogridge L *et al*. Mood disorders in the year after first stroke. *Br J Psychiat* 1991; **153**: 83–92.
6. Cummings JL, Masterman DL. Depression in patients with Parkinson's disease. *Int J Geriat Psychiat* 1999; **14**: 711–18.
7. Evans JG. Commentary: curing is caring. *Age Ageing* 1989; **18**(4): 217–18.
8. Evans JG. High hopes for geriatrics. *J R Coll Physicians* 1994; **28**: 392–3.
9. Pattie A. Measuring levels of disability—the Clifton Assessment Procedures for the Elderly. In Wattis JP, Hindmarch I, eds, *Psychological Assessment of the Elderly*. Edinburgh: Churchill Livingstone, 1988; 61–88.
10. Millard PH. Meeting the needs of an ageing population. *Proc R Coll Physicians Edinb* 1994; **24**: 187–96.
11. Bergmann K. Neurosis and personality disorder in old age. In Isaacs AD, Post F, eds, *Studies in Geriatric Psychiatry*. Chichester: Wiley, 1978; 41–76.
12. Pitt B. *Psychogeriatrics*, 2nd edn. Edinburgh: Churchill Livingstone, 1982.
13. Hodkinson HM. Rehabilitation of the elderly. In *Medicine in Old Age*, 2nd edn. London: British Medical Association, 1985.
14. Hemsi L. Psychogeriatric care in the community. In Levy R, Post F, eds, *The Psychiatry of Late Life*. London: Blackwell Scientific, 1982; 252–87.
15. Bennett DH. The mentally ill. In Mattingly S, ed., *Rehabilitation Today*, 2nd edn. London: Update Books, 1981; 119–22.
16. Department of Health. *The Hospital Discharge Workbook: A Manual on Hospital Discharge Practice*. London: HMSO, 1994.
17. Department of Health. *Better Services for Vulnerable People*, EL (97) 62, CI (97) 24. London: HMSO, 1997.
18. Shah A *et al*. Physical dependency and dementia in the NHS continuing care wards and contracted NHS beds in voluntary nursing homes. *Int J Geriat Psychiat* 1994; **9**: 229–32.
19. Kane RA, Kane RL. *Long-term Care*. New York: Springer, 1987.
20. Turrell AR, Castleden CM, Freestone B. Long-stay care and the NHS: discontinuities between policy and practice. *Br Med J* 1998; **317**: 942–4.
21. Wattis J, Fairbairn A. Towards a consensus on continuing care for older adults with psychiatric disorder. *Int J Geriat Psychiat* 1996; **11**: 163–8.
22. Social Information Systems. *A State of Confusion: A Report to the Alzheimer's Disease Society*. Knutsford: Social Information Systems, 1997.
23. National Mental Health Association. *Summary of the 1987 Omnibus Budget Reconciliation Act (OBRA)*. Washington, DC: NMHA, 1988.
24. McGrath M, Jackson GA. Survey of neuroleptic prescribing in residents of nursing homes in Glasgow. *Br Med J* 1996; **312**: 611–12.

25. Thacker S, Jones R. Neuroleptic prescribing to the community elderly in Nottingham. *Int J Geriat Psychiat* 1997; **12**: 833–7.

26. Thacker S, Jones R. Use of neuroleptics in dementia—a review of recent concerns. *Res Pract Alzheim Dis* 1998; suppl.

27. Snowdon J. The epidemiology of affective disorders in old age. In Chiu E, Ames D, eds, *Functional Psychiatric Disorders of the Elderly*. Cambridge: Cambridge University Press, 1994.

28. Samuels SC. Depression in the nursing home. *Psychiat Ann* 1995; **25**: 419–24.

29. Ames D. Depression in nursing and residential homes. In Chiu E, Ames D, eds, *Functional Psychiatric Disorders of the Elderly*. Cambridge: Cambridge University Press, 1994.

30. Marshall M, ed. *Working with Dementia: Guidelines for Professionals*. Birmingham: Venture, 1990.

31. Marshall M. "They should not really be here"—people with dementia in the acute sector. *Age Ageing* 1999; **28–52**: 9–11.

32. Sutcliffe BJ. Improving quality of life: psychogeriatric units. In Denham MJ, ed., *Care of the Long-stay Elderly Patient*. London: Croom Helm, 1983; 185–205.

33. Head DM, Portnoy S, Woods RT. The impact of reminiscence groups in two different settings. *Int J Geriat Psychiatry* 1990; **5**(5): 295–302.

34. Lilley S-J, Brook L, Bryson C et al. *British Social Attitudes and Northern Ireland Social Attitudes. 1996 Surveys: Technical Report*. London: Social Community and Planning Research, 1998.

35. Smith CW, Wattis JP. Medical students' attitudes to old people and career preferences: the case of Nottingham Medical School. *Med Educat* 1989; **23**: 81–5.

36. Arie T, Jones R, Smith C. The educational potential of psychogeriatric services. In Arie T, ed., *Recent Advances in Psychogeriatrics*, vol 1. Edinburgh: Churchill Livingstone, 1985; 197–208.

37. Wattis JP. Old age psychiatrists in the United Kingdom—their educational role. *Int J Geriat Psychiat* 1989; **4**(6): 361–4.

Anaesthetics and Mental State

David Gwyn Seymour

University of Aberdeen, UK

The anaesthetist uses many drugs that directly or indirectly affect mental status and, as is discussed below, age-related changes in drug handling tend to increase the risk of adverse cognitive effects. The multiplicity of drugs used in modern anaesthesia also increase the risk of drug interactions, and at the same time make it more difficult to decide the cause of any adverse effect that occurs. For instance, a typical general anaesthetic might involve premedication drugs, intravenous induction agents, gases and volatile agents, competitive neuromuscular blockers, drugs to reverse the neuromuscular blockade, opiate and non-opiate analgesics (which may be given pre-, intra- or postoperatively) and major and minor tranquillizers.

It might be thought that a "regional" anaesthetic (such as a local, spinal or epidural anaesthetic), where the patient maintains consciousness, would be free from central nervous system effects. However, premedication is often given prior to a regional anaesthetic and sedatives and analgesics may be administered during and following the operation. All of these may have a prolonged effect on mental status. Regional anaesthesia might also influence postoperative outcome, for good or ill, by affecting the ability to mount a "stress" response.

Apart from the expected pharmacological effects of anaesthetic agents on mental status, there are also unwanted reactions to be considered, such as the increased tendency of anticholinergic drugs to precipitate acute delirium in older patients. Secondary drug effects may also be important, such as the disturbance of sleep pattern by opiates, which has been hypothesized as a cause of late postoperative hypoxaemia. Many of these individual effects are discussed below.

It should also be appreciated that an acute or chronic change in cognitive state which follows an anaesthetic may have nothing to do with that anaesthetic. Acute delirium can be precipitated by a variety of "stresses", including acute illness and non-anaesthetic drugs, and also by withdrawal from drugs, such as alcohol and tranquillizers, which were being taken prior to surgery[1,2]. Neurological damage following operation may result from hypotension or cardiac arrhythmias, which had nothing to do with the anaesthetic, hypocarbia may reduce cerebral blood flow, and the patient who appears demented for the first time following emergency surgery may have been dementing quietly and unobserved for many months before.

In an attempt to bring some structure to the above complexity, the following discussion will be divided into three parts: first, age-related changes in drug handling which are of particular importance to the anaesthetist; second, major direct and indirect mechanisms by which anaesthetic agents might affect mental function; and third, short-term and long-term studies of psychometric testing before and after anaesthesia (including the effects of clinical risk factors and type of anaesthetic, and the findings of the ongoing ISPOCD studies). It should be recognized, however, that the list is not exhaustive. For example, an operation under anaesthesia, like any other major life event, may precipitate anxiety and other changes in mental status[3].

Cognitive changes that occur after open heart surgery have also been well studied in the literature. However, in this group of patients, the cerebral effects of the cardiac bypass procedure add another layer of complexity to the analysis of the postoperative outcome, and they have not been further discussed in the present brief account, although part of the recent comprehensive review into postoperative cognitive dysfunction by Dodds and Allison[4] deals with this subject.

AGE CHANGES IN DRUG HANDLING THAT ARE OF PARTICULAR RELEVANCE TO THE ANAESTHETIST

As a broad generalization, Dodson[5] has subdivided anaesthetic drugs into two classes:

1. Drugs to which the elderly patient tends to demonstrate *increased sensitivity*. This class embraces most of the drugs that affect the central nervous system, including sedatives and analgesics. Such drugs usually have a more profound and long-lasting effect in the elderly. There may also be an increased incidence of side-effects of drugs in old age, such as muscle rigidity following fentanyl, and delirium following anticholinergic agents.
2. Drugs that act on the autonomic nervous system, where the elderly patient tends to demonstrate *decreased sensitivity* at receptor sites. Thus, the effects of autonomic blockade by anticholinergic drugs or β-blockers may be less dramatic, as may be the effects of vagal and sympathetic stimulants.

While the above classification is a useful conceptual framework, dosage regimens in individual elderly patients need to take into account individual differences in drug susceptibility, age-associated illness and physiological status. In most cases, however, the anaesthetist will need to give smaller doses of drugs to elderly patients[5,6].

In a more recent review, Dodds[7] has described anaesthesia as "applied clinical pharmacology with enough patho-physiology to confuse the picture". He lists nine key points, three of which are of direct relevance to mental function, and six of which are of potential relevance:

1. The minimum alveolar concentration (MAC) is that concentration of an anaesthetic gas which suppresses movement in

response to a surgical stimulus in 50% of subjects. MACs tend to fall with age.

2. Because of reduced neuronal density and a reduced metabolic rate, the elderly may be more sensitive to a given amount of anaesthetic drug. In elderly patients with a delayed circulation time, there is an added potential for overdosage when intravenous agents are given too fast, because a delayed response may be mistaken for a lack of therapeutic effect, so that when the drug eventually reaches the brain, too much drug has been given. Smaller doses, slower rates of infusion or repeated small boluses are recommended in the elderly.

3. The elderly appear to have an increased sensitivity to opiates.

4. Where there is pre-existing ischaemic heart disease, the patient may be vulnerable to the cardiac depressant effects of some anaesthetics. There is also a theoretical risk that some anaesthetic agents can "steal" blood from ischaemic myocardium by increasing vasodilation in normal vessels.

5. With increasing age there is a tendency to increased shunting in the lungs and decreased cardiac output. These pathophysiological changes have complex effects on the uptake of volatile gases, as a low cardiac output favours rapid uptake, while a decreased lung function produces the opposite effect. Such effects are less with the more insoluble gases.

6. Hepatic metabolism and/or clearance of drugs tends to be affected by age, although there is considerable interindividual variability. Insoluble anaesthetic agents which require no hepatic metabolism should be safer than soluble agents. Some anaesthetics, such as halothane, are also potentially hepatotoxic.

7. Renal clearance of drugs tends to fall with age in some, but not all older people. Some anaesthetics, such as sevoflurane, are potentially nephrotoxic.

8. Neuromuscular blocking agents can be classified into depolarizing types and non-depolarizing types. The non-depolarizing agents are usually favoured in old age.

9. Non-steroidal anti-inflammatory agents are increasingly being used for analgesia in younger patients, but may present increased hazards in the elderly because of nephrotoxicity, fluid retention and tendency to gastric irritation.

MECHANISMS BY WHICH INDIVIDUAL ANAESTHETICS MIGHT AFFECT MENTAL FUNCTION

A fuller discussion of this topic can be found in the review of Dodds and Allison[4], but major potential mechanisms are as follows:

Direct Cerebral Effects

Trace amounts of general anaesthetic agents can have effects on alertness and concentration after patients recover consciousness. Experiments involving young volunteers have also documented the effects of subanaesthetic doses of drugs on mental function, behaviour and motor skills[8,9], and have also studied the effects of prolonged general anaesthesia in the absence of surgery[10]. None of these studies involved old subjects, but it would be expected that the central effects of anaesthetics would become more marked with age.

Hypoxaemia

In recent years, pulse oximeters have provided a convenient, non-invasive means of monitoring postoperative hypoxaemia[11]. The new technology produced some unpleasant surprises: many elderly patients who appear to be stable and well-perfused experience profound and prolonged episodes of nocturnal hypoxaemia several days after surgery. Such episodes might explain some of the "unexpected" episodes of confusion, cardiac abnormality and sudden death that can occur up to a week following operation. However, as discussed in the review of Dodds and Allison[4], some researchers are not convinced that hypoxaemia is a major cause of temporary or permanent postoperative cerebral dysfunction (POCD), and the ISPOCD1 Study (see below) failed to find a correlation between hypoxaemia and postoperative cognitive status, even though it set out with the hypothesis that such a relationship existed.

The mechanisms by which anaesthetic agents, particularly opiates, might cause postoperative hypoxaemia are reviewed by Jones and his colleagues[11]. It appears that postoperative hypoxaemia is caused by the interaction of two major factors. The first of these factors is a gas exchange abnormality induced during anaesthesia, which tends to be most marked in the first few postoperative hours but which may persist longer. The second factor is episodic obstructive sleep apnoea, which may occur several nights after anaesthesia. The episodes of obstructive breathing seem to be precipitated by the *return* of rapid eye movement (REM) sleep, which had been abolished for a few days by drugs, particularly opiates, given around the time of operation, and by the stress of operation itself. This late hypoxaemia, once recognized, can be alleviated by giving oxygen, but in high risk patients a week of oxygen administration may be required.

Anticholinergics

As has already been explained, anticholinergic drugs tend to be less effective in blocking cholinergic function in old age. Much more important, however, are the direct central effects of anticholinergic drugs (such as atropine) that can cross the blood–brain barrier. In some cases excessive drowsiness results, while in others hallucinations and delirium occur, and some authors refer to a "central anticholinergic syndrome". A number of drugs that are not primarily anticholinergic agents also have anticholinergic properties, including phenothiazines, pethidine, thiobarbitone, flurazepam and tricyclic antidepressants. Two decades ago, in a small group of open heart surgery patients aged 29–75, Tune et al.[10] reported that the presence and severity of postoperative delirium was correlated with the level of anticholinergic drug activity in the blood. More recently, O'Keeffe and Chonchubhair[13] have reviewed the potential contribution of anticholinergic drugs to postoperative delirium, and have considered their importance relative to other pharmacological and non-pharmacological mechanisms.

While the evidence is not absolutely conclusive, it would seem prudent to minimize anticholinergic use in older surgical patients. One way to achieve this would be to avoid anticholinergics in premedication regimens, or perhaps to avoid premedication altogether. If an anticholinergic drug is thought essential, then glycopyrrolate, which does not cross the blood–brain barrier, would appear to have advantages over atropine[14].

COGNITIVE TESTING IN YOUNG AND OLD PATIENTS BEFORE AND AFTER SURGERY

Postoperative Delirium

Before considering the more subtle cognitive effects that can occur postoperatively, the syndrome of acute postoperative *delirium* will be discussed. The causes of postoperative delirium, as in delirium in other settings, include acute illness, drugs and drug withdrawal[1,2,13,15] but the incidence tends to rise with age. Estimates of the incidence of postoperative delirium in the over-65s range between 7% and 50%, depending on the definitions used and the clinical circumstances[2,13,15]. The incidence tends to rise with age, the urgency of surgery, the use of sedative and anticholinergic drugs and the degree of preoperative mental impairment. Factors (such as sepsis) that favour the development of delirium in a non-surgical situation[12] may also be of relevance postoperatively.

Recent advances in the study of postoperative delirium have included attempts to standardize definitions[13] and a large study in the USA by Marcantonio et al.[15], which attempted to develop a clinical prediction rule in 1341 patients aged 50+ having major non-cardiac surgery. The latter authors found that seven preoperative factors (age over 70, alcohol abuse, poor cognitive status, poor functional status, serum electrolyte/glucose disturbances, thoracic surgery and aneurysm surgery) had an independent relationship with postoperative delirium. However, the effect of intraoperative events, including anaesthesia, was not studied, as the aim was to produce a preoperative rule.

O'Keeffe and Chonchubhair[13] have concluded that, in at least 90% of cases of delirium following general surgery, it is postoperative medical or surgical complications that are to blame, which implies that the appearance of delirium should lead to a diligent search for underlying physical medical problems. The increased incidence of postoperative delirium with age is likely to be due to causes such as these, rather than effects arising from age-related differences in handling anaesthesia[16].

Postoperative Changes in Psychometric Tests in Older People

Delirium is an important postoperative syndrome, but more worrying is the possibility that *dementia* could occur for the first time as the direct result of *routine* surgery and/or anaesthesia (as opposed to the mental changes that might arise from an intraoperative catastrophe, such as cardiac arrest). In 1955, Bedford[17] published a much-quoted retrospective study in which he sought to trace those patients in the Oxfordshire area who had "never been the same again" after an elective or emergency anaesthetic. Over a 5 year period he was able to identify 18 cases where there was reasonable evidence that dementia had appeared for the first time after surgery and anaesthesia. In interpreting this data, it is important to realize that a detailed assessment of preoperative mental function was not available, and that even in cases where dementia was reported immediately following surgery, it did not necessarily imply that anaesthetic drugs were the cause.

In a subsequent study, Simpson et al.[18] attempted the very difficult task of replicating Bedford's findings in a prospective study. As formal preoperative psychological assessment was part of Simpson's study design, only elective patients could be included. After considerable efforts, 678 elderly patients having surgery were evaluated, two-thirds of whom underwent general anaesthesia. This major undertaking yielded only one patient in whom there was good evidence that a permanent deterioration in mental function occurred immediately after anaesthesia.

These two reports[17,18] stimulated many psychometric studies of short- and long-term postoperative cognitive outcome. Tables 137.1 and 137.2 summarize the results of 17 such studies[19-35], which have looked at psychometric test performance in ageing patients before and after surgery. Follow-up periods have ranged from a few days to over 3 months, and many different types of psychometric tests have been used. Table 137.1 contains 13 studies in which older patients have been randomized to receive general or regional anaesthesia, while Table 137.2 summarizes four alternative study designs that have given an insight into the effect of age on postoperative cognitive problems. These include the ISPOCD1 study, which is discussed in detail below.

There are major methodological problems in carrying out clinically meaningful psychometric testing in elderly elective surgical patients[35]. These problems become almost insuperable in patients who are admitted as emergencies, and only two of the studies listed in Tables 137.1 and 137.2 considered non-elective patients. Unfortunately, there is ample evidence that it is non-elective patients who have the highest incidence of postoperative mental events, although in many emergency cases non-anaesthetic factors, such as acute illness, are probably more culpable than anaesthetic drugs.

The 13 studies in Table 137.1 compared the psychometric effects of general anaesthesia with those associated with "regional" techniques (local, spinal or epidural anaesthesia). Four of the earlier studies reported that the general anaesthetic group performed more poorly, but even here the effect was seen only during the immediate postoperative period.

The studies that make up Tables 137.1 and 137.2 contain a wealth of detail, but some broad overall conclusions can be drawn. As might be expected, the major effects on mental function are seen in the first postoperative day, but some of the studies report minor effects on some tests for up to 7 days. The studies that specifically compared young and old patients found that the older group performed slightly worse than the younger during the early postoperative period.

While *short-term* mental impairment following surgery is of importance, especially in these days of increasing day surgery provision[36], it is *long-term* mental impairment that is feared most by patients, their relatives and their doctors. In the first edition of this textbook[37], comfort was drawn from the fact that the best-designed of the long-term studies up to that date had reported no objective evidence of mental impairment 1 month or more after surgery. It was noted, however, that 16% of the patients of Jones et al.[21] had complained of subjective changes in memory and concentration at 3 months after surgery, and that these authors had commented that these patients might have had minor intellectual changes which had been missed by the chosen psychological tests. Since that time, the study of Williams-Russo et al.[19] has similarly reported long-term postoperative cognitive changes in 5% of patients. Further concern has been raised by the finding of long-term cognitive deficit in the ISPOCD1 study[32], which, unlike the Williams-Russo et al. study, included a group of non-operated control patients to meet the criticism that some of the effects reported in early studies reflected the progression of coincidental dementia, unrelated to surgery or anaesthesia. The ISPOCD1 study and its successor, ISPOCD2, will now be described in some detail.

The ISPOCD Studies

The first International Study of Post-operative Cognitive Dysfunction (ISPOCD1) collected data between 1994 and 1996 on 1218 patients aged 60+ who were undergoing major non-cardiac surgery in 13 hospitals in eight European countries and the USA[32]. This was a major undertaking, which was intended to answer many of the questions about early and late postoperative cognitive dysfunction in older people that had been raised in the literature over the previous 30 years. In the event, the results of the ISPOCD1 study, published in 1998[32], still left several unanswered questions which are being addressed in a further study (ISPOCD2), which is due to report in May 2001.

Table 137.1   Randomized studies comparing the psychometric effects* of general anaesthesia (GA) and regional anaesthesia** (RA)

Reference	Number of patients	Age (years)	Type of surgery [anaesthesia]	Timing of postoperative tests	Main findings	Difference between GA/RA?	Long-term cognitive deficit?
19	262	>40, median 69	knee replacement (TKR) [Epidural vs. general anaesthesia]	7 days, 6 months	Delirium occurred in 11%. Complex changes in psychometric tests, but there was a general reduction at 7 days with return to baseline (or better) by 6 months. However, Trail Making A and B worse at 6 months	No	5% Showed significant deterioration at 6 months, but there were no untreated controls
20	169	65–98	Cataract [GA vs. local]	1, 14 days, 3 months	Reduction in verbal recall/learning, psychomotor speed and tactile naming on day 1 only	No	No
21	146 patients, 50 controls (patients on waiting list)	60+	hip (THR) or knee replacement [GA vs. epidural]	3 months	No decreases on tests in patients or controls at 3 months. Tests included Choice Reaction Time (which *increased* in GA group), object learning, digit copying, critical flicker fusion, and cognitive difficulties scale	No	No *measurable* decrease, but 11/56 GA and 10/60 RA patients thought concentration and memory were poorer
22	64	60–86	TKR [GA vs. spinal]	3 months	Tests tended to improve at 3 months (? practice effect)	No	No
23	40	60–80	Transurethral resection of prostate (TURP) [GA vs. epidural]	4, 21 days	Day 4 only: reduced paired associate learning, visual memory and visual recall	No	No
24	105	25–86	Hysterectomy, TURP, THR/TKR	1–7 days, 3 months	Modest decrease in memory and cognitive tasks in early period. Later tests usually better than baseline	No	No
25	30	50–80	THR [GA vs. spinal]	1, 2, 7 days	Spinal group had worse word recall/recognition on day 1, no differences on later days	Yes	Not tested
26	44	60–93	TURP, pelvic floor surgery [GA vs. spinal]	6 h, 1, 3, 5 days, 1 month	At 6 h GA group had reduced Mini-Mental Status. No later differences on Mini-Mental or Geriatric Mental Assessment	Yes	No
27	57	65–92	Hip fracture [GA vs. epidural]	1, 7 days	38–50% Delirium (even though patients excluded if Organic Brain Syndrome Scale abnormal preoperatively)	No	Not tested
28	40	>60	Hip fracture [GA vs. spinal]	7 days, 3 months	Abbreviated Mental Test *improved* at 1 week (no other test was used)	No	No
29	30	>60	THR [GA vs. epidural vs. both]	2, 4, 7 days, 3 months	Assessment by psychologist. Various tests impaired for 2–4 days, then recovered	No	No
30	60	>65	Cataract [GA vs. local + sedation]	7 days	Wechsler Memory Scale and Luria tests reduced relative to baseline	Yes (LA *worse*, Luria only)	Not tested
31	60	56–84	THR [GA vs. epidural]	1, 3, 7, 12 days	No formal psychological tests; 7 out of 31 in GA group (0 out of 29 epidural group) said to have mental changes in first 7 days	Yes	5 out of 31 GA patients reported mental changes 4–10 months after surgery

*For full details of psychometric tests, see references 4, 37.
**Regional anaesthesia includes local, spinal and epidural anaesthesia.

A key feature of the ISPOCD studies has been the use of the European psychometric test battery (EUPT battery), which has been designed as a sensitive and standardized research tool for the detection of postoperative neuropsychological deficits and which can be administered over a 45 min period. This battery uses the Mini-Mental State Examination (MMSE) as a screening test, with patients scoring 23 or less being excluded from further testing. The remaining tests (used in ISPOCD1 and in a slightly modified form in ISPOCD2) comprise a Verbal Learning Test, a Concept Shifting Test, the Stroop Colour Word interference test, a Letter Digit substitution task, a four boxes test, the Broadbent Cognitive Failure Questionnaire, and a Zung Depression Score Questionnaire (the Geriatric Depression Scale being used in ISPOCD2). The definition of postoperative cognitive dysfunction (POCD) has been reached by comparing changes in the normalized (Z) scores of individual patients with age-matched controls who were not undergoing surgery, who were studied at the same time intervals.

ISPOCD1[32] was particularly concerned to test the hypothesis that hypoxaemia and/or hypotension were causative factors in POCD. Accordingly, oxygen saturation was measured by

Table 137.2 Other studies of general anaesthesia and postoperative cognitive dysfunction

Reference	Age (n)	Type of surgery	Type of psychometric tests	Timing of post-operative tests	Results	Long-term change?	Comments
32	>60 (1218 patients, plus 321 community controls)	Major non-cardiac surgery (if preoperative Mini-Mental Status was 24 or more)	EUBT (see text for details)	7 days 3 months	Postoperative cognitive dysfunction (defined after comparisons with untreated controls) in 25.8% at 7 days and 9.9% at 3 months (controls 3.4%, 2.8%)	Yes	Age, duration of anaesthesia, less education, and respiratory and other complications (but *not* hypoxaemia) correlated with dysfunction at 7 days. Age was *only* risk factor correlating with cognitive dysfunction at 3 months
33	48–88 (112)	Transurethral resection of prostate	Choice reaction time	1, 2, 3 days	Increased variability in choice reaction time, day 1 only	Not tested	Increased variability associated with previous low CAPE (Clifton Assessment Procedure for the Elderly), extent of surgery, postoperative pain/sedation
16	25–83 (40)	Cholecystectomy	Mini-Mental, digit symbol/span, trail making	1, 2, 3, 4 days, 1 month	Changes on day 1 only: digit symbol (all), trail making (old only)	No	Concluded there was no major difference in rate of recovery between young and elderly groups
34	Two groups: young, mean age 50; old mean age 69 (n=85)	Orthopaedic, gynaecological and general surgery	17 Questions (orientation/concentration), plus object learning test	2 days	Memory deficits (young and old). Orientation and concentration deficits (old only)	Not tested	Correlation between postoperative deficits and poor preoperative cognitive function

continuous pulse oximetry before surgery, throughout the day of surgery, and for the next three nights. Blood pressure was recorded by oscillometry during the operation and every 30 min for the rest of the operative day and night. Patients received general anaesthesia but no restriction was placed on anaesthetic or surgical technique, which conformed to local practice in the study centers. However, to avoid the cerebral vasoconstrictor effects of hypocapnia, capnography was a requirement during surgery, so that normocapnia could be maintained.

Analysis of the data from ISPOCD1[32] showed that 25.8% patients had POCD 7 days after surgery and that 9.9% of all patients still had evidence of POCD on the repeat neuropsychological tests carried out at 3 months (corresponding values for controls were 3.4% and 2.8%). Contrary to expectations, no relationship was found between hypoxaemia and/or hypotension and the development of early or late POCD. Indeed, despite analyses of the effects of more than 25 other clinical parameters, only age showed a statistically significant correlation with late POCD. Age was also positively correlated with early POCD, as were duration of anaesthesia, a lesser level of education, a second operation, postoperative infections and respiratory complications.

The overall conclusion of the ISPOCD1 investigators[32] was that their study had demonstrated a measurable degree of postoperative cognitive change in a minority of older patients 3 months after surgery (in about 10% of patients vs. about 3% of non-operated controls) and that the risk increased with age. However, the expected relationship between hypoxaemia and/or hypotension and POCD did not emerge in the study. It was also disappointing that, despite a large number of statistical analyses, the study failed to find any specific risk factors that were amenable to therapeutic or preventive intervention. In addition, the hope that the study would give better insight into the pathophysiology of POCD was not fulfilled.

Because the ISPOCD1 study did not provide the expected answers in regard to the prevention or treatment of POCD, ISPOCD2 is now under way, coordinated from Copenhagen by J. T. Moller and L. S. Rasmussen. I am very grateful to Dr Christopher Hanning, a member of the ISPOCD2 steering committee, for the following information. ISPOCD2 comprises a linked group of multicentre projects which will ask a dozen major research questions in a variety of patient populations. A major task of ISPOCD2 will be to follow up patients for a prolonged period, to see whether the 3 month postoperative neuropsychological changes persist, and to test whether these changes produce measurable effects on Activities of Daily Living and Quality of Life. Other research tasks addressed by ISPOCD2 include: an investigation of the effects of outpatient anaesthesia; a comparison of the effects of regional anaesthesia with those of general anaesthesia; a comparison of POCD incidence in patients aged 40–60 years and in older patients; a test of the hypothesis that there might be a genetic predisposition to POCD related to the apolipoprotein E allele, which is known to have an association with the development of Alzheimer's disease; a correlation of blood levels of benzodiazepines and their metabolites with the development of POCD; an examination of the role of cholinergic and other neurotransmitters in POCD, using an animal model and positron emission tomography (PET) in humans; the study of possible protected effects of ondansetron; a study of structural cerebral changes by both MRI and SPET scanning; correlations of POCD with neurone specific enolase and protein S100; and the investigation of the relationship between POCD and "stress", particularly prolonged hypercortisolaemia.

CONCLUSION

While the great majority of older people undergoing surgery and anaesthesia will emerge without any cognitive sequelae, absolute guarantees cannot be given. Indeed, since the last edition of this book, the previous consensus that routine anaesthesia *per se* had essentially no long-term effect on postoperative function has been challenged by large carefully designed studies. It is to be hoped that the ISPOCD2 study and similar large-scale investigations will allow us to give more authoritative advice to older patients undergoing surgery in the first decade of the twenty-first century.

REFERENCES

1. Seymour DG, Rees GAD, Crosby DL. Introduction—demography, prophylaxis, surgical diagnosis, pathophysiology, and approach to anaesthesia. In Crosby D, Rees G, Seymour DG, eds, *The Ageing Surgical Patient: Anaesthetic, Operative and Medical Management*. Chichester: Wiley, 1992; 1–90.
2. Lipowski ZJ. *Delirium: Acute Confusional States*. New York: Oxford University Press, 1990.
3. Adams B. Psychiatric aspects of surgical operations. In Kaufman L, ed., *Anaesthesia: Review 5*. Edinburgh: Churchill Livingstone, 1988, 34–53.
4. Dodds C, Allison J. Postoperative cognitive deficit in the elderly surgical patient. *Br J Anaesth* 1998; **81**: 449–62.
5. Dodson ME. Modifications of general anaesthesia for the aged. In Davenport HT, ed., *Anaesthesia and the Aged Patient*. Oxford: Blackwell Scientific, 1988; 204–30.
6. Dodson ME, Seymour DG. Surgery and anaesthesia in old age. In Brocklehurst J, Tallis RC, Fillit HM, eds, *Textbook of Geriatric Medicine and Gerontology*, 4th edn. Edinburgh: Churchill Livingstone, 1992: 942–68.
7. Dodds C. Anaesthetic drugs in the elderly. *Pharmacol Ther* 1995; **66**: 369–86.
8. Bruce DL, Bach MJ, Arbit J. Trace anesthetic effects on perceptual, cognitive, and motor skills. *Anesthesiology* 1974; **40**: 453–8.
9. Bruce DL, Bach MJ. Effects of trace anaesthetic gases on behavioural performance of volunteers. *Br J Anaesth* 1976; **48**: 871–6.
10. Davison LA, Steinhelber JC, Eger EL, Stevens WC. Psychological effects of halothane and isoflurane anesthesia. *Anesthesiology* 1975; **43**: 313–24.
11. Jones JG, Sapsford DJ, Wheatley RG. Postoperative hypoxaemia: mechanisms and time course. *Anaesthesia* 1990; **45**: 566–73.
12. Tune LE, Damlouji NF, Holland A *et al*. Association of postoperative delirium with raised serum levels of anticholinergic drugs. *Lancet* 1981; **ii**: 651–3.
13. O'Keeffe ST, Chonchubhair AN. Postoperative delirium in the elderly. *Br J Anaesth* 1994; **73**: 673–87.
14. Simpson KH, Smith RJ, Davies LF. Comparison of the effects of atropine and glycopyrrolate on cognitive function following general anaesthesia. *Br J Anaesth* 1987; **59**: 966–9.
15. Marcantonio ER, Goldman L, Mangione CM *et al*. A clinical prediction rule for delirium after elective noncardiac surgery. *J Am Med Assoc* 1994; **271**: 134–9.
16. Chung F, Seyone C, Dyck B *et al*. Age-related cognitive recovery after general anesthesia. *Anesth Analg* 1990; **71**: 217–24.
17. Bedford PD. Adverse cerebral effects of anaesthesia on old people. *Lancet* 1955; **ii**: 259–63.
18. Simpson BR, Williams M, Scott JF, Crampton Smith A. The effects of anaesthesia and elective surgery on old people. *Lancet* 1961; **ii**: 887–93.
19. Williams-Russo P, Sharrock NE, Mattis S *et al*. Cognitive effects after epidural vs. general anesthesia in older adults. A randomised trial. *J Am Med Assoc* 1995; **274**: 44–50.
20. Campbell DNC, Lim M, Kerr Muir M *et al*. A prospective randomised study of local versus general anaesthesia for cataract surgery. *Anaesthesia* 1993; **48**: 422–8.
21. Jones MJT, Piggott SE, Vaughan RS *et al*. Cognitive and functional competence after anaesthesia in patients aged over 60: controlled trial of general and regional anaesthesia for elective hip or knee replacement. *Br Med J* 1990; **300**: 1683–7.
22. Nielson WR, Gelb AW, Casey JE *et al*. Long-term cognitive and social sequelae of general vs. regional anesthesia during arthroplasty in the elderly. *Anesthesiology* 1990; **73**: 1103–9.
23. Asbjorn J, Jakobsen BW, Pilegaard HK *et al*. Mental function in elderly men after surgery during epidural analgesia. *Acta Anaesthesiol Scand* 1989; **33**: 369–73.
24. Ghoneim MM, Hinrichs JV, O'Hara MW *et al*. Comparison of psychologic and cognitive functions after general or regional anesthesia. *Anesthesiology* 1988; **69**: 507–15.
25. Hughes D, Bowes JB, Brown MW. Changes in memory following general or spinal anaesthesia for hip arthroplasty. *Anaesthesia* 1988; **43**: 114–17.
26. Chung F, Meier R, Lautenschlager E *et al*. General or spinal anesthesia: which is better in the elderly? *Anesthesiology* 1987; **67**: 422–7.
27. Berggren D, Gustafson Y, Eriksson B *et al*. Postoperative confusion after anesthesia in elderly patients with femoral neck fractures. *Anesth Analg* 1987; **66**: 497–504.
28. Bigler D, Adelhoj B, Petring OU *et al*. Mental function and morbidity after acute hip surgery during spinal and general anaesthesia. *Anaesthesia* 1985; **40**: 672–6.
29. Riis J, Lomholt B, Haxholdt O *et al*. Immediate and long-term mental recovery from general vs. epidural anaesthesia in elderly patients. *Acta Anaesth Scand* 1983; **27**: 44–9.
30. Karhunen U, Jonn G. A comparison of memory function following local and general anaesthesia for extraction of senile cataract. *Acta Anaesth Scand* 1982; **26**: 291–6.
31. Hole A, Terjesen T, Breivik H. Epidural vs. general anaesthesia for total hip arthroplasty in elderly patients. *Acta Anaesth Scand* 1980; **24**: 279–87.
32. Moller JT, Cluitmans P, Rasmussen LS *et al*. Long-term postoperative cognitive dysfunction in the elderly: ISPOCD1 study. *Lancet* 1998; **351**: 857–61.
33. Smith C, Carter M, Sebel P, Yate P. Mental function after general anaesthesia for transurethral procedures. *Br J Anaesth* 1991; **67**: 262–8.
34. Smith RJ, Roberts NM, Rodgers RJ, Bennett S. Adverse cognitive effects of general anaesthesia in young and elderly patients. *Int Clin Psychopharmacol* 1986; **1**: 253–9.
35. Ghoneim MM, Ali MA, Block RL. Appraisal of the quality of assessment of memory in anesthesia and the practice of psychogeriatric medicine psychopharmacology literature. *Anesthesiology* 1990; **73**: 815–20.
36. Tzabar Y, Asbury AJ, Millar K. Cognitive failures after general anaesthesia for day case surgery. *Br J Anaesth* 1996; **76**: 194–7.
37. Seymour DG. Anaesthetics and mental state. In Copeland JRM, Abou-Saleh MT, Blazer DC, eds, *Principles and Practice of Geriatric Psychiatry*, 1st edn. Chichester: Wiley, 1994: 995–1004.

Nutritional State

D. N. Anderson[1] and M. T. Abou-Saleh[2]

[1]*Mossley Hill Hospital, Liverpool, and* [2]*St George's Hospital Medical School, London, UK*

Dietary surveys of elderly people in the UK and Sweden have shown that a substantial proportion of subjects had intakes below recommended standards. Two US National Health and Nutrition surveys showed that 50% of the population, especially the elderly, were deficient in one or more nutrients. In 1979, a Department of Health and Social Security (DHSS) survey in the UK suggested that 7% of those aged 65+ may be undernourished and twice this proportion of those aged 80+[1]. A survey in Sydney found that intakes of nutrients by old people in Australia were similar to those recorded in the UK[2] and concluded that a significant proportion of this population may be at risk. Depending on definitions and diagnostic criteria, undernutrition in community-based elderly people is in the range 0–82% and in hospital 5–63%[3].

High-risk groups include the housebound and those with impaired cognitive function, a history of depression, chronic pulmonary disease and partial gastrectomy. Poor dentition, swallowing difficulties and not having regular cooked meals are further factors placing people at greater risk of malnutrition.

The reasons for poor nutrition are various and the cause often multifactorial. Nutritional deficiency rarely occurs in isolation but is usually consequent upon ill-health or poverty. The UK DHSS survey of 1968[4] found 3% of 1000 elderly people to be malnourished, largely because of untreated underlying medical conditions or socioeconomic disadvantage. Poor financial reserves, isolation, physical handicap, dental problems and mental disorder all contribute, and the effects of disease, disability and ageing can combine to change a marginally sufficient diet into a grossly deficient one[5]. The prevalence of malnutrition is certainly higher in old people than in younger groups, attributable in the main to higher proportions of the elderly living in poverty and a greater prevalence of disease in old age. The diet of lower socioeconomic groups provides cheap energy and is lower in essential nutrients, such as calcium, iron, magnesium, folate, other B vitamins and vitamin C[6].

Methods of food preparations and a lack of knowledge about daily requirements are also important. It must be cause for concern that elderly people in residential care and long-stay hospital wards have been found to be at greatest risk of undernutrition, although naturally, they represent some of society's oldest and most frail individuals. Burns *et al.*[7] found a group of elderly dementing people in institutional care to be more undernourished than those living alone in the community, even though they were no more cognitively impaired. Kennedy and Henderson[8] found the risk of nutritional deficiency to be greater in residential than in hospital care.

Classical single deficiency states are rare in the UK and USA elderly, but there is a strong suspicion that suboptimal nutrition frequently contributes to ill-health in old age. Malnutrition leads to lowered physical strength, greater inactivity and risk of accidents, a weaker immune system and osteoporosis[6]. Poor vision, macular degeneration and cataracts are being linked to diets lower in fruit, vegetables and antioxidants[9]. Subclinical vitamin deficiency is more common in the elderly, particularly those with psychiatric disorders. Hancock *et al.*[10] compared nutritional indices of healthy and mentally ill elderly women and reported lower levels of vitamin C, riboflavine and pyridoxine among the elderly mentally ill. Of 255 psychogeriatric admissions with organic and functional disorders, Bober[11] found low concentrations of ascorbic acid in over 50% and low plasma folate in approximately 20% of subjects.

A study in England conducted by the Health Advisory Service 2000, commissioned by the Secretary of State for Health, identified feeding and nutrition in acute hospital wards for the elderly to be deficient in many respects[12]. Malnutrition is largely unrecognized in British hospitals and is particularly common in old age[13]. In one study of adult hospital admissions, the overall average weight loss was 5.4% and was greatest in those initially most undernourished. Nutritional status was infrequently recorded[14].

There are difficulties in the assessment of nutritional status and establishing accepted recommendations for daily requirements. Commonly used reference data in the UK may not be appropriate for all populations of elderly people, and contemporary reference data that are widely applicable, with clinically defined criteria for undernutrition, are needed[15]. Furthermore, it is not clear how illness may alter these requirements. The assessment of nutritional status is complex and a single measure usually insufficient; however, anthropometric measurements are the preferred clinical tool for routine use and can provide practical and valid indices of nutritional status[16]. Preferably, evidence of undernutrition is established from a combination of history and examination, anthropometry, haematological and biochemical indices[17,18]. Of the 10 risk factors described by Davies[19], depression, loneliness and alcoholism feature, in addition to social variables and factors reflecting dietary intake and weight change. Bender[20] points out that tables of nutrient requirements are of limited value, as individuals' energy and nutritional needs vary.

Although discussions of nutrition tend to focus on deficiencies, it should be remembered that the commonest nutritional disorder affecting old people in developed countries is obesity. The problem of obesity, which is often difficult to remedy, has established implications for physical illnesses such as hypertension, heart disease, diabetes mellitus and arthritis. Drugs used in the treatment of mental illness in old age not infrequently lead to weight gain.

Principles and Practice of Geriatric Psychiatry, 2nd edn. Edited by J. R. M. Copeland, M. T. Abou-Saleh and D. G. Blazer

Low body weight is associated with an increased mortality of elderly people living at home[21] and admitted to hospital[22]. Poor nutrition increases the risk of falls and hip fractures[23] and is associated with excess winter deaths[24], the development of pressure sores[25] and infections[26].

Undernutrition may arise from quantitative and qualitative dietary inadequacy, leading to mixed nutrient deficiency. If old people meet their energy requirements by taking a good mixed diet their needs for nutrients will be met. Some elderly people lead such sedentary lives that their energy requirement is very low[27] and they become at risk of taking inadequate protein, minerals and vitamins. As life becomes more sedentary and energy intake declines, then diet needs to become more nutrient-dense. Asplund et al.[28] found that 30% of 91 patients, with a variety of diagnoses, admitted to psychogeriatric inpatient care were undernourished. A high prevalence of thiamine deficiency has been reported, especially among the housebound, solitary and confused[29] but also among admissions to psychiatric units[30]. Alcoholism is commonly associated with deficiencies in thiamine but also riboflavine, pyridoxine, vitamin B_{12} and folic acid. Subnormal levels of vitamin C, thiamine and pyridoxine were found by MacLennan et al.[31] in long-stay elderly patients who were also protein-deficient. Inadequate intake of vitamin C has been shown for 75% of elderly men and over 80% of women, not always reflected by leucocyte ascorbate levels or laboratory parameters[31,32]. Vitamin D levels have been shown to be very low in long-stay elderly populations[33], almost certainly secondary to inadequate exposure to sunlight[34]. Evidence of multiple vitamin deficiencies has been reported in elderly day hospital attenders and residents of local authority residential homes[8].

Vitamin deficiency is rarely sought in clinical practice, when only B_{12} and folate estimations tend to be performed with any regularity. Yet any deficiency, particularly involving the B group, can present with apathy, anorexia, weight loss, mood changes, acute and chronic confusional states and occasionally hallucinations and paranoia[35]. Depression and alcoholism seem to be the characteristic disorders associated with vitamin B and folate deficiencies, while organic psychosyndromes are typical of B_{12} deficiency[30]. Thiamine deficiency can produce a wide variety of mental disturbance and ascorbic acid deficiency is usually linked with apathy and depression. Irritability, aggressive behaviour and personality change were reported in healthy volunteers undergoing thiamine restriction[36]. Vitamins and minerals are intimately involved in cell metabolism, neurotransmitter synthesis and cell membrane stability. Mineral and electrolyte deficiencies, including iron, calcium, potassium and magnesium, are also common findings among elderly populations[3], with obvious implications for health.

TREATMENT

The immediate significance of single deficiency states is confined to few specific circumstances, e.g. thiamine and the Wernicke–Korsakoff syndrome, B_{12} and folate with certain dementias and pseudodepressive states. In most instances, the import of nutritional status is less obvious and the effects of deficiency probably more subtle. Although nutritional supplementation is unlikely to be curative in these situations, there are few studies of the effects of nutritional intervention in elderly populations with mental disorder and more information is needed before drawing firm conclusions. While the real significance of nutritional manipulation is awaited, a pragmatic position recommending dietary supplementation and adjustment with efforts to prevent undernutrition is advised.

In many circumstances, treating an underlying mental disorder or physical illness effectively will restore appetite and drive, thereby correcting deficiency by the resumption of a normal diet. The admission of a confused elderly person to hospital or care may provide the opportunity to re-establish a normal eating pattern. In specific deficiency disorders the prescription of necessary supplements will be an essential part of treatment. The possibility that nutrient supplementation may enhance the response to conventional psychotropic medication[37] is an interesting possibility that requires further exploration.

The correction of deficiency does not necessarily involve prescribed medication but may be possible by simple measures, such as supplementing the diet with fruit juices to provide more vitamin C. Low levels of vitamin D are found in up to 40% of the elderly living at home or in hospital. Diet is an inadequate source of vitamin D, which depends on exposure to ultraviolet light for its formation. A greater exposure to natural sunlight is the most important preventive measure, but because the elderly are at special risk it is recommended they receive vitamin D supplementation to achieve a daily intake of $10 \mu g$[38].

The overwhelming priority in the management of undernutrition among the elderly population is prevention. A major impetus must ultimately come from a change in public policy that improves the elderly person's social, material and financial position in society and ensures the efficient provision of services to those in need.

The market-led approach to nutrition that operates in many food-rich countries has been found to increase the disparity between the nutrition and health of the rich and poor[39]. The provision of domiciliary care services is inequitably distributed, often inefficiently organized and frequently determined by demand rather than need[40]. Consequently, invaluable services, like meals-on-wheels and home helps (often the only people to provide food to isolated mentally ill old people), may not reach those most at risk. Little attention or imagination has been given to the meals service, potentially an important resource, which suffers from a complex, multi-agency organization, inflexibility in delivering meals of a type or at a time to suit individuals and often arriving cold. Only half the recipients find the meals at least moderately satisfactory[41] while 15% never eat them and 15% eat only half those delivered[42]. There is little evidence that they are targeted at those most at risk of undernutrition and some evidence that the meals, themselves, are nutritionally inadequate[40]. This has led some to suggest that the service acts only as a symbol of concern for elderly people[43].

Often the supervision of meal times is as important as the meal itself. Confused elderly people may eat voraciously in the company of their family yet put meals aside when left to eat alone. Altering the timing of home help or family visits or attendance at a day centre or luncheon club may be the intervention required.

The prevention of undernutrition may be possible by simple measures, e.g. providing meals in a form that is appealing and easily edible. Kennedy and Henderson[8] demonstrated the importance of noting the food returned after meals by the elderly in residential care. Fruit, vegetables and meat were often left because they were difficult to chew. For seriously impaired individuals, maximizing food intake during the times of day when cognitive abilities are at their peak can improve dietary intake[44]. The time allowed for meals is normally less in institutions than at home[45], meal times are inflexible and little consideration is given to personal choice. Some patients will take food from family members and not care staff, or only from certain members of staff. Obviously adequate staffing levels will affect success when large numbers of disabled or resistive patients are eating together.

The recent practice in UK hospitals of extending menus to include less traditional dishes may be appreciated by the young, but experience suggests many elderly people are happier with local dishes and attempting radical alterations of lifelong dietary habits can be difficult and may be counterproductive. Changes of this sort may actually reduce the opportunity to provide a nutritious diet to elderly hospitalized patients at a time when it is most needed. Fresh fruit is often difficult to obtain in institutions and modern methods of mass food preparation have been criticized. It may not be appreciated that less mobile elderly people have a fast protein flux that requires a higher, not lower, daily requirement for protein[17,18] and the protein intake of long-stay elderly patients can be inadequate[31].

Poor dentition is associated with undernutrition[46] and the fitting of dentures to old people in institutional care has been shown to increase the consumption of raw vegetables[47]; 78% of independent elderly patients examined by MacEntee et al.[48] believed their oral health to be good but only 17% had clinically healthy mouths. A study of hospitalized patients aged 61–99 years found that 60% had disease of the oral soft tissue[49].

Medication can impair the absorption and reduce the availability of essential nutrients, impair appetite, cause dry mouths and constipation or directly promote the loss of minerals, as with diuretics and potassium[50].

For those living in the community, preventive health care with early recognition and treatment of illness is essential. The elderly population may benefit from greater education and advice about healthy and affordable eating, issues normally targeted at younger age groups. The judicious use of fruit juices, frozen vegetables and some convenience foods might ease the burden of food preparation. Realizing that visual impairment and arthritic joints can prevent shopping and the opening of packets and tins may point the way to practical interventions, such as the provision of domestic aides or arranging for someone to collect shopping. One survey found that 22% of elderly people who had difficulty opening screw-top jars had to ask non-household members to do it for them[51]. The teaching of culinary skills is particularly relevant to the older bereaved male who never cooked when his wife was alive. Men, although age-for-age fitter than women, are twice as likely to say they are unable to cook a main meal[52].

In the modern era shops themselves are often large, impersonal, confusing places and sited some distance from home, making effective shopping difficult for physically and mentally disabled people. Low income and disability not only restricts ability to afford a protective diet but also limits access to retailers where healthy food can be purchased more cheaply. Local shops are less prevalent and can be significantly more expensive than more distantly sited supermarkets[53].

Finally, unless people are aware of the possibility of undernutrition and able to make an assessment, little progress will be made for the sick and vulnerable. Sadly, doctors and nurses frequently fail to recognize undernourishment because they are not trained to look for it[54] and medical students' knowledge of the issue of nutrition is poor[55]. Improved education is greatly needed. The Royal College of Nursing[56] provides clear guidelines for the assessment of nutritional status in older people.

CONCLUSION

A great deal needs to be known about the fundamentals of diet, nutrition and mental health in old age. The evidence connecting nutrition and morbidity suggests this is an area of importance to all professionals working with elderly people and a strong case could be made for the regular involvement of a dietician in the psychogeriatric team.

Establishing roles for nutritional intervention offers prospects of simple and economic measures that may improve the treatment and prognosis of mental disorders in old age, enhance clinical recovery and reduce morbidity.

At the present time, it cannot be claimed that vigorous dietary intervention offers curative treatment for mental illness but attention to diet may, at least, reduce the physical complications of mental disorder, hospitalization and ageing. However, there is accumulating interest in the role of antioxidants in the treatment of dementia [see Nutritional Factors in Dementia] and the possible significance of omega polyunsaturated fatty acids for maintaining the development and integrity of neuronal function has obvious relevance to severe mental illness[57]. Schizophrenic patients taking additional omega 3 polyunsaturated fatty acids may experience milder symptoms[58] and a recent study of community residing schizophrenic patients aged 20–79 years demonstrated nutritional deficiency, despite most being overweight, with a high intake of saturated fat and low intake of antioxidant[59].

Further exploration of the relationship between dietary constituents and the course of mental illness may yet yield information significant to the management of mental illness in old age.

REFERENCES

1. Department of Health and Social Security. *A Nutrition Survey of the Elderly*. London: HMSO, 1979.
2. Stuckey SJ, Darnton-Hill I, Ash S *et al*. Dietary patterns of elderly people living in inner Sydney. *Hum Nutrit Appl Nutrit* 1984; **38A**: 255–64.
3. Lipski PS, Torrance A, Kelly PJ. A study of nutritional deficits in long stay geriatric patients. *Age Ageing* 1993; **22**: 244–55.
4. Department of Health and Social Security. *A Nutrition Survey of the Elderly*. Reports on Health and Social Subjects, No. 3. London: HMSO, 1972.
5. MacLennan WJ. Nutrition of the elderly in continuing care. In Caird FI, Grimley Evans J, eds, *Advanced Geriatric Medicine 3*. London: Pitman Press, 1983: 9–20.
6. Philip W, James T, Nelson M *et al*. The contribution of nutrition to inequalities in health. *Br Med J* 1997; **314**: 1545–9.
7. Burns A, Marsh A, Bender DA. Dietary intake and clinical, anthropometric and biochemical indices of malnutrition in elderly demented patients and non-demented subjects. *Psychol Med* 1989; **19**: 383–91.
8. Kennedy RD, Henderson J. Nutrition in the elderly in residential care. In Caird FI, Grimley Evans J, eds, *Advanced Geriatric Medicine 3*. London: Pitman Press, 1983.
9. McLaughlan WR, Sanderson J, Williamson G. Antioxidants and the prevention of cataracts. *Biochem Soc Trans* 1995; **23**: 257S.
10. Hancock MR, Hullin RP, Aylard PR *et al*. Nutritional state of elderly women on admission to mental hospital. *Br J Psychiat* 1985; **147**: 404–7.
11. Bober MJ. Senile dementia and nutrition. *Br Med J* 1984; **288**: 1234.
12. Health Advisory Service 2000. Not because they are old: an independent enquiry into the care of older people on acute wards in general hospitals. London: Health Advisory Service, 1999.
13. Potter J, Klipstein K, Reilly JJ, Roberts M. The nutritional states and clinical course of acute admissions to a geriatric unit. *Age Ageing* 1995; **24**: 131–6.
14. McWhirter JP, Pennington CR. Incidence and recognition of malnutrition in hospitals. *Br Med J* 1994; **308**: 945–8.
15. Bannerman E, Reilly JJ, MacLennan WJ *et al*. Evaluation of validity of British anthropometric reference data for assessing nutritional state of elderly people in Edinburgh: cross sectional study. *Br Med J* 1997; **315**: 388–41.
16. Gibson RS. *Principles of Nutritional Assessment*. Oxford: Oxford University Press, 1990.
17. Lehmann AB. Nutrition in old age: an update and questions for future research: part I. *Rev Clin Gerontol* 1991; **1**: 135–45.
18. Lehmann AB. Nutrition in old age: an update and questions for future research: part 2. *Rev Clin Gerontol* 1991; **1**: 231–40.
19. Davies J. Risk factors for malnutrition. In Horwitz A, Macfadyean DM, Munro H *et al*., eds, *Nutrition in the Elderly*. Oxford: Oxford University Press, 1989.
20. Bender ARE. Institutional malnutrition. *Br Med J* 1984; **288**: 92–3.

21. Matilla K, Haavisto M, Rajala S. Body mass index and mortality in the elderly. *Br Med J* 1986; **292**: 867–8.

22. Bienia R, Ratcliff S, Barbour GL, Kummer M. Malnutrition in the hospitalised geriatric patient. *J Am Geriat Soc* 1982; **30**: 433–6.

23. Farmer ME, Harris T, Madans JH *et al.* Anthropometric indicators and hip fracture. The NHANES-I epidemiological follow-up study. *J Am Geriat Soc* 1989; **37**: 9–16.

24. Keating W. The medical problems of cold weather. *J R Coll Physicians Lond* 1986; **20**: 283–7.

25. Pinchofsky-Devlin GD, Kaminski MV. Correlation of pressure sores and nutritional status. *J Am Geriat Soc* 1986; **34**: 435–40.

26. Chandra RK. Nutritional regulation of immunocompetence and risk of disease. In Horwitz A, Macfadyean DM, Munro H *et al.*, eds, *Nutrition in the Elderly*. Oxford: Oxford University Press, 1989.

27. Lonergan ME, Milne JS, Maule MM, Williamson J. A dietary survey of older people in Edinburgh. *Br J Nutrit* 1975; **34**: 517–27.

28. Asplund K, Mormark M, Patterson V. Nutritional assessment of psychogeriatric patients. *Age Ageing* 1981; **10**: 87–94.

29. MacLeod CC, Judge TG, Caird FI. Nutrition of the elderly at home II. Intakes of vitamins. *Age Ageing* 1974; **3**: 209–19.

30. Carney MWP. Vitamin deficiency and mental symptoms. *Br J Psychiat* 1990; **156**: 878–82.

31. MacLennan WJ, Coombe NB, Martin P, Mason BJ. The relationship of laboratory parameters to dietary intake in a long-stay hospital. *Age Ageing* 1975; **4**: 189–94.

32. Milne JS, Lonergan ME, Williamson J *et al.* Leucocyte ascorbic acid levels and vitamin C intake in older people. *Br Med J* 1971; **iv**: 383–6.

33. Corless D, Beer M, Boucher BJ *et al.* Vitamin D status in long-stay geriatric patients. *Lancet* 1975; **1**: 1404–6.

34. MacLennan WJ. Vitamin D metabolism in the elderly. *J Clin Exp Gerontol* 1979; **1**: 1–11.

35. Lishman WA. Vitamin deficiencies. In *Organic Psychiatry*, 3rd edn. London: Blackwell Scientific, 1998; 570–93.

36. Word B, Gysbert A, Grode A *et al.* A study of partial thiamine restriction in human volunteers. *Am J Clin Nutrit* 1980; **33**: 848–61.

37. Godfrey PSA, Toone BK, Carney MWP *et al.* Enhancement of recovery from psychiatric illness by methylfolate. *Lancet* 1990; **336**: 392–5.

38. Committee on Medical Aspects of Food Policy. *Report of the Panel on Dietary Reference Values. Dietary Reference Values for Food, Energy and Nutrients for the United Kingdom*. London: HMSO, 1991.

39. Milio N. Nutrition and health: patterns and policy perspectives in food-rich countries. *Soc Sci Med* 1989; **29**(3): 413–23.

40. Sinclair I, Parker R, Leat D, Williams J. *The Kaleidoscope of Care: a Review of Research on Welfare Provision for Elderly People*. London: HMSO, 1990.

41. Sinclair I, Crosbie D, O'Connor P *et al. Bridging Two Worlds: Social Work and Elderly Living Alone*. Aldershot: Gower, 1988.

42. Bebbington AC, Charnley H, Davies BP, Ferlie EB *et al. The Domiciliary Care Project: Meeting the Needs of the Elderly*. Interim Report to the Department of Health and Social Security, University of Kent, UK.

43. Johnson ML, Gregorio S, Harrison B. *Ageing, Needs and Nutrition: a Study of Voluntary and Statutory Collaboration in Community Care for Elderly People*. London: Policy Studies Institute, 1981.

44. Suski NS, Nielsen CD. Factors affecting food intake of women with Alzheimer's-type dementia in long-term care. *J Am Dietet Assoc* 1989; **12**: 1770–3.

45. Hu T, Huang L, Cartwright WS. Evaluation of the costs of caring for the senile demented elderly: a pilot study. *Gerontologist* 1986; **26**: 158–63.

46. Department of Health and Social Security. *Nutrition and Health in Old Age*. Reports on Health and Social Subjects, No. 16. London: HMSO, 1979.

47. Anderson EL. Eating patterns before and after dentures. *J Am Dietet Assoc* 1971; **58**: 421–6.

48. MacEntee MI, Stolar E, Glick N. Influence of age and gender on oral health and related behaviour in an independent elderly population. *Commun Dental Oral Epidemiol* 1993; **21**: 234–9.

49. Sweeney MP, Shaw A, Yip B, Bagg J. Oral health of elderly institutionalised patients. *Br J Nurs* 1995; **4**: 1204–8.

50. Dickerson JWT. Nutrition and drugs. In Davis SH, ed., *Symposium on Nutrition*. Edinburgh: Royal College of Physicians (Edinburgh), 1980.

51. Office of Population Censuses and Surveys. *General Household Survey*. London: HMSO, 1980.

52. Hunt A. *The Elderly at Home*. London: HMSO, 1978.

53. Piachaud D, Webb J. *The Price of Food: Missing Out on Mass Consumption*. London: Sticerd, 1996.

54. Lennard-Jones JE. *A Positive Approach to Nutrition as Treatment*. London: King's Fund, 1992.

55. Parker D, Emmett PM, Heaton KW. Final year medical students knowledge of practical nutrition. *J R Soc Med* 1992; **85**: 338.

56. Royal College of Nursing. *Nutrition Standards and the Older Adult*. London: Royal College of Nursing, 1993.

57. Peet M, Laugharne J, Rangarajan N. Depicted red cell membrane essential fatty acids in drug treated schizophrenic patients. *J Psychiat Res* 1995; **29**: 227–32.

58. Peet M, Laugharne JD, Mellor J. Essential fatty acid deficiency in erythrocyte membranes of chronic schizophrenic patients and the clinical effect of dietary supplementation. *Prostaglandins Leukot Essent Fatty Acids* 1996; **55**: 71–5.

59. McCreadie R, MacDonald E, Blacklock C *et al.* Dietary intake of schizophrenic patients in Nithsdale, Scotland; case-control study. *Br Med J* 1998; **317**: 784–5.

Mental Illness in Nursing Homes and Hostels in Australia

David Ames

Royal Melbourne Hospital, Parkville, Victoria, Australia

Australia has a population of over 19 000 000 people. Less than 2% are descended from the original inhabitants and over 12% are aged 65+. The probability of using nursing home care at some point in one's life is currently estimated to be around 25% at birth, rising to 60% from when aged 80 and 95% from when aged 90. As the life expectancy of those aged 65 now extends well beyond 80 years, the majority of older Australians can expect to have some experience of residential care before their lives end[1]. In recent years Australian government policy has directed funding away from residential provision towards community care, and has acted to blur the distinction between nursing homes providing full nursing care 24 h/day and hostels that offer accommodation, meals, supervision and some assistance with activities of daily living but do not furnish residents with 24 h/day nursing care[2,3].

In 1993 there were 74 494 nursing home beds in Australia and by 2011, if the intended planning ratio of 40 beds/1000 persons aged 70+ has been reached, there will be 78 600 beds[4]. The policy direction for hostels is to increase the level of supply from a 1993 level of 40 places/1000 persons aged 70+ to a projected level of 52.5 by 2011. There were 54 429 hostel places in Australia in 1993.

By early 1999, 140 000 nursing home and hostel places were available in Australia, with 2500 new places being established each year, mostly in hostels[1]. These places serve 2 154 000 Australians aged 65+, of whom 129 600 were thought to have dementia in 1995[5].

Few residential facilities offer specialized care for the elderly with mental illness. In the State of Victoria a small number of nursing homes subsidized by the State Government, called "Psychogeriatric Nursing Homes", offer specialized care to elderly people with mental health problems (usually dementia), associated with behaviour too challenging to be managed in mainstream facilities. Long-term care in large mental hospitals and state geriatric centres is virtually a thing of the past[6].

A small number of researchers have examined the prevalence of psychiatric disorders among elderly people in Australian nursing homes and hostels. At least 50% and possibly 80% of nursing home residents have dementia[5–7]. Around 40% of hostel residents have cognitive impairment consistent with dementia[6,8]. Although the more severely demented residents cannot be assessed, it is unusual for an assessable resident to have no symptoms of depression at all and at least 10% suffer a depressive disorder at any time[9,10]. No detailed statistics are available for the numbers of individuals with schizophrenia and related disorders living in nursing homes in Australia. The four specialist psychogeriatric nursing homes in the author's own catchment area, which serve a population of over 120 000 elderly, have 120 beds, of which around 30 are occupied by individuals with a primary diagnosis of schizophrenia and related disorder. Most of these residents are former long-term inmates of psychiatric facilities, so this percentage is likely to fall in future as fewer individuals with schizophrenia will experience long-term incarceration. The percentage of individuals with schizophrenia and related disorders in ordinary nursing homes and hostels would be far lower than this.

Despite high levels of depression and dementia, a recent study by Reberger, Hall and Criddle[11] revealed that entering a hostel can lead to an overall improvement in quality of life, although the size of the study was small, assessing only 50 subjects.

General practitioners are responsible for the medical care of the vast majority of individuals in nursing homes and hostels, as few residents see a psychiatrist once, let alone on a regular basis. A well-conducted study of over 2000 residents in 46 Sydney nursing homes revealed very high levels of psychotropic drug prescribing to this population[12]. Psychotropic drugs were taken regularly by 58.9% of residents and another 7% were prescribed such drugs on an "as-required" basis. Antipsychotic drugs were taken regularly by 27.4% and on an "as-required" basis by a further 1.4%. These drugs were more likely to be given to residents with greater cognitive impairment and more disturbed behaviour. Benzodiazepines were prescribed to 32.3%, hypnotics to 26.6% and antidepressants to 15.6%. At least half the antidepressant doses were subtherapeutic.

As in other countries, one major concern has been the underdetection and undertreatment of depression in residential care. An innovative and painstaking series of studies were done in North Sydney by Llewellyn-Jones et al.[13]. This project included a randomized, controlled trial, with control and intervention groups studied sequentially and blind follow-up after 9.5 months of 220 depressed residents in a large residential facility. The interventions consisted of multidisciplinary consultation and collaboration, training of general practitioners and carers in the detection and management of depression, and depression-related health education and activity programmes for residents. The control group received routine care. There was significantly more movement to less depressed levels of depression, as measured by the Geriatric Depression Scale (GDS) at follow-up, in the intervention than the control group. Multiple linear regression analysis found a significant intervention effect after controlling for possible confounders, intervention groups showing an average improvement of 1.87 points on the GDS. Although the impact of this study on total GDS scores was not huge, small movements in depressive symptomatology in populations are likely to be associated with significant decrease in morbidity among some individuals. In the past it has been hard to show that intervention programmes in these populations can be efficacious[10], but the work of Llewellyn-Jones' team suggests that the future may not be as bleak as some of us had feared.

There is no doubt that mental illness is common among individuals who live in residential care in Australia. The challenge for our health professionals is to improve the detection and management of these conditions. A multifaceted approach is required, with improved medical education for both undergraduates and general practitioners, education for care staff and an overall improvement in the quality of residential provision for older people. Slow, relative economic decline in Australia[6], which continues apace, will make this a difficult challenge to rise to, but Australia's track record in this area suggests that the goal is not an unachievable one.

REFERENCES

1. Howe A. Future directions for residential care. *Australas J Ageing* 1999; **183**(suppl): 12–18.
2. Howe AL. From states of confusion to a national action plan for dementia care: the development of policies for dementia care in Australia. *Int J Geriat Psychiat* 1997; **12**: 165–71.
3. Flynn E, Ames D, LoGiudice D. Dementia service provision in Australia. In O'Brien J, Ames D, Burns A, eds, *Dementia*. London: Edward Arnold, 2000.
4. Gibson D, Liu Z. Planning ratios and population growth: will there be a shortfall in residential aged care by 2021? *Aust J Ageing* 1995; **14**: 57–62.
5. Henderson AS, Jorm AF. *Dementia in Australia*, 4th edn. Canberra: Australian Government Publishing Service, 1998.
6. Ames D, Flynn E. Dementia services: an Australian view. In Burns A, Levy R, eds, *Dementia*. London: Chapman and Hall, 1994.
7. Phillips-Doyle CJP. Social interventions to manage mental disorders of the elderly in long term care. *Aust Psychol* 1993; **28**: 25–30.
8. Rosewarne R, Carter MG, Bruce A. *Hostel Dementia Care: Survey of Programs and Participants (Victoria)*. Canberra: Commonwealth Department of Community Services and Health, 1991.
9. Phillips CJ, Henderson AS. The prevalence of depression among Australian nursing home residents: results using draft ICD-10 and DSM-IIIR criteria. *Psychol Med* 1991; **21**: 739–48.
10. Ames D. Depressive disorders among elderly people in long-term institutional care. *Aust N Z J Psychiat* 1993; **27**: 379–91.
11. Reberger C, Hall SE, Criddle RA. Is hostel care good for you? Quality of life measures in older people moving into residential care. *Aust J Ageing* 1999; **18**: 145–9.
12. Snowdon J, Baughan R, Miller R et al. Psychotropic drug use in Sydney nursing homes. *Med J Aust* 1995; **163**: 70–2.
13. Llewellyn-Jones RH, Baikie KA, Smithers H et al. Multi-facteted, shared care intervention for late life depression in residential care: randomised, controlled trial. *Br Med J* 1999; **319**: 676–82.

Caregivers and Their Support

Kathleen C. Buckwalter[1], Linda Garand[2] and Meridean Maas[3]

[1]*University of Iowa,* [2]*University of Pittsburgh School of Nursing, and* [3]*University of Iowa College of Nursing, USA*

As this book clearly demonstrates, Alzheimer's disease and related dementias (ADRD) are tragic, debilitating, chronic illnesses with an unpredictable clinical course. The tragedy is compounded by the consequences associated with caregiving, such as impaired mental and physical health, and disruption of normal activities and social relationships of the caregiver. Cognitively impaired elders are often placed in long-term care facilities when family caregivers are either no longer available or are unable to continue home caregiving because of inability to manage behavioral problems, unremitting stress or caregiver illness. This chapter highlights the importance of the caregiver role, as well as costs to, and support for, family caregivers in the community and throughout the process of relocating the recipient to an institutional setting. Research on caregiver stress and the positive and negative effects of caregiving is reviewed, with attention to both psychosocial and physiological outcomes, as well as variables that may moderate stressors inherent in the caregiving role.

IMPORTANCE OF THE CAREGIVER ROLE

Most older adults requiring assistance reside in the community, including those with dementia[1]. The main reason why persons with dementia are able to reside in the community is because they receive care from their families[2]. Of the more than 4 million Americans with ADRD, over 70% are cared for by family members, and spouses typically are the primary caregivers[3].

Families play a paramount role in the provision of care to persons with dementia and most families want to retain the role of caregiver, since their efforts can forestall institutionalization[4]. Consequently, dementia caregiving has emerged as one of the most serious healthcare issues facing our society today[5].

Who Are Family Caregivers?

There is no precise definition of family caregiving to guide researchers and health professionals[6,7]. Caregiving is a truly heterogeneous concept. Family members define caregiving and care-receiving differently, depending upon their relationship to the care recipient, gender, and whether or not residence is with the care recipient.

Informal caregiving typically falls to women, who provide 72% of family caregiving, with adult daughters providing 29% and wives 43%[8]; 80% of caregivers of persons with dementia are women, 55% are spouses, 35% are adult offspring and 5% are siblings; the remainder are other relatives or paid providers. Thus, family caregiving is more often a career for women[9]. Wives and daughters provide more activities of daily living (ADL) and instrumental activities of daily living (IADL) assistance to family members than do husbands and sons[10,11]. The preponderance of customary IADL assistance, viewed as "women's work", may result in the underestimation of the amount of caregiving of persons with dementia that is borne by women. However, there is evidence that men and women caregivers do not differ in length of caregiving service, hours per day spent in caring for relatives, and the perceived stress of caring for persons with dementia. Both perceive the most stress from dealing with behavioral problems, a common precipitant of institutionalization[12].

Public Policy and Cost Implications of Caregiving

Factors such as the aging of the population, the increase in dependency with age, and the scope of care provided by family members are especially important in understanding dementia care. Policy makers are increasingly aware of the fact that family caregiving is not cost-free. Caregivers incur numerous expenses, including home modifications, assistive devices, special food, high utility costs, and the cost of foregoing paid employment. This type of family support is estimated to be the equivalent of full-time work in about one-third of households providing dementia care. According to Day[13], the cash value of services performed by family caregivers far exceeds the combined cost of government and professional services to both the elderly who live in the community and those who live in institutions. Current estimates indicate that dementia family caregivers save the US healthcare system $196 billion/year[14]. Therefore, the importance of family caregivers will increase in the future, as the number of persons with dementia, and the costs of their care, increase.

Society at large benefits from the willingness and ability of families to care for their members who have dementia. Were it otherwise, persons with dementia would be institutionalized sooner and in larger numbers than is currently the case. This, in turn, would impose a far greater economic burden on society in providing long-term care to persons with dementia. Importantly, monetary estimates of dementia care in no way reflect the human costs of this devastating disease. Although family caregiving helps to contain costs to society as a whole, it often results in serious costs that are concentrated in caregiving families. As noted, the breadth and magnitude of these costs cannot be calculated solely in economic terms. A large body of research has established that there are also profound effects of caregiving associated with poor health-related outcomes[15,16], as detailed later in this chapter.

CAREGIVER STRESS AND BURDEN AND ITS IMPACT ON CAREGIVER WELL-BEING

Concomitant with an increase in the prevalence of dementia is an escalation of the physical, emotional and economic burdens of dementia care. The concept of caregiver burden has been advanced as an all-encompassing term that refers to the financial, social, physical and emotional effects of caring for a family member with dementia[17]. Subjective burden, the caregiver's perception of the caregiving experience, is distinguished from objective burden, the actual changes in the caregiver's home situation[18]. Studies of the burden and stress of caring for a person with dementia, the resulting effects on mental and physical health outcomes of family caregivers, and the use of a variety of interventions to relieve adverse effects of caregiving burden are numerous. More recent research also has focused on the positive aspects associated with caregiving. Major findings from this body of research are summarized throughout this chapter.

Family caregivers of persons with ADRD experience numerous stressors that affect their health and well-being and precipitate institutionalization of the care recipient. Hence, the notion of "stress" has emerged as an important concept in dementia caregiver research[3]. The words "stress", "burden" and "distress" are often used interchangeably and are conceptualized to have similar meaning. George and Gwyther[19] defined the concept of dementia caregiver stress as: "the physical, psychological or emotional, social and financial problems that can be experienced by family members caring for impaired older adults" (p. 243). A variety of factors related to the symptoms associated with ADRD cause caregiver stress, including cognitive changes, loss of ability to function in daily activities, and behavioral disturbances. Spouses of persons with dementia may be at greatest risk for caregiver stress, since they are often elderly themselves. They may also have physical, psychological and financial challenges that could decrease their ability to respond to the demands of caregiving[20,21].

Models of Caregiver Stress

A number of theoretical frameworks have been used to guide studies of persons with dementia, their family caregivers and the effects of interventions on outcomes for both[22-28]. Stress models, in particular, have guided much of this research. However, models that predict a simple positive linear relationship between caregiver stress and the care recipient's level of impairment, such that caregivers providing assistance to the most behaviorally impaired persons report the greatest degree of burden, are not supported by the literature[29,30]. Rather, research indicates that caregiver stress is related to a number of care recipient and caregiver variables[31] and, as such, is a multivariate phenomenon.

Caregiver stress is moderated by many factors, including the caregiver's available resources, such as good physical health, social support, financial assets, coping abilities and personality

$$\text{Distress} = \frac{\text{Exposure to stressors} + \text{Vulnerability}}{\text{Psychological resources} + \text{Social resources}}$$

Figure 138b.1

traits[17]. Although a number of multivariate models of caregiver distress exist, space limitations preclude a review of extant models in this chapter. Rather, Vitaliano's model of distress[32] (Figure 138b.1) is set forth as an example of one useful model for understanding caregiver stress, because the variables of interest are well grounded in the caregiving and theoretical stress literature. Additionally, the model allows for the stratification of resources and vulnerability variables, which improves the chances of detecting relationships among stressors, resources and burden. In Vitaliano's model, both caregiver and care recipient variables, as well as psychological and social resources of the caregiver, are postulated to contribute to caregiver distress[32].

The underlying assumption of research on caregiving stress and health outcomes is that the chronic stress of caregiving can lead, via vulnerabilities and limited resources, to psychological or physiological distress and illness. Vitaliano's model, for example, considers both psychological and biological markers of distress. Since data overwhelmingly suggest negative psychological consequences of caregiver stress, biological outcomes allow for assessment of the impact of the psychological distress on major physiological systems. As noted earlier, in caregiver research, multivariate models provide a more comprehensive picture of a caregiver's level of distress than either psychological or physiological variables alone[32]. Moreover, since Vitaliano's model of distress is expressed as a mathematical formula, a caregiver's level of distress (burden) may improve by decreasing undesirable variables or by increasing desirable variables.

STRESSORS ASSOCIATED WITH FAMILY CAREGIVING

Providing care for a family member with dementia is conceptualized as a chronic stressor[33]. Symptoms of dementia that the caregiver must contend with include (but are not limited to) progressive loss of: memory; judgment; the ability to interpret abstractions; language and motor deficits; and altered personality. Dementia results in profound cognitive and behavioral changes that culminate in an inability to perform instrumental activities of daily living, such as cooking and managing money, as well as basic activities of daily living (ADLs), such as bathing and toileting. The level of functional (ADL and/or IADL) impairment in care recipients was related to caregiver burden in one study[15], although a larger number of studies found no association between these variables[34-41]. Similarly, no evidence of a relationship exists between the care recipient's level of cognitive impairment and the caregiver's level of burden[34,35,39,42-44].

The course of the illness is unpredictable, as is the rapidity of decline; the only certainty is that the progressive cognitive impairments that characterize dementia will lead to an increasing need for supportive care and eventual death for the person with dementia. As the illness progresses, caregivers must be increasingly vigilant, since dementia patients may elope from home or injure themselves. In the final stages, patients are often completely dependent on their caregivers and need to be fed, bathed, toileted, transferred and dressed. Providing care to a person with dementia eventually becomes an all-consuming 24-h job, which may extend for 10 years or longer[45,46].

Behavioral Impairments in Care Recipients

The stress of providing 24 h care for a person with dementia is complicated by the development of episodic, problematic (or catastrophic) behaviors, when the person with dementia becomes increasingly agitated, stressed or disorientated. The most commonly reported behavioral changes associated with dementia include neurovegetative symptoms (e.g. lethargy, social withdrawal), sleep disturbance, restlessness, wandering, assault, aggression, destroying property, verbally disruptive behavior (e.g. screaming), and inappropriate sexual behavior[47-51]. Behavioral problems are extensive in persons suffering from dementia, appearing in up to 67% of care recipients upon diagnosis[52], approximately 65% of demented persons who are institutionalized[49], and 70–90% of persons with advanced dementia[53,54]. They worsen with disease progression and may be related to fatigue, change, overstimulation, excessive demands or physical stressors[23]. Problematic behaviors appear to have a profound effect on caregivers' stress, and a number of investigators have concluded that these secondary symptoms are the most stressful to manage from a caregiving perspective[46,55,56]. In fact, the one care recipient characteristic that overwhelmingly predicts caregiver distress is the degree to which the care recipient demonstrates behavioral problems[15,34,37,44,47,50,51,57]. Many investigators also report that behavioral problems are strong predictors of institutionalization[47,57,58].

Other Factors that Influence Caregiver Stress

As noted earlier, researchers typically theorize the stress of caregiving as chronic because caregivers face many years of continuous exposure to the daily demands of caregiving. However, over the disease trajectory, the intensity and/or frequency of a caregiver's level of distress may vary widely. In an effort to better understand this variability, investigators have identified a number of factors associated with differing levels of morbid outcomes. Of special interest are a number of variables that appear to moderate, or render less harmful, the effects of caregiving among some individuals.

It appears that the amount of stress is influenced by whether or not the caregiver is co-resident with the care recipient, the abruptness of onset of the care recipient's disease, kinship relationship with the care recipient, and the coping strategies used by caregivers[59,60]. Seltzer and Li[61] found that daughters in later stages of caregiving had a more distant relationship with the care recipient and more subjective burden than daughters in the earlier stages, while wives evidenced the opposite pattern. Wives who had provided care for a longer time reported less burden and a closer relationship with their husbands if they perceived themselves to be in the later stages of caregiving. This finding is supported by the longitudinal studies of Schulz and Williamson[40], which suggest that caregivers have successfully adjusted to the rigors of caregiving and have learned to cope with the demands of the task. Evidence is mixed as to gender differences in the stress experienced once the caregiving role is undertaken[62]. Overall, the literature suggests that stress-related gender differences are more pronounced for caregivers of non-demented persons[12].

Social support has been examined both as a correlate of distress (a main effect) and as a modifier of the relationship between stressful experiences and distress (an interaction effect). In the broader stress and coping literature, social support has been a consistent moderator of stress-related outcomes[63], in that the presence of a strong social network and satisfaction with support is a powerful predictor of positive outcomes. Caregiving studies suggest a direct effect of social support on measures of burden, but evidence for a buffering effect has been less clear[32].

In sum, research has identified potential exposure (care recipient behaviors), vulnerability (e.g. age, gender, neuroticism, pre-existing hypertension) and resource (social support) variables that may either moderate or mediate relationships of caregiving psychological distress with measures of physiological impairment and illness. In spite of overwhelming evidence that caregiving is stressful, factors contributing to caregiver distress have not yet been delineated in a way that can effectively direct interventions or preventive strategies.

Dementia vs. Non-dementia Caregiving

There is evidence that family caring for a person with dementia is more stressful than caring for a person who is not demented or who has a physical limitation[64]. For example, Clipp and George[65] found that family members caring for a person with a dementia were more adversely affected by their role than family members caring for a relative with cancer. This relationship was not explained by the duration of the illness or by whether or not the caregiver was employed; however, younger spouse caregivers were more adversely affected than older caregivers. In a review of studies of caregiving in different types of illnesses, Biegel et al.[66] observed different patterns of distress. They concluded that the pattern of a peak distress period after initial diagnosis of acute onset, followed by a reduction in distress as time passes, was not observed in family caregivers of persons with gradual onset illness where no relief of distress was observed[67]. Co-resident caregivers of persons with stroke and of persons with dementia experienced similar degrees of burden and high levels of psychological distress, with psychiatric aspects of care resulting in greater stress than physical aspects[36].

POSITIVE AND NEGATIVE OUTCOMES OF FAMILY CAREGIVING FOR PERSONS WITH DEMENTIA

Although family caregiving of persons with dementia is usually regarded as stressful and includes a variety of negative outcomes, there is growing consensus that this is not always the case[68]. Some caregivers may receive satisfaction from the role[69,70]. Caregivers can gain satisfactions, emotional uplifts, gains in self-esteem and self-efficacy, optimism, and growth and meaning from their roles[71-74].

Impact of Caregiving on Health of Caregivers

Findings of studies are inconsistent as to the effects of caring for persons with dementia on family caregivers' mental and physical health. Some report no changes in emotional and physical health and a decrease in depression over time, although far more report worsening of depression and physical health[45,75-79]. Based on the findings from several studies[44,59,60,80] Wright[81] suggests that these inconsistent findings may be due to differences in coping strategies employed by caregivers.

Mental Health Outcomes

There is extensive documentation that caregivers are at risk for high levels of psychological distress (e.g. burden, stress, depression, perceived hassles). Despite gaps in the literature and differences in research methods used, caregiver studies have overwhelmingly pointed to the adverse effects that caregiving for someone with troublesome behavioral symptoms can have on the caregiver's mental health[16,82,83]. A number of studies have also revealed negative changes due to the strains of direct care, grief associated with the deterioration of their loved ones, social isolation, and the role changes of caregiving, including care at home, following institutionalization, and when the care recipient dies[20,41,66,83–85].

Depression

Depressive symptoms are among the most frequently examined mental health effects on family caregivers of persons with dementia. Several studies document a greater prevalence of depression among caregivers of persons with dementia, compared to other age and gender group norms and persons who are not caregiving[43,86–88].

Prevalence rates of depressive symptomatology among caregivers range from 30%[87] to 46% among community caregivers[86]. Moreover, depression among caregivers is associated with intensity of their reactions to the patients' memory and behavior problems[89,90] and to other adverse outcomes, such as increased physical burden[36], subjective burden[91–93], and use of psychotropic medications[15,65].

Depression is also noted to be greater among females than males[10] and appears to increase over time among residential caregivers and decrease over time following institutionalization and bereavement[83,87]. However, younger spouse caregivers were found to have higher levels of depression than older spouses in a study of residential and institutional caregiving[94]. There were positive relationships between depression and health status and depression and days unable to work among residential caregivers, but only between physical health characteristics and health status among the institutional spouse caregivers, and no significant difference in depression between genders. Compared to non-caregiving men, male spouse caregivers have been shown to have higher levels of depression, respiratory symptoms and poorer health habits, but the groups did not differ on other measures of physical and mental health[95].

Although no subjects were clinically depressed, Wright[81] found spouse caregivers of demented persons to have significantly greater dysphoric moods than a comparison group of non-caregiving spouses, with sadness of subsequently widowed spouses significantly greater than for non-widowed spouses. Widowed spouses also had poorer health outcomes over time and used fewer positive coping strategies, regardless of whether they placed their loved one in an institution.

Anxiety

Several investigators incorporated self-report measures of anxiety into their studies of depression. Mohide et al.[96] found that 22/23 individuals found to have significant symptoms of depression also reported significant symptoms of anxiety. Similarly, Vitaliano et al.[30] found 35.4% of their sample to have significant symptoms of anxiety. Neundorfer[93] reported much lower rates of both anxiety (15%) and depression (25%) among her sample of caregivers, although their scores were somewhat higher than population norms for elderly individuals.

Overall, there is strong evidence suggesting that caregivers exhibit higher levels of psychiatric symptomatology than comparison groups. Yet caution must be exercised when interpreting the generalizability of these findings, since many of the samples may be biased toward the more distressed members of the caregiving community. For example, the majority of caregivers are recruited from local chapters of the Alzheimer's Association, caregiver support groups, or through referrals by healthcare professionals. Individuals who have little difficulty with the caregiving role or who are so distressed or constrained that they are unable to participate in supportive programs or visit healthcare professionals may be underrepresented in research.

Some authors have also questioned the clinical significance of psychiatric symptoms reported in caregiver distress studies. There remains a criterion problem of distinguishing normal distress from psychiatric illness[84]. Transient periods of grief, despair, helplessness and hopelessness may be much more common than a diagnosable depression among family caregivers. Becker and Morrissey[84] argue that the severe and chronic stressors associated with dementia caregiving are unlikely to precipitate a major depressive disorder, except in predisposed individuals. They suggest that the depressive-like symptoms among caregiving spouses should be categorized under Code V: Conditions Not Due to a Psychiatric Disorder[84]. This view is consistent with the conclusion reached by Fitting et al.[97] who state: "It is our impression that most caregivers reporting depressive symptomatology are experiencing a 'transient dysphoric mood' and not major depression" (p. 250).

To summarize, the literature on mental health outcomes of caregiving is suggestive but not conclusive[98]. There is strong evidence for increased symptom reports for depression, anxiety and increased psychotropic drug use among caregivers in these studies, as well as support for increased clinical psychiatric illness among some caregivers.

Physical Health Outcomes

Most of the literature examining the physical effects of caregiving has used one or more indicators of caregiver health: (a) self-reported health status; (b) self-reported incidence of illness-related symptoms; (c) self-reported utilization of health-care services; (d) self-reported medication use; and (e) biological indicators as a measure of susceptibility to disease. Reported predictors of poor physical health outcomes for caregivers include older age, being a spouse rather than adult child or other relative, and being female rather than male[15,79]. Interestingly, a relationship between the positive aspects of caregiving and physical health has also been reported. Emotional uplifts in family members with coronary heart disease (CHD), who are caring for persons with dementia, mediates the severity of metabolic signs that predict CHD[99].

Although there are fewer reported studies, the psychoneurological and immunological effects of caregiving are receiving increased attention. A decrease in measures of cellular immunity, and more days of infection following long-term residential caregiving of persons with dementia compared to controls also has been demonstrated, with caregivers who reported less social support and more stress having the greatest adverse immune function effects 13 months later[87]. Alterations in physiological function as a result of exposure to stress have been found to increase the probability of illness[100].

Similarly, psychological stress can increase caregiver vulnerability to disease by compromising the integrity of the immune system[101]. Kiecolt-Glaser et al.[101] have examined depression and distress as immunological modifiers. Their research team has also documented poorer immune response, in particular changes in the percentages of helper T-lymphocytes and natural killer (NK) cells, in caregivers of persons with dementia, while controlling for nutritional intake and illness-related variables[101].

Caregivers in this study also reported nearly three times as many stress-related symptoms and higher rates of psychotropic drug use than controls, especially those who were living with the person with dementia. Other studies comparing psychotropic drug use in caregiving and non-caregiving samples have also reported that caregivers use more psychotropic medications than non-caregiving controls[15,87,102]. Reports of somatic medication use among caregivers are less consistent, but most studies do not demonstrate a significant difference in the use of these medications between caregiving and non-caregiving samples[42,87,103].

In summary, the findings for physical health effects of caregiving are more equivocal than those for mental health outcomes. Although a number of investigators report significant health effects among subsets of caregivers, patterns of findings across studies are not as consistent. Evidence linking caregiving to physical health indicators, such as reported illness, physical symptoms, healthcare utilization or health-related behaviors, is generally weak[15]. This may be due to different definitions of health, health outcome measures, caregiving and control samples (varying levels of vulnerability and resources), care recipient samples (functional vs. behavioral impairments) and the fact that some self-report measures of physical health may primarily reflect life satisfaction[104].

Evaluating links between caregiver distress and health outcomes will ultimately require complex, multivariate models that are tested prospectively, over an extended period of time. Despite methodological challenges inherent in the evaluation of caregiving outcomes, data from several laboratories lend weight to the argument that chronic stressors contribute to affective disorders and may alter caregivers' sympathetic, neuroendocrine and immunological function.

FAMILY CAREGIVING: RELOCATING THE CARE RECIPIENT

Placing a relative in a nursing home is a stressful event for both the family caregiver and the patient. Caregiving places substantial burdens upon the caregiver and these burdens increase with the progression of the disease. Yet demented persons are usually placed in nursing homes only when all other avenues have been tried and other resources are exhausted[105-107]. Generally, the decision is postponed long past the time when more objective persons see it as appropriate[108]. Or decisions may be crisis-driven, e.g. the care recipient wanders off, sets the stove on fire, or overdoses on pills. One reason this delay occurs is that some caregivers, especially spouses, believe that their role obliges them to sole caregiving responsibility and to never institutionalize their relative[109]. Others may have promised, "I'll never put you in a nursing home", or "... til death do us part". Children, while more likely than spouses to rely on formal services and less enduring than spouse caregivers, nevertheless delay placement decisions because of reluctance to reverse roles and take charge of a parent's life[110].

Overall, the literature indicates that the care recipient's extent of cognitive impairment, loss of self-care abilities, and disruptive behaviors; mediated by caregiver age, employment status, health, stress and burden, relationship with the care recipient, duration of caregiving, and support and moderation by caregiver minority status, kinship relationship with the care recipient, and use of in-home services and resources, are predictive of institutionalization. Cohen et al.[105] described seven variables that affect a caregiver's decision to institutionalize a dependent elder with dementia: use of services; enjoyment of caregiving; caregiver burden and health; caregiver rating; reaction to care receiver behavior and memory problems; and presence of troublesome behaviors. Six variables predicted actual institutionalization: caregiver health; caregiver burden; use of services; care receiver cognitive function; troublesome behaviors; and caregiver reaction to behaviors. Montgomery and Kosloski[110] compared predictors of placement for adult child caregivers and spouse caregivers. Higher income, eligibility for Medicaid, lower morale and age of the elder were associated with placement for both groups, but other predictors of placement were different.

Notably, level of affection predicted placement for children, but not for spouses, while sense of obligation was predictive for spouses, but not for children, who were more likely to place the care recipient in a nursing home at all points in time. The probability of placement declined with time for a while, then leveled off, then rose as caregiving duration exceeded 30 months, with the probability increasing more sharply for child caregivers than for spouses.

Although the number of community services has increased to support family caregiving in the home, the extent to which these services are meeting the needs of caregivers is questioned[111-113]. Collins et al.[114] found that 40% of family caregivers who had placed their loved one with dementia in a nursing home, reported that the availability of at least one additional community service would have delayed the institutionalization. The assumptions that family members know how to provide all of the care that is needed and that they have access to the resources to assist them with provision of needed care in the home are not valid, according to current research[112]. As a result, studies by Archbold et al.[115], Brennan et al.[116] and Buckwalter et al.[117] have evaluated interventions to assist family caregivers in the home with skills, anticipation of decisions and role changes and access to resources.

The consideration of relocation raises the prospect of sharp role transition. For most spouses, relocation changes a longstanding pattern of living together and providing for the other. For children it can mean the restoration of a pattern in which the child is not living with, and/or is not directly responsible for, the care of the parent. Roles that were previously reversed from parent parenting child to child parenting parent are again reversed. Interviews conducted during the Family Involvement in Care research[118] revealed that adult child caregivers of persons with dementia found the decision to put parents in a nursing home very distressing. Frequently reported comments were: "... the worst time in my life"; "... it about killed me to do it"; "... it really bothered me because I knew she would be angry with me", or "... my brothers didn't agree with me and that was a worry". While spouses reported some of these feelings, they tended to be more concerned with the loss of spouse and of the role of caring for the mate. Comments included: "... I knew I would miss him"; "... I hated thinking about not being able to take care of him"; or "... I kept thinking about how he would probably miss me and the things I do for him".

Persons with dementia placed in nursing homes may be highly resistant and fearful of the change. Given their diminished capacity for reasoning, it can be impossible to convince them that they require institutionalization. This presents a very stressful dilemma for family caregivers. It may be more difficult for child caregivers than for spouses, because of the need to reverse roles. Constant requests to be taken home are especially stressful to families. On the other hand, spouses may find it more difficult if their long-term close relationship has been affectionate and loving. In Family Involvement in Care interviews[118], the majority of children, spouses and other relatives noted that it was very hard to actually place the relative in a nursing home. Comments were: "... I cried all the way home"; "... it was so empty at home and I felt so lonely"; "... I knew she would miss her things, so I took as much along as I could, pictures and such. She had so much and then so little, it didn't seem fair"; or "... he kept saying he wanted to go home and tried to leave with me ... it was so sad". Many of the same family members' comments, however, indicated that they also were relieved, but ambivalent: "... it was hard, but I felt like a weight had been lifted"; "... I feel guilty saying so, but I was so glad it was finally done"; "... I felt free to do some things for myself again"; or "... it was hard to do but I knew it was best for my family".

When caregivers lack the necessary skills to manage problematic behaviors effectively, care recipient behaviors often escalate, leading to increased levels of confusion and agitation[23,103] that have been cited as the primary reasons for institutionalizing a family member with dementia[46,119,120]. Considering the psychological and financial expense associated with placing a person with dementia in an institutional setting, interventions which help caregivers in the prevention and/or management of behavioral problems are both timely and significant. In support of this position, the 1993 *Report of the Advisory Panel on Alzheimer's Disease* recommends that emphasis be directed toward health services research that focuses on reducing the burdens of care for family members of persons with dementia.

Although our understanding of the dementias and the severe negative consequences of caregiving for this population has grown, too little research has focused on the development, implementation and evaluation of interventions, especially for family caregivers. The American Association for Geriatric Psychiatry, the Alzheimer's Association and the American Geriatrics Society, in consensus, state: "Interventions that reduce the risk of caregiver depression and improve tolerance and the capacity to care for patients in the home, including educational materials, counseling support groups, day care and respite care, are among the most promising areas for future research"[121].

CONCLUSION

Caring for a person with cognitive impairment is chronically stressful. For persons with dementia, caregiving can last an average of 15 years, with the task being a demanding and often overwhelming experience[62]. This chapter has summarized the research on family caregiving of persons with dementia in the community setting. Informal caregiving, mostly by family members, of elders with chronic illnesses and disabilities has increased during the past two decades due to growth in the proportion of elders in the population, shorter hospital stays, advancing technologies that forestall mortality, and continuing higher costs of health care, with limited reimbursement of caregiving by professionals in the home. As a result, the impact of informal caring on family members quickly became a concern of health professionals and social and behavioral researchers, especially in the context of dementia caregiving. After two decades of extensive attention by the public and researchers, there is some consensus that, while there are both negative and positive effects of informal caregiving, outcomes are different depending upon characteristics of the caregiver and the care recipient. Moreover, different interventions are effective in ameliorating negative caregiver outcomes for specific caregiver and care recipient contingencies.

REFERENCES

1. Doty P. Family care of the elderly: the role of public policy. *Milbank Quarterly* 1986; **64**: 34–75.
2. Daniels M, Irwin M. Caregiver stress and well-being. In Light BDLE, ed., *Alzheimer's Disease Treatment and Family Stress: Directions for Research*. New York: Hemisphere, 1990; 292–309.
3. Grant I, Patterson T, Hauger R, Irwin M. Current research on dementia and Alzheimer's disease. *Arch Psychiat* 1992; **4**(suppl): 77–80.
4. Mittelman MS, Ferris SH, Shulman E *et al*. A family intervention to delay nursing home placement of patients with Alzheimer's disease. *J Am Med Assoc* 1996; **276**: 1725–31.
5. Buckwalter KC. Report of the advisory panel on Alzheimer's disease. *Arch Psychiat Nurs* 1989; **3**: 358–62.
6. MaloneBeach EE, Zarit SH. Current research issues in caregiving to the elderly. *Int J Aging Hum Dev* 1991; **32**: 103–4.
7. Walker AJ, Pratt CC, Eddy L. Informal caregiving to aging family members: a critical review. *Fam Relat* 1995; **44**: 402–11.
8. Horowitz A. Family caregiving to the frail elderly. In Eisdorfor, ed., *Annual Review of Gerontology and Geriatrics*. New York: Springer, 1985; 194–246.
9. Kramer BJ, Kipnis S. Eldercare and work-role conflict: toward an understanding of gender differences in caregiver burden. *Gerontologist* 1995; **35**: 340–8.
10. Miller B, Cafasso L. Gender differences in caregiving: fact or artifact? *The Gerontologist* 1992; **32**: 498–507.
11. Tennstedt SL, Crawford S, McKinley JB. Determining the pattern of community care: is coresidence more important than caregiver relationship? *J Gerontol* 1993; **48**: 574–83.
12. Ford GR, Goode KT, Barrett JJ *et al*. Gender roles and caregiving stress: an examination of subjective appraisals of specific primary stressors in Alzheimer's caregivers. *Aging Ment Health* 1997; **1**: 158–65.
13. Day AT. Who cares? Demographic trends challenge family care for the elderly. *Populat Trends Publ Policy* 1985; **9**: 1–17.
14. United States Administration on Aging (AOA). *Aging Research & Training News*. Silver Springs: Business Publishers, 1999.
15. Baumgarten M, Battista RN, Infante-Rivard C *et al*. The psychological and physical health of family members caring for an elderly person with dementia. *J Clin Epidemiol* 1992; **45**: 61–70.
16. Schulz R, Visintainer P, Williamson GM. Psychiatric and physical morbidity effects of caregiving. *J Gerontol* 1990; **45**: 181–91.
17. Dunkin JJ, Hanley CA. Dementia caregiver burden: a review of the literature and guidelines for assessment and intervention. *Neurology* 1998; **51**(suppl 1): S53–60.
18. Montgomery RJV, Gonyea JG, Hooyman NR. Caregiving and the experience of subject burden. *Fam Relat* 1985; **34**: 19–26.
19. George LK, Gwyther LP. Caregiver well-being: a multidimensional examination of family caregivers of demented adults. *Gerontologist* 1986; **26**: 253–9.
20. Kuhlman GJ, Wilson HS, Hutchinson SA, Wallhagen M. Alzheimer's disease and family caregiving: critical synthesis of the literature and research agenda. *Nurs Res* 1991; **40**: 331–7.
21. Pushkar-Gold D, Reis MF, Markiewicz D, Andres D. When home caregiving ends: a longitudinal study of outcomes for caregivers of relatives with dementia. *J Am Geriat Soc* 1995; **43**: 10–16.
22. Chick N, Meleisa. *Nursing Research Methodology: Issues in Implementation*. Rockville: Aspen, 1986.
23. Hall GR, Buckwalter KC. Progressively lowered stress threshold: A conceptual model for care of adults with Alzheimer's disease. *Arch Psychiat Nurs* 1987; **1**: 399–406.
24. Kahana E. *A Congruence Model of Person–Environment Interaction*. Washington, DC: Gerontological Society, 1975.
25. Hardy M, Conway M. *Role Therapy: Perspectives for Health Professionals*. New York: Appleton-Century-Crofts, 1978.
26. Lawton M. *Competence, Environmental Press, and the Adaptation of Older People*. Washington, DC: Gerontological Society, 1975.
27. Parr J. The interaction of persons and living arrangements. In Poon LW, ed., *Aging in the 1980's: Psychological Issues*. Washington, DC, 1980.
28. Pearlin LI, Mullan JT, Skaff MM. Caregiving and the stress process: an overview of concepts and their measures. *Gerontologist* 1990; **30**: 583–94.
29. Hadjistavropoulos T, Taylor S, Tuokko H, Beattie BL. Neuropsychological deficits, caregivers' perceptions of deficits and caregiver burden. *J Am Geriat Soc* 1994; **42**: 308–14.
30. Vitaliano PP, Russo J, Young HM *et al*. Predictors of burden in spouse caregivers of individuals with Alzheimer's disease. *Psychol Aging* 1991; **6**: 392–402.
31. Stephens MAP, Kinney JM. Caregiver stress instruments: assessment of content and measurement quality. *Gerontol Rev* 1989; **2**: 40–54.
32. Vitaliano PP, Maiuro RD, Ochs H, Russo J. *A Model of Burden in Caregivers of DAT Patients*. DHHS Publication No. (ADM)89-1569. Bethesda, MD: National Institutes of Health, 1989.
33. Light E, Lebowitz BD. *Alzheimer's Disease Treatment and Family Stress: Directions for Future Research*. Rockville: National Institute of Mental Health, 1989.

34. Boss P, Caron W, Horbal J, Mortimer J. Predictors of depression in caregivers of dementia patients: boundary ambiguity and mastery. *Family Process* 1990; **29**: 245–54.

35. Cattanach L, Tebes JK. The nature of elder impairment and its impact on family caregivers' health and psychosocial functioning. *Gerontologist* 1991; **31**: 246–55.

36. Draper BM, Poulos CJ, Cole AMD et al. A comparison of caregivers of elderly stroke and dementia victims. *J Am Geriat Soc* 1992; **40**: 896–901.

37. Hinrichsen GA, Niederehe G. Dementia management strategies and adjustment of family members of older patients. *Gerontologist* 1994; **34**: 95–102.

38. Morrissey E, Becker J, Rubert MP. Coping resources and depression in the caregiving spouses of Alzheimer's patients. *Br J Med Psychol* 1990; **63**: 161–71.

39. Russo J, Vitaliano PP, Brewer DD et al. Psychiatric disorders in spouse caregivers of care-recipients with Alzheimer's disease and matched controls: a diathesis-stress model of psychopathology. *J Abnorm Psychol* 1995; **104**: 197–204.

40. Schulz R, Williamson GM. A 2-year longitudinal study of depression among Alzheimer's caregivers. *Psychol Aging* 1991; **6**: 569–78.

41. Wallhagen ME. Caregiving demands: their difficulty and effects on the well-being of elderly caregivers. *Scholar Inqu Nurs Pract Int J* 1992; **6**: 111–27.

42. Brodaty H, Hadzi-Pavlovic D. Psychosocial effects on carers of living with persons with dementia. *Aust NZ J Psychiat* 1990; **24**: 351–60.

43. Dura JR, Stukenburg KW, Kiecolt-Glaser JK. Anxiety and depressive disorders in adult children caring for demented parents. *Psychol Aging* 1991; **6**: 467–73.

44. Pruchno RA, Potashnik L. Caregiving spouses: physical and mental health in perspective. *J Am Geriat Soc* 1989; **37**: 697–705.

45. Brody EM. *Women in the Middle: Their Parent-Care Years*. New York: Springer, 1990.

46. Teri L. Behavior and caregiver burden: behavioral problems in patients with Alzheimer's disease and its association with caregiver stress. *Alzheim Dis Assoc Disord* 1997; **11**: S35–8.

47. Chenoweth B, Spencer B. Dementia: the experience of family caregivers. *Gerontologist* 1986; **26**: 267–72.

48. Folstein MF, Bylsma FW. Non-cognitive symptoms of Alzheimer's disease. In Terry RD, Katzman R, Bick KL, eds, *Alzheimer's Disease*. New York: Raven, 1994; 27–40.

49. Nasman B, Bucht G, Erikson S. Behavioral symptoms in the institutionalized elderly: relationship to dementia. *Int J Psychiat* 1993; **8**: 67–73.

50. Rabins P, Mace NL, Lucas MJ. The impact of dementia on family. *J Am Med Assoc* 1982; **248**: 333–5.

51. Teri L, Traux P, Logsdon R, Uomoto J. Assessment of behavioral problems in dementia: the revised memory and behavior problems checklist. *Psychol Aging* 1992; **7**: 622–31.

52. Cacabelos R. Diagnosis of Alzheimer's disease: defining genetic profiles. *Acta Neurol Scand* 1996; **93**: 572–84.

53. Swearer JM, Drachman DA, O'Donell BF, Mitchell AL. Troublesome and disruptive behaviors in dementia: relationships to diagnosis and disease severity. *J Am Geriat Soc* 1988; **36**: 784–90.

54. Teri L, Larson E, Reifler BV. Behavioral disturbance in dementia of the Alzheimer's type. *J Am Geriat Soc* 1988; **36**: 1–6.

55. Advisory Panel on Alzheimer's Disease. *Second Report of the Advisory Panel on Alzheimer's Disease*. NIH Publication No. 93-3520. Washington, DC: Superintendent of Documents, US Government Printing Office, 1991.

56. Smith GC, Smith MF, Toseland RW. Problems identified by family caregivers in counseling. *Gerontologist* 1991; **31**: 5–22.

57. Cohen-Mansfield J. Agitated behaviors in the elderly: preliminary results in the cognitively deteriorated. *J Am Geriat Soc* 1986; **34**: 722–7.

58. Zimmer J, Watson N, Treat A. Behavioral problems among patients in skilled nursing facilities. *Am J Publ Health* 1984; **74**: 1118–21.

59. Quayhagen MP, Quayhagen M. Alzheimer's stress: coping with the caregiving role. *Gerontologist* 1988; **28**: 391–6.

60. Zarit SH, Birkel RC, MaloneBeach E. Spouses as caregivers: stresses and interventions. In Goldstein MY, ed., *Family Involvement in Treatment of the Frail Elderly*. Washington, DC: American Psychiatric Press, 1989; 26–62.

61. Seltzer MM, Li LW. The transitions of caregiving: subjective and objective definitions. *Gerontologist* 1996; **36**: 614–26.

62. Schulz R, O'Brien AT, Bookwala J, Fleissner K. Psychiatric and physical morbidity effects of dementia caregiving: prevalence, correlates, and causes. *Gerontologist* 1995; **35**: 771–91.

63. Lazarus RS, Folkman S. *Stress, Appraisal, and Coping*. New York: Springer-Verlag, 1984.

64. Browning JS, Schwirian PM. Spousal caregivers' burden: impact of care recipient health problem and mental status. *J Gerontol Nurs* 1994; **20**: 17 22.

65. Clipp EC, George LK. Psychotropic drug use among caregivers of patients with dementia. *J Am Geriat Soc* 1990; **38**: 227–35.

66. Biegel DE, Sales E, Schulz R. *Family Caregiving in Chronic Illness: Alzheimer's Disease, Cancer, Heart Disease, Mental Illness, and Stroke*. Newbury Park, CA: Sage, 1991.

67. Reese DR, Gross AM, Smalley DL, Messer SC. Caregivers of Alzheimer's disease and stroke patients: immunological and psychological characteristics. *Gerontologist* 1994; **34**: 534–40.

68. Gatz M, Bengtson VL, Blum MJ. Caregiving families. In Birren JE, Schaie KW, eds, *Handbook of the Psychology of Aging*. New York: Academic Press, 1990; 405–26.

69. Silliman RA, Fletcher RH, Earp JL, Wagner EH. Families of elderly stroke patients: effect of home care. *J Am Geriat Soc* 1986; **34**: 643–8.

70. Zarit SH, Todd PA, Zarit JM. Subjective burden of husbands and wives as caregivers: a longitudinal study. *Gerontologist* 1986; **26**: 260–6.

71. Farran CJ, Keane-Hagerty T, Salloway S, Kupferer S. Finding meaning: an alternative paradigm for Alzheimer's disease family caregivers. *Gerontologist* 1991; **31**: 483–9.

72. Kinney JM, Stephens MAP. Hassles and uplifts of giving care to a family member with dementia. *Psychol Aging* 1989; **4**: 402–8.

73. Shifren K, Hooker K. Stability and change in optimism: a study among spouse caregivers. *Exp Aging Res* 1995; **21**: 59–76.

74. Stephens MAP, Franks MM. Spillover between daughters' roles as caregiver and wife: interference or enhancement? *J Gerontol* 1995; **50**: 9–17.

75. Cox C, Monk A. Minority caregivers of dementia victims: a comparison of black and Hispanic families. *J Appl Gerontol* 1990; **9**: 340–54.

76. Liptzin G, Grob MC, Eisen SV. Family burden of demented and depressed elderly psychiatric inpatients. *Gerontologist* 1988; **28**: 397–401.

77. Schulz R, Tompkins CA, Rau MT. A longitudinal study of the psychosocial impact of stroke on primary support persons. *Psychol Aging* 1998; **3**: 131–41.

78. Townsend A, Noelker L, Deimling G, Bass D. Longitudinal impact of interhousehold caregiving on adult children's mental health. *Psychol Aging* 1989; **4**: 393–401.

79. Young RF, Kahana E. Specifying caregiver outcomes: gender and relationship aspects of caregiving strain. *Gerontologist* 1989; **29**: 660–6.

80. Barusch AS. Problems and coping strategies of elderly spouse caregivers. *Gerontologist* 1988; **28**: 677–85.

81. Wright LK. Spousal caregivers: longitudinal changes in health, depression, and coping. *J Gerontol Nurs* 1994; **20**: 33–45, 48.

82. Cohen D, Eisdorfer C. Depression in family members caring for a relative with Alzheimer's disease. *J Am Geriat Soc* 1988; **36**: 885–9.

83. Collins C, Stommel M, Wang S, Given C. Caregiving transitions: Changes in depression among family caregivers of relatives with dementia. *Nursing Res* 1994; **43**: 220–5.

84. Becker J, Morissey E. Difficulties in assessing depressive-like-reactions to chronic severe external stress as exemplified by spouse caregivers of Alzheimer's patients. *Psychology and Aging* 1988; **3**: 300–306.

85. Given B, Given CW. Family caregiving for the elderly. In Fitzpatrick J, Taunton R, Jacox A, eds., *Annual Review of Nursing Research*. New York: Springer, 1991; 77–101.

86. Gallagher D, Rose J, Revera P et al. Prevalence of depression among family caregivers. *Gerontologist* 1999; **29**: 449–56.

87. Kiecolt-Glaser JK, Dura JR, Speicher CE et al. Spousal caregivers of dementia victims: longitudinal changes in immunity and health. *Psychosom Med* 1991; **53**: 345–62.

88. Moritz DJ, Kasl SV, Berkman LF. The health impact of living with a cognitively impaired elderly spouse. *J Gerontol* 1989; **44**: S17–27.

89. Kiecolt-Glaser JK, Dyer CS, Shuttleworth EC. Upsetting social interactions and distress among Alzheimer's disease caregivers: a replication and extension. *Am J Commun Psychol* 1988; **16**: 825–35.

90. Pearson J, Teri L, Wagner A, Traux P, Logsdon R. The relationship of problem behavior in dementia patients to the depression and burden of caregiving spouses. *Am J Alzheim Dis Rel Disord Res* 1993; **8**: 15–22.

91. Drinka TJ, Smith J, Drinka PJ. Correlates of depression and burden for informal caregivers of patients in a geriatrics referral clinic. *J Am Geriat Soc* 1987; **35**: 522–5.

92. Gaynor SE. The long-haul: the effects of home care on caregivers. *Image—J Nurs Scholarship* 1990; **22**: 208–14.

93. Neundorfer MM. Coping and health outcomes in spouse caregivers of persons with dementia. *Nurs Res* 1991; **40**: 260–5.

94. Bergman-Evans G. A health profile of spousal Alzheimer's caregivers: depression and physical health characteristics. *Caregiver Health* 1994; **32**: 25–30.

95. Fuller-Jonap F, Haley WE. Mental and physical health of male caregivers of a spouse with Alzheimer's disease. *J Aging Health* 1995; **7**: 99–118.

96. Mohide EA, Pringle DM, Streiner DL *et al*. A randomized trial of family caregiver support in the home management of dementia. *J Am Geriat Soc* 1990; **38**: 446–54.

97. Fitting M, Rabins P, Lucas MJ, Eastham J. Caregivers for dementia patients: a comparison on husbands and wives. *The Gerontologist* 1986; **26**(suppl 3): 248–252.

98. Schulz R, O'Brien AT. Alzheimer's disease caregiving: an overview. *Semin Speech Lang* 1994; **15**: 185–93.

99. Vitaliano PP, Scanlan JM, Siegler IC *et al*. *Caregiving Exacerbates the Metabolic Syndrome Associated with Coronary Heart Disease*. Presented at the American Psychosomatic Medicine Society Annual Meeting, Santa Fe, New Mexico, 1997.

100. Brantley P, Garrett V. *Psychobiological Approaches to Health and Disease*. New York: Plenum Press, 1993; 647.

101. Kiecolt-Glaser J, Glaser R. Psychosocial moderators of immune function. *Ann Behav Med* 1987; **9**: 16.

102. Grafstrom M, Fratiglioni L, Sandman PO, Winblad B. Health and social consequences for relatives of demented and non-demented elderly: a population-based study. *J Clin Epidemiol* 1992; **45**: 861–70.

103. Vitaliano PP, Young HM, Russo J *et al*. Does expressed emotion in spouses predict subsequent problems among care recipients with Alzheimer's disease? *J Gerontol* 1993; **48**: 202–9.

104. Hooker K and Siegler IC. Separating apples from oranges in health ratings: Perceived health includes psychological well-being. *Behavior, Health and Aging* 1992; **2**: 81–92.

105. Cohen C, Gold D, Shulman K *et al*. Factors determining the decision to institutionalize demented individuals: a prospective study. *Gerontologist* 1993; **33**: 714–20.

106. Tipton-Smith S, Tanner G. Coping with placement of a parent in a nursing home through preplacement education. *Geriat Nurs* 1994; **15**: 322–6.

107. Zarit S, Whitlatch C. Institutional placement: phases of the transition. *Gerontologist* 1992; **32**: 665–72.

108. Ade-Ridder L, Kaplan L. Marriage, spousal caregiving, and a husband's move to a nursing home: A changing role for the wife. *J Gerontol Nurs* 1993; **19**: 13–23.

109. Dellasega C, Mastrian K. The process and consequences of institutionalizing an elder. *West J Nurs Res* 1995; **17**: 123–40.

110. Montgomery R, Kosloski K. A longitudinal analysis of nursing home placement for dependent elders cared for by spouses versus adult children. *J Gerontol* 1994; **49**: S62–74.

111. Applebaum R, Phillips P. Assuring the quality of in-home care: the "other" challenge for long-term care. *Gerontologist* 1990; **30**: 444–50.

112. Kelley LS, Buckwalter KC, Maas ML. Access to health care resources for family caregivers of elderly persons with dementia. *Nursing Outlook* 1998; **47**: 8–14.

113. Kane R. The noblest experiment of them all: learning from the National Channeling Evaluation. *Health Serv Res* 1988; **23**: 189–98.

114. Collins C, King S, Kokinakis C. Community service issues before nursing home placement of persons with dementia. *Western Journal of Nursing Research* 1994; **16**(suppl 1): 40–56.

115. Archbold P, Stewart B, Miller L *et al*. The PREP system of nursing interventions: A pilot test with families caring for older members. *Res Nurs Health* 1995; **18**: 3–16.

116. Brennan P, Moore S, Smyth K. Alzheimer's disease caregivers' use of a computer network. *West J Nurs Res* 1992; **14**: 662–73.

117. Buckwalter KC, Hall GR, Kelly A *et al*. PLST model: effectiveness for rural ADRD caregivers. Unpublished NIH/NINR Grant, University of Iowa, Iowa City, IA, 1992.

118. Maas M, Swanson E. *Nursing Interventions for Alzheimer's: Family Role Trials*. Research Grant, National Institute of Nursing Research, R01-NR01689. Rockville: National Institutes of Health, 1992.

119. Pruchno RA, Michaels JE, Potashnik SL. Predictors of institutionalization among Alzheimer's disease victims with caregiving spouses. *J Gerontol* 1990; **45**: S259–66.

120. Potter JF. Comprehensive geriatric assessment in the outpatient setting: population characteristics and factors influencing outcome. *Exp Gerontol* 1993; **28**: 447–57.

121. Small GW, Rabins PV, Barry PP *et al*. Diagnosis and treatment of Alzheimer's disease and related disorders. Consensus statement of the American Association for Geriatric Psychiatry, the Alzheimer's Association, and the American Geriatrics Society. *J Am Med Assoc* 1997; **278**: 1363–71.

122. Miller B, McFall S. Gender differences in caregiving: fact or artifact? *Gerontologist* 1991; **32**: 498–507.

The Sydney Dementia Carers' Training Program

Henry Brodaty

School of Psychiatry, University of New South Wales, Little Bay, Australia

In 1983, when we devised the Sydney Dementia Carers' Training Program, previously named the Prince Henry Hospital Dementia Caregivers' Training Program[1] and the Dementia Carers' Programme[2], we aspired to provide state-of-the-art caregiver intervention. Our aims were to reduce caregiver distress by addressing, where possible, all factors known to aggravate caregiver distress and to delay nursing home admission of persons with dementia.

A number of facts were already well known about caregivers. Caregivers had high levels of psychological morbidity and negative affect, and were more likely to be depressed and experience low morale. Caregivers most vulnerable to adverse psychological effects were women, spouses, care providers (rather than care managers) and those who were physically unwell, used immature coping mechanisms and were socially isolated. Lack of support from family and friends, critical comments from those

EXACERBATING FACTORS

Social isolation

Lack of knowledge

Poor skills

Immature coping

Guilt

Poor marital relationship

High expressed emotion

PROTECTIVE FACTORS

Practical support

Family help

Problem-focused coping

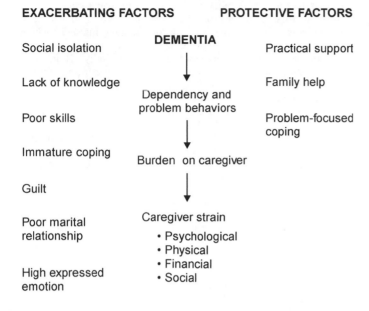

DEMENTIA

Dependency and problem behaviors

Burden on caregiver

Caregiver strain
- Psychological
- Physical
- Financial
- Social

Figure 1 Model of the effects of dementia on caregivers

close to the caregiver and past history of psychological ill-health were other risk factors[3–6].

By the early 1980s, several intervention techniques had been described. These were designed to enhance the skills of caregivers in coping by cognitive-behavioural approaches, training in problem solving, educational therapy, meditative relaxation, training in social skills, supportive counselling of individuals or families, and the management of stress (see reviews[7,8]).

The outcomes of studies were limited by a number of methodological difficulties. The numbers of subjects were small, the period of follow-up was insufficient, the interventions were limited in scope, the baseline level of morbidity in subjects was often low, making it impossible to demonstrate improvement, and patient outcome was inadequately evaluated. Even so, there were some positive outcomes demonstrated: reduced family burden, decreased psychological morbidity, greater knowledge about dementia and more assertiveness and tolerance by caregivers[7].

A number of events, some unique, led to the development of the Sydney Dementia Carers' Training Program. First was the content, which was based on addressing factors known to exacerbate caregiver distress and indirectly potentiate nursing home admission. Second, there was a period of low occupancy on the psychiatric ward of a general hospital which, if not remedied, meant that some of the beds were under threat of closure. Third, the author, as the director and superintendent of that ward, was able to utilize a variety of staff to assist in the program. Fourth, a pilot program had proved feasible and anecdotally effective and facilitated a grant from the Australian Commonwealth Department of Health.

In the model underpinning the program (Figure 1), dementia leads to increasing dependency and a number of problem behaviours. These impose a burden on the caregiver, which can manifest as psychological, physical, financial and social strain.

Exacerbating factors drive the reaction towards more psychological strain; protective factors ameliorate this.

CONTENT OF THE PROGRAM[a]

The content of the 10 day intensive residential program can be conceptualized under 10 rubrics [discipline of professional(s) conducting the session; number of sessions and duration of sessions are indicated in parentheses]:

1. *Reducing caregiver distress* (social worker/occupational therapist; 2×2 h $+ 1 \times 1.5$ h). These sessions were scheduled first, as we found that caregivers were unable to acquire new knowledge until their psychological distress had been dealt with. Sessions were informal, supportive and expressive in nature, with caregivers encouraged to unburden themselves. Discussion in the first session included topics such as caregivers' stories, the stresses of caring, associated feelings, setting limits for the person with dementia and caregiver, coping with caring, and role changes. The second session explored the additional themes of acceptance of the disease and how dementia affects relationships with family, friends and community. The third session focused on caregiver burnout and how to look after one's individual needs.

2. *Combating isolation* (psychiatrist; 1×1 h). We aimed to reduce caregivers' social isolation by the group interaction, residential setting and bringing together four caregivers for 10 days. This often led to mini-support groups forming and was a rehearsal for participation in other support groups. After the intensive residential program, telephone conference calls and hospital follow-up visits strengthened the bonds between groups of four caregivers. Extended formal family sessions brought together an expanded network of potential caregivers. For many families it was the first time they had all gathered to discuss ways of assisting with care. Sometimes geographically distant families participated on speaker telephones.

3. *Guilt and separation.* Caregivers previously trapped by their role, guilt or their partner's insecurity or suspiciousness were separated from their charges for most sessions, and encouraged to enjoy a number of activities, such as excursions to the local shopping centre or coffee shop. This provided a rehearsal for more separateness when at home.

4. *New ways of thinking*
   (a) *Assertiveness training* (psychologist or occupational therapist; 2×1.5 h). Participants were provided with a working knowledge of assertive, non-assertive and aggressive behaviours, with their own "Bill of Rights", and with strategies for coping with criticism. Sessions were concrete and used role-play extensively.
   (b) *Re-roling* (psychologist; 1×2 h). This focused on roles—concept, definition (mainly by gender), expectations and responsibilities—and how these were affected by dementia. Many caregivers had considerable difficulty taking over roles relinquished by the dementing person, such as driving, organizing the family and dealing with bureaucracy. Required skills were identified and their development promoted.
   (c) *Relaxation and stress management* (occupational therapist; 8×30 min, daily). Techniques for relaxation, meditation, use of physical imagery and progressive muscular relaxation, complemented by two half-hour discussions on the theory of relaxation and stress response, were very popular. Caregivers obtained audiotapes to practise techniques themselves and with their partners.

5. *New coping skills*
   (a) *Communication* (psychologist; 1×2 h). The first half of this component was theoretical. It focused on:
   - How to communicate with a dementing person.
   - The functions and expectations of communication.
   - How communication processes can be disrupted.
   - Information on language impairment that occurs in dementia, such as receptive and expressive dysphasia.
   - Techniques for clear communication, e.g. the four Ss— keep it simple, slow, short and specific[9].

   In the second half, techniques were practised by each patient–caregiver dyad while being videotaped and/or observed by the group through a one-way mirror. Caregivers were able to review the videotape and analyse their performance and communication techniques.
   (b) *Reality orientation* (occupational therapist; 1×1 h). This was based on a 24 h environmental reality orientation model with use of verbal techniques, signs, pictures, clocks, diaries and other strategies.
   (c) *The therapeutic use of activities* (occupational therapist; 1×1 h). This introduced the concepts of activity as being goal-directed use of time, energy and attention. *Activity analysis* was explained as breaking tasks into small steps, then modifying, eliminating or replacing steps that prevented the dementing person from completing the task (e.g. having a bath, playing golf, cooking). There was also much discussion on appropriate leisure pursuits.
   (d) *Reminiscence* (occupational therapist; 1×1 h). Caregivers were taught how to compile a "This Is Your Life" book, comprising mementos and photographs that described the past life of the patient. This proved to be a positive experience and subsequently provided a good stimulus for conversation and reminiscing.
   (e) *Coping with physical frailty* (various; 3×1 h). First, a physiotherapist discussed back care, walking and mobility aids. Second, an occupational therapist discussed the use and abuse of aids to daily living; caregivers tried out many of these aids in a modified kitchen, bathroom and bedroom in the occupational therapy department. Third, a registered nurse outlined the care of bed-bound, chair-bound and incontinent persons.
6. *Fitness, diet, organizing the day and home* (various; 3×1 h).
   (a) A physiotherapist encouraged fitness and flexibility in caregivers as well as patients. For example, a daily routine of walking after lunch was established.
   (b) A dietitian outlined the principles of a healthy, balanced diet and discussed time-saving kitchen techniques as well as food fads and eating problems associated with dementia.
   (c) In a session on *work simplification*, and *organization and safety in the home*, the occupational therapist explored techniques of how to prioritize and simplify tasks and how and when to recruit outside assistance. The aim was to help caregivers achieve a balance between work, leisure and rest in their lives. Safety issues pertinent to the older person and the dementing process were discussed and a safety checklist for the home and garden was provided.
7. *Medical aspects of dementia* (psychiatrist; 2×1 h). These sessions provided medical information on dementia and its different types, principles of management, psychiatric complications and behavioural changes, use and abuse of medication, the interaction of dementia and other illnesses, and prognosis. As with all of these sessions, much time was given to answering individual concerns.
8. *Using community services* (welfare officer; 1×1.5 h). This very practical session included procedures and eligibility for social securities, provision of useful contact persons, and access to and availability of services. For some caregivers it was a novelty to adopt the role of *care manager*, e.g. organizing other people, such as domiciliary nurses, to help with provision of care, rather than that of *care provider*, where the caregiver undertook tasks personally. Reinforcement was given that use of services did not represent failure or dereliction of duty. Numerous pamphlets were provided on domiciliary nursing care benefits, pensions, methods of assessing nursing homes and hostels and mechanisms for complaints about services.
9. *Planning for the future* (psychiatrist; 1×1 h). The last formal session was fairly open and considered *how to plan for emergencies*, e.g. should something happen to the caregiver. Other issues, such as driving, medications, safe use of alcohol, smoking, legal, medical and financial matters and other emergency contingencies were discussed.
10. *Coping with problem behaviours*. There was no time set to discuss these specifically, although each session was structured to allow discussion of current or potential problems, such as aggression or wandering. The aim was to give caregivers a broad education on the possible reasons for the emergence of problems and a repertoire of skills to prevent their occurrence or to deal with them if they occurred.

THE PATIENT PROGRAM

For caregivers to be able to learn in a relaxed setting, they needed to know that their partners were receiving satisfactory care. Patients had their own program, which consisted of: (a) general ward activities, such as occupational therapy, outings and relaxation classes; and (b) specific programs—group discussion of their frustrations with their memory loss, reminiscence therapy and a memory retraining program. Given a forum for honest and open discussion, patients established strong bonds with each other, were able to discuss their feelings surprisingly frankly and often became protective of each other. Memory techniques included use of visualization and one-tracking (focusing on one task to be remembered at a time). While we were unable to demonstrate any improvement in cognitive function[10], our impression was that patient morale improved.

Process

The course was residential and for a variety of (non-essential) reasons, as explained above, took place in the psychiatric ward of a general teaching hospital, with caregiver and patient couples sharing individual rooms. An advantage of this setting was the availability of facilities and staff. A disadvantage was the inappropriateness of some interactions with psychiatric patients, yet there was no attrition among the 96 participants who attended the program. The 10 day program began on a Tuesday and finished on the Thursday of the following week (Table 1). Our 5 day, Monday to Friday, pilot programs proved too congested and caregivers requested that a weekend be included. This allowed caregivers time to spend talking together, having fun, such as a picnic, and consolidating some of the knowledge previously presented.

A major aim of the course was for participants to enjoy themselves. Sadly, fun and spontaneity are often lacking from caregivers' lives. Leisure pursuits, such as walks, table games like "Trivial Pursuit", carpet bowls, singalongs, dances and going out for a drink, were included as part of the evening and weekend program. During these activities, caregivers would practise their

Table 1 Timetable of Dementia Caregivers' Training Program

	Morning	Afternoon	Evening
Day 1	Admission procedures Welcome and orientation	"Getting to know you" Reducing carer distress 1	Socializing
Day 2	Stress management and relaxation "Telling your story" Reducing carer distress 2	Healthy eating for older people	Film night
Day 3	Relaxation Re-roling	Reminiscence Keeping fit and healthy	Carer outing
Day 4	Relaxation Assertiveness training 1	Therapeutic use of activities and activity analysis Medical aspects of dementia 1	Socializing
Day 5	Relaxation practice with tape Picnic outing		Socializing
Day 6	Relaxation practice with tape Church	Sunday drive	Socializing
Day 7	Relaxation Communication	Assertiveness training 2 Medical aspects of dementia 2	Extended family sessions
Day 8	Stress management and relaxation Reality orientation	Work simplification and organization in the home Combating burnout	Extended family sessions
Day 9	Relaxation Use of community services	Coping with physical frailty	Socializing
Day 10	Relaxation "What if"—planning for the future	Farewell afternoon tea and presentation of diplomas	

skills of communication, activity analysis, reality orientation and reminiscence.

Patients and caregivers were given name tags and briefed daily after breakfast to review the previous night and to confirm each day's arrangements. Less threatening sessions were scheduled for the first week of the program; those that required more self-examination or were more confronting about the realities of the dementia were left until the second week. At the end of the program there was an afternoon tea graduation ceremony and presentation of a diploma.

Follow-through

Follow-through was an essential part of the program. While the 10 day program was both intensive and comprehensive and supplemented by take-home written materials and audiotapes, it was felt that the lessons would be lost without reinforcement. Telephone conferences were arranged with the coordinator at increasing time intervals over 12 months, starting at 2 weekly and finishing at 6 weekly intervals. The coordinator's input was gradually diminished on these telelinks. Towards the end of the year, the coordinator would absent herself from teleconference calls. Cohorts of caregivers attended the hospital for follow-up assessments at 3, 6 and 12 months after the completion of the program, thus providing opportunities for reunions. Relationships among cohorts of caregivers varied, with some establishing quite close friendships and continuing to meet informally at each other's houses. After the first year, annual telephone follow-ups were conducted. Two long-term outcomes were monitored, nursing home admission and death. Data on these endpoints were obtained for all patients.

THE TRIAL

We recruited subjects by seeking referrals from doctors, aged care and healthcare providers or by having articles in the media. While the pilot programs had been heavily subscribed, once the research proper began, the well-known "disappearing subjects" phenomenon was evident. Of the 96 caregivers who entered the study, 40 did so of their own initiative, 16 were referred by local doctors, 15 through the Alzheimer's Disease and Related Disorders Society, eight after media publicity, and 17 through other sources.

To be eligible, we required that patients be less than 80 years old (for follow-up purposes) and have mild to moderate dementia, defined by the *Diagnostic and Statistical Manual of Mental Disorders*, 3rd edn[11]. The patients had to live in a private home with a supporter, be able to understand English, not be a wanderer and not be aggressive. We stipulated that patients had to have dementia of mild to moderate severity defined as a score on the basic Activities of Daily Living of 0 or 1. All subjects agreed to random allocation to either a memory-retraining program (for patients only) or a dementia caregivers' program (as described above). Subjects were told that neither program offered a cure, but both offered the possibility of improvement in function. Institutional ethics committee approval was received prior to the trial and all subjects gave written informed consent.

Procedures

Prospective applicants for the program were sent questionnaires and the postal date on the envelope of the questionnaire determined which group eligible subjects were assigned to. Importantly, no systematic bias could have occurred because the time when caregivers sent their application was purely random and therefore meant that their allocation was not biased by any selection procedure. Subjects were assigned in turn to one of three treatment groups: *memory retraining program, immediate dementia caregivers' program*, or *wait-list or delayed dementia caregivers' program*. In the *memory retraining program*, patients were admitted for 10 days and received the patient component of the dementia caregivers' program, while their caregivers had 10 days' respite. Those in the *delayed training group* received the dementia caregivers' program after approximately 6 months. We calculated a sample size of over 30 for each of the three groups as necessary for an intervention of moderate power (estimate 0.6) to produce a relevant effect size (estimate 0.67) for $\alpha = 0.5$.

Assessment

Patients were assessed on the Orientation Information Memory Concentration scale [OIMC, range 0–37 (37 = maximum cognitive functioning)[12]; the Dementia Scale [range = 0–27 (higher score indicates worse function)[12]; the Mini-Mental State Examination [range 0–30 (30 = maximum cognitive function, < 17 indicated important deterioration)[13]; the 21 item Problem Behaviour Checklist[14] [range 0–42 (0 = no problems, 42 = all problems occurring frequently)]; the Activities of Daily Living [range 0–6 (0 = completely independent, 6 = completely dependent)[15]; the Instrumental Activities of Daily Living [range 1–4 (1 = complete independence, higher scores indicate increasing dependence)[16]; the 21 item Hamilton Rating Scale for Depression [range 0–64 (> 16 indicates important depression)[17]; the Geriatric Depression Scale [range 0–20 (> 10 indicates possible depression)[18]; and the Clinical Dementia Rating Scale for Dementia [range 0–3; (0 = healthy, 3 = severely demented)[19].

Carers completed the General Health Questionnaire [range 0–30 (those with scores > 4 probably were considered to have significantly psychological morbidity)[20]; and the Zung Depression Scale [range 20–80 (⩾ 40 indicated important depression)[21] and were rated on the Hamilton Depression Rating Scale. They were asked to keep a health diary of all the healthcare visits made and medications taken by them and the patient over the 12 months of follow-up. They were also asked to keep a record of all visits to day centres and any days in residential care. Completion of the diaries was encouraged at the regular telephone conference sessions. Demographic data on all participants were collected and included the position on the Congalton scale for socioeconomic status [range 1–7 (1 = highest status occupation, 7 = lowest)[22].

RESULTS

The Sample Defined

One hundred and one pairs of patients and caregivers entered the trial. Three of the 36 pairs in the *immediate carers' program* had insufficient follow-up data, and one of the 32 patients in the *memory retraining group* (MRP) changed caregivers during the follow-up period. These four pairs were excluded from further analyses. Two pairs in the *delayed carers' program* (DCP) completed intake and pretraining assessments but elected not to proceed with the training. Their data from the initial two assessments were included in the analyses at 0 and 6 months, but not subsequently. Otherwise all patients and caregivers who began the programs completed them.

This left 33 pairs in the immediate DCP, 32 in the wait-list DCP and 31 in the MRP. Of the 96 carers, 89 were spouses, four were siblings and three were children of patients. Forty-four caregivers were men and 30 of the 87 who completed the question affirmed their membership of the Alzheimer's Disease and Related Disorders Society. The caregivers' mean age was 67.7 (SD = 8.2 years).

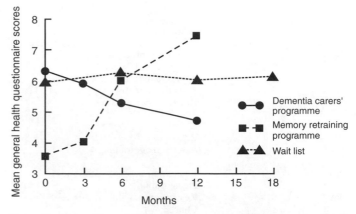

Figure 2 Mean General Health Questionnaire scores for carers in all three groups. Standard deviations of each group at zero, three, six, and twelve months respectively were 6.2, 5.8, 6.2, and 5.6 for the dementia carers' programme group; 6.3, 7.1, 8.4, and 9.4 for the memory retraining group; and 6.1, not available, 6.7, 6.6, and 7.7, at 18 months, for the wait list group. From Brodaty and Gresham[2], by permission of the BMJ Publishing Group

Of the 96 patients, 50 were men, 70 had probable Alzheimer's disease, 19 had multi-infarct dementia, and seven had other causes of dementia. Their average age was 70.2 (SD = 6.5 years; range 49–79 years) and they had had 10.4 (3.6) years' education and had mild-moderate dementia [Clinical Dementia Rating Scale score 1.1 (0.5)]. The duration of dementia, a mean of 3.8 (3.8) years, was similar in the three groups. The sample was predominantly middle-class (n = 52), with 16 from the upper socioeconomic classes and 25 from the lower socioeconomic classes. Data from three patients were missing. There were no significant differences between the three groups, for caregivers or patients, on any socioeconomic variable or initial measure of outcome at entry into the trial.

In later reports from the study, three subjects were excluded. One subject did not decline and he was subsequently rediagnosed as having benign forgetfulness; another subject who had undertaken the *memory retraining program* was excluded because he and his wife subsequently undertook a caregiver training program; and a third subject from the wait-list group did not provide sufficient data. Otherwise, all subjects declined over time, confirming their diagnosis of a progressive dementia. Diagnoses were able to be refined over time, so that of the 93 patients, 65 were subsequently diagnosed with probable Alzheimer's disease, 21 with multi-infarct dementia, three with Pick's disease and four with other uncertain cause of dementia (two subcortical dementia, one carbon monoxide poisoning and one diagnosis deferred). There were some slight differences in the baseline characteristics of patients and caregivers once these three pairs had been excluded, but these were trivial. Details can be found in the report from Brodaty et al.[1]

Caregivers' Outcome

Caregivers' psychological morbidity, as judged by the General Health Questionnaire (GHQ-30) declined significantly over 12 months in the immediate intervention but rose steadily in the memory retraining group. GHQ scores of those in the delayed training program remained steady (Figure 2). Scores on the Zung Depression Scale did not show this differential effect, probably reflecting the low initial scores on that scale and the biological nature of many of its items[21].

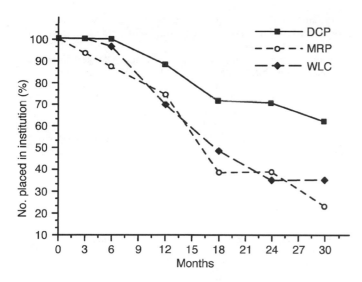

Figure 3 Survival curve showing percentage of patients not placed in an institution over time in the three programme groups. From Brodaty and Gresham[2], by permission of the BMJ Publishing Group

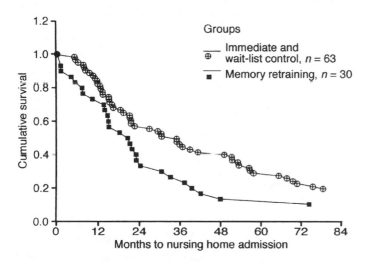

Figure 4 Kaplan–Meier survival functions for nursing home admission comparing the combined training groups with the memory retraining group. From Brodaty *et al.*[1], with permission. Copyright John Wiley & Sons Ltd

Patients' Outcomes

Over the 12 months there was a steady decline in all measures of patient cognition and function (Figure 2). Thus for the total sample, the MMSE scores declined from 17.1 (6.5) at baseline to 16.2 (7.3) at 6 months and 15.2 (7.6) at 12 months. Similarly, the Blessed dementia scale score increased from 7.0 (2.9) to 8.2 (4.3) and 10.4 (5.4) over the 12 months. Activities of Daily Living declined from 0.3 (0.6) to 1.1 (1.4) and 1.7 (1.7) over the 12 months. There were no differences between the three groups in the rate of patient decline. Patients were not depressed clinically. Fewer than six at any assessment over the 12 months had a Hamilton score of $\geqslant 16$. Their mean Hamilton and Geriatric Depression scale scores remained low and stable over time.

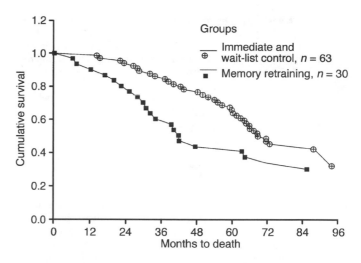

Figure 5 Kaplan–Meier survival functions for death comparing the combined training groups with the memory retraining group. From Brodaty *et al.*[1], with permission. Copyright John Wiley & Sons Ltd

Nursing Home Admission and Mortality

In the first 30 months, there was a marked difference between the groups in the percentage of patients still at home (Lee-Desu statistic = 6.19, df = 2, $p < 0.05$) (Figure 3). At 8 years follow-up, the rates of nursing home admission in the immediate and delayed carer training groups were similar and were combined, allowing for a comparison of the effect of caregiver training in general to the memory retraining group (Figure 4). Using Kaplan–Meier survival functions, there was a significant difference between the groups in survival at home and mortality. The rates of death of patients at 30 month and 8 year reviews were lower where caregivers had had training (Figure 5).

Costs

Program Costs and Institutional Costs

As the program was conducted within the psychiatric unit of a general teaching hospital, it was more expensive than may have been necessary. Even so, we were able to demonstrate that the costs of training were more than counterbalanced by the delay in nursing home admission. By 39 months follow-up, there were only 32 patients still alive at home: 17 of 31 (55%) from the immediate carers' program, 11 of 29 (38%) from the delayed carers' program and 4 of 30 (13%) from the memory retraining program. At the time, the average cost of a nursing home bed was *$92.23/day. We calculated the total institutional costs for the three groups as $19 918 for immediate carers' training patients, $27 375 for delayed carers' program patients, and $36 753 for memory retraining program patients. The cost of the training was estimated in 1991 as $8868, including the hospital stay and 12 months' follow-up. This represented a saving of $7967 (Australian) ($5975 US) per couple in the immediate training program (compared to those in the memory training program) in the first 39 months of the program.

---

*Costs quoted in Australian dollars throughout. $1 Australian = $0.75 US at that time.

Health Care and Lost Employment Costs

We found that over the first 12 months of follow-up there were no appreciable differences between the groups in the number of visits to all doctors, general practitioners or non-medical health practitioners; or in the use of medication or of hospitals. In the second 6 months of the first year, memory retraining patients spent more nights in institutional care than the other two groups.

Prediction of Nursing Home Admission and Death

By 5 years follow-up, 75.8% of patients had entered a nursing home and 41.8% had died. Dementia severity and rate of deterioration and carer psychological morbidity significantly influenced rates of nursing home admission and death. These rates were comparable to previous reports[23,24].

Carer training had a significant protective effect against nursing home admission and, surprisingly (and independently of nursing home admission), against death. There was an association between earlier nursing home admission and caregiver distress, as measured by the GHQ; index measures of dementia severity and problem behaviours; more rapid decline in cognitive function; more rapid decline in overall dementia severity; and increase in problem behaviours.

COMMENTS

Carer intervention programs have considerable potential. They can improve the quality of life of the carers and probably that of patients[1]. We have recently reviewed 35 controlled studies of carer intervention and found that a minority of them demonstrated clinically significant beneficial effects[8].

Limitations to previous studies included: heterogeneity of patients and of carers in the sample; variety of recruitment methods; ceiling and floor effects as regards the outcome measures; low number of numbers and insufficient power; lack of blindness; insufficient duration of follow-up; and lack of specificity in matching interventions with carer needs[8].

The Sydney Carer Training Program study overcame many of these limitations and demonstrated psychological improvement in carers, delay in nursing home admissions and cost savings. The delay in institutionalization was not at the expense of increased carer distress.

There were a number of unanswered questions from the study. It was not possible to know which components of the package of interventions were effective. We provided a broad-spectrum intervention—something for everybody. This was confirmed at exit interviews after 12 months' follow-up, where each component of the program was identified by at least one carer as being helpful to him/her.

The program was unnecessarily expensive in that it was conducted within a hospital setting. While this provided many advantages, it was very costly, and the cost analyses allowed for 20 hospital bed-days per patient–carer couple. We do not know whether the program needed to be residential, although this did provide some advantages. The advantages of residential programs are that they promote more cohesive bonding and allow for observation of behaviours not easily accessible within a day program. Clearly, residential programs could be conducted in less expensive settings.

The ideal number of couples per training cohort is unknown, but our impression was that numbers greater than 10 would impede the group process. Also, our experience suggested that the earlier the intervention, the better, and that matching carer cohorts, e.g. spouses, younger people with dementia, socioeconomically and geographically, may have advantages.

Future research might benefit from a more targeted, selective approach—matching the needs of carers with appropriate interventions. The questions of which carer interventions benefit which carers for which patients at what time in the course of the dementia are complex. Finally, the advent of specific drug treatments for Alzheimer's disease begs the question of whether carer interventions plus drug treatments are superior to either alone.

REFERENCES

1. Brodaty H, Gresham M, Luscombe G. The Prince Henry Hospital dementia caregivers' training programme. *Int J Geriat Psychiat* 1997; **12**: 183–92.
2. Brodaty H, Gresham M. Effect of a training programme to reduce stress in carers of patients with dementia. *Br Med J* 1989; **299**: 1375–9.
3. Morris RG, Morris LW, Britton PG. Factors affecting the emotional well-being of the caregivers of dementia sufferers. *Br J Psychiat* 1988; **153**: 147–56.
4. Brodaty H. Dementia and the family. In Bloch S, Hafner J, Harari E, Szmukler GI, eds, *The Family in Clinical Psychiatry*. Oxford: Oxford University Press, 1994: 224–46.
5. Brodaty H, Green A. Family caregivers for people with dementia. In O'Brien J, Ames D, Burns A, eds, *Dementia*, 2nd edn. London: Chapman & Hall, 2000.
6. Donaldson C, Tarrier N, Burns A. Determinants of carer stress in Alzheimer's disease. *Int J Geriatr Psychiat* 1998; **13**(4): 248–56.
7. Brodaty H. Carers: training informal carers. In Arie T, ed., *Recent Advances in Psychogeriatrics 2*. Singapore: Churchill Livingstone, 1992.
8. Green A, Brodaty H. Evidence-based dementia: caregiver interventions. In Qizilbash N, Schneider L, Chui H *et al.*, eds, *Evidence-based Dementia Practice: a Practical Guide To Diagnosis and Management*. Oxford: Blackwell Science (in press).
9. Ball J. Communicating with people with dementia. In Bowden F, Squires B, eds, *Dealing with Dementia—A Self Study Course for Carers*. Continuing Education Support Unit, University of New South Wales, Kensington, 1987.
10. Christiansen H. Lack of cognitive benefit from a memory training program. Unpublished manuscript, 1988.
11. American Psychiatric Association. *Diagnostic and Statistical Manual of Mental Disorders*, 3rd edn, revised (DSM-III-R). Washington, DC: American Psychiatric Association, 1987.
12. Blessed G, Tomlinson BE, Roth M. The association between quantitative measures of dementia and of senile change in the cerebral grey matter of elderly subjects. *Br J Psychiat* 1968; **114**: 797–811.
13. Folstein MF, Folstein SE, McHugh PR. "Mini-Mental State". A practical method for grading the cognitive state of patients for the clinician. *J Psychiat Res* 1975; **12**: 189–98.
14. Gilleard CJ. Problems posed for supporting relatives of geriatric and psychogeriatric day patients. *Acta Psychiat Scand* 1984; **70**: 198–208.
15. Katz S, Apkom CA. A measure of primary sociobiological functions. *Int J Health Ser* 1976; **6**: 493–507.
16. Lawton MP, Brody EM. Assessment of older people: self-maintaining and instrumental activities of daily living. *Gerontologist* 1969; **9**: 179–86.
17. Hamilton M. A rating scale for depression. *J Neurol Neurosurg Psychiat* 1960; **23**: 56–62.
18. Yesavage JA, Brink TL, Rose TL, Adey M. The geriatric depression rating scale: comparison with other self-report and psychiatric rating scales. In Crook T, Ferris S, Bartus R, eds, *Assessment in Geriatric Psychopharmacology*. New Canaan, CT: M. Dowley, 1983.
19. Hughes CP, Berg L, Danzieger WL *et al.* A new clinical scale for the staging of dementia. *Br J Psychiat* 1982; **140**: 566–72.

20. Goldberg D. *The Detection of Psychiatric Illness by Questionnaire.* New York: Oxford University Press, 1972.
21. Zung WWK. Depression in the normal aged. *Psychosomatics* 1967; **8**: 287–92.
22. Congalton AA. *Status Ranking List of Occupations in Australia. Appendix B to Status and Prestige in Australia.* Melbourne: FW Cheshire, 1969.

23. Bird M, Llewellyn Jones R, Smithers H *et al.* Challenging behaviour in dementia: a project at Hornsby/Ku-Ring-Gai Hospital. *Australas J Ageing* 1998; **17**: 10–15.
24. Brodaty H, McGilchrist C, Harris L, Peters K. Time until institutionalization and death in patients with dementia: role of caregiver training and risk factors. *Arch Neurol* 1993; **50**: 643–50.

Elder Abuse—
Epidemiology, Recognition and Management

Martin J. Vernon

South Manchester University Hospitals NHS Trust, Manchester, UK

During the 1980s, elder abuse emerged as a health and social issue of international importance[1]. It is defined as "a single or repeated act or lack of appropriate action occurring within any relationship where there is an expectation of trust which causes harm or distress to an older person"[2]. While most authorities include self-neglect within the broad definition, acts which threaten an elder's well-being as a consequence of their competently made decisions are specifically excluded.

Abuse may occur in one of two settings. Domestic abuse is perpetrated within the home of the victim or a caregiver by either a relative or other care provider. Institutional abuse occurs within a designated care facility (residential or nursing home or hospital), perpetrated by one or more individuals having an obligation to care for and protect the victim.

Five major categories of abuse have been identified[3,4]:

1. *Physical*: any activity involving force to generate bodily injury or pain, including striking or burning and the use of physical or pharmacological restraint.
2. *Sexual*: any form of non-consensual sexual contact, including unwanted touching, rape, sodomy and coerced nudity.
3. *Psychological*: the infliction of distress through verbal or non-verbal acts, including insults, threats, humiliation, infantilization and harrassment.
4. *Financial*: the improper use of an elder's property or assets, including theft, deception, coercion and misuse of authority to act, such as power of attorney.
5. *Neglect*: the refusal or failure to fulfil care obligations, including the provision of food, water, clothing, medication, comfort and protection.

PREVALENCE AND INCIDENCE

Variability in case definition obscures direct comparison, although the prevalence of elder abuse is broadly similar throughout Europe and North America. To date there are few data from developing countries (Table 138c.1). With the exception of the USA, a lack of national incidence data reflects widespread absence of formal mechanisms for case reporting and validation. American data estimate the incidence of domestic abuse at 450 000 elderly people/year, of which only 16% are reported to statutory agencies[5].

VICTIM CHARACTERISTICS

Likelihood of being abused increases with age[6]. Elders aged over 85 are at particular risk of neglect[7], financial abuse[8] and abuse by designated carers[9]. There is some evidence that minority ethnicity and non-White race represent risk factors for abuse[6,10]. Women are more likely than men to be victims[11] but this observation may be confounded by greater likelihood of living alone, which is associated with financial abuse[8]. In contrast, victims of physical, sexual or psychological abuse are likely to live with others, particularly a spouse or child[12]. Poverty elevates the risk of abuse[6].

The role of cognitive impairment is complex. Factors predicting abuse of dementia patients include behavioural disturbance, poor premorbid relationship with a carer and psychological or physical abuse by the patient[13]. The severity of cognitive impairment does not appear to be associated with abuse. Spouses caring for dementia patients are at particular risk of psychological and physical abuse[33]. In one series, one-third of carers reported physical abuse by the patient, which in turn was associated with abuse of the patient by the carer[14].

Vulnerability to abuse has been associated with certain personality traits[15]. Victims of psychological abuse have less ability to control problem situations and tend to react aggressively when feeling anger or frustration. In contrast, physical abuse victims pursue passive or avoidant behaviour, while financial abuse victims possess negative beliefs of self-efficacy and turn aggression or frustration on themselves.

ABUSER CHARACTERISTICS

Greater understanding of abusive situations has focused attention on those perpetrating abuse. Carers who suffer social isolation, feel unsupported and are financially dependent are at risk of abusing[13,16,17]. Men are more likely to abuse than women, and more likely to cause physical abuse[18]. Psychological abuse is more likely to be caused by women. Abusers tend to suffer declining health and mental illness increases the risk of perpetrating abuse[19]. In particular, depression and anxiety among carers are associated with abusive behaviour[20,21].

The role of drug and alcohol misuse is controversial. Abusers identified as misusing substances are likely to be male children of the victim, less likely to provide care and more likely to cause physical or psychological abuse than financial abuse[22]. However, in one study of referrals to a community psychiatric service, consumption of alcohol by the carer was not associated with abuse[13].

Principles and Practice of Geriatric Psychiatry, 2nd edn. Edited by J. R. M. Copeland, M. T. Abou-Saleh and D. G. Blazer
©2002 John Wiley & Sons, Ltd

Table 138c.1 Prevalence (%) of elder abuse (aged 65+)

Abuse type	UK[1]	The Netherlands[2]	USA[3]	Canada[4]	Sri Lanka[5]*
Physical	1.5	1.2	2.0	0.5	1.5
Psychological	5.4	3.2	1.1	1.4	1.5
Financial	1.5	1.4	–	2.5	1.0
Neglect	–	0.2	0.4	0.4	5.6

[1]Ogg and Bennett[32].
[2]Comjis et al.[31].
[3]Pillemer and Finklehor[12].
[4]Podnieks[33].
[5]Lekamwasam and Chandanee[34].
*Aged 60+.

Table 138c.2 Risk factors for abuse

Victim
  Age >75
  Living alone (financial abuse)
  Living with spouse or child (physical, sexual or psychological abuse)
  Low income
  Cognitive impairment
  Poor pre-morbid relationship with carer
  Abusive, passive or avoidant behaviour

Abuser
  Male (physical abuse)
  Female (psychological abuse)
  Social isolation
  Financial dependency
  Impaired physical or mental health
  Substance abuse
  History of receiving or perpetrating abuse

Table 138c.3 Abuse signals[29]

Caregiver personal problems
Caregiver interpersonal problems
Care receiver social support shortage and history of abuse

Table 138c.4 Symptoms and signs of abuse[4]

Physical abuse
  Carer refusal to permit examination
  Reports of being hit, kicked or mistreated
  Unexplained behavioural disturbance
  Presence of unexplained bruises, lacerations, ligature marks, fractures
  Untreated injuries in various stages of healing
  Inappropriate use of prescribed medication

Sexual abuse
  Reports of sexual assault or rape
  Bruising of breasts or genital area
  Torn, stained or bloody underclothing
  Unexplained genital infection or bleeding

Psychological abuse
  Reports of verbal or emotional mistreatment
  Withdrawal, non-communication or non-responsiveness
  Unexplained or unusual agitation or behavioural disturbance

Financial abuse
  Reports of financial exploitation
  Unauthorized or unexplained changes in banking practice
  Abrupt, unauthorized or unexplained changes to financial documentation
  Unexplained disappearance of assets
  Unmet care needs in the presence of adequate financial resources
  Sudden appearance of individuals asserting their rights to an elder's assets

Neglect
  Reports of mistreatment
  Failure to provide food and hydration
  Failure to meet clearly identified care needs
  Hazardous or unsanitary living conditions

NATURAL HISTORY OF ABUSE

Those who have suffered abuse are themselves likely to become abusers[23] and carers who have violent elders express more violence to their dependants[24]. In one follow-up study, 20% of victims suffered physical or financial damage following abuse, although 70% were able to stop abuse either themselves or with the help of others[31]. Corroborated abuse is associated with greater risk of death for elderly victims (odds ratio 3.1; 95% CI, 1.4–6.7) after adjusting for co-morbid and demographic factors[25]. However, abuse rarely leads to homicide: in one study only 2% of elderly homicides could be attributed to abuse[26].

RECOGNITION

Diagnosis of elder abuse requires a high index of suspicion. Professionals should be alert to the presence of one or more risk factors for abuse (Table 138c.2) and sensitive to principal abuse signals (Table 138c.3). In cases of suspected abuse, a coordinated multi-agency approach must identify all care needs and deficiencies. Corroborated history must be obtained from all participants, including victim, alleged abuser and designated carers, with careful verification of information obtained from cognitively impaired individuals.

Symptoms and signs of abuse must be elicited during a comprehensive clinical assessment to which the victim consents (Table 138c.4). Accurate documentation, including note keeping, radiology and photography, will facilitate future management planning. The presence or absence of particular features do not alone confirm or exclude the diagnosis of abuse. Nevertheless,
defensiveness and irritability by caregivers are predictive of abuse, poor physical care predicts physical abuse and psychosocial stress or exploitation predict psychological abuse[27].

MANAGEMENT

Denial, resistance to intervention, ignorance of intervention protocols, confidentiality and fear of reprisal have all been cited as professional barriers to the management of elder abuse[28]. Central to effective management is the establishment of a single coordinating agency, providing education, advice and access to resources. Intervention models should be low-cost, multidisciplinary, collaborative and capable of evaluating outcomes[29]. The key elements of such a model may include:

- Educational resources.
- Mechanisms for accurate case identification.
- Professionals to identify and deal with health, social, financial and legal issues.
- Workers to support and monitor victims and their care networks.
- Victim empowerment and advocacy groups.

Identification of incipient abuse should generate a brisk response to avoid escalation. Management must aim to preserve autonomous choice for the victim and avoid paternalistic action that seeks to provide a speedy resolution, perhaps through institutionalization. Accurate identification of unmet care needs should generate planned and effective care strategies, which engender safety without intrusion. Given that abuse may be multidirectional, attention may need to be focused on both victim and abuser.

While overtly criminal activity, such as theft or assault, may be dealt with by prevailing criminal law, most countries have eschewed a legislative approach to elder abuse, relying instead upon health and social service agencies to develop locally applicable policies and procedures. In the USA mandatory reporting laws have achieved only limited success and professionals remain unfamiliar with reporting procedures[30]. Of greater potential benefit for the future is the emergence of national organizations, aiming to prevent the abuse of older people by disseminating research, informing public policy and providing specialist advice to both professionals and the general public[3].

REFERENCES

1. Bennett G, Kingston P. *Elder Abuse: Concepts, Theories and Interventions*. London: Chapman and Hall, 1993.
2. Action on Elder Abuse. *Definition*. London: Action on Elder Abuse, 1995.
3. Jenkins G, Asif Z, Bennett G. *Listening is Not Enough*. London: Action on Elder Abuse, 2000.
4. National Center on Elder Abuse. *Briefing Papers*. Washington, DC: National Aging Information Center, 2000.
5. Takamura C, Golden O. *National Elder Abuse Incidence Study*. Washington, DC: National Aging Information Center, 1998.
6. Lachs MS, Williams C, O'Brien S *et al.* Older adults: an 11 year longitudinal study of adult protective service use. *Arch Intern Med* 1996; **156**(4): 449–53.
7. Pittaway E, Gallagher E. *Services for Abused Canadians*. Centre on Aging, University of Victoria, 1995.
8. Penning MJ. *Elder Abuse Resource Centre. Research Component—Final Report*. Winnepeg: Centre on Aging, University of Manitoba, 1992.
9. Vinton L. Services planned in abusive elder care situations. *J Elder Abuse Neglect* 1992; **4**(3): 85–99.
10. George J. Racial aspects of elder abuse. In Eastman M, ed., *Old Age Abuse*, 2nd edn. London: Age Concern England/Chapman and Hall, 1994.
11. Wilson G. Abuse of elderly men and women among clients of a community psychogeriatric service. *Br J Soc Work* 1994; **24**: 661–70.
12. Pillemer K, Finklehor D. The prevalence of elder abuse: a random sample survey. *Gerontologist* 1988; **28**(1): 51–7.
13. Compton SA, Flanagan P, Gregg W. Elder abuse in people with dementia in Northern Ireland: prevalence and predictors in cases referred to a psychiatry of old age service. *Int J Geriat Psychiat* 1997; **12**(6): 632–5.
14. Coyne A, Reichman WE, Berbig LJ. The relationship between dementia and elder abuse. *Am J Psychiat* 1993; **150**(4): 643–6.
15. Comjis HC, Jonker C, van Tilburg W, Smit JH. Hostility and coping capacity as risk factors of elder mistreatment. *Soc Psychiat Psychiat Epidemiol* 1999; **34**(1): 48–52.
16. Cooney C, Mortimer A. Elder abuse and dementia—a pilot study. *Int J Soc Psychiat* 1995; **41**(4): 276–83.
17. Kurrle SE, Sadler PM, Lockwood K, Cameron ID. Elder abuse: prevalence and outcomes in patients referred to four aged care assessment teams. *Med J Aust* 1997; **166**(3): 119–22.
18. Segstock MC. Sex and gender implications in cases of elder abuse. *J Women Aging* 1991; **3**(2): 25–43.
19. Wolf RS, Pillemer KA. *Helping Elderly Victims: the Reality of Elder Abuse*. New York: Columbia University Press, 1989.
20. Homer A, Gilleard CJ. Abuse of elderly people by their carers. *Br Med J* 1990; **301**: 1359–62.
21. Paveza GJ, Cohen D, Eisdorfer C *et al.* Severe family violence and Alzheimer's disease: prevalence and risk factors. *Gerontologist* 1992; **32**(4): 493–7.
22. Hwalek MA, Neale AV, Goodrich CS, Quinn K. The association of elder abuse and substance abuse in the Illinois Elder Abuse System. *Gerontologist* 1996; **36**(5): 674–700.
23. Penhale B, Kingston P. Elder abuse: similarities, differences and synthesis. In Kingston P, Penhale B, eds, *Family Violence and the Caring Professions*. London: Macmillan, 1995: 245–61.
24. Pillemer K, Suitor JJ. Violence and violent feelings: what causes them among family caregivers? *J Gerontol* 1992; **47**(4): 165–72.
25. Lachs MS, Williams CS, O'Brien S *et al.* The mortality of elder mistreatment. *J Am Med Assoc* 1998; **280**(5): 428–32.
26. Falzon AL, Davis GG. A 15 year retrospective review of homicide in the elderly. *J Forens Sci* 1998; **43**(2): 371–4.
27. Mendonca JD, Velamoor VR, Sauve D. Key features of maltreatment of the infirm elderly in home settings. *Can J Psychiat* 1996; **41**(2): 107–13.
28. Krueger P, Patterson C. Detecting and managing elder abuse: challenges in primary care. *Can Med Assoc J* 1997; **157**(8): 1095–100.
29. Reis M, Nahmiash D. When seniors are abused: an intervention model. *Gerontologist* 1995; **35**(5): 666–71.
30. Jones JS, Veenstra TR, Seamon JP, Krohmer J. Elder mistreatment: national survey of emergency physicians. *Ann Emerg Med* 1997; **30**(4): 473–9.
31. Comjis HC, Pot AM, Smit JH *et al.* Elder abuse in the community: prevalence and consequences. *J Am Geriat Soc* 1998; **46**(7): 885–8.
32. Ogg J, Bennett GCJ. Elder abuse in Britain. *Br Med J* 1992; **305**: 998–9.
33. Podnieks E. National Survey on abuse of the elderly in Canada. The Ryerson Study. Toronto: Ryerson Polytechnical Institute.
34. Lekamwasam S, Chandanee H. Elder maltreatment, Sri Lankan experience. Communications to the Spring Meeting of the British Geriatrics Society, London, 1999; 7.
35. Levin E, Sinclair I, Gorbach P. *Families Services and Confusion in Old Age*. Aldershot: Gower, 1989.
36. Reis M, Nahmiash D. Validation of the indicators of abuse (IOA) screen. *Gerontologist* 1998; **38**(4): 471–80.

The Care of the Dying Patient

Robert E. Nelson and Keith G. Meador

Duke Institute on Care at the End of Life, Durham, NC, USA

The care of the older dying patient is provided in many settings, including homes, tertiary care hospitals, nursing care facilities and inpatient hospices. The issues relevant to psychiatry are relatively consistent across these contexts. This chapter provides an overview of the major psychiatric syndromes and therapies that are covered more thoroughly in the primary palliative care literature.

PSYCHIATRIC SYNDROMES IN PALLIATIVE CARE

Depression

Depression is common in terminal illness. The prevalence of a major depressive syndrome in late-stage cancer patients has been estimated at 23–58%, varying by diagnostic criteria and methodology[1]. The diagnosis of depression is sometimes difficult to make in the setting of medical illness, because many of the symptoms of the patient's condition may overlap with those of depression, such as fatigue, loss of energy and altered sleep and appetite. Furthermore, many of these same symptoms can be side effects of medications, such as corticosteroids or chemotherapeutic agents. The general approach to this diagnostic problem is to rely more on the psychological and cognitive symptoms of depression, such as worthlessness, hopelessness, excessive guilt and suicidal ideation[2]. One method used to clarify the distinction between depression and medical illness is the substitution of physical symptoms of uncertain etiology with psychological counterparts. An example of this approach is found in the Endicott Substitution Criteria[3], which replaces physical symptoms as follows: (a) change in appetite and weight is replaced by tearfulness and depressed appearance; (b) sleep disturbance is exchanged for social withdrawal and decreased talkativeness; (c) fatigue and loss of energy are substituted with brooding, self-pity and pessimism; and (d) diminished concentration and indecisiveness are replaced by lack of reactivity.

Another complexity in diagnosing depression in dying older adults is the question of how much of a patient's symptoms should be attributed to the normal difficulties of adjusting to the terminal nature of his/her diagnosis. When interviewing the patient, each of the clinical symptoms of depression should be explored in detail, with special attention to its pervasiveness and its interference in functioning. For example, hopelessness may be understandable with regards to hoping for a cure or recovery, but patients who are not depressed may be able to maintain hope for other improvements, such as better symptom control, or a better connection with their loved ones before their death. Hopelessness that is accompanied by despair or suicidal ideation is highly associated with a depressive syndrome and usually merits treatment[4]. While the multitude of issues relevant to its discussion is beyond the scope of this chapter, the assisted suicide movement heightens the need for careful assessment of depressive symptoms in the elderly dying patient.

The treatment of depression in terminally ill older patients often includes pharmacotherapy and is similar to other geriatric settings in its attention to managing symptoms and side effects. For this reason, selective serotonin reuptake inhibitors (SSRIs) are widely used in this setting because of their tolerability and their ability to also address anxiety. However, the principal side effect of SSRIs, gastrointestinal upset, can lead to weight loss, which is particularly detrimental to debilitated, medically fragile patients. Special care needs to be taken regarding drug interactions of the cytochrome P450 system with this class of drugs. Venlafaxine, a serotonin–norepinephrine reuptake inhibitor (SNRI), is less likely to interact with other medications because of its low protein binding (35%). Terminal illness makes a second variable relevant in medication choice, that of likely duration of treatment. In the setting of a life expectancy of days to weeks, an SSRI will not have time to take effect. For this reason, many clinicians favor the shorter-acting SSRIs, such as sertraline or citalopram. Bupropion has a similarly low side-effect profile as the SSRIs and also has some of the same dopamine agonist properties as the psychostimulants (see below), which may make it a good alternative in this setting. Tricyclic antidepressants are useful as adjuvant pain control and for sleep, but their side-effect profile and drug interactions make them a second-line choice.

Psychostimulants are a well-studied alternative for treating depression in terminally ill patients. While they are less useful in general populations because of tolerance and abuse potential, patients at the end of life can tolerate stimulants for up to a year without significant abuse problems[2]. Particularly helpful in the depressed patient with psychomotor retardation and mild cognitive impairment, stimulants such as methylphenidate and dextroamphetamine have been shown to reduce sedation from narcotic analgesics and also have adjuvant analgesic effects in cancer patients[5]. Pemoline is a less potent stimulant with a lower abuse potential than methylphenidate, and therefore has the advantage of being less regulated by the federal government. Also, it is available in a chewable form that can be advantageous for patients who have trouble swallowing or have intestinal obstruction[6].

Anxiety

As with depression, anxiety must be viewed as part of a normal spectrum in the patient's reaction to a life-shortening illness. Death can be seen as a model for human feelings of abandonment and separation[7] and therefore brings with it the likelihood of anxiety that needs to be addressed. Such anxiety can often interfere with interpersonal relationships and impair the patient's ability to understand and make decisions about his/her treatment. The range of etiologies for anxiety in the terminally ill is wide, and includes the full range of psychiatric disorders (adjustment disorder, panic, generalized anxiety disorder, phobia) but also covers a number of medical conditions such as hypoxia, sepsis, pain, akathisia, and withdrawal from alcohol, barbiturates or benzodiazepines[8]. One must also consider the restlessness and agitation that can be part of delirium. Each patient's anxiety must be assessed with empathy and a special care toward building rapport with the patient, since open discussion in itself can be very therapeutic in the patient who fears abandonment at the end of life.

When a patient's level of distress is sufficiently intense, treatment is warranted. In mild cases, cognitive–behavioral techniques, such as progressive muscle relaxation, can be very effective[9]. With more serious anxiety in terminally ill patients, pharmacotherapy is indicated. Benzodiazepines are a mainstay of anxiolytic treatment in the population, especially because of the decreased concern regarding abuse potential. Short-acting agents, such as lorazepam and alprazolam, are favored for older adults over their longer-acting counterparts, such as diazepam and clonazepam, because of the potential for the impaired metabolism in many elderly individuals to lead to toxic accumulation of drugs or their metabolites. Several of these medications are available parenterally, as is a rectal form of diazepam, which is widely used in the hospice setting. Neuroleptics, such as haloperidol and risperidone, tend to be favored when the etiology of anxiety is suspected to be due to corticosteroids or delirium, or if there are psychotic symptoms associated with the anxiety[2]. Hydroxyzine is an antihistamine which is an effective sedative, anxiolytic and also has some analgesic properties and has minimal side effects[10,11]. Lastly, opiates are very effective in reducing anxiety, especially when it is associated with pain. Their use, however, is limited by respiratory depression.

Delirium

Delirium is a disorder of arousal and cognition caused by a medical condition that has relatively rapid onset and fluctuating course. Delirium has a prevalence of one-quarter to one-half of patients at the end of life[12]. This condition greatly complicates the treatment of the patient's other symptoms, such as pain, and causes great concern in family members and staff. In many cases delirium is reversible, even in relatively advanced terminal illness. Therefore, an investigation into reversible causes of delirium should be considered, including complete blood count, electrolyte studies, including calcium level and coagulation panel to rule out sepsis, dehydration, hypercalcemia and disseminated intravascular coagulation.

The diagnostic work-up of delirium in the terminally ill differs from that of the general population, in that special consideration must be made regarding the patient's or the family's wishes for invasive procedures to diagnose or treat the underlying cause of the delirium. The cause of terminal delirium most often is multifactorial or may not be found. Furthermore, when a distinct cause is found, it may be irreversible (such as hepatic failure or brain metastasis)[2]. In one study, an etiology was discovered in less than 50% of terminally ill patients with delirium[13]. Lastly, it should be noted that in the last 24–48 h before death, cognitive changes are usually irreversible and are attributable to multiple organ failure.

Treatment of delirium involves correction of any reversible underlying causes that can be found; supportive therapies, such as fluid, nutrition and vitamins are often helpful. Non-pharmacolo-gic interventions to help reduce anxiety and disorientation include a quiet, well-lit room with familiar objects, a visible clock or calendar and the presence of family[12]. When these measures are insufficient, neuroleptics are the treatment of choice, especially in patients with an agitated presentation. Haloperidol in low doses is still favored by many clinicians; intravenous administration can hasten the onset of action, and may be less apt to cause extrapyramidal side effects than the oral form. If sedation is necessary, a short-acting benzodiazepine can be added.

PSYCHOSOCIAL INTERVENTIONS IN PALLIATIVE CARE

Even in the absence of serious psychiatric morbidity, the end of life can be a period of considerable intrapsychic and interpersonal conflict for the patient. In many cases, psychotherapeutic interventions can offer considerable benefits to a palliative care setting. The fact that this area of intervention is not better studied may reflect anxieties in therapists who are forced to confront their own mortality in providing palliative care[14]. Methods vary in the treatment of dying patients, but some common elements unite the different approaches. In general, psychotherapy with patients with terminal illness should seek to:

1. *Allow the patient to openly communicate his/her feelings about death.* The dying patient experiences many fears, and often feels isolated because there is no-one with whom they can be shared[15].
2. *Strengthen the interpersonal bonds with those who will survive the patient.* This serves to alleviate the sense of abandonment that accompanies dying and allows the patient a sense of having "put affairs in order". It is also important for the survivors and their eventual grieving process, since ambivalent feelings toward the deceased are a risk factor for complicated bereavement[16].
3. *Establish hope while gently confronting denial.* While hope of cure may not be realistic, it can be replaced by the hope to live to be present at certain near-term events such as a graduation. Similarly, patients can hope for dignity in their final days, for freedom from pain or for their personal understanding of an afterlife.
4. *Help the patient find existential meaning and coherence in his life and in his death.*

Kubler-Ross

Any discussion of the psychology of dying owes a debt to Ellen Kubler-Ross and her seminal book, *On Death and Dying*[17]. Kubler-Ross interviewed hundreds of patients with terminal illness and described the process of dying in five stages: (a) *denial and isolation*, in which the patient refuses to believe he/she is terminally ill and feels suddenly alienated from the rest of the population that is not acutely dying; (b) *anger*, which can be expressed either overtly or in subtle, passive ways, depending on the personality of the individual; (c) *bargaining*, in which the patient seeks to prolong life by making promises to a higher power; (d) *depression*, the sense of existential loss upon realizing that death is unavoidable; (e) *acceptance*, in which the patient achieves a serenity and grace even in the face of death and comes to terms with the inevitable. Kubler-Ross herself states that these stages may recur several times and vary in order throughout the patient's terminal illness, and any one stage may be missing altogether. Therefore, these stages should only serve as guideposts to anchor one's clinical assessment and interpretation of the dying patient. Any attempt by the therapist to impose the stages as a structure can be an undue burden placed on the dying.

Psychotherapeutic Care

Psychotherapeutic approaches vary widely but, in general, the psychodynamic modes employ open-ended methods through which the patient gains insight. Underlying this approach is the belief that by better understanding the emotional pain of terminal illness, the patient will gain some relief from it[15]. The therapist pays careful attention to the patient's defenses, such as denial, displacement, counterdependency and dependency, and those that are felt to be adaptive are gently reinforced. If the defense is maladaptive, the question becomes whether the patient could tolerate an attempt to change it. Denial is felt to be the most common defense encountered in clinical practice, and it can be the most difficult to navigate for those who do not commonly work with the dying. The decision of whether or not to confront denial plagues psychiatrists, primary physicians and families alike. Stedeford[15] recommends that denial is a problem only when it is the sole or prominent defense. It then blocks communication with family and friends and prevents making suitable plans for the future. Often denial serves an important role in allowing the patient time to assimilate gradually information that would be overwhelming if absorbed all at once. Connor[18] believes that most denial is used to preserve interpersonal relationships. In this model, patients use denial primarily to cope with guilt about the effect of their condition on others, to protect others from the emotional stress they might feel if the patient were to openly acknowledge his/her condition and feelings, or out of fear of abandonment. He devised an intervention for this type of denial through a structured set of questions displayed in Table 138d.1.

Some other techniques are especially appropriate with dying older patients. Problem-solving therapy is a brief treatment that attempts to alleviate emotional symptoms by focusing on the social and practical difficulties faced by patients[19]. These problems are linked to the patient's symptoms, and the patient is helped to solve the problem by breaking it down into stages as follows: (a) clarification and definition of the problem; (b) setting of achievable goals; (c) consideration of alternative solutions; (d) selection of a preferred solution; (e) clarification of the necessary steps to implement the solution; (f) evaluation of progress. The advantages of this therapy are its brief format, which is sometimes necessary to fit the time frame of dying patients, as well as its accessibility to patients, who are sometimes uncomfortable with the jargon of psychotherapy. Cognitive and behavioral techniques are widely used to address specific symptoms, such as anxiety and phobias, through progressive muscle relaxation, imagery exercises or cognitive restructuring[9]. Guided imagery and trance states have also been successfully used to treat cancer pain. Education is often overlooked as a highly therapeutic tool to combat anxiety, since much of a dying patient's fear is generated by the unknown. The resources to assist in this education of the patient and family are growing exponentially and are available through varied media.

Psychological Benefits of Hospice Care

The first modern hospice was founded in 1967 in England to address concerns about the poor training of physicians to deal with terminal illness. Since then, the hospice movement has grown and spread to the USA, where roughly 20% of all deaths are now accounted for by patients who use hospices. The hospice approach seeks to improve the quality of the end of life by focusing on the whole patient, including his/her medical, pain relief, emotional and spiritual needs. Hospices employ a number of the above described therapeutic interventions through varied disciplines with a distinctive commitment to a team-based approach. Along with the psychological benefits for the dying patient in receiving this interdisciplinary, psychologically sensitive care at the end of life, there appears to be a psychological benefit to survivors of patients who use hospices; McNeilly and Hillary found survivors of hospice patients less likely to regret not having more openly expressed feelings to the person they cared for than those who used a home health care group[20]. Hospices can be seen as an intentional aid to the patient in his/her psychological journey at the end of life in its explicit commitment to helping the patient "die well", as he/she understands and interprets it, while maintaining an abiding commitment to the family and other survivors.

Although psychiatric care of the dying older patient embodies many challenges, it is full of rewards for the physician, patient and the patient's families. The reciprocity inherent within the relationship with dying patients is profound in its implications for educating us about life, suffering and adaptation. The more capable we become of caring well for the dying during this transition in their lives, the better we will be at understanding and caring for all of our patients.

Table 138d.1 Structured psychosocial intervention for denial

1. Different people experience different kinds of difficulties when they are ill. What, for you, have been some of the most difficult aspects of having your illness?
2. Are there any things you do, or that other people do, that make these difficulties easier to deal with?
3. Is there anything you or other people do, that make these difficulties harder to deal with?
4. Do you believe you will or will not recover from this illness?
5. Have you had any close encounters with death?
6. What effect has your illness had on your family and close friends, and how have they reacted to it?
7. How do you feel about the way in which your family and friends have been affected by or have reacted to your illness?
8. Is there anything good that has come out of your having your illness?
9. Are there any other thoughts or feelings about your illness or the questions I've asked that you'd like to talk more about?

From Connor[18], with permission.

REFERENCES

1. Breitbart W, Bruera E, Chochinov H, Lynch M. Neuropsychiatric syndromes and psychological symptoms in patients with advanced cancer. *J Pain Sympt Managem* 1995; **10**: 131–41.
2. Breitbart W, Jacobsen PB. Psychiatric symptom management in terminal care. *Clin Geriat Med* 1996; **12**: 329–47.
3. Endicott J. Measurement of depression in patients with cancer. *Cancer* 1984; **53**: 2243–9.
4. Massie MJ, Holland JC. Depression and the cancer patient. *J Clin Psychiat* 1990; **51**: 12–17.
5. Bruera E, Chadwick S, Brennels C *et al*. Methylphenidate associated with narcotics for the treatment of cancer pain. *Cancer Treatm Rep* 1987; **71**: 67–70.
6. Breitbart W, Mermelstein H. Pemoline: an alternative psychostimulant for the management of depressive disorders in cancer patients. *Psychosomatics* 1992; **33**: 352–6.
7. Schwartz AM, Karasu TB. Psychotherapy with the dying patient. *Am J Psychother* 1977; **31**: 19–33.
8. Holland JC. Anxiety and cancer: the patient and family. *J Clin Psychiat* 1989; **50**: 20–25.

9. Holland JC, Morrow G, Schmale A *et al.* A randomized clinical trial of alprazolam versus progressive muscle relaxation in cancer patients with anxiety and depressive symptoms. *J Clin Oncol* 1991; **9**: 1004–11.

10. Stambaugh JE Jr, Lane C. Analgesic efficacy and pharmacokinetic evaluation of meperidine and hydroxyzine, alone and in combination. *Cancer Invest* 1983; **1**: 111–17.

11. Runmore MM, Schlichting DA. Analgesic effects of antihistaminics. *Life Sci* 1985; **36**: 403–16.

12. Breitbart W, Strout D. Delirium in the terminally ill. *Clin Geriat Med* 2000; **16**: 357–72.

13. Bruera E, Miller L, McCalion S. Cognitive failure in patients with terminal cancer: a prospective longitudinal study. *Psychosoc Asp Cancer* 1990; **9**: 308–10.

14. Clarke PJ. Exploration of countertransference toward the dying. *Am J Orthopsychiat* 1981; **51**: 71–7.

15. Stedeford A. Psychotherapy of the dying patient. *Br J Psychiat* 1979; **135**: 7–14.

16. Gonda TA, Ruark JE. *Dying Dignified: The Health Professional's Guide to Care.* Menlo Park, CT: Addison-Wesley, 1984: 40.

17. Kubler-Ross E. *On Death and Dying.* New York: Macmillan, 1969.

18. Connor SR. Denial in terminal illness: to intervene or not to intervene. *Hospice J* 1992; **8**: 1–15.

19. Wood BC, Mynors-Wallis LM. Problem-solving therapy in palliative care. *Palliat Med* 1997; **11**: 49–54.

20. McNeilly DP, Hillary K. The hospice decision: psychosocial facilitators and barriers. *Omega* 1997; **35**: 193–217.

Prevention in Mental Disorders of Late Life

Barry D. Lebowitz and Jane L. Pearson

National Institute of Mental Health, Bethesda, MD, USA

INTRODUCTION

In its influential 1994 report, *Reducing Risks for Mental Disorders: Frontiers for Preventive Intervention Research*, the Institute of Medicine (IoM) of the US National Academy of Sciences[1] assessed the state of knowledge in prevention research and identified directions for future scientific development. The index of this substantial volume contains no entries for "aging", "aged", "elderly", "geriatric" or "gerontological". In a section on illustrative preventive intervention research programs, examples are given of two service programs, one for caregivers of patients with Alzheimer's disease and one for widows, that are considered to have relevance to prevention. The authors could identify no randomized controlled preventive trials in the area of aging.

Prevention in the mental health field has been seen, traditionally, as an area that has been implicitly restricted to those concerns designed for application to issues in childhood and adolescence. If anything, prevention in geriatrics was seen as an oxymoron. Very simply, prevention was taken to mean youth. Theory and research in prevention were restricted to issues of child development and intervention early in the life course.

Why be concerned with prevention in late life? As is well covered in other sections of this text, there is the demographic imperative brought about by the overall aging of the world population and, in particular, by the aging of the older population. As pointed out in the classic papers by Gruenberg[2] and Kramer[3], the same dynamics—public health measures, technological development and lifestyle changes—that created this growth in the overall population were also relevant to growth of the population of those with chronic illnesses and disabilities. They conclude that, in the absence of cures or effective preventive strategies, we will see an explosion in the number of older persons with serious and persistent disabling illnesses, particularly mental disorders. The availability of more efficacious treatments and the accessibility of appropriate services in the community combined to produce huge gains in the life expectancy of those with mental disorders who, in earlier times, would have died long before reaching old age. This demographic imperative leads to the conclusion that prevention must be an important part of the agenda of geriatric psychiatry.

The traditional public health view derives from infectious disease and is divided into primary, secondary and tertiary prevention. Primary prevention is directed toward maintaining health by isolating the causes of disease and eliminating or counteracting them. Secondary prevention is directed toward enhancing recovery by case identification and prompt intervention early in the course of illness. Tertiary prevention is directed toward those already ill and emphasizes treatment and rehabilitation[4].

There is a growing consensus that the traditional public health view is not optimal. The components of this approach, including, for example, concepts such as pathogens, risk factors, disease vectors and definitions of caseness, do not translate easily into psychopathology or chronic disease. The 1994 IoM report[1] adapts a scheme developed by Gordon[5] to characterize preventive interventions as universal (targeted to a general population), selective (targeted at individuals at increased risk) or indicated (targeted to individuals with minimal levels of signs or symptoms).

Universal interventions are broad public health measures intended for an entire population or for significant geographic, socioeconomic or categorical subgroups within it (e.g. rural residents, low-income older persons, or pregnant women). Universal interventions (e.g. iodizing salt) may reduce risk for a large segment of a population but in all likelihood do not have impact on those already at high risk or those who would not have been at risk at all. Cost–benefit assessment is a clear decision criterion for the development and implementation of universal interventions, since they would, by necessity, involve exposure of many individuals not at risk for development of an illness.

Selective interventions are targeted toward those individuals at significantly increased risk of developing the particular illness or condition. Genetic loading and positive family history, other illnesses, or psychosocial or environmental transitions are all examples of factors that might be used to target selectively preventive interventions. Although selective interventions may seem easy, careful efforts are needed to assure proper identification and to avoid stigmatization or unnecessary fear.

Indicated interventions are targeted on those individuals who are already symptomatic and in whom early intervention may alter the longitudinal course or optimize the outcome of the illness. The underlying assumption is that significant advantage is gained when preventive interventions are extended to concerns with function and disability in those who already have an illness. Interventions directed at minimizing post-treatment relapse or recurrence would also fit within this category[41].

Following recommendations of the National Advisory Mental Health Council[6], this chapter is based on assumptions that an appropriate approach to prevention must: (a) be tied closely to treatment; (b) have strong connections to service systems and services; and (c) be based upon models of etiology, pathophysiology and risk. Following Kraemer *et al.*[7] we use "risk" and "risk factor" narrowly to indicate an empirically demonstrated agent or exposure that influences the likelihood of an event in a defined population. Preventive interventions are those directed at reducing risk of the development, exacerbation or adverse consequences of mental disorders.

Principles and Practice of Geriatric Psychiatry, 2nd edn. Edited by J. R. M. Copeland, M. T. Abou-Saleh and D. G. Blazer
©2002 John Wiley & Sons, Ltd

PREVENTIVE INTERVENTIONS IN THE CONTEXT OF TREATMENT

Prevention of Relapse and Recurrence

Establishment of the efficacy of treatments is one of the major accomplishments of geriatric psychiatry research. As outlined in other sections of this text, many studies have demonstrated that older patients respond robustly to treatments that are appropriately applied with adequate intensities. These data are, largely, based on relatively brief, randomized controlled trials addressing the short-term efficacy of treatments to manage the symptoms of serious illnesses like depression[8] and Alzheimer's disease[9,10]. More recently, the prevention of relapse and recurrence has emerged as a major orientation in the treatment of the older patient. As the recognition has grown that most mental disorders in late life are chronic, recurring illnesses with substantial residual disability[11], so too has the acknowledgement that treatment must be approached with a much longer-term perspective[12]. An intervention is preventive if acute treatment response is the starting point, with the major purpose of preventing relapse or recurrence and not managing symptoms.

Prevention of Side Effects and Adverse Reactions

Co-morbidity and the associated polypharmacy that comes from treatment of multiple conditions are characteristic of older patients. New information on the genetic basis of drug metabolism and on the action of drug-metabolizing enzymes now provide us with important perspectives on clinically significant alterations in drug concentration levels or on complex drug interactions[13]. For example, many of the newer antidepressant agents, the selective serotonin reuptake inhibitors (SSRIs), compete for the same metabolic pathway used by β-blockers, type 1 C antiarrhythmics and benzodiazepines.

Many older patients require antipsychotic treatment for the management of behavioral disturbance in schizophrenia, depression and Alzheimer's disease. Movement disorders are common side effects of the older types of these medications, the conventional neuroleptics. Although doses tend to be quite low compared to doses used in young or mid-life adults, age and length of treatment represent major risk factors for the development of movement disorders[14]. Recent data suggest the possibility that the newer antipsychotics present a much lower risk and that the development of tardive dyskinesia may be preventable through use of different medication[15]. Trials of agents (e.g. antioxidants) hypothesized to treat these side effects have been proposed, although the data from some of the early studies have been inconsistent[16,17].

Many drugs affect body sway and postural stability, although there is substantial variability within classes of drugs[18]. In older patients, where the prevention of falling is a major concern, a preventive strategy would reflect a differential selection of treatments or development of fall-specific preventive interventions[19].

PREVENTIVE INTERVENTIONS IN THE CONTEXT OF SERVICES

Prevention of Suicide

Recognition of mental illness in older patients is highly variable. Changes in cognition, affect, thinking, sleep, etc. are often attributed to normal processes of age-related change by older people themselves, their spouses and close family members, and even by their family doctors and primary care physicians. The most tragic result of the failure to recognize illness is suicide. Suicide rates increase with age, and men always outnumber women in suicide completion. In most countries, older men generally are at the greatest risk of suicide. In the USA, for example, old White men have a rate of suicide six times that of the general population. Psychological autopsy studies show that depression is common among these men but that it is rarely recognized. Nearly 40% of the men who kill themselves see their primary care doctors in the week of their death; nearly 70% in the month of their death[20]. An uncontrolled field experiment on the island of Gotland in Sweden suggested that a depression-orientated educational intervention directed toward primary care physicians could reduce suicide[21]. Other approaches to the prevention of suicide, using aggressive outreach and case-finding techniques, have been developed in the context of community-based mental health or aging services[22,23].

Prevention of Premature Institutionalization

Nursing home placement typically comes at the end of a long and difficult period of caregiving by the families of patients with Alzheimer's disease. The burden of this caregiving in terms of stress, depression and quality of life has been extensively documented[24]. It is only the rare (and very wealthy) family that can provide the care necessary to maintain a patient with Alzheimer's disease at home; institutional care is required for virtually all patients who survive to the end-stage of the disease. From a public health perspective, delay of institutional placement until it was absolutely necessary could have significant impact. In an important randomized controlled trial of a family-based counseling intervention, Mittelman et al.[25] demonstrated clear benefit: a delay of over 300 days in nursing home admission for patients whose families were randomized to receive the treatment. The counseling intervention also resulted in a significant reduction in depressive symptoms in these caregivers. Clinical drug trials in Alzheimer's disease have begun using institutionalization as a primary outcome[26] or as an outcome from open-label follow-up after the trial had ended[27].

Prevention of Excess Disability

The concept of excess disability is a classic one in geriatrics[28] and refers at its core to the observation that many older patients, particularly those with Alzheimer's disease, are more functionally impaired than would be expected on the basis of the stage or severity of their mental disorder. There are many sources of this excess disability: some are medical, some are psychosocial and some are environmental. A generation of research has clearly demonstrated that attention to these issues, and aggressive intervention where appropriate, will prevent excess disability and will optimize levels of function.

MODELS OF ETIOLOGY, PATHOPHYSIOLOGY AND RISK

Biological Models

Improved understanding of the etiology and pathophysiology of mental disorders can potentially lead to interventions that will prevent the onset or progression of disease. A useful model here is the large simple trial in a broad population; incident cases represent the primary outcome. The state of our knowledge is not yet sufficiently well developed to support this type of research.

Nonetheless, there are some interesting possibilities developing as we learn more about oxidative and inflammatory processes, apoptotic mechanisms, hormonal correlates and genetic factors in disease. One possible example is the area of vascular depression. Several different lines of evidence are now supporting the conclusion that one form of late-onset depression has a cerebrovascular etiology[29]. Trials of vascular agents could use incident depression as outcomes.

Genetic Models

The genetics of mental disorders is an area of expanded activity[30]. Notably, several genes are now implicated in different forms of Alzheimer's disease. At present, the genetic correlates of mental disorders are not sufficiently specific to be used for purposes of population screening. It is entirely conceivable, however, that trials directed at delaying onset of disease, or directed at minimizing excess disability, could be launched using some of this genetic information as a basis for subject selection.

Clinical Models

Co-morbidity is one of the hallmarks of mental disorders throughout the life course. In late-life mental disorders, the most frequently observed co-morbidities are physical illness and brain disease. This provides a possible opportunity for preventive interventions; we present a few examples.

Visual impairment is common among older people; there is a high frequency of depression among older persons with impaired vision, and the depression is more strongly predictive of disability than is the vision loss[31]. The vision clinic would seem to be an appropriate location for the development of programs orientated to the prevention of depression in older patients. Similarly, aggressive intervention in depression has the potential for minimizing disability and optimizing function. This latter point is supported by a broad range of studies demonstrating that depression compromises the outcome of rehabilitation in stroke, Parkinson's disease, heart disease, pulmonary disease and fractures[32]. Research has also demonstrated that treatment of depression can significantly improve outcome of treatment and rehabilitation for the co-morbid physical illness or condition[33,34].

Complex programmatic interventions have been shown to have efficacy in the area of prevention as well. Ray et al.[19], for example, show how an intervention directed at safety with appropriate use of wheelchairs, psychotropic drugs and provision for transfer and ambulation, has a significant impact on the reduction of falls in nursing homes. In the outpatient setting, multidisciplinary comprehensive assessment resulted in significant improvements in the detection of depression and cognitive impairment and resulted in substantially reduced risk for nursing home placement[35,36].

Psychosocial Models

Bereavement is perhaps the prototypical psychosocial risk factor in late-life mental disorders[37]. Considerable research has been devoted to the exploration of bereavement-related depression, complicated grief, traumatic grief and similar constructs[38–40]. It is entirely conceivable that preventive interventions for those with complicated grief could have major impact on both mental and physical health. It is also conceivable that greater understanding of the correlates and predictors of complicated or traumatic grief may lead to the design of earlier-stage interventions, directed at modifying the likelihood of developing the risk factor in the first place. Interventions directed toward risk factors, rather than toward disorders, may be properly considered to be primary prevention.

CONCLUSION

In this chapter we have presented the broad parameters of a programmatic approach to prevention in late-life mental disorders. There is no established approach to prevention research that could be easily adapted to meet the needs of the field. Approaches to prevention need to be based in the deep foundation of knowledge in treatment and services research. They must be built upon improved models of etiology, pathophysiology and risk. A new approach to prevention holds the promise to be a significant development for the field. We have no doubt that success is achievable.

REFERENCES

1. Mrazek PI, Haggerty RI, eds. *Reducing Risks for Mental Disorders: Frontiers for Preventive Intervention Research*. Washington, DC: National Academy Press, 1994.
2. Gruenberg EM. The failure of success. *Health Soc Milbank Memorial Fund Qu* 1977; **55**: 3–23.
3. Kramer M. The rising pandemic of mental disorders and associated chronic diseases and disabilities. *Acta Psychiat Scand* 1980; **62**(suppl 285): 382–97.
4. Burns B. Prevention of mental disorders in old age. In Copeland JRM, Abou-Saleh MT, Blazer DG, eds, *Principles and Practice of Geriatric Psychiatry*, 1st edn. Chichester: Wiley, 1994; 1011–16.
5. Gordon R. An operational definition of disease prevention. *Publ Health Rep* 1983; **98**: 107–9.
6. National Advisory Mental Health Council. *Priorities for Prevention Research at NIMH*. NIH Publication No. 98-4321. Bethesda, MD: NAMHC, 1998.
7. Kraemer HC, Kazdin AE, Offord DR *et al.* Coming to terms with the terms of risk. *Arch Gen Psychiat* 1997; **54**: 337–43.
8. Schneider LS. Pharmacological considerations in the treatment of late life depression. *Am J Geriat Psychiat* 1996; **4**(suppl 1): S51–65.
9. American Psychiatric Association. Practice guidelines for the treatment of patients with Alzheimer's disease and other dementias of late life. *Am J Psychiat* 1997; **154**(suppl): 1–39.
10. Small GW, Rabins PV, Barry PV *et al.* Diagnosis and treatment of Alzheimer's disease: consensus statement of the American Association for Geriatric Psychiatry, the Alzheimer's Association, and the American Geriatrics Society. *J Am Med Assoc* 1997; **278**: 1363–71.
11. Lebowitz BD, Pearson IL, Schneider LS *et al.* Diagnosis and treatment of depression in late life: consensus statement update. *J Am Med Assoc* 1997; **278**: 1186–90.
12. Reynolds CF, Frank E, Kupfer DI *et al.* Treatment outcome in recurrent major depression: a post hoc comparison of elderly ("young-old") and midlife patients. *Am J Psychiat* 1996; **153**: 1288–92.
13. Nemeroff CB, De Vane CL, Pollock BG. Newer antidepressants and the cytochrome P450 system. *Am J Psychiat* 1996; **153**: 311–20.
14. Paulsen JS, Caligiuri MP, Palmer B *et al.* Risk factors for orofacial and limbtruncal tardive dyskinesia in older patients: a prospective longitudinal study. *Psychopharmacology* 1996; **123**: 307–14.
15. Katz IR, Jeste DV, Brecher M *et al.* Comparison of risperidone and placebo for psychosis and behavioral disturbances associated with dementia: a randomized, double-blind trial. *J Clin Psychiat* 1999; **60**: 107–115.
16. Lohr LB, Lavori P. Editorial: whither vitamin E and tardive dyskinesia? *Biol Psychiat* 1998; **43**: 861–2.
17. Adler LA, Edson R, Lavori P *et al.* Long-term treatment effects of vitamin E for tardive dyskinesia. *Biol Psychiat* 1998; **43**: 868–72.
18. Laghrissi-Thode F, Pollock BG, Miller MC *et al.* Double-blind comparison of paroxetine and nortriptyline on the postural stability of late-life depressed patients. *Psychopharm Bull* 1995; **31**: 659–63.

19. Ray WA, Taylor IA, Meador KG et al. A randomized trial to reduce falls in nursing homes. *J Am Med Assoc* 1997; **278**: 557–62.

20. Conwell Y, Duberstein PR, Cox C et al. Age differences in behaviors leading to completed suicide. *Am J Geriat Psychiat* 1998; **6**: 122–6.

21. Rihmer Z, Rutz W, Pihlgren H. Depression and suicide in Gotland: an intensive study of all suicides before and after a depression training programme for general practitioners. *J Affect Disord* 1995; **35**: 147–52.

22. Raschko R. Spokane community mental health center elderly services. In Light E, Lebowitz BD, eds, *The Elderly with Chronic Mental Illness*. New York: Springer, 1991; 232–44.

23. DeLeo D, Carollo G, Buono MD. Lower suicide rates associated with a Tele-Help/Tele-Check service for the elderly at home. *Am J Psychiat* 1995; **152**: 632–4.

24. Light E, Niederehe G, Lebowitz BD, eds. *Stress Effects on Family Caregivers of Alzheimer's Patients*. New York: Springer, 1994.

25. Mittelman MS, Ferris SH, Shulman E et al. A family intervention to delay nursing home placement of patients with Alzheimer's disease: a randomized controlled trial. *J Am Med Assoc* 1996; **276**: 1725–31.

26. Sano M, Ernesto C, Thomas RG et al. A controlled trial of selegiline, α-tocopherol, or both as a treatment for Alzheimer's disease. *N Engl J Med* 1997; **336**: 1216–22.

27. Knopman D, Schneider LS, Davis K et al. Long-term tacrine (Cognex) treatment effects on nursing home placement and mortality. *Neurology* 1996; **47**: 166–77.

28. Kahn R. Psychological aspects of aging. In Rossman I, ed., *Clinical Geriatrics*. Philadelphia, PA: J. B. Lippincott, 1971; 107–13.

29. Alexopoulos GS, Meyers BS, Young RC et al. The "vascular depression" hypothesis. *Arch Gen Psychiat* 1997; **54**: 915–22.

30. Risch NI, Merikangas KM. The future of genetic studies of complex human disease. *Science* 1996; **273**: 1516–17.

31. Rovner BW, Zisselman PM, Shmuely-Dulitzki Y. Depression and disability in older people with impaired vision: a follow-up study. *J Am Geriat Soc* 1996; **44**: 181–4.

32. Katz IR. On the inseparability of medical and physical health in aged persons: lessons from depression and medical comorbidity. *Am J Geriat Psychiat* 1996; **4**: 1–16.

33. Borson S, McDonald GI, Gayle T et al. Improvement in mood, physical symptoms, and function with nortriptyline for depression in patients with chronic obstructive pulmonary disease. *Psychosomatics* 1992; **33**: 190–201.

34. Mossey IM, Knott KA, Higgins M et al. Effectiveness of a psychosocial intervention, interpersonal counseling, for subdysthymic depression in medically ill elderly. *J Gerontol Med Sci* 1996; **SIA**: M172–8.

35. Silverman M, Musa D, Martin DC et al. Evaluation of outpatient geriatric assessment: a randomized multisite trial. *J Am Geriat Soc* 1995; **43**: 733–40.

36. Stuck AE, Aronow HU, Steiner A et al. A trial of annual in-home comprehensive geriatric assessments for elderly people living in the community. *N Engl J Med* 1995; **333**: 1184–89.

37. Institute of Medicine. *Bereavement: Reactions, Consequences, and Care*. Washington DC: National Academy Press, 1984.

38. Horowitz MJ, Siegel B, Holen A et al. Diagnostic criteria for complicated grief disorder. *Am J Psychiat* 1997; **154**: 904–10.

39. Prigerson HG, Frank E, Kasl SV et al. Complicated grief and bereavement-related depression as distinct disorders: preliminary empirical validation in elderly bereaved spouses. *Am J Psychiat* 1995; **152**: 22–30.

40. Prigerson HG, Bierhals Al, Kasl SV et al. Traumatic grief as a risk factor for mental and physical morbidity. *Am J Psychiat* 1997; **154**: 616–23.

41. Smyer MA. Prevention and early intervention for mental disorders of the elderly. In Gatz M, ed., *Emerging Issues in Mental Health and Aging*. Washington, DC: American Psychological Association, 1995.

A Damning Analysis of the Law and the Elderly Incompetent Patient—Rights, What Rights?

Peter Edwards

Peter Edwards & Co.,* Hoylake, UK

Does the legal process provide a framework in the UK for protecting the rights of those who lack the capacity to make their own decisions? In what way should the law impact on families, professionals and carers? Surely you, the practitioner, you the carer, you the family member take decisions on what you believe to be in that person's best interests? You are there to do a good job exercising sound judgements. You are motivated by a desire to protect, to support and to make safe decisions in the best interests of the incapacitated person. You surely do not want to be impeded by considerations of an incapacitated person's legal rights. But what if the person him/herself wishes to make a different decision? You may consider it unwise or even risky for him/her to follow his/her desires. On what legal basis does one citizen override the ability of another to exercise choice? Who decides?

DOES THE LAW HAVE A ROLE?

Why is the law of incapacity/incompetence so important when it comes to protecting rights? For a person with capacity, the law recognizes the right to take responsibility for decisions. However, we must then bear the consequences of those decisions. Incapacity equates with society's view that incompetent adults may have to be protected. They may lack the ability to realize the consequences of the exercise of their decisions and that could place them at risk.

The dilemma is therefore apparent. At some point we cross that invisible divide between capacity and incapacity; between the right to make unsafe decisions and the right to be protected from them; between taking responsibility and the loss of the power to exercise our own judgement; between having enforceable rights and not.

For those who are deemed to lack capacity, the responsibility for deciding what is in their "best interests" may lie with those for whom there is a conflict of interest. They may be going to inherit the estate or they may even be those who are perpetrating abuse. The state of UK law leaves the incapacitated ripe for exploitation. Proposals for a change in the law appear to have stalled.

Perhaps when it comes to making a will, preparing an enduring Power of Attorney or protecting someone's financial affairs from fraud or exploitation, it is easy for us to accept the need for a protective framework. However, what about the concept of enforceable human rights? When should the elderly be allowed to take risks?

We, ourselves, have rights and we can take steps to enforce them. But if we have lost the capacity to fight for or defend our rights, what then? When we have lost capacity, is there a right that restrains the distribution of our confidential information? "I don't want to go into a nursing home." "I want to choose with whom I live and with whom I have a personal/sexual relationship." "No, whatever they say, I do not believe that my children are acting in my best interests." Who will enforce my rights now? Who will listen?

On 2 October 2000, the UK Government belatedly brought into force the Human Rights Act 1998 in England. It sets out the rights and responsibilities of the citizen and provides a framework based on the European Convention of Human Rights and Fundamental Freedoms. It provides a baseline of rights below which the citizen should not be allowed to fall and introduces a rights culture laid on our domestic legislation. The indications are that it could have far-reaching effects on the practice of old age psychiatry, as well as impacting on the causes of action open to an increasingly aged population when their rights and opportunities are infringed.

The greatest impediment to the development of a rights-based system is the identification of the individual who will act on behalf of the incompetent client. Who will make the bridgehead to the lawyer? Who will blow the whistle? How does the incompetent client get to know of his/her rights in the first place? What happens when we cannot trust the families? The questions are easier to identify than the answers.

ROLE OF THE LAW

The role of the law must be viewed within the context within which it prevails. At present there is no doubt that in the UK[a] the percentage of the population reaching the traditional retirement age[b] is increasing and has done so since the post-war boom of the 1950s and 1960s. This, of course, has both political and financial ramifications. Linked to this has been a gradual increase in income, disposable assets such as homes, cars and other property, as well as a notable increase in the number of elderly people with their own assets.

---

*A specialist mental health law firm.
[a]Unlike the Republic of Ireland, where the average age of the population is 28 years of age.
[b]65 for men and 60 for women.

Principles and Practice of Geriatric Psychiatry, 2nd edn. Edited by J. R. M. Copeland, M. T. Abou-Saleh and D. G. Blazer

In examining a rights-based culture, it is relevant to remind ourselves that a notable shift emerged during the Conservative/Thatcherite years from 1979 onwards, when notions of solidarity and community waned and a "self" culture emerged.

What does all this mean in the context of the law, elderly people and incapacity? What does it mean within a society focused on "self" and where there are a greater number of assets and a greater number of people who need to have their rights protected?

Capacity is a concept based in our common law. Therefore, those with the final say are the judiciary. However, rarely is the law asked to be the arbiter of individuals' capacity. Where there is dispute, it is always possible to seek a declaration from the courts. In practice, however, the final decision is taken by the myriad of individuals who come into contact with the incapacitated person. It could be the doctor, the nurse, the social worker, the staff in the nursing home or even the family. When it comes to medical treatment, the doctor who is in charge of treatment has the responsibility to make that decision. Some believe that only psychiatrists can perform this task. Psychiatrists get called in unnecessarily by other doctors (e.g. general practitioners, surgeons or anaesthetists) who do not seem to realize that they themselves are responsible. Usually those who are deciding on capacity have no concept of the test to be applied and merely assert that the individual will now have decisions made for him/her. It is a chilling scenario, particularly as many of us may eventually be in this predicament.

It is worrying that at times, medical staff, without any consideration of capacity, seek to obtain consent to a medical intervention from a person who does not have the capacity to consent. If that patient declines to agree with the treatment, then it is not given. It could perhaps have been justified by the common law doctrine of necessity. Failure to treat under those circumstances could amount to negligence.

Any process that purports to be based on a rights-based system must not be arbitrary. There should be a clear framework within which decisions are made. This should particularly be so when the essence of the decision is to strip away from the individual the right of autonomous decision making.

OBJECTIVES

What should be the guiding objectives and principles upon which any such decisions are to be based? Further, how is capacity to be assessed and what are the tests that the law will endeavour to apply?

When the citizen turns to the law to find an answer, it soon becomes apparent that in the UK it is a mess. There is not one separate body of law established to deal with elderly incapacitated people. However, what can be determined from the case law and statutes that do exist, is that the law has constructed a number of overriding objectives.

First, there are the means by which the duties that are owed to those who lack capacity are enforced. This can be illustrated in financial and property matters, where the Court of Protection can be invited to intervene[c]. A Receiver can be appointed to take control of a person's financial affairs and the Receiver is answerable to the Court. The great weakness here is that professionals and others who have concerns about the possible exploitation of an incapacitated individual will often know little of this remote and distant Court. It only has one base, and that is in London. What is more, those who are aware that exploitation is taking place may be the very people who are perpetrating it. Who then will activate the process?

Whilst we have capacity, it is possible to make plans that would result in avoiding the costly involvement of the Court of Protection. It is possible to complete a simple document called an Enduring Power of Attorney. This must be completed whilst a person still has capacity and allows one to appoint the individual(s) who will control one's financial affairs when and if one loses capacity. The simplicity of the process can allow those determined to abuse to prevail on the vulnerable person, who may even lack the capacity to execute the document. The principle is that, as we have capacity, we have the right to make unwise decisions. When capacity is lost, the Enduring Power of Attorney becomes effective by registering it with the Court of Protection. This is essentially an administrative task.

Second, the law can be invited to consider what is in the "best interest" of the incapacitated person. This can involve the right to be supported and to be legally represented. However, if the criteria for appointing a receiver under the Court of Protection are met, then the incapacitated person cannot instruct a solicitor or bring legal proceedings in his/her own right. This role must be undertaken by a "litigation friend"[1]. This objective is further endorsed by the Human Rights Act 1998 which sets out to promote the fundamental rights, freedoms and liberties of UK citizens. Article 6 protects the right to a fair trial. The difficulty arises when seeking a mechanism to achieve this. Yet again, the process of protection is entirely dependent on someone making the link between the incapacitated person and the judicial process.

Third, and perhaps most significantly, is the role of the law to protect individuals from ill-treatment, abuse, neglect and exploitation. The forms that these take are endless and nauseating, as we see in the range of daily media reports illustrating that people know no bounds in gratifying their excesses against vulnerable people, in areas such as money, possessions and physical and sexual abuse. The obvious difficulty in using the criminal justice system is that the abused person may not have sufficient capacity to give evidence. Unless there is separate, corroborative evidence the perpetrator may go unpunished.

PRINCIPLES

The above objectives are not, and in fact cannot be, freestanding. They are guided by a set of prevailing principles that are transferable to the development of the law itself.

In exploring the principles, it should be noted that much research was done by the Law Commission[2] and the Lord Chancellor's Department[3] in the area of Capacity.

In UK law, all adults are presumed to be competent and as such will have the same rights and opportunities as others. The burden of proof therefore lies on those who seek to assert the citizen's lack of capacity. Where there is the need to interfere in the lives of those who lack capacity, any such intervention should be the minimum required in the circumstances. Where an individual has been found not to have capacity, nevertheless, he/she should be encouraged to take the kind of decisions that he/she might have taken before capacity was lost. This may sound like an effective set of principles. However, they need to be set in their practical context.

Sadly, it may be in the interests of everyone concerned that the individual should be treated as if he/she were no longer capable of making his/her own decisions. After all, an elderly person may want to make a decision that we might consider unwise, foolish or

---

[c]Court of Protection is an Office of the Supreme Court and the provisions cited are to be found in s. 93 of the Mental Health Act 1983.

even dangerous. That person could be your mum or dad, who may want to give money away or enter into a close relationship with someone many years younger; your inheritance might be threatened. Asserting his/her incapacity could protect your finances. Or a situation might arise where the elderly person does not like the rules and regulations in the nursing home. He/she may find him/herself being treated as a child. "No, you cannot go out; here is your medicine you must take it; it is time for bed now; what we are doing is in your best interests." Who has proved his/her incapacity? Who has even thought about it? Rights can be very uncomfortable.

The courageous professional who correctly asserts that a person has capacity and that he/she may take responsibility for his/her own decisions may be left vulnerable to criticism and even attempts at litigation. Defending the decision when some damage or loss has ensued against an irate family member or community can be an uncomfortable business. This takes knowledgeable and confident professionals.

Therefore, the confidence of professionals and others who are called upon to exercise these judgements is crucial, as is the extent and timing of the intervention. The law has a further role in determining whether and to what extent the intervention by the state has been *proportionate* to the presenting facts and evidence. A proportionate response is an important concept in the Human Rights Act.

Before concluding this section on the role of the law within the context of incapacity, there is an often-overlooked area, namely the role of the lawyer. The role of the lawyer can become confused if the lawyer has not posed to him/herself the vital questions: who is my client?; who am I actually acting for?; to whom do I owe my professional responsibility?; is it the vulnerable elderly person or the family member? The lawyer has to be alert to the situation in which he/she is requested to advise the family who are trying to use the law to exploit the incapacitated individual, e.g. by assisting the family in obtaining an Enduring Power of Attorney (see above) from someone who, had the proper enquiries been made, would have been found to lack capacity (and therefore unable to execute the deed).

WHO LACKS CAPACITY?

Most decisions about capacity are made without any thought at all about objective criteria. Doctors, nurses, social workers, families, or nursing home owners will simply assert it as a fact in order to justify overriding the wishes of the individual.

As indicated above, the Court is the ultimate arbiter of the issue of capacity. However, in those rare cases where it is asked, it is misleading to believe that the judge will arrive at some clear and objective decision when the very criteria for analysis are based partly on the shrouded mystic of clinical analysis and partly on societal attitudes. Essentially there are no clear criteria and it is not good enough simply to assert that each case will be decided on its own facts. The Human Rights Act should cause a shift in emphasis, where the starting point will be the rights of the citizen. Article 6 guarantees the right to a fair trial. The problem may be, who is going to enforce this? The judiciary will have to be alert.

THE BURDEN OF PROOF

When making this decision, the law asserts that a person is presumed at common law to have legal capacity unless it is shown that they do not. However, it is the medical practitioner who may seek to assist or convince the court of the lack of capacity. If such a question comes before the Court, the law at present places the burden of proving such incapacity on the person who asserts it (on

a balance of probabilities, e.g. 51/49). In itself this is worrying, as a diagnosis of incapacity may lead to the loss freedoms, rights and liberties which, our society says in other contexts, namely criminal justice, require that a much higher standard of proof should be reached. Bearing in mind the consequences of a finding of incapacity, surely the standard of proof to rob a person of the control of his/her own affairs should be a much higher one (i.e. beyond all reasonable doubt).

THE HERE AND NOW TEST

An important principle needs to be understood. In assessing a person's capacity, the law will seek to do so at the relevant time in respect of the particular activity/transaction that the person is about to enter into. Anyone assessing an individual's capacity must apply this test. It is possible that a loss of capacity may be transient or episodic. In the early stages of dementia it may be the subject of partial remission.

What is more, a person may both have and lack capacity at the same moment in time. There are differing tests to be applied, e.g. when making a will, entering into a contract, consenting to marriage or sexual activity, making an Enduring Power of Attorney or consenting to medical treatment. When looking at the statutory test of incapacity to be applied when applying to the Court of Protection to appoint a Receiver to manage the property and (financial) affairs of an incapacitated person, it is required that the person must be incapable "by reason of mental disorder". This is defined at Section 1 of the Mental Health Act 1983.

A person may lack the capacity to make a will but possess sufficient capacity to go shopping or vote. Unless it really is the case, we should refrain from defining a person generally as "incapacitated".

There are various ways of approaching the assessment of capacity. The three key methods were usefully outlined in the Law Commission Consultation Paper[4]. The three approaches are:

- *Outcome.* Capacity is determined by the content of the individual's decision.
- *Status test.* May apply in respect of age/diagnosis, etc. without further consideration of the individual's actual competence.
- *Test of understanding.* This concerns an assessment of whether the particular individual is able to make a particular decision at a particular time.

It is the last of these that applies in our common law and which in fact was proposed by the Law Commission in its *New Jurisdiction* publication of 1991 to form the basis of a statutory test.

As can be seen above, a range of different specific tests exists for particular instances, but normally general principles apply which substantively are based upon the individual's understanding, rather than the exercise of his/her judgement. If we were to be judged by the appropriateness of the decisions we make, incapacity would be a far more common concept!

Having noted the very variable application of the framework, it is disturbing to note that little if any research has been undertaken to determine the skills and abilities necessary to establish capacity[5].

EVIDENCE

Regardless of the above criteria, from an evidential position mental incapacity is a question of fact and there can be no doubt that the correct legal test must be applied. That, as alluded to above, will vary according to the circumstances. The role of the judge within the court proceedings is seeking to determine capacity as a lay person, influenced by personal observations and on the strength of evidence submitted from doctors and others who know of the individual[d]. In the words of His Honor Mr Justice Nicholas Wall:

> Expert witnesses need to remember that most judges do not have any more medical expertise than the average intelligent lay person...it is for this reason that they rely upon the integrity of expert witnesses[6].

THE "NEXT OF KIN"

Our nearest blood relative. Our kind and loving family. Those who are only capable of acting in our best interest. Surely, in the legal lacunae of decision making they are the legal rock on which we can build. If we are incapable of making decisions for ourselves, then surely professionals must turn to them to sanction actions. They know the best way to spend our money, they know when we should be going into a home, they know what is best. Really? Are you sure?

IN WHOSE BEST INTERESTS?

The UK law confers no legal rights on the "next of kin" *per se*. The matrix of decision making for a person who lacks capacity is our common law doctrine of necessity. This involves four basic elements:

- The person must lack capacity in relation to that particular decision at that time.
- It must be sufficiently necessary to make that decision.
- The person making it must be reasonable.
- It must be in the best interests of the incapacitated person (not the next of kin and not the professional).

All too often the professionals may feel powerless in the face of families who are demanding admission to a nursing home, or a discharge from hospital. They may be trying to insist on a particular form of treatment or withholding their consent to what the medical team is proposing. The professionals know that no "reasonable person" could possibly believe that certain decisions were in the incapacitated person's best interests. But, the family want it, so how can I possibly prevent it? The lawyer would point out that if the professionals capitulate and damage ensues, that it could be called professional negligence.

TREATMENT

To have capacity gives us the right to refuse any treatment that we do not wish to receive, even if death would be the result. Only in the case of people detained under the Mental Health Act can a competent adult be treated against his/her wishes, and then only for his/her mental disorder.

Clearly drawn and unambiguous "advance refusals" (otherwise known as living wills or advance directives) allow persons with capacity to bind the hands of the doctors. They can indicate that in the event of them becoming incapacitated, there would be certain treatments that, had they retained capacity, they would not have consented to. These have emerged through our case law, notably the case of *Airedale NHS Trust v. Bland* [1993] 1 All E.R. 821 and are a common law concept. An advance refusal could only be overridden if either it was not sufficiently clear or the

person was then "sectioned" under the Mental Health Act because he/she required treatment in a hospital for mental disorder. Our statute law always takes precedence over common law principles.

WHEN TO "SECTION" UNDER THE MENTAL HEALTH ACT

From my own experience of training mental health professionals for many years, few professionals working with the elderly seem to realize that the Mental Health Act provides a framework of protective powers for those who lack capacity and have a mental disorder. This term includes the mentally ill. Dementia is of course a form of mental illness.

The Act allows a person to be "sectioned" when his/her mental disorder is of a nature or degree that requires either assessment (section 2) or treatment (section 3) in hospital and his/her health, safety or the protection of others require it. Once sectioned it allows the professionals to impose their will on the patient but certain boundaries are proscribed. It gives the individual certain rights of appeal, and these can be triggered simply on the basis that the right has not been exercised.

Since the House of Lords judgement in the case of *R v. Bournewood Community and Mental Health NHS Trust ex parte L 1998 3 W.L.R. 107*, the incompetent patient need only be sectioned if it is necessary to treat him/her in hospital for a mental disorder and he/she demonstrates actual objection by word or deed. Because statute law (that passed by Parliament) takes precedence over our common law, the person should be sectioned, and if he/she is not, then any treatment given under the common law doctrine of necessity would amount to unlawful imprisonment and assault. You cannot use the defences available under common law if you are obliged to apply the statute law. At present, it would seem to me that few medical and nursing professionals realize this. The guidance issued by the Department of Health[7] following the Bournewood judgement tells us that if there is doubt as to whether the action amounts to an objection, then it is to be treated as if it were an objection. The incapacitated person who is trying to leave the ward or is objecting to medication (e.g. spitting it out), where there is doubt, should be considered for a Mental Health Act section. This would then accord him/her rights under that Act. It would then follow that further treatment for mental disorder under common law would be unlawful.

What about the person who is "required" to go into a nursing or residential home and does not wish to go? The Code of Practice to the Mental Health Act, Chapter 13 paragraph 13.10.b., indicates that, under these circumstances, Guardianship under the statutory powers in the Mental Health Act should be seriously considered.

> Where an adult is assessed as requiring residential care, but owing to mental incapacity is unable to make a decision as to whether he/she wishes to be placed in residential care, those who are responsible for his/her care should consider the applicability and appropriateness of guardianship for providing the framework within which decisions about his/her current and future care can be planned.

Few professionals seem to realize this.

A Guardianship Order allows a guardian to require a person to "reside in a particular place", attend various places for occupation, education or treatment or to allow access to the person on Guardianship by specified third parties or the guardian.

---

[d]This proposition is strongly supported in the High Court Judgement of Wall J in Re: G (Minors) (Expert Witnesses) [1994] 2 FLR 291, 298.

Although the use of Guardianship is increasing with the elderly (Mental Health Act Commission 7th Biennial Report[8]), it is still used infrequently. There were 804 Guardianship cases current at 31 March 1998 compared with 335 in 1992. This, however, includes all age groups and mental disorders. There are no statistics available specifically for the over-65s. Usually the common law doctrine of necessity is invoked and this allows reasonable force to be used where necessary, either to prevent a person leaving or to restrain him/her for medication or other reasons. This is likely to be subject to challenge under the Human Rights Act 1998. There is a strong possibility that the Bournewood case will be overturned by a decision of the European Court of Human Rights. This is because, under Article 5, there is a Right to Liberty and Security of the Person. This states under Article 5(4) that:

> Everyone who is deprived of his liberty...shall be entitled to take proceedings by which the lawfulness of his detention shall be decided speedily by a court and his release ordered if the detention is not lawful.

For those who lack capacity and are "detained" under common law there is not a mechanism that allows this challenge in English law.

THE NEW ERA OF HUMAN RIGHTS

With the passage of the Human Rights Act 1998 we are entering a new era for the concept of human rights in the UK. With the partial incorporation of the European Convention of Human Rights and Fundamental Freedoms there is the opportunity for the citizen to take proceedings against public bodies for alleged breaches of human rights. Public Bodies would include state and private hospitals, social service authorities, doctors and social workers who can carry out specific functions under the Mental Health Act where any of these bodies are carrying out a public function. As appears usual in the legal process, the mechanism by which the incapacitated can seek to assert their rights is far from clear. Yet again it will require the identification of the individual who will take the proceedings on their behalf.

The most relevant Articles to the European Convention of Human Rights and Fundamental Freedoms are:

- Article 2 enshrines the right to life. This includes the right to be protected by those who are caring for the vulnerable from risks that may lead to death.

- Article 3 protects the citizen from torture, inhuman or degrading treatment or punishment.
- Article 5 states that there is a Right to Liberty and Security of the Person.
- Article 6 protects the right to a fair trial when, for example, the Court of Protection is considering removing a person's right to control his/her own financial affairs.
- Article 8 provides for respect for a person's home and family life. This would include decisions about confidentiality of information, where a person lives or with whom he/she has contact.
- Article 12 provides for the right to marry (despite one's age!).

IN CONCLUSION

With an inadequate legal framework, extensive abuse taking place in many guises, with those working with the elderly often unaware of what the law permits, with the government apparently unwilling to legislate, the future looks bleak. The Human Rights Act could and should be about changing our culture. It should affect the way that we conceptualize the exercise of decisions that affect the rights of the citizen. My fear is that in all other areas of society this may well be the case. However, for the elderly confused incapacitated person, who will take on responsibility for this awesome responsibility?

REFERENCES

1. Civil Procedure Rules 1998, Rule 21, Statutory Instrument 3132, 1998.
2. Law Commission. *Mentally Incorporated Adults and Decision Making.* Consultation Papers Nos. 128–130. London: HMSO, 1993.
3. Lord Chancellor's Department. *Who Decides? Making Decisions on Behalf of Mentally Incapacitated Adults.* London: HMSO, 1997.
4. Law Commission. *Mentally Incapacitated Adults and Decision Making: An Overview.* Paper 119 (May). London: HMSO, 1991.
5. Ashton G. *Elderly People and the Law.* London: Butterworth, 1995.
6. A Handbook for Expert Witnesses in Children Act Cases. *Family Law 2000.*
7. Department of Health. HSC 1998/122 NHS Executive, 1998.
8. Mental Health Act Commission. *The Biennial Report 1995–1997.* London: The Stationery Office.

Older People, Clinicians and Mental Health Regulation

Elaine Murphy

Queen Mary College, University of London, London, UK

The Mental Health Act 1983 (England and Wales) made no mention of age, applying to children and those of advanced years just the same as to younger adults. Similarly, the Mental Health Act Commission created by the 1983 Act to "keep under review the operation of the Act" as it related to detained patients also had no responsibilities specific to older people. The old Commission had an awkwardly circumscribed role with few real powers. It visited hospitals and registered nursing homes to meet patients and ensure that the conditions in which they were detained were of an acceptable standard. The Commission also investigated complaints relating to detained patients and monitored the consent to treatment safeguards in Part IV of the Act, appointing independent doctors to give second opinions.

In December 2000, after 10 years of discussion and consultation about the failings of the 1983 Act, the government published proposals for a new Mental Health Act[1], which will have a very significant impact on the practice of geriatric psychiatrists. It contains new safeguards for the care and treatment of people with long-term mental disorders in institutional care, providing obligatory second opinions for those who are unable, through mental incapacity, to consent to treatment. In effect, this will cover all those with dementia in long-term care and many other older psychiatric patients. The new Act also replaces the old Commission with a new Commission for Mental Health, which will have wide powers in relation to overseeing the new legislation but will not be a visitorial or inspectorial body. For the first time, the new Commission will have a responsibility to ensure that professionals are trained properly in the legislation. This will surely require far closer working relationships with professional training and accreditation agencies. The old visitorial function, however, will be handed over to the new National Care Standards Commission and the Commission for Health Improvement. Thus, clinicians can expect even more inspection and regulation, rather than less, under the new regulations.

The central regulatory system is usually dated back to 1833, when the Factory Inspectorate was established. *The Times*[2] pronounced that this new system contained "the seeds of mighty changes", although the Editor was "no enthusiast" for central regulation but acknowledged that an inspectorate offered advantages "if inspectors or visitors of strong capacity, of enlightened humanity and moral courage" were appointed. The Lunacy Commission of 1845, chaired by the indefatigable 7th Earl of Shaftesbury for 40 years until his death in office, achieved considerable influence with government and changes in local asylums and workhouses because the Commission remained small, elite and adopted a coherent, unifying set of policies in its early years[3].

Modern mental health commissions are similar to the Lunacy Commission in being only as effective as their members are. Ministers have not always been convinced of this simple truth and have sometimes seen Commission appointments as a convenient reward for other fields of endeavour or as an opportunity to promote other laudable government objectives. Since its inception in 1984, the old Commission, a multiprofessional body, struggled to attract members of distinction from the professions of psychiatry and law and yet, to achieve credibility and respect from psychiatric services, the quality, training and behaviour of members was crucial. Over the years there was a steady improvement in the administrative efficiency of the organization and a significant step up in quality of the recruits. The new Commission will need to learn some of the lessons learnt if it is to achieve early credibility. Being a good commissioner requires enormous tact, humility and an ever-present awareness that a nurturing, developmental, encouraging approach achieves far more and is less alienating to professional staff than a heavy-handed "policing" approach.

The notion underpinning regulatory bodies dies hard. The idea is that the Secretary of State employs a team of quasi-independent "eyes and ears" to act as the conduit for information to central government and to channel edicts from the centre to the field. The proliferation of statutory commissions and non-statutory regulatory bodies (so-called QUANGOS) in the late twentieth and early twenty-first centuries would suggest that faith in these institutions as movers and shakers of social improvement remains undimmed in governments today. The zeal with which agencies are established falls away as soon as it is realized that inspectors and monitors cannot substitute for good local managers. In mental health services, good hospital unit management and improvements of standards of training and clinical work through professional bodies, such as the Royal College of Psychiatrists and the National Boards for nursing education, are more likely to effect permanent improvements in standards of care. "Watchdogs" and Commissions inevitably disappoint ministers and the usual cycle of events is that a commission's powers are progressively reduced and in due course frequently disbanded on the grounds of economy. As the numbers of factories grew beyond what it was reasonable to inspect, the Factory Inspectorate's sweeping powers to make statutory regulations and act as local magistrates were abolished in 1844. The Board of Control similarly found its powers diminished from those of its predecessor, the old "dead duck" Lunacy Commission, and was

Principles and Practice of Geriatric Psychiatry, 2nd edn. Edited by J. R. M. Copeland, M. T. Abou-Saleh and D. G. Blazer
©2002 John Wiley & Sons, Ltd

finally abolished in 1959. More recently, the Health Advisory Service, established by Richard Crossman's health ministry in the 1960s, was perceived to be unable to stop hospital scandals and was gradually denuded of its powers and eventually extruded from agency status to make a living from consultancy as best it could. Now the Mental Health Act Commission predictably gives way to a new-style Commission, with more circumscribed, focused powers, and it remains to be seen whether the new one will fare any better in the eyes of services and the government than the old one.

It has been estimated that there are approximately 44 000 informal admissions to institutions annually in England and Wales of mentally incapacitated patients who are compliant with treatment but lack the capacity to consent to treatment[4]. This far exceeds the 13 000 detained under formal powers. The new Act will provide them with extra safeguards, the right to a second opinion for long-term treatment and the right to appeal to a Tribunal. Some psychiatrists will regard an extension of legal powers to informal incapacitated patients as an unwelcome extra burden of work on them and their clinical teams. On the other hand, the new provisions will ensure that older people will receive greater attention from the regulatory bodies and their legal rights to decent care and treatment will be enhanced.

When they work well, central regulatory Mental Health Commissions can be strong allies to clinicians seeking to improve their patients' lives. Psychiatrists need to understand the role and remit of the Commission and be willing to serve during part of their career. The effectiveness of the new Commission will be greatly enhanced if the profession adopts a strategy of supporting and involving itself in its work and also ensures that the needs of older people are kept firmly in the forefront of the regulators' considerations.

REFERENCES

1. Reforming the Mental Health Act. *Part I. The new legal framework*. Cm5016-I; 6, 7, 49–51.
2. *The Times*. Leading Article, 21 September 1833.
3. Shaftesbury, Lord. *Minutes of Evidence to the Select Committee on Lunatics*. 25 May 1860; BPP 495.XXII.349: 22–36.
4. Mental Health Act Commission. *Petition to the House of Lords to intervene in the Bournewood Case and submissions*. London: Mental Health Act Commission, 1998.
5. Mental Health Act Commission. *Eighth Biennial Report 1997–1999*. London: Stationery Office, 1999; 73.

140

Training Requirements for
Old Age Psychiatrists in the UK

Susan M. Benbow

Wolverhampton Health Care NHS Trust, Wolverhampton, UK

In the UK over the last 20 years, increasing numbers of psychiatrists have specialized in working with older adults. Various terms have been used to describe this area of work: "psychogeriatrics", "geriatric psychiatry" and "old age psychiatry" are probably the most common. In 1978 the Royal College of Psychiatrists formed a Section (now Faculty) of Old Age Psychiatry and just over 10 years later, in 1989, old age psychiatry became recognized as a specialty by the Department of Health. The Royal Colleges of Physicians and Psychiatrists produced a Joint Report in 1989, which devoted a chapter to education and training in the psychiatry of old age[1]. At that time there was no accepted training programme for psychiatrists aiming for a career in the developing specialty. Things have changed considerably over recent years.

BACKGROUND: GROWTH OF THE SPECIALTY

In the early 1980s, two surveys of psychogeriatric services[2,3] showed considerable growth in the developing specialty, such that over 200 consultants were identified by late 1983. At that time the Joint Committee on Higher Psychiatric Training of the Royal College of Psychiatrists required higher trainees to spend 12–18 months in posts where the bulk of the work was in the subject; 28 senior registrar placements were identified. The authors predicted ongoing growth in old age psychiatry and a need to expand available training.

By 1990 there were 360 consultants working mainly in old age psychiatry and in 1993 the total had increased to 405[4]. Figures collected by the Faculty of Old Age Psychiatry show that the total has continued to rise, although there is still a high vacancy rate of approximately 14%.

UNDERGRADUATE EDUCATION

The first Joint Report[1] recommended that each medical school should have a senior academic in old age psychiatry and that all medical undergraduates should receive training in the subject. Faire and Katona[5] surveyed undergraduate teaching in the UK and reported a considerable expansion of academic posts in the specialty, but noted that more than half of all departments lacked a senior old age psychiatry academic. Almost all medical schools offered formal lectures in the subject, but there was great variation in the amount of clinical experience on offer and the authors felt that there was a strong case for all medical students having clinical experience in old age psychiatry, as recommended by the Joint Report. Gregson and Dening[6] surveyed teaching hospital psychiatrists and found that many teachers set no formal learning objectives in old age psychiatry. Most respondents wanted their teaching to impart enthusiasm for the subject, a sense of hope in working with mentally ill older adults, and an awareness of issues specific to ageing and ageism.

Although there are now chairs or readerships at a number of medical schools in the UK, gaps remain[7] and the second Joint Report, published in 1998, recommends that the characteristics of mental disorders among older people and the principles of good quality care should be included in the core curricula of all schools of medicine and nursing.

POSTGRADUATE TRAINING

The total minimum duration of specialist training in old age psychiatry is 6 years, of which 3 years will be in general professional or basic specialist training and 3 years in higher training (as a specialist registrar).

Basic Specialist Training

Part II of the Membership examination of the Royal College of Psychiatrists (MRCPsych) can normally only be taken after 30 months of training in psychiatry and is a requirement for entry into higher training, so basic training normally lasts for about 3 years. The first 12 months may include 6 months in old age psychiatry, provided that the experience offered is broad and includes the assessment and treatment of people with functional mental illness. Experience in old age psychiatry during basic training is regarded as important because of the increasing elderly population and the high rate of mental illness in older people, but the College *Basic Specialist Training Handbook*[8] states that trainees should be exposed to acute and functional mental disorders in late life and not solely to organic brain diseases. Old age psychiatry placements can often offer good community experience for trainees and the opportunity to attract young psychiatrists into the specialty.

Basic training concentrates on providing a range of experience in the specialties and subspecialties of psychiatry, aiming to develop history taking, formulation and case presentation skills, therapeutic skills and clinical judgement, relationships with

Principles and Practice of Geriatric Psychiatry, 2nd edn. Edited by J. R. M. Copeland, M. T. Abou-Saleh and D. G. Blazer
©2002 John Wiley & Sons, Ltd

colleagues, patients and relatives/carers, basic psychiatric knowledge and appropriate knowledge of general medicine.

By the time the trainee is ready to move into higher training, he/she will have completed a minimum of 3 years in approved training placements and will hold the MRCPsych[9]. He/she will also have some idea of his/her eventual career intentions. General psychiatry and old age psychiatry Specialist Registrar posts may be advertised separately, but trainees may opt to undertake training jointly in both specialties (see below).

Higher Specialist Training

Higher training aims to provide an educational programme to prepare a trainee for independent practice in old age psychiatry. The number of higher trainees is determined by the number of national training numbers (NTNs) and this is fixed centrally by the NHS Management Executive or equivalent body. The Specialist Training Committee of the Royal College of Psychiatrists (STC) sets the standard for training schemes and, under the aegis of the Specialist Training Authority (STA), sets the standard for award of certificates of completion of specialist training (CCSTs), which indicate that specialist training has been successfully completed. Since 1997 a CCST has been mandatory before taking up an NHS consultant post. Old age psychiatry falls within the remit of the Royal College of Psychiatrists' General and Old Age Psychiatry Specialist Advisory Committee (GOAPSAC)[10].

General and old age psychiatry higher training schemes may offer two options for aspiring old age psychiatrists. Single accreditation involves training for 3 years to gain a CCST in old age psychiatry. Currently these trainees may spend 1 year in general psychiatry or one of its subspecialties if they so wish. Single accreditation therefore necessitates a total of at least 6 years in psychiatric training. Many trainees (probably about 60%) opt to complete dual training, which aims at dual certification in general and old age psychiatry. These trainees complete a 4 year higher training programme, with 2 years in each specialty. They must have been appointed to their specialist registrar posts by an appropriately constituted appointments committee and will hold a NTN in old age psychiatry. Dual certification will require a total of at least 7 years in psychiatric training.

During their training, specialist registrars are expected to develop their professional attributes, core knowledge and skills, and are set goals in research and audit, teaching and supervision, and management. Currently, six "core" sessions are devoted to experience in old age psychiatry (or other specialty). "Core" experience involves working with a multidisciplinary team to provide a service to a defined population. Two further sessions are available for research, audit and personal study, and another two can be used to develop special interests. Old age psychiatry trainees are expected to gain experience of geriatric medicine at some stage of their training, and this is usually achieved either on a short-term attachment or using special interest sessions.

CONTINUING PROFESSIONAL DEVELOPMENT

Loane and Barker[11] surveyed newly appointed old age psychiatrists' views of their higher training. Overall clinical experience was felt to be satisfactory, but management experience was lacking in a number of areas and experience in dealing with complaints, dealing with difficult professional relationships, recruitment and disciplinary proceedings were all identified as areas where training was insufficient. Higher trainees are expected to get training in management but it can be difficult to pitch it at the right level.

The emphasis today is on lifelong learning[12], which is regarded as essential for all healthcare professionals. Old age psychiatrists are no different and are likely to see continuing developments in their field throughout their working lifetimes. Learning does not stop at the transition from higher trainee to consultant, and some might say that this is the point at which learning really starts. Consultants increasingly plan their CPD programmes[13], although these need to be flexible and to evolve with the specialty, the individual and the job. Increasingly too, consultants change their interests, disciplines and posts as their careers progress. This may be a way to re-energize and deal with the stresses of their multiple roles[14]. Continuing professional development should be a positive supportive opportunity for consultants to continue learning throughout their working lives.

LIFELONG LEARNING

Learning about old age psychiatry starts in medical school and continues throughout the working life of an old age psychiatrist. The context within which the specialty operates is constantly changing. There are various threats and opportunities on the horizon, including changes to the Mental Health Act[15], new ways of dealing with people unable to consent[16] and the National Service Framework for older adults. Old Age Psychiatry and its practitioners cannot stand still. The enthusiasm which teaching hospital psychiatrists aim to impart to their medical undergraduates can be maintained during specialist training and boosted throughout a consultant's career by continuing professional development and the challenge of working within a constantly changing health and social service context.

REFERENCES

1. Royal College of Physicians of London and Royal College of Psychiatrists. *Care of Elderly People with Mental Illness: Specialist Services and Medical Training*. London: Royal College of Physicians, 1989: 29.
2. Wattis JP, Wattis L, Arie T. Psychogeriatrics: a national survey of a new branch of psychiatry. *Br Med J* 1981; **282**: 1529–33.
3. Wattis J, Arie T. Further developments in psychogeriatrics in Britain. *Br Med J* 1984; **289**: 778.
4. Benbow SM, Jolley DJ. A specialty register: uses and limitations. *Psych Bull* 1996; **20**: 459–60.
5. Faire GM, Katona CLE. Survey of undergraduate teaching of old age psychiatry in the United Kingdom. *Psychiat Bull* 1993; **17**: 209–11.
6. Gregson CA, Dening T. Teaching old age psychiatry to medical schools in England. *Int J Geriat Psychiat* 1995; **10**: 883–6.
7. Working Party of the Royal College of Psychiatrists and Royal College of Physicians. *The Care of Older People with Mental Illness: Specialist Services and Medical Training*. London: Royal College of Psychiatrists, 1998: 40.
8. Royal College of Psychiatrists. *Basic Specialist Training Handbook*. London: Postgraduate Educational Services Department, Royal College of Psychiatrists, 1999: 17.
9. Royal College of Psychiatrists. *Educational Policy*. Occasional Paper OP36. London: Royal College of Psychiatrists, 1997: 57.
10. Royal College of Psychiatrists. *Higher Specialist Training Handbook*. Occasional Paper OP43. London: Royal College of Psychiatrists, 1998; 55.
11. Loane R, Barker A. Newly appointed consultants in old age psychiatry and the adequacy of higher training. *Psychiat Bull*, 1996; **20**: 388–90.
12. Department of Health. *A First Class Service: Quality in the New NHS*. London: Department of Health, 1998: 86.

13. Royal College of Psychiatrists. *Policy for the Continuing Professional Development of Psychiatrists*. Council Report CR58. London: Royal College of Psychiatrists, 1997: 32.
14. Benbow SM, Jolley DJ. Psychiatrists under stress. *Psychiat Bull*, 1998; **22**: 1–2.

15. Department of Health. *Reform of the Mental Health Act 1983. Proposals for Consultation*. London: The Stationery Office, 1999: 93.
16. Lord Chancellor's Department. *Making Decisions. The Government's Proposals for Making Decisions on Behalf of Mentally Incapacitated Adults*. London: HMSO, 1999.

Old Age Psychiatrists and Stress

Susan M. Benbow

Wolverhampton Health Care NHS Trust, Wolverhampton, UK

Stress, and its effect on the workforce, is a matter of increasing concern in the Health Service. Stress levels in health professionals generally are high[1]. Doctors as a group have increased rates of cirrhosis, road traffic accidents and suicide, compared with the general population[2]. They are prone to symptoms of anxiety and depression, and are more likely to misuse alcohol or other substances[3].

WHY WORRY ABOUT SERVICES FOR OLDER PEOPLE?

Working with older people, especially those with mental health problems, might be particularly stressful, for various reasons. This client group is more likely to exhibit challenging behaviours. They are subject to the increasing disadvantages, disabilities and progressive loss of independence associated with increasing age, and are approaching death. Consultants (and other staff) in geriatric medicine and geriatric psychiatry are working in so-called "Cinderella specialties", which struggle to compete for resources with the more "sexy" acute specialties. The stigma of being old, mentally ill and cognitively impaired is contagious and affects attitudes towards the staff who work in these specialties[4]. In addition, staff will have to confront their own beliefs and fears about ageing, dementia and death for themselves and members of their own families[5].

It is not surprising, in this context, that psychiatrists are retiring earlier[6] and recruitment to the specialty is inadequate to maintain consultant numbers[7]. Stress is an important issue for the workforce.

WHAT DO WE KNOW?

Studies of the work patterns of old age psychiatrists have found that they have long working days with little opportunity for recreation, family life, personal study and research[8,9]. More than 40% of old age psychiatrists do extra work at home on every day of the working week except Friday, and more than 30% do so on Saturdays and Sundays[9]. Most of the stresses identified by old age psychiatrists relate to work overload or organizational structure and climate[10]. Many of these factors are equally applicable to staff working in geriatric medicine.

WHAT CAN BE DONE?

Appointment as a consultant brings long working hours and a number of different, often conflicting, roles (including responsible clinician, manager, budget holder, counsellor, researcher, teacher, team member, perhaps team leader) in various settings (wards, day hospitals, community and others). The result is role ambiguity, conflict and overload. Doctors could be better trained for the demands of consultanthood. The means by which consultants are supported, supervised and valued could be radically revised[11]. Individuals need to be able to change and develop their interests and work patterns over time, in order to allow re-energization. Time allocated to clinical work, teaching, research, family and other interests will vary at different stages of a person's working life. Organizations need to accept and support the evolving careers of their staff members.

REFERENCES

1. Caplan RP. Stress, anxiety and depression in hospital consultants, general practitioners and senior health service managers. *Br Med J* 1994; **309**: 1261–3.
2. Margison FR. Stress in psychiatrists. In Payne R, Firth-Cozens J, eds, *Stress in Health Professionals*. Chichester: Wiley, 1987: 107–24.
3. Holmes J. Mental health of doctors. *Adv Psychiat Treatm* 1997; **3**: 251–3.
4. Benbow SM, Reynolds D. Challenging the stigma of Alzheimer's disease. *Hosp Med* 2000; **61**: 174–7.
5. Turner SJ, Benbow SM. Dementia, stigma and the general practitioner. *Update* (in press).
6. Kendell RE, Pearce A. Consultant psychiatrists who retired prematurely in 1995 and 1996. *Psychiat Bull* 1997; **21**: 741–5.
7. Storer D. Prematurely retiring consultant psychiatrists. *Psychiat Bull* 1997; **21**: 737–8.
8. Benbow SM, Jolley DJ, Leonard IJ. All work? A day in the life of geriatric psychiatrists. *Int J Geriat Psychiat* 1993; **8**: 1019–22.
9. Jolley DJ, Benbow SM. The everyday work of geriatric psychiatrists. *Int J Geriat Psychiat* 1997; **12**: 109–13.
10. Benbow SM, Jolley DJ. Old age psychiatrists: what do they find stressful? *Int J Geriat Psychiat* 1997; **12**: 879–82.
11. Benbow SM, Jolley DJ. Psychiatrists under stress. *Psychiat Bull* 1998; **22**: 1–2.

141

Developing and Maintaining Links between Service Disciplines: the Program for Organizing Interdisciplinary Self-education (POISE)

John A. Toner

Columbia University Stroud Center, New York, USA

The need for effective and systematic education of geriatric specialists in the field of psychiatry has been widely recognized[1]. Current shortages of general and child psychiatrists are gradually being surpassed by the shortages of geriatric psychiatrists[2]. The field of geriatric psychiatry education began to expand only recently, and this expansion was a direct result of funding of postgraduate specialty training programs in geriatric mental health by the National Institute of Mental Health[3].

Another major development in the field of psychiatry that has led to increased interest in, and expansion of, geriatric psychiatry training programs has been the evolution of subspecialization in geriatric psychiatry through Added Qualifications (Board Examinations) and the accreditation of geriatric psychiatry residency/ fellowship programs. However, as the specialty field of geriatric psychiatry has evolved, it has become more apparent than ever that general practitioners, rather than geriatric psychiatrists, will provide the bulk of care to mentally ill older people. Although guidelines for developing curricula in geriatric psychiatry have been developed[1,3], these guidelines focus primarily on the clinical skills necessary for the psychiatrist or general practitioner to treat geriatric patients, and not on the leadership skills necessary for the psychiatrist or general practitioner to facilitate and lead the interdisciplinary healthcare team. The curriculum guidelines also neglect to emphasize the role of the geriatric psychiatrist as the key link between service disciplines on the mental healthcare team.

For some time, the interdisciplinary healthcare team approach has been well established in specialty areas, such as rehabilitation, surgery and dentistry; however, the fields of psychiatry and and general medicine, specifically geriatric psychiatry, have been slow to realize the important role of the geriatric psychiatrist as part of the mental healthcare team approach to care of the geriatric patient. The field has been even slower to recognize the central role the geriatric psychiatrist can and should play in facilitating cohesive team function and linking treatment goals of different service disciplines. The purpose of this chapter is to describe a model interdisciplinary team leadership training program, which exists within the curriculum of a geriatric psychiatry fellowship program sponsored by the New York State Office of Mental Health. This model program is unique in that it focuses on training geriatric psychiatrists in the skills required to develop, lead and maintain interdisciplinary treatment teams in inpatient and outpatient settings.

Schmitt *et al.*[4] indicate that the term "interdisciplinary teams" in healthcare settings has a variety of meanings, depending on usage. Thus, it is important to establish criteria that define the term. For the purpose of this chapter, we have adopted the criteria set out by Schmitt and her colleagues[5]. These criteria require at a minimum that the healthcare team: (a) includes a variety of disciplines in the care of the same patient; (b) encompasses a diversity of dissimilar knowledge and skills required to treat the patient; (c) plans care by establishing an integrated set of goals shared by the providers of that care; and (d) shares information and coordinates their services through a systematic communication process.

PROGRAM BACKGROUND

The interdisciplinary team training program described in this chapter is the outcome of 15 years of work devoted to the development of a durable, cost-effective method of linking and coordinating mental health services within the institutional setting. The program evolved, in part, from an educational philosophy that focuses on a participative model of self-education. The assumption is that the healthcare staff of an institution already have the technical skills required to function in their particular position, but need to enhance their understanding of how their roles in their particular discipline relate to the roles of other team members from different disciplines, and how the team as a whole relates to other staff and teams. A system by which the staff can work collaboratively to deliver effective treatment to patients is regarded as essential.

This concept was first applied in assessment training programs and subsequent related studies involving mental healthcare teams at state psychiatric centers in New York[6–8]. The results of these evaluation studies and the favorable response of staff to the interdisciplinary mental healthcare team leadership training[9–11] led to a request by the Deputy Commissioner of the New York State Office of Mental Health to adapt the program for implementation in other psychiatric centers throughout New York State. In subsequent discussions, it was determined that the training would be most successful and relevant if it was conducted with the key member of the mental healthcare team who most often is responsible for team leadership, namely the psychiatrist. In this way, a culture of learning would be established and the psychiatrist trainees would then go on to work on interdisciplinary treatment teams elsewhere, and bring with them to their new work setting this culture of learning. Thus, the psychiatrist trainees would

Principles and Practice of Geriatric Psychiatry, 2nd edn. Edited by J. R. M. Copeland, M. T. Abou-Saleh and D. G. Blazer
©2002 John Wiley & Sons, Ltd

disseminate to other staff members from other disciplines the knowledge they obtained during the team leadership training. This adaptation of the original model program was applied to the development of the Columbia University Geriatric Psychiatry Residency and Fellowship Programs, which are sponsored by the Stroud Center and the Department of Psychiatry of the Columbia University Faculty of Medicine, Binghamton Psychiatric Center of the New York State Office of Mental Health. This program is accredited by the Accreditation Council for Graduate Medical Education. The Geriatric Psychiatry Residency and Fellowship Programs bring together the clinical resources of the Binghamton Psychiatric Center and the educational and clinical research resources of the Stroud Center/Center for Geriatrics and Gerontology of Columbia University.

Since its inception, the Geriatric Psychiatry Residency and Fellowship Programs has included, as a core ingredient of the long-term care component of the curriculum[12], the training of psychiatrist-fellows in the methods of interdisciplinary team leadership. Additionally, every fellow is required, during his/her fellowship, to develop and/or lead an interdisciplinary treatment team under direct and regular supervision of fellowship faculty.

PROGRAM DEVELOPMENT

Rationale

All clinicians need a good system for identifying patients' symptoms, making informed treatment decisions regarding the patients, and managing stress that is related to providing care. All members of the treatment team need practical tools to guide them in eliciting, classifying, recording, and interpreting information on patients' health status and functioning—in short, a system that will help them to evaluate each patient's status, identify the appropriate treatment, predict possible outcomes, and plan the patient's care. This system must also include methods to assist the interdisciplinary team in functioning as a team and managing their own stress.

A program designed to train interdisciplinary mental health care team members at psychiatric centers within the New York State Office of Mental Health was developed, implemented and evaluated[8,10]. The purpose of the program was to upgrade the functioning of the multidisciplinary/interdisciplinary mental healthcare treatment team and to train staff to identify and manage the stress that developed as a result of caring for older psychiatric patients, many of whom are demented. The Program for Organizing Interdisciplinary Self-education (POISE), the name by which the program is officially known, is a multi-disciplinary/interdisciplinary approach to improving the assessment of patients in psychiatric hospitals and the treatment planning decisions based on those assessments. The program also provides training of staff in current methods of stress management. POISE currently focuses on the training of the geriatric psychiatrist as the central member of the interdisciplinary mental healthcare team.

The geriatric psychiatrist is a key figure in the treatment and management of geriatric patients in both inpatient and outpatient psychiatric facilities. The geriatric psychiatrist is also a core member of the interdisciplinary treatment team and is a key link between service disciplines on the team in psychiatric settings. Regardless of the level of functioning of the team, the geriatric psychiatrist is often viewed by team members as the primary care physician who is ultimately responsible for leading the team and thus coordinating the treatment of geriatric patients. However, most geriatric psychiatrists receive little or no training that will enable them to work effectively as a core member of the inter-disciplinary team and key link between team members.

The geriatric psychiatrist and other members of the inter-disciplinary team require special training to enable them to work effectively together[13,16]. Training, which can be accomplished either formally or informally on and/or off the unit, can be directed at facilitating and encouraging a team approach to patient care. This training must be durable in as much as it can be replicated throughout an entire system of care to achieve objectives; in that its effects last beyond the period of training; in that it concentrates on developing team cohesiveness and increased productivity; and in as much as it is based on teaching the team how to continue and maintain self-learning processes (including monitoring of own performance to achieve objectives). The training must be directed at a key member of the team (e.g. geriatric psychiatrist), who then goes on to train other members of the team. In this way, team functioning can continue, even in the absence of the facilitator, the geriatric psychiatrist.

The Columbia University Geriatric Psychiatry Residency and Fellowship Programs includes training in interdisciplinary team leadership as a core component of its training of geriatric psychiatrists. This training component, POISE, is described below. Details regarding the specific interdisciplinary treatment team training approaches used in the training of geriatric psychiatrists are given in Toner et al.[14] and Miller and Toner[15], who have outlined the steps in developing and implementing a geriatric team.

Program Description

POISE is a durable, cost-effective approach to teaching geriatric psychiatrists (i.e. residents and fellows in training) methods of self-learning which serve as ongoing tools for planning treatment for patients. It is durable and cost-effective, in as much as the geriatric psychiatrist, and ultimately other members of the interdisciplinary team, learn methods of effectively working with one another by collaboratively setting goals and arriving at appropriate treatment decisions for the patient. After the geriatric psychiatry resident/fellow receives core training in interdisciplinary team development and leadership, he/she is assigned to an existing interdisciplinary team, where he/she imparts the core training to the members of the team. The team then continues to apply these methods on an ongoing basis and the geriatric psychiatrist continues to provide guidance and leadership as the group leader/facilitator. This approach to staff training is untraditional because, instead of relying on conventional didactic approaches to learning or the charismatic qualities of the group leader, the core training focuses on teaching the geriatric psychiatrist the methods of self-learning in regard to assessment[16]. Geriatric assessment serves as the unifying theme of the training, because most staff conduct assessment in one way or another—including the nursing aides, who generally do not view themselves as assessors—and because most staff feel they need additional training in assessment. Furthermore, although most team members assess patient functioning, no single discipline considers assessment as their exclusive domain. In this way, while team members are organized and ultimately conditioned to focus on the theme of assessment, interdisciplinary conflict revolving around disciplinary territorial issues is avoided, since no one discipline or individual has exclusive rights to the theme. The theme of assessment also serves as a springboard for discussing more general group functioning issues.

In POISE, the concept of self-learning is applied directly to the training of the geriatric psychiatrist resident/fellow in a long-term care setting serving the elderly. Thus, the geriatric psychiatrist resident/fellow and other members of the inter-disciplinary team are trained to develop their own skills and strengths in regard to the identification, classification and treatment of patient problems, rather than superimposing a costly didactic approach which, at best, can expect to yield only short-term effects because of frequent staff turnover and administrative changes.

More concretely, the geriatric psychiatrist is trained in the methods of team leadership, using geriatric assessment as a central theme, and the methods of facilitating interdisciplinary team collaboration among the kinds of people associated with the chain of patient care, the treatment team. The geriatric psychiatrist also receives, as part of his/her core training, instruction in a method of developing with the team the universe of management decisions available to them in that particular setting (i.e. the Treatment Decision Guide). By using case examples, review of patient records, videotapes of case conferences, admission interviews, etc., the geriatric psychiatrist (as facilitator) and the team arrive at an understanding of good and bad management decisions, what problems exist in making treatment decisions, how these problems develop, what treatment options are (or might be) available, what methods team members use in arriving at appropriate treatment decisions, and what possible alternatives exist in arriving at a diagnosis. By establishing with the team the criteria that must be met in order to arrive at a particular treatment decision, the geriatric psychiatrist and other team members establish goals and objectives for any specific treatment decision available to them and discuss how assessment can be used to better link patient problems to the appropriate treatment decision. Through this process, the Treatment Decision Guide[14,15] is developed. This Treatment Decision Guide identifies the dynamic pathway for use of information regarding the patient in planning, implementing and monitoring treatment. The Treatment Decision Guide provides team members with a guide for using assessment and is also a useful, cost-effective and durable recipe for planning treatment.

Clinical Applications

POISE sensitizes the geriatric psychiatrist to the psychosocial problems that have a high frequency in the elderly long-term care patient population. It provides the geriatric psychiatrist with a program for upgrading the interaction process between interdisciplinary team members through group process exercises and lectures, which emphasize the role of the geriatric psychiatrist and other team members in assessing the well-being of patients and linking that assessment to treatment. The program then goes on to train the geriatric psychiatrist to lead teams and train other team members in team leadership.

POISE also improves the quality of staff interaction and team functioning by: (a) setting up systematic approaches and procedures for making appropriate treatment decisions; and (b) once this system has been set up, providing a device by which professionals and paraprofessionals relate to one another in operating the ongoing system themselves. This is done primarily through the use of the Treatment Decision Guide and Systematic Problem Solving. In addition, POISE enhances patient care by improving staff knowledge and skills in regard to assessment. This is accomplished through group exercises designed to build the geriatric psychiatrist's and other team members' skills in observing patients and formulating decision plans based on those observations. In this way, the geriatric psychiatrist is trained to be a facilitator, who provides the team with a mechanism by which the group does its own learning on an ongoing basis.

SUMMARY

The Program for Organizing Interdisciplinary Self-education, POISE[16], is one program that has demonstrated that the principles of interdisciplinary collaboration and team training can be applied successfully in a geriatric psychiatry residency/fellowship program[13]. The learning process involved in POISE covers the skills, knowledge and attitudes of team members regarding the following program components: team development, management, and maintenance; and program needs assessment.

POISE focuses on the training of geriatric psychiatrist fellows in the following areas[13]:

1. The role each member of the team plays in assessing the patient.
2. Linking each member's assessment to a treatment plan.
3. Systematic approaches and procedures for making appropriate treatment decisions. This includes methods of defining and negotiating team members' roles; case study approaches to prioritizing treatment goals; and systematic approaches to problem solving.
4. The Treatment Decision Guide (TDG): a guide designed by the interdisciplinary team members specifically for patient management in their particular institution, the TDG provides a key to arriving at available treatment alternatives in that institution.

After the geriatric psychiatrist is trained in POISE, he/she is trained in the method of teaching other interdisciplinary treatment team members the POISE method and thus provides the team members with the crucial techniques for maintaining the ongoing team themselves. Once the geriatric psychiatrist is assigned to the interdisciplinary team, the emphasis of the training is on shared leadership functions of all team members, with designated leaders, experiential learning to facilitate team functioning and problem solving, and ongoing orientation of new team members (to team objectives and norms).

REFERENCES

1. Kennedy G, Goldstein M, Northcott C et al. Evolution of the geriatric curriculum in general residency training: recommendations for the coming decade. Acad Psychiat 1999; 23: 187–97.
2. Shulman K. The future of geriatric psychiatry. Can J Psychiat 1994; 39(suppl 1): S4–8.
3. Colenda CC. Essential curriculum in geriatric psychiatry for general internal medicine residency and geriatric medicine fellowship. Am J Med 1994; 97(suppl): 4A, 15–18S.
4. Schmitt M, Watson N, Feiger S, Williams T. Conceptualizing and measuring outcomes of interdisciplinary team care for a group of long-term, chronically ill institutionalized patients. In Bachman J, ed., Interdisciplinary Health Care: Proceedings of the Third Annual Interdisciplinary Team Care Conference. Center for Human Services, MI: Western Michigan University, 1982.
5. Schmitt MH, Farrell MP, Heinemann GD. Conceptual and methodological problems in studying the effects of interdisciplinary geriatric teams. Gerontologist 1988; 26: 753–64.
6. Toner J, Gurland B, Gasquoine P. Measuring depressive symptomatology in an inpatient psychogeriatric population. Gerontologist 1984; (abstr)24: 196.
7. Toner J, Gurland B. Interdisciplinary team training for geriatric health care providers. Gerontologist 1983; (abstr)23: 191.
8. Toner J, Meyer E. Multidisciplinary team training in the management of dementia: a stress management program for geriatric staff and family caregivers. In Mayeux R, Gurland B, Barrett V et al., eds, Alzheimer's Disease and Related Disorders: Psychosocial Issues for the Patient, Family, Staff and Community. Springfield, IL: Charles C. Thomas, 1988: 81–102.
9. Toner J, Gurland B, Leung M. Chronic mental illness and functional communication disorders in the elderly. Am Speech–Language–Hearing Assoc Rep 1990; 19: 54–64.
10. Toner J. Interdisciplinary treatment team training: A training program in geriatric assessment for health care providers. In

Nicholson CK, Nicholson JI, eds, *The Personalized Care Model for the Elderly*, 2nd edn. New York: Nicholson & Nicholson, 1982: 25–37.

11. Ricco-Schwartz S, Gasquoine P, Toner J. Communication deficits in an inpatient psychogeriatric population: implications for programmatic trends. *Gerontologist* 1983; **23**: 146.

12. Toner J. The continuum of long term care: an educational guide for faculty in the health sciences. *Phys Occ Therapy Geriat* 1990; **8**: 93–117.

13. Nadelson C. Medical education: a commentary on historical and contemporary issues. *Am J Psychiat* 1996; **153**(suppl): 3–6.

14. Toner J, Miller P, Gurland B. Conceptual, theoretical and practical approaches to the development of interdisciplinary teams: a transactional model. *Educ Gerontol* 1994; **20**: 53–69.

15. Miller P, Toner J. The making of a geriatric team. In Meyers W, ed., *New Techniques in the Psychotherapy of Older Patients*. New York: American Psychiatric Press, 1991.

16. Gurland B, Toner J, Mustille A *et al*. The organization of mental health services for the elderly. In Lazarus L, ed., *Essentials of Geriatric Psychiatry*. New York: Springer, 1988: 189–213.

Appendix—
International Psychogeriatric Association (IPA)

Barry Reisberg (former IPA President) and Fern F. Finkel (Executive Director)
New York University School of Medicine, New York, USA

The International Psychogeriatric Association is a worldwide, multidisciplinary group of healthcare professionals dedicated to the advancement of mental health in the elderly and the field of psychogeriatrics.

The organization was proposed by Imre Fejer and Hans Reichenfeld in 1980, following a very popular course in psychogeriatrics that had been developed by Professor Tom Arie in Nottingham, UK. The organization's founding meeting was held in Cairo, Egypt, in November 1982. Subsequently, IPA congresses have been held every 2 years. Early congresses were held in Umeå, Sweden (1985), Chicago, USA (1987), Tokyo, Japan (1989) and Rome, Italy (1991). The organization has maintained these widely geographically dispersed settings for its congresses until the present time (Table 142.1). In its early years, the growth of the organization was shepherded by Manfred Bergener (Cologne, Germany), President and Sanford Finkel (Chicago, USA), Secretary–Treasurer. A measure of the influence that Sanford Finkel has had on the organization includes his unique role in having served as IPA President (Table 142.2), as well as Secretary–Treasurer and chair of many important IPA committees and task forces.

From the outset, IPA has been successful in contributing to major developments in the field of psychogeriatrics. The organization has done this in large part through its very successful conferences. IPA's Board of Directors has also contributed very significantly. Currently, there are 25 directors and five officers from around the world serving on IPA's Board. From the very beginning, the Board decided that no more than two directors can represent any single country. Consequently, IPA's Board is a disparate and geographically diverse group. Many of the outstanding scientific and medical leaders in our field have served on IPA's board. Examples include Sir Martin Roth (UK), Luigi Amaducci (Italy) and Kazuo Hasegawa (Japan). IPA has also, from the outset, had regularly scheduled regional meetings at intervals of approximately 6 months. These meetings have also been held in diverse locations around the world (Table 142.1). A great advantage of these meetings is that, unlike the IPA congresses, they are generally held in conjunction with a local organization with a neuropsychogeriatric interest. This has enabled IPA to have fertile interchanges with many local professional groups. These include joint meetings with ongoing local or regional groups, such as the Turkish Society of Psychogeriatrics, the Institute of Mental Health of Beijing Medical University, the Royal College of Psychiatrists' Faculty of Old Age and the Brazilian Association of Geriatric Neuropsychiatry.

Table 142.1 IPA congress and meeting dates and locations

November 22–25, 1982	1st Congress; Cairo, Egypt
October 18–20, 1984	Cologne, Germany
August 28–31, 1985	2nd Congress; Umeå, Sweden
September 5–6, 1986	Paris, France
March 26–28, 1987	Baden/Vienna, Austria
August 23–31, 1987	3rd Congress; Chicago, USA
April 28–29, 1988	Lausanne, Switzerland
August 25–27, 1988	Budapest, Hungary
May 18–19, 1989	Modena, Italy
September 5–8, 1989	4th Congress; Tokyo, Japan
September 21–22, 1990	Gothenburg, Sweden
April 2–5, 1991	Cambridge, UK
August 18–23, 1991	5th Congress; Rome, Italy
February 15–17, 1992	San Francisco, USA
October 29–30, 1992	Lille, France
April 16–18, 1993	Toronto, Canada
September 5–10, 1993	6th Congress; Berlin, Germany
June 5–8, 1994	Amsterdam, The Netherlands
February 17–20, 1995	Cancun, Mexico
October 29–Nov 3, 1995	7th Congress; Sydney, Australia
March 9–10, 1996	New Delhi, India
October 4–5, 1996	Reykjavik, Iceland
April 25–27, 1997	São Paulo, Brazil
August 17–22, 1997	8th Congress; Jerusalem, Israel
May 21–23, 1998	Istanbul, Turkey
September 13–18, 1998	Munich, Germany
April 12–14, 1999	Beijing, China
August 15–20, 1999	9th Congress; Vancouver, Canada
April 4–7, 2000	Newcastle upon Tyne, UK
October 13–15, 2000	Pôrto Alegre, Brazil

Table 142.2 IPA Presidents

M. Bergener, Germany (1982)
G. Bucht, Sweden (1987)
K. Hasegawa, Japan (1989)
S. Finkel, USA (1991)
B. Steen, Sweden (1993)
R. Levy, UK (1995)
B. Reisberg, USA (1997)
E. Chiu, Australia (1999)

The regional meetings and congresses have been the lifeblood of the organization and have brought together diverse professionals who are interested in our field. These include geropsychiatrists, neurologists, geriatric general and family

Principles and Practice of Geriatric Psychiatry, 2nd edn. Edited by J. R. M. Copeland, M. T. Abou-Saleh and D. G. Blazer
©2002 John Wiley & Sons, Ltd

physicians, psychologists, geropsychiatric nurses, social workers, occupational therapists and others with an interest in our field. Presidents of the organization have until now been drawn from the disciplines of psychiatry and geriatric medicine.

Although these meetings and congresses have been sufficient to serve the growth of our organization, IPA has also created initiatives which have independently served our discipline. One of these initiatives concerns the coveted IPA Research Awards in Psychogeriatrics. The research awards were conceived through the vision of Manfred Bergener and were supported through the generosity of Bayer AG for the first decade, from 1989. These awards, for which submissions are solicited from throughout the world, are given for the best unpublished research submission. Since its inception, the Research Awards Committee has been chaired by Barry Reisberg, with referees from many nations who devote their time, energy and expertise to the exceedingly rigorous review process for these awards.

Winning papers over the course of the years have provided a significant contribution to the body of knowledge and progress in our field. For example, in the first Awards in Tokyo, 1989, subsequently famous research studies on behavioral and psychological symptoms of dementia (BPSD) by Alistair Burns (UK) and on reduction of Alzheimer's disease caregiver stress by Henry Brodaty (Australia) were awarded, in addition to seminal research by Barry Rovner (USA) on agitation in nursing home settings in the USA. Each of these award-winning research entries provided a stimulus for numerous subsequent papers and, more importantly, major changes in the structure of our field. For example, in part as a result of Alistair Burns' work, we now know much more regarding the nature of BPSD and pharmacologic and non-pharmacologic treatments of BPSD. As a result, in part, of Henry Brodaty's award-winning research, Alzheimer's organizations and associated support groups have now proliferated throughout the globe. Barry Rovner's findings led, in part, to changes in the quality of care provided to nursing home residents.

This astoundingly important work, singled out for accolades in IPA's first series of research awards, has resulted in commensurate effects on the careers of these scientists. For example, Alistair Burns is currently the President-elect of IPA and Henry Brodaty is presently the medical director of Alzheimer Disease International. The research awards have remained similarly successful from 1989 to the present, and have clearly not only stimulated the growth of our field but also served to advance the mental health quality of the elderly.

Another modality that IPA has chosen to coalesce growth in our field has been the convening of special meetings. These meetings have typically brought together leading scientists, leading clinicians, government officials, representatives of regulatory agencies and others to coalesce knowledge around a particular subject in our field. For example, a meeting was held in 1994 on "Methodology for drug trials in mild, moderate and severe Alzheimer's disease". This meeting, held in New York, helped to stimulate the approval and understanding of pharmacologic treatments for Alzheimer's disease which have now been approved in many nations around the world.

Another timely special meeting concerned behavioral and psychological symptoms of dementia (BPSD) in 1996. This meeting stimulated worldwide trials of drugs for the treatment of BPSD and subsequent demonstrations of efficacy. An update special meeting on BPSD was held in 1999. Yet another special meeting, which was held in Geneva in 1996, pulled together current knowledge regarding the diagnosis of Alzheimer's disease from diverse clinical and psychologic, electrophysiologic, neuroimaging, pathologic and biomolecular perspectives. This meeting helped foster the understanding that Alzheimer's disease, like all other major illnesses, is a diagnosis of inclusion as well as of exclusion.

IPA has published a journal, *International Psychogeriatrics*, since 1989, which is an Index Medicus publication and is a leading organ for research and information regarding worldwide activities in psychogeriatrics. Apart from regularly scheduled quarterly issues, *International Psychogeriatrics* has published groundbreaking and syncretic special issues. The special issues have included the proceedings of IPA's special meetings as well as comprehensive issues on other topics, such as a special issue on suicide in the elderly.

Another important publication of IPA is the *Bulletin*, a newsletter which serves as a less formal organ of communication for psychogeriatricians around the world. The IPA also publishes modules, pamphlets and slides on topics of special interest, such as BPSD. The publications further serve IPA's broad educational mission.

Other special and noteworthy activities of IPA include an international visiting junior scholar pilot program, sponsored by Pfizer, which enabled junior psychiatrists and neurologists from less financially endowed research nations to visit wealthier research institutions. For example, physician scholars from Argentina, Brazil, PR China, ROC Taiwan and Russia, were able to work at research centers in the USA, UK and Australia and absorb the most up-to-date methodologies for scientific research.

Yet another important initiative of IPA is its affiliate organization program, which is enabling regional and national organizations to have more ready access to international opportunities and resources and also enable IPA to reach physicians at the "grass roots" level. Equally important in terms of IPA's individual reach is its excellent website (www.ipa-online.org).

Apart from the activities listed in this brief summary, IPA has been involved in numerous other activities and communications in psychogeriatrics. The net result of these activities at the present time was reflected in part by IPA's outstanding Ninth Congress, which was held in Vancouver in 1999. This meeting was the largest meeting ever held in the field of psychogeriatrics. It brought together colleagues from 50 countries that represent IPA's diverse constituency, currently encompassing 75 of the world's nations.

In coming years, IPA seeks to further develop governmental consulting activities in psychogeriatrics, and to further develop its website and affiliate organization program, while maintaining, expanding and improving upon its numerous other activities on behalf of our field.

In summary, through a series of outstanding initiatives and activities, IPA has served the growth of psychogeriatrics worldwide for the past two decades. The goals of these activities continue to be improved mental health as people age, and consequently improved health more generally, throughout the world.

Index

Abbreviated Mental Test   127, 128, 169
acetylcholine in Alzheimer's disease
      229–30
acetylcholine receptor proteins   62
active life expectancy   72
activity theory   21
acute stress disorder (ASD)   553, 556
adjustment disorder   418, 538, 579
   clinical features   581
   with depressed mood   372–3
   therapy   581
adoption studies, genetics of affective
      disorders   376
α₂-adrenergic binding   399
adult day center (ADC) movement   706
Africa, dementia and depression in   649
age-associated cognitive decline (AACD)
      49, 303–4, 305–6
age-associated memory impairment
      (AAMI)   49, 237, 303–4, 305, 308
AGECAT   161
aging-associated cognitive decline
      (AACD)   305
aging clock   19–20
aging, theories of
   biological   19–20
   healthy vs. pathological   65–7
   psychological   20–1
   social   21
agoraphobia without history of panic
      disorder (AWORD)   551–2
AIDS dementia complex   365
akathisia   522–3
alcohol
   prevalence of heavy drinking   608–9
   prevalence of use   607–8
   see also alcohol abuse
alcohol abuse   601–4
   characteristics   602
   effects in the elderly   601–2
   epidemiology   607–11
   factors association with   609–10
   identification   609
   offending and   628
   onset   610
   outcomes   610–11
   recognition   602–3
   in South America   651
   treatment   603–4
alcoholic dementias   285–6
alcoholic neuropathy   342
alprazolam   565
Alzheimer's disease
   age and   205–6
   antemortem markers in   233–5

apolipoprotein E in   214
autosomal genes with dominant
      expression in   213–14
cholinergic system   233
cholinergic approaches to
      treatment   230–1
clinical features   237–9
concurrent in Parkinson's disease   259
CT in   353
depression in   239, 373
disease modification   325–6
Down's syndrome and   219–20
early-onset   273
eating disorders in   245
environmental factors   234
epidemiology   205–7
familial   185
genetics   206, 213–15, 273
histopathological changes   223–5,
      229–30
incidence/prevalence   196, 273
inflammation in   234
international criteria for   221–2
cf MHD   347
mild   310
mixed pathologies   307
moderate   310
moderately severe   310–11
neurochemical changes   229–30, 233–4
neuroimaging   230, 233, 234–5
neuropathology   223–5, 230
neurotransmission in   230, 233–4
noradrenergic system   233
PET in   360
cf Pick's disease   346
presenilins in   217–18
prevention   318–19, 325–6
prognosis   309–11
protein abnormalities   234
retrogenesis   31
risk factors   205–6
serotonergic system   233–4
severe   310–11
SPECT   365
staging   142–3
systemic pathology   234
treatments   317–21
   current   317–18
   future   325–6
Alzheimer's Disease Assessment Scale
      (ADAS)   298
Alzheimer's Disease Diagnostic and
      Treatment Centers (ADDTC)   249
Alzheimer's Disease Societies   10
Alzheimer's Society   334

ambulatory psychiatric care   697–702
   admission to hospitals   701
   beginning of the relationship   699
   family involvement   700
   influences on private practice   697–8
   in-hospital treatment   701–2
   inpatient hospital treatment   701
   office planning and design   699
   private practice as a business   698
   range of services   699–700
   relations with hospitals   701
   relationships with physicians   700
   relationships with professionals   700–1
   relationships with psychiatrists   700
amnesia, dissociative   581–2
amyloid angiopathy   225
amyloid β protein (Aβ)
   in Alzheimer's disease   223–4
   prevention of deposition   320–1
amyloid precursor protein (APP)   224
   in Alzheimer's disease   218
amyotrophic lateral sclerosis–
      Parkinson–dementia complex of
      Guam   295
anaesthetics   743–8
   effect on mental function   744
antemortem markers in Alzheimer's
      disease   233–5
anticholinergics, anaesthetics and   744
anticipatory grief   465
anti-dementia drugs   318
antidepressants   566–7
antihistamines   568
antipsychotics
   in acute mania   487
   classical   63
   newer   63
antistage theory of aging   21
anxiety/anxiety disorder   538
   acute management   559–61
   adult studies   564
   clinical features   551–4
   in dementia   553
   differential diagnosis   563–4
   due to a medical condition   553, 556
   in family caregivers   758
   not otherwise specified   553
   in palliative care   775–6
   pharmacological management   559–60
   prognosis   555–7
   psychological management   560
   psychopharmacological treatment
      563–8
   social   552, 555, 560
   special adaptations   564

anxiety/anxiety disorder *continued*
    substance-induced 553, 556
apolipoprotein E (APOE) 218–19, 299
apolipoprotein E gene (*APOE*)
    in Alzheimer's disease 214
apoptosis 19
assessment
    basic issues 137
    of carers 170
    of depression 170
    of depressive states 153–6
    of environment 170
    of morale 170
    multidisciplinary 111
    non-computerized 138–40
    problems in 133–5
    procedures 37–8
    selection of tools 138–40
Assessment of Daily Living 165–7
attitudes towards older people 741
atypical antipsychotics 523–5, 528–9
audit 668
Australia
    nursing homes in 752–3
    Sydney Dementia Carers' Training
        Program 762–8
autoimmune theory of aging 20
autonomy, patient 715

Barthel's Index of ADL 166
Beck Depression Inventory (BDI) 155,
    298
Behaviour Rating Scale 169
benign senescent forgetfulness (BSF) 49,
    237, 303–4
benzodiazepines 63, 564–8
    correlated 615
    dependence and withdrawal 565
    detection of use 616
    efficacy 565
    gender and age 615
    misuse in the community 619
    pharmacokinetics 565
    prevalence of use 614–15
    psychiatric morbidity 615
    selection 566
    side effects 565–6
bereavement 465–7
    early phases 466–7
    later phases 467
    pathological 407–8
    pre-bereavement situation 465–6
    at time of death 466
β-blockers 567–8
Binswanger's disease 247, 270
biological models 780–1
biological programming 19
biological theories of aging 19–20
biomarkers of aging 71
bipolar disorder 371–2
    epidemiology 477
    genetics 473
    natural history 100
    prognosis 481–2
    risk factors 477–8
    symptoms 408–9
    treatment 440, 456

Blessed Dementia Rating Scale 169, 298
blood oxygenation level-dependent
    (BOLD) contrast 357
blood pressure in dementia 256–7
bovine spongiform encephalopathy (BSE)
    277
brain
    adult neurogenesis 48
    aging, normal 308
    in Alzheimer's disease at autopsy 223
    anatomy 25–41
    atrophy, MRI in measurement of
        355–6
    collateral sprouting 47–8
    CSF spaces, changes in size of **34–8**
    hippocampus 49
    linear measurements **26**
    literature review 26–41
    neural transplantation 48
    neuroimaging studies 23, 25–6
    non-specific structural abnormalities in
        schizophrenia 506
    parenchyma, changes in size **27–33**
    post-mortem studies 23–4
    potential regeneration 47–8
    quantitative MRI 39–40
    quantitative structural changes 45–9
    regenerative sprouting 48
    subcortical hyperintensities, incidence
        of **39**
    tropic support 48
    see also hippocampus
brain–body weight theory 20
brain electrical activity mapping (BEAM)
    347
brain tumours 335–7
Brief Agitation Rating Scale 170
Brief Assessment Schedule 734
    depression cards 170
Burden interview 170
buspirone 566

CADASIL (cerebral autosomal sominant
    arteriopathy with subcortical infarcts
    and leukoencephalopathy) 248, 251
CAGE questionnaire 603, 609
caloric restriction and aging 20
CAMCOG 162
CAMDEX (Cambridge Examination for
    Mental Disorders of the Elderly) 162
CANTAB (Cambridge Neuropsycho-
    logical Test Automated Battery)
    148–9
capacity, concept of 784
carbamazepine (CBZ) in acute mania
    484–5
cardiovascular disease 319–20
    risk factors, Alzheimer's disease and 206
care *see* caregiving; carers/caregiving;
    community care; daycare; family
    caregiving; nursing homes
Caregiver Activity Survey 170
caregiving
    adverse effects 331–2
    for carers 332
    cost 755–6
    definition 331

dementia vs. non-dementia 757
    patterns of formal/informal 81
    policy background 331
    types 332
    in USA 689–95
    see also family caregiving
carers/caregivers
    caring for 332
    importance of role 755–6
    informal 331, 671
    stress and burden 756
    support for 686
    see also family caregiving
Caretaker Obstreperous-Behaviour Rating
    Assessment (COBRA) 170
CARITAS 655, 664
carpal tunnel syndrome (CTS) 344
case-control studies 199–201
    conducting 199
    of dementia 199–200
case identification 105
Cavalieri method 45
Center for Epidemiologic Studies Depres-
    sion Scale (CES-D) 158, 159, 170
central nervous system (CNS) malignancies,
    psychiatric manifestations 335–7
cephalization, index of 20
CERAD (Consortium to Establish a
    Registry for Alzheimer's Disease)
    228
cerebral amyloid angiopathy 253
cerebrovascular disease 270
Charles Bonnet syndrome 127, 505
cholecystokinin-B receptor antagonists
    63
cholesterol metabolism, dementia risk
    and 319–20
chronological aging 71–3
Clifton Assessment Procedures for the
    Elderly (CAPE) 169, 733
Clinical Dementia Rating (CDR) 143
clinical models 781
Clock Drawing Test 169
clonazepam 565
    in acute mania 486–7
clozapine 523
COGDRAS (Cognitive Drug Research
    Computerized Assessment System)
    149
Cognitive Assessment Scale 169
cognitive behavioral therapy (CBT)
    447–8, 454
cognitive dysfunction
    computer methods of assessment
        147–9
    depression and 430
    non-computerized assessment 138–40
cognitive psychology 20–1
cognitive regression hypothesis 21
cognitive tests before and after surgery
    744–5
cohort studies 68–9
communication 641
    in multidisciplinary teamwork 667
community care
    background 671–3
    backup from geriatric psychiatry 671–2

community care *continued*
  informal carers 671
  interventions 328
  normal aged in 79–81
  political and economic factors 672–3
  primary health care 671
  psychogeriatric services in 662
community-living elderly
  hallucinations in 511
  paranoid ideation in 511
  psychosis diagnosed in 511–12
community services
  clinical roles 706
  clinicians as geriatric specialists 706
  community roles 706–7
  educational roles 707
  need for mental health services 705–6
  psychiatrist's role in 705–7
co-morbidity 105
Compensation Theory 379
compliance 456
Comprehensive Assessment and Referral evaluation (CARE) 174–5
Comprehensive Psychopathological Rating Scale (CPRS) 159
compression of morbidity 72–3
computed tomography (CT) 346–7, 351–3
  in Alzheimer's disease 234, 353
  in assessment of delirium 129
  in assessment of dementia 130
  in clinical practice 351
  clinico-radiological correlations 353
  diagnostic ability of 353
  differential diagosis using 351–3
  in schizophrenia-like psychosis 508
confusion/confusional state
  acute *see* delirium
  chronic *see* dementia
Confusion Assessment Method 179, 180
congophilic angiopathy 225
consent to ECT 435
consultation rates 731
continuity theory 21
conversion disorder 581, 582
Convoy Model of Social Relations 379
coping 97, 379–80, 545–6
  neurotic disorders and 546–7
Cornell Scale for Depression in Dementia (CS) 155, 170, 298
cortical infarcts 251–2
cortico-basal degeneration 279
cost
  of Alzheimer's disease treatment 318
  of caregiving 755–6
Creutzfeldt–Jakob disease (CJD) 260, 277, 296, 346
  new variant 278
  SPECT 365
Crichton Behavioural Rating Scale (CBRS) 169
crises 313
crying, pathological 425
CSF spaces, changes in size of **34–8**
cultural awareness 641
culture-bound syndromes 641–2

cyclothymia 372
cystathionine *β*-synthase (CBS) 319

day care/day centers 681–3
  aims 681–2
  cost-effectiveness 682
  day hospitals vs. 682
  development of 677–9
  effectiveness 682
  functions 678–9
  models 681
  problems and issues in 682–3
  psychogeriatric services in 662
day hospitals
  vs. day centers 682
  development of 677–9
  functions 678–9
  see also day care
delirium (acute confusion) 179–81, 293
  assessment scales 180
  clinical features 179–80
  diagnosis 128–9
  incidence 179
  investigations 180
  neuropathogenesis 180
  in palliative care 776
  in paranoid psychoses 497
  post-operative 744–5
  prognosis 183
  risk factors 179, 181
  role of physician in assessment 127–9
  treatment 180–1
delusional disorders/delusions
  depression and 430
  in paranoid psychoses 498
dementia (chronic confusion)
  acute management 313–15
  in Africa 649
  alcoholic 285–6
  anxiety/agitation in 553
  assessment scales 169, 186
  blood pressure in 256–7
  case-control studies 199–200
  clinical presentation 297–8
  concurrent depression and 300
  cortical cf subcortical 348
  culture and 642
  decompensated 129
  depression cf 297–301
  diagnosis, cross-national inter-rater reliability 189–90
  differential diagnosis 293–6
  Down's syndrome and 624
  due to single infarcts 247
  early detection 191–2
  early-onset (EOD) 273–5
  EEG 299
  epidemiology 195–7
  of the frontal lobal type 281, 295
  genetics 299
  in ICD-10 113–14
  incidence 196–7, 200–1
  in Indian subcontinent 647
  laboratory evaluation 299
  lacking specific histological features 279
  of the Lewy body type 259–60, 268, 295

neurochemistry 397
neuroimaging 299–300
neuropsychological assessment 298–9
nosology 185–8
nutritional factors in 210
offending and 628
in paranoid psychoses 497–8
prevalence 195–6
prognosis 308–11
pseudodementia and depression as a prodrome to 300
reversible 289–91
role of physician in assessment 129–30
in South America 651
staging 142–4
subcortical 188, 269–70, 295
subcortical white matter 255–6
telecare and 686
types 185–8
see also Alzheimer's disease; frontotemporal dementia; pseudodementia; vascular dementia
dementia care mapping (DCM) 327, 328
Dementia Mood Assessment Scale 155
Dementia Questionnaire for Persons with Mental Retardation 219
Dementia Rating Scale (DRS) 139
Dementia Scale for Down Syndrome 219
dementia syndrome of depression 410
demography
  age and sex 88
  components of population aging 88
  gender differences 90
  global trends and prospects 87–90
  population 87–8
  recent trends 90–1
  support structures 88–9
dentatopallido–Luysian atrophy 278
dentition 751
dependence syndrome 613
depersonalization–derealization syndrome 539
depression/depressive states 361, 641–2
  acute management 429–30, 453–4
  age and 381
  in Alzheimer's disease 239, 373
  assessment 153–6
  assessment scales 170
  atypical forms 409–10
  biological changes in aging and 397
  clinical features 297–8, 407–11
  cognitive decline 384, 430
  co-morbidity 154
  compliance 456
  continuation treatment 440
  delusional vs. non-delusional, neurochemistry 397
  delusions and 430
  dementia and 130, 300
  dementia cf 297–301
  diagnosis 393–4, 417
  early-onset, neurochemistry 397
  EEG 299
  epidemiology 389–91, 417
  etiology 381–4
  in family caregivers 758

depression/depressive states *continued*
  family history, genetic liability and past
      psychiatric history   383–4
  in Finland   416
  gender and   381–2
  general medical condition and   410
  historical trends   390–1
  history taking   154
  in the Indian subcontinent   645
  laboratory evaluation   155, 299
  life events   382–3
  lithium therapy   455–6
  long-term management   453–8
  longitudinal outcome   413–14
  marital status and   381–2
  medical work-up   155
  medication history   155
  morbidity and mortality   417–18
  natural history   453
  neuroimaging   299–300, 403–4
  neurochemistry   397
  neuropsychological assessment   298–9
  in palliative care   775
  in paranoid psychoses   498
  in personality disorder   589
  pharmacological treatment   439–41
  physical disability and   382, 427–8
  physical illness and   417–21
      conundrums   423
      hospitalization   430–1
      liaison in   419
      primary care and   429
      prognosis   420
      service implications   420–1
      suicide   420, 429–30
      treatment   419–20
  post-stroke (PSD)   386–7, 425–6
      prevalence   386
      risk factors   386–7
  pretreatment   439
  prevalence/prevalence   393, 389–91
  primary, neurochemistry   397
  prognosis   410–12
  prophylactic treatment   440, 454–5
  pseudodementia and, as a prodrome to
      dementia   300
  psychological tests   155
  psychotherapy of   445–9
      under diagnosis and   445–6
      under treatment   446
  secondary, neurochemistry   397
  social class, income and education   383
  social factors   96
  socioeconomic status and   96
  somatized   419
  in South America   651
  subsyndromal   410
  support social and the buffer hypothesis
      383
  symptoms of   408
  treatment-resistant   440–1, 442–3, 449
  vascular   300
  vascular dementia and   373
depressive (major depressive) episode
    371
depressive pseudo-dementia *see* pseudo-
    dementia

Dexamet   155
dexamethasone suppression test (DST)
    53, 299, 461–3
  diagnostic value   461–2
  methodological considerations   461
  prognostic value   462
  in psychogeriatric practice   463
diabetic amyotrophy   342
diabetic neuropathy   341–2
Diagnostic and Statistical Manual (DSM)
  DSM-III   117
  DSM-III-R   117
  DSM-IV   117–21
      axis I   118, 119–20
      axis II   120
      axis III   120
      axis IV   120
      axis V   120–1
      cognitive disorders   118–19
      criteria for Alzheimer's disease   221–2
      in neurotic disorder   537–8
      in personality disorder   593, 596
      vascular dementia   249
dialectical behavior therapy (DBT)   448
disability
  depression and   382, 427–8
  excess, prevention   780
  measure of   72
disability-free life expectancy   72
disengagement theory   21
disposable soma theory   20
Disruptive Behaviour Rating Scale   170
dissector method   45
dissociative amnesia   581–2
dissociative disorder   538, 581
  of movement and sensation   582
dissociative fugue   582
divalproex sodium   456
donepezil   231, 318
dopamine   62
Down's syndrome
  Alzheimer's disease and   219–20
  dementia and   624
drug absorption   61
drug distribution   61
drug excretion   62
drug history   127
drug metabolism   61–2
drug misuse   613–17
  detection   616
  illicit   615
  polysubstance   615–16
  prevalence and correlates   614
  psychological interventions   617
  treatment   616–17
drug sensitivity   743–4
dual process phenomenon conception
    21
duty of care   715
dying patient, care of   775–7
dyskinesia, risk factors for   527–31
dysthymia   153, 372
  clinical features   407–11
  prognosis   410–12
  psychotherapy   445–9
  symptoms of   408
dysthymic disorder *see* dysthymia

early-onset dementias   273–5
eating disorders in Alzheimer's disease
    239
ECT   420, 433–6
  in acute mania   487–8
  administration   434–5
  consent   435
  continuation therapy following   454
  contraindications   434, 487
  efficacy   454
  indications   433–4
  maintenance (M-ECT) and continuation
      (C-ECT)   435
  side effects   435–6, 487–8
education
  Alzheimer's disease and   206
  depression and   383, 384
  see also training
EEG   345–8
  in assessment of delirium   129
  changes with aging   57–8
  cognitive and CT scan changes   346–7
  computerized (CEEG)   347
  in dementia   346
  in diagnosis of dementia and depression
      299
  in healthy aging   345–6
  normal   58
  origin   57
  principles of interpretation   345
  routine   57
  in unhealthy aging   346
eight-stage theory of aging   21
elder abuse   771–3
  abuser characteristics   771–
  management   772–3
  natural history   772
  prevalence and incidence   771, 772
  recognition   772
  victim characteristics   771
ELDRS   170
Emotional Medical Service (EMS)   657
emotionalism   425
  cultural presentations   641
endocrine function, neural control of   52
environmental factors   379–80
Epidemiological Catchment Area studies
  of mood disorders   392
  neurotic disorders and   542
epidemiology
  of alcohol abuse   607–11
  of Alzheimer's disease   205–7
  of bipolar disorder   477
  of dementia   195–7
  of depression   389–91, 417
  of hypochondriacal disorder   576
  life satisfaction   75
  of mania   477
  of neurotic disorders   541–2
  of obsessive-compulsive disorder   571–2
  of personality disorder   588–9
  of psychotic disorder   521
  of schizophrenia   511–12
  of suicidal behaviour   469
  of vascular dementia   511–12
epilepsy   336
EPISTAR   357

erectile failure 635
EURO-D scale 159–60
EURODEM collaboration on incidence of dementia 199–200
EURODEP 393
event-related potentials (ERPs) 347–8
  aging and 58
  brainstem 348
  cognitive 348
  endogenous 58–9
  exogenous 58
  in healthy aging 348
  long latency, effect on age on 59
  types 348
  visual 348
Evercare Demonstration Project 694, 695
Everyday Memory Battery 147–8
exchange theory of aging 21

FAIR 357
familial spastic paraparesis 279
family caregiving 755
  impact on health of caregiver 757
  mental heath outcomes 757–8
  physical health outcomes 758–9
  positive and negative outcomes 757–9
  relocating the care recipient 759–60
  stressors associated with 756–7
  in USA 700
family studies
  Alzheimer's disease and 213
  genetics and 375
Finland, depression in 416
free radical theory 20
Friedreich's ataxia 295
frontal lobe degeneration 261
frontal lobe dementia 270
frontal variant frontotemporal dementia (FV FTD) 281
frontotemporal dementia 188, 261, 281–2, 295
  cf Alzheimer's disease 346
  frontal variant (FV FTD) 281
  management 282
  neuroradiological findings 282
  temporal lobe variant 281–2
fugue, dissociative 582
functional aging 71–3
  disease vs. 71–2
Functional Assessment Staging (FAST) 144, 308
functional health status 71
functional magnetic resonance imaging (fMRI) 357

gabapentin 480, 486
galantamine 231, 318
gender
  Alzheimer's disease and 205–6
  benzodiazepines and 615
  demographic differences in aging 90
  depression and 381–2
  schizophrenia and 96, 504
  tardive dyskinesia and 529
General Health Questionnaire 733
genetic models 781

genetics
  aetiology of bipolar disorder and 473–4
  of affective disorders 375–7
  of aging 19
  of Alzheimer's disease and 206, 213–15
Geriatric Behavioural Scale 170
Geriatric Depression Scale (GDS) 155, 157, 170, 298, 733
Geriatric Education Retreat (GER) 707
Geriatric Mental State (GMS) 161
  GMS/AGECAT 159
  GMS–HAS–AGECAT package 161
geriatric psychiatry as subspeciality 8
Gibson Maze 169
Global Deterioration Scale (GDS) 143, 308
glutamate
  in Alzheimer's disease 230
  NMDA receptors 62
granulovacuolar degeneration 224–5
grief 407–8
  anticipatory 465
group therapy 448

Hachinski Ischemic Score 186, 294
hallucinations
  in Alzheimer's disease 239
  in community-living elderly 511
  in paranoid psychoses 498
Halstead–Reitan battery 139
Hamilton Rating Scale for Depression (HAM-D) 298
head trauma, Alzheimer's disease and 206
health expectancy 74
health status of normal aged 80–1
help seeking 97
Henry Ford Aging Program 39–40
Hierarchic Dementia Scale 144
Hirano bodies 225
historical views of aging 3–5
  before nineteenth century 3
  during nineteenth century 4
  involutional melancholia 6
  nineteenth century views on mental decay 4
  notion of brain sclerosis 4
  senile dementia 4–5
History and Aetiology Schedule (HAS) 161
history-taking 123–6
  from depressed patient 154
  elements 123–4
  execution 124–5
  purpose 123
HIV infection, subcortical dementia in 270
HMPAO SPECT 365
^{99m}Tc-HMPAO SPECT 364–5
homocysteine, vascular disease and 319
homocysteinuria 319
honeymoon palsy 344
hormone replacement therapy (HRT) 319
hospital/hospitalization
  management in 314
  psychogeriatric services in 662

see also medical psychiatry inpatient units
Human Rights Act 787
Huntington's disease (HD) 188, 260–1, 270, 279, 295, 346
  PET of basal ganglion function in 360–1
  SPECT 365
hydrocephalus 270
hypertension, dementia and 256–7
hypochondriasis 154, 409, 417, 575–6
hypophysis naviculare 52
hypothalamic–pituitary peripheral endocrine axis 52
hypothalamo–hypophyso–thyroid (HPT) axis 52
hypothalamo–pituitary–adrenal axis (HPA) 52–3, 398
hypothalamo–pituitary–gonadal (HPG) axis 52
hypothalamo–somatotroph–somatomedin axis 52
hypoxaemia, anaesthetics and 744

imaging see neuroimaging
^{3}H-imipramine binding 399
income, depression and 384
incontinence in Alzheimer's disease 238–9
index of cephalization 20
Indian subcontinent
  dementia 647
  depression in 645
institutionalization
  effects on schizophrenic patients 514
  premature, prevention of 780
Instrumental Activities of Daily Living Scale (IADL) 169–70
International Classification of Diseases, Tenth (ICD-10) 113–15
  criteria for Alzheimer's disease 221–2
  dementia in 113–14
  uses 113
  vascular dementia 249
International Psychogeriatric Association (IPA) 799–800
interpersonal psychotherapy (IPT) 440, 447, 454
interview in paranoid psychoses 498–9
intracranial lesions 295
IQCODE 141–2
ISPOCD studies 745–7
ITHACA project 685

Katz Index of ADL 166, 167
Kendrick Battery 169
Kluver–Bucy syndrome 295
Korsakoff's psychosis 365
Kraepelin 6, 493
Kubler-Ross, Ellen 776–7
kuru 277

lacunar infarction 252
lamotrigine 486
Landry–Guillain–Barré–Strohl syndrome (AIDP) 341

language impairment in Alzheimer's
   disease   237–8
laughing, pathological   425
law, capacity and
   burden of proof   785
   evidence   785–8
   here and now test   785
   human rights and   787
   lack of capacity   785
   next of kin   786
   objectives   784
   principles of   784–5
   role of   783–4
   sectioning   786–7
   treatment   786
learning disability   623–5
   care in the family home   624–5
   causes of death   623
   community teams   625
   day care   625
   frequency of dementia   623–4
   medical contribution to diagnosis   624
   multihandicapped person   625
   rehabilitation into the community   624
   services for   624
   social background   623
   terminal care   625
leukoaraiosis   23, 252–3
Lewy body dementia   188
life events   82, 379–80
Life Events and Difficulties Schedule
   (LEDS)   382
life expectancy, measurement of   72–3
life review   446–7
life satisfaction   75–7
   definition   75
   determinants   75–6
   epidemiology   75
   explanatory mechanisms   76
lithium therapy   63, 440
   in acute mania   479, 483–4
   in affective disorders   440
   depression and   455–7
   drug interactions   458, 484
   optimum plasma levels   457–8
   response to   456
   side effects   457, 484
     renal   457
     subjective   457
     thyroid   457
living arrangements   88–9, 313–15
   alone   313–14
   of normal aged   79–80
   with others   314
   see also hospitalization; long-term care;
     nursing homes
long-term care   717–20
   psychiatric services in   717–20
   rehabilitation and   741
long-term outcome studies   105–7
   case identification   105
   co-morbidity   105
   choice of comparison groups   106
   follow-up   106–7
   measurement of outcomes   106
   measures of intervening variables
     106

sample representativeness and attrition
   106
lorazepam in acute mania   487
lumbar puncture (LP) in assessment of
   delirium   129
Lundby Study   208–9
Luria–Nebraska battery   139

magnetic resonance imaging (MRI)
   in Alzheimer's disease   234–5
   brain atrophy   355–6
   functional (fMRI)   357
   in geriatric psychiatry   355
   at Henry Ford Aging Program
     39–40
   in schizophrenia-like psychosis   508
magnetic resonance morphometry   355
magnetic resonance spectometry (MRS)
   403–4
maintenance therapy   448–9
major depressive disorder (MDD), natural
   history   99–100
mania
   clinical features   479–80
   early-onset (EOM)   100
   epidemiology   477
   genetics   473–4
   after head injury   482
   late-onset (LOM)   100
   management   479–80, 483–8
   in paranoid psychoses   498
   risk factors   477–8
   secondary   481
   treatment goals   483
manic episode   371
MAO-A inhibitors   63
MAOIs   439, 441
Marital Intimacy Scale   170
Measurement of Morale in the Elderly
   Scale   170
Medicaid   692
medical psychiatry inpatient units   709–12
   clinical and patient characteristics
     710–11
   organizational features   710
   problems, advantages and caveats
     711–12
   structure and organization   709–10
Medicare   691–2
Medicare Economic Index (MEI)   692
MELAS (mitochondrial encephalomyopathy with lactic acid and stroke-
   like episodes)   251
Mental Health Act 1983 (England and
   Wales)   789–90
   sectioning under   786–7
Mental Status Examination (MSE)
   125–6, 154–5, 499
Mental Status Questionnaire (MSQ)
   169
Mental Test Score   733
meralgia paresthetica   344
methylene tetrahydrofolate reductase
   (MTHFR)   319
metrifonate   231
mild cognitive impairment (MCI)   49,
   304, 305–6, 308

Mini-Mental State Examination (MMSE)
   127, 128, 140–1, 143, 144, 169 180,
   298, 733
Minimum Data Set (USA)   728
mirtazapine   567
mixed anxiety depressive disorder   553
MMPI   593
modernization theory   21
monoamine oxidase (MAO), platelet
   activity   398
monoamine oxidase inhibitors (MAOIs)
   567
mononeuritis multiplex   342
mononeuropathies   343–4
Montgomery–Asberg Depression Rating
   scale (MADRS)   155, 298
mood disorders
   Epidemiological Catchment Area studies
     392
   longitudinal studies   415
   mood-incongruent paranoid states
     511–12
   nosology and classification   371–3
morale, assessment   170
mortality
   cause of death   103–4
   community-based studies   103
   death certificate studies   103
   methodological studies   104
   patient-based studies   103
motor neurone disease   278
motor neurone disease inclusion dementia
   261
MRC Cognitive Function and Ageing
   Study (MRC CFAS)   202–4
multi-chemical networking profile,
   brain   62
multidisciplinary team   111, 667–9
   audit   668
   communication in   667
   effectiveness in treatment of depression
     in physically disabled   427–8
   future development   668–9
   leadership in   667–8
   morale   668
   in psychogeriatric services   662
multi-infarct dementia (MID)   186–7,
   247 255–6, 346
   cf Alzheimer's disease   347
Multiphasic Environment Assessment
   Procedure   170
multiple sclerosis, subcortical dementia in
   270
multiple systems atrophy (MSA)   270
multiprocess phenomenon conception   21
multisystem atrophy   278

National Health Service
   origins   658
   reforms   658, 659
necrosis   19
nefazodone   567
nerve growth factor (NGF) therapy   320
neurasthenia (fatigue syndrome)   582–3
neuritic plaques   223
neurochemistry   397–9
neuroendocrinology   51–4

neurofibrillary tangles (NFT) 224
neuro-imaging 23, 25–6
  in Alzheimer's disease 230, 233, 234–5
  in dementia 299–300
  in depression 299–300, 403–4
  justification in older people 404–5
  see also computed tomography; magnetic resonance imaging; positron emission tomography; single photo emission computed tomography
neuroleptic induced parkinsonism (NIP) 522
neuroleptic malignant syndrome (NMS) 523
neuroleptics 522–3, 567
neuronal loss in Alzheimer's disease 225
neurotic disorders
  coping and 546–7
  diagnostic features 538–40
  epidemiology 541–2
  findings from Epidemiological Catchment Area surveys 542
  in ICD-10 and DSM-IV 537–8
  nosology and classification 537–40
  social support and 546–7
  stress and 546–7
neurotransmitter receptors in Alzheimer's disease 230
neurotransmitters in Alzheimer's disease 229–30
NINCDS–ADRDA criteria for Alzheimer's disease 221–2
NINDS–AIREN criteria 187–8
  for vascular dementia 249
nocturnal myoclonus 632
non-fluent progressive aphasia 282
noradrenaline depletion 62
noradrenergic function 399
normal pressure hydrocephalus 278–9, 295
Nottingham Model of Health Care 673–5
NSAIDs, Alzheimer's disease and 206
Nurses' Observation Scale for Inpatient Evaluation (NOSIE) 170
nurses, rating scales designed for 169–70
Nursing Home Behaviour Problem Scale 170
nursing homes 97–8, 314
  in Australia 752–3
  clinical psychiatry in 717–18
  as mental health care environment 718–19
  psychiatrist in 713–14
  quality and life and care in 727–9
  regulatory environment, USA 719–20
nutritional factors in dementia 210
nutritional state 749–51

OARS (Older Americans Resources and Services) 173
obsessive-compulsive disorder 538, 552
  aetiology 572
  clinical assessment 571
  clinical features 571
  diagnostic criteria 571
  differential diagnosis 571

epidemiology 571–2
  prognosis 555
  treatment 572
offenders 627–9
  affective disorders and 627–8
  assessment 628
  clinical aspects 627–8
  extent and pattern 627
  mental abnormality and 627
  within the criminal justice system 628–9
olanzapine 524
Older American Research and Service Center (OARS) instrument 167
olivopontocerebellar atrophy (OPCA) 278
OPTIMA (Oxford Project to Investigate Memory and Ageing) 227
Overt Aggression Scale 170
over-the-counter medication 615

PACE 694, 695
palliative care 775–7
panic disorder with/without agoraphobia (PD/PDA) 551
  prognosis 555
panic disorder, psychological management 560
paraneoplastic disorders, brain tumours and 336
paraneoplastic encephalomyelitis (PEM) 336
paranoid personality disorder 498
paranoid psychoses
  assessment 498–9
  differential diagnosis 497–8
parenchyma, changes in size **27–33**
Parkinson's disease 188, 295, 365
  concurrent Alzheimer's disease 259
  dementia and 259–60, 265–7
    cause 266–7
    clinical features 265
    development of 266
    likelihood of 265–6
    neuropathological correlates 266
    organic disorders 265
  innominato-cortical dysfunction 259
  neuronal loss in pigmented brainstem nuclei 259
  subcortical dementia 270
pathological laughing and crying 425
Performance test for Activities of Daily Living (PADL) 169, 170
periodic leg movement in sleep (PLMS) 632
peripheral neuropathy 341–4
  examination of patient with 342–3
personality disorders
  aetiology and genetics 587–8
  assessment 588, 593–6
    DSM criteria 593, 596
    organicity 595
    outcome measures 595–6
    self-report vs. informant data 595
    state–trait problems and co-morbidity 594–5
    time-frame considerations 595
  in community settings 588–9
  co-morbid disorders 596

depression and 589
  epidemiology 588–9
  in institutional settings 589
  in outpatient settings 589
  pharmacotherapy 596
  prognosis 589
  psychotherapy 597
  treatment 596–7
personality theories of aging 21
pharmacodynamics 62
pharmacokinetics 61–2, 565, 613–14
phenelzine 439
phenothiazides 522
Philadelphia Geriatric Center Morale Scale 170
phobias 538
  acute management 559–61
  pharmacological management 559–60
  psychological management 560
  see also simple (specific) phobia
Physical and Mental Impairment of Function Evaluation in the Elderly (PAMIE) 170
physical illness
  depression and 417–21
  suicidal behavior and 420, 470
Physical Self-maintenance Scale 169
physician, role in assessment 127–30
physostigmine 231
Pick's disease see frontotemporal dementia
pituitary, posterior 53
pneumoencephalography (PEG) 25–6
polyneuropathy 341–3
polypharmacy, prevention of side effects 780
Poor Law 657
positron emission tomography (PET) 359–61
  activation studies 360
  in Alzheimer's disease 235
  basal ganglion function in Huntington's disease 360–1
  blood flow and metabolism in Alzheimer's disease 360
  of depression 361, 403–4
  sources of variation in 359–60
  tracer substances 359
post-hospital treatment 702
post-operative changes in psychometric tests 745
post-operative delirium 744–5
post-stroke depression (PSD) 386–7, 425–6
post-traumatic dementia 279
post-traumatic stress disorder (PTSD) 540, 552–3, 579
  clinical features 580
  delayed onset 580
  differential diagnosis 580
  prognosis 556
  therapy 580–1
poverty 81
presenilins in Alzheimer's disease 217–18
prevention in mental health 779–81
primary health care, community care 671
Problem Checklist and Strain scale 170
problem-solving therapy (PST) 447–8

Professional Environmental Assessment Protocol (PEAP) 728
Program for Organizing Interdisciplinary Self-education (POISE) 795–7
progressive subcortical gliosis 279
progressive supranuclear palsy (PSP) 270, 278, 365
propranolol 568
PS-1 protein in Alzheimer's disease 217–18
pseudobulbar palsy 295
pseudodementia 130, 289, 290, 293–4, 419
psychiatric hospitals, private 723–5
psychiatrists
　in community services 705–7
　in nursing home 713–14
　stress and 792
　training for 791–2
psychneuroendocrine markers 53–4
psychoanalysis, age and 7–8
psychodynamic therapy 446
Psychogeriatric Assessment Scales (PAS) 146
psychogeriatric consultation–liaison service
　need for 733–4
　education and 737
Psychogeriatric Dependency Rating Scale (PGDRS) 170
psychogeriatric services 661–3
　in Britain 9–10
　education and entry to 10
　guidelines 663
　international developments 10
　key components 662
　organization 664–5
　origins 9, 15–16
　primary vs. secondary care 661
　reality 663
　specialist services 663
　theoretical basis 661
psychological interventions 327–8
psychometric tests, post-operative changes 745
psychopharmacologic drugs 564
psychopharmacological approach 7
psychosocial interventions 327–8
psychosocial models 781
psychotherapy 7–8
　interpersonal (IPT) 447
　in palliative care 777
　special issues 445–6
psychotic disorders
　1940–1970 493–4
　1970–present 494
　differential diagnosis 521–2
　early history 493
　epidemiology 521
　neurochemical hypothesis 521
　nosology and classification 493–5
　toward a consensus 494–5
　treatment 521–5

quality of care
　defining 727–8
　in institutions 727–9

quality of life
　assessment 134–5
　care 686
　defining 728–9
　in institutions 727–9
quetiapine 524

raloxifene 319
rapid cycling 372
Rating Scale for Aggressive Behaviour in the Elderly (RAGE) 633
reality orientation 327, 328
recurrence, prevention of 780
referral rates 731–3
rehabilitation 739–41
　of elderly with psychiatric disorder 739–41
　long-stay care and 741
　rating scales in 519
　in schizophrenia 518–19
relapse prevention 448–9, 780
Relatives' Stress Scale 170
religious participation 97
REM sleep behavior disorder (RSBD) 631–2
reminder devices 686
reminiscence therapy 446–7
Repeatable Battery for the Assessment of Neuropsychological Status (RBANS) 139
retrogenesis 311
reversible dementias 289–91
　classification 289
　investigation protocols 291
　prevalence 289
　response to treatment 290
risperidone 63, 524
rivastigmine 231, 318
Ryden Aggression Scale 170

Saturday night palsy 344
scaling theory of aging 20
Schedule for Affective Disorders and Schizophrenia–Lifetime (SADS-L) 105
schizophrenia
　care 514–15
　cognitive impairment 513
　early-onset (EOS)
　　natural history 100–1
　　social factors 95
　epidemiology, prevalence, incidence and course 511–12
　environmental. social and cultural factors and outcome 518
　gender 96, 504
　genetics 503–4
　institutionalization, effects of 514
　late-onset
　　gender difference 96
　　natural history 100–1
　　social factors 95–6
　long-term outcome 513, 517
　mortality 514
　non-specific structural brain abnormalities 506

　offending and 628
　organic factors 506
　in paranoid psychoses 498
　premorbid characteristics 504–5
　rehabilitation and 518–19
　sensory deficits 505–6
　social isolation 505
　stress and 96
schizophrenia-like psychosis, brain imaging in 508
scrapie 277
Secondary Dementia Schedule 161
secondary dementias 188
secretases 224
sectioning 786–7
seizures, brain tumors and 336
Selective Optimization 379
selective serotonin reuptake inhibitors (SSRIs) 567
Self Care (D) 170
semantic dementia 281–2
senile dementia of the Alzheimer type (SDAT) 237
senile plaques 223
senile squalor syndrome 571
serotonin 398
serotonin reuptake sites 62
sexual disorders 635
shell-shock 582
sheltered housing 314
Short Michigan Alcohol Screening Test (SMAST) 609
Short Orientation–Memory–Concentration Test 169
Short Portable Mental Status Questionnaire (SPMSQ) 298
SHORT-CARE 159
Shy–Drager syndrome 278
silent infarcts, MRI in diagnosis of 356
Simmonds' disease 66
simple (specific) phobia 552
　prognosis 555–6
　psychological management 560
single photo emission computed tomography (SPECT) 359, 363–6
　of depression 403–4
　normal subjects and normal aging 363–4
　principles and techniques 363
　in schizophrenia-like psychosis 508
　studies in dementia 364
　^{99m}Tc-HMPAO SPECT 364–5
sleep
　abnormalities 299
　disorders and management 631–2
　EEG patterns in healthy aging 345–6
sleep apnoea 631
smart housing 686
social class, depression and 384
social contact of normal aged 80
social health maintenance organizations (S/HMO) 694–5
social inequality 81
Social Network Assessment Scale 170
social networks of normal aged 80
social phobia (social anxiety disorder) 552
　prognosis 555
　psychological management 560

social support 96–7, 546
    depression and 384
    neurotic disorders and 546–7
socioeconomic status 96
Socio-emotional Selectivity Theory 379
somatization 409, 417, 575–6
somatoform disorders 538 9
South America, mental illness in 651–2
specific phobia *see* simple phobia
spinocerebella ataxias (SCA), subcortical
        dementia in 270
spinocerebellar atrophy associated with
        dementia 279
spontaneous dyskinesia 531
SSRIs 439–40
staging
    axial and multi-axial 143–4
    dementia 142–4
    global 143
Steele–Richardson–Olszewski syndrome
        278
steroidal hormones, Alzheimer's disease
        and 206
Stockton Geriatric Rating Scale 169, 170
stress 53, 545
    acute stress disorder (ASD) 553, 556
    life events and 82
    neurotic disorders and 546–7
    psychiatrists and 793
    schizophrenia and 96
    see also post-traumatic stress disorder;
        stress reaction
stress reaction 538, 579–80
stroke 319–20
    post-stroke depression (PSD) 386–7,
        425–6
Structured Interview for Disorders of
        Personality scale (SIDP-R) 588
subcortical dementia 188, 269–70, 295
subcortical hyperintensities, incidence of
    39
subcortical white matter dementia 255–6
substance-induced anxiety 553, 556
suicidal behavior/suicide 469–71
    biological factors 470
    epidemiology 469
    physical illness and 420, 470
    prevention 470–1, 780
    psychiatric illness 469–70
    rates 469
    social factors 469
sundowning 154
support networks 83–4
Support/Efficacy Model 380
supranuclear palsy 188
Sydenham's chorea 571
Sydney Dementia Carers' Training Program
        762–8

tacrine 231
tardive dyskinesia (TD) 523

acute extrapyramidal side effects 530–1
advancing age 527–8
affective disorder and 529
akathisia 530–1
antipsychotic medication 528–9
clinical features 527
dementia and 530
gender 529
organicity 529
parkinsonism 530–1
prevalence, incidence and natural history
    527
psychiatric diagnosis 529–30
risk factors 527–31
schizophrenia and 530
TCAs 439–40, 441
technology, changes in 7
telecare
    concepts and applications 685–6
    dementia and 686
    ethical issues 686
teleconsultation 685
telemedicine 685
temporal lobe variant frontotemporal
        dementia 281–2
terminal drop 21
30 stage theory of adult cognitive devel-
        opment 21
TIDE 686
Tourette's syndrome 571
toxic dementias 286
toxic metabolic abnormalities 295 6
training
    community services 707
    for psychiatrists 791–2
    psychogeriatric services 10, 737
triazolam 565
tricyclic antidepressants 63, 566–7
twin studies
    of Alzheimer's disease genetics 213
    genetics of affective disorders 375–6

UK
    community care in 672
    day hospital and day care in 677–9
    history of health and social services
        657–9
    psychogeriatrics in 10
    research in 10
undernutrition 750–1
unipolar disorder 371–2
USA
    1600–1900 13–14
    acute inpatient hospitalization 691
    ambulatory psychiatric care 697–702
    community mental health centers 690
    financing mental health care 691–4,
        694
    future of integrated services and finan-
        cing 694
    mental care managed care 692–4

nursing home 690–1, 719–20
outpatient psychiatric service settings
        689–90
primary care 689
private psychiatric hospitals 723–5
psychiatric service settings 689–91
structure and organization of mental
        health services 689–91
system of care in 689–95

valproate (valproic acid) 63, 440
    in acute mania 485–6
    drug interactions 486
    in mania 480
    side effects 485–6
vascular cognitive impairment (VCI)
        249
vascular dementia 186–8, 294
    Alzheimer's disease and 373
    assessment 253
    assessment scales 187
    clinical types 251–3
        cerebral amyloid angiopathy 253
        cortical infarcts 251–2
        lacunar infarction 252
        leukoaraiosis 252–3
    early-onset (EOVD) 274
    epidemiology 251
    international criteria for 249
    investigation 253–4
    management 253–4
    pathology 247 8
    prevalence 196
    risk factors 251
    subgroups 255–6
    treatment 254
vascular disease, homocysteine and
        319
venlafaxine 567
visual impairment 781
vitamin deficiency 750
voluntary organizations in Great Britain
        10

wandering 238, 637–8
waste, accumulation of 20
Ways of Coping Check List 170
wear and tear view of aging 3
Wernicke–Korsakoff syndrome 210,
        285
white matter changes
    in Alzheimer's disease 225
    dementia due to 247
white matter lesions (WMLs) 186–7
Wilson's disease 295
Wisconsin Card Sorting Test 281
WPA/WHO consensus statements 655

ziprasidone 524–5
Zung Self-rating Depression Scale (ZSDS)
        159

Index compiled by Annette Musker